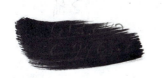

WOMEN'S HEALTH: BODY, MIND, SPIRIT

An Integrated Approach to Wellness and Illness

Marian C. Condon, R.N., D.Ed., HNC
York College of Pennsylvania
York, Pennsylvania

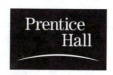

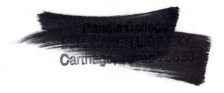

Prentice Hall

Upper Saddle River, New Jersey 07458

Library of Congress Cataloging-in-Publication Data

Condon, Marian C.
    Women's health : an integrated approach to wellness and illness / Marian C. Condon.
       p. ; cm.
    Includes bibliographical references and index.
    ISBN 0-8385-9648-7
      1. Women—Health and hygiene. 2. Health.
      3. Holistic medicine. I. Title.
      [DNLM: 1. Women's Health. 2. Women's Health
      Services. WA 309 C746w 2001]
    RA778 .C73 2001
    613'.04244—dc21   2001053105

Publisher: *Julie Levin Alexander*
Executive Editor: *Maura Connor*
Editorial Assistant: *Sladjana Repic*
Marketing Manager: *Nicole Benson*
Director of Production and Manufacturing: *Bruce Johnson*
Managing Production Editor: *Patrick Walsh*
Manufacturing Buyer: *Pat Brown*
Production Liaison: *Julie Li*
Production Editor: *Lynn Steines*
Creative Director: *Cheryl Asherman*
Cover Design Coordinator: *Maria Guglielmo*
Cover Designer: *Joseph Sengotta*
Composition: *Carlisle Production Services*
Printing and Binding: *Courier Westford*

Pearson Education LTD.
Pearson Education Australia PTY, Limited
Pearson Education Singapore, Pte. Ltd
Pearson Education North Asia Ltd
Pearson Education Canada, Ltd.
Pearson Educación de Mexico, S.A. de C.V.
Pearson Education—Japan
Pearson Education Malaysia, Pte. Ltd
Pearson Education, Upper Saddle River, New Jersey

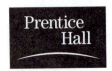

10 9 8 7 6 5 4 3 2 1
ISBN 0-8385-9648-7

This book is dedicated to the memory of H. Walter Condon

—

Contents

SECTION III

The Emerging Healthcare Delivery System 163

Chapter 9 Traditional Healthcare 164

Chapter 10 Nontraditional Healthcare: Emerging into Integrative Healthcare 182

Chapter 11   Holistic Health: Complementary Therapeutic Disciplines and Remedies   195

SECTION IV

Physical Health   227

Chapter 12   Cardiovascular Wellness and Illness   228

Chapter 22 Sexual Wellness and Illness 445

Chapter 23 Pregnancy and Childbearing 463

Foreword

Only in the past few decades have the differences between men's and women's health been recognized and addressed specifically by either health care professionals or researchers. Previously, clinical studies focused almost exclusively on male subjects unless the topic dealt with a condition unique to women. Scientists used the rationale that women's menstrual cycles, pregnancies or menopause would add uncontrollable variables and interfere with studies' results. They also assumed, incorrectly, that men and women were basically the same in terms of human response and function and that diseases of various body systems, organs and tissues varied little if at all. Today scientists and the public alike realize that past assumptions that the health of men and women is indistinguishable are erroneous.

The importance of explicitly addressing women's health and health care needs emerged with the growth of the women's movement and accompanying legislation that today requires all research funded by the National Institute of Health to include women as subjects unless the study targets a problem exclusive to men, e.g, prostate cancer. The consumer movement as well has contributed to demands by women and men for more health information, and access to previously unavailable data is now obtainable via the internet.

Women's Health: Body, Mind, Spirit—An Integrated Approach to Wellness and Illness, by Marian Condon, is a comprehensive test for both health care professionals and lay consumers. The health of women is presented in the context of society, and the book illustrates how present-day practices have emerged from the past. Dr. Condon describes important differences between men's and women's health care, and she explains why those differences often have been ignored.

Several strengths make this text valuable and functional. First, Dr. Condon embeds her discussion of women's health in the social and economic realities of today's world. Wellness and illness are not viewed on a continuum, but rather as interrelated states of health. Also she considers women's health within a holistic framework, including mind-body relationships and women's spiritual well-being. Although she presents extensive information about traditional Western medicine's approach to illness, Dr. Condon offers information about alternative and complementary methods as well, content often neglected in many health-related texts. Finally, in spite of the complexity of the information included, it is presented in an interesting and easily understood way; few words are wasted.

Content included in this text is useful to all women and those raising or teaching female children, lay and professionals alike. The book bridges the gap between technical books and publications designed for the public. It can serve as a textbook for students, a health manual for consumers and a reference for both. This is one book that students will keep long beyond completion of their course.

Navigating the maze of the American health care system is made easier by the explanations offered in this book. Both consumers and professionals will find that content useful. While it is virtually impossible to write a text that keeps up with the latest research findings and practice guidelines, *Women's Health: Body, Mind, Spirit* suggests future directions in research and treatment. Self-assessment questionnaires are included in many chapters. Questions for reflections and discussion can be used by readers on their own or by students in a classroom. Resources include up to date as well as classic videos, websites, organizations, and references from scientific sources and the popular press.

Marian Condon's work is a welcome addition to the literature on women's health. Armed with the information contained here, health care professionals will be better prepared to deal with the complex and often interrelated health problems of women and to help them to achieve a state of wellness even in the presence of illness. Women consumers, too, will be knowledgeable and thus able to partner with their health care providers.

Eleanor J. Sullivan, PhD, RN, FAAN
Professor, School of Nursing
University of Kansas

Preface

I put this book together for a very practical reason: I needed a textbook for a course on women's health, and I could not find one with all the features I wanted. For example, because the course is open to both healthcare majors and nonhealth majors, I wanted a text that would be engaging and worthwhile for *both* sets of students and for the general public as well. I knew that many traditional and older college students had little knowledge of how to go about evaluating, preserving, and/or improving their health and that even women majoring in nursing, or another health-related discipline sometimes know more about taking care of other people than about caring for themselves. Therefore, I wanted a text that would spell out what it means to be *well*—for example, to have a healthy cardiovascular system, lungs, and kidneys. Thus, *Markers of Wellness* sections in this book came into being, and, of course, my desire for a book that would help readers foster their own wellness led to the promoting wellness sections. It was obviously also necessary that the nature of the various illnesses that women commonly experience, and the signs and symptoms that betray their presence, be described. For those purposes, I devised the sections on illnesses and problems. Because I have a *holistic* philosophy of health, however, I also wanted a book that would address more than just physical health. I wanted one that would convey the interrelated and interdependent nature of *physical*, *mental*, and *spiritual* health and would provide information on evaluating and improving health status in all three of those areas. Another wish was for a book that would address the *integrated* healthcare delivery system that is emerging in this country. I knew that readers would need information that would help them choose wisely from among the wide range of available *traditional* and *nontraditional* healthcare-related *products* and *providers*. Last, but perhaps most important, I wanted a book that would acknowledge the often-ignored link between *women's health* and their *status and roles* in the society in which they live and would address the ways in which *socioeconomic variables,* such as age, ethnicity, socioeconomic status, disability and sexual orientation, affect women's health.

Women's Health: Body, Mind, Spirit—An Integrated Approach to Wellness and Illness meets all the aforementioned criteria. First, it is suitable for both healthcare majors and persons without a formal background in healthcare. It is worthwhile reading for students majoring in nursing and other healthcare professions, as it addresses topics and details pertinent to women's health that, due to space limitations, are *not included* in more general texts. In all discussions of illness diagnosis and treatment, *areas of disparity between men's and women's experience* (symptoms, accuracy of diagnostic indicators, treatment efficacy, and so on) are highlighted. Lay readers will appreciate the *definitions* that accompany all medical terms used, as well as the clear *explanations* of physiological processes, medical interventions, and the like. The *wellness self-assessments* sections found in most chapters are designed to assist readers in evaluating their own health status. The *resources,* including books, journals, videotapes, websites, and organizations, listed at the end of each chapter will be of general interest, as well the information in the New Directions sections on trends in research, prevention, diagnosis, and treatment. The information in the New Directions sections also remind readers of the fluid and ephemeral nature of "knowledge" and the need for lifelong inquiry and critical thinking.

No book intended to assist people in managing their health is complete without a section on *accessing and interacting with* our rapidly evolving healthcare delivery system. Readers need information about providers and systems, as well as on their own roles as consumers, to be able to get good care with which they are satisfied. Readers will appreciate the information pertaining to dealing with *managed care* (such as HMOs and PPOs) and the importance of *advance directives* (such as living wills and medical powers of attorney) included in Chapter 9, as well as the guidelines for communicating effectively with providers and seeking and evaluating sources of health-related information.

Women's Health: Body, Mind, Spirit—An Integrated Approach to Wellness and Illness meets my need for a *holistic* text in that it acknowledges and explains the *interconnectedness* among the physical, mental/emotional, and spiritual aspects of our being, and therefore our health. In it, *health* is defined as a continuum ranging from wellness to illness, and it is conceptualized as multidimensional: *physical* (organ systems), *psychological* (thought patterns, attitudes, feelings, and moods), and *spiritual* (the process of creating meaning in one's life through a sense of connection to something that transcends the self). The book makes the point that each dimension of health influences, and is influenced by, the others. For example, Chapter 27 contains a section on *psychoneuroimmunology,* a relatively new science that investigates the connections between mental/emotional states and physical manifestations of health and illness. Also, psychological, emotional, and spiritual factors known to play a role in physical illnesses are highlighted. For example, considerable attention is paid to *hostility* as a potential factor in the development of coronary artery disease. In Chapter 28, concrete information on dealing optimally with the physical, psychological, and spiritual aspects of dying and death is presented.

Addressing psychological wellness and spiritual wellness in their own right is also important. For one thing, there is evidence that both can be actively *promoted,* just as physical wellness can. Also, some of the *markers* of psychological wellness may be different in women and men. For example, it has been suggested that women are happiest when embedded in a *web of relationships,* whereas men seem to do well without this. Including information about spiritual wellness for women is important, because research suggests that persons who have developed the spiritual dimension of their being enjoy a higher level of physical and emotional health than persons who do not. Although most women describe themselves as having religious or spiritual faith, the patriarchal nature of the major religions is problematic for many. Therefore, resources related to both the growing movement to make mainstream religions more woman-friendly and alternative women-centered spiritual practices are provided.

Women's Health: Body, Mind, Spirit—An Integrated Approach to Wellness and Illness meets my need for an *integrated* text in that it addresses not only traditional healthcare but also what has been seen as *alternative,* or *complementary,* healthcare. The inclusion of material on nontraditional healthcare is important, because it has been estimated that the general public spends more money on alternative therapies than on mainstream remedies and services. Readers must have information on the nature, efficacy, and safety of the most commonly used alternative therapies in order to make intelligent choices as healthcare consumers. Chapter 10 addresses what is referred to as the *holistic paradigm,* the set of beliefs and values that distinguishes alternative healthcare systems from traditional Western healthcare. In Chapter 11, alternative *systems,* such as traditional Chinese medicine, Ayurveda, homeopathy, and naturopathy, and *treatment modalities,* such as acupuncture, healing touch, aromatherapy, and herbs, are discussed in terms

of the beliefs about health and healthcare that underlie them and their demonstrated efficacy or lack of it. All chapters with an illness section contain information about alternative treatments that are commonly used for the malady under discussion. For example, Chapter 12 addresses not only the American Heart Association's dietary recommendations but also those of Dean Ornish (author of *Dr. Dean Ornish's Program for Reversing Heart Disease*). The section on treatment options for depression contains information about the herb St. John's wort, as well as standard drugs, such as Prozac. A brief synopsis of the research literature on all newer treatment options is included.

No book on women's health is complete without a discussion of the implications of the *female gender* for healthcare. The content in this area addresses historical and contemporary cultural beliefs and attitudes toward women, as well as women's relationships with the healthcare establishment. It has been well documented that decisions in such areas as medical research, insurance reimbursement policies, and diagnostic and treatment protocols are influenced by societal views of women. Readers must have sufficient information about the *past* to think critically about the *present.* The ways in which *socioeconomic variables* such as age, ethnicity, socioeconomic status, disability and sexual orientation affect women's health are addressed primarily in Chapter 2, as well as alluded to in other chapters.

It is my hope that the existence of this book will stimulate faculty in departments of nursing and other healthcare disciplines to offer courses on women's health that are open to students from all majors. Educators in health-related disciplines have an obligation to support the health of the student body at large, and to establish themselves as expert sources of information about health and healthcare.

Finally, it is my hope that you, the reader, will consider this book to have been worth your investment in time and money. I hope *Women's Health: Body, Mind, Spirit—An Integrated Approach to Wellness and Illness* will stimulate you to maximize your wellness and will equip you to cope better with illness. I hope that, after having read it, you will be more aware of the ways in which the physical, psychological, and spiritual aspects of your being interact to affect your overall health. I hope also that you are dazzled by what you learn about the wonders of your body and the strength, stamina, resiliency, and tenacity of your female kind. Finally, I wish you health and happiness in body, mind, and spirit.

Marian C. Condon

Acknowledgments

I am so very grateful to the many people who helped me in ways large and small to complete this manuscript. First and foremost, I wish to convey my heartfelt gratitude to all the contributors for their excellent work. Without you, friends, there would be no book. And, I wish to thank the reviewers, many of whom made very useful suggestions for improvement. Special thanks are in order for contributors Elva Winter, Lindy Harrison, and Kay Huber, who helped with the editing. And I would be remiss if I did not publicly commend Dr. Barbara Barski-Carrow for her amazing patience and forbearance.

I also wish to thank Maura Connor, Beth Romph, and Sladjana Repic at Prentice Hall and Lynn Steines at Carlisle Publishing Services for lending me their invaluable assistance, expertise, and support. Debra DeBord has to be the finest copyeditor on the planet and I do so appreciate her acumen and eagle eye.

Others to whom I am indebted for rendering assistance when it was needed include Linda Avillo, who also did some editing; Marge Duraski, who organized source materials; Debby Barton who acted as a shutterbug, computer maven, and all-around helpful person; and York College reference librarians Vicci Kline, Sue McMillan, and Zehao Zhou who can find absolutely anything on the Web.

Finally, I would never have gotten through this project without the ongoing support of my personal TLC Squad—Annette, Diane, and Robert. Thanks, Pals!

Contributors

Jeanie Bachand, Ed.D., R.N.
York College of Pennsylvania
York, PA

Barbara Barski-Carrow, Ph.D.
U.S. Department of Health and Human Resources
Office of Equal Employment Opportunity
Washington, DC

Kathleen M. Blade, M.S., R.N., C.S.
St. Joseph's Hospital School of Nursing
North Providence, RI

Lorraine W. Bock, R.N., M.S.N., C.R.N.P., C.E.N.
Widener University School of Nursing
York Hospital
York, PA

Lynn Bradley, M.S., C.N.M.
Johns Hopkins Medical Services Corporation
Johns Hopkins School of Nursing
Baltimore, MD

Joan Davenport, Ph.D., R.N.
York College of Pennsylvania
York, PA

Ruth E. Davis, D.Ed., R.N.C., C.R.N.P., N.P.-C.
Department of Nursing
Millersville University
Millersville, PA

Eric Doerfler, M.S.N., C.R.N.P.
Nightingale Health Centers, Inc.
Harrisburg, PA

Elaine R. Feeney, Ph.D., R.N.C., C.A.R.N.
York College of Pennsylvania
York, PA

Normandie J. Gaitley, S.S.J., Ph.D.
Formerly at York College of Pennsylvania
York, PA

Christine L. Gold, M.S.N., R.N., C.R.N.P.
York Women's Health Center
York, PA

Jacqueline Harrington, D.Ed., R.N.
York College of Pennsylvania
York, PA

Aline Harrison, Ph.D.
York College of Pennsylvania
York, PA

Rhada Artz Hartmann, R.N., B.S.N.
York Hospital
York, PA

Kathryn Van Dyke Hayes, D.N.Sc., R.N.C.
Shenandoah University
Winchester, VA

James Heindel, B.S., R.R.T.
York College/York Hospital School of Respiratory Care
York, PA

Joanne Hessmiller, Ph.D., A.C.S.W.
Marywood University
Scranton, PA

Marilyn J. Horan, M.Ed., R.N.C.
St. Joseph's Hospital School of Nursing
North Providence, RI

Kay Huber, D.Ed., R.N., C.R.N.P.
Messiah College
Grantham, PA

Karl W. Kleiner, Ph.D.
York College of Pennsylvania
York, PA

Linda Ledray, Ph.D., R.N., F.A.A.N.
Sexual Assault Resource Service
Minneapolis, MN

Deborah Lessard, Esq.
Pennsylvania State Nurses' Association
Harrisburg, PA

Valerie Lincoln, Ph.D., R.N., H.N.C.
Minnesota State University
Minneapolis, MN

Nancy Mann, R.N., M.S.N.
York Hospital
York, PA

Patricia Molloy, M.S.N., R.N.
Rhode Island Department of Health
Providence, RI

Teresa Nardontonia, M.S.N., R.N.C., C.R.N.P.
Hershey Medical Center of the Pennsylvania State University
Hershey, PA

Oma Reilly-Giomariso, Ph.D., R.N., C.C.R.N., C.R.N.P.
York College of Pennsylvania
York, PA

Mark Simmons, M.S., R.R.T.
York College/York Hospital School of Respiratory Care
York, PA

Marta Smith, M.S., R.D.
Formerly at York Health System
York, PA

Susan Sponsler, M.S.
York College of Pennsylvania
York, PA

Lynn Warner, Ph.D., R.N.C.
York College of Pennsylvania
York, PA

Elva J.S. Winter, Ph.D., R.N.C.S., M.P.S.S.C.
York College of Pennsylvania, Ret.
York, PA

Victoria Zeiler, B.S., R.R.T.
York Hospital
York, PA

Reviewers

Christine Hoyle, A.R.N.P., M.N.
University of Washington
Seattle, WA

Robin Webb Corbett, Ph.D., R.N.C.
East Carolina University
Greenville, NC

Mary Ann Kelley, R.N., M.S.N.
Mississippi University for Women
Columbus, MS

Marjorie Thomas Lawson, Ph.D., R.N.C.S., F.N.P.
University of Southern Maine
Portland, ME

Lois Montiero, Ph.D.
Brown University
Providence, RI

Marjorie Muecke, R.N., Ph.D., F.A.A.N.
University of Washington
Seattle, WA

Shirley Murphy, R.N., Ph.D., F.A.A.N.
University of Washington
Seattle, WA

Ann Niculescu, R.N., M.S.N.
J. Sargeant Reynolds Community College
Chester, VA

Susan Rawlins, M.S., R.N.C.
University of Texas Southwestern Medical School
Pottsboro, TX

Carol Roehrs, Ph.D., M.S.N., B.S.N.
University of Northern Colorado
Greeley, CO

Jane C. Walton, Ph.D., R.N., C.S.
Rush University
Chicago, IL

SECTION I

Health and Healthcare: Implications of Female Gender, Ethnicity, and Socioeconomic Status

1

Women, Society, Health, and Healthcare: Historical Roots and Contemporary Perspectives

Marian C. Condon

CHAPTER OUTLINE

Objectives

1. *Identify beliefs about women that affect women's health and healthcare.*
2. *Discuss ways in which societal views of women affect women's health and healthcare.*
3. *Contrast historical beliefs about women with the contemporary empirical literature on women's nature.*
4. *Define* social construction of health *and identify examples of the phenomenon.*
5. *Identify reasons that most medical research has been done on men.*

Introduction

Contemporary American women enjoy a level of social status and health that equals or surpasses that of most other women in the world. They have equal rights with men under the law, can pursue any occupation or profession for which they are prepared, and are serving in government at higher levels and in greater numbers than ever before. American women also live longer and are generally healthier than women in many other cultures, yet vestiges of their historical subordination remain and have implications for their health status. In this chapter, we will explore historical beliefs about and attitudes toward women that continue to influence women's lives and health. We will briefly review the status and circumstances of women in ancient Europe, colonial America, and eighteenth- and nineteenth-century America in terms of relevance to contemporary women's health and healthcare. We will also review outdated, yet still influential, theories about women's psychology and development and explore contemporary insights into the overall strength that characterizes women's biology and psychology. Current theories regarding the emergence of patriarchy will be briefly addressed, as will selected social phenomena relevant to women's health, such as the social construction of health and the medicalization of women's health. Finally, we will examine an overview of the efforts that have been made by women and their male advocates to procure better health and healthcare for women.

Revisiting the Past to Better Understand the Present: Historical Beliefs About and Attitudes Toward Women

An understanding of the relationship between women's place in the larger culture and their health during the colonial and later periods provides a perspective from which to view contemporary American women's health and its relationship to gender. In order to understand how early attitudes toward and policies pertaining to women came into being, it is necessary to examine briefly the early European societies that were the forebears of young America.

A Brief History of Women's Rights and Status

Because women have been historically viewed as physically and psychologically inferior to men, they have been denied rights and privileges granted routinely to men. Social policies based on the devaluing of women had serious implications for women's well being, both in the Old World and the New.

WOMEN IN ANCIENT EUROPE

Pre-Christian Greek, Roman, Germanic, Celtic, and Hebrew societies were intensely **patriarchal.** The extent to which women in those societies were undervalued, discriminated against, restricted, and persecuted can hardly be exaggerated. The Greek philosopher Aristotle, whose ideas dominated European science until well into the sixteenth century, is the author of the following: "The male is by nature superior, and the female inferior; and the one rules and the other is ruled" (from *Politics*). Aristotle believed that women exist only to *reproduce* and supply the world with more men. The Roman orator Cicero, who lived during the first century B.C.E., had beliefs similar to Aristotle's; he decreed that women must be ruled by men because women have *inherently weaker intellects* (Okin, 1979). In Celtic Ireland, women were considered legally "senseless," a category that also included drunks, prisoners, and slaves (Anderson & Zinsser, 1988). The belief that women are not as intellectually capable as men would greatly affect women's lives and women's health in colonial and nineteenth-century America.

The belief in females' inferiority was often fatal to them. Fewer female than male children were raised to adulthood in both ancient Greece and Rome because **female infanticide** was common (as it is in China and some other countries today), and little girls were weaned sooner and given less to eat than boys (Blaffer-Hrdy, 1999). Adult women could be *murdered* at will by their husbands—Roman law, for example, allowed a man to kill his wife for committing adultery or drinking wine (Anderson & Zinsser, 1988). Men's license to kill their wives was mitigated somewhat in colonial America (Kerber & DeHart-Mathews, 1987), where the law allowed men to merely beat their wives with any instrument no larger in circumference than their thumbs (the origin of the term **rule of thumb**). Its echo lives on, however, in contemporary America, in which thousands of women are killed each year by their spouses or male companions.

In the ancient world, women's **sexuality** was seen as belonging not to women themselves, but to men. Whereas men were free to copulate with any woman who did not belong to another man, women were expected to "save" their virginity for their husbands and then remain faithful to them after marriage. The Greek word for adultery referred specifically to sexual intercourse between a married woman and a man other than her husband. Unmarried women's sexuality belonged to men, too. For example, in Athens, the cultural center of the Greek world, women could be sold into brothels by their nearest male relative, and women who had sex with men other than their husbands could be put to death (Anderson & Zinsser, 1988).

The idea that women's sexuality is the property of men is by no means an anachronism. Even in the modern age, women thought guilty of adultery are still executed in some parts of the world. In America, rape is all too common and, until recently, a defense of "justifiable homicide" could be used in some states to shield men who had killed their unfaithful wives.

WOMEN IN COLONIAL AMERICA

The earliest, or colonial, period in American women's history began in 1607 (early seventeenth century), when white settlers from England established the first permanent colonies on the eastern seaboard of what would become the United States of America. It ended in 1781, when the colonists won the Revolutionary War and established America as a free republic. The colonies the **Puritans** established were considered territories of England, and the colonists were subject to English law. Women were still considered morally and intellectually inferior to men and were given virtually no rights under the law. Most of the text discussion that follows applies specifically to *white* women. The black women in colonial America were indentured or enslaved, and the Native American women were part of the indigenous culture.

Religion   The Puritans who settled America were intensely religious people, and the writings contained in the Christian Bible had great influence in their culture. Since about 3000 B.C.E., the dominant religions of the world, of which Christianity is one, have been intensely patriarchal. In patriarchal religions, God is conceptualized as male, and women are seen as inferior, less worthy beings. In the pre-Christian Hebrew culture from which the Bible's Old Testament came, women were placed in the same inferior classification as children and slaves, and their words were given no legal weight (Anderson & Zinsser, 1988). Both the Old and New Testaments contain many passages in which women are depicted as *weak* and *naturally subordinate* creatures. This view of women has been accepted as the word of God and has been used to justify male supremacy. According to the Bible, "as the church is subject to Christ, so let wives also be subject in everything to their husbands" (Ephesians 5).

Interestingly, some theologians (Fox, 1988) assert that, in the New Testament, **misogynist** (antiwomen) passages are always attributed to someone other than Jesus Christ and that there was no language and imagery damaging to women in the teachings of Jesus himself. According to this view, Jesus actually had a most unusual and enlightened view of women for a man of his time and culture. For example, in Luke 10:38–42, it is recorded that Jesus fraternized with women (very much against the customs of the time) and exhorted them to become more active in public life. After his crucifixion and death, Jesus appears not to one of his male disciples, but to Mary Magdalene, a woman (Eisler, 1988).

The Ideal Woman   White colonial women were burdened by a legacy of European cultural mores, which dictated how they should think, act, and dress. According to European middle- and upper-class beliefs, the ideal woman was a wife and mother who was faithful to her husband, hard-working, prolific, pious, and devoted to her family and her domestic duties. Above all, she was willingly *subordinate* to the men in her family. Seventeenth-century English men wanted obedient, docile wives who would be faithful to them, bear their children, obey them unquestioningly, and never compete with them (Riley, 1986). Among the English upper and middle classes, women were considered inherently delicate in body and mind and constitutionally unfit for anything physically or intellectually rigorous. This characterization kept wives of wealthy men idle and ignorant. It had little relevance to the lives of the much more numerous working class and poor people, among whom both sexes toiled constantly and had little access to education

Jean-Jacques Rousseau, a prominent eighteenth-century French philosopher whose works have been widely read in England, summed up the life's work of the ideal woman in his book *Emile:*

> To please, to be useful to us [men], to make us love and value them, to Educate us when young, and take care of us when grown up, to advise, console us, to render our lives easy and agreeable; these are the duties of women. (Okin, 1979, p. 31)

As he wrote in *Emilius and Sophia*, Rousseau also believed that women should, at an early age, be conditioned for a life of *subjugation:* "This daily constraint will produce the docility that women need all their lives. . . . She must learn to submit uncomplainingly" (Okin, 1979, p. 34).

The English model of the ideal woman was altered somewhat in colonial America. The idea that women are incapable of hard physical labor was of necessity suspended in that harsh wilderness environment—to be resurrected later as the country became more civilized. The rest of the model, particularly the part that mandated subservience and obedience, persisted. It must be remembered that Colonial women were as inculcated with English values as were the men. The extent to which they accepted their role is revealed in the phrases with which they commonly closed their letters:

> Your faithful and obedient wife. . . . Your sister to command. . . . Thy everloving and kind wife to command in whatsoever thou pleasest. (Kerber & DeHart-Mathews, 1987, p. 209)

Legal Rights   The English practice of denying women the rights that men enjoyed was continued, with some modification, in colonial America. Women were barred from town meetings and provincial legislatures and thus could not participate in their governance. When a woman married, she lost her **individual legal rights** under the law. She could no longer own property, make a will, or enter into a contract, as a single woman could. A married couple were considered to have **one identity**—that of the husband. When Sybilla Masters, a colonial woman who lived in Philadelphia, invented a new way of cleaning and curing corn in 1715, the patent was granted to her husband instead of to her. Married women had no legal right to **custody** of their children and were not even accorded the dignity of being held responsible for their own conduct; a man was legally responsible for any crimes his wife committed (Kerber & DeHart-Mathews, 1987).

The concept that women were the **property** of their husbands influenced laws related to sex crimes. Rape was punished by death only if the woman was married, engaged, or under the age of 10. Adultery was defined as intercourse between a married woman and a man other than her husband. As it involved the usurpation of one man's property by another, adultery was punished more severely than fornication, which was defined as sexual congress between a man, married or otherwise, and an unmarried woman (Kerber & DeHart-Mathews, 1987). The gradual repeal of laws upholding men's right to regard their wives as property has proceeded at a glacial pace. Until very recently, men had the right to force sex on their wives, and an English law that permitted men to forcibly restrain their wives from leaving the marriage remained in effect until 1973 (Wilson & Daly, 1992).

Unmarried colonial women were somewhat better off than their married sisters in terms of legal rights, in that they were recognized as independent individuals under the law. Even so, most had to join the households of their nearest male relatives, where they became unpaid household help. They did much spinning and weaving, which is reflected in the word *spinster,* slang for "unmarried woman." Some single women were able to pursue occupations, and a number were quite successful. There are even records of unmarried women having been allowed to argue for their own interests in court (Kerber & DeHart-Mathews, 1987).

In spite of severe social and legal consequences, most women of the time did marry. It was considered shameful to remain a single person when the colonies were in dire need of a larger population. This was particularly true for females, who might become burdens on male relatives if they did not marry. Women were taught that their proper destiny lay in *marriage* and *motherhood;* any other role was considered anomalous. The following quote from a newspaper dated 1764 illustrates the degree to which single women, or "old maids," were scorned:

> *An old maid is one of the most cranky, ill-natured, maggoty, peevish, conceited, disagreeable, hypocritical, fretful, noisy, gibing, canting, never-to-be-pleased, good for nothing creatures. (Kerber & DeHart-Mathews, 1987, p. 307)*

There is still in existence a card game for children called Old Maid. One loses the game of Old Maid if, at the end of the game, one is stuck with the Old Maid card, which has on it the cartoon image of a cranky elderly woman.

Work   The daily lives of colonial women were characterized by an output of physical labor that it is difficult for their con-temporary descendants to imagine. Women worked inside their homes and often outside as well. Inside, they were responsible for providing all of the food and clothing for their families. They cured meat, pickled and preserved vegetables and fruits, and tended gardens, cowherds, and chickens. They spun thread, wove cloth, and sewed clothes and rag rugs. And, of course, women did all of the cleaning and childcare—still mostly true, 300 years later. In addition to those duties, colonial women did many other kinds of outside work that they had not been allowed to do in England. Some women in the colonies were shopkeepers, innkeepers, teachers, printers, midwives, tanners, butchers, shipwrights, blacksmiths, gunsmiths, barbers, printers, publishers, and more (Kerber & DeHart-Mathews, 1987).

Providing healthcare for their families was also part of women's domestic responsibilities. Information about the use of medicinal plants was passed from mothers to daughters and—after 1700, when written material became widely available—was supplemented by information contained in a few popular medical guides. Licensing laws were not yet in existence and medical practice was undefined and unregulated. Anyone could use the title Doctor, including people with no formal training. A few doctors were graduates of European medical schools (which did not admit women), but many more had gained their experience through apprenticeship to an experienced practitioner. There were no medical schools in the colonies until the 1760s (Weisman, 1998).

Women's and men's lives were really quite similar in colonial times, as was their general health. Their mortality rates, however, were different. Women died *prematurely* more often and at an *earlier age* than men (the reverse of the present pattern), and the reason was childbirth.

Childbearing   Women's unending physical labor was punctuated regularly, at two-year intervals, by labor of another sort—childbearing. Women faced the hazards of childbirth, on average, **eight times** during their lifetimes. Reliable forms of contraception did not become available until the twentieth century; like millions of women before and after them, colonial women were *pregnant* or *lactating* throughout most of their adult lives. Although such a prospect seems daunting to many today, demographic evidence from New England and Pennsylvania indicates that most colonists, male and female, desired large families. Folk remedies thought to promote fertility and prevent miscarriage were popular. Contraception was frowned upon because the population was so small. Abortions, always dangerous and uncertain, were attempted to prevent illegitimate births, but not to control the size of families (Apple, 1990).

Childbirth was an almost totally natural process in colonial times. Although professional birth attendants, called **midwives,** were frequently used, their medical knowledge and skills would not be considered significant today. Tracts written specifically for pregnant women recommended that they meditate on the possibility of death. Although morbid, this was not unrealistic; *1 out of every 30* deliveries resulted in maternal death (Apple, 1990). The pain and danger of childbirth were seen as divinely ordained retribution for the "sins of Eve."

Laboring women were surrounded by female relatives and friends. Men generally did not witness births, and male physicians, scarce in the early colonial period, did not begin to supplant midwives until the late 1700s. When they did, they had a mixed effect on women's health. Physicians frequently provided **opium** to ease birth pangs and used **forceps** to aid difficult births; however, women attended by physicians were in greater danger of dying from **infection** than were women attended by midwives. The concept of germs was unknown, and doctors would go from the beds of patients suffering from infections to the beds of women in labor without washing their hands in between. Also, the prohibition against the display of the female body was so strong that medical education did not include the direct observation of childbirth until 1850 (Weisman, 1998). Thus, a typical midwife would have been considerably more experienced than the average physician. Nevertheless, the wealthier women, who could afford their services, frequently chose to have physicians attend them during childbirth.

Education Although it did not earn them equal rights under the law, women's indispensable work alongside men did gain them a measure of respect and worth. Even so, professions such as law, medicine, government, and the clergy were closed to them. For that reason, it was not deemed necessary that colonial women be educated to the degree that men were. Those who were schooled at all were usually taught to read, so that they could study the Bible and correspond with friends and relatives, but they were exposed to only rudimentary mathematics and little science and philosophy. It was expected that women would be accomplished only in music, sewing, and the social graces. In 1732, an 11-year-old girl named Betty Pratt complained of her inferior education in a letter to her younger brother:

> *I find you have got the start of me in learning very much, for you write better already than I can expect to do as long as I live and you are got as far as the rule of three in arithmetic, but I can't cast up a sum in addition cleverly, but I am striving to do better everyday. I can perform a great many dances . . . but I cannot speak a word of French. (Kerber & DeHart-Mathews, 1987, p. 389)*

The belief that women cannot achieve intellectually became a **self-fulfilling prophecy.** Deprived of the learning they needed to develop their minds, women had their inevitable lack of sophistication used against them as "proof" of their inborn intellectual inferiority. The fact that women were generally poorly educated and, with a few exceptions, barred from professional schools guaranteed that most women would be attended by male physicians, who, in most cases, did not question prevailing beliefs about women's inferior nature. Most physicians endorsed women's exclusion from higher education on the theory that mental efforts weakened women's reproductive organs and caused disease (Apple, 1990).

Black Women The first black women to arrive in the colonies were indentured servants, individuals, both black and white, who agreed to work for another individual for a given period of time in exchange for a given sum of money. When their period of indenture was over, they were free. Later, other black women were forcibly imported as slaves— West Africans brought to the colonies in chains aboard slave ships. The first "slaver" landed in the New World in 1690. Most of its slaves were male, but one-third of the human cargo of later ships consisted of women. Enslaved women were as brutally treated as enslaved men. They were forced to work long hours, were bought and sold like cattle, and were whipped and branded if they tried to escape (Mellon, 1990). The degree to which men controlled female sexuality in the colonial and later periods is illustrated by the fact that, although slave women were raped and/or punished if they resisted sexual advances from white men, antiamalgamation laws (first enacted in Maryland in 1664) enjoined white women from having sexual relationships with black men (Hooks, 1981). After slavery was abolished, black women went from being enslaved to being poor and suffered the same health consequences as poor women of other races.

Native American Women The native inhabitants of the New World were American Indians, who had lived there for thousands of years before the arrival of the first white settlers. They had a well-established culture markedly different from that of the European immigrants—particularly in the status accorded women. Among the people of the six Iroquois Nations (Cayuga, Tuscarora, Seneca, Onondaga, Oneida, and Mohawk), for instance, female as well as male tribal elders served on the most powerful ruling body, the Tribal Council. Indian women as well as men served as shamans—the medical practitioners and religious leaders of the tribe—and there are records of women having led warriors into battle. Some Indian peoples were **matrilocal** and **matrilinial**—married couples went to live in the wife's village, and lines of descent were traced through women. Among the Algonquin tribes, rape, though very rare, was punishable by death. Native American women resembled European women in that they did most of the domestic work in their villages, but they were not confined to that sphere; they also bartered and traded with each other and with white settlers. The gender-based division of labor, plus the fact that Indian women usually ate apart from men and remained in their huts during menstruation, led colonial historians to assume incorrectly that Indian women had no status in their society (Ehrenreich & English, 1978).

Contact with the white immigrants had a negative effect on the social and health status of women in Native American culture. The influence of female tribal leaders was undermined when the colonists would not accept them as representatives of their people (Ehrenreich & English, 1978), and female, as well as male, Native Americans died in great numbers from *diseases* introduced by white settlers.

INDEPENDENCE FOR MEN

The Revolutionary War was won and the American Republic established in 1783. The arguments that were used to justify replacing a monarchy with a republic could have been used also to justify an expansion of women's rights, but they were not. In their Declaration of Independence from Great Britain (which was printed by a woman newspaper publisher, Mary Katherine Goddard), the founding fathers had stated their belief that "... all *men* are created equal. ...." That sentiment was all too evident in the new Constitution of the United States. It not only failed to redress any of the previous legal wrongs done to women, but it also perpetrated a new one: It restricted the right to vote to *free white males* only. Nearly 150 years would pass before American women would be allowed to participate in the governance of their country.

WOMEN IN NINETEENTH-CENTURY AMERICA

After the colonial period, America industrialized rapidly. As factories were built and businesses were set up in cities, more and more men moved their families there to take advantage of employment opportunities. An urban culture developed, in which men left their property to go to work rather than working on their property, as most had done in the colonial period. Women remained on their property and attended to childrearing and the domestic tasks that remained. The original productive labor of women—food production, weaving, and sewing—became *centralized* in factories. Although some women, particularly poorer, unmarried women, followed their customary tasks into the factory as employees, they lost their authority over the process. Because childcare and domestic duties were still exclusively women's responsibility, married women remained in their homes. In wealthy families, it was no longer necessary for the woman of the house to carry out domestic duties, as servants were available. Wives of rich men became more and more irrelevant to the actual running of their households and came to be valued for their *reproductive* and *ornamental* qualities only. The old European "ideal woman" was reborn in America (Ehrenreich & English, 1978).

Upper-Class Women: Corsets and the Fainting Couch

The ideal woman was physically and mentally delicate, submissive, and completely dedicated to her family and home. She also had an exaggeratedly feminine figure, with a wasp waist and a generous bossom and derriere. To achieve that ideal to the greatest degree possible, wealthier women wore heavy (up to 20 pounds) whalebone **corsets,** which cinched their waists tightly and elevated their breasts. The tight lacing that was the norm exerted pressure on internal organs, which caused some women to develop minor or major health problems. Constriction of the lower chest caused corseted women to breathe shallowly. This led to frequent bouts of shortness of breath and dizziness, thus necessitating the presence of a **fainting couch** in every fashionable home and reinforcing the notion that women are physically weak. Downward pressure on abdominal and pelvic contents caused the uteri of some women to descend gradually into the vagina and even actually protrude from it—a condition called **vaginal prolapse** (Ehrenreich & English, 1978).

There was a tremendous amount of rather vaguely defined illness among middle- and upper-class women in nineteenth-century America. Historians have referred to it as a "wave of invalidism" (Ehrenreich & English, 1978). Women suffering from these indispositions exhibited various combinations of symptoms, including headache, loss of appetite, frequent bouts of crying, marked fatigue, insomnia, digestive complaints, and bizarre emotional outbursts. Doctors had a number of diagnostic labels, such as nervous prostration, neurasthenia, and, most famous of all, hysteria.

The term *hysteria* comes from a Greek word meaning **wandering uterus.** Ancient Greek physicians had believed that the uterus is the root of many, if not all, diseases in women. Their descendants in the nineteenth century clung to that belief and associated women's ailments, particularly mental disorders, with inherent pathology in the uterus and ovaries. **Hysterectomy,** the surgical removal of the uterus, and **oophorectomy,** the removal of the ovaries, were common treatments for depression and other emotional illnesses (Ehrenreich & English, 1978). The term *hysteria* was reserved for the more spectacular manifestations of emotional upset, and the word *hysterical* is still used to describe "fits" or outbursts. Modern historians have a number of theories about the true nature and origin of hysteria and invalidism, and there is likely some element of truth in all of them.

One of the most persuasive theories is that invalidism and hysteria were essentially **stress-related** disorders caused by a combination of the actual circumstances of women's lives and the gendered cultural myths they, and their physicians, internalized. Nineteenth-century middle- and upper-class white women were seen as, and believed themselves to be, passive, and emotionally and physically delicate. They may well have had low self-esteem and a fragile sense of self and self-efficacy. Thus, they would have been ill equipped to face the realities of daily life, which included the illness and the death of loved ones to a greater extent than is common today. For example, the risk of dying in childbirth was very real, as was the risk of **gynecological complications** following it. **Tuberculosis,** called the "white plague," raged at epidemic proportions and killed twice as many women as men for reasons that are poorly understood. **Child mortality** was high, and it was not uncommon for parents to experience the deaths of several of their children (Apple, 1990). Contemporary insights into the relationship between stress and physical and emotional symptoms lend strength to the gender role-stress hypothesis. Many authorities accept the theory that stress plays a part in the etiology and/or progression of coronary heart disease, hypertension, psoriasis, and a host of other disorders (see Chapter 7).

Others have described hysteria and invalidism as manifestations of *women's resentment of the confined nature of their lives.* This interpretation is supported by the work of **Charlotte Perkins Gilman,** a nineteenth-century woman who had insight into her own illness. In a short story titled *The Yellow Wallpaper,* Gilman described her "hysterical" depression as a consequence of her frustrated desire to be an artist, and recorded that when she finally left her home to pursue a career, her depression lifted. It has also been suggested that women used invalidism, consciously or unconsciously, to avoid unwelcome sexual encounters and too frequent pregnancies.

Hysteria and invalidism in general have also been attributed to the increasing numbers of physicians and their need for patients. Upper-class women's supposed constitutional weakness fit nicely with doctors' need for a class of affluent patients whose leisure allowed for lengthy periods of illness and whose socialization would assure their submission to medical authority. Some consider it no accident that poor women, who had neither the money to pay for medical care nor time to spend in invalidism, were considered *immune* to invalidism and hysteria (Apple, 1990). Physicians attributed that seemingly odd difference to lower class (especially nonwhite) women's supposed *primitive* nature, which was thought to endow them with stronger constitutions.

Working-Class Women Working-class women, a group that included almost all immigrant and nonwhite women, suffered health problems related to poverty and overwork. Poor women's inferior *nutritional status* made them more vulnerable to communicable diseases, as did the lack of *sanitation* in the tenements in which many lived. Constant childbearing drained their strength, as contraception was almost never available and was actually against the law from 1873 to the beginning of the 1930s (Apple, 1990). There was little healthcare available to poor people, who could not pay for it.

To bring in enough money to keep their children from starving, many poorer married women worked outside their homes, in addition to doing all the domestic labor inside them. Most of those who did not leave their homes to go to work took in laundry or sewing. Poor single women and widows had to work; there were no wealthy relatives to take them in. Female, as well as male, factory workers worked long hours for little pay. They developed many work-related health problems, such as **lung disease** from the lint in textile factories, and many were maimed or killed in accidents involving machinery. There was no time off for pregnancy or recovery from childbirth. The following description of a woman who worked in a New England factory is from an 1889 survey on the health of women who worked outside their homes:

> *Constant application to work, often until 12 at night and sometimes on Sundays affected her health and injured her eyesight. She . . . was ordered by the doctor to suspend work . . . but she must earn money, and so she has kept on working. Her eyes weep constantly, she cannot see across the room. . . . She owed when seen three months board for self and children. (Ehrenreich & English, 1978 p. 114)*

Prior to the passage of child labor laws, it was not uncommon for female and male children as young as six to work 14-hour days in filthy, unsafe conditions. Also, many young women were forced into **prostitution** by their impoverishment. Although poor women did not suffer from invalidism, they sometimes suffered because of it. Dr. Marion Sims, known as the father of gynecology, specialized in the surgical treatment of female emotional disorders. He kept female slaves for the sole purpose of practicing his techniques on them and operated on one unfortunate woman 30 times in four years. Later, he continued his experiments on poor Irish women in the indigent wards of New York Women's Hospital (Ehrenreich & English, 1978).

Women and Health Research

Overall, less is known about women's health than men's. Until recently, almost all the medical research pertaining to nongynecological problems was conducted using male subjects, whether animal or human. Major clinical trials, intended to determine the efficacy of drugs and procedures, were conducted on cohorts of male subjects. Thus, findings relevant to the prevention, detection, and treatment of problems such as coronary heart disease and cancer, which afflict both men and women, were derived from research on men but *generalized* to women. There are a number of much discussed examples of medical research bias toward men. In the 1977 Mr. Fit (Multiple Risk Factor Intervention Trial) study, which tested the efficacy of various strategies for reducing the incidence of coronary heart disease, 15,000 men, but no women, were studied (Hales, 1999). The Physician's Health Study, begun in 1982, evaluated aspirin as a possible protective agent against coronary heart disease and included more than 2,000 male physician subjects, but no female ones (Hales, 1999). The Coronary Drug Project, a large study that evaluated drugs used in coronary heart disease, also excluded women (Dickerson & Schnaper, 1996). The Baltimore Longitudinal Study of Aging followed more than a thousand men but no women—despite the fact that more women than men live to reach old age (Weisman, 1998). A particularly egregious aspect of this study was that the publication to which it led, a 1984 document titled *Normal*

Human Aging, clearly exposed the authors' assumption that *"normal" equals male.*

A number of explanations for the neglect of women in medical research have been put forward. Feminists have argued that the general *overvaluing of men* and concomitant devaluing of women in Western culture, and the characterization of male as normal and female as "other" and abnormal, are the most salient underlying factors. The preponderance of men in the research sciences, including medicine, and on government committees that oversee research funding, has also been mentioned. However, others (Legato, 2002) have argued that, at least in the past, large cohorts of men, such as men in the military, have been easier for researchers to access. Also, researchers have been loathe to expose women who might be or might become pregnant to the effects of drugs and other experimental conditions. The dearth of information about women's health, ironically, sometimes resulted in women being excluded from studies. The designers of the Mr. Fit trial said they omitted women from their study because they considered coronary heart disease a problem of middle-aged men (Weisman, 1998). It is now known that coronary heart disease kills more women than any other health problem (see Chapter 12).

Other problems related to women and health research have been identified. When women *are* included in studies, they are sometimes present in insufficient numbers to ensure statistically valid findings about their response to the treatment under study. Also, women have had much less input than men into decision making about research funding and design. Finally, research on women's health is too often justified in terms of its benefits to women's children or family members, rather than to women themselves. For example, early studies on women and AIDS focused on the danger that infected women might pose to their children and partners, rather than on the symptoms and problems of the women themselves (Weisman, 1998).

Androcentric Theories of Women's Psychology and Development

The inaccurate and pejorative beliefs about women handed down to modern European and American culture resulted in the development of many theories of psychology and human development that were based on men's experience alone. Because those theories equated that which was typically *male* as *normal,* that which was typically female was seen as abnormal and inferior. The incorporation of those theories into the "common knowledge" of female nature and their application in clinical psychology have done a disservice to generations of women. The following sections discuss such theories.

Freud

Sigmund Freud, the founder of **psychoanalysis** and a towering figure in the history of the social sciences, was very much a product of the turn-of-the-twentieth-century, patriarchal, Viennese society in which he lived. Most of Freud's ideas about the nature of women have been proven incorrect; nevertheless, they have been exceedingly persistent, and some continue to be defended by contemporary psychoanalysts. Freud theorized that basic gender differences, rooted in biology and therefore inescapable, exist. One of his most famous dictates is "anatomy is destiny" (Starr, 1991). Freud believed that normal women are inherently docile and passive and that women who harbor "masculine strivings," such as a desire for education and accomplishment outside the home, suffer from a disorder called **penis envy.** Freud also believed and taught that women are **masochistic**—that they have an unconscious need for, and actually enjoy, suffering and humiliation. Additionally, Freud thought that normal women experience sexual orgasm **vaginally** and that to do so via the **clitoris** is evidence of immature or incomplete psychological development. It is now known that clitoral orgasms are the norm for most women (see Chapter 22).

Although Freud's groundbreaking concept of the **unconscious** assures his continued place in the pantheon of science, his theories about women merely echo the traditional patriarchal bias against women. This bias is captured perfectly in a statement by Greek philosopher **Plato:** "The female is a female by virtue of a certain lack of qualities; we should regard the female nature as afflicted with a natural defectiveness" (Mahowald, 1994, p. 13).

Erikson

Until recently, *male* life-cycle development was accepted as a synonym for *human* development. Women, whose lives often diverged from "normal" male patterns, were seen as **developmentally abnormal.** The major theories of life-cycle development can be divided into two basic categories, or models: One is the **timing of events** model, in which it is supposed that people will undergo certain experiences at certain times in their lives. The other is the **normative crisis** model, in which it is assumed that, in order to develop fully, individuals must successfully negotiate, in the proper order, certain predictable "crises" of living.

Erik Erikson was one of the most influential of the normative crisis theorists, and his theory is still taught in most colleges and universities today. Writing in the 1950s and heavily influenced by Freud, Erikson developed a theory of human development, which he articulated in his book *The Eight Stages of Man.* Erikson theorized that growth arises out of a series of eight developmental crises, which occur in a predictable order over a person's lifetime. Normal development requires the successful resolution of each of these crises as it occurs. Two of Erikson's crises, the fifth and the sixth, are problematic in terms of their implications for women: During the fifth crisis, **identity versus role confusion,** adolescents must develop a sense of personal identity by committing to a philosophy of life and to a career path. Failure to do this leaves them floundering in aimlessness and confusion. Because, in

Erikson's day, most women did not work outside their homes, *career* for women meant marriage and commitment to a man. According to Erikson, then, single women and lesbian women are *abnormal* by definition. During the sixth crisis, **intimacy versus isolation,** young adults must commit to a partner of the opposite sex or face a barren, isolated existence without spouse and family. Because Erikson's model is linear and the sixth crisis follows the fifth, the capacity for intimacy cannot be developed until identity has been established. For women, however, *career* means marriage, which is associated with intimacy. Thus, in Erikson's model, the fifth and sixth stages are conflated for women, and a woman's identity is incomplete until she meets and mates with the man whose name she will carry and whose status will determine her own.

Erikson's beliefs about the nature of women are further revealed by his comments regarding women whose children are grown. Erikson saw such mothers as often having excessive and deleterious influence on their adult offspring: "Mom is a woman in whose life cycle remnants of infantility join advanced senility to crowd out the middle range of mature womanhood, which thus becomes self-absorbed and stagnant" (Ehrenreich & English, 1978, p. 237).

Vaillant and Levinson

Many timing of events models are equally biased against and problematic for women. Theorists such as **George Vaillant** and **Daniel Levinson** maintained that the phases of "normal" people's lives unfold in an *orderly and predictable* sequence: childhood, schooling, work, marriage, childrearing, retirement, and death. This, however, is a much more typically *male* than female sequence. Women's lives, certainly modern women's lives, are seldom so linear. Some women become mothers while in their twenties, but others do so in their forties, and still others have babies at both ages. Many women drop out of college to raise families and then drop back in again, years later. Many women do education and career, or education and childrearing, *at the same time,* and many do all three at the same time.

How Wrong They Were: Modern Insights into Women's Nature

That women are not, and have never been, the frail, flawed creatures described in patriarchal mythology is obvious. Even in the historically darkest times, a few exceptional women soared above social expectations to remarkable achievement. Hildegard of Bingen was a twelfth-century mystic, philosopher, musician, and healer whose exquisite chants have been rediscovered and are selling well today. Hypatia, a fifth-century teacher and mathematician, invented scientific instruments and wrote texts in algebra and geometry in the city of Alexandria. In the early 1700s, Maria Gaetana Agnesi wrote a text on mathematical analysis and calcu-

lus. So superior was her work that she was awarded a diploma by the University of Bologna in Milan and invited to join its faculty. Chinese Empress Shi Dun invented paper, using the bark of mulberry trees. Early British Queen Boadicea led troops against Roman invaders, and, in the 1500s, Queen Elizabeth I ruled England and Ireland for over 40 years. More recently, women have invented such indispensable innovations as Macintosh computer icons, bulletproof vests, laser optics used in CD players and the heat-resistant ceramic tiles used in the space shuttle (Hales, 1999).

Many more women in contemporary American society have distinguished themselves in virtually all walks of life. They are astronauts, tycoons, scientists, judges, and politicians. More women than men now earn baccalaureate degrees (Hales, 1999) and, in recent national elections, women have cast the deciding vote. Nevertheless, thousands of years of antiwoman propaganda have left their mark. Some women and men today still say they would not patronize a woman physician or cast a vote for a woman running for high office because "women are just not cut out for that sort of thing." Unjustified concerns about women's overall robustness, intelligence, and emotional stability remain. The truth is that women and men are quite similar in many ways. Differences that exist are just that—differences, rather than evidence of an innate superiority of one gender over another.

Health and Longevity

Each gender has both strengths and weaknesses in terms of overall fitness and vitality. Men *suffer less illness* than women, but women *live longer* than men. It is an unchallenged fact that, on average, women in developed countries live from five to seven years (between 5 and 10 percent) longer than men. The average life expectancy is 79.5 years for white American women and 74.5 years for black women. For white men, it is 74.3 years and, for black men, 67.2 years. Mortality rates for women are lower than for men even *before birth*. About 115 male babies are conceived for every 100 female babies; however, because males are miscarried more than females, only 104 boys are born for every 100 girls (Why Women Live Longer Than Men, 1999). Women have not always outlived men, however. Women's advantage in life expectancy has emerged over the past 50 years, likely because of increased access to birth control and advances in obstetrical technology (Cross, 1997).

Various explanations have been offered for women's longer life span, but there is no clear answer as to what explains the phenomenon. Some argue that evolution favors female longevity to ensure the continuation of the species because human infants are dependent on their mother's milk and care for a relatively long period. Women do seem to have a **genetic advantage** in that they have two X chromosomes, whereas men have only one. This "spare" X chromosome is important because a number of inherited diseases, such as muscular dystrophy and hemophilia, are carried on the X chromosome. If one of a woman's X chromosomes carries such a gene, the body can shut it down and allow the other one to take over, thus preventing the gene from being expressed. In addition, the X chromosome contains a gene responsible for repairing damaged DNA. If a man's X chromosome fails in this function, he is more vulnerable to cancer, whereas women have a backup.

Another aspect of women's genetic protection is the **estrogen** produced in their bodies. Estrogen decreases women's vulnerability to coronary heart disease by decreasing levels of harmful forms of cholesterol, elevating beneficial forms of it, and maintaining the flexibility and elasticity of blood vessels. Women also have a slower metabolic rate, which causes them to produce fewer damaging **free radicals** (see Chapter 3), which speed the aging process and increase susceptibility to disease. Moreover, estrogen is a natural **antioxidant.** Finally, women have more competent **immune systems** than men and are therefore less susceptible to communicable disease and cancer (Kimura, 1999).

Some argue that women live longer than men because they have less *stress* and *work* in their lives. This is debatable, however, as more women than men suffer the stress associated with being **poor,** and the majority of women with families work outside their homes, and doing most of the work inside their homes as well (see Chapter 7). However, stress may take a lesser toll on women than men because estrogen, present in higher levels in women, ameliorates physiological stress responses, whereas **testosterone,** present at higher levels in men, exacerbates them (Hazzard, 1994). Testosterone also seems to make men more impulsive and aggressive and probably accounts, in part, for their higher rate of accidents, homicides, and drug overdoses. At ages 15 to 34, men die at three times the rate that women do—often because of reckless behavior and violence. However, gender roles likely bear on this phenomenon also. In this culture, **masculinity** is synonymous with aggression, daring, and fearlessness, among other things. Many men remain trapped in the macho paradigm exemplified by characters played by John Wayne, Sylvester Stallone, and Clint Eastwood.

Failing to transcend their gender role, as women are increasingly doing, harms men in other ways, too. Men still define themselves primarily in terms of their work, and much of their self-image and self-esteem is tied to their **work role** (Doyle & Paludi, 1997). Women, in contrast, derive their self-concept from **multiple roles**—spouse, worker, parent, caretaker, and so on. The painful loss of identity many men suffer on retirement may explain why their risk of suffering from **depression** rises with age, whereas women's does not. Men's gender role orientation toward work and competition, and the "silent loner" stereotype, makes men less likely than women to form deep, intimate **friendships** in which they can express their feelings and obtain support. This may further undermine men's longevity, as intimacy and love have been found in a number of studies to be protective against the development of coronary heart disease (Ornish,

1998). Although women generally outlive men, they have more nonfatal health problems, which will be discussed in more detail in Chapter 2.

Intelligence

Intelligence is a multifaceted construct. One form of intelligence, **general intelligence,** is reflected in scores on I.Q., or **intelligence quotient,** tests, such as the Wechsler Adult Intelligence Scale. Other aspects of intelligence, such as **musical intelligence, artistic intelligence,** and **interpersonal intelligence,** have been described by Sternberg (1994). Most recently, Goleman (1995) has brought to national attention the importance of what he calls **emotional intelligence.** The form of intelligence in which women have been seen as deficient, however, has been general intelligence. In centuries past, it was assumed that brain size correlates with intelligence; since men's brains outweigh women's by an average of about 10 percent (Hales, 1999), men were assumed to be more intelligent than women. Although it is now generally accepted that there is **no** overall intelligence gap between women and men, there is disagreement among modern scientists as to the actual significance of the approximately 4 billion more neurons (Kimura, 1999) possessed by the average man. Some argue that there is little or no practical significance and point out that men may need more cells because men's brain cells die faster as they age (*Women's Health Advisor,* 1999). What is currently agreed on, given the available literature, is that males tend to be better at some specialized skills and females tend to be better at others.

Men are often considerably better than women at a spatial skill that involves the mental rotation of a three-dimensional figure. That may explain why men tend to be better at map reading and often give directions in terms of cardinal points—for example, "Go south on Rt. 84 and then East on Rt. 70." Women as a group have more trouble with maps and tend to give directions in terms of landmarks—such as "Go left at the church and then turn right at the Kentucky Fried Chicken." Women tend to be much better than men at a mental process called **disembedding;** they can, for example, usually find all the *p*'s in a paragraph faster than men (Kimura, 1999). In general, men score higher on tests of math aptitude and math reasoning, but women score higher on mathematical computation and do better in math in school. Nevertheless, males who achieve nearly perfect scores on sophisticated math tests outnumber females seven to one, and men outnumber women in fields in which mathematical reasoning is important, such as physics and engineering. Men can throw more accurately and are better at finding hidden figures (where's Waldo?), but women outdo them on tests of fine motor skills and memory for location of objects. Women are also better at visual perceptual speed—which means they can more easily find identical figures in a large field of figures. They also are much more attuned to facial expression and tone of voice and can read body language in general better than men. Women also do better than men on some aspects of verbal intelligence. They tend to be better spellers and tend to be better at grammar and color naming. Women also have better recall of verbal material. They do not, however, have better vocabularies (in adulthood), and they do not speak more fluently than men. These sex-linked strengths appear to be related to differences in hormone levels and brain anatomy.

The sex hormones estrogen and testosterone influence brain organization prior to birth and brain function after birth. By the fourth month of gestation, for example, the absence or presence of testosterone has determined whether a fetus's brain will develop female or male features. The subtle anatomical differences between men's and women's brains, in addition to size, are found mainly in the **hypothalamus** and the **corpus collosum,** which is the bridge between the right and left hemispheres. Women have a larger corpus collosum, and that may explain why they are able to use both hemispheres to process language, whereas men use only the left hemisphere. Why nature conferred this ability on women and not on men is unknown, but women who suffer damage to the left side of the brain are more likely to retain their ability to speak than are men with similar damage (*Women's Health Advisor*, 1999). It has been theorized that sex-linked anatomical differences in the brain are a result of the differing **gender roles** that emerged as the human species evolved. The human brain is still structurally the same as it was 50,000 years ago. Male brains may have become somewhat specialized for tasks associated with hunting, scavenging, and defense, whereas female brains may have adapted to allow women to excel at tasks related to caring for infants and searching for food and other needed materials (Kimura, 1999). The exact functions related to all of the small differences in brain anatomy between females and males have not been mapped out yet, but it is likely that they are related to the sex-linked differences in cognitive functioning.

The effects of sex hormones on the brain do not doom women and men to a narrow range of respective abilities. For one thing, the prenatal hormone levels that influence sex-linked differentiation in brain structure are influenced by such factors as **maternal stress** and **nutrition.** It cannot be assumed that these hormones will exert their full potential effects on the brains of all female and male fetuses. Moreover, later in life, men's spatial ability can vary with fluctuating testosterone levels, and fluctuations in estrogen levels can affect women's perceptual speed and manual dexterity. Influences other than brain organization and hormone levels are also significant in determining the ultimate cognitive ability profile of a given woman or man. If individuals are not willing, or are denied the opportunity, to develop whatever inborn aptitudes they have, they are likely to lose them because brain structures tend to become more robust with use and to atrophy (shrink) with disuse (Hales, 1999). Thus, women who take courses in higher mathematics and pursue careers in which they must use mathematical reasoning will

do better in mathematical reasoning than men who do not develop their ability in that realm. **Gender socialization** often causes individuals to develop, or fail to develop, specific abilities. For example, women who are socialized to believe they cannot excel at math may avoid math courses and other situations in which they might develop mathematical ability, thus creating a self-fulfilling prophecy. Because of the many variables that affect aptitude and ability, there is a greater range of aptitudes *within* the sexes than *between* them. Whereas some men are good at map reading, others are not; whereas some women are not very good at it, others are terrific. Overall, there is *much more similarity than dissimilarity* in overall cognitive functioning between the sexes.

Emotion

The idea that women are more emotional than men has been a staple of gender lore for a long time; however, surprisingly little research has been done on emotion in comparison with cognition, perhaps because emotion is associated with **femininity.** Modern researchers are finally beginning to study emotion and much more is now known about how emotions are experienced and expressed by women and men.

GENERAL EMOTIONAL EXPERIENCE AND EXPRESSION

Both women and men experience the complete range of emotions—sadness, joy, love, anger, and so on. It does seem to be true, though, that women experience their emotions more *intensely* than men and to manifest them more *openly*, in many situations (Goleman, 1995). Differing gender socialization may explain that, at least partially. For example, crying is generally more socially acceptable for women than men, although that is slowly changing. Also, there may be differences in the frequency with which the genders experience certain emotions. For example, whether women experience *anger* as often as men is open to question. Some researchers, such as Grossman and Wood (1995), report that men become angry more often than women do and are more likely to express their anger as aggression. Others believe that women experience anger as often as men but are more likely to express it in other ways or to not express it at all (Brody, 1997). Some researchers have found that women do seem to be more likely than men to keep their anger bottled up and seething beneath the surface (Hales, 1999).

Women are better able than men to "read" emotions in others, a knack that is present as early as the preschool years and that is refined over time (Hales, 1999). Interestingly, men can detect sadness more easily in other men's faces than in women's, although they detect sadness in both genders less well than women. Women seem also to be more affected by disharmony and conflict than men, at least in some situations. In one study of long-married couples, the women, but not the men, had higher levels of stress hormones and a lowered immune response after a quarrel (Kiecolt-Glasser et al., 1997). Women also experience more *guilt* than men. Society programs women to see themselves as caregivers and nurturers and to believe that they should put the needs of others—spouses, children, aging parents—ahead of their own. Indeed, it is the tyranny of the countless "shoulds" related to women's multiple roles that feed women's guilt. Women tend to internalize myriad guilty feelings and brood about them, whereas men focus their contrition briefly on a single act of commission or omission and then move on (Hales, 1999).

Some researchers have identified **physiological differences** between women's and men's brain functioning, which may play a part in their tendency to display different patterns of emotional expression. When neuroimaging scans (Gur, 1994) were done on brains in a state of relaxation (not being stimulated externally or attending to any volitional task), the men's brains were more likely to show activity in an ancient region of the limbic system responsible for unsubtle, active expressions of emotion, such as aggression. The resting female brains, however, most often showed a pattern of activity in a different, more recently evolved part of the limbic system, in which more symbolic manifestations of emotion, such as words, gestures, and facial expressions, are controlled. The sex differences were not absolute; about a third of the men tested and 17 percent of the women tested had brain activity patterns more typical of the opposite gender. Some men do seem to be more evolved emotionally than others, whereas some women lag behind the rest of their gender in this regard.

Another difference in the physiology of women's and men's brains is related to the way the emotion *sadness* affects cerebral blood flow. When a group of men and women were asked to recall sad incidents or circumstances in their lives, positron emission tomography (PET) scans of their brains revealed eight times as much activity in the "sadness centers" of the women's brains as in the men's. Because almost all the sad memories recalled by the subjects had to do with people—family, friends or other loved ones—the women's greater sadness may have had to do with the importance *relationships* seem to have for women.

EMOTIONAL INTELLIGENCE

Daniel Goleman (1995) has written that success in modern society depends more on emotional intelligence than on any other form of intelligence. *Emotional intelligence* is defined as being in touch with, managing, and valuing one's feelings as a source of information about the self. People who possess emotional intelligence are able to consider short- and long-term consequences before taking action. They are better able to reach goals and better at *compromise* and *collaboration* with others. Women may possess more of this essential form of intelligence than men, and emotional intelligence may underlie women's increasingly recognized ability as managers. Recent studies from the world of business suggest that women are more flexible, better able to deal with ambiguity,

and more oriented toward supporting and maintaining relationships than are men and that they are strong in idea generation and innovation. In a study that matched percentages of women managers with the overall success of businesses, Shrader, Blackburn, and Illes (1997) found that the financial performance of firms with relatively more women in management positions was higher than that of companies with fewer women managers.

EMOTIONAL STABILITY

Another staple of gender lore is that women are *emotionally unstable* and more likely than men to collapse or become nonfunctional in a crisis. Anyone who has seen contemporary women paramedics, nurses, physicians, and air-traffic controllers in action would find this proposition ludicrous; however, research suggests that the way in which women respond to the short-term stress of a crisis depends on a number of factors. The way in which people, female or male, respond to challenging and stressful situations depends to a great extent on how *powerful* or *powerless* they believe themselves to be. Martin Seligman (1991) has written extensively about what he calls "learned helplessness." In early experiments on animals, Seligman found that, when dogs were confined in a series of secure enclosures from which they could not escape, they eventually came to believe that escape was impossible and stopped attempting it. When the same dogs were later placed in boxes from which escape was possible, they still made no attempt. Seligman went on to establish that learned helplessness occurs in human beings as well and that it is a precursor of depression.

Women's historical reputation for emotional frailty was related to the confined, circumscribed lives so many of them led; being unable to cope can be seen as an expression of learned helplessness. The learned helplessness–depression connection is supported by the demographics of depression. Worldwide, women are still considerably less empowered than men, and they suffer more depression than men. Moreover, the rates at which women become depressed vary inversely with the degree to which their societies are egalitarian; the more freedom and agency women have, the less likely they are to be depressed (Hales, 1999). There is no evidence that women are *intrinsically* less emotionally stable than men. In fact, some women, under some circumstances, have proven to be *more* stable than men. In World War II, psychologists studied the impact of unrelenting stress on Londoners who were being bombed day and night during the blitz. To their astonishment, the men who became psychiatrically disturbed outnumbered women by 70 percent (Hales, 1999).

Women's Development

Contemporary social scientists are developing theories that more accurately reflect women's lives. **Qualitative, or naturalistic, research methods,** which allow subjects to present information in their own words, have yielded much information about women's realities—as well as men's. Social scientists at Wellesley College's Stone Center have developed a **relational** theory of women's development. According to this theory, women's identities are formed within the context of relationships, although not just heterosexual romantic relationships, as Erikson would have it. Relational theory holds that women form their identities as a function of the interactional process in all its manifestations. Beginning with the earliest attachment to mothers or primary caregivers and continuing with intimate friendships, sexual relationships, and relationships with others in the wider community, relationship is a primary source of meaning and identity in women's lives (Jordan, 1991). According to this theory, whereas most men are socialized to *compete with each other* and value *autonomy* and *power* over others, women are more likely to value *harmony* and a sense of *connection* with others (Hales, 1999). According to this theory, the goal of connection for women tends to be **mutual empowerment,** rather than winning or gaining control over another person.

Indeed, most women make deep, long-lasting friendships that allow them to confide in, and receive support from others. Hite (1989) found that almost 90 percent of the women in her study reported having their deepest emotional relationship with a woman friend. It is also generally women who are most active in maintaining family ties. Women are considerably more likely than men to have large social support networks—friends and relatives who will provide various kinds of help when needed (Paludi, 1992). This may be yet another reason that widowed women usually do better, physically and psychologically, than widowed men (Matlin, 1993).

Patriarchy: Natural and Inevitable?

How did the pervasive and long-standing pattern of prejudice and discrimination against female persons come to be? Is patriarchy "natural" and therefore perhaps inevitable? Painstaking and ongoing investigations conducted in scientific fields, such as biology and archeology, have yielded intriguing and conflicting answers to those questions.

Biological Theories

Some theorists from the field of **sociobiology,** the study of how genetic predispositions and social factors interact to determine human behavior, have suggested that men's tendency to dominate women is at least partly a function of **natural selection,** the mechanism of evolution. According to evolutionary theory, the genes that are **selected**—that is, passed to succeeding generations—are the genes of individuals who have succeeded at reproducing and whose off-

spring have also reproduced. Some have interpreted evolutionary theory as suggesting that men who controlled women and restricted their access to other men were more successful in passing on their genes than men who did not. In men, then, tendencies toward aggression and a desire for control were selected as human beings evolved (Blum, 1997). Sociobiologists are quick to point out, however, that the existence of a gene that fosters a certain trait does not guarantee that the trait will emerge in every individual. In order for a genetic possibility to become a behavioral reality, the *environment* must be conducive to it. For example, a person who possesses a gene that will allow her to grow to be six feet tall will not realize that potential unless she is adequately nourished during her growth years. Interestingly, male domination over females is not ubiquitous in primate (ape and monkey) societies. In rhesus monkeys, for example, females dominate the much larger males. Chimpanzee society, however, more closely resembles human society in that males tend to dominate females. Blum (1997) suggests that the secret to one sex's having power over the other in a given society may lie in that sex's propensity for forming the right kinds of **alliances** for the right reason. Male humans, male chimpanzees, and female rhesus monkeys, which share the characteristic of being **dominant** in their societies, all tend to form alliances with same-sex individuals for the purpose of acquiring and maintaining *power.* Bonds are formed on the basis of an individual's ability to contribute to the coalition's overall strength, and personal quarrels do not break linkages within coalitions. In contrast, female humans and female chimpanzees, which share the characteristic of being **subordinate** in their respective societies, tend to form alliances for the purpose of garnering *social support* rather than political power. Moreover, disputes disrupt alliances among females fairly frequently in human and chimpanzee societies (Blum, 1997).

Theories Derived from Archeological Discoveries

Whereas biologists have argued that natural selection during human evolution fostered men's dominance over women, some archeologists maintain that patriarchy is *not* the only gender/power schema that has characterized human culture and that it is, in fact, a relatively recent schema in terms of the total span of human history. Evidence that prepatriarchal societies, in which women and men were on a much more equal footing, existed throughout most of the world has been found. The locations of these sites include present-day Turkey, France, Greece, the Near and Far East, Siberia, India, and North America. The earliest societies in which women appear to have played a central role were the **Goddess Cultures** of the **Paleolithic** era (30,000–5,000 B.C.E.). Artifacts such as wall paintings, figurines, carved bones, and other items from cave sanctuaries and burial sites have been seen by modern scientists as evidence of "some form of early religion in which feminine representations and symbols played a central part" (Eisler, 1988, p. 6). The much more plentiful artifacts from the (7000–3500 B.C.E.) **Neolithic** era provide additional evidence that cultures characterized by a **gynocentric** (Goddess-based) religion and equality between the sexes not only existed but were the norm.

Neolithic Egalitarian Cultures

It was in the Neolithic period that agriculture (the domestication of wild plants as well as animals) began to be developed. During the height of Neolithic civilization in what is known as Pre-Indo-European or "Old" Europe, villages such as Catal Huyuk, Hacilar, Vinca, Butmir, Cucuteni, Lengyel, Gumelnita, Karanovo, Tisza, Hamangia, and Petresti flourished. From the very large number of artifacts brought to light (clothing, furniture, food, containers, tools, wall paintings, pictures, and engravings on seals and jewelry), multidisciplinary archeological teams have been able to discern many details about these early human societies. In stark contrast to later civilizations, Neolithic culture is believed to have been Goddess-centered, amazingly *egalitarian* in terms of gender and social class, and peaceful (Gimbutas, 1989).

Archeologists such as Marija Gimbutas interpret the archeological evidence as suggesting that there was great respect and reverence for the feminine in Neolithic cultures. The **Great Goddess** seems to have been the central object of religious devotion; multifaceted images of her were fashioned into clay objects and carved onto walls, jewelry, and so on. Approximately 97 percent of the figurines found in excavated houses, temples, and shrines are female; most male images were carved into walls or painted on objects. Neolithic culture was matrilinear and matrilocal; lines of descent were traced through the **mother** (matriliniar descent) and men went to live with the clan or family of their **wives** (matrilocality). Despite the apparent primacy of the Goddess, however, there is no evidence that a **matriarchy,** in which women dominated and oppressed men, existed. The available evidence suggests that women and men lived and worked together on an approximately equal basis; no lavish tombs for great rulers or persons of special importance of either sex have been found. Of course, there is not universal agreement that a Goddess-centered religion translates into equality for women. Some (Blaffer-Hrdy, 1999) have argued that representations of female deities are common in the dominant religions of patriarchical societies, such as India, and do not necessarily imply gender equity within a culture.

The Rise of Patriarchy

Beginning in about 3500 B.C.E., the Great Goddess cultures were slowly but inexorably overrun by wave after wave of cattle-herding, patriarchal, Indo-European tribes. Those

tribes, which Gimbutas dubbed the "Kurgans," were ruled by powerful male warriors and priests, and they imposed their ideology and their male gods on the inhabitants of the lands they conquered. This process began in East-Central Europe and later spread to more western areas. The **Minoan** Goddess culture on the Mediterranean Island of Crete persisted until about 1400 B.C.E.

The Goddess-centered religion lasted much longer than the patriarchal ones that supplanted it. The Goddess ruled for approximately 25,000 years—the greater part of human history. If it is indeed true that human females had equal status with males in the Goddess-worshiping Neolithic period, it follows that it is not "natural" and not inevitable that women occupy a subordinate position in human societies. The great strides that American and European women have made toward equality over the past century suggests that the wheel of change is at last returning women to the position of respect and influence they once enjoyed.

The Social Construction of Health

By now it should be evident that *biological factors,* such as inherited predisposition to disease and the presence of disease-causing microorganisms, are not the only factors that affect health and illness. **Social factors,** such as gender, ethnicity, class, and age, influence not only the amount and quality of healthcare members of a group will likely receive, but also the very *nature* of the health problems they are likely to develop. For example, as a group, black Americans have less access to healthcare and suffer more from certain health problems than do white Americans. This pattern began in the past, when black people were enslaved and denied access to education, and it continued after slavery ended. Persistent negative attitudes toward and beliefs about blacks barred them from truly equal educational and employment opportunities and locked them into the cycle of poverty, with its attendant health problems and lack of access to healthcare. The relationship between societal attitudes and practices pertaining to specific groups and the health status of members of those groups reflects what is known as the **social construction of health.**

Society's beliefs about various groups are often more **normative** than **descriptive** and reflect the views of the dominant social group, rather than the views of the society as a whole. For example, white men were the dominant group in nineteenth-century America (as they are today), and their beliefs about people of color and women were based on assumptions, not facts. There is no basis for the belief that black persons have primitive natures and that women's reproductive organs cause them to be mentally and physically weak. However, the views of the dominant group tend to be **internalized** by many members of the subordinate groups, even when those views are unflattering and damaging to the very people who hold them. Most (not all) women in nineteenth-century America believed themselves mentally and physically inferior to men—and acted the part. Similarly, the effects of centuries of racist thinking on the psyches of African Americans are still being felt. Fortunately, societal views change in response to scientific advances and pressures brought to bear by subordinate group members who perceive injustice.

Gender is one of the most potent of the social influences that affect patterns related to health, illness, and healthcare. The term *gender* is not to be confused with the term *sex*. Sex refers to biological femaleness or maleness, whereas *gender* is defined as "the socially prescribed roles and statuses that attach to the sexes within a given cultural and historical context . . ." (Weisman, 1998). Gender, like much about health and healthcare, is socially constructed and can differ from culture to culture. In mainstream American and European society today, for example, it is considered appropriate only for women to wear elaborate wigs, silks, ruffles, and hose. In seventeenth- and eighteenth-century Europe, however, men wore them, too. Social factors influencing health and illness, such as gender, socioeconomic status, ethnicity, and age, interact with each other, and some factors have the power to mitigate the effects of others. The effects of ethnicity, for example, may be tempered by the effect of wealth. Gender, however, is such a powerful factor that its influence persists regardless of age, ethnicity or socioeconomic status (Apple, 1990). The health of all women is affected by their gender. Who gets what kind of healthcare is not, and has never been, determined simply by the rational application of medical science and technology to existing health problems. The allocation of healthcare is determined by complicated social negotiations based on the perceptions and beliefs, interests, and relative power of various groups. Other social factors highly relevant to health and healthcare (socioeconomic status, ethnicity, age, sexual orientation, and disability) are addressed in more depth in Chapter 2.

Another social phenomenon of importance is the **medicalization of women's health.** The term *medicalization* refers to the expansion of the medical domain into an area not previously considered to be within the purview of physicians. An example is the "sin to sickness" transformation of explanatory models related to addiction. Once viewed as problems of will and morals, addictions are now seen as **diseases** best responded to by medical treatment rather than punishment (see Chapter 4). The process of medicalization begins with a reconceptualization of the phenomenon in question as a *medical problem*. Next, *institutions* spring up to support the now imperative medical case finding and delivery of care and to educate new providers. Simultaneously, institutions and providers convey the new concept to society at large through provider-patient encounters and public health campaigns. The medical establishment becomes the ultimate *authority* on the phenomenon, and individuals and groups that resist the new orthodoxy are viewed as *problematic* (Morgan, 1998).

Women's health, more than men's, has been medicalized; that is, processes intrinsic to women's natural functioning have come to be seen as rendering women in need of physicians' care. For example, childbearing and menopause, once seen as natural processes, are now highly medicalized. Women are monitored throughout their pregnancies, and most give birth in a hospital under medical supervision. Menopause is seen as a hormone deficiency disease, treatable by drug therapy, and estrogen is one of the most frequently prescribed "drugs" in the country. Women, on average, seek advice and assistance from healthcare providers considerably more often than men (*Women's Health Advisor*, 1999), and, fairly recently, a syndrome related to women's reproductive functioning, PMS, has emerged. Various theories have been put forward as to why women's health has been so medicalized, and there has been debate over how this has affected women overall.

One factor that may have contributed to the medicalization of women's health is that women have been *intimately connected with healthcare* from the earliest periods of human civilization. It was women, no doubt as a logical extension of their childcare activities, who nursed ill or injured family members. Some became proficient in the use of herbs and at assisting at childbirth and became village herbalists and midwives (Ehrenreich & English, 1978). In modern America, it is still women ("Dr. Mom") who monitor the health of their spouses and children, as well as that of aging relatives, and it is women who most often interact with medical providers on behalf of others. Another theory holds that society has a relatively greater interest in women's reproductive health because, due to the demands of pregnancy and birth, a reasonable level of health in women is necessary to ensure the propagation of the human species. Still others have argued that women of the new millennium, like their nineteenth-century forebears, are merely acting out their roles in a societal play in which they have been cast as inherently weak and sick because of their sex.

Women Working for Change

Throughout American history, women have played pivotal roles in a succession of movements aimed at improving their own health and healthcare. Specific causes taken up by specific groups of women have been related to broader social movements and controversies.

The Popular Health Movement

In the nineteenth century, physicians began to constitute a larger percentage of healthcare providers, they ushered in what was known as the age of "Heroic Medicine." In lieu of the traditional herbal remedies and other treatments offered by midwives, homeopaths, and other lay healers of the time, physicians used an array of invasive and usually painful procedures, such as surgery, bloodletting, blistering, and purging. Physicians also attempted to get laws passed establishing themselves as the only legitimate practitioners of medicine. The **Popular Health Movement** arose as a protest against heroic medicine and physicians' attempts to disenfranchise other practitioners, and white, middle-class women played pivotal roles in it (Weisman, 1998). The movement's activists promoted a *healthy lifestyle* as a way of avoiding disease and the ministrations of physicians. They gave public lectures on such topics as nutrition and hygiene. Mary Grove Nichols spoke on the benefits of exercise and the dangers of corseting. The movement also espoused limiting the size of families as a way of improving women's health, although not by means of contraception. As women were thought to be fundamentally disinterested in sex, anyway, the movement endorsed decreasing the frequency of marital intimacy in order to postpone pregnancy and spare women unwelcome encounters with their spouses.

The Popular Health Movement succeeded, temporarily, in reviving interest in traditional medical specialties, such as herbology and homeopathy, and in promoting women as *providers of medical care*. It founded its own medical schools, to which women were encouraged to apply, and infirmaries in which women could work. The movement also stimulated public discussion about women's health and women as healthcare providers. Also, although it did not support artificial contraception, the movement's widely circulated texts on women's anatomy and physiology no doubt aided those who did. Under attack from the movement, physicians founded the **American Medical Association** in 1847 and barred women, as well as nonphysician healthcare providers, from membership. Eventually, M.D.s established themselves as the only legitimate providers of medical care and relegated other types of practitioners to the fringe.

The Women's Medical Movement

The term *Women's Medical Movement* has been applied to efforts made by late nineteenth-century women physicians to establish themselves as experts in women's health. In the second half of the nineteenth century, women had more access to higher education and began entering medical schools in significant numbers. In 1900, women comprised 6 percent of all physicians in the United States.

Medical dogma held that women are biologically different from men and that women's physiology is controlled by their reproductive organs. In 1870, for example, a highly regarded professor of medicine proclaimed that "the Almighty, in creating the female sex, had taken the uterus and built up a woman around it" (Weisman, 1998, p. 49). Many women physicians of the time challenged this view of women. They saw menstruation and menopause as natural functions, rather than debilitating conditions that require extended periods of rest, if not medical treatment, and

promulgated these views in their own practices, as well as in health education literature and presentations. Women physicians advocated exercise, education, and useful work for women and recognized the dangers of too frequent childbearing. Mary Putnam Jacobi, M.D., not only alluded to physicians' economic motives for medicalizing women's health but also conducted research showing that the *least* ill health was to be found among the *best educated* women. Women physicians believed that their status as women made them more able to identify with women patients and that women were more willing to reveal their bodies, and to speak frankly, to another woman. Although a few women gained admission to "regular" medical schools, female physicians of the nineteenth century were likely to be graduates of women-only medical schools and to be employed in women's hospitals and clinics (Office on Women's Health, 2002).

Margaret Sanger and the Battle for Birth Control

By the late 1800s, laws had been passed making both abortion and the dissemination of information and devices related to birth control illegal. Not even physicians could advise women as to how to go about limiting their pregnancies. Although wealthier families sometimes had access to such banned devices as condoms, the situation in which poor women found themselves was dire. They, and their numerous children, suffered from malnutrition and disease. Furthermore, it has been estimated that, at the turn of the twentieth century, complications related to pregnancy and childbirth were the *second leading cause of death* among American women (tuberculosis was the first). It was also known that many women were dying as a result of illegally performed abortions. A public health nurse named **Margaret Sanger** became the founder of, and dominant figure in, the movement to legalize birth control. Sanger opened a birth control clinic for poor immigrant women in 1916 and founded the Birth Control League in 1921. She faced opposition from many forces in society, including organized medicine, the Catholic Church, and conservative women's groups, and she endured imprisonment, expatriation, and many other hardships for her cause. Sanger based her arguments in favor of legalizing birth control not only on the premise that doing so would obviate deaths from illegal abortion and result in healthier mothers and children but also on the more radical notion that women have a right to social justice and to sexual enjoyment unspoiled by fear of pregnancy. Sanger eventually triumphed and lived to see a string of birth control clinics nationwide (Weisman, 1998). Margaret Sanger also induced her wealthy husband—and, later, heiress Katherine McCormick—to finance the research that led to the development of the first **birth control pill**. As methods of birth control became more sophisticated, physicians became even more involved with women's reproductive healthcare.

Our Bodies, Ourselves: The Women's Health Movement of the 1960s

During the years between 1960 and 1975, the antiwar and women's liberation movements challenged the status quo in the United States. Liberal feminists demanded that women be recognized not as fundamentally different from men—more moral, self-sacrificing, and delicate—but as essentially the *same* as men and entitled to equal rights and opportunity. Feminists who focused on the reform of women's healthcare demanded that women be given more control over the healthcare they received. They directly challenged the power of physicians (92 percent of whom were male) and documented their overuse of surgery—including hysterectomy, mastectomy, and cesarean section (Weisman, 1998). Two other problems targeted by the Women's Health Movement were the total medicalization of childbirth and women's lack of access to legal abortion.

Most of the leaders of the Women's Health Movement were white, middle-class, educated women in their twenties and thirties. They depended on physicians for fertility control as well as delivery of their children and, so, were in more continuous contact with physicians than their foremothers had been. Feminism had taught them that they need not submit to overbearing medical authority. One of the most powerful strategies they used to empower female healthcare consumers was to provide them with information about how their bodies worked and about self-treatment of common illnesses and problems. Feminist activists held healthcare conferences, documented medical abuses, and published a vast amount of literature aimed at the lay public. The most famous of the healthcare manuals produced by the movement was the book *Our Bodies, Ourselves*. It was published in 1970 by the Boston Women's Health Care Collective, and updated versions are still available and in demand. Another highly effective strategy used by the Women's Health Movement was the creation of new, women-friendly healthcare facilities as alternatives to the traditional ones. For example, the **Feminist Women's Health Centers,** which originated in California and had numbered 48 by 1976 (Weisman, 1998) offer gynecological care and contraceptive services. The centers are staffed by sympathetic physicians (of both sexes) and nurses and are distinguished by an egalitarian atmosphere in which women can be active participants in their care.

Another kind of alternative women's healthcare organization that grew out of the Women's Health Movement was the free-standing **birthing center.** Traditional childbirth practices of the time were entirely physician-centered and impersonal. It was the physician who delivered the child, not the woman. Mothers were seldom educated about or prepared for childbirth and were routinely restrained on delivery tables and/or anesthetized. Birthing centers provide childbirth education and support for mothers throughout labor, and they allow fathers, and even other family members, to be present during births. Births are sometimes attended by certified nurse midwives instead of physicians. Birthing centers are popular with both feminist women and more traditional women, who want greater family involvement in the birthing process.

Perhaps the most hard-fought and passionately opposed battle fought by the feminist reformers of the Women's Health Movement of the 1960s and 1970s was the campaign for **abortion rights.** Women's right to control their fertility by all means necessary was seen as absolutely essential if women were to take advantage of equal rights and equal opportunity under the law. Laws that had been enacted in the late 1800s (in most states) forbade physicians from performing abortions unless necessary to save a woman's life. Whether a woman would be granted an abortion was decided by therapeutic abortion boards set up in hospitals and controlled by physicians. Two events are generally considered to have galvanized the abortion rights movement in the United States: the Sherri Finkbine case and an outbreak of rubella that exposed many pregnant women to a virus known to cause fetal abnormalities.

Sherri Finkbine had used the drug **Thalidomide** in 1962 to control nausea associated with her pregnancy. Shortly after Finkbine began taking the drug, it was recalled because it had been shown to cause serious fetal deformities. Finkbine applied for a therapeutic abortion and was turned down. She traveled to Sweden, where a badly deformed fetus was aborted. Around the same time, many pregnant women were exposed to the rubella (a form of measles) virus, which had reached epidemic proportions in some parts of the country. A number of those women applied for therapeutic abortions and, like Finkbine, were turned down. They eventually bore severely deformed infants. Both the Finkbine case and the rubella cases received wide press coverage. Abortion rights activists succeeded in having the circumstances under which a woman can obtain an abortion widened (in some states) to include pregnancy due to rape or incest, likely fetal deformity, or the preservation of the mental or physical health of the mother. These changes, however, still left decisions regarding abortion up to physicians and not women themselves. The supporters of abortion rights pressed on, and eventually, in 1973, Supreme Court decisions in the case *Roe v. Wade v. Bolton* decriminalized abortion and made it much more widely available to women (Weisman, 1998).

The Women's Health Movement of the 1960s had far-reaching implications for contemporary women. In addition to expanding women's rights to control their fertility, it focused national attention on *medical biases against women* and established **alternative services,** which eventually served as models for the improvement of traditional services. For example, childbirth education, natural childbirth, and family-centered childbirth are commonplace today, and patient education is the norm rather than the exception. Also, the movement motivated women to join the ranks of physicians and prompted legislation that made it possible for them to do so. In 1970, only 9 percent of medical students were female; women had not been encouraged to enter the professions, and medical schools had an informal **quota system,** which limited the number of women accepted. As a result of the movement, medical matters pertaining to women were demystified in feminist clinics and literature, and a provision of the 1972 Civil Rights Act prohibited sex discrimination in educational institutions. By 1980, the percentage of women in medical school had risen to 25 percent (Weisman, 1998). It is estimated that, by 2010, women will constitute 30 percent of all physicians and 50 percent or more of all medical students (About Women in Medicine, 1999).

More Research on Women's Health

Demands from women researchers, healthcare providers, and patients have resulted in a gratifying increase in the amount of research being done on women's health. Influential organizations, such as the Society for the Advancement of Women's Health Research, and an assortment of advocacy groups for women with problems such as breast cancer came into being and put pressure on government officials and legislators. In July 1990, the Women's Health Equity Act (WHEA) was introduced into Congress and ultimately passed. It contained 20 bills addressing access to health services, health screening initiatives, and research policy and funding. As a result of WHEA, the National Institutes of Health (NIH) created the **Office of Research on Women's Health** (ORWH). In addition, Dr. Bernadine Healy, M.D., became the first woman director of the NIH.

Ghosts of the Past That Continue to Haunt Women

Although there is no question that women, as well as men, have benefited enormously from the social and medical advances that have occurred over the past century, problematic vestiges of the past remain. Women have still not achieved equal power with men in American society, due to lingering attitudes and beliefs. As women are known to be more concerned than men with issues related to social justice (Hales, 1999), their relative lack of influence in society contributes to the substandard medical care poor women receive (see Chapter 2) and likely to women's higher rate of depression (see Chapter 26). There is evidence that women's reproductive organs are still seen, to some extent, as more pathological than they really are and that some opportunistic providers still see women as sources of revenue. The rates of both hysterectomy and cesarian section in this country have been criticized as unnecessarily high (see Chapter 17). There is evidence also that the hoary view of women as hysterical still lingers—the symptoms of coronary heart disease in women are sometimes misinterpreted as evidence of emotional upset (see Chapter 12).

Problems and concerns pertaining to men's health are still sometimes seen as more urgent and important than problems and concerns relevant to women—some insurance plans that still do not cover birth control pills for women cover the Viagra prescribed for men. Women's right to control their own reproduction remains controversial. There is still no easy access to drugs that can prevent conception after intercourse, and the dispensing of drugs that produce very early, nonsurgical abortions has been restricted by various legislative actions. Finally, although men's use of violence as a means of controlling women is no longer formally sanctioned by our society, male violence in the form of intimate abuse and rape continues to be a significant source of mental and physical trauma for women (see Chapter 25).

QUESTIONS FOR REFLECTION AND DISCUSSION

1. *Certain factors are seen as having been related to the nineteenth-century phenomenon known as hysteria. Do any of those factors pertain to modern women's lives?*
2. *To what extent do social factors that affected poorer women's health in the past impact it in the present?*
3. *Are modern women more in control of their health and healthcare than nineteenth-century women were?*
4. *Are societal factors that negatively impact women's health related to beliefs and attitudes held by men, women, or both?*
5. *Discuss the pros and cons of the medicalization of women's health.*

REFERENCES

About Women in Medicine (1999, http). American Women's Medical Association. [Online]. Retrieved June 25th, 2001. Available: www.amwa-doc.org/abouta.html

Anderson, B., & Zinsser, J. (1988). *A history of their own: Women in Europe.* New York: Harper & Row.

Apple, R. D. (Ed.). (1990). *Women, health, and medicine in America.* New York: Garland.

Blaffer-Hrdy, S. B. (1999). *Mother nature: A history of mothers, infants, and natural selection.* New York: Pantheon.

Blum, D. (1997). *Sex on the brain.* New York: Penguin.

Brody, L. (1997). Gender and emotion: Beyond stereotypes. *Journal of Social Issues, 53*(2), 369.

Cross, R. (1997). *Why women live longer than men: And what men can learn from them.* San Francisco: Jossey-Bass.

Dickerson, K., & Schnaper, L. (1996). Reinventing medical research. In Moss, K. (Ed.), *Man-made medicine.* Durham, NC: Duke University Press.

Doyle, J., & Paludi, M. (1997). *Sex and gender.* Burr Ridge, IL: McGraw-Hill.

Ehrenreich, B., & English, D. (1978). *For her own good: 150 years of the experts' advice to women.* New York: Anchor Books, Doubleday.

Eisler, R. (1988). *The chalice and the blade*. San Francisco: Harper San Francisco.

Fox, M. (1988). *The coming of the cosmic Christ*. San Francisco: Harper & Row.

Gimbutas, M. (1989). *The language of the Goddess*. San Francisco: Harper San Francisco.

Goleman, D. (1995). *Emotional intelligence*. New York: Bantam Books.

Grossman, M., & Wood, W. (1995). Sex differences in intensity of emotional experiences. *Journal of Personality and Social Psychology, 65*(5), 1010.

Gur, R. (1994). Effects of emotional discrimination tasks on cerebral blood flow. *Brain & Cognition, 25,* 271–73.

Hales, D. (1999). *Just like a woman*. New York: Bantam.

Hazzard, W. R. (1994). The sex differences in longevity. In W. L. Hazzard, E. L. Bierman, J. P. Blass, W. H. Ettinger Jr., & J. B. Halter (Eds.), *Geriatric medicine and gerontology*. (3rd ed.). New York: McGraw-Hill, pp. 248–257.

Hite, S. (1989). *Women & Love*. New York: St. Martin's Press.

Hooks, I. (1981). *Ain't I a woman?* Boston, MA: South End Press.

Jordan, J. V. (Ed.). (1997). *Women's growth in diversity: more writings from the Stone Center*. New York: Guilford Press.

Kerber, L. K., & DeHart-Mathews (Eds.). (1987). *Women's America*. New York: Oxford University Press.

Kiecolt-Glaser, J., Glaser, R., Cacioppio, J. T., MacCallum, R. C., Snydersmith, M., Kim, C., & Malarkey, W. B. (1997). Stress hormones and marital conflict in older adults: endocrinological and immunological correlates. *Psychosomatic Medicine, 59*(4), 339–449.

Kimura, D. (1999). *Sex and cognition*. Cambridge, MA: Bradford Books.

Legato, M. J. (2002). *Eve's rib*. New York: Harmony Books.

Mahowald, M. B. (1994). *Philosophy of woman*. Indianapolis: Hackett.

Matlin, M. (1993). The psychology of women (2nd ed.). Orlando, FL: Holt, Rhinhart & Winston.

Mellon, J. (Ed.). (1990). *Bullwhip days: The slaves remember*. New York: Weidenfeld & Nicolson.

Morgan, K. P. (1998). Contested bodies, contested knowledges: Women, health, and the politics of medicalization. In Susan Sherwin (Ed.), *The politics of woman's health* (pp. 83–121). Philadelphia: Temple University Press.

Office on Women's Health U.S. Dept. of Human Services (2002). *A century of women's health 1900–2000*. Washington, D.C.: DHHS Office on Women's Health.

Okin, S. M. (1979). *Women in western political thought*. Princeton, NJ: Princeton University Press.

Ornish, D. (1998). *Love and survival*. New York: HarperCollins.

Paludi, M. (1992). *The psychology of women*. Saddle River, NJ: Prentice Hall.

Riley, G. (1986). *Inventing the American woman*. Chicago, IL: Harlan Davidson.

Seligman, M. (1991). *Learned helplessness*. New York: Alfred A. Knopf.

Shrader, C. B., Blackburn, V., & Illes, P. (1997). Women in management and firm performance: an exploratory study. *Journal of Managerial Issues, 9*(3), 355–73.

Starr, T. (1991). *The natural inferiority of women: Outrageous pronouncements by misguided males*. New York: Poseidon Press.

Sternberg, R. (1994). *Encyclopedia of human intelligence*. New York: Macmillan.

Tavris, C. (1992). *The mismeasure of woman*. New York: Simon & Schuster.

Weisman, C. (1998). *Women's health care*. Baltimore: Johns Hopkins University Press.

Why Women Live Longer Than Men (June, 1999). *Women's Health Advisor, 3*(6), 4.

Wilson, M., & Daly, M. (1992). The man who mistook his wife for a chattel. In M. Wilson & M. Daly (Eds.), *The adapted mind* (pp. 289–326). New York: Oxford University Press.

2

Class, Ethnicity, Age, Physical Status, and Sexual Orientation: Implications for Health and Healthcare

Ruth Davis and Kay Huber

CHAPTER OUTLINE

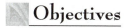
Objectives

1. *Discuss the influence of societal views on the health of poor, ethnic minority, elderly, disabled, and lesbian women.*

2. *Describe the overall health differences in morbidity and mortality among women in different ethnic and age groups.*

3. *Demonstrate an understanding of the ways in which culture influences health beliefs and practices.*

4. *Discuss the implications of the growing number of older American women for entitlement and other social support programs.*
5. *Identify potential problems in the healthcare system that may interfere with the equitable care of growing numbers of persons with disabilities.*

Introduction

This chapter focuses on the nonbiological factors, such as socioeconomic status, ethnicity, age, physical status, and sexual orientation, that affect women's health. Poorer women are known to have more health problems and less access to healthcare than wealthier women (Office on Women's Health, 1998d). Thirty-five million, or 26 percent, of American women belong to minority ethnic groups—groups other than Euro-American (Office on Women's Health, 1998d). Ethnic minority women are disproportionately represented among the poor, and their poverty gives rise to some, but not all, of the social problems that adversely affect their health. Age is another factor that strongly influences health. Older women face different health problems than younger women, and many must also contend with the health-related consequences of poverty. Women with physical disabilities or chronic health disorders face a host of personal and social challenges, and many lesbian women lack preventive healthcare because they are often alienated by insensitivity on the part of healthcare providers.

Socioeconomic Status

All adult women are more likely than men to be **poor** at any age. Single women, particularly single mothers, are statistically at risk for becoming poverty-stricken during their lifetimes. Almost half of all single Latina and African American women either are poor or are on the verge of poverty (Council of Economic Advisers for the President's Initiative on Race, 1998). The burdens of childcare often prevent young mothers from obtaining higher-paying jobs with greater security. Single mothers tend to have fewer sources of social support and, thus, more difficulty fulfilling the responsibilities of a job or professional position. Furthermore, when single mothers fall into poverty, they are often unable to find a way out. Current statistics show that, although Welfare recipients in general are decreasing in number, the majority of those in need of assistance include Latinas, older women with their children, and those women who receive no assistance from any other source (U.S. Department of Health and Human Services, 2000). Wright (1988) was one of the first researchers to investigate the association between single mothers and poverty. He found that most homeless families consist of single mothers and their children. The downward spiral that living in poverty engenders can be tena-

cious and long lasting and can bring with it a lifetime of **poor health** for women and their children.

Low income is a strong predictor of who does not use healthcare services and is associated with poor health outcomes. Low socioeconomic status is cited as the single most powerful contributor to illness and premature death (Lantz et al., 1998). Some of the health conditions that disproportionately affect poor women include breast cancer, cervical cancer (National Cervical Cancer Coalition, 2000), depression, and alcohol and other drug abuse (National Women's Health Resource Center, 2000). Most poor women are uninsured and lack the funds to obtain health services or to engage in health-promoting activities (Jacobs Institute of Women's Health, 1998). In addition, poor women often have low self-worth, a history of poor self-care, and feelings of powerlessness (Leenerts, 1998). A lack of preventive services and delayed treatment for potentially curable conditions contribute to the poorer health of economically disadvantaged women. The majority of the more than 43 million individuals who are considered to be medically underserved are poor, young, and female, and many are ethnic minority women (Gaston, Barrett, Johnson, & Epstein, 1998).

Ethnicity

Poverty, discrimination, and lack of social support all contribute to the poorer health that ethnic minority women experience in comparison with Euro-American women (Evans & Herr, 1991). Ethnic women also receive lower-quality healthcare, and less healthcare overall, than do wealthier, better-educated, higher-status Euro-American women. Most ethnic minority women use public clinics, rather than private healthcare providers, and many factors preclude poor ethnic minority women from availing themselves of even public clinics. These factors are referred to as **barriers to healthcare.**

The barriers to healthcare experienced by the medically underserved include a lack of health insurance, transportation, and childcare, as well as language barriers (Leenerts, 1998). Ethnic minority women, who tend to have lower-paying jobs and more unemployment, are much more likely to be uninsured than Euro-American women (Office on Women's Health, 1998d). Poor people without health insurance, childcare, or transportation are understandably reluctant to seek treatment for health problems that are not presently incapacitating. Failing to seek treatment early in the course of diseases, however, plays a significant role in the development of chronic illness and poor health. Other barriers to effective healthcare include gender inequalities, distrust of the healthcare system, perceptions of the healthcare system as insensitive, and poor satisfaction with healthcare received (Office on Women's Health, 1998d). Ethnic minority women frequently experience discrimination from healthcare providers (Davis, 1993, 1996). Discriminatory behaviors include lack of respect, inattention, and judgmental remarks. Such unprofessional behavior often causes ethnic women to decide not to return for continued care.

Ethnicity in America

The United States is a country made up of myriad ethnic groups. Sowell (1981), in his landmark exploration of America's ethnicity, found that the most prominent ethnic groups, the English and German, make up only about 28 percent of the total population. The 2000 census found that approximately 75 percent of the American population identified themselves as being of European descent, or "white," including the Irish, Eastern Europeans, Italians, Greeks, and others. However, when the German and English groups are combined, particularly when associated with Protestant religions, they are known as **WASPS** (white, Anglo-Saxon, Protestants). WASPS constitute the dominant culture in America and largely control all aspects of social and political life, including healthcare policy and reform, yet WASPS are **not** in the majority. In fact, by the next generation, 2020, it is projected that no actual majority population will exist in the United States (Giger & Davidhizar, 1995). If, however, the members of all minority ethnic groups were counted together, they would outnumber the Euro-American WASPS. Ethnic groups in this country have not been part of the power structure and have had little input into health policy decisions.

TERMINOLOGY

People belonging to groups other than the Euro-American have been traditionally referred to as **minorities,** but that term is now considered outmoded and incorrect. Many agencies and institutions have now adopted the term **ethnic group,** which is more accurate. The term **races,** also widely and incorrectly used to refer to ethnic groups, properly refers only to humanity as a whole. There is the human race, just as there is the canine race (dogs) and the equine race (horses). According to Montagu (1997), the longstanding use of the term *race* to refer to subsets of humans is actually a social construct intended to differentiate WASPS from others, particularly individuals whose physical appearance includes darker pigmentation. In the remainder of this chapter, terms taken from the U.S. Census, such as *African American, Latino, Native American,* and *Asian American,* will be used. The general term *ethnic minority* will be used to refer to non-Euro-American people and groups.

STEREOTYPING VERSUS GENERALIZING

Giving importance to superficial differences among people by unnecessarily referencing them contributes to the divisiveness that has plagued our society since its inception. Often, in our everyday conversations, we provide descriptors such as "black," "white," and "gay" without thinking very much about it. For example, we might say, "I was talking with my black friend, Ted, today." Specifying a person's ethnicity, however, is important only if one believes that something can be assumed on the basis of it. Assumptions based on such factors as ethnicity and sexual orientation are called **stereotypes.** Stereotypes assume that all persons belonging to a certain group have certain characteristics, often negative ones. When we think critically about scenarios in which ethnicity or sexual orientation is mentioned unnecessarily, we begin to understand how often we allow stereotypes to distort our simplest activities.

In examining the health concerns and issues surrounding the health of ethnic minority women, we will be seeing some generalizations about certain groups. That is not the same as stereotyping them. A generalization describes a trait or trend common in a given group; it does not assume that the generalization applies to every member of the group. Generalizations are starting points that allow us to explore further the commonalties as well as the differences (Galanti, 1997).

CULTURE

All ethnic groups have their own **culture,** as does the Euro-American group. *Culture* is defined as a system of rituals, traditions, ideas, symbols, and customs practiced within a group. Individuals express their beliefs through their culture. The music, art, and food of a given group are all part of its culture. Beliefs about health and illness are also part of a group's culture. Responses to illness, pain, and treatment are often linked to traditions that are hundreds of years old.

Most ethnic minority groups share cultural similarities that are different from those of Euro-Americans. For example, extended family ties are extremely important for all ethnic minority groups. Families consist of aunts, uncles, cousins, godparents, and even neighbors. During times of illness, it is not unusual for all members of a family to visit a sick relative. This sometimes conflicts with hospitals' limited visiting policies. Ethnic minority groups also tend to have different views regarding a desirable body type; they find slenderness unappealing and ampleness appealing. For the majority of ethnic minority people who immigrated to the United States over the past 40 years, severe poverty was a way of life; in developing countries, individuals rarely have enough food to provide adequate daily nutrition. Slenderness is the norm and is a sign of poverty. Being overweight, or even obese, is seen as evidence of wealth—that one has so much to eat that one is able to gain weight. Poor immigrants new to this country are mystified at the obsession with thinness in a land where food is so plentiful, and it can be hard for them to see being overweight as a threat to their health.

HEALTH BELIEF PARADIGMS

Ethnic groups and Euro-Americans subscribe to one of the three major health belief–health practice paradigms: the magico-religious, the holistic, and the biomedical. Often, elements of other paradigms exist along with the major one.

The **magico-religious paradigm** is thousands of years old and is supernatural and spiritual. Individuals rely on divine intervention for assistance in daily living, as well as for healing during illness. Those who ascribe to this belief system may view illness as a punishment from God. The supernatural realm can play a major role in practices related to health and illness. For example, many ethnic groups believe that spirits can interfere in life activities of living human beings and cause illness, death, and misfortune. Spirits are appeased through incense, prayer, sacrifice, and other similar types of practices. Spiritual healers may be called on to relieve suffering or provide guidance. In the Puerto Rican culture, these **espiritistas** use the good spirits of the supernatural world to cure and heal.

The **holistic paradigm** is the oldest known. It is based on ancient Chinese philosophy (as well as other traditions), with Taoism a primary influence. In the holistic paradigm, it is of primary importance that human beings remain in balance with nature and the environment. In order to be in balance with nature, humans themselves must be in balance. For many groups, this implies a balance between light and dark, female and male, and hot and cold. The holistic paradigm is important in the Chinese culture and in the cultures of groups from Mexico, Central and South America, and the Caribbean. The Asian and Latino groups, for example, base much of their therapeutic regimens on balancing "hot" conditions with the use of cold substances, and vice versa.

Native American health-related beliefs are based on a unique combination of the holistic and the magico-religious paradigms. Highly spiritual traditional Native Americans use healing ceremonies for the treatment of disease, particularly if the situation seems critical. Native Americans also seek harmony with nature and view the earth as a sacred place, rather than just a usable commodity. For Native Americans, harmony with nature, the spiritual world, and other people promotes good health and well-being.

The **biomedical paradigm** is relatively new. The biomedical belief system, based on the scientific model, emphasizes cause and effect in illness. For example, smoking is believed to cause lung disease. The germ theory, a major construct in the biomedical paradigm, stipulates that, if a person harbors disease-causing bacteria in sufficient numbers, that person will become ill. Until very recently, with the advent of integrative healthcare (see Chapters 10 and 11), there was no place in the biomedical paradigm for the supernatural or the spiritual, and no particular importance was placed on harmony.

Ethnicity, Health, and Healthcare

Health statistics are traditionally reported in terms of morbidity and mortality. **Morbidity** rates refer to numbers of people diagnosed with a disease, whereas **mortality** rates reflect actual deaths caused by a disease. Of all ethnic minority

groups, African Americans continue to experience the most coronary heart disease (Crawford, 1998), whereas Asians experience the least. In addition, women in all ethnic minority groups are more likely to develop depression than are Euro-American women. This tendency is thought to be related to the stress of poverty, higher rates of physical and emotional trauma, and inequities in social roles (Agency for Health Care Policy and Research, 1999). HIV/AIDS affects the health of more African American and Latina women than women in all other groups (Council of Economic Advisers for the President's Initiative on Race, 1998).

The life expectancy for all Americans has been steadily increasing, although ethnic minority individuals die at a younger age than Euro-Americans. The life expectancy of a Euro-American woman born in 2000 is 79.5 years. For Latina women it is 77.1 years and for Native American women it is 76.2 years. African American women can expect to live only 74.5 years on average (National Center for Health Statistics, 2000a).

The rate of **infant mortality,** or deaths within the first year of life, is considered to be a reliable predictor of the general health of a country's people. Although the United States is considered to be the richest nation in the world, it has the highest infant mortality rate among industrialized nations (Council of Economic Advisers for the President's Initiative on Race, 1998). African Americans and Native Americans have higher rates of infant mortality than other groups. The infant mortality rate for African Americans is more than twice that of all other groups in the United States (National Center for Health Statistics, 2000b). **Prenatal care** is well known to prevent complications of pregnancy and support the birth of healthy babies. Unfortunately, not all women are able to receive the same quality and quantity of healthcare during a pregnancy. Over 40 percent of African American, Native American, and Latina women do not obtain prenatal care during the first trimester of pregnancy (Office on Women's Health, 1998d). African American women are more likely than other women to experience labor and delivery complications and to give birth to low birth weight infants. The National Maternal and Infant Health Survey of 1988 found that over 78 percent of Euro-American women have access to private healthcare, compared with only 51 percent of Mexican American, 44 percent of African American, and 37 percent of Puerto Rican women (Gardner, Cliver, McNeal, & Goldenberg, 1996).

With the exception of Asian American women, who are healthier overall than women from other ethnic minority groups, ethnic minority women are at higher risk than Euro-American women for developing chronic illnesses and suffering their long-term effects. Ethnic minority women (and poor women) do not avail themselves of **preventive health services,** such as pap smears and mammograms, as readily as Euro-American, wealthier women do. This is unfortunate, as it is well known that such services assist in the early identification of two prevalent cancers in women.

Health Status of Women from Selected Ethnic Minority Groups

With the exception of Asian Americans and Pacific Islanders, the women in most ethnic minority groups tend to have poorer health than Euro-American women do. Although some of the reasons for this vary among minority groups, poverty and lack of education are usually implicated.

LATINA WOMEN

The largest ethnic category in the United States, constituting 12.5 percent of the population, is the group commonly known as the **Hispanics.** Most of the groups in this category originated in Latin American countries. Many individuals belonging to this group find that the term *Hispanic* does not apply to them. *Hispanic* comes from the Spanish word *hispania,* or Spain. However, many Hispanics come from countries other than Spain (Perez-Stable, 1987). The broader term **Latino** denotes those individuals who originated in Latin America (Hayes-Bautista & Chapa, 1987), which includes Central America, Mexico, and the Caribbean nations. Latino women are referred to as *Latinas.* Latin Americans have a rich heritage, which historically includes Spanish and Indian ethnic groups. Some Caribbean groups—the Puerto Rican, for example—also include African ethnic groups as part of their ancestry.

Over 35 million people living in the United States in 2000 identified themselves as Latino (U.S. Census Bureau, 2001) of these, the Mexican Americans comprise the largest group, followed by immigrants from Central and South America, Puerto Rico, and Cuba.

Mexican Americans are known for persistence of culture and have resisted **acculturation** to the Euro-American way of life. The urban centers of California, Texas, New York, Florida, and Illinois have the largest Mexican American populations. One of the major reasons for Mexican American immigration to the United States is the limited number of employment opportunities in Mexico. Conditions related to high degrees of poverty affect the health of Mexican Americans and include **poor nutrition** and increased incidence of **infectious disease,** including sexually transmitted diseases, such as syphilis, gonorrhea, chlamydia, and HIV/AIDS (Purnell & Paulanka, 1998).

The only ethnic minority group whose members are U.S. citizens by birth (besides Native Americans) is the Puerto Rican group. As the island of Puerto Rico is a territory rather than a state, Puerto Ricans enjoy all the privileges of American citizenship except representation in Congress. Puerto Rico has been part of the United States since the Spanish-American War ended in 1898. Puerto Rican ethnicity consists of a combination of Indian, Spanish, and African groups.

Cuban Americans immigrated to the United States in two major waves. The first wave of immigration occurred in 1959, when Fidel Castro overthrew the existing government, causing many middle- and upper-class professional Cubans to flee to the United States. The second wave occurred during the 1980s, when more than 120,000 Cubans released from jails and mental institutions came to the United States during the Mariel boat lift (EthnoMed, 1998). As can be imagined, vast cultural and socioeconomic differences exist between these two groups of Cuban immigrants.

The leading cause of death for Latina women is **coronary heart disease,** or disease of the heart and blood vessels (National Women's Health Information Center, 2000). This is particularly true for Puerto Rican women, who suffer a 15 percent higher incidence of coronary heart disease (Office on Women's Health, 1998b & d). Many of the risk factors associated with cardiovascular disease, such as hypertension, diabetes, obesity, and physical inactivity, are prevalent among Latina women, yet the death rates from coronary heart disease for Mexican American and Cuban American women are actually lower than that for Euro-American women.

An increasingly frequent cause of death among Latina groups is **HIV/AIDS.** In those Latinas ages 25–44, it is the leading cause of death (U.S. Department of Health and Human Services, 1997a). Over the past decade, HIV/AIDS cases increased from 30 to 60 percent (U.S. Bureau of the Census, 1998). Latinas now represent 18 percent of all HIV/AIDS cases (Office on Women's Health, 1998). Puerto Rican women, in particular, are at far greater risk for acquiring HIV/AIDS disease than women from other Latina groups, and their risk is 20 times that of Euro-American women. Puerto Rican women's higher risk is associated with an increase in intravenous drug use, as well as exposure during unprotected heterosexual sex (Menendez, 1990). It can be difficult for Latinas to persuade their partners to use condoms.

In general, Latina women use screening tests, such as mammography and clinical breast examination, less often than Euro-American women (Tortolero-Luna, Glober, Villarreal, Palos, & Linares, 1995). Although these screening tests do not prevent disease, they do allow for early case finding, which can help decrease morbidity and mortality from breast cancer. **Breast cancer** is on the rise among Latina women, and Latinas experience poorer survival rates than Euro-American women (Office on Women's Health, 1998a). An interesting study completed with Mexican American women found that those women with the strongest traditional family beliefs actually participated more often in breast cancer screening (Suarez & Pulley, 1995).

The most recent Cuban immigrants to the United States suffer from conditions associated with poor living conditions, such as tuberculosis, hepatitis B, and parasites. Dengue fever, a disease of epidemic proportions in many tropical countries, is a major concern for **Haitians.** In addition, many Haitians lack immunizations to childhood illnesses, such as measles, chicken pox, and rubella.

Even though the United States has no national language, it is assumed that all individuals should speak English. However, as we enter the new millennium, the number of persons fluent in Spanish may exceed the number of those who speak English. Most Latina women are Spanish-speaking, with En-glish as their second language. Lack of fluency in English prevents many Latinas from participating fully in healthcare services. Research indicates that Puerto Ricans become frustrated with the healthcare system when health information materials are not available in Spanish (Davis, 1996).

African American Women

African Americans constitute 12.3 percent of the population and by a way small margin make up the **second largest** ethnic minority group in the United States (U.S. Census Bureau, 2001). The African American category includes people of African, Haitian, and West Indian origin.

Many African American women carry heavy social burdens that make it difficult for them to obtain preventive healthcare and early treatment for health problems. Unless a condition or an illness is severe, they may not seek outside professional healthcare at all. African American women, many of whom are single mothers, struggle to make ends meet financially while caring for their children and sometimes their grandchildren as well. In one study, in which African American women were asked to discuss their feelings about health screening, they indicated that they had little energy to devote to problems that *might* develop (Davis, 1998).

African American women experience more deaths from **coronary heart disease** and **stroke** than Euro-American women do. Also, **cancers** of the breast, cervix, and colon cause more mortality among African Americans (National Women's Health Information Center, 2000). Although African American women experience less breast cancer overall than Euro-American women, they are far more likely to die of the disease (Tessaro, Eng, & Smith, 1994). Breast cancer rates for African American women have increased 16 percent over a 10-year period, yet they decreased 5 percent for Euro-American women (Office on Women's Health, 1998d). The reasons for this include lack of access to healthcare—particularly for mammography screening, which can detect treatable cancer lesions. In addition, African American women are less likely to receive clinical breast examinations or to perform self-breast examinations (Bowen, Hickman, & Powers, 1997). Finally, African American women's death rate from **HIV/AIDS** is approximately 5 times that of Euro-American women.

Other health concerns that significantly impact African American women's lives include trauma related to **violence, teen pregnancy,** and **substance abuse** (U.S. Department of Health and Human Services, 1997a). **Obesity** and associated diseases, such as coronary heart disease and diabetes, are found to a greater degree among African

American women (Bowen et al., 1997; Walcott-McQuigg, Logan, & Smith, 1995). **Sickle-cell anemia** is an inherited trait common among African Americans. Sickle-cell anemia causes infections and joint and muscle pain, and it results in a significantly lower life expectancy. The Agency for Health Care Policy and Research (1999) has recommended a national screening process for this potentially preventable illness.

Asian American Women

The large umbrella group designated by the U.S. Census Bureau as *Asian Americans and Pacific Islanders* contains dozens of ethnically diverse groups. Some of these are the Chinese, Japanese, Korean, Filipino, Malaysian, Vietnamese, Cambodian, Hmong, Mien, and Thai. It is predicted that, by the year 2010, the population of Asian Americans and Pacific Islanders will have increased by more than 100 percent (U.S. Department of Health and Human Services, 1997a). Overall, Asian women in the United States have far fewer risk factors for major chronic illness than other ethnic minority groups (Hahn, Teutsch, Franks, Chang, & Lloyd, 1998). These differences take into account socioeconomic status, yet little is known about the reasons that Asian American women have fewer health problems than their counterparts in other ethnic groups. It has been suggested that their traditional **diets,** heavy in vegetables and soy products and low in fat, may play a part.

The most rapidly growing ethnic minority groups are those from Southeast Asia. Of these, the Vietnamese will be the third largest Asian group by the end of the 21st century. More than 1 million refugees from Southeast Asia now reside in the United States. Although the Vietnamese, Cambodian, and the Hmong, Mien, and Laotians from Laos constitute different ethnic groups, they do share some commonalities. For example, the belief that the body is holistic and should therefore always be kept in balance is the foundation of all health treatments, many of which found their way into Southeast Asian villages over the past 2,000 years.

One of the difficulties in discussing the specific health concerns of Asian Americans and Pacific Islanders is that one heading represents many ethnic groups. It is to be hoped that the U.S. Department of Health and Human Services will recognize this situation and encourage disaggregation in future research studies, so that each group's problems can be enumerated and its concerns addressed.

Asian Americans have less mortality from common chronic illnesses than Euro-Americans. The leading cause of death for Asian American women is **cancer.** Koreans have five times more stomach cancer than the total U.S. population (National Women's Health Information Center, 2000). The Vietnamese have significantly higher rates of liver cancer. Hepatitis B rates are higher for Asian Americans and Pacific Islanders—two to three times the national average (U.S. Department of Health and Human Services, 1997a). This high incidence of hepatitis is thought to be a contributing factor to high liver cancer rates.

Vietnamese women are much less likely to have annual Pap smears than Euro-American women, and their mortality rate from cervical cancer is three times higher (Office on Women's Health, 1998d). One of the primary reasons Southeast Asian women do not commonly obtain Pap smears is the high value placed on **modesty** and **virginity** in their culture. Unmarried women, regardless of their age, are discouraged from having gynecological examinations.

Asian American women experience a number of **cultural barriers** to optimum healthcare. For example, many older women do not speak English and must rely on their children for the translation of very personal information in healthcare situations. Also, the holistic health-related beliefs typical of Asian cultures can create problems in the solidly biomedical U.S. healthcare system. For example, Southeast Asians see postpartum women as being in a state of recovery that is considered "cold" and that requires "hot" treatments to prevent further cooling. Consequently, many Southeast Asian women do not shower, bathe, or drink cold fluids for a period of time following childbirth. Such beliefs and practices can cause friction between maternity patients and healthcare providers who are not familiar with Southeast Asian culture.

NATIVE AMERICAN WOMEN

Native Americans were not considered citizens of the United States until 1924, even though they were the original inhabitants of the North American continent. More than 2 million Native Americans constitute more than 500 federally recognized tribes (U.S. Department of Health and Human Services, 1997a). Many individuals prefer to be referred to as American Indians or by the name of their specific tribe. The largest Native American tribes in the United States today are the Cherokee (369,035), Navaho (225,298), Sioux (107,321), and Chippewa (105,988) (Spector, 1996). Native Americans constitute the smallest of the major ethnic groups and have significantly poorer health status. Indian Health Services, a branch of the Department of Health and Human Services, supplies healthcare for approximately 60 percent of the Native American population (Public Health Services Agencies, 1995).

Native Americans lived throughout the United States for over 30,000 years. In 1830, the U.S. government forcefully relocated all Native Americans from the East Coast to states west of the Mississippi River. Once there, they were herded into military encampments known as **reservations.** Many tribes, such as the Cherokee, were almost extinguished over the course of brutal forced marches. Today, Native Americans live freely either on or off reservations in 34 states, most in the West. **Poverty** due to high unemployment rates is high among Native Americans, as are rates of illness, disease, and addiction. Inadequate sewage disposal and contaminated water on reservations, together with the poor nutritional status associated with poverty, have resulted in high rates of **infectious disease. Diabetes** and diabetes-related coronary heart disease are major causes of morbidity, possibly because Native Americans are unable to handle the relatively large amount of **sugar** found in the Euro-American diet. Native Americans are also thought by some to be genetically susceptible to **alcoholism,** which is a major problem among them.

Native American women are much more likely to die from **injuries** or **accidents** than are women from other ethnic minority groups and almost twice as likely to die from those causes as Euro-American women. Native Americans also suffer from higher rates of diabetes, heart disease, liver disease, and cancer of the lung, colon, rectum, and gall bladder (National Women's Health Information Center, 2000). These cancers are thought to be associated with higher rates of **cigarette smoking** among Native American individuals; Native Americans smoke more than all other groups, including Euro-Americans, and the rate of tobacco use continues to escalate.

Alcoholism is considered to be the most widespread problem in Native American communities. Alcoholism is implicated as a contributing factor in many health problems, such as motor vehicle fatalities, domestic violence, fetal alcohol syndrome and liver disease. The rate of alcoholism among Native Americans is seven times that of the total U.S. population (U.S. Department of Health and Human Services, 1997b). It has been theorized that Native Americans are genetically susceptible to alcoholism because they metabolize alcohol differently. Other forces may also push Native Americans toward addiction. The historic displacement of Native Americans may have damaged their identity and sense of place and purpose in society. Table 2–1 lists the major causes of death for Native Americans.

REFUGEES

The term **refugee** refers to "those who have fled their countries because of a well-founded fear of persecution for reasons of race, religion, nationality, political opinion or membership in a particular group, and who cannot or do not want to return" (United Nations High Commissioner for Refugees, 1998, p. 1). The United States is historically a country of refugees and immigrants. Early immigrants include European groups such as Germans, Irish, and Italians. At the turn of the twentieth century, groups from Asia—the Japanese and Chinese—began to arrive. World War II triggered another major influx of refugees from Europe.

The end of the twentieth century saw an influx of refugees from **Eastern Europe.** Due to the wars that consumed much of Yugoslavia after the fall of the communist regime, thousands of individuals from Bosnia and Kosovo were displaced from their homes. Between January and June

TABLE 2-1   Five leading causes of death among women in the major ethnic groups.

Euro-American	Latina	African American	Native American	Asian American or Pacific Islander
Coronary heart disease	Coronary heart disease	Coronary heart disease	Coronary heart disease	Cancers
Cancers	Cancers	Cancers	Cancers	Coronary heart disease
Stroke	Stroke	Stroke	Injuries/accidents	Stroke
Lung disease	Diabetes	Diabetes	Diabetes	Injuries/accidents
Pneumonia and influenza	Injuries/accidents	Injuries/accidents	Stroke	Pneumonia and influenza

1999, more than 200,000 citizens of Yugoslavia, most of them Kosovo Albanians, filed asylum applications (United Nations High Commissioner for Refugees, 1999). Although the majority of Kosovo refugees sought asylum in Austria and Switzerland, many immigrated to the United States. Also, over the past 20 years, famine and drought have driven from their home individuals from **African** countries such as Ethiopia, Somalia, and Nigeria.

These newest refugees from Bosnia and Yugoslavia are now interacting with the American healthcare system. As would be expected, many Bosnian women suffer from **post-traumatic stress disorder** and **depression** as consequences of war. Some of the other major health problems found in Bosnian refugees and others from Eastern Europe include **poor nutrition, tuberculosis,** and **hepatitis** (EthnoMed, 1998). Bosnians are accustomed to taking advantage of preventive healthcare, as it was common in their home country. Bosnian women are much more likely to undergo gynecological examinations than are their Muslim counterparts in the Middle East (EthnoMed, 1998).

Refugees from African countries experience a multitude of health problems due to conditions associated with poor hygiene, lack of sanitary water, and poor nutrition. These include parasites and tuberculosis (EthnoMed, 1998).

Female genital mutilation (FGM) involves the removal of portions of the external genitalia. Also known as female circumcision, FGM effects an estimated 130 million women and girls worldwide, and an estimated 2 million new procedures are carried out each year (World Health Organization, 1998). FGM has been performed in the Sudan, Sierra Leone, Somalia, Ethiopia, Kenya, and other African countries for over 1,500 years. In Somalia and Sudan, over 95 percent of girls undergo some form of the procedure, and it is practiced in a number of Middle Eastern countries as well (World Health Organization, 1998). FGM is one of the few cultural practices that cause absolute injury to women. It can include one or more of the various forms of circumcision and the more severe procedure known as infibulation.

Circumcision involves one or more of the following procedures: removal of the clitoral hood, removal of the cli-

toris itself, and removal of the labia minora. In **infibulation,** most or all of the external genitalia are removed and the wound is sewn closed in a way that narrows the vaginal orifice; a small opening is left for the passage of urine and menstrual blood (World Health Organization, 1998). On marriage, the opening is made slightly larger to accommodate intercourse. The opening is enlarged to accommodate childbirth and then resewn after delivery.

Procedures involving genital mutilation are usually done as part of **initiation rituals.** They are most often performed on girls between the ages of five and eight but may also be done to infants. In some cultures, they are performed prior to marriage (World Health Organization, 1998). The women who actually carry out the genital surgery (excisors) earn their income by performing initiation rituals that include it. They are usually revered and feared individuals believed to possess supernatural powers. Often, they are members of a secret society of women, such as the Sande society of Sierra Leone, where 90 percent of women are genitally mutilated (Affara, 2000).

Unsterile instruments, such as razor blades or pieces of glass, are used to carry out the procedures and no anesthesia is administered. Some girls and young women die of shock and infection. The more mutilating operations can also cause severe ongoing health problems; **ectopic pregnancies** are common after infibulation, as are **complications of childbirth** (Arbesmen, Koller, & Buck, 1993). **Urinary tract infections** related to urinary retention are also problematic, as it can take an infibulated woman as long as 15 minutes to empty her bladder (Affara, 2000). Adverse psychological consequences, such as **post-traumatic stress disorder** and **panic attacks,** have been reported (World Health Organization, 1998) and may be more likely to occur if the girl was deceived, coerced, or intimidated by trusted parents and relatives.

Although the origin of the practice is unknown, it is believed that female genital mutilation was originated in Egypt by a small sect associated with the Islamic religion. There is, however, no stipulation in the Koran, the Islamic holy book, that mandates female circumcision, and some Islamic cultures (such as Saudi Arabia) do not practice it (Heise, 1993). Nevertheless, among some Islamic groups, circumcision has become deeply associated with female *purity*. Uncircumcised women are considered unclean and dangerous, and men will not consider marriage to them. Marriage is highly valued in most ethnic cultures in which women's lives are restricted in terms of gender role, and women have limited access to economic and social resources. In such cultures, marriage is the only way for a woman to secure her future, and to be unmarriageable is seen as a catastrophe in which a woman is doomed to live her life unfulfilled—without companion, caretaker, or children (Affara, 2000). Other cultural rationales for FGM are as follows: female genitalia are aesthetically displeasing; FGM guarantees chastity before marriage and prevents promiscuity afterward, thus safeguarding the honor of the family; FGM enhances male sexual pleasure and boosts fertility (Affara, 2000).

The parents who allow FGM to be performed on their daughters and the villagers—or, in some cases, medical personnel—who carry out the procedure believe it to be in the best interests of the female child. Although Westerners usually view the procedure as barbaric and cruel, it is not seen as such within the cultures that practice it, and it is supported as fully by women as men. The very term *FGM* may be offensive to women who have undergone the procedure and they themselves may refer to it as *traditional female surgery, ritual female surgery, cutting,* or *circumcision*. Women who leave their culture of origin and move to areas where FGM is not accepted may feel alienated and shamed if their healthcare providers openly condemn the procedure.

Efforts to eradicate FGM are underway on the international, national, and local levels. The United Nations, the World Health Assembly, and other international organizations have all adopted resolutions opposing it (Affara, 2000). In 1984, African women formed the Inter-African Committee on Traditional Practices Affecting the Health of Women and Children (IAC). The IAC lobbies other organizations and fosters local efforts to eradicate FGM. In 1998, it organized a conference of Christian and Islamic leaders from 11 African countries, which resulted in the drafting of a statement that neither Christianity nor Islam permits the destruction of a healthy human organ for any reason (Affara, 2000). The IAC has also set up national committees in 26 African countries that promote antimutilation campaigns; educational programs for birth attendants, excisors, healers, and religious and community leaders; alternative initiation ceremonies; and other means of self-support for excisors (Affara, 2000).

The International Council of Nurses, as well as some other professional provider organizations, firmly opposes any effort to "medicalize" FGM by participating in excisions done as surgical procedures under sterile conditions, because to do so would be to legitimize the procedures and to undermine the message that genital mutilation is bad for the health of girls and women (Affara, 2000).

 # Age

Age is yet another factor that influences women's health. Although there are many similarities among the health problems and needs experienced by women of all ages, there are also differences. These differences are based on biology and culture.

Adolescence

Adolescence is a major life stage. It encompasses the ages 11 through 21 years and is divided into three stages (Lewis & Bernstein, 1996):

- Early adolescence: 11–14 years
- Middle adolescence: 15–17 years
- Late adolescence: 18–21 years

Young women undergo major physical changes during adolescence. These include the development of secondary sexual characteristics, such as mature breasts, the initiation of the menses, and the growth of pubic hair. Adult height and weight are reached during this stage, although height can continue to be gained until long bone growth subsides at age 25. Adolescence involves social changes as well. Experimentation and risk taking often accompany the process of developing a unique self. Risk-taking behaviors underlie the statistically high levels of accidents and injuries among adolescents.

An important developmental milestone in the life of an adolescent girl is **menarche,** the onset of menstruation, and traditionally that term is used to identify the age of a young woman at her first menstrual period (Sloane, 1993). The average age of menarche for women in the United States is 12 years of age (Dains, Baumann, & Scheibel, 1998), while the range is between 9 and 17 years of age. Variations in the age of menarche have been linked to nutritional status (Houppert, 1999). The age of menarche, the duration and frequency of menstrual periods, and the potential implications of hormonal influence during medical and surgical interventions have been poorly studied to date (Koblinsky, Campbell, & Harlow, 1993), however. Recently, it has been proposed (Herman-Giddens et al., 1997) that girls are now entering puberty and menarch at an earlier age than their forebears, possibly due to the ubiquity of environmental xenoestrogens which are compounds that mimic the effects of estrogen in the body (see Chapter 5).

The beginning of menstruation signals a woman's ability to conceive and have children for the next 30 years of her life. Although menstruation is a natural and inevitable part of every young woman's development, it can be influenced by cultural, ethnic, and family values related to issues associated with reproduction. Mothers' perceptions of menstruation can have a long-lasting influence on how daughters view their menstruation experiences throughout their lives. For example, in Davis's (1993) study of Puerto Rican women and their health beliefs and practices, girls that received information about menstruation from their mothers in anticipation of the event described their present experiences in a more matter-of-fact way than did those whose mothers never broached the subject.

Accidents are the major causes of morbidity and mortality among adolescents in all age ranges, and most involve motor vehicles. Female adolescents, however, are far less likely to be involved in a life-threatening accident than their male counterparts. Problems that commonly beset girls are **eating disorders, pregnancy, sexually transmitted diseases,** and **substance abuse.** Such difficulties are seen as related to adolescent experimentation, in conjunction with low self-esteem.

Low Self-Esteem

That adolescent girls' self-esteem tends to be lower than boys' has been documented in a number of published works (Brown & Gilligan, 1992; Greenburg-Lake Staff & Analysis Group Staff, 1994). Adolescent girls are socialized to be *nice,* yet the development of niceness is an insidious process through which girls give up much of their self-hood (Pipher, 1994). Carol Gilligan's (1982) study of adolescent girls demonstrated that girls are not encouraged to state what is on their minds but, rather, to avoid confrontations, arguments, and nonconformity. Although conformity may encourage connections between individuals, it also discourages autonomy, or being oneself. In order to form a solid sense of self, girls need to be able to develop boundaries; that is, they must be able to distinguish their own feelings, beliefs, and wishes from those of other people. Girls must be supported in learning to identify and defend their interests. Girls' unwillingness and inability to do so make them vulnerable to a host of social problems, from unintended pregnancy and sexually transmitted diseases to workplace discrimination, domestic abuse, and rape.

Eating Disorders

Eating disorders, such as **anorexia** and **bulimia** (see Chapter 26), are serious problems that occur with much greater frequency in adolescent girls than in boys of the same age. Dieting for weight loss is one of the major factors in the development of eating disorders in adolescents (Pesa, 1999). Dieting is associated with cigarette smoking and the use of alcohol and other drugs and can lead to irritability, sleep disturbances, and difficulty with concentration. Amenorrhea, delayed sexual maturation, and growth retardation are closely associated with extreme forms of dieting. The causes of eating disorders have not been definitively identified, but factors such as low self-esteem, poor family relationships, and poor body image may be involved.

Pregnancy

Almost 1 million teen pregnancies, 80 percent of which are unintended, occur every year in the United States (The Na-

tional Campaign to Prevent Teen Pregnancy, 2001). The teen birth rate peaked in 1991 at 62.1 births per 1,000 teens (The National Campaign to Prevent Teen Pregnancy, 2001). Since then, teen birth rates have been steadily declining and are lower now than when first recorded in the 1940s. The decline has been particularly impressive among teenagers ages 15 to 17 and among black teens (Curtin & Martin, 2000). Various factors have been credited with contributing to the decline in teen pregnancy, including fear of AIDS and other sexually transmitted diseases, school sex education programs, and campaigns promoting abstinence. Nonetheless, teen pregnancy remains a critical issue in the United States. Almost a million teens still give birth every year, and it is not uncommon for 11- to 13-year-old girls to become pregnant and subsequently give birth to a child.

Studies have yielded information as to why pregnant teens fail to protect themselves against conception. The pregnant teen participants in one qualitative study (Burns, 1999), reported that they feared losing the relationships with their boyfriends if they insisted on using condoms or other birth control methods. Maintaining the relationship took precedence over concerns about pregnancy and its long-term social effects. Many participants also reported having strongly doubted that a pregnancy could occur. Others said they had been willing to allow *fate* to determine whether they would conceive. A few reported that pregnancy, once it occurred, was desirable.

Adolescents are not physically or emotionally prepared to engage in a mature sexual relationship, nor are they prepared to cope with pregnancy. Nevertheless, new sexual feelings, the tendency toward experimentation, and working parents' inability to supervise their children effectively all contribute to the still unacceptably high rate of teenage pregnancy in this country. Multipronged efforts to reduce the teen birth rate further must continue, and more education regarding the health and social risks of pregnancy must be provided during the adolescent years.

Sexually Transmitted Diseases

Sexually active adolescent girls are at risk for contracting sexually transmitted diseases. Two means of protection exist: **abstinence** and **condom use.** The few studies that have investigated the use of contraceptives among adolescents suggest that condom use is infrequent. Chlamydia and gonorrhea (see Chapter 22) are two sexually transmitted diseases that can have dire consequences for young women who contract them and yet are preventable through the persistent and consistent use of condoms. If left untreated, both are associated with the development of **pelvic inflammatory disease** and consequent infertility due to scarring and adhesions. Unfortunately, in their early stages, these diseases typically cause few signs and symptoms that would cause a woman to seek healthcare.

CERVICAL CANCER

Cervical cancer is a preventable disease. It is caused by changes in the cells of the **cervix,** or the neck of the uterus (womb). During adolescence, the cells located in and on the cervix are extremely vulnerable to changes in their environment. Since the environment of the cervix is the **vagina,** anything introduced there can potentially harm the changing cells of the cervix. Engaging in sexual intercourse during the adolescent years greatly increases the risk of developing cervical cancer. Semen can carry the human papilloma (wart) virus, which can cause cancer. The mechanical pounding to which the cervix is subjected during intercourse heightens this possibility and may itself cause cancerous changes to occur, even in the absence of virus. The risk factors for the development of cervical cancer are as follows:

- Sexual intercourse before age 18
- Multiple sexual partners
- Cigarette smoking
- A history of genital warts

The **Pap smear** (see Chapter 17) is a way of detecting changes in the cells of the cervix. This is a relatively painless procedure whereby some cells are scraped from the surface of the cervix and placed on a slide. These slides are then sent to a laboratory, where they are examined for any abnormalities. Young women should have their first Pap smear when they become sexually active or at age 18—whichever comes first. Sexually active women should continue to have Pap tests every year. Women who are not sexually active and not on a hormonal birth control method should have Pap smears every 3 years.

SUBSTANCE ABUSE

Adolescents may experiment with a wide variety of substances, including alcohol, marijuana, anabolic steroids, cigarettes, smokeless tobacco, over-the-counter medications, and inhalants, such as paint and household chemicals.

Cigarette smoking is the most common form of substance abuse among adolescent girls. Even though the risks of cigarette smoking are well known, and many antismoking campaigns are used in schools, the rate at which teenage girls take up cigarette smoking continues to rise. Adolescent girls who smoke are at higher risk for alcohol and other drug abuse and, if they become pregnant, are more likely to experience complications of pregnancy and give birth to low birth weight babies. Moreover, girls who smoke greatly increase their risk of developing lung cancer, the leading cause of cancer deaths in the United States. Ninety percent of all lung cancers are caused by cigarette smoking (Young Women and Smoking, 2000).

Middle-Aged Women

Midlife, or middle age, encompasses approximately the years between age 45 and age 65. This is a life stage, rather than a chronological period, during which women often experience a growing recognition that their lives are changing irrevocably. During this time, women often experience a burst of new energy, termed **menopausal zest** by anthropologist Margaret Mead, as well. At midlife, women often refocus on their own desires rather than those of their children or other loved ones. They pursue new interests, acquire new skills, refine old skills, seek employment outside the home, spend time with persons outside the family, and enjoy time for reflection (The Boston Women's Health Collective, 1998).

The middle years can also be a time of **losses,** such as losses that change self-concept and self-image, losses of parents, loss of fertility at menopause (see Chapter 24), and loss of children leaving home. Other important relationships may change as well, as this is a time when women may have to cope with divorce and severed relationships, as well as with the death of aging loved ones. Middle-aged women also are part of the **sandwich generation,** and many face the dual demands of caring for children and aging parents (Morris, 1996). It is critical for women to initiate dialogue with their parents about the future and about potential role reversals. Women who are caregivers must learn about support services both for their aging parents and for themselves. Spouses or lovers may resent the time and attention women focus on their parents, and this may make an already stressful situation worse. Joining a support group for both support and nurturing may be valuable. More information about the stresses associated with caring for aging relatives can be found in Chapter 7.

Seventy-five percent of women between the ages of 45 and 64 who are employed work in service, administrative support, or professional specialty roles. Opportunities for employment are clearly linked to education and are reduced by the lack of it (Stone & Griffith, 1998). Middle-aged women who work in service occupations, where low wages and poor benefits are the norm, generally have no more than a high school education and may lack even that. Women in administrative support roles are typically better educated than women who work in service occupations; nearly 70 percent have some education beyond high school. The most highly educated middle-aged women are in professional specialties, where over 70 percent have at least a baccalaureate degree (U.S. Bureau of the Census, 1995a). Higher education increases the likelihood that women will be employed, and, on average, a woman with at least a bachelor's degree earns more at every age than a woman with less education.

Women at midlife must cope with signs of **aging** that require the development of a new body image. Many women feel more confident when they delay outward signs of aging by using cosmetics and hair dyes, yet growing numbers of women feel entitled to their gray hair, wrinkles, or other signs of aging. A way of approaching midlife changes positively is to see them as opportunities to experiment with new styles, colors, and ways of presenting oneself.

TABLE 2–2 Personal income of women and men age 65 and over by income level, 1995 (percent distributions).

Personal Income	Women (%)			Men (%)		
Without income			2.2			1.3
$1–$4,999	55.5%	{	14.2	24.3%	{	3.8
$5,000–$9,999			39.1			19.2
$10,000–$14,999			19.6			21.2
$15,000–$24,999			14.9			27.1
$25,000–$34,999			5.3			12.2
$35,000–$49,999			2.7			6.2
$50,000–$74,999			1.4			5.1
$75,000 or more			0.6			3.9
Total percentage			100.0			100.0
Total number (in thousands)			18,398			13,260

Source: US Bureau of the Census. (1995). *Money Income in the United States.* Washington, DC: U.S. Government Printing Office.

Older Women

The population of older adults in America is overwhelmingly female, and many of these women are poor, have multiple health problems, and are outliving their support systems. Many older women find themselves suffering the consequences of having had a low income or no income during their youth and middle years. Additional factors that contribute to the **high poverty rates** among older women include ethnicity, discriminatory Social Security benefits, and lifelong histories of gender bias. Older women (and men) with chronic health problems who need community-based services learn that Medicare reimburses for few such services. Such factors as aging, poor health, low income and poverty, inadequate healthcare, entrenched social and political structures, and continuing lack of sensitivity to gender differences combine to create an interactive network of problems for older women. The issues of aging are mostly women's issues, and that will not change in the near future.

DEMOGRAPHICS OF AGING WOMEN IN THE UNITED STATES

The total population of the United States is approximately 250,000,000. According to the 2000 census, 1 in every 10 persons is a woman 60 years of age or older (U.S. Administration on Aging, 2001). The percentage of widowed Euro-American women and African American women is about equal, even though African American women constitute only about 1.5 million of the total number. Proportionally, more older African American women than older Euro-American women are living without spouses. Women currently make up 70 percent of the population age 85 and over, and women will continue to outnumber men in the twenty-first century. By 2025, there will be approximately 2.5 times more women than men who are age 85 or older (U.S. Administration on Aging, 2001). Women continue to have a longer life expectancy than men, no matter their race or ethnicity, with women expected to live into their late seventies and men expected to live only into their early seventies. The female majority is concentrated in the upper age ranges, with older women living alone, without a spouse, and in poorer health than men (U.S. Administration on Aging, 2001).

ECONOMIC CONSIDERATIONS

Women who were always poor or nearly poor will most likely be living at or near the poverty level in old age. Women who live on fixed incomes that do not increase along with increases in the cost of living are also economically vulnerable. **Median personal income** is lower for women than for men, at every age (Costello, Miles & Stone, 1998). In 1995 (see Table 2.2), more than half (55.5 percent) of the women over age 65 had personal incomes of less than $10,000, compared with less than a quarter of the men (U.S. Bureau of the Census, 1995c). Almost all the older persons living below the poverty level are women. Poverty is especially liable to afflict older ethnic minority women and all women who live alone (U.S. Administration on Aging, 2001).

Older women are likely to have fewer sources of personal income than men. In comparison with men over 65, relatively few older women have income from earnings. Both the amount of money women receive from Social Security and the amount of money they receive from pensions are generally much smaller than for men. Only about 1 in 12 older women has income from a survivor's benefit based on a deceased spouse's employment. The income of older ethnic minority women is much lower than that of Euro-American women and it comes from fewer sources. Although African American women who receive pensions average considerably more income from this source than Euro-American women, they are less likely to have income from Social Security.

Social Security is the most common source of income for Americans over the age of 65. Most female recipients receive a wife's or widow's benefit. This is because about two in five women find that the benefit to which they are entitled as retired workers is smaller than that to which they are entitled based on their spouse's employment. Women who are entitled to pension benefits based on both their own work and that of a spouse are known as **dually entitled** beneficiaries. Dually entitled beneficiaries receive an amount based on their own work record (the primary benefit) plus an amount equal to the difference between the primary benefit and the usually larger benefit to which they are entitled as the spouse or widow of a covered worker (Stone & Griffith, 1998).

Poverty rates for women over age 65 have declined less than the poverty rates for men over age 65, and significant numbers of older women are poor. The Bureau of the Census reports that, in 1995, 75 percent of the elderly poor were female. In 1998, the yearly income that qualified a person over age 65 and living alone for the designation "poor" was $7,818 or less.

Poor women are typically older than poorer men, with larger proportions being African American or *Latina*. In addition to the approximately 2.5 million older women with incomes below the poverty level, there are about 3.1 million on the borderline of poverty.

LIVING ARRANGEMENTS

Less than one-third of women between ages 65 and 75 live alone in the community; however, for women over age 75, living alone is the norm. Women in both these age groups, however, are more than twice as likely to live alone as their male counterparts, and the millions of older women who live alone are the ones most likely to be in difficult financial straits.

According to the 2000 census, 80 percent of all older persons who live alone are women. Older women are three times as likely as older men to be living alone. Three out of five older African American and two out of five older Latina women who live alone have incomes below the poverty level (U.S. Administration on Aging, 2001).

Older women are more likely than older men to live in a nursing home, home for the aged, or a similar institution. On average, four of every five residents over the age of 85 in such institutions are women (U.S. Administration on Aging,

2001). Women predominate in the nursing home population both because they tend to live longer and because they are more likely than men to have chronic and disabling health problems that make independent living difficult or impossible.

MARITAL STATUS

The older a woman is, the more likely she is to lack the companionship and support of a husband. Although the overwhelming majority of older women have been married at some point in their lives, women over age 75 are quite likely to be widows. Whereas nearly 7 of every 10 men over age 75 is living with a spouse, more than 6 of every 10 women over age 75 are widows (Stone & Griffith, 1998). The risks for financial burdens and social support problems grow as women age.

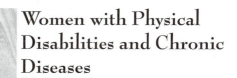

Women with Physical Disabilities and Chronic Diseases

The sophistication of the healthcare system in the United States and other developed countries means that there are increasing numbers of people with chronic physical health problems and disabilities. The word *chronic* denotes the slow and persistent development of a health problem over a period of time, often for the remainder of a person's life. Many chronic problems eventually result in impairment and subsequent disability. The reverse is also true; women with physical disabilities report chronic conditions more often than do women without disabilities, and they do so at a younger age (Nosek, Howland, Rintala, Young, & Chanpong, 1997). The World Health Organization defines *disability* as any restriction or lack of an ability to perform an activity in the manner or within the range considered normal for human beings (Lubkin, 1998). The Americans with Disabilities Act of 1990 uses the term *disability* to denote physical or mental impairment that limits one or more major life activities. In this section, only physical disabilities will be addressed.

Incidence and Nature of Physical Disability in Women

Women and girls with physical disabilities make up an estimated 21.3 percent of the female population (Jans & Stoddard, 1999). One in five Americans has a disability, and more than half the physically disabled population is female. Of the 129.3 million noninstitutionalized women in the United States, about 15.4 percent have activity limitations. This is a slightly higher percentage than for men; it is believed that women's higher rate of activity limitation is due to their greater longevity and the fact that activity limitations increase sharply with age. Women have higher disability rates than men in all of the major ethnic groups except the Native American, in which males have disability rates comparable with that of females. **Native American women** have the highest disability rate of any female population group, and **African American** women have the second highest (Jans & Stoddard, 1999).

Back disorders are the most prevalent cause of physical disability in the United States for both genders. Women, who get arthritis twice as often as men, most often develop either osteoarthritis or rheumatoid arthritis (The Boston Women's Health Collective, 1998). Rheumatoid arthritis is usually crippling and debilitating, and osteoarthritis causes joint pain as cartilage in weight-bearing joints decreases (see Chapter 14). Physical disability in immigrant women is sometimes nutritional in origin. Girls and women in many cultures are more likely than boys and men to experience nutritional deficiencies. Other causes of disability in immigrant women include preventable childhood diseases, pelvic inflammation, female genital mutilation, and complications of labor and childbirth (Smyke, 1991).

Social Consequences

Women with disabilities may find themselves in a socially devalued role, experience changes in social relationships or interactions, or limit the number of social activities in which they participate (Falvo, 1999). Environmental barriers, prejudice, and stereotyping may prevent persons with disabilities from being socially active and engaged in relationships with others.

Women with physical disabilities have lower rates of marriage than do women without such disabilities. They also have lower rates of marriage than men with disabilities. Only about 50 percent of the women with minor or moderate disabilities and 44 percent of the women with severe disabilities are currently married. Women with physical disabilities have higher rates of divorce than women without disabilities (Jans & Stoddard, 1999). Women with disabilities have endured a long history of medical treatment without consent, including involuntary and concealed contraception, sterilization, and abortion (Gill, 1997).

Immigrant women with activity limitations often have particular difficulties. In families whose cultural roots lie in countries in which the causes of disability are less well understood, disability may lead to shame or even complete isolation or abandonment. Educational opportunities for girls with disabilities may be decreased; in many areas of the world, the assumption is made that a male with a disability should learn a skill or profession, but the same assumption is not made about women with disabilities (Smyke, 1991). Universally, women with disabilities may find the attitudes of society more difficult to handle and more disabling than the disability itself.

The treatment and rehabilitation of women with disabilities involves not just the healthcare system and issues of accessibility but also support for initiatives that provide aid, education, and employment opportunities. Women with disabilities face the same potential discrimination from healthcare providers as men, because healthcare professionals share the same values and expectations as the rest of society. In this country, most healthcare providers share the American dream of achievement, attractiveness, and a cohesive, healthy family (Lubkin, 1998). These shared values may influence the ways in which persons who are disabled or impaired or are perceived by persons who are not disabled or impaired. Gill (1997) points out that women with disabilities encounter all the problems other women do, and then some, when seeking healthcare access. More and more women with disabilities are becoming politically active in an effort to have their health needs heard as a minority community. The health needs and concerns of women with disabilities are, in fact, women's health issues.

Lesbian Women

The term **lesbian** refers to a woman who is sexually or romantically oriented to other women. Although no reliable data exist, it is presumed that gays, lesbians, and transgender persons make up approximately 6 to 10 percent of the population (Wojciechowski, 1998). The lesbian population is as diverse as the population at large and crosses all ethnic, religious, and economic boundaries.

Less is known about the health of lesbian women than about that of women from other minority groups (Lee, 2000). Researchers have difficulty differentiating records of lesbian patients from those of heterosexual patients because lesbian women are often reluctant to be candid about their sexual orientation with healthcare providers who may be prejudiced against them (Price, Easton, & Telljohann, 1996). Homosexual people, both gay men and lesbian women, have been treated as social outcasts by the larger culture, and, until quite recently, homosexuality was classified as a mental disorder. Unions between committed gay people still cannot be recognized as legal marriages in most states. Gay men and lesbian women have had to disguise their true sexual orientation in order to evade legal and social discrimination, including violent assaults. Lesbians are at risk for many of the same health problems that beset heterosexual women, such as sexually transmitted diseases, breast cancer, and issues related to pregnancy. Societal prejudice against them is a major barrier to optimal healthcare.

Preventive Healthcare

As a group, lesbians tend to seek preventive healthcare less often than heterosexual women do (Roberts, Dibble, Scanlon, Paul, & Davids, 1998). On a recent national survey, only 54 percent of the lesbian and bisexual respondents reported having been screened for cervical cancer during the past year (Diamont, Schuster, McGuigan, & Lever, 1999). The underutilization of screening health services jeopardizes the early detection of sexually transmitted diseases, as well as cancers of the breast, cervix, and endometrium. Like sexually active heterosexual women, sexually active lesbian women are at risk for infection with the human papilloma virus and subsequent cervical cancer. In one study (Marrazzo et al., 1998), 14 percent of the female subjects who reported never having had sex with a man were found to have precancerous or cancerous cervical lesions.

Whether lesbian women undergo mammography as often as heterosexual women is unclear, as the results of studies on that subject are conflicting (Lee, 2000). A recent study of 534 lesbian women (Koh, 2000), however, found them to be less likely than heterosexual women to get mammograms and cholesterol screening. One factor that may prevent lesbian women from receiving preventive healthcare is lack of **insurance.** Few lesbians enjoy the benefits of spousal health coverage.

Perhaps the most critical factor in lesbian women's failure to seek preventive healthcare is related to the perceptions and reactions of healthcare providers. Many providers, as well as members of the general public, are not personally acquainted with any women who have divulged a lesbian sexual orientation and therefore tend to assume that all women are heterosexual. They often routinely ask all sexually active women questions such as "What kind of birth control do you use?" instead of asking whether the woman is interested in birth control. The *assumption of heterosexuality* is offensive to many lesbian women and gay men. It serves as a signal that the provider is not accepting of homosexuality, and forces lesbian clients either to misrepresent themselves or to risk rejection or disapproval. The assumption of heterosexuality and overt hostility toward lesbian clients are major reasons that lesbian women tend to undergo less screening and preventive healthcare (Roberts et al., 1998). In a study involving 53 lesbian women, only 31 percent had disclosed their sexual orientation to their healthcare providers. Of the women who had been frank about their orientation, 27 percent reported that their disclosure had had a negative effect on their healthcare (Lehmann, Lehmann, & Kelly, 1998).

Mental Health

The results of the few recent surveys done on the prevalence of emotional/mental health problems generally suggest that gay adults are no more likely to suffer from a mental disorder than are heterosexual people. An analysis of the data from the 1996 National Household Survey of Drug Abuse did reveal a *slightly* higher past-year incidence of psychiatric morbidity and use of mental health services among the sexually active gay people surveyed than among the heterosexual people surveyed (Cochran & Mays, 2000). In the most comprehensive survey of lesbians' health done to date (Bradford, Ryan, & Rothblum, 1994), however, over half the

1,925 respondents indicated they had thought of committing suicide at some point in their lives, and 75 percent disclosed that they had received counseling because of sadness or depression. Information as to the respondents' ages when those incidents occurred was not elicited.

Unfortunately, *adolescent* lesbians and gay males are at considerably higher risk than heterosexual young people for depression and suicide (Lock & Steiner, 1999). For example, according to one estimate, 40 percent of lesbian, gay, or transgender adolescents have either seriously considered or attempted suicide, and lesbian adolescents are twice as likely as heterosexual adolescents to attempt suicide (Gibson, 1994).

Sexually Transmitted Diseases

There is evidence that lesbian women have the lowest incidence of gonorrhea and syphilis of any group except women who have never had sexual relations (Lee, 2000). There is also some evidence that lesbian women are somewhat more likely than heterosexual women to practice safer sex (Koh, 2000). Nevertheless, lesbian women can and do contract sexually transmitted diseases (STDs) through exclusively homosexual relations (White, 1997). A number of **pathogens** capable of causing infection are shed in vaginal secretions. Sex between women can be the means of transmission for chlamydia, trichomoniasis, and the bacteria that cause bacterial vaginosis (Berger, 1995). Hepatitis B and C, herpes, genital warts, and AIDS can all be transmitted during lesbian sex as well (Lynch & Ferri, 1997). Recent research revealed that HIV/AIDS is a risk factor in a lesbian relationship if either partner ever had a relationship with a male with HIV/AIDS or with a female who used intravenous drugs (Norman, Perry, Stevenson, Kelly, & Roffman, 1996). The virus that causes AIDS has been detected in cervical and vaginal secretions as well as in menstrual blood, and the likelihood of transmitting hepatitis and HIV/AIDS is especially high during the menstrual period (Lynch & Ferri, 1997). Only women who are in a long-term, monogamous relationship should forgo routine screening for AIDS and other sexually transmitted diseases.

Pregnancy

Lesbian and bisexual adolescents are as much at risk for unwanted and unintended pregnancy as heterosexual adolescents. A 1999 analysis of a fairly large-scale study of adolescent behavior revealed that lesbian or bisexual respondents not only were almost as likely as heterosexual respondents to have had intercourse but also were significantly more likely to become pregnant when they did (Saewyc, Bearinger, Blum, & Resnick, 1999).

Some lesbian women wish to become pregnant and rear a child. It is not unusual for lesbian couples to seek **artificial insemination** for one partner in order to create a family together. This can pose a health risk, however, as lesbian women who fear judgment and discrimination on the part of healthcare providers often go outside the medical system for sperm donors. They may use semen from men who have not been tested for HIV and other sexually transmitted diseases (Lynch & Ferri, 1997).

Breast Cancer

There is no evidence that the incidence of breast cancer is higher in lesbian than heterosexual women. However, in one study (Roberts et al., 1998), the lesbian women had more *risk factors* (more breast biopsies, greater body mass, and fewer pregnancies) than the heterosexual women, but no more actual cases of breast cancer. The authors speculated that the reason little cancer occurred in either group might have been that all the women in the study were relatively young.

Substance Abuse

The preponderance of evidence from literature analyses (Lee, 2000) and studies (Cochran & Mays, 2000) to date suggests that adult lesbian women do not abuse drugs, such as alcohol and cocaine, significantly more than heterosexual women. Tobacco use, though, does seem to be more frequent among lesbian women. According to a 1990 survey, 43 percent of the lesbians and 22 percent of the heterosexual women queried reported having smoked cigarettes in the previous month (Skinner, 1994). Unfortunately, lesbian *girls* are at considerably greater risk for substance abuse than heterosexual girls. Lesbian girls younger than 13 are more likely than their heterosexual counterparts to smoke tobacco and marijuana and to use cocaine (Savin-Williams, 1994).

New Directions

The health of women in general, and ethnic minority and lesbian women in particular, has been underresearched. There is much that is not known about ethnic minority and lesbian women's health and how it can be improved. For example, studies that will determine more clearly how and why ethnic minority women suffer from poorer health status are needed. The impact of lack of resources must be further explored (Pearlman, 1998), as must ethnic minority women's beliefs about and attitudes toward health and healthcare and their actual experiences within the healthcare system. The need for more research on ethnic minority women's health has been recognized at the federal level. In 1994, the National Institutes of Health developed guidelines for research that emphasized the importance of including ethnic women in health-related studies (Caban, 1995). Researchers must

now provide clear rationales for excluding ethnic minority women from federally funded studies.

More programs specifically created to meet the healthcare needs of ethnic minority women are also needed. It is known that community-based outreach programs with integrated preventive services have proven effective at improving the health of Latina and African American women (Vellozzi, Romans, & Rothenberg, 1996). Such programs work because women do not have to leave their own communities to obtain care. More ethnic minority healthcare providers are also needed. Providers who are members of the same communities as the women they serve more easily establish trust and connection.

More research is needed on lesbian women's health. Little is known about the actual rates at which diseases are transmitted in the course of sexual relations between women. The rate at which lesbian women develop breast cancer must also be more specifically determined. Finally, more qualitative research into lesbian women's health must be done, so that more issues of concern to lesbian women will be raised.

The population of older adults, especially women, will soon be higher than ever before in the history of the United States. Many of the existing research studies about the health of older Americans have been conducted on males, but there are several large-scale longitudinal studies now underway that will provide information about the health of women as they age. Additional studies and subsequent programs will be needed to provide education and information for older women in the next several decades.

QUESTIONS FOR REFLECTION AND DISCUSSION

1. *One of the most valuable ways to foster peace and fairness in the world is to develop self-awareness. What are your biases and prejudices regarding poor people, people from different ethnic groups, older people, people with disabilities, and lesbians? What are some changes you could make in your attitude and behavior toward people from these groups?*

2. *How can we, on the individual, community, and societal levels, assist and empower disadvantaged women regarding preventive healthcare?*

3. *What factors do you think are most responsible for the recent decline in teenage pregnancy rates?*

4. *What research questions could be developed that would be culturally sensitive and yield needed information about ethnic minority and lesbian women's health?*

5. *What changes in social policy and/or the healthcare delivery system would most benefit women with physical disabilities?*

Resources

Books and Videotapes

Alcena, Valerie, M.D. (2001). The African-American Woman's Health Book: A Guide to the Prevention and Cure of Illness. Barricade Books.

Delgado, J. (1997). *Salud: A Latina's guide to total health-body, mind, and spirit.* Scranton, PA: HarperCollins.

Organizations

Caribbean Women's Health Association, Inc.
2725 Church Avenue
Brooklyn, NY 11226

Center for Research on Women with Disabilities
3440 Richmond Ave., Suite B
Houston, TX 77046
Phone: 1-800-44-CROWD
Web: www.bcm.tmc.edu/crowd

Female Genital Mutilation Education and Networking Project
P.O. Box 6597
Albany, CA 94706
Phone: 510-234-4779
E-mail: fmg@fmgnetwork.org
Web: http://www.fgmnetwork.org

Gay and Lesbian Medical Association (GLMA)
459 Fulton St., Suite 107
San Francisco, CA 94104
E-mail: info@glma.org
Web: http://glma.org/indexmain.html

Gay and Lesbian National Hotline—toll free peer counseling and referrals
Phone: 1-888-843-4564

Initiative to Eliminate Racial and Ethnic Disparities in Health
Web: http://raceandhealth.hhs.gov/

Lesbian Health—On-line articles related to lesbian health and other topics
Web: http://www.lesbian.org/lesbian-moms/health.html

National Asian Women's Health Organization
250 Montgomery St., Suite 410
San Francisco, CA 94104
Phone: 415-989-9747
Web: http://www.nawho.org/contactframe.html

National Center for Children in Poverty
Joseph L. Mailman School of Public Health of Columbia University
154 Haven Avenue
New York, NY 10032
Phone: 212-304-7100
Fax: 212-544-4200 or 212-544-4201
Web: http://cpmcnet.columbia.edu/dept/nccp/cpf598.html

National Institute on Disability and Rehabilitation Research
Web: www.ncddr.org/doorways/women

National Women's Health Information Center (Women with Disabilities)
8550 Arlington Blvd., Suite 300
Fairfax, VA 22031
Phone: 1-800-994-9662
TDD: 888-220-5446
Web: www.4women.gov/wwd/index.htm

Native American Women's Health Education Resource Center
P.O. Box 572
Lake Andes, SD 57356
E-mail: nativewoman@igc.apc.org
Phone: 605-487-7072

Office of Minority Health
Division of Information and Education
Rockwall II Bldg, Suite 100
5600 Fishers Lane
Rockville, MD 20857
Phone: 1-800-444-6472
Web: http://www.omhrc.gov/

Public Health Service
Agency for Health Care Research and Quality (formerly Agency for Health Care Policy and Research)
P.O. Box 8547
Silver Spring, MD 20907-8547
Phone: 301-594-1364
Web: http://www.ahcpr.gov

Research, Action, and Information Network for the Bodily Integrity of Women (RAINBO)
915 Broadway, Suite 1109
New York, NY 10010-7108
Phone: 212-477-3318
E-mail: info@rainbo.org
Web: http://www.rainbo.org

U.S. Public Health Service Office on Women's Health
Department of Health and Human Services
200 Independence Ave., SW, Rm 730B
Washington, DC 20201

World Health Organization
Department of Women's Health
E-mail: whd@who.ch
Web page on female genital mutilation: www.who.int/frh-whd/FGM/index.htm

References

Affara, F. (2000). When tradition maims. *American Journal of Nursing, 100*(8), 52–61.

Agency for Health Care Policy and Research. (1999). Some Latino children are more likely to have asthma than others. *Research Activities, 226*(11), 44–46.

Arbesman, M., Koller, H., & Buck, G. M. (1993). Assessment of the impact of female circumcision on the gynecological, genitourinary, and obstetrical health problems of women from Somalia to Poland: Literature review and case series. *Women's Health, 20*(3), 27–42.

Berger, B. J. (1995). Bacterial vaginosis in lesbians: a sexually-transmitted disease. *Clinical Infections and Diseases, 21*(6), 1402–1405.

Bowen, D., Hickman, K., & Powers, D. (1997). Importance of psychological variables in understanding risk perceptions and breast cancer screening of African American women. *Women's Health, 3,* 227–242.

Bradford, J., Ryan, C., & Rothblum, E. D. (1994). National lesbian health care survey: Implications for mental health care. *Journal of Consulting Clinical Psychology, 62*(2), 228–242.

Brown, L. M., & Gilligan, C. (1992). *Meeting at the crossroads: Women's psychology and girl's development.* Cambridge, MA: Harvard University Press.

Burns, V. E. (1999). Factors influencing teenage mothers' participation in unprotected sex. *Journal of Obstetrical, Gynecologic and Neonatal Nursing, 28*(5), 493–500.

Caban, C. (1995). Hispanic research: Implications of the National Institutes of Health guidelines on inclusion of women and minorities in clinical research. *Journal of the National Cancer Institute Monograph, 18,* 165–169.

Cochran, S. D., & Mays, V. M. (2000). Relations between psychiatric syndromes and behaviorally defined sexual orientation in a sample of the US population. *American Journal of Epidemiology, 151*(5), 516–523.

Costello, C., Miles, S., & Stone, A. (Eds.). (1998). *The American woman: 1999–2000.* New York: W. W. Norton.

Council of Economic Advisers for the President's Initiative on Race. (1998). *Changing America: Indicators of social and economic well-being by race and Hispanic origin.* Washington, DC: Author.

Crawford, V. (1998). African American women in the twenty-first century: The continuing challenge. In C. Costello, S. Miles, & A. Stone (Eds.), *The American woman 1999–2000* (pp. 102–132). New York: W. W. Norton.

Curtin, S. C., & Martin, J. (2000). Birth: Preliminary data for 1999. *National Vital Statistics Reports [On-line], 48*(14). Available: http://www.cdc.gov/nchs/data/nvs48_14.pdf

Dains, J., Baumann, L., & Scheibel, P. (1998). *Advanced health assessment and clinical diagnosis in primary care.* St. Louis: Mosby-Year Book.

Davis, R. (1993). *A phenomenological study of adult Puerto Rican women's health beliefs and health practices: Implications for adult educators in health care settings.* Unpublished doctoral dissertation, The Pennsylvania State University, University Park.

Davis, R. (1996). The perceptions of Puerto Rican women regarding health care experiences. *Journal of the American Academy of Nurse Practitioners, 8*(1), 21–25.

Davis, R. (1998). Coming to a place of understanding: The meaning of health and illness for African American women. *Journal of Multicultural Nursing and Health, 4*(1), 32–41.

Diamant, A. L., Schuster, M. A., McGuigan, K., & Lever, J. (1999). Lesbians' sexual history with men: Implications for taking a sexual history. *Archives of Internal Medicine, 159*(22), 2730–2736.

EthnoMed. (1998). *Features of major refugee and immigrant groups seen at Central Seattle health clinics* [On-line]. Available: http://healthlinks.washington.edu/clinical/ethnomed/features

Evans, K., & Herr, E. (1991). The influence of racism and sexism in the career development of African American women. *Journal of Multicultural Counseling and Diversity, 19*(3), 130–135.

Falvo, D. (1999). *Medical and psychosocial aspects of chronic illness and disability* (2nd ed.). Gaithersburg, MD: Aspen.

Galanti, G. (1997). *Caring for patients from different cultures.* Philadelphia: University of Pennsylvania Press.

Gardner, M., Cliver, S., McNeal, S., & Goldenberg, R. (1996). Ethnicity and sources of prenatal care: Findings from a national survey. *Birth, 23*(2), 84–87.

Gaston, M., Barrett, S., Johnson, T., & Epstein, L. (1998). Health care needs of medically underserved women of color: The role of the Bureau of Primary Health Care. *Health and Social Work, 23*(2), 86–95.

Gibson, P. (1994). Gay male and lesbian youth suicide. In G. Remafedi (Ed.), *Death by denial: Studies of suicide in gay and lesbian teens* (pp. 15–88). Boston: Alyson.

Giger, J., & Davidhizar, R. (1995). *Transcultural nursing: Assessment and intervention.* St. Louis: Mosby-Year Book.

Gill, C. (1997). The last sisters: Health issues of women with disabilities. In S. Ruzek, V. Olesen, & A. Clarke (Eds.), *Women's health, complexities and differences* (pp. 96–111). Columbus: Ohio State University Press.

Gilligan, C. (1982). *In a different voice.* Cambridge, MA: Harvard University Press.

Gold, S. (1994). Mental health and illness in Vietnamese refugees. *The Western Journal of Medicine, 157,* 290–294.

Greenburg-Lake Staff & Analysis Group Staff. (1994). *Short-changing girls, shortchanging America* (2nd ed.). Washington, DC: American Association of University Women.

Hahn, R., Teutsch, S., Franks, A., Chang, M., & Lloyd, E. (1998). The prevalence of risk factors among women in the United States by race and age, 1992–1994: Opportunities for primary and secondary prevention. *Journal of the American Women's Association, 53*(2), 96–104, 107.

Hayes-Bautista, D., & Chapa, J. (1987). Latino terminology: Conceptual bases for standardized terminology. *American Journal of Public Health, 77*(1), 61–68.

Heise, L. (1993). Violence against women. In M. Koblinsky, J. Timyan, & J. Gay (Eds.), *The health of women: A global perspective* (pp. 171–195). Boulder, CO: Westview Press.

Herman-Giddens, M. E., Slora, E. S., Wasserman, R. C., Bourdony, C. J., Bhapkar, M. V., Koch, G. G., & Hasmeier, C. M. (1997). Secondary sexual characteristics and menses in young girls seen in office practice: A study from the Pediatric Research in Office Settings Network. *Pediatrics, 99*(4), 505–12.

Houppert, K. (1999). *The curse.* New York: Farrar, Straus & Giroux.

Jacobs Institute of Women's Health. (1998). *Medicaid managed care: The challenge of providing care to low-income women.* [On-line]. Available: http://www.jiwh.org/insights/jan98no6.htm

Jans, L., & Stoddard, S. (1999). *Chartbook on women and disability in the United States. An InfoUse Report.* Washington, DC: United States National Institute on Disability and Rehabilitation Research.

Koblinsky, M., Campbell, O., & Harlow, S. (1993). Mother and more: A broader perspective on women's health. In M.

Koblinsky, J. Timyan, & J. Gay (Eds.), *The health of women: A global perspective* (pp. 33–62). San Francisco: Westview Press.

Koh, A. S. (2000). Use of preventive health behaviors by lesbian, bisexual, and heterosexual women: Questionnaire survey. *Western Journal of Medicine, 172*(6), 379–384.

Lantz, P., House, J., Lepkowski, J., Williams, D., Mero, R., & Chen, J. (1998). Socioeconomic factors, health behaviors, and mortality: Results from a nationally representative prospective study of US adults. *Journal of the American Medical Association, 279*(21), 1703–1708.

Lee, R. (2000). Health care problems of lesbian, gay, bisexual and transgendered patients. *Western Journal of Medicine, 172*(6), 403–408.

Leenerts, M. (1998). Barriers to self-care in a cohort of low-income white women living with HIV/AIDS. *Journal of the Association of Nurses in AIDS Care, 9*(6), 22–26.

Lehmann, J. B., Lehmann, C. U., & Kelly, P. J. (1998). Development and health care needs of lesbians. *Journal of Women's Health, 7*(3), 379–387.

Lewis, J., & Bernstein, J. (1996). Women's health: a relational perspective across the lifes cycle. Sudbury, MA: Jones and Bartlett.

Lock, J. R., & Steiner, H. (1999). Gay, bisexual, and lesbian youth risks for emotional, physical, and social problems: Results from a community-based survey. *Journal of the Academy of Child and Adolescent Psychiatry, 38*(3), 228–242.

Lubkin, I. (1998). *Chronic illness, impact and interventions* (4th ed.). Boston: Jones and Bartlett.

Lynch, M. A., & Ferri, R. S. (1997). Health needs of lesbian women and gay men. *Clinical Reviews, 7*(10), 85–112.

Marrazzo, J. M., Koutsky, L. A., Stine, K. L., Kuypers, J. M., Grubert, T. A., Galloway, D. A., Kiviat, N. B., & Handsfield, H. H. (1998). *Journal of Infectious Disease, 178*(6), 1604–1609.

Menendez, B. (1990). AIDS-related mortality among Puerto Rican women in New York City, 1981–87. *Puerto Rican Health Sciences Journal, 9*(1), 43–45.

Montagu, A. (1997). *Man's most dangerous myth: The fallacy of race* (6th ed.). Walnut Creek, CA: AltaMira.

Morris, V. (1996). *How to care for aging parents.* New York: Workman.

National Cervical Cancer Coalition. (2000). *Legislation (H.R. 1070) will expand treatment coverage for uninsured cervical cancer program* [On-line]. Available: http://www.nccc-online.org/

National Women's Health Information Center (2000). [On-line]. *The Health of Minority Women.* Retrieved: August 26, 2002. Available: http://www.4women.gov/own/pub/minority/Table 1.html

National Women's Health Resource Center. (2000). *Healthy women* [On-line]. Available: http:www.healthywomen.org/

Norman, A. D., Perry, M. J., Stevenson, L. Y., Kelly, J. A., & Roffman, R. A. (1996). Lesbian and bisexual women in small cities—At risk for HIV? *Public Health Reports, 111*(4), 347–352.

Nosek, M., Howland, C., Rintala, D., Young, M., & Chanpong, G. (1997). *National study of women with physical disabilities.* Houston: Center for Research on Women with Disabilities.

Office on Women's Health. (1998a). *Breast cancer: Increasing 5-year survival rates in Hispanic women.* Washington, DC: U.S. Public Health Service.

Office on Women's Health. (1998b). *Cardiovascular disease in Hispanic women.* Washington, DC: U.S. Public Health Service.

Office on Women's Health. (1998d). *The health of minority women.* Washington, DC: U.S. Public Health Service.

Pearlman, D. (1998). Slipping through the safety net: Implications for women's health. *Journal for Health Care of the Poor and Underserved, 9,* 217–221.

Perez-Stable, E. (1987). Issues in Latino health care. *Western Journal of Medicine, 146,* 213–218.

Pesa, J. (1999). Psychosocial factors associated with dieting behaviors among female adolescents. *Journal of School Health, 69*(5), 196–201.

Pipher, M. (1994). *Reviving Ophelia: saving the lives of adolescent girls.* NY: Ballentine Books.

Price, J. H., Easton, A. N., & Telljohann, S. K. (1996). Perceptions of cervical cancer and pap smear screening behavior by women's sexual orientation. *Journal of Community Health, 21,* 89–105.

Public Health Services Agencies. (1995). *Healthy people 2000 progress report for: American Indians and Alaska natives.* Washington, DC: Author

Purnell, L., & Paulanka, B. (1998). *Transcultural health care.* Philadelphia: F. A. Davis.

Roberts, S., Dibble, S., Scanlon, J., Paul, S., & Davids, H. (1998). Differences in risk factors for breast cancer: lesbian and heterosexual women. *Journal of the Gay and Lesbian Medical Association, 3,* September.

Saewyc, E. M., Bearinger, L. H., Blum, R. W., & Resnick, M. D. (1999). Sexual intercourse, abuse and pregnancy among adolescent women: Does sexual orientation make a difference? *Family Planning Perspectives, 31*(3), 127–131.

Savin-Williams, R. C. (1994). Verbal and physical abuse as stressors in the lives of lesbian, gay male, and bisexual youths: associations with school problems, running away, substance abuse, prostitution, and suicide. *Journal of Consulting and Clinical Psychology, 62*(2), 261–269.

Skinner, W. F. (1994). The prevalence and demographic predictors of illicit and licit drug use among lesbians and gay men. *American Journal of Public Health, 84*(8), 1307–1310.

Sloane, E. (1993). *Biology of women* (3rd ed.). Albany, NY: Delmar.

Smyke, P. (1991). *Women and health.* London: Zed Books.

Sowell, T. (1981). *Ethnic America.* New York: Basic Books.

Spector, R. (1996). *Cultural diversity in health and illness.* Stamford, CT: Appleton & Lange.

Stanley, M., & Beare, P. (1995). *Gerontological nursing* (2nd ed.). Philadelphia: F. A. Davis.

Stone, A., & Griffith, J. (1998). *Older women: The economics of aging.* Washington, DC: Women's Research & Education Institute.

Suarez, L., & Pulley, L. (1995). Comparing acculturation scales and their relationship to cancer screening among older Mexican-American women. *Journal of the National Cancer Institute Monograph, 18,* 41–47.

Tessaro, I., Eng, E., & Smith, J. (1994). Breast cancer screening in older African American women: Qualitative research findings. *American Journal of Health Promotion, 8,* 286–293.

The Boston Women's Health Collective (1998). *Our bodies ourselves for the new century*. NY: Touchstone.

The National Campaign to Prevent Teen Pregnancy (2001). Online. Facts and stats. Retrieved August, 2001. Available: http://www.teenpregnancy.org/factstats.htm

Tortolero-Luna, G., Glober, G., Villarreal, R., Palos, G., & Linares, A. (1995). Screening practices and knowledge, attitudes, and beliefs about cancer among Hispanic and non-Hispanic white women 35 years old or older in Nueces County, Texas. *Journal of the National Cancer Institute Monograph, 18*, 49–56.

United Nations High Commissioner for Refugees. (1998). *UNHCR and refugees* [On-line]. Available: http://www. unhcr.ch/

United Nations High Commissioner for Refugees. (1999). *Kosovo crisis update* [On-line]. Available: http://www.unhcr.ch/news/media/kosovo

U.S. Administration on Aging (2001). [On-line]. Meeting the needs of older women: A diverse and growing population. Retrieved August 28, 2002. Available: http://www.aoa.dhhs.gov/factsheet/ow.html

U.S. Bureau of the Census. (1995a). *Educational attainment in the United States*. Washington, DC: U.S. Government Printing Office.

U.S. Bureau of the Census. (1995b). *Marital status and living arrangements*. Washington, DC: U.S. Government Printing Office.

U.S. Bureau of the Census. (1995c). *Money income in the United States*. Washington, DC: U.S. Government Printing Office.

U.S. Bureau of the Census. (1995d). *Poverty in the United States*. Washington, DC: U.S. Government Printing Office.

U.S. Bureau of the Census. (1995e). *Statistical abstracts of the United States* (115th ed.). Washington, DC: U.S. Government Printing Office.

U.S. Bureau of the Census. (1998). *Poverty thresholds by size of family and number of related children under 18 years*. Washington, DC: U.S. Government Printing Office.

U.S. Census Bureau (2001). Population by race and hispanic or Latino origin, for all ages and 18 years and over for the United States: 2000. Retrieved August 6, 2002. Available: http://www.census.gov/population/cen2000/phc-ti/tab01.pdf

U.S. Department of Health and Human Services. (1997b). *Trends in Indian health*. Washington, DC: Author.

U.S. Department of Health and Human Services. (2000). *Temporary assistance for needy families (TANF) program. Third annual report to Congress*. Washington, DC: Author.

Vellozzi, C., Romans, M., & Rothenberg, R. (1996). Delivering breast and cervical cancer screening services to underserved women: Part I. Literature review and telephone survey. *Women's Health Issues, 6*(2), 65–73.

Walcott-McQuigg, J., Logan, B., & Smith, E. (1995). Preventive health practices of African American women. *Journal of the National Black Nurses Association, 7*(2), 49–59.

White, J. C. (1997). HIV risk assessment and prevention in lesbians and women who have sex with women: Practical information for clinicians. *Health Care of Women International, 18*(2), 127–138.

Wojciechowski, C. (1998). Issues in caring for older lesbians. *Journal of Gerontological Nursing, 27*(7), 28–33.

World Health Organization. (1998). *Classification and definitions of female genital mutilation* [On-line]. Available: http://www.who.int/frh-whd/FGM/f-defini

Wright, J. (1988). The worthy and unworthy homeless. *Society, 25*(5), 64–69.

Young Women and Smoking (2000). [online]. Department of Health and Human Services. Retrieved Aug. 10th, 2001. Available: http: //www.inwat.org/young.htm

SECTION II

Environmental/Lifestyle Factors That Affect Health

3

Nutrition

Marta L. Smith and Laura A. Filippelli

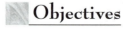

Objectives

1. Discuss the role of diet in the maintenance of health and in the prevention of disease.
2. Identify the major nutritional components of a healthful diet.
3. Demonstrate the ability to evaluate nutritional claims in literature and on food labels.
4. Compare and contrast the characteristics of nutritious foods and "junk" foods.
5. Identify issues related to the use of nutritional supplements.

6. *Explore current issues related to food safety, organic foods, and bioengineered foods.*
7. *Discuss strategies for achieving safe, long-term weight loss.*

Introduction

Women make dietary decisions not only for themselves but also for their families. They have the potential to impact the eating habits of our nation by demanding healthful foods in restaurants, grocery stores, schools, farms, and factories—everywhere food is purchased, prepared, or produced. The information in this chapter will help ensure that women are educated nutrition consumers and that they can assume leadership roles in actively improving the nutritional health of our country.

Dietary Patterns in America

Millions of Americans are starving for good nutrition, even though our country has the most abundant food supplies in the world. Many diets are high in animal proteins and the sugars, fats, and alcohol that supply empty calories, but they are low in fiber and other essential nutrients. An ironic acronym for the Standard American Diet is SAD (Lark, 2000). The SAD is one of the **major causes** of **adult morbidity** and **mortality,** including coronary heart disease, cancer, diabetes, hepatitis, arthritis, and osteoporosis. Poor diets and lack of exercise are major contributors to chronic illness and premature death. Other than tobacco use, no other element of lifestyle has a greater impact on an individual's overall health.

Because the consequences of poor dietary habits develop gradually, it is never too late to make a change and reap the benefits of a more healthful diet. Unfortunately, the quest for a healthful diet can be made more difficult by confusing, contradictory, and often sensational claims promoted by manufacturers of dietary supplements and specialty food products. The public is led to believe that certain dietary components or practices will ensure high energy levels; thick, shining hair; blemish-free skin; and freedom from chronic diseases. The accompanying testimonials are compelling, and the consumer is attracted to the simplistic rationales for the product's efficacy. Each year, consumers who wish to preserve or improve their health are duped into spending impressive amounts of money on unnecessary and often valueless products; sales of vitamins and nutritional supplements exceed $10.3 billion per year (*F-D-C Reports, Inc.,* 1997). The irony is that Americans' food consumption patterns are out of sync with this supposed interest in health. Americans eat on the run at fast-food restaurants and wash down handfuls of vita-

mins with their sodas. The false belief that supplement use can mitigate the effects of a poor diet is a major barrier to an improved standard of nutritional health.

The American diet has changed over the past two decades and is continuing to do so. According to a recent United States Department of Agriculture (USDA) report (Putnam & Allshouse, 1997) on food consumption, prices, and expenditures, we are purchasing less beef, eggs, and whole milk, and that is a positive change. The same study reports that we are also consuming more chicken, sugar, cheese, fats, oils, and soft drinks—a not so healthy change. And we have an insatiable sweet tooth, with each person's consuming over 150 pounds of sweeteners—primarily as sucrose and high fructose corn syrup (Putnam & Allshouse, 1997). On a daily basis, that translates to over 1 cup of sugars per day. This quantity is significantly higher than the USDA dietary guidelines recommendation of 6 teaspoons (1,600 calorie diet) or 12 teaspoons (2,200 calorie diet). In addition, we are consuming 10 more pounds of fat per person than in 1970, and much of that fat is from shortening, an unhealthy, artery-clogging transfat (Putnam & Allshouse, 1997). It is no wonder that **obesity** is the major nutritional problem facing Americans today, with approximately 50 percent of adult Americans classified as overweight or obese (Blackburn & He, 1999). In addition to consuming too much sugar and fat, we fail to get recommended amounts of healthful, nutrient-rich foods. Although the National Cancer Institute's Five-a-Day campaign (begun in October 1991) recommended that adults consume at least five servings of fruits and vegetables a day, a recent study revealed that only 24 percent of adults consume the recommended two servings of fruit. Only 12 percent consume the recommended three servings of vegetables (Krebs-Smith, Cook, Subar, Cleveland, & Friday, 1995).

Positive changes in dietary choices continue to be counterbalanced by negative ones. Despite all of the information that is available about the components of a healthful diet, truly significant dietary changes have not been made.

The Basics of Sound Nutrition

Food supplies the energy that we need to function, as well as the nutrients needed to build body tissue and catalyze biochemical processes. There are two broad categories of nutrients: macronutrients and micronutrients. **Macronutrients**—carbohydrate, protein, and fat—provide the body with energy in the form of calories, as well as the building blocks needed for growth and the repair of body structures. **Micronutrients**—vitamins, minerals, and trace elements—are required in small amounts. Although they do not provide energy, they play a critical role in the regulation of biochemical processes. Fiber and water are also important components of a healthy diet.

Macronutrients

PROTEIN

Protein is the structural component of body tissues. Proteins are nitrogen-containing compounds that are comprised of amino acids. Plant and animal proteins are made up of varying combinations of about 20 common amino acids. Each food protein source has its own unique combination of amino acids, and all food proteins contain all of the amino acids but in varying amounts. Our bodies use the amino acids from food to create new proteins for use in the body. The body needs proteins to build new tissues during growth and to rebuild and replace worn-out tissues. The body is extremely efficient at recycling degraded protein and using the amino acids for new structures; however, not all of the protein is saved. Some protein is lost during metabolism and some in body secretions, such as urine, feces, and sweat, and in the sloughing of hair, skin, and nails. Protein stores must be continually replenished from dietary protein, and nine of the amino acids **(essential amino acids)** must be obtained from dietary sources because the body cannot manufacture them.

Not all food proteins are created equal. In general, protein from animal sources, such as milk, meat, eggs, fish, and cheese, is of higher quality because it is a **complete protein**—it supplies all of the essential amino acids in adequate amounts. Plant sources of protein (primarily grains, legumes, and vegetables) contain varying levels of amino acids and are referred to as **incomplete proteins.** One or more of the essential amino acids is present in lower amounts than the other amino acids and is the **limiting amino acid** for that food. By balancing foods that are low in a particular amino acid with foods that are high in it, a high-quality protein diet can be obtained from incomplete plant proteins alone.

The Recommended Dietary Allowance (RDA) for **protein** is **0.75 g of protein/kg of body weight per day** for both men and women (National Academy Press Food and Nutrition Board, 1989). For example, a woman who weighs 135 lb, or 61 kg, needs to consume approximately 46 g (61 kg body weight × .75 g protein/kg body weight) of protein per day to achieve this recommended level. This level is fairly easy to obtain during the course of a day; a 3 oz cheeseburger on a bun supplies approximately 32 g of protein, already 70 percent of the woman's daily requirement. Protein intake is usually excessive in the typical American diet, in which 20 percent of the total calories consumed are from protein sources. When dietary protein intake exceeds the level necessary for the synthesis of body proteins, the additional protein is not stored as protein but is used as energy or is eventually converted to fat.

CARBOHYDRATES

Dietary **carbohydrates** consist of either sugars or starches. Sugars are referred to as simple carbohydrates and include **monosaccharides,** such as glucose and fructose (fruit sugar), and **disaccharides,** such as sucrose (table sugar), maltose, and lactose (milk sugar). Starches are referred to as **complex carbohydrates** and are derived primarily from cereals, grains, fruits, and vegetables. All carbohydrates are metabolized in the intestinal tract and converted to glucose by the liver. Glucose is the cellular fuel of choice. Any excess glucose that is not needed for cellular functions is either stored in the muscles and liver as **glycogen** or converted to fat. Glycogen is used as an energy source when the body switches to anaerobic metabolism during times of strenuous exercise (such as running a marathon). Once the glycogen stores are depleted, any additional glucose not used for energy is converted to fat.

The current USDA recommendations for a healthful diet suggest that 55 percent of total caloric intake be comprised of carbohydrates. From a nutritional standpoint, complex carbohydrates are preferred over simple sugars because foods that contain them also provide vitamins, minerals, and fiber. From a health standpoint, excess consumption of refined and highly processed carbohydrates (such as white bread, cookies, pasta, and candy) may have a deleterious effect. There is some speculation that a diet high in these carbohydrates may increase a woman's risk for coronary heart disease, obesity, and diabetes; however, additional research is needed before a direct cause and effect relationship can be established. The **glycemic index** is a scale that rates foods according to how much they raise blood sugar levels. In one study (Frost, Leeds, Trew, Margara, & Dornhurst, 1998), it was found that high glycemic index foods, such as potatoes and white bread, triggered unhealthy lipid changes in the blood, whereas foods that had lower glycemic indexes, such as whole fruits and whole grains, did not. Although the relationship between simple carbohydrate consumption and risk of certain diseases, such as diabetes and coronary heart disease, is not yet clear, it is apparent that whole grains and cereal fibers play a protective role against the development of diabetes in older women (Meyer, Kushi, Jacobs, Slavin, & Sellers, 2000). The overall recommendations for a diet based on carbohydrates is still sound, as long as the majority of those carbohydrates are in the complex form (such as whole grains, flours, cereals, and fresh fruits and vegetables) instead of simple sugars and refined flours.

FAT

More than one-third of the calories in the standard American diet come from **fat.** Fat contributes to the flavor and texture of foods, and foods that are high in fat typically have a creamy, smooth mouth feel. Because of this, we are attracted to foods that contain fat; nevertheless, as with many things in life, one can have too much of a good thing. A diet that is chronically high in fat contributes to obesity, coronary heart disease, and some forms of cancer. Avoiding fat entirely, however, is neither necessary nor nutritionally sound. Healthy fats are essential components of a healthy diet.

Dietary fat is the most concentrated source of calories, containing more than *double* the caloric concentration of either protein or carbohydrate. Fat provides *9 calories per gram,* whereas carbohydrate and protein each provide only *4 calories per gram.* In addition to being an excellent source of energy, fat also facilitates the absorption and transfer of fat-soluble vitamins. Fats are comprised of fatty acids, which are chemical chains of carbon, hydrogen, and oxygen. Two of the fatty acids, **linoleic** and **linolenic,** are considered essential fatty acids. In nutritional parlance, that means two things: They are essential for proper health and functioning, and, because the body cannot manufacture them, they must be provided by dietary sources.

Fatty acids are classified as saturated, monounsaturated, or polyunsaturated, depending on the type of bonds that exist in the chemical chains and the number of hydrogen atoms present. **Saturated fatty acids (SFAs)** contain no double bonds between the carbon atoms and carry all the hydrogen atoms the chain can hold; the chain is saturated with hydrogen atoms. Most saturated fats, such as butter and lard, are derived from animal products and are solid at room temperature. The exception to this generalization is that several tropical oils—namely, coconut, palm, and palm kernel oils—are vegetable sources of saturated fat. SFAs are the fatty acid "bad guys" because they raise blood **cholesterol** levels, which in turn increase the risk for coronary heart disease.

Monounsaturated fatty acids (MUFAs) contain one double bond between two carbon atoms because they are missing one pair of hydrogen atoms. Monounsaturated fats are liquid at room temperature but will solidify if chilled. The best sources of monounsaturated fats are olive, canola, and peanut oils and avocados. MUFAs, when they replace SFAs, can result in lower blood cholesterol levels (Golub, 1999a).

Polyunsaturated fatty acids (PUFAs) contain more than one double bond and are the primary fatty acids in corn, safflower, sunflower, and cottonseed oils. Like MUFAs, PUFAs are liquid at room temperature and lower blood cholesterol levels when they replace dietary SFAs. PUFAs can be further distinguished as either omega-3 or omega-6 fatty acids. The **omega-6 fatty acids,** found in vegetable oils, seeds, and nuts, contain the essential fatty acids necessary for proper growth and functioning of the body and may also have a pro-inflammatory effect to help fight infection (Margolis, Cheskin, & Wilder, 2000). **Omega-3 fatty acids,** which are found primarily in fish and fish oils, may confer such health benefits as reducing triglyceride levels, lowering blood pressure, and preventing cardiac arrhythmias (Margolis et al., 2000). At this point, nutrition experts recommend increased consumption of dietary sources of omega-3 fatty acids, by selecting fish entrees several times per week.

In the 1950s and 1960s, studies showed that replacing SFAs with PUFAs resulted in lower serum cholesterol levels (Putnam & Allshouse, 1997). Health-conscious consumers switched from butter to stick margarine because margarine is made from polyunsaturated vegetable oils. This recommendation was relatively short-lived, however. In 1993, health concerns about trans fats were making headlines (Putnam & Allshouse, 1997), leaving the same health-conscious consumers who had shunned butter for years feeling frustrated and confused. Stick margarine was found to be an even more artery-clogging fat than butter. The following explanation will help clarify issues pertaining to a healthful dietary fat choice.

In order to create a margarine that is solid at room temperature, liquid vegetable oil undergoes a process called **hydrogenation.** Hydrogen atoms are added to the double bonds of the monounsaturated or polyunsaturated fat, and the resulting fat has a higher melting point and a firmer, more creamy texture. Hydrogenated fats help make French fries crispier and pie crusts flakier. Food manufacturers like them because they are more stable and can be reused more times in deep fat frying. Unfortunately, this process of hydrogenation creates a heart-unfriendly substance known as **trans fatty acid (TFA).** Trans fatty acids are structurally more similar to saturated fatty acids than to polyunsaturated fatty acids, and they pack a double whammy in that they not only raise LDL levels—the "bad" cholesterol but also lower HDL levels—the "good" cholesterol (Judd et al., 1994; Katan et al., 1994). See Chapter 12 for a discussion of LDL and HDL. Stick margarine has no cardiovascular health benefit over butter (Zock & Katan, 1997).

Currently, there is no way to identify foods that are heavily hydrogenated and therefore contain high amounts of trans fatty acids. Food manufacturers are required to list on their products' nutrition labels only the *original* source of the fat and the amount of total fat, saturated fat, and cholesterol; currently, the disclosure of trans fatty acid content is voluntary. What this means to the consumer is that a food, such as French fries, may be advertised as fried in 100 percent vegetable *oil* when it was really fried in partially hydrogenated vegetable *shortening.* The nutrition brochures from fast-food restaurants, and the nutrition labels placed on commercially prepared foods, while not inaccurate, are nonetheless misleading. They do not divulge the presence of cholesterol-raising trans fatty acids, and unsuspecting consumers who are trying to make healthy food choices are easily hoodwinked into selecting foods that are more damaging than they appear to be.

The following points summarize the SFA, PUFA, MUFA, and TFA effects on cardiovascular health:

- SFAs raise blood cholesterol levels.
- Replacing SFAs with PUFAs results in lower LDL cholesterol (the bad cholesterol) and lower HDL (the good cholesterol).
- Replacing SFAs with MUFAs lowers LDL cholesterol but leaves HDL cholesterol stable.
- TFAs not only cause an increase in LDL cholesterol but also lower HDL cholesterol.

The key to enjoying fatty foods without damaging one's health is *moderation.* The American Heart Association, the

American Cancer Society, the American Dietetic Association, and the American Diabetes Association all concur on the following dietary guidelines for the inclusion of fat in the diet:

- No more than 30 percent of calories from all types of fat
- Between 7 and 10 percent (less than 10 percent) of total calories from saturated fat
- No more than 10 percent of total calories from polyunsaturated fat
- No more than 10 percent of calories from monounsaturated fat
- Dietary cholesterol limited to 300 milligrams per day

Reducing the consumption of fried foods and foods high in fat will effectively reduce both total fat and saturated fat and trans fatty acid intake. A further reduction of trans fatty acid intake can be achieved by selecting liquid or tub vegetable spreads (softer fats have a lower percentage of hydrogenated oil and are therefore lower in TFAs) instead of stick margarine, avoiding foods that contain vegetable shortening or partially hydrogenated vegetable oils, and choosing mono-unsaturated fats, such as olive oil or canola oil, instead of butter or margarine.

Micronutrients: Vitamins, Minerals, and Trace Elements

Research conducted within the last 10 years suggests that some vitamins, minerals, and trace elements may play an even more important role in nutrition than previously thought. Much controversy remains, however, about the amounts necessary for optimum health, and even whether the same amounts are indicated for everyone.

VITAMINS

The Latin roots of the word *vitamin* means "essential for life." Vitamins are substances that either cannot be manufactured by the body or cannot be produced in sufficient amounts to sustain good health and prevent vitamin-deficiency diseases. Vitamins are needed in only minute amounts to prevent vitamin-deficiency diseases, such as scurvy (vitamin C deficiency), beri-beri (vitamin B-1 deficiency), pellagra (vitamin B-2 deficiency), and rickets (vitamin D deficiency). Vitamins function primarily as enzymes, or **catalysts,** for biochemical reactions in the body. Although vitamins are involved in many energy-producing processes, they themselves do not provide the body with calories.

The Recommended Dietary Allowance (RDA) is the amount of a vitamin necessary to meet the needs of a healthy population and to prevent vitamin-deficiency diseases. The RDAs were first established in 1941 by the Food and Nutrition Board (FNB). They were intended for use in planning to meet the food needs of populations, for establishing standards for food-assistance programs, and for designing nutrition education programs. It is important to be cognizant of the value of the RDAs, as well as their limitations. The RDAs are not meant to be guidelines for either the minimal intake or the optimal intake of nutrients. The requirements for given individuals, based on their needs and health status, may be higher or lower than the RDAs; however, the RDAs are safe and adequate for most individuals and take into account the bioavailability of the individual nutrients (National Academy Press Food and Nutrition Board, 1989).

There are 13 vitamins essential for good health. They are categorized as either water-soluble or fat-soluble. The nine **water-soluble vitamins** are vitamin C and eight B vitamins (thiamin, riboflavin, niacin, vitamin B-6, pantothenic acid, vitamin B-12, biotin, and folic acid). They function primarily as catalysts for many metabolic reactions in the body, including the normal digestion and metabolism of food. One of the B vitamins, vitamin B-12, is unique in that it is found only in animal flesh and by-products of animals (such as eggs, milk). These water-soluble vitamins are transported in the bloodstream, they are not stored in the body in any appreciable amounts, and any surpluses are excreted in the urine. Therefore, water-soluble vitamins are usually not *toxic*.

The **fat-soluble vitamins** (A, D, E, and K) are generally found in fat and oily parts of food. Because they are stored in body tissues, primarily in the liver, excess vitamins can *accumulate* in the body and cause toxicity. The benefit of this ability of the body to store fat-soluble vitamins is that it can take a long time, sometimes months, for deficiency symptoms to appear. However, the downside of this storage capacity is the risk of vitamin overload, which can lead to serious health consequences, including liver damage and even death.

See Table 3–1 for basic information on each of the 13 vitamins: the RDA levels for adult women (not pregnant, not breast-feeding), the function in the body, and the best food sources.

Determining the amount of a given vitamin that a given individual needs at a given point in time is not a straightforward matter. For example, the amount of vitamin C required to prevent scurvy is well known to be 10 milligrams per day (Ausman, 1999). The goal of most Americans, however, is not the mere prevention of scurvy but optimum health. The current RDA for vitamin C has recently been increased from a level of 60 mg per day to 75 mg/day for women and 90 mg/day for men (Food and Nutrition Board and Institute of Medicine, 2000). This level can easily be achieved by drinking one 8 oz glass of orange juice per day. Although this level can prevent scurvy and provide the individual with several weeks of reserve, this amount may be less than desirable for optimal health. It is known that body tissues do not become fully saturated with vitamin C until between 200 and 1,000 mg per day are consumed. At levels greater than 1,000 mg per day, the body compensates by decreasing absorption and simultaneously increasing renal excretion.

As with many dietary components, there is a tendency to promote the concept that, if a relatively small amount of vitamin is good, more must be better. There has long been

TABLE 3–1 Functions and sources of vitamins.

Vitamin	RDA	Functions in the Body	Best Food Sources
Vitamin A	800 micrograms RE—retinol equivalents	Eyesight—protects against night blindness; healthy skin and mucous membranes; resistance to infection	Retinol—from liver, oily fish, whole and fortified milk, egg yolk; beta-carotene—from orange-colored fruits and vegetables and dark, leafy green vegetables, such as sweet potatoes, carrots, mangoes, spinach, cantaloupe, dried apricots
Thiamin (vitamin B-1)	1.1 milligrams	Metabolism of carbohydrate; normal appetite and digestion; proper functioning of heart and nervous system	Brewer's yeast, wheat germ, wheat bran, unrefined cereal grains, organ meats, lean pork, legumes, seeds, nuts
Riboflavin (vitamin B-2)	1.3 milligrams	Healthy skin and eyes; metabolism of carbohydrate, protein, and fat; release of energy from food; functioning of vitamin B-6 and niacin	Milk and other dairy products, meat, poultry, fish, whole grain breads and flours, green vegetables
Niacin (vitamin B-3)	15 milligrams NE—niacin equivalents	Metabolism of carbohydrate and fat; release of energy from food	Lean meat, liver, yeast, wheat bran, peanuts, tuna, salmon, kidney, fortified breakfast cereals
Pyridoxine (vitamin B-6)	1.6 milligrams	Metabolism of protein; formation of red blood cells; prevention of anemia	Kidney, liver, poultry, fish, yeast, soybeans, nuts, whole grains
Cyanocobalamin (vitamin B-12)	2.0 micrograms	Formation of red blood cells; prevention of anemia; formation of nerve cells and DNA	Found only in animal foods—liver, kidney, lean meat, oysters, fish, seafood, eggs, milk
Folic acid (folate)	180 micrograms	Formation of enzymes and red blood cells; prevention of anemia; metabolism of DNA; prevention of neural tube defects	Yeast extract, leafy vegetables, whole grains, legumes, nuts, organ meats (liver, kidney, heart)
Biotin	30 to 100 micrograms (estimated safe and adequate intake—no RDA set)	Metabolism of fat, carbohydrate, and protein	Egg yolk, liver, kidney, heart, oats, whole grains, sardines
Pantothenic acid	4 to 7 milligrams (estimated safe and adequate—no RDA set)	Metabolism of carbo-hydrate, fat, and protein	Yeast extract, liver, fish, lean meat, sardines, nuts, eggs, vegetables, breads and cereals
Ascorbic acid (vitamin C)	60 milligrams	Healthy gums, teeth, and bones; wound healing and resistance to infection; formation of collagen; assistance in iron absorption; antioxidant properties	Fruits and vegetables: green and red peppers, collard greens, broccoli, spinach, tomatoes, potatoes, strawberries, citrus fruits

(continued)

TABLE 3–1 (Continued)

Vitamin	RDA	Functions in the Body	Best Food Sources
Vitamin D (calciferol)	10 micrograms or 400 IU (International Units)	Strong bones and teeth; prevention of rickets; absorption of calcium and phosphorus	Milk fortified with vitamin D, fish liver oils, oily fish, eggs, table margarine, butter
Vitamin E (tocopherols)	8 milligrams	Antioxidant properties; maintenance of healthy cell membranes; prevention of neurological defects	Vegetable oils (soybean, corn, cottonseed, safflower), wheat germ, nuts, leafy green vegetables
Vitamin K	65 micrograms	Formation of prothrombin—necessary for blood clotting	Leafy green vegetables

Source: Reprinted with permission from *Recommended Dietary Allowances,* 10/e. Copyright 1989 by the National Academy of Sciences. Courtesy of the National Academy Press, Washington, DC.

a minority of health scientists who promote **megadoses** of various vitamins for the optimization of health and treatment of disease. Vitamin C, like some other micronutrients, has been thought by some to have therapeutic effects in high doses.

In the early 1970s, Dr. Linus Pauling, a Nobel scientist in the field of chemistry, advocated very high intakes of vitamin C as a prevention for the common cold. Pauling recommended daily intakes in the range of two to four grams (2,000–4,000 mg) per day, which is more than 200 percent of the RDA. He also suggested daily dosages of as much as 10 grams (10,000 mg) a day for individuals with cancer (Pauling, 1980). Subsequent research has been unable to confirm the efficacy of high dose vitamin C in *preventing* colds, although a decrease in their severity and duration has been observed (Douglas, Chalker, & Treacy, 1999). In terms of vitamin C's role as an anticarcinogen, the studies are promising. Vitamin C is a powerful antioxidant (see the next section for more information on antioxidants) and has been found to inhibit tumor growth and genetic damage caused by carcinogens (cancer-causing agents) in laboratory animals (Ausman, 1999).

Although vitamin C, like most water-soluble vitamins, is relatively nontoxic at high levels, megadoses (doses of more than 1,000 mg/day) can cause nausea, abdominal cramps, and diarrhea in some individuals (Jacobs, 1999). Another downside of megadosing is that the body may adjust to the high levels and experience what is known as **rebound scurvy** if dosages are decreased suddenly. In the case of rebound scurvy, the individual experiences deficiency symptoms at a level that would be considered adequate for the average person.

The debate regarding the optimal intake of vitamin C continues and, as with other nutrients, that level seems to be an amount somewhere between the level needed to prevent a deficiency and the amount that causes toxicity (Golub, 1999a). Other factors complicate the process of making recommendations for the public. Two issues that must also be considered include the body's ability to digest and absorb the nutrient (bioavailability) and the level of nutrient actually present in the food (this can vary significantly with growing conditions, food processing, and cooking and storage conditions). In the example of vitamin C, there can be losses in the concentration of the vitamin up to 40 percent even before the food reaches the grocery store, and losses as great as 80 percent during the cooking process, especially if the food is boiled (Ausman, 1999).

MINERALS AND TRACE ELEMENTS

Minerals are **inorganic** nutrients that are needed to perform various structural and cellular functions necessary for life. Some of these functions include the regulation of body fluids and the maintenance of acid-base balance. Unlike vitamins, minerals are extremely stable, even on exposure to light and air, and, as is the case with fat-soluble vitamins, excess intake can be toxic. Most minerals that are consumed are derived from food sources, and the mineral content in foods can vary, depending on the mineral content of the soil in which the foods are grown. Minerals can also be derived from cooking utensils, which can add small amounts of minerals to the food during the cooking process. For example, foods cooked in cast iron pans absorb extra iron from the pan, particularly if they are acidic (such as tomato sauce).

There are 7 major minerals and 10 minor minerals, which are known as **trace elements.** The minerals most commonly found in food, and required in the largest quantities, are those that contribute to the formation of the bones of the skeletal system—namely, calcium, phosphorus, and magnesium. Table 3–2 lists RDAs, functions, and sources for the most common minerals and trace elements.

TABLE 3–2   Minerals and trace elements.

Mineral or Trace Element	Requirements for Adult, Nonpregnant, Nonlactating Women	Function in the Body	Food Sources
Calcium	19–24 yr: 1,200 mg 25–51+ yr: 800 mg	Skeletal formation; nerve conduction; blood clotting; muscle contraction	Milk and other dairy products, leafy green vegetables, calcium precipitated tofu, soft bones of fish
Phosphorus	19–24 yr: 1,200 mg 25–51+ yr: 800 mg	Essential component of bone mineral	Widely present in most foods, protein-rich foods, cereal grains
Magnesium	280 mg	Numerous biochemical and physiological processes; nerve conductivity; component of bone	All unprocessed foods with the highest concentrations in seeds, nuts, legumes, unmilled grains
Iron	19–50 yr: 15 mg 51+ yr: 10 mg	Structural component of hemoglobin, myoglobin, and several enzymes	Meat, eggs, vegetables, fortified cereal products
Zinc	12 mg	Constituent of enzymes required for most metabolic pathways; immune function; sensations of smell and taste; sexual maturation	Meat, liver, eggs, seafoods (oysters), whole grains
Iodine	150 mcg	Part of the thyroid hormones; prevention of goiter	Concentrations in foods varies widely, depending on soil concentrations and food processing; iodized salt
Selenium	55 mcg	Antioxidant properties	Seafood, kidney, liver

Source: Reprinted with permission from *Recommended Dietary Allowances,* 10/e. Copyright 1989 by the National Academy of Sciences. Courtesy of the National Academy Press, Washington, DC.

One of the most important trace elements for women is *iron.* Iron is an important component of hemoglobin and is necessary for the transport of oxygen to body tissues. Eighty percent of the body's iron is found in the **blood;** therefore, blood loss will result in losses of iron as well. Because of regular blood loss during menstruation, women's iron requirements are twice as high as that of men up until menopause. The typical American diet provides 5 to 6 mg of iron per 1,000 kilocalories (kcal). As the recommended intake for menstruating women is 18 mg/day, a young woman eating a typical diet would have to take in approximately 3,000 kcal per day to meet her iron requirements. Because many women consume only 2,000 kcal or fewer per day, it is important for women to emphasize *iron-rich* foods. Not all food sources of iron are created equal; iron found in meat, fish, and poultry products is known as **heme-iron** and is more readily absorbed than iron from vegetable sources (**non-heme iron**). Most of the iron from the diet is in the form of non-heme iron. Eating meat, fish, or poultry with vegetables maximizes the absorption of the non-heme iron

the vegetables contain. Meat, fish, and poultry contain what is known as **MFP** factor, substance that promotes the absorption of iron from other foods that are eaten at the same time. Another way to increase the absorption of iron is to add foods high in vitamin C; as the level of vitamin C increases, so does the absorption of iron. This relationship is consistent up to a vitamin C dose of 1,000 milligrams (Cook & Monsen, 1977). Foods and beverages that contain substances known as phytates, such as soy, coffee, and tea, can inhibit iron absorption.

Calcium is another mineral of great importance to women. The recommended calcium intake for women varies according to age. Higher intakes are required during the growth years to support skeletal development and build adequate **bone mass.** Higher intakes are also needed after menopause to offset bone demineralization (see Chapter 24). Unlike many other nutritional deficiencies, most cases of calcium deficiency cause no immediate signs and symptoms to alert the individual that something is wrong. The gradual bone demineralization that occurs over decades of inadequate calcium intake is "silent" and, by the sixth or seventh decade of life, can result in bone weakening, which leads to fractures, reduction in height, and pain. This condition, known as **osteoporosis** (see Chapter 14), has been described as a disease of the young that begins in childhood and manifests itself in late adulthood.

Population studies of girls and young women 12–19 years of age reveal that their calcium intake averages only 900 mg per day (National Institutes of Health [NIH], 1994). This is well below the optimal level of 1,200–1,500 mg per day. It is critical that during childhood, adolescence, and early adulthood enough calcium is consumed to build strong bones for two reasons: First, during periods when dietary intake of calcium is inadequate, the body steals the calcium it needs to carry out metabolic functions from the body's calcium bank, the skeleton. Second, women who do not have dense bones are at particular risk for osteoporosis after menopause, especially if they do not take estrogen.

Once peak bone mass is achieved, bone stores are relatively stable until menopause. Healthy women between the ages of 25 and 50 years need a calcium intake of 1,000 mg/day (NIH, 1994). After menopause, women who take estrogen need 1,000 mg/day, and women who do not take estrogen need 1,500 mg/day. Calcium absorption and use depend on several dietary cofactors. One of the most important of these cofactors is vitamin D, which is needed for the absorption of calcium in the intestinal tract. In the absence of the active form of vitamin D, less than 10 percent of dietary calcium may be absorbed (NIH, 1994). This is one of the reasons that milk is fortified with vitamin D. Phosphorus also affects calcium absorption. The ideal ratio of dietary calcium to phosphorus is 2:1. This ratio promotes maximum calcium absorption and is the ratio naturally present in milk. Other nutrients, including magnesium, fluoride, and vitamin A, are also essential for skeletal integrity, as they play a role in forming and stabilizing the structure of the bones. Some foods contain binders, which chemically combine with calcium in the intestinal tract and make it unavailable for absorption; therefore, a diet high in these foods negatively affect calcium absorption. Two such binders that render calcium unavailable for absorption are **phytic acid,** found in whole grain cereals, and **oxalic acid,** found in beet greens, rhubarb, and spinach. In addition, high intakes of both protein and sodium promote the renal excretion of calcium. The typical American diet is usually high in both protein and sodium.

Milk and other milk products, such as cheese, cottage cheese, and yogurt, provide some of the highest concentrations of dietary calcium, and the calcium from these sources is very well absorbed. In addition to calcium, milk and other milk products provide other essential nutrients, such as riboflavin (vitamin B-2) and vitamin D, which are not as concentrated in other foods. Unfortunately, some people are allergic to milk or have an intolerance to lactose (the carbohydrate in milk). True milk **allergy** is caused by the protein in milk. Cooking milk to denature the protein may abol-

TABLE 3–3 Sources of calcium.

Food	Quantity	Mg of Calcium
Yogurt, plain nonfat	1 cup	452
Milk, skim	1 cup	302
Orange juice, calcium-enriched	1 cup	293
Swiss cheese	1 ounce	272
Cheddar cheese	1 ounce	204
Sardines, canned	2 ounces	185
Tofu, processed with calcium	3 ounces	150
Turnip greens, cooked	½ cup	99
Low-fat cottage cheese	½ cup	77
Bread, whole wheat	2 slices	47
Pinto beans, cooked	½ cup	41
Broccoli, cooked	½ cup	36
Sweet potato, baked	1 medium	32

Source: Adapted from USDA nutrient database for standard reference (1999). Washington, DC: U.S. Government Printing Office.

ish the allergic reaction. Switching from cow's milk to goat's milk may be tolerated because the proteins in goat's milk differ from those in cow's milk. Individuals who have **lactose intolerance** can drink milk to which digestive enzymes, such as *LactAid,* have been added. Lactose-free milk is also available. Fermented dairy products, such as yogurt or aged cheese, may also be well tolerated; the bacteria used in the fermentation process use lactose as their energy source; therefore, these food products contain lower amounts of lactose. Many individuals with lactose intolerance are able to tolerate milk in smaller quantities with no adverse side effects.

Calcium is also present in other classes of foods—namely, green vegetables and fish and shellfish; however, in the case of green vegetables, the calcium is less well absorbed than is the calcium in milk. Many calcium-fortified food products are available, including calcium-fortified cereals, breads, and fruit juices. Individuals who avoid animal flesh and animal products (total vegetarians, or **vegans**) can obtain calcium by consuming green vegetables, tofu that has been processed with calcium, canned fish, seeds, nuts, and some legumes (see Table 3–3).

Two Essential Noncaloric Nutrients: Fiber and Water

Fiber

Fiber is the indigestible structural component of plants. There are basically two categories of fiber, those that dissolve in water—soluble fibers—and those that do not dissolve in water—insoluble fibers. Both types of fiber are recommended for a healthful diet. **Water-soluble fibers** (pectins, gums, and mucilages) are found primarily in citrus fruits, apples, dried peas and beans, oatmeal, and oat bran. These types of fiber help lower blood cholesterol levels and stabilize blood sugar levels by slowing down the digestion of carbohydrates. **Water-insoluble** fibers (cellulose and lignin) are found in whole wheat and other whole grains, vegetables, and fruits. These types of fiber add bulk to the stool by absorbing water in the intestinal track. This helps speed the passage of waste through the intestinal tract.

The standard American diet (SAD) is highly refined and processed; therefore, the average intake of fiber is well below the recommended level of 25–30 grams per day. The major dietary sources of fiber are fruits, vegetables, and whole grain. Whole grain consumption has been linked to reduced risk for coronary heart disease, cancer, diabetes, obesity, and other chronic diseases (Slavin, Martini, Jacobs, & Marquat, 1999). Although further study is required to determine which component or components of whole grains provides these protective effects, fiber is certainly a likely suspect.

Water

The human body is approximately 55 to 60 percent water, and all body processes occur in this aqueous environment. Body fluids serve many functions, including the following:

- Transporting vitamins, minerals, glucose, and amino acids throughout the body
- Lubricating joints
- Cushioning vital organs, such as the eyes and the spinal cord
- Maintaining the body's temperature

The body's fluid status is delicately balanced through excretion and intake. Thirst and satiety regulate intake; however, thirst can sometimes lag behind a water deficiency and dehydration can result. The best way to monitor hydration status is through checking the color of the urine. Very yellow urine generally indicates a need to increase fluid intake. Paler urine usually indicates adequate hydration. Water excretion is regulated by the hypothalamus in the brain and by the kidneys. When salt concentration in the blood is too high, the hypothalamus stimulates the pituitary gland to secrete **antidiuretic hormone (ADH).** This hormone causes the kidneys to retain water and return it to the circulatory system, rather than excreting it.

Water requirements vary with diet, physical activity, and environmental conditions, such as temperature and altitude. The National Academy of Sciences recommends an intake of 7 to 11 cups per day (Margolis et al., 2000). A daily intake of approximately 2½ quarts of fluid is required daily to maintain fluid balance and replace fluids lost through urination, defecation, perspiration, and respiration (breathing). An adequate daily water intake reduces the risk of bladder cancer, kidney stones, and colon cancer (Welland, 1999).

Although many foods and beverages are high in water content, the best source of fluid for the maintenance of adequate hydration is plain water. Some beverages contain alcohol or caffeine and may actually promote dehydration because of their **diuretic** (water-losing) effect on the body. Although beverages containing caffeine do have a diuretic effect, the amount of fluid lost is usually equal to or less than the amount consumed, so the net effect is usually a slight fluid gain. With alcoholic beverages, however, the situation is somewhat different. Alcohol exerts a dehydrating effect on the body through two mechanisms: It both acts as a diuretic and inhibits the action of ADH, thereby causing even more body water to be excreted. Therefore, alcohol has a significant dehydrating effect on the body; alcoholic beverages are not a good choice for quenching thirst or for rehydrating the body.

Antioxidants

Most nutrition experts favor the consumption of foods rather than the intake of supplements to achieve dietary health. Foods provide the most biologically available source of nutrients as well as fiber and important phytochemicals, which may not be present in the supplement. **Phytochemicals,** or **phytonutrients** are, as the names imply, chemicals or nutrients that are found in plants. A subset of the phytonutrients is the antioxidants.

Antioxidants are chemicals that limit the activity of cellular and molecular damage from substances known as **free radicals.** All cells require oxygen to metabolize protein, fat, and carbohydrates for energy. A by-product of that metabolic process is the formation of free radicals in the form of oxygen molecules that have lost an electron and therefore are very unstable. These molecules steal electrons from other, nearby molecules, in an effort to stabilize themselves. This process can cause a chain reaction of cellular damage. Fortunately, our bodies have a natural defense mechanism in the form of antioxidant compounds. Such compounds are able to give up an electron to the unstable oxygen molecule without themselves becoming unstable. By doing so, antioxidants block free radicals' deleterious effects. The body produces some antioxidant compounds naturally; others are provided by the foods we eat, with fruits and vegetables being particularly rich sources. Many compounds have antioxidant properties, including many of the vitamins and minerals. Among these are vitamin E, vitamin C, beta-carotene, and selenium. Compounds that provide color to fruits and vegetables, such as lycopene (the red matter of tomatoes), carotenes (contained in yellow or orange foods)—act as antioxidants, as do another group of substances found in foods called flavonoids. A method for measuring the antioxidant power of a particular food is the **oxygen radical absorbance capacity (ORAC)** developed by Guohua Cao, a principal researcher investigating the phytochemical activity of foods at Tufts University Phytochemical

TABLE 3–4	Top antioxidant foods, ORAC units per 100 grams (3.5 ounces).		
Fruit	**Amount**	**Vegetable**	**Amount**
Blueberry	2,400	Garlic	1,900
Blackberry	2,100	Kale	1,700
Strawberry	1,550	Spinach	1,275
Raspberry	1,200	Brussels sprouts	975
Plum	950	Beets	840
Red grape	750	Red bell pepper	725

Source: Antioxidant Foods, April 1999 (online). United States Department of Agriculture. Available: www.ars.usda.gov/is/np/fnrb/.

Research Laboratory (*ORAC of Selected Fruits and Vegetables,* 2000). Some of the richest food sources of antioxidants are listed in Table 3–4.

Making Sound Nutritional Decisions

The first section of this chapter focused on the fundamental principles of nutrition. In this section, we will examine additional information that can aid consumers in making everyday decisions related to nutrition. The following topics are addressed: supplementation with vitamins and minerals, and planning a healthful diet.

Vitamin and Mineral Supplementation

A visit to the supplement section of the grocery store or local pharmacy can be an enlightening experience. At one time, only a few food supplements were available—mostly multivitamins in tablet form for adults and chewable form for children. Now, an often bewildering array of supplements is available: multivitamins, vitamins with minerals, all-natural vitamins, and special vitamin formulas for men, women, children, and older adults. Isolated nutrients, often in megadoses, are available as well. Many preparations contain combinations of nutrients designed to address specific concerns, such as stress, bone health, extra energy, and aging. Making a selection from all of these can be as challenging as deciding which stocks or mutual funds to buy, yet keeping the fundamentals of nutrition in mind can narrow the choices considerably and increase one's chances of making a wise investment in nutritional health.

Most health authorities, including the American Dietetic Association and the American Medical Association, support the concept that nutritional requirements should be met through a *well-balanced diet*. Nonetheless, 25 to 30 percent of Americans report taking a vitamin or mineral supplement daily, and 70 percent take nutritional supplements on a regular basis (*Vitamin and Nutritional Supplements,* 1997). Supplement sales are booming. The question is, are vitamin and mineral supplements a wise investment, a waste of money, or a potential health risk? The following information will help answer that question and provide guidance regarding the intelligent use of vitamin and mineral supplements.

SAFETY AND QUALITY

Most consumers assume that the same rules that apply to medicinal products sold as drugs apply to food supplements, that the manufacturer has to prove a supplement's safety, quality, and effectiveness before it can be sold, and that the Food and Drug Administration (FDA) prevents any unsafe products from reaching the market. This is not the case, however, and whether food supplements should be treated as drugs is a subject about which there is much disagreement.

Manufacturers and consumers of products (such as vitamins and minerals) now classified as food supplements have long contended that food supplements are generally much safer than the much more powerful prescription and nonprescription drugs and should be exempt from FDA premarket testing requirements, as premarket testing is an extremely expensive and lengthy process. Nevertheless, in the 1970s, the FDA attempted to classify vitamin supplements as prescription drugs and thereby render them subject to such testing. This plan was vehemently opposed by proponents of the safety and efficacy of vitamin dietary supplementation, and it was ultimately defeated. Two decades later, the FDA attempted to classify all amino acids, and some minerals, as prescription drugs—again unsuccessfully (*A History of Victories over the FDA,* 2000). In 1994, Congress passed the Dietary Supplement Health and Education Act (DSHEA), which created a category for dietary supplements separate from food and drugs (see Chapter 11). This act, which limited the power of the Food and Drug Administration to oversee products such as vitamins and herbs without removing the FDA's power entirely, has been controversial. Manufacturers and consumers of food supplements, although wary of any regulation of vitamins, herbs, and so on, saw the act as giving them a measure of protection against the powerful drug lobby, which they feared might influence the FDA to make it unduly difficult to market products that compete with prescription drugs. Mainstream health organizations, on the other hand, feared that the dietary supplement industry would become totally unregulated, resulting in consumers' being harmed by dangerous products. The act, however, does confer some protection to consumers: Although food supplements are not subject to premarket safety evaluation by the FDA, manufacturers are still responsible for ensuring that the products are safe and properly labeled, as is the case with manufacturers of food products. Moreover, the secretary of Health and Human Services has the right to declare that a dietary ingredient or supplement poses an **imminent hazard** to public health or safety and to protect the public by removing it from the market (*Dietary Supplement Health and Education Act of 1994, 1995*). However, as most evaluations of specific food supplements' safety have been triggered after the fact by consumer complaints and adverse outcomes, it behooves buyers to use caution when purchasing dietary supplements.

One indication of quality is the presence of the **United States Pharmacopoeia (USP)** seal. The USP is an independent organization that ensures that products meet **dissolution standards,** which means that the supplements will dissolve sufficiently to be absorbed. Solubility can be evaluated by putting the pill into a cup of white vinegar. At least 75 percent of the pill should be dissolved within 30 minutes. Pills that do not meet this standard may not dissolve in the gastrointestinal tract. In that case, the nutrients listed on the label would not be absorbed and would essentially pass through the digestive system undigested. Another indication of product quality is the presence of an **expiration date** on the label. Vitamins and minerals have a limited shelf life, and the potency of the supplement cannot be guaranteed if the product is outdated. The product label should also indicate the lot number in order to identify clearly the product batch if recall is necessary. The manufacturer's name, address, website, and so on should also be present, so that consumers can inquire about quality-control standards and can report any adverse outcomes. It is wise to select established companies, which are more likely to have the resources to ensure that quality and safety standards are adhered to and that the supplement contains the ingredients that are listed on the label. It is best to avoid products with fillers and additives.

Risks Consuming supplements carries with it potential health risks and the risk of financial expenditure with no benefit as well. Most health risks are associated with the fat-soluble vitamins, which are stored in the body and can build up to toxic levels. Vitamin A overdoses can lead to liver damage or death, and excess vitamin D causes increased calcium absorption, with subsequent deposition in soft tissues. High levels of beta-carotene can cause the palms of the hands and whites of the eyes to turn yellow; fortunately, this condition is easily reversed when intake of vitamin A is lowered.

For water-soluble vitamins, the downside has been assumed to be only a financial one, as generally any excess intake is excreted in the urine and flushed down the toilet. Newer research, however, indicates that the chronic excess intake of water-soluble vitamins can have negative health consequences as well. Excess levels can result in toxicity, can interfere with the absorption of other nutrients, and can mask a deficiency in another nutrient. For example, excess niacin (vitamin B-3) causes flushing and interferes with liver function; overdoses of vitamin B-6 can damage sensory nerves and produces a loss of sensation in the body's extremities. Vitamin C increases iron absorption, whereas excess calcium decreases iron absorption. The excess supplementation of folate or folic acid is not suggested. Intakes beyond the UL of 1,000 mcg folic acid have not been researched; however, such high levels could mask vitamin B-12 deficiency, paving the way to crippling, irreversible nerve damage (Grodner, Anderson, & DeYoung, 2000).

Benefits Research into current eating patterns indicate that 28 percent of Americans skip meals frequently, and, in 1997, away-from-home snacks and meals captured 45 percent of the U.S. food dollar (Putnam & Allshouse, 1997). Only 1 person in 10 regularly consumes the recommended five servings of fruits and vegetables per day (*Vitamin and Nutritional Supplements,* 1997). Despite these less than desirable patterns, most individuals are able to select a varied diet and obtain adequate amounts of vitamins and minerals from foods, if they are *motivated* to do so. Obtaining vitamins and minerals from food rather than supplements is much preferred because of the other nutrients found naturally in foods. Fiber and phytochemicals are two very important food ingredients that are difficult to obtain in supplement form. There are also thousands of other substances (many of which are not yet identified or studied) in whole foods that may be important for good health. Also, by consuming a well-balanced diet, one is more likely to obtain vitamins and minerals in biologically available forms and less likely to consume toxic amounts through supplementation. Finally, no one would dispute that the pleasure of eating a variety of foods, with their array of colors, textures, flavors, and aromas, far surpasses the swallowing of tasteless supplements. There are, however, exceptions to this whole foods first rule. The following is a list of individuals for whom, and instances in which, vitamin and/or mineral supplementation is often recommended:

- Pregnant women
- Patients recovering from illness or surgery
- Older adults with decreased appetites and reduced ability to absorb certain nutrients
- Individuals with food intolerances that may limit dietary variety
- Individuals with chronic diseases or with conditions of the gastrointestinal tract that may limit the absorption of nutrients
- Individuals purposefully restricting calories in order to lose weight
- Instances in which a limited amount of a particular nutrient is available in commonly consumed foods

TABLE 3–5 Vitamin and mineral supplement guidelines.

Nutrient	Daily Value	Maximum Dosage (No Observed Adverse Effect at this Level)
Vitamin A	5,000 IU	10,000 IU
Vitamin C	75 mg	1,000 mg
Vitamin D	400 IU	800 IU
Vitamin E	30 IU	1,200 IU
Vitamin K	80 mcg	30 mg
Vitamin B-1 (thiamin)	1.5 mg	50 mg
Vitamin B-2 (riboflavin)	1.7 mg	200 mg
Vitamin B-3 (niacin)	20 mg	500 mg
Vitamin B-6 (pyridoxine)	2 mg	200 mg
Folic acid	400 mcg	1,000 mcg
Vitamin B-12 (cobalamin)	6 mcg	3,000 mcg
Biotin	300 mcg	2,500 mcg
Pantothenic acid	10 mg	1,000 mg
Calcium	1,000 mg	2,000 mg
Iron	18 mg (for women up to menopause), 0 mg (for men and postmenopausal women)	65 mg
Phosphorus	1,000 mg	1,500 mg
Iodine	150 mcg	1,000 mcg
Magnesium	400 mg	700 mg
Zinc	15 mg	30 mg
Selenium	70 mcg	200 mcg
Copper	2 mg	9 mg
Manganese	2 mg	10 mg
Chromium	120 mcg	1,000 mcg
Molybdenum	75 mcg	350 mcg
Chloride	3,400 mg	Not established (plentiful in diet)
Potassium	3,500 mg	Not established (plentiful in diet)

Source: Adapted from Golub, C. (1999). Making Sense of the Supplement Scene. Environmental Nutrition 22(11) 1, 4–5. Hathcock, J. N. (1997). Vitamin and Mineral Safety. Council for Responsible Nutrition, Washington, D.C.

RDAs are based on the needs of specific populations, with a margin of safety built in to ensure that the needs of most healthy individuals are met. The RDAs may not be adequate for persons undergoing illness or surgery or for those who have digestive problems that may effect nutrient absorption. A supplement can serve as a little extra insurance that all of the requirements are being met. On the other hand, it is wise to remember that supplements are just that—*supplements.* They are not intended to replace food or to make up for a chronically poor diet (Golub, 1999b).

WISE SUPPLEMENT USE

In those all too common instances when a well-balanced diet is not being consumed, a multivitamin can help ensure an adequate daily intake of essential vitamins and minerals. It is best to choose a multivitamin and mineral supplement that con-

tains 100 percent of the Daily Value (DV) of each nutrient listed in the ingredient list. The DV is the same thing as the RDA. A maximum of 300 percent of the DV may be taken. Beyond that level, toxicities may develop. See Table 3–5 for guidelines for recommended and maximum safe dosages.

Supplements should be taken with a meal and at least 8 ounces of fluids. This allows more time for the stomach to break down the pill and ensures that it will be thoroughly dissolved in order to maximize absorption in the intestinal tract. Including a small amount of fat with the meal will facilitate the absorption of fat-soluble vitamins. It is not necessary to select *natural* supplements instead of *synthesized* supplements. Generally speaking, the body cannot distinguish the chemical structure of a natural vitamin from that of a manufactured vitamin; therefore, they are of equal potency. The one exception to this rule is vitamin E, which is more readily absorbed in its natural form (alpha-tocopherol) than in the synthetic form (dl-tocopherol).

Women may need more of certain nutrients than the amount typically found in multivitamin/mineral supplements. One such nutrient is the mineral calcium, which if it were included in adequate amounts in the multivitamin/mineral supplement it would result in a pill too large to swallow. The preferred method for achieving optimal calcium intake is through dietary sources; however, for some individuals calcium supplementation may be necessary in order to attain the desired daily intake. There are a variety of calcium supplements to choose from, and deciphering the label can be quite challenging. The goal is to understand how much **elemental calcium** (the calcium mineral itself without other compounds) each supplement provides to determine how many supplements to take. Calcium is not stable by itself and therefore is combined with various salts, such as citrate, carbonate, or lactate, to render it stable in pill form. The amount of elemental calcium varies from supplement to supplement, depending on the amount of calcium combined with the salt. Generally, the label will list the amount of calcium or elemental calcium. Sometimes, however, only the weight of the supplement is listed; if that is the case, some simple math can determine exactly how much elemental calcium is in each dose. Calcium carbonate is 40 percent calcium by weight (multiply the weight by the percentage of calcium to determine the amount of calcium); thus, a 500 mg tablet contains 200 mg of calcium (500 mg × .40). Other common calcium compounds are calcium citrate (21 percent calcium by weight), calcium lactate (13 percent calcium by weight), and calcium gluconate (9 percent calcium by weight). In order to ensure maximum absorption, most calcium supplements should be taken in dosages of 500 mg or less and taken between meals, because foods may contain certain compounds that reduce the bioavailability of the calcium (NIH, 1994). Calcium carbonate, however, should be taken with certain foods, particularly those that are acidic in nature, because the acids improve the bioavailability of the calcium. In the case of meeting calcium requirements, it may be beneficial to combine supplements with a calcium-rich diet in order to ensure adequate intake.

Planning a Healthy Diet

Tools such as the food guide pyramids and nutrition information labels can be used to help in choosing foods that will ensure a healthy diet. A vegetarian diet offers a healthy alternative for those who choose not to consume dairy products or meat. Other alternative diets must be viewed with caution, however, as their efficacy and safety have, for the most part, not been empirically demonstrated.

The goal of nutritionists is to ensure that the American diet is optimal in terms of promoting health and longevity. Their task is made more difficult, however, by the fact that research on the effects of various foods and food combinations on the human body is ongoing and the recommendations regarding what to eat for optimal health are subject to change. Over the years, a number of models of healthy eating have been used to guide the public in making wise food choices.

USDA Food Guide Pyramid

In 1956, the U.S. Department of Agriculture (USDA) developed its Basic Four Food Group Plan. This model of a healthy diet relied heavily on meat and its alternatives, such as dairy products. Fruits, vegetables, bread, and cereal (currently seen as the foundations of a good diet) played only a supportive role in this early attempt to better the public health through diet. Nevertheless, misguided as it may now appear to have been, the Basic Four campaign convinced the public that health and diet are connected and introduced the now ubiquitous concept of *"eating right."* In 1992, after 20 years of additional research, the USDA reevaluated the Basic Four Plan and replaced it with the Food Guide Pyramid, a more healthful, easy-to-understand model of good nutrition. (See Figure 3–1.) Its reduced emphasis on fat-laden foods and clear portrayal of nutrient needs have made it a favorite among dietitians and wellness professionals. In its

Figure 3–1   USDA Food Guide Pyramid

The pyramid is an outline of what to eat each day. It's not a rigid prescription, but a general guide that lets you choose a healthful diet that's right for you. The pyramid calls for eating a variety of foods to get the nutrients you need and at the same time the right amount of calories to maintain a healthy weight.

The Food Guide Pyramid emphasizes foods from the five food groups shown in the three lower sections of the pyramid.

Each of these food groups provides some, but not all, of the nutrients you need. Foods in one group can't replace those in another. No one food group is more important than another—for good health, you need them all.

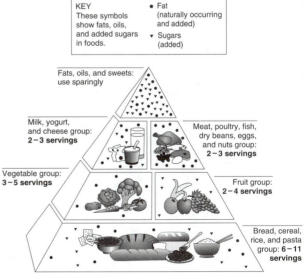

U.S. Department of Agriculture & U.S. Department of Health and Human Services.

Figure 3-2   Food Group Serving Recommendations

Food Group	Servings per day	Sample serving sizes
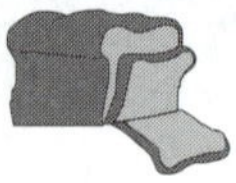 Bread, cereal, rice, and pasta	1,600 calories = 6 2,200 calories = 9 2,800 calories = 11	• 1 slice whole grain bread • 1/2 bagel, English muffin, hamburger roll, or pita bread • 1/2 cup cooked rice or pasta, 1 cup ready-to-eat cereal
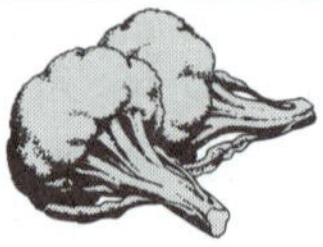 Vegetable	1,600 calories = 3 2,200 calories = 4 2,800 calories = 5	• 1/2 cup chopped raw, nonleafy vegetables • 1/2 cup cooked vegetables • 1 small baked potato—3 ounces • 3/4 cup vegetable juice
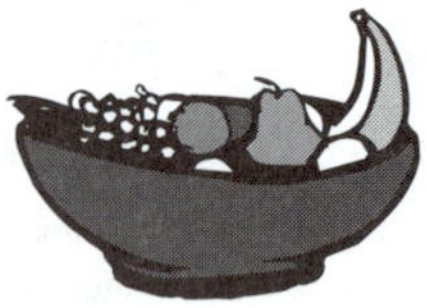 Fruit	1,600 calories = 2 2,200 calories = 3 2,800 calories = 4	• 1 medium fruit (apple, orange, peach, banana) • 3/4 cup fruit juice • 1/2 cup cooked, canned, or frozen fruit
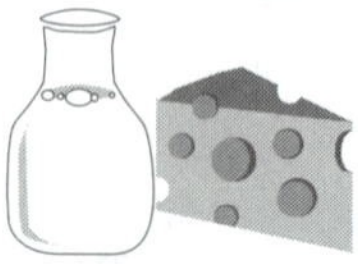 Milk, yogurt, and cheese	1,600 calories = 2–3 2,200 calories = 2–3 2,800 calories = 2–3	• 1 cup milk, buttermilk, or yogurt • 1 1/2 ounces natural cheese (cheddar, mozzarella, swiss) • 1 cup frozen yogurt
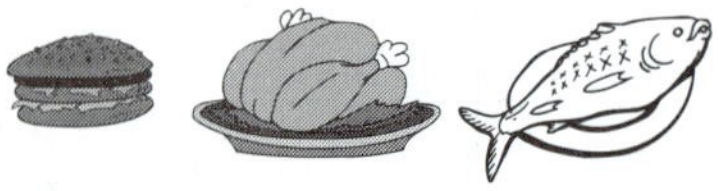 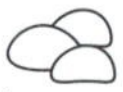 Meat, poultry, fish, dry beans, eggs, and nuts	1,600 calories = 2–3 2,200 calories = 2–3 2,800 calories = 2–3	• 2–3 ounces cooked lean meat, poultry, or fish • 1/2 cup cooked legumes (equals 1 ounce of meat) • 1 egg (equals 1 ounce of meat)
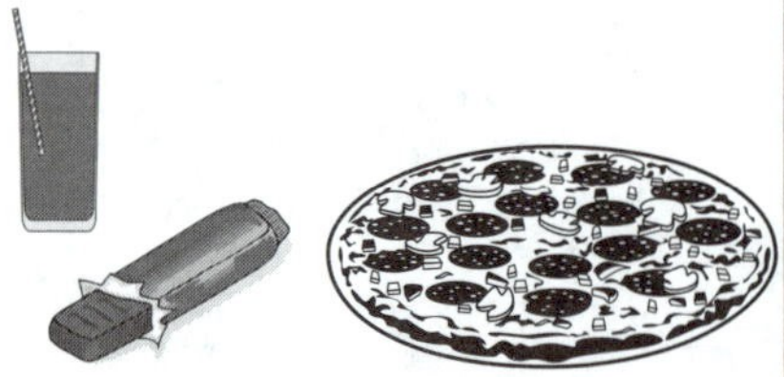 Fats, oils, and sweets	Use sparingly.	• Sugars • Salad dressings • Oils • Cream • Butter • Soft drinks

Source: Adapted from *The American Dietetic Association's Monthly Nutrition Companion: 31 Days to a Healthier Lifestyle* (1997). Chronimed Publishing. Reprinted by permission of John Wiley & Sons, Inc.

current incarnation, it is one of the foundation tools that can be used in planning a well-balanced, nutritious diet. The pyramid is formed in sections, or blocks, each of which depicts a food group. The lowest, widest block represents the group of foods that should provide the greater portion of daily calories. The middle blocks represent groups of foods that should be consumed in moderation, and the uppermost, smallest blocks symbolize the food groups from which the least number of calories should be derived.

A *strength* of the Food Guide Pyramid is that it does not seek to ban specific types of foods. It is not dogmatic in that it does not dictate a hard-and-fast diet but, rather, appears to adhere to the age-old adage "everything in moderation." Individuals can include most of the things they like in their diets, provided they do not exceed the amounts recommended in the model. The pyramid is divided into six sectors, each listing the name of a food group and the corresponding recommendation for the number of servings to be consumed daily (see Figure 3–2).

In accordance with its nondictatorial nature, the guide lists *ranges* of serving specifications. Adherence to the low-end specifications will result in a daily intake of approximately 1,600 calories, whereas adherence to the high end will result in an intake of 2,500 to 3,000 calories daily. Small circular shapes, strewn about all the levels of the pyramid, denote the amount of fat contained in the foods that constitute each group. Similarly, the small triangles that appear represent the added sugars present in each group. The foods to be eaten in greatest quantities are those with the lowest concentration of fat and sugars.

The USDA pyramid is not without *weaknesses*, however. An individual could conceivably drink three glasses of whole milk and consume over a half a pound of high-fat red meat and still be in compliance, technically, with its guidelines. Such a meal plan would be unacceptably high in fat, particularly heart-unhealthy saturated fats and cholesterol—clearly incongruent with the intention of the pyramid's creators. Another flaw of the USDA model is that it fails to distinguish *healthy* fats from *unhealthy*, artery-clogging fats. Protein-rich foods, such as red meat, poultry, legumes, eggs, and nuts, are all lumped into one category, with no clear guidelines to assist the individual in making more healthful, lower-fat selections. Other weaknesses of this pyramid include the failure to recommend *low-fat* milk and dairy products or to specify the selection of high-fiber whole grains over refined grains. Finally, although the USDA pyramid does specify a range of daily servings in each category, the specifications are not consistent. In some instances, the number of servings recommended is intended to represent the *minimum* number of daily servings allowed; in others, the *maximum*. For example, in the fruit and vegetable categories, the three to five servings of fruit and the two to four servings of vegetables recommended represent the *minimum* recommendation. In the meat, poultry, fish, dry beans, eggs, and nuts category, however, the number of servings recommended (two to three per day) represents

the *maximum* number of servings allowed. This inconsistency can create confusion for the individual and result in a less than desirable selection of foods.

Nonetheless, the USDA Food Guide Pyramid has been so successful that others have copied its format and have attempted to rectify some of its identified weaknesses. Two of these iterations are the Mediterranean Diet Pyramid and the Vegetarian Diet Pyramid.

MEDITERRANEAN DIET PYRAMID

The World Health Organization, Harvard School of Public Health, and Oldways Preservation and Exchange Trust developed the Mediterranean Diet Pyramid in 1993 as an alternative to the USDA pyramid. Diets congruent with the Mediterranean plan are associated with a lower risk of coronary heart disease (CHD), hyperlipidemia (high blood fat), colon cancer, and hypertension (high blood pressure). This is thought to be due to their abundant fiber and healthy sources of fat. The Mediterranean model mirrors the typical diet consumed in the countries that border the Mediterranean Sea, such as Italy, Greece, and France (see Figure 3–3).

An individual living in the United States may have the same high blood pressure as an individual living in Italy, but

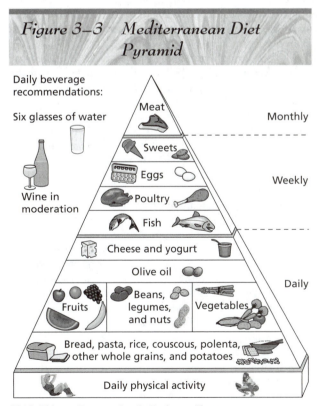

Figure 3–3   Mediterranean Diet Pyramid

2000 Oldways Preservation & Exchange Trust.

the American is three times more likely to die of a heart attack. The evidence suggests that diet is responsible for this difference. The Mediterranean diet contains less meat and dairy products and more fish, fruits, vegetables, and whole grains versus the meat-laden, high-saturated-fat, high-refined-carbohydrate, low-fiber Western diet. Although genetics play a small role in these differences, researchers relate that lifestyle continues to be the greatest factor in preventing cardiac illness (MacMahon, 1999).

Individuals who have survived a heart attack can also benefit from instituting the Mediterranean diet. Researchers in Lyon, France, studied the effects of a Mediterranean diet in 600 men and women who had suffered a heart attack. The study results revealed that the heart attack patients eating the Mediterranean diet had a 50 to 70 percent lower risk of recurrent coronary heart disease than patients eating a Western diet. The heart patients also consumed more oleic and alpha-linolenic fatty acids, or omega-3 fatty acids, than did the Western group (DeLorgeril et al., 1999).

The Mediterranean diet may also support memory. Researchers in Italy (Solfrizzi et al., 1999) reported that this diet may retard age-related memory loss. During the aging process, there appears to be an increasing demand for unsaturated fatty acids, and the researchers suggest that fatty acids may help maintain the structure of the brain. In the study, the participants reported consuming 46 grams of olive oil—a monounsaturated fat—per day. The more monounsaturated fatty acids they consumed, the greater the protection they received from cognitive decline.

There are striking similarities between the Mediterranean pyramid and the USDA pyramid. Both encourage the consumption of a variety of foods, with an emphasis on more foods from the grain, fruit, and vegetable categories. Both are similarly flawed, in that each fails to recommend lower-fat dairy products and high-fiber, whole grain products.

The Mediterranean model does differ somewhat from its USDA counterpart. Structurally, it allows a bit more flexibility in overall eating patterns. It is not a guide to daily food choices, or even serving sizes, but, rather, a unique plan for daily, weekly, and monthly food-group intake levels. Substantively, it allows for lesser amounts of meat, poultry, and seafood in the diet and more vegetables, seeds, nuts, and legumes. Consequently, it is higher in fiber. The Mediterranean pyramid also emphasizes protein sources that are plant-based, rather than animal-based, thereby promoting a diet that is lower in saturated fat and cholesterol. The Mediterranean pyramid also scores points with dietitians and nutritionists because it emphasizes fish (high in omega-3 fatty acids) over red meat (high in saturated fat and cholesterol). Other distinctions are the recommendations for regular exercise, the daily use of olive oil, and the inclusion of wine in moderation. Olive oil is considered a particularly healthy fat because of its properties as a monosaturated fat. Recent studies have shown that monounsatu-

rated oils, such as olive and canola, do not increase the level of "bad" LDL cholesterol and do not lower the level of "good" HDL cholesterol. The polyunsaturated fatty acids found in oils such as corn and safflower do not confer these benefits. However, the total emphasis on one kind of oil may be a shortcoming: A variety of plant oils is necessary to ensure an adequate intake of the essential fatty acids, linolenic acid (found in soybean and canola oils) and linoleic acid (found in nuts, seeds, and safflower oil). The recommendation that wine be consumed in moderation may be more appropriate for some women than others. Some studies suggest a direct correlation between the quantity of alcohol consumed and the risk of breast cancer (Smith-Warner et al., 1998), so total avoidance of all forms of alcohol may be the best course of action for women with a personal or family history of breast cancer. Medical problems may limit the variety of foods that an individual can tolerate. In such instances, a registered dietitian (RD) can be an invaluable source of information and advice.

VEGETARIAN DIET PYRAMID

Still another version of the pyramid food selection guide is the Vegetarian Diet Pyramid developed by the Oldways Preservation Trust in conjunction with Harvard and Cornell Universities. This pyramid is particularly intriguing because of the compelling health benefits of a vegetarian lifestyle. Vegetarians who live in developed countries enjoy unusually good health; they have low rates of cancer and coronary heart disease, as well as decreased mortality overall (Willett, 1999).

Among the strengths of this model is that the elimination of red meats provides the opportunity for increased consumption of grains, fruits, and vegetables, resulting in a diet that is naturally low in saturated fat and cholesterol and high in fiber. Unlike the USDA and Mediterranean pyramids, the Vegetarian Diet Pyramid recommends specifically that whole grains be consumed at each meal. It also recommends *daily* physical activity as opposed to the *regular* exercise called for in the Mediterranean pyramid. However, even the Vegetarian Diet Pyramid allows for unhealthy food selections; for example, one could make a meal of pizza and ice cream and wash it down with a cola beverage. (See Figure 3–4.)

The fact that the consumption of fruits and vegetables confers a substantial health benefit is acknowledged by many prestigious institutions. A noteworthy research report by the American Institute for Cancer Research (AICR) further emphasizes the fact that diets high in fruits and vegetables, even those that include small amounts of meat, provide protection against cancer, similar to that provided by total vegetarian diets (Expert Panel of the AICR-WCRF Diet & Cancer Project, 1997). A plant-based diet does not necessarily imply a vegetarian diet. A primarily plant-based diet emphasizes vegetables, fruits, and whole grain products. Daily meals, therefore, are mostly comprised of plant foods—such as vegetables and fruits, grains and whole grains (whole grain

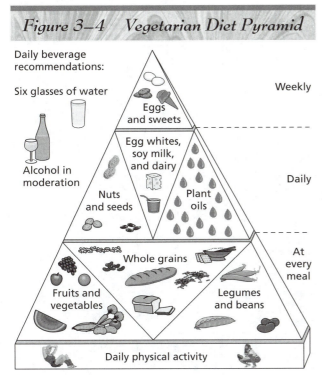

Figure 3–4   Vegetarian Diet Pyramid

Daily beverage recommendations:

Six glasses of water

Alcohol in moderation

Weekly

Eggs and sweets

Egg whites, soy milk, and dairy

Nuts and seeds

Plant oils

Daily

Whole grains

Fruits and vegetables

Legumes and beans

At every meal

Daily physical activity

2000 Oldways Preservation & Exchange Trust.

bread and cereal, rice, and pasta), tubers (including potatoes—yellow, red, and traditional as well as sweet potatoes and yams), and legumes (including a variety of beans, peas, and lentils). AICR's expert report clearly states that there is convincing evidence that diets high in vegetables and fruits can decrease the risk of certain cancers, including cancers of the colon, rectum, lung, stomach, mouth, pharynx, and esophagus. The report also suggests that plant-based diets probably offer protection against cancers of the breast, bladder, larynx, and pancreas, although more research is needed to confirm a cause and effect relationship. Because vegetables, fruits, and other plant foods are potent sources of antioxidant nutrients (including vitamins C and E, beta-carotene and other carotenoids), they may protect cells from damage by cancer-causing agents, thus halting the earliest mutating processes that lead to cancer (Expert Panel of the AICR-WCRF Diet & Cancer Project, 1998). Consuming an abundance of fruits, vegetables, and other plant foods not only offers protection against certain cancers but in addition may protect against coronary heart disease, stroke, diabetes, hypertension, and obesity. Soluble fiber from grains and legumes may also have a favorable impact on lowering blood cholesterol.

Because of this demonstrated correlation between vegetarian diets and reduced risk for disease, growing numbers of health-minded individuals, as well as those who object to animal slaughter, eat a plant-based diet, with or without eggs and milk. There are a variety of vegetarian subclassifications. **Vegans** consume only plant foods, whereas **lacto-vegetarians** eat dairy products as well. The **ovo-vegetarian** diet includes eggs and plant foods, and **lacto-ovo-vegetarians** consume all dairy products and eggs along with plants. Finally, **semi-vegetarians** eat fish and poultry but no red meat.

Vegetarian diets, even if totally plant-based, can be safe if the appropriate dietary guidelines are followed. However, even vegetarian diets can be unhealthy if high-fat foods, such as olives, avocados, nuts, peanut butter and other spreads, and salad dressings, are eaten to excess, and there are specific vitamin and mineral requirements that may be more challenging for a vegetarian to meet. One of the vitamins is vitamin B-12, which is found only in foods of animal origin or in nutritional supplements. A lacto- or lacto-ovo-vegetarian will have no problem getting enough vitamin B-12; however, a total vegan will need to find a suitable B-12–fortified food (such as a soy meat replacement or a fortified soymilk). Vitamin D is another vitamin that is not readily available from plant sources. Vegetarians who consume milk will be protected, but total vegans will require a supplement—especially if their exposure to sunlight is limited. Two minerals of concern to the vegetarian are iron and calcium. By consuming foods rich in vitamin C, a vegetarian can improve iron absorption from foods eaten at the same meal. The lacto variants of the vegetarian lifestyle are at greatest risk for iron deficiency, because milk and other dairy products are poor sources of iron. Finally, by consuming calcium-fortified products and nondairy foods that are rich in calcium, vegans can solve the problem of a low calcium intake. Infants and young children, however, may be in precarious nutritional positions, because their stomach capacity is limited. They may not be able to consume enough foods in sufficient quantities to meet all of their nutritional requirements. All too often, the careful planning needed to ensure proper nutritional balance of the vegetarian diet becomes overlooked, which can be critical especially with the more restrictive vegetarian diets. (See Table 3–6.)

Vegetarians must choose their foods wisely and remember to consult a registered dietitian about any special questions or concerns, especially when food intolerances or certain chronic diseases limit food choices.

General Dietary Guidelines

The USDA and the Department of Health and Human Services have drawn up a list of nutritional guidelines (Johnson & Kennedy, 2000) that consumers can use in conjunction with the food guide pyramids. This list—intended for those two years of age and older—has recently been revised to include the latest scientific findings,

1. *Aim for fitness.*
   - *Aim for a healthy weight.*
   - *Be physically active each day.*

TABLE 3–6 Nutrients to consume daily.

✓	Nutrients	Food Sources
✓	Protein	Peanuts, almonds, cashews, walnuts, tofu, tempeh, kidney beans, garbanzo beans, black-eyed beans, refried beans, milk, yogurt, cheese, eggs
✓	Calcium	Calcium-processed tofu, almonds, broccoli, kale, beet greens, collards, mustard greens, legumes, calcium-fortified juice and cereals, milk, yogurt, cheese
✓	Vitamin B-12	Vitamin B-12–fortified breakfast cereal, soy milk products and beverages, vegetarian garden patties, milk, yogurt, cheese
✓	Vitamin D	Vitamin D–fortified cereal and soy milk, Vitamin D–fortified milk
✓	Iron	Iron-fortified cereals and grains, tofu, legumes, spinach, beet greens, kale, cashews, almonds, dried fruit, prune juice, egg yolk
✓	Zinc	Whole wheat bread, whole grain products, tofu, cashews, almonds, peanuts, seeds, milk, yogurt, cheese, eggs

2. *Build a healthy base.*
   - *Let a pyramid guide your food choices.*
   - *Eat a variety of grains daily, especially whole grains.*
   - *Eat a variety of fruits and vegetables daily.*
   - *Do not eat spoiled or moldy food.*
3. *Choose sensibly.*
   - *Choose a diet that is low in saturated fat and cholesterol and moderate in total fat.*
   - *Choose beverages and foods low in sugars.*
   - *If you drink alcoholic beverages, do so in moderation.*

Food Labels

The **nutrition facts label** found on processed food packages is an invaluable tool for health-conscious consumers. It lists the amounts of key nutrients contained in the food followed by the **percent daily value (PDV)** number. These numbers refer to the percentage (based on a 2,000 calorie diet) of nutrient that is present in one serving. For example, a commercial brand of orange juice lists the serving size as 8 fluid ounces and the PDV for vitamin C as 130 percent. Thus, an individual consuming a 2,000 calorie diet would have already met—and, in fact, exceeded—the recommended level of vitamin C intake with a glass of this orange juice. Consumers can easily decide whether a given food fits their dietary plans by comparing its fat, cholesterol, sodium, and sugar content to the suggested allowances for their particular daily caloric limits. There may be an additional footnote on the label reminding consumers that nutrient requirements vary with calorie levels. See Figure 3–5 for a sample nutrition facts label.

Figure 3–5 Nutrition Facts Label

Nutrition Facts

Serving Size 1/2 cup (114g)
Servings Per Container 4

Amount Per Serving

Calories 90	Calories from Fat 30
	% Daily Value*
Total Fat 3g	**5%**
Saturated Fat 0g	**0%**
Cholesterol 0mg	**0%**
Sodium 300mg	**13%**
Total Carbohydrate 13g	**4%**
Dietary Fiber 3g	**12%**
Sugars 3g	
Protein 3g	

Vitamin A	80%	•	Vitamin C	60%
Calcium	4%	•	Iron	4%

* Percent Daily Values are based on a 2,000 calorie diet. Your daily values may be higher or lower depending on your calorie needs:

	Calories	2,000	2,500
Total Fat	Less than	65g	80g
Sat Fat	Less than	20g	25g
Cholesterol	Less than	300mg	300mg
Sodium	Less than	2,400mg	2,400mg
Total Carbohydrate		300g	375g
Fiber		25g	30g

Calories per gram:
Fat 9 • Carbohydrate 4 • Protein 4

More nutrients may be listed on some labels.

Source: U.S. Department of Health and Human Services Food and Drug Administration.

TABLE 3–7 Health claims permitted on food labels.

Health Claim Link	What's the Connection?
Calcium and osteoporosis	A calcium-rich diet has been directly correlated to a reduced risk of osteoporosis, a condition that renders bones soft or brittle.
Fat and cancer	A diet low in total fat is linked to a reduced risk of certain cancers—breast cancer, in particular.
Saturated fat and cholesterol and coronary heart disease	A diet low in saturated fat and cholesterol can be a major help in reducing the risk for coronary heart disease.
Fiber-containing grain products, fruits, and vegetables and cancer	A diet rich in high-fiber whole grain products, fruits, and vegetables can reduce the risk for certain cancers—cancer of the colon, in particular.
Sodium and high blood pressure	A low-sodium diet may help reduce the risk hypertension, which is a risk factor for heart attack and stroke.
Fruits and vegetables and some cancers	A low-fat diet rich in fruits and vegetables is linked to a reduced risk of certain cancers—especially foods that are low in fat and high in dietary fiber, vitamin A, and vitamin C.
Folic acid and neural tube birth defects	Women of childbearing age who intake 0.4 mg of folic acid a day reduce their risk of giving birth to a child with a neural tube defect.

Source: Adapted from "Label Talk." The U.S. Food and Drug Administration and the International Foods Information Council (IFIC) Foundation at http://ific.org; document URL—http://www.ific.org/proactive/newsroom/release.vtml?id=18306.

Food packages typically display two types of messages: (1) health claims and (2) nutrient content claims or descriptors. The government strictly regulates both of these.

HEALTH CLAIMS

Health experts are in agreement that what you eat can affect your well-being. A healthful diet promotes health and wellness and may offer help in lowering risks for certain diseases. In order to help consumers learn how food choices can affect health, certain health claims now appear on food labels. A health claim describes how a food or food nutrient—such as fat, calcium, iron, or fiber—relates to a disease or health-related condition. Currently, only health claims that are supported by scientific evidence are allowed on labels. Eight health claims have been approved by the FDA, as shown in Table 3–7.

NUTRIENT CONTENT CLAIMS

The nutrient content claims found on food packaging give the consumer a quick and basic idea of the amount of a particular nutrient in a food serving. A "low-fat" nutrient content claim, for example, lets the consumer know that the food contains no more than 3 g of fat per standardized serving size. The term *low-fat* has the same meaning regardless of the product or brand it appears on. For example, a box of fruit and grain cereal bars may display a label stating the product is low in fat.

The meanings of such claims as "fat free," "low fat," etc., are provided in Table 3–8. Manufacturers may also claim that certain food products are "heart healthy," or imply that they do not raise blood pressure. If such claims are made, however, additional criteria (also listed in Table 3–8) must be met. To know more precisely how much fat, sodium, etc. is in a serving, however, the consumer must read the **Nutrition Facts** section on the package. Specific claims are defined in Table 3–8.

The Problem of Overweight and Obesity

Currently, more than 50 percent of all American adults are overweight (Centers for Disease Control, 2002), and the number of adults who are obese (sufficiently overweight to threaten health) has increased by 50 percent over the past 20 years (Flegal, Carroll, Kuczmarski, & Johnson, 1998). The Centers for Disease Control (CDC) report that *one in five* adults is obese. This represents a 50 percent increase in less than a decade, and we are continuing to get fatter as a nation. Whereas a survey conducted between 1976 and 1980 revealed that only 25 percent of U.S. adults were overweight, a similar survey done between 1988 and 1994 showed that 35 percent of the population was overweight (*Fastats A to Z*, 1999). Those surveys were the second National Health and Nutrition Examination Survey (NHANES II), conducted on

TABLE 3–8 Nutrient claim definitions.

Nutrient Claim	Definition
Free	A product contains literally none of the nutrient. This is usually used in conjunction with the following terms preceding the word *free*: *calorie, sugar, sodium, salt, fat, saturated fat,* and *cholesterol.*
Low	A product contains a low enough amount of a nutrient to allow frequent consumption without concern about going over dietary recommendations.
Low sodium	A product has no more than 140 mg per standardized serving.
Low calorie	A product has no more than 40 calories per standardized serving.
Low fat	A product has no more than 3 g of fat per standardized serving.
Low saturated fat	A product has no more than 1 g of sat fat per standardized serving.
Low cholesterol	A product has no more than 20 mg of cholesterol per standardized serving.
Very low	This refers to sodium only: A product contains no more than 35 mg per standardized serving.
Reduced or *less*	A product has at least a 25 percent reduction in a nutrient, compared with one-third the regular product.
Light or *lite*	A product has fewer calories than a comparable product or 50 percent of the fat in a similar product.
Good source	A product has 10 to 19 percent of the Daily Value for a nutrient.
High, rich in, or *excellent source*	A product has at least 20 percent of the Daily Value for a nutrient.
More	A product has at least 10 percent more of a desirable nutrient than does a comparable product.
Lean	This refers to meat or poultry products with less than 10 g of fat, less than 4 g of saturated fat, and less than 95 mg of cholesterol per 100 g serving size.
Extra lean	This refers to meat or poultry products with less than 5 g of fat, less than 2 g of saturated fat, and less than 95 mg of cholesterol per 100 g serving size.

Source: Adapted from "Label Talk." The U.S. Food and Drug Administration and the International Foods Information Council (IFIC) Foundation at http://ific.org; document URL—http://www.ific.org/proactive/newsroom/release.vtml?id=18306.

a sampling of 20,322 individuals ages 6 months to 74 years, and the NHANES III study, conducted from 1988 to 1994 on a sampling of 33,994 individuals ages 2 months and older. Sales of weight-loss products, low-fat foods, and diet plans have skyrocketed, yet with each decade we get fatter and fatter.

FAT VERSUS LEAN WEIGHT

Obesity and overweight are usually determined by using a scale to weigh an individual. This can present some challenges, because *weight* is determined by the pull of gravity against the body. The number on the scale does not distinguish fat weight from bone weight, water weight, or muscle weight. From a health standpoint, body *fat* has greater implications than body weight, and, according to the definition of *obesity,* it is body *fat* that must be meas-

ured (Bray & James, 1998). Unfortunately, it is not that easy for the average person to determine her percent of body fat. The most accurate method is underwater weighing—which requires a special apparatus and trained evaluators—in which the body's weight on land is compared with the body's weight in water. Because fat is lighter than water, a fatter individual will weigh significantly less in water, in comparison with her land weight, than will a leaner individual. Another mechanism for determining body fat involves the use of calipers. These calipers measure the width of **subcutaneous** (under the skin) **fat** stores, which are then compared with data in standard tables.

There is also a mathematical calculation that correlates highly with more direct measures of body fat, and that can be used to distinguish between overweight and obesity. This calculation is known as the **body mass index (BMI)**

TABLE 3–9 Classifications of overweight and obesity by body mass index (BMI).

Description	Obesity Classification	BMI
Underweight		<18.5
Normal		18.5–24.9
Overweight		25.0–29.9
Obese	I	30.0–34.9
	II	35.0–39.9
	III	≥40

Source: Adapted from Bray, G. A., & James, W. P. T. [Eds.], *Handbook of obesity*. (1998). By courtesy of Marcel Dekker, Inc.

TABLE 3–10 Getting a feel for BMI.

BMI	Level
10–12	Lowest level believed to support life
16	BMI of fashion models
25	Definition of *overweight*, according to National Institutes of Health
26.5	Average U.S. adult, according to NHANES III study
30	Definition of *obesity*; FDA approves use of antiobesity drugs at this level
35	Surgery for obesity approved in patient with obesity-related complications
40	Classification of morbid obesity; surgery justified even without complications
43.7	Average BMI of Sumo wrestlers

Source: Allison, D. B., & Rha, S. S. (1998, July/Aug). Getting a feel for body mass index (BMI). *The Weight Control Digest*, pp. 740–41.

(Allison & Rha, 1998). BMI is calculated by dividing the individual's weight (without clothes) in kilograms by the square of her height (without shoes) in meters. BMI can be also calculated by dividing weight in pounds by height in inches squared and then multiplying that number by the factor 703. Criteria established by the National Heart, Blood, and Lung Institute and the World Health Organization are used to classify individuals as underweight, normal, or overweight. Obesity can also be established (see Table 3–9). Table 3–10 can put BMI into perspective and aid understanding of the various BMI levels.

According to the newsletter *Miss America News,* the BMI for 13 of 41 responding Miss America contestants in 1999 was *below* 19 (Pawling, 1999). A review of Table 3–10 reveals that these women were *underweight.* Over the past eight decades, the average Miss America has gotten steadily thinner; whereas the average height for the contestants has *increased* by 2 percent, the average weight has *decreased* by 12 percent (Pawling, 1999). However, many normal-weight women look to these contestants as examples of ideal body weight.

Although the icons of femininity are underweight, according to the NHANES III survey (*Fastats A to Z*, 1999), the "average" American woman is overweight at a height of 5 feet 3¾ inches and a weight of 152 pounds. The BMI for this "average woman" is 26 (152 pounds divided by 63.75 inches squared, times 703). The average woman would be assigned to the "normal" weight category, however, if she were to lose only 10 pounds of fat. Achieving a normal weight is highly desirable, because BMIs greater than 25 have been linked to adverse health consequences.

HEALTH RISKS OF OBESITY

Obesity is second only to smoking as the foremost cause of preventable death in the United States. It is responsible for approximately 325,000 deaths per year (Allison, Fontaine, Manson, Stevens, & VanItallie, 1999). Obesity increases the risk of certain chronic diseases, including coronary heart disease, high blood pressure, stroke, dyslipedemia (high blood fat levels), osteoarthritis, certain kinds of cancer, and diabetes (Must et al., 1999). The location of the fat stores has even greater implications for health.

Extra weight in the *abdominal* region (apple shape) is less healthy than weight deposited *below the waist* (pear shape), in the hip and thigh region (Margolis & Cheskin, 1999). Most men seem to be wider in the abdominal and chest region (apple shaped), whereas most women are pear-shaped, with wider circumferences in the hips and thighs. *Apples* have a far greater risk of coronary heart disease, high blood pressure, high blood sugar, and insulin resistance than do *pears*. Pears, on the other hand, seem to suffer more from varicose veins and knee problems from supporting heavier hips. Although it is not possible to switch body **morphology** (shape) easily, it is possible to lower health risks by becoming a thinner apple or a thinner pear.

Body shape is a function of what is known as **waist to hip ratio.** To determine this, use a tape measure and measure your waist (it is the smallest measurement between your rib cage and the **umbilicus,** or "belly button") and your hips where they are widest. Divide the waist measurement by the hip measurement to arrive at the waist to hip ratio. The goal for women is a ratio below 0.95 and for men a ratio below 0.85. Newer studies are showing that waist measurement alone can be an accurate indicator of health risk. For women, a waist measurement greater than 35 inches and for men a waist measurement greater than 40 inches is linked to increased health risks, particularly cardiovascular risks (Lean, Han, & Seidell, 1998).

FUNCTIONAL ROLE OF FAT

In an overzealous attempt to lose weight quickly, some dieters eliminate almost entirely the nutrient with the highest concentration of calories—fat. That strategy is unwise because of the vital role that fat plays in the body. Appropriate amounts of fat in our diets and in our bodies are essential to good health. Fat is stored in the cells as an energy reserve and is present as a structural component of the cell membrane. Cholesterol, a kind of fat, is found in cell membranes and is a structural component of steroid hormones and bile acids. The body very efficiently stores excess calories as **adipose tissue** (body fat). This is a survival mechanism intended to allow the individual to sustain life during times of famine. This mechanism is of little use to most Americans, however, to whom a rich abundance of foods is available. In addition to providing portable calories, fat helps cushion and protect vital organs, absorb and transport fat-soluble vitamins, prevent fatty acid deficiencies, and provide the body with many essential biochemicals, such as hormones. However, the average American woman has an excess of body fat, which fosters ill health rather than survival.

ENERGY METABOLISM AND CALORIC BALANCE

In order to understand the relationship among calories, fat, and obesity, it is essential to understand the concepts of energy metabolism and caloric balance. One's weight is a reflection of one's long-term **caloric balance.** Positive caloric balance occurs when the consumption of calories exceeds the body's energy requirements. The body stores these excess calories as body fat, and weight increases. If, on the other hand, more calories are used than are consumed, the body taps this stored energy (primarily adipose tissue) and fat weight in the body decreases.

Calories are essential for three primary functions: to support basal metabolic rate, to digest food, and to provide energy for physical activity. The **basal metabolic rate (BMR)** is the amount of energy that the body needs to maintain the functions of its organs and for cellular metabolic processes. BMR varies with sex, age, and amount of muscle mass. There is a positive correlation between muscle mass and BMR, and, because men generally have more muscle mass than women, their BMR is higher. Clinicians typically use the Harris-Benedict Equation to calculate the basal energy expenditures (BEE—a term similar to BMR) for men or women:

Harris-Benedict Equation

For women: BEE = 655 + (9.6 × weight in kg) + (1.8 × height in cm) − (4.7 × age in yr)

For men: BEE = 66 + (13.7 × weight in kg) + (5 × height in cm) − (6.8 × age in yr)

For example, a man and a woman—each of whom is 5′6″ (167.6 cm) tall, 135 pounds (61.3 kg), and 20 years of age—have different calorie requirements. The man would require approximately 1,600 calories/day, whereas the woman would require only approximately 1,450 calories/day. BMR also declines with age, with an estimated decrease of 10 percent per decade. That means that, if calorie consumption and energy expenditure remain constant, individuals gain weight as they age.

The body also needs calories to digest and metabolize food. This is known as the **thermic effect of food** and is estimated to account for approximately 10 to 15 percent of the body's total energy expenditure (Margolis & Cheskin, 1999). However, the level of physical activity is the primary determinant of calorie variations between individuals. Sedentary individuals obviously require fewer calories than moderately active people do, because activity increases caloric requirements. An individual who weighs 110 pounds burns approximately 100 calories per hour sleeping, 240 calories per hour walking, and 490 calories per hour jogging or running (see Table 3–11).

Body weight is simply a reflection of caloric balance. One pound of body fat represents 3,500 calories in storage. Imagine four sticks of butter or margarine to get a visual concept of the size of a pound of fat. Many Americans are overfat and have more fat in storage than they need. To lose a pound of fat, the energy balance needs to be negative; one must use 3,500 calories more than one consumes. A 500 calorie per day reduction in intake will result in a deficit of 3,500 calories (and a weight loss of 1 pound) within one week.

Calories from food are units of energy that help fuel all of the body's processes, contribute to the digestion of food, and support varying levels of physical activity. Calories are derived from the foods we consume. The three macronutrients—carbohydrates, proteins, and fats—contain calories. Carbohydrates and proteins provide a caloric concentration of 4 calories per gram. Fat is a highly concentrated caloric source, containing a whopping 9 calories per gram. As a point of reference, 1 g is equal to 0.04 oz. One-half cup of cooked vegetables is about 100 g, or 3½ oz. (Whitney, Cataldo, & Rolfes, 1998). Calculating calories from foods involves nothing more than adding up the number of calories obtained from fat, carbohydrate, and protein.

Calculating caloric intake can be fairly simple when the particular food is pure fat (such as vegetable oil), pure carbohydrate (such as table sugar), or pure protein (such as egg white). It becomes considerably more complicated, however, when the food consists of a combination of protein, fat, and carbohydrate, as most foods do. This is where food labels and food composition tables come in handy.

A given individual's weight is not always entirely a reflection of the balance between the number of calories consumed and the number of calories burned. Other factors also come into play—factors that can leave the obese individual discouraged and her primary healthcare provider frustrated.

FACTORS THAT DETERMINE BODY WEIGHT

Excess caloric intake is one of the major factors contributing to obesity. Some studies have reported that obese individu-

TABLE 3–11	Calorie expenditure chart: Time in minutes required to burn 100 calories.		
		Weight	
Type of Activity	125 pounds	150 pounds	175 pounds
Sitting quietly and watching television	100	84	72
Standing quietly	84	70	60
Typing at a computer	67	56	48
Grocery shopping	44	36	31
Walking, slow pace (2 miles per hour)	40	34	28
Walking, moderate pace (3 miles per hour)	30	26	22
Walking, brisk pace (4 miles per hour)	20	17	14
Hiking with a 10 pound load	14	11	10
Jogging (12 minute mile)	12	10	9
Jogging (10 minute mile) or swimming freestyle, fast	10	8	7

Source: Adapted from "How Long Does it Take to Burn 100 Calories?" Tufts University Health & Nutrition Letter, 8/00.

als seem to eat no more than their lean counterparts. The results of these studies are questionable, however, because many were based on self-reported food intake, and obese individuals tend to underestimate how much they consume. Most obese individuals are not gluttons; they do not eat very much more than normal-weight people. Unfortunately, small caloric excesses over time contribute to weight gain. This process is insidious and at times imperceptible. A small caloric excess of *100 calories per day* (two extra pats of butter or margarine) can result in an excess of 36,500 calories at the end of one year. Because there are 3,500 calories in 1 pound of fat, this translates into a 10-pound weight gain. However, there is no single cause of obesity, and to point to excess calorie intake as *the* cause is simplistic. There are factors that cannot be modified by the individual, and new research may provide some promising treatments, especially for individuals who are obese (BMI ≥ 30).

It is estimated that 70 percent of the variability in human body weight can be attributed to *genetic factors* (Yanovski & Yanovski, 1999), and researchers are now able to identify several genes that affect the regulation of body weight. One of the newest discoveries is the existence of a hormone, **leptin,** which is manufactured in adipose tissue. Obese mice have been found to have low levels of circulating leptin, and injections of leptin cause obese mice to decrease their consumption of food (Halaas, Gajiwala, Maffei, & Cohen, 1995). Studies to determine the significance of leptin in the etiology of human obesity are underway, as are other investigations regarding genes that may affect the storage of fat and the use of energy by lean tissues. One of the most interesting unsolved mysteries is why some individuals tend to be resistant to fat weight gain, despite calorie intakes that would normally result in weight increases. As more is learned about the underlying metabolic and genetic factors affecting body weight regulation, obesity will become more

amenable to effective treatment. In the meantime, there is strong evidence that ". . . increased physical activity, in conjunction with a healthful diet, are the best hope for Americans to achieve and maintain a healthy weight" (Yanovski & Yanovski, 1999, p. 1505).

EVALUATING ALTERNATIVE WEIGHT-LOSS THEORIES

Over the past 20 years, a plethora of alternative dietary plans that challenge the basic principles accepted by the USDA, the American Dietetic Association, and other mainstream organizations have been aggressively marketed to the public. Most were developed as solutions to common, chronic problems such as obesity and atherosclerosis (see Chapter 12) and described in books for the lay public that quickly ascended the best-seller lists. Some—such as *Dr. Atkins' New Diet Revolution* (1998), Barry Sears' *Enter the Zone* (1995), and the Eades' *Protein Power* (1996)—advocate a diet relatively high in either fat or protein or both, and they claim that the consumption of excess carbohydrate, particularly refined carbohydrate, is fundamentally detrimental to health. Others, such as the Pritikin (2000) and Ornish (1996) plans maintain that the amounts of fat allowed in the USDA and Mediterranean pyramids is too great and that adherence to a very low-fat diet would greatly enhance the health of the nation.

A central argument put forth by proponents of the *high-fat/protein, low carbohydrate* dietary plans is that the human body is not designed to metabolize refined carbohydrates (flour and sugar) because early hominids had no access to them (Eaton, 1988). A corollary of this theory is that many overweight individuals suffer from **insulin resistance** caused by years of excessive carbohydrate intake. Insulin resistance exists when the cells lose their sensitivity to insulin and increasingly high blood levels of insulin are needed to allow the metabolism of glucose to take place. According to proponents of the insulin-resistance theory of obesity, this metabolic imbalance causes rising blood sugar levels, water retention, increased fat storage, and cholesterol synthesis and is the primary cause of high blood pressure, coronary heart disease, and adult onset diabetes (*High-Protein, Low-Carb Diets,* 2000). Mainstream nutritional authorities dispute this. They maintain that the chronic diseases rampant today stem not from the overconsumption of carbohydrates per se, but from the fat content that is so frequently consumed along with them. The excess intake of saturated fat and calories overall, plus an insufficient expenditure of calories through exercise, is considered by most experts to be the actual culprits in diet-induced ill health. Dietary plans similar to those advocated by Atkins and the Eades have been roundly criticized in mainstream journals (*Eat Fat, Get Thin?* 2000) because they are high in fat and/or protein and low in beneficial complex carbohydrates and because the claims they make have not been supported by published empirical evidence. High saturated fat intake has been associated with higher cholesterol levels and the risk of coronary heart disease. However, in a small study (Westman et al., 2002) subjects placed on a relatively high-fat, Atkins-like diet lost weight and *lowered* their LDL cholesterol and triglyceride levels. Diets high in protein have been associated with increased uric acid levels, which can lead to the formation of kidney stones in susceptible people (*Eat Fat, Get Thin?* 2000) and the heightened excretion of calcium (NIH, 1994).

Proponents of *very low-fat* dietary plans maintain that only small amounts of unsaturated fat are needed in the diet and that anything beyond that contributes to atherosclerosis and other disease processes. Ornish has demonstrated through objective medical testing that patients with coronary heart disease can reduce the amount of plaque in their arteries through adherence to a plan that includes exercise, stress reduction, and a very low-fat diet. He has also demonstrated that plaque deposits continue to *increase* in size when patients adhere to the USDA plan, which allows 30 percent of dietary calories to come from fat (Ornish, 1996). Critics, however, contend that the success of the Ornish plan may be due, at least in part, to factors other than diet.

A successful solution to the problem of obesity in this country either remains to be discovered or already exists and remains to be adopted. As with the decisions regarding vitamin and mineral supplementation, there is no universal right answer, and each individual is challenged to make an intelligent choice that will meet her needs. Obviously, the more one understands about nutrition and metabolism, the easier it will be to examine many of these new weight loss theories with a critical eye.

SAFE WEIGHT LOSS AND WEIGHT MANAGEMENT

Since there is no simple *cause* of overweight and obesity, it stands to reason that there is no magic solution for their *treatment.* The most effective long-term treatment consists of a three-pronged approach: modifying dietary patterns, increasing physical activity, and changing behavioral patterns. Although the sales of diet products are a multibillion-dollar industry, and books on quick, easy methods for weight loss climb to the top of the best-seller lists, the results of embarking on most of the popular weight loss regimens are disappointing. Many of the diets are not well balanced or healthy for the long term, and individuals are not able to follow them long enough to experience adverse physical outcomes. Unfortunately, individuals who try to lose weight with a quick-loss scheme end up losing only money, time, and self-esteem. Some tips for instituting the behavioral changes that will result in safe, long-term, weight loss are as follows:

1. Check with your healthcare provider before making major dietary and exercise changes. *Your physician or nurse practitioner can help ensure that the changes you are planning to make are the right ones for you and identify any conditions that would require special attention or assistance from other healthcare professionals (such as a registered dietitian or an exercise physiologist).*

2. Monitor your food intake and activity level. *It is always helpful to understand what your current habits are. You may be surprised to learn how much you eat and how little you exercise. This initial evaluation will help you to make appropriate decisions about what to change in order to achieve your goal.*

3. Set realistic goals. *It is best to strive for a weight loss of 1 to 2 pounds per week to ensure that fat, rather than muscle tissue, is lost.*

4. Obtain support from your family and friends. *Studies show that people who receive social support are more successful in changing their behaviors. Communicate to those whose support you are seeking exactly what you are trying to do, and tell them how they can help you. This may head off well-meaning but demotivating behaviors, such as nagging you to walk or making statements such as "Why are you eating that?" and "I thought you were on a diet!" Guiding family and friends as to how best to support you will take some assertiveness on your part, but the results will be worth it. Remember also to recognize your supporters for their help and keep them apprised of your progress along the way.*

5. Be patient and make changes gradually *in order to prevent yourself from feeling overwhelmed or frustrated. It may take up to three weeks for a new behavior to become a habit.*

6. Think positively. *Rather than focusing on what you cannot have, or what you are sacrificing, look at what you can have—such as more fruits and vegetables—and appreciate how much better you feel when you are not overstuffed with fat-laden calories.*

7. Eat slowly. *Eating more slowly helps you consume fewer calories as well as learn to appreciate the flavors and*

textures of your food. Putting your fork down between bites, thoroughly chewing each mouthful before swallowing, and eating with your nondominant hand are all methods of slowing down your rate of food consumption.

8. Plan for snacks. *Eating something every couple of hours prevents intense hunger from developing. Skipping meals can increase the likelihood that you will overeat.*

9. Exercise. *Exercise goes hand in glove with any effective weight-loss/maintenance program. Exercise not only burns calories but also helps you feel better and manage stress more effectively.*

10. Check your progress. *Many successful weight losers find that daily (or regular) weight checks can be very effective in helping them stay on track. Remember, however, that the scale has its limitations. There may be daily fluctuations in your weight due to other causes, such as fluid retention. What you are interested in is* fat loss. *Your healthcare provider can help you find other signs of progress, such as lower blood pressure and lower cholesterol, to help you to appreciate your efforts.*

11. Pay attention to portion sizes. *Since most of us do not travel with a food scale or measuring spoons and cups, use the following guide to estimate portions. A 3 oz portion is approximately the size of the palm of an adult woman's hand or the size of a standard deck of playing cards. A 1 oz portion is thumb-size or the size of a slice of prewrapped American cheese. A 1 cup portion is equivalent to the size of one's fist. One teaspoon is approximately the size of the tip of the thumb, and a 2 tbsp portion is equivalent to a golf ball. One piece of medium fruit is the size of a baseball (hardball, not softball), and a small baked potato is the size of a computer mouse.*

12. Reward yourself for your progress. *This critical step is often overlooked. Remember that making lifestyle changes is hard work and you need to celebrate your successes. This attention to rewards will help to compensate for the "all to common" tendency to focus on failures. "Slip-ups" are a normal part of the process, and should be anticipated, but they are not an excuse for giving up. Expect that there will be some slips, but as with any new skill, practice makes perfect.*

GUIDELINES FOR EVALUATING WEIGHT-LOSS PROGRAMS

A myriad of weight-loss plans and supplements are marketed aggressively to consumers. Jenny Craig and Nutrisystems are examples of popular weight loss plans. Guidelines for weight loss are also included in the many alternative dietary plans not endorsed by the USDA, ADA, and so on. Whereas some plans advocate a balanced, albeit calorie-restricted diet, others promote diets that are decidedly *unbalanced* and inherently lacking in vital nutrients. Supplements used to promote weight loss include, but are not limited to, Citramax, Metabolife, chromium, ephedra, caffeine, and phenylalanine. Some of the

dietary supplements touted as supporting weight loss have been studied and found to be worthless and/or dangerous. **Hydroxycitric acid (HCA),** an herbal supplement derived from the rind of an Indian fruit, *Garcinia cambogia,* is a main ingredient in the weight-loss supplement Citramax. It is claimed to increase fat oxidation (burning) and metabolic rate. However, a 1999 randomized, blinded study (Kriketos, Thompson, Greene, & Hill, 1999) found no difference in energy expenditure, either at rest or during exercise, between subjects who took HCA and those who did not. **Chromium,** an essential trace element marketed as supporting weight loss and muscle building, *has not* been demonstrated to do either of those things. Moreover, new studies suggest that it may cause DNA mutations, and this possibility is being further investigated (*New Study Tarnishes Chromium,* 1999). The popular herbal weight-loss product Metabolife contains **guarana,** a caffeine source, and **ephedra,** in addition to other herbs. Both caffeine and ephedra raise blood pressure and heart rate and can be dangerous for people with high blood pressure, palpitations, coronary heart disease, and other cardiovascular problems commonly associated with obesity. Both drugs can also cause nervousness and insomnia, particularly when taken together. Withdrawal headaches are common when the use of both drugs (singly or together) is stopped. Although the combination of caffeine and ephedra has been demonstrated to raise metabolic rate slightly and support loss of fat tissue as opposed to lean body mass, the benefits are modest in comparison with the risks (Barrette, 2000).

Quick-fix diet plans that rely on the use of supplements or chemical imbalances in the body, or that urge consumers to "Eat whatever you want, whenever you want it," just don't work. Although sometimes effective in the short term, such plans almost always lead to a rapid regain of any weight that may have been lost, and a gain of additional weight as well (Korkeila, Rissanen, Kaprio, Sorensen, & Koskenvuo, 1999).

Some of the weight-loss programs marketed to the public, however, are safe and effective. Any approach, such as the Weight Watchers program, that uses a balanced diet, plus exercise, and does not require any potentially harmful supplements is acceptable. Diets used to achieve weight loss should be congruent with the principles of good nutrition discussed previously in this chapter. Use the checklist shown in Table 3–12 to assess the safety and effectiveness of weight-loss programs you may be considering. The goal is to have all of the checkmarks in the "yes" column.

IMPLEMENTING A WEIGHT-LOSS PLAN

Carrying out a weight loss plan need not be a grim exercise in self-deprivation. By following the suggestions presented below, women can lose weight and still enjoy food, as well as better health.

General Guidelines The key to following a weight-loss plan and making choices is *balance*. Attempting to adhere

TABLE 3–12 Characteristics of a safe weight-loss program.

Does Your Plan Measure Up?

Weight Loss Component	Yes	No
Daily calorie level is not less than 1,000–1,200 calories per day.		
A variety of foods are recommended from all major food groups (grains, fruits, vegetables, meats, and other high-protein foods, dairy products).		
It allows you to include your favorite foods.		
It requires no special foods or products.		
It encourages weight-loss rates of 1 to 2 pounds per week.		
It recommends the inclusion of regular activity.		
It is adaptable and flexible to be used long term.		
It recommends physician (primary care provider) involvement to evaluate health status prior to the program start.		

TABLE 3–13 Low-fat, low-calorie snacks.

- Air-popped popcorn drizzled with no-fat butter-flavored cooking spray and sprinkled with herbs (or lightly salted)
- Breadsticks
- Bagels
- English muffins
- Fresh fruit
- Gingersnaps
- Graham crackers
- Saltines
- Pretzels
- Rye crisps
- Rice cakes (there are flavored ones that are quite tasty)
- Pita chips with salsa
- Dry-roasted soybeans
- Raw vegetables
- Hard candy or Gummy Bears

perfectly to one's basic plan fails to acknowledge the psychological appetite we all seem to have for goodies of one sort or another. Occasional indulgence has its place in even the most ambitious healthy-eating regimen. We can offset a meal or snack that is high in fat, sugar, salt, or calories by choosing foods extra low in fat, sugar, and so on for the rest of the day or the next day. Striving for balance and consistency and making *"eating right"* a way of life are the keys to maintaining a normal weight and a healthy body.

Balance is not only the key to eating healthfully; it is the key to achieving and maintaining optimal weight as well. **BALANCE** can be used as an acronym for the following additional principles of healthy eating:

Breakfast
Award
Liquids
Acknowledge
Nothing
Calm
Exercise

Breakfast—Breakfast is indeed the most important meal of the day. Those who eat a healthful, substantial breakfast that includes a food high in protein will feel less hungry during the remainder of the day.

Award (reward)—An occasional (weekly or monthly) reward for sticking to your plan, such as indulging in a favorite food, is psychologically beneficial. Even better than a food reward is a treat such as a massage or facial.

Liquids—Always drink plenty of fluids, especially water. A cup of tea or a tall glass of water before a meal can also help bridle the appetite and reduce the desire to overeat.

Acknowledge—Acknowledge the fact that there will be overindulgences. Don't be dismayed; realize what has happened, accept it, and get back on your plan.

Nothing—Nothing distasteful should be included in your plan. If you can't stand tofu, don't eat it; think rice cakes are bland?—avoid them. Furthermore, no food is totally forbidden; remember that moderation is the key.

Calm—Eating in a calm, relaxed atmosphere is key to proper digestive functioning. Don't eat on the run. Sit down, preferably at a table; relax and eat slowly. Enjoy the social aspects of dining.

Exercise—Exercise not only burns calories; it suppresses appetite. No healthy diet strategy is complete without it. Brisk walking is a safe, effective form of exercise, and there are many others as well (see Chapter 6).

Additional strategies can help dieters in their quest to lose weight safely and permanently. For example, to assuage the hunger that commonly arises between meals, dieters can choose from among the low-fat, low-calorie snacks listed in Table 3–13. Strategies for coping with restaurant eating and the summer ice cream season can also be very helpful.

Eating Out Eating out is both a pleasure and a necessity for many people, whether in the form of fine dining with friends and family or a quick stop at a fast-food restaurant. Eating out frequently can pose a challenge for those committed to eating right, particularly if they are also trying to lose weight. Responding wisely to the questions and statements that follow can help reconcile the inherent conflict between eating out and eating right:

"Will there be an appetizer?" Ordering a well-chosen appetizer can take the edge off hunger without adding excessive calories to the meal. Fresh fruit, raw vegetables, shrimp or crab cocktail, broth-based soups, and bread minus the butter are all good choices.

"And for the entrée?" Wise choices are dishes that are steamed, roasted, broiled, or baked. It is best to avoid anything fried or sautéed. Fish and chicken without skin are usually better choices than red meat.

"That comes with a hollandaise sauce." Restaurants will hold sauces if asked. Avoid thick, rich gravy mixtures. Red pasta sauce contains less fat than white.

"The vegetable choices are . . ." Steamed vegetables are lowest in calories.

"What dressing would you like on your salad?" It is best to order dressings on the side and use them sparingly.

"Would you like a take-out container?" Saving a portion of the meal for later is a strategy that can do wonders for both the waistline and the budget. Eating slowly will give the satiety center in the brain enough time to register a feeling of fullness before the entire meal has been eaten.

"Would anyone care for dessert?" Having dessert, but sharing it with a companion, can stave off both feelings of deprivation and weight gain. It is important to learn to be satisfied with small portions of sweet, rich foods.

Most table service restaurants will accommodate these suggestions.

Summer Treats In warm weather, frozen treats, such as ice cream cones and milkshakes, are all too tempting. Healthier warm-weather choices, however, are available. Delicious milkshakes can be made from low-fat cow's milk (or soymilk) and frozen fruit. Frozen yogurt comes in a wide variety of flavors, is a great replacement for ice cream, and is available in fat-free form.

An added bonus when opting for yogurt instead of ice cream is the boost yogurt can give to your immune system while helping ward off infection. Researchers believe that certain bacterial cultures found in yogurt, such as *Lactobacillus bulgaricus,* help increase the body's production of disease-fighting cells (Webb, 1999). Frozen yogurt is also a calorie and fat bargain when compared with the same serving size of soft-serve ice cream. A ½ cup serving of full-fat soft-serve frozen yogurt contains 114 calories and 4.0 grams of fat, whereas the soft-serve ice cream weighs in at 185 calories and 11.2 grams of fat (Pennington, 1998). Sorbet is also a tasty, low-fat alternative to ice cream. Frozen fruit-juice bars can also nicely satisfy cool treat craving, as can frozen lemonade cups. Chocolate syrup makes a great topping for low-fat sundaes and banana splits. Low-fat fudge and caramel toppings are also available.

Food Safety

In recent years, a number of concerns have been raised about the safety of our food supply. Outbreaks of bacterial infections traced to contaminated foods have led to the practice of irradiating foods to destroy microorganisms. Concerns about pesticide residues on food have led to a boom in the organic produce industry, and advances in biotechnology have made it possible to manipulate the genetic properties of plants, and even animals, used for food.

According to the Centers for Disease Control and Prevention (CDC), as many as 70 million cases of food-borne illnesses are reported each year in the United States, and thousands of Americans die from them. The number one cause of bacterial food-borne illness is *E. coli,* a type of bacteria found in chicken, beef, lettuce, alfalfa sprouts, and unpasteurized apple juice. In 1993, *E. coli* was responsible for an outbreak of food poisoning that sickened hundreds and killed four children who had ingested tainted hamburgers. In 1996, another bacterium, *Cyclospora,* which had made its way into imported raspberries, caused more than 1,300 people to develop fever, vomiting, fatigue, and diarrhea. Salmonella, perhaps the best-known culprit in food-borne illnesses, is sometimes found in raw eggs and chicken and has been around so long that it is often resistant to antibiotics.

The Department of Health and Human Services predicts that food-borne illnesses, and even deaths from such, will *increase* over the next 10 years. A potential hindrance to the management of this problem is that not just one, but a number of, government agencies are involved: The U.S. Department of Agriculture (USDA) inspects meat and poultry, whereas the Food and Drug Administration (FDA) is responsible for the safety of all other foods. The Environmental Protection Agency (EPA) sets tolerances for chemicals in food. Overall, 12 federal agencies and more than 30 laws govern food safety and inspection functions. Another problem is inconsistency in the degree to which various food sources are monitored for safety. For example, whereas the USDA inspects meat and poultry processing facilities frequently, the FDA, which is responsible for foods considered to be high-risk (seafood and eggs), surveys facilities in its jurisdiction only once every 10 years, on average (Brophy & Schardt, 1999).

Though the United States has the safest food supply of any country in the world, a need for improvement has been identified and action may be pending. The Center for Science in the Public Interest (CSPI) has begun a project in conjunction with the Safe Food Coalition called The Recipe for Safe Food. This is a legislative campaign intended to provide the government with better tools to clean up America's food supply. The Safe Food Act of 1999 (S.1281 or H.R. 2345), introduced on June 24, 1999, proposes that all U.S. food safety functions be assigned to a single new agency—the Food Safety Administration—in order to eliminate waste and confusion and to increase accountability. The intent is to consolidate in a single agency of the executive branch the responsibilities for food safety, labeling, and inspection that currently are divided among several federal agencies. As of this writing, the last major action taken was on July 7, 1999, when The Act was referred to House subcommittees on agriculture and commerce.

Individuals and families can take a number of precautions to lessen the chance that they will contract a foodborne illness. The following tips are adapted from the Food Safety Inspection Service of the United States Department of Agriculture (*Gateway to Government Food Safety Information*, 2000).

Store Food Safely

- Maintain refrigerator temperatures at 40°F or lower—many of the bacteria that cause illness can grow at temperatures found in home refrigerators.
- Thaw frozen foods in the refrigerator in cold, water-proof wrapping or in the microwave—but *never* on the kitchen counter. Once food is thawed, it is best to cook it immediately or refrigerate it.
- Keep meat, fish, poultry, and eggs refrigerated until ready to be cooked. Bacteria thrive in a warm (such as room temperature) environment where they can multiply rapidly.

Clean Work Habits

- Clean the sink, kitchen countertops, and utensils before you begin to cook.
- Wash hands before, during, and after food preparation. Use hot, soapy water.
- Wash all cutting boards, knives, and other utensils immediately after using.
- Avoid food handling if you are suffering from any infection, sore throat, or diarrheal illness.
- Wash all vegetables and fruits in cool water before eating or cooking. There are also safe commercial solutions available in your supermarket to help rid food of bacteria and pesticide residues that might be on the surface.
- Rinse raw poultry with cool water before cooking
- Marinate meats in the refrigerator, and do *not* reuse marinade.
- Avoid tasting raw or partially cooked meat, poultry, egg mixtures, fish, or shellfish.

Cook Foods Thoroughly

- Cook red meat to an internal temperature of at least 160°F. Look at the color; meat cooked to the correct temperature should be gray or brown—no pink juices should be seen. For thicker cuts of meat, use a meat thermometer to check the temperature.
- Cook whole poultry to 180°F—juices should run clear and flesh should be tender.
- Use roasting bags or covered containers if cooking poultry in the microwave. This lets steam ensure more even cooking.
- Cook fish until its flesh is flaky and opaque. Do not eat raw fish or shellfish.
- Cook eggs until the yolk is firm, not runny. The white should be firm as well.
- Cook in one uninterrupted cooking period. Never hold a roast or casserole to finish cooking it later—this will only encourage bacterial growth.

IRRADIATION

Food irradiation is the practice of exposing foods to **radiant energy** for the purpose of reducing or eliminating bacteria—thus making the food safer and more resistant to spoilage. The Radura symbol (see Figure 3–6) is the international sign for irradiation and must be visible on all irradiated foods sold at retail level in the United States. In the symbol, the petals represent the food, and the surrounding broken circle depicts the rays from the energy source. The words *treated by* [or *with*] *irradiation* must also be present. Food irradiation is often referred to as "cold pasteurization" because, unlike heat pasteurization, it does not cause a loss of nutrients or affect taste.

Food irradiation has been used in the United States for over 30 years. After World War II, the U.S. Army began experimenting with irradiation as a method of rendering fresh foods safer for field troops. Since 1963, the FDA has allowed the use of irradiation for the purpose of reducing the number of insects and microorganisms in spices and for slowing decay in fruits and vegetables. Food irradiation has been approved in 40 countries around the world, for more than 35 products, and has been supported by several national and international food and health organizations. Additional con-

Figure 3–6   The Radura Symbol

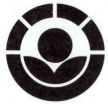

http://www.fda.gov/opacom/catalog/irradbro.html. Source: U.S. Department of Health and Human Services Food and Drug Administration.

sumer items treated with ionizing energy include medical bandages, dressings, and sanitary products.

In recent years, the irradiation of pork and chicken has also been approved. In 1985, the FDA approved the use of irradiation to control *Trichinella spiralis,* the organism that causes trichinosis in pork. In 1992, the Food Safety and Inspection Service (FSIS) of the USDA approved guidelines for the use of irradiation in raw packaged poultry, and in December 1997 the FDA deemed the use of irradiation to be safe on raw meat. Both the American Dietetic Association and the American Medical Association have endorsed food irradiation as a safe method of reducing the incidence of food poisoning (American Dietetic Association [ADA], 2000).

The irradiation of foods does not increase human exposure to radiation. The amount of energy used to irradiate the food is not sufficient to cause the food itself to become radioactive, and irradiated meat and poultry products *do not* give off radiant energy. Food irradiation facilities are regulated and monitored for worker and environmental safety.

Although food irradiation enhances food safety, it does not obviate the need for proper food handling and safety procedures because food can become contaminated after it has been irradiated. The International Food Information Council Foundation (IFICF), which develops science-based education programs dealing with topics of food safety and nutrition, is an excellent source of information on food irradiation and other topics related to food safety (see the Resources section at the end of this chapter).

FOOD BIOTECHNOLOGY

The term **food biotechnology** refers to the science of using genetic engineering to manipulate the properties of plants and animals used for food. More work in this area has been done on plants than animals. A variety of techniques involving gene manipulation are currently used to produce plants with desirable characteristics: **Genetically engineered organisms (GEOs)** and **genetically modified organisms (GMOs)** are plants and animals whose DNA has been somewhat altered but whose properties remain basically intact. **Transgenic** plants and animals are those that contain DNA from a completely unrelated plant, animal, or bacterium.

Through these forms of technology, growers have produced vegetables that are naturally resistant to diseases, as well as better tasting, faster ripening, and more nutritious. Vividly red tomatoes that are ripened on the vine and remain flavorful for longer periods of time are available, as are soybeans that are lower in saturated fats and higher in oleic acid, and that offer better frying stability when turned into oil. Peppers that have been modified to be crisper and sweeter are also to be found in the produce sections of grocery stores. The projected benefits of biotechnology include the development of fruits and vegetables that contain higher levels of vitamins C and E and beta-carotene, as well as plants that are more tolerant of extremes of heat and cold. The removal of allergy-causing proteins from foods may also be possible, and smaller, sweeter

peas; seedless, single-serving melons; and bananas with delayed ripening qualities may soon be available.

The FDA, the USDA, and the EPA have all endorsed the genetic modification of foods as safe, as have the AMA and the ADA. As early as 1991, the American Medical Association issued a report stating, among other things, that it is the policy of the AMA to "actively participate in the development of national programs to educate the public about the benefits of agricultural biotechnology" (Council on Scientific Affairs American Medical Association, 1991, p. 1432). In 1995, the American Dietetic Association (ADA) issued a position statement entitled "Biotechnology and the Future of Food," which it updated in February, 2000. It is the ADA's position that biotechnology techniques have the demonstrated potential to be useful in enhancing the quality, nutritional value, and variety of food available for human consumption, as well as in increasing the efficiency of food production, food processing, food distribution, and waste management.

Biotechnology has its critics, however. For example, groups such as the Center for Science in the Public Interest (CSPI) have repeatedly voiced concern over genetically engineered foods. On August 11, 2000, Michael F. Jacobson, the executive director of CSPI, issued a statement to Dr. Jane Henney, commissioner of the Food and Drug Administration, urging the agency to tighten its regulations concerning genetically engineered foods. Most recently, Mildred Cody, an associate professor of nutrition at Georgia State University, represented the ADA before the FDA in Washington, DC. Dr. Cody's remarks included the following statement: "The coordinated oversight of biotechnology by FDA, USDA, and EPA needs to be strengthened by the contributions of scientists and industries, health care professionals and educators, consumer organizations and others, into a concerted national information initiative. No one group—not government or industry, not scientists or consumer advocates—can successfully address the information and trust gaps developing around biotechnology" (Cody, 1999).

Proponents of agricultural biotechnology maintain that the processes used are not unlike the cross-breeding techniques used for centuries to create plants with different characteristics. Concerns, however, have been raised about potential problems, such as allergic reactions that may develop in response to foods that contain proteins from other species, as well as increased antibiotic resistance due to the incorporation of antibiotics into plants themselves (Ikramuddin, 1999). Other potential consequences are the evolution of superweeds and superbugs that have become resistant to the herbicides and pesticides engineered into plants. There is the possibility that unforeseen harm will be done to nontarget insect and animal species; pollen from plants genetically engineered to contain insecticide has been shown to be toxic to monarch butterfly caterpillars (*BT Corn Pollen from Iowa Fields Kills Monarch Caterpillars,* 2000). Finally, there is concern that some genetically modified foods may pose a threat to human health due to increased cancer risk (Marshall, 1999). The British Medical Association has recommended that further tests be done before more genetically modified crops are developed (Fox, 1999), and a growing list of agricultural and environmental organizations in the United States have called for stronger regulation of the biotech industry and mandatory labeling of bioengineered foods (Ikramuddin, 1999).

One of the most hotly debated issues involving food biotechnology is that of *labeling*. Currently, there are no laws mandating that bioengineered foods be labeled as such, and producers do not do so voluntarily. Environmentally oriented consumer groups, such as Mothers and Others for a Sustainable Planet (see Resources section), maintain that the public has a right to know what it is eating and demand that biotech foods be labeled. The FDA, however, disagrees, maintaining that current laws require labeling only if the food poses a possible health or safety risk. The FDA requires that a food be labeled if it meets the following criteria:

- The food contains a potential food allergen.
- The nutritional content of the product has been altered.
- The product is significantly and profoundly so different from the same type of non-bioengineered food that it cannot be called the same product.

The FDA's position is that all new food products, whether created through conventional means or genetic engineering, are evaluated for their individual safety, allergenicity, and toxicity and that the genetically engineered foods currently in the marketplace are safe.

ORGANIC FOODS

The term **organic** means that a food source or food product is free of chemical fertilizers, pesticides, and additives. In lieu of artificial fertilizers and toxic pesticides, organic farmers use cover crops (crops to be plowed into soil) and animal manure to fertilize their soils, and they rotate their crops to ensure that the soil does not become depleted of specific nutrients. Organically grown produce contains minimal or no levels of pesticides and other toxins. Organic farmers who raise food animals do not feed them hormones or antibiotics. The manufacturers of organic foods use only organically grown food sources and no additives (Mellon, 1997). In recent years, consumers concerned about environmental contamination and the potentially toxic effects of food additives, pesticides, hormones, and antibiotics on the human body (see Chapter 5) have created an increased demand for organic food products.

The position of the USDA, the FDA, the ADA and most mainstream agricultural organizations is that the presence of chemicals and additives in food is not inherently bad. They maintain that chemicals are added to food to enhance its flavor, texture, and color; to retard spoilage; and to discourage contamination by insects and that it is foolhardy to argue that the mere presence of chemicals in food is cause for

concern. The federal government maintains that the levels of herbicides, pesticides, hormones, and antibiotics that currently exist in plant and animal foods are safe. The Environmental Protection Agency (EPA) regulates pesticide use and establishes the maximum levels permitted. However, the present daily limits set for 19 organophosphate pesticides (see Chapter 5) do not reflect recent research suggesting that those substances can negatively affect the nervous system (Neville, 1999).

The EPA has until 2006 to set standards for new pesticides and to make sure that the standards for current pesticides meet the tougher standards recommended by the Food Quality Protection Act of 1996. In the meantime, consumers can protect themselves by buying organic when possible, washing all produce under running water, discarding the outer leaves of greens, and peeling vegetables and fruits as appropriate. A new food label, *USDA Organic*, began appearing on organic foods as of summer, 2002.

Nutritional Wellness Self-Assessment

Read the questions below and honestly answer them yes or no. The more yes answers you have, the higher your level of nutritional wellness.

1. *My weight is within the recommended range for my height and build.*
2. *I eat at least five servings of fruits and vegetables every day.*
3. *I avoid trans fats and limit saturated fats.*
4. *I include small amounts of mono- and polyunsaturated fats in my diet.*
5. *I drink at least eight glasses of water every day.*
6. *I choose whole grain breads, rolls, and cereals.*
7. *I eat a variety of foods, rather than the same foods every day.*
8. *I read food labels.*
9. *I limit my consumption of pie, cake, doughnuts, candy, and other high-fat, high-sugar foods.*
10. *I limit my consumption of red meat, pork, ham, and bacon.*
11. *I select at least three low-fat, calcium-rich foods each day.*
12. *I eat breakfast most days of the week.*
13. *I choose fish as an entrée at least once a week.*
14. *I add nuts to foods or use them as a snack three times a week.*
15. *I include soy products and beans and use these products to replace meat several times a week.*
16. *I trim fat from meats and remove skin from poultry products before cooking whenever possible.*

17. *I prepare foods by baking, broiling, steaming, or microwaving instead of frying in fat.*
18. *I select at least one food high in vitamin A each day (such as yellow or orange fruits or vegetables, and dark green, leafy vegetables)*
19. *I include a cruciferous vegetable (such as broccoli, cauliflower, cabbage, kale, or brussels sprouts) every other day.*
20. *I select a vitamin C–rich food daily (such as citrus fruits, kiwis, strawberries, or broccoli).*
21. *If I did not answer "yes" to questions 18–20, I take a multivitamin and mineral supplement daily.*

New Directions

Although nutritionists have long recommended that consumers eat vegetables, fruits, and unrefined, unprocessed foods in general as a method of enhancing health, until recently no one food source has been promoted as a potential weapon in the war against specific diseases and conditions. Now, however, **soy** is being promoted as a food that quells the symptoms of menopause and combats coronary heart disease, breast cancer, and osteoporosis. Although the health claims made for soy are exciting and provocative, there is more empirical evidence for some of these claims than for others.

The protective ingredients in soy are thought to be **isoflavones.** Isoflavones are phytoestrogens (see Chapter 5) that compete with the body's own estrogens for space on cell receptor sites. Isoflavones are thought to trigger the good reactions to estrogen, such as preventing coronary heart disease and maintaining bone, without triggering the bad ones, such as fostering the development of breast cancer. The literature to date, however, is not definitive regarding the exact effects of isoflavones in the body or the optimal isoflavone dosage. Soy isoflavones do seem to exert a protective effect against coronary heart disease. The evidence for this is sufficiently compelling that the FDA is now allowing manufacturers of soy products to claim in their advertising that eating 25–50 grams of soy protein per day may reduce the risk of coronary heart disease. Soy provides its cardiovascular benefits by lowering blood cholesterol. In one study (Washburn, Burke, & Morgan, 1999), adding 20 grams of soy protein containing 34 milligrams of phytoestrogens to the participants' daily diets significantly lowered their total and LDL (bad) cholesterol levels and reduced their blood pressure. The evidence that soy lessens the risk for cancers, however, is less compelling.

The observation that rural Asian women who consume a traditional soy and vegetable–based diet have much lower rates of breast and other cancers than American women led to the interest in soy's potential as an anticarcinogenic food. Nevertheless, the studies on this subject to date, have yielded mixed results. A recent review of the literature on soy isoflavones and malignancy identified no consistent, positive correlations between intake of isoflavones and either the prevention or the treatment of breast, uterine, and colon cancers (Lu, Anderson, Grady, Kohen, & Nagamani, 2000). There is suggestive, but not conclusive, evidence that soy confers some protection against endometrial cancer. One study (Goodman et al., 1997) found that women who ate phytoestrogen-rich foods experienced a 54 percent reduction in their risk of endometrial cancer. Preliminary evidence also suggests that an intake of 25–50 grams of soy per day may help protect women against osteoporosis. Although soy isoflavones are available in concentrated form in powders and pills, some physicians are concerned about the possible health risks of adding large amounts of phytoestrogens to the daily diet. This is especially of concern in women who have or have had hormonally dependent cancers, such as breast, ovarian, or uterine cancer (*Phytoestrogens—Hormones from Plants,* 2000).

Until questions surrounding soy can be more thoroughly answered via further research, a prudent recommendation may be to discuss adding soy to your diet with a registered dietitian or medical doctor (American Institute for Cancer Research, 2000). Soy appears to be a safe and beneficial food for women when consumed in typical amounts. It may be wise to substitute soy products for some or all of the meat in our diets, but not for beneficial whole grains, beans, fruits, and vegetables. As is true regarding other aspects of nutrition, *balance* is the key to the wise use of soy as a dietary adjunct to health.

Also new to the market—or at least new to the parlance of nutrition—are **functional foods.** Functional foods are defined as foods with added ingredients that provide a health benefit to consumers beyond the gain rendered by the food itself. Iodized salt and vitamin-fortified milk and cereal are examples of foods whose nutritional value is enhanced by additives. Newer enhanced foods have been developed recently and more are in the planning stage. Other terms commonly used to describe functional foods are **nutraceuticals** and **designer foods.**

As more is learned about the relationship between diet and disease, researchers are striving to uncover the exact substances in particular foods that appear to provide protection against various ailments. Hot cereal with added soy and orange juice laced with calcium are but a couple of the enhanced foods currently available. The research community is committed to developing designer foods that will reduce the risk of disease, strengthen the body, and perhaps ward off, to some degree, the effects of aging.

The process of ascertaining that a given food additive is both effective and safe is a long one, however, and both merchants and consumers are sometimes too eager for the new miracle food. Thus, products of dubious benefit about which exaggerated claims are made may be allowed to prosper. It is important that consumers look for convincing and thorough scientific evidence supporting the value of neutraceutical products before purchasing them. In an interesting and informative article, Brophy and Schardt (1999) identified some of the newer functional foods and discussed potential consumer concerns with these products. One of the key issues is that there currently is no guarantee regarding either product safety or its effectiveness. One cannot assume that all functional foods foster good health. For example, some of the popular power or energy snack bars available in supermarkets today are comprised largely of water, sugar, fat, and some protein—and in that order. The authors wisely suggest that, no matter how healthful- and impressive-looking a functional food's packaging and health claims may be, consumers should check the Nutrition Facts label before deciding to buy. An enriched or fortified junk food is still a junk food. On July 18, 2000, the CSPI issued a press release urging the FDA to halt the sale of functional foods and beverages containing potentially dangerous ingredients (CSPI Press Release, 2000). CSPI listed as an example, Snapple's Moon Tea Drink, which contains kava kava, which is claimed to "enliven your senses." According to CSPI, kava is a sedating herb which has been implicated in several driving while intoxicated (DWI) arrests.

Until more is learned about functional foods, consumers would be wise to choose nature's functional foods—fresh fruits, vegetables, whole grains, legumes, and low-fat dairy products. These foods come naturally equipped with nutrients and phytochemicals that may reduce the incidence of cancer, coronary heart disease, hypertension, eye disease, and other health concerns. The foods listed below are but a few of those that confer exceptional health benefits:

- Broccoli: Broccoli is loaded with cancer-fighting fiber, beta-carotene, and vitamin C, as well as folic acid and potassium.
- Blueberries: Blueberries are chock full of flavonoids, which may prevent cancer and coronary heart disease. They also contain concentrated proanthocyanidins, which are believed to ward off urinary tract infections.
- Barley: Barley is packed with magnesium and may aid in the deterrence of osteoporosis.
- Spinach: New studies suggest that this antioxidant-rich food may improve memory and slow the rate at which the brain declines with age. It can also reduce the risk of macular degeneration, another age-related illness.
- Apples: Flavonoids in apples have been found to reduce the risk of lung cancer.
- Garlic: Well-known for its ability to fight coronary heart disease by lowering cholesterol, garlic can also prevent blood clots and battle infections. Its source of power is a photochemical called allicin.
- Rosemary: Brimming with cancer-preventing antioxidants, rosemary has also been known to ease indigestion.

- Tomatoes: Tomatoes are laden with lycopene (a very potent antioxidant). One extensive study spanning six years and 48,000 male subjects found that those who ate more than 10 weekly servings of cooked tomato-based foods (such as spaghetti sauce) had the lowest risk of prostate cancer.

(*Adapted from "Super Foods That Act Like Medicine" by Donna Webb, Ph.D, R.D. as found in the February 16, 1999 issue of *Family Circle* magazine.)

QUESTIONS FOR REFLECTION AND DISCUSSION

1. *What factors account for the generally poor quality of the standard American diet (SAD)?*
2. *What factors, if any, keep you from improving your diet?*
3. *Do you take a vitamin/mineral supplement? Why or why not?*
4. *How much of a role in human health would you say diet plays?*
5. *Do you think genetically altered foods should be labeled as such? Why?*
6. *Do you consume organic foods? Why or why not?*
7. *Where would you go for credible current nutrition information?*

RESOURCES

Books

Duyff, R. L. (1998). *The American Dietetic Association's complete food and nutrition guide*. Wiley.

Havala, S. (1999). *The complete idiot's guide to being vegetarian*. Alpha Books.

Kirby, J., & American Dietetic Association. (1999). *Dieting for dummies*. IDG Books Worldwide.

Sizer, F., & Whitney, E. (1997). *Nutrition concepts and controversies* (7th ed.). West/Wadsworth.

Newsletters

Environmental Nutrition, Inc.
P.O. Box 420451
Palm Coast, FL 32142-0451
Phone: 1-800-829-5384

Nutrition Action Health Letter
Centers for Science in the Public Interest
1875 Connecticut Ave. NW, Suite 300
Washington, DC 20009-5728
Phone: 202-332-9110

Vegetarian Nutrition Health Letter
1711 Nichol Hall, School of Public Health
Loma Linda University
Loma Linda, CA 92350
Phone: 1-888-558-8703

Organizations

American Dietetic Association
216 West Jackson Blvd.
Chicago, IL 60606-6995
Phone: 1-800-877-1600
Web: http://www.eatright.org

Council for Responsible Nutrition
1300 19th Street NW, Suite 310
Washington, DC 20036-1609
Phone: 202-872-1488
Web: http://www.crnusa.org

Food and Drug Administration
5800 Fishers Lane
Rockville, MD 20857
Phone: 1-800-332-0178
Website: http://www.vm.cfsan.fda.gov

Mothers and Others for a Livable Planet
40 West 20th Street, 9th floor
New York, NY 10011
Phone: 212-242-0010 or 1-888-ECO-INFO
Web: http://www.mothers.org/mothers

Organic Consumers Association
6114 Highway 61
Little Marais, MN 55614
Phone: 218-726-1443
Web: http://www.purefood.org

Organic Trade Association
P.O. Box 1078
Greenfield, MA 01302
Phone: 413-774-7511
Web: http://www.ota.com

Union of Concerned Scientists
2 Brattle Square
Cambridge, MA 02238
Phone: 617-547-5552
Web: http://www.ucsusa.org

Websites

www.ConsumerLab.com This site was founded by a physician and former natural-products chemist from the FDA and is funded by private investors. It sponsors independent analyses of various supplements and reports on their ingredients and potency. Testing does not extend to evaluations of product efficacy or bioavailability.

www.cyberdiet.com This site offers support and counseling for those who are dieting.

www.navs-online.org Sponsored by the North American Vegetarian Society, this site offers information about planning healthy vegetarian diets.

www.dash.bwh.harvard.edu This site offers detailed information about the DASH diet.

www.eatright.org. This site is sponsored by the American Dietetic Association. It offers daily nutrition tips and answers questions about nutrition. You can also use this site to locate a dietitian near you.

www.fda.gov This is the official website of the Food and Drug Administration. It contains information about a wide range of topics related to foods, drugs, and medical devices.

www.ificinfo.health.org Maintained by the International Foods Information Council, this site provides information on science-based education programs addressing topics in food safety and nutrition.

www.LearnEducation.com BMI calculators can be obtained at this site.

www.mayohealth.org This site is sponsored by the Mayo Clinic. By clicking on "Nutrition," consumers can access nutrition topics, a library of Q and A's, and an on-line cookbook.

http://www.usda.gov/cnpp/dietary—guidelines.htm This USDA site includes information about the new *Dietary Guidelines for Americans,* 5th ed., plus healthy nutrition and diet recommendations formulated by government experts.

www.navigator.tufts.edu Maintained by Tufts University, this on-line rating and review guide is designed to help consumers sort through the myriad of nutrition information available on the Internet and find accurate, useful nutrition information.

www.niddk.nih.gov/health/nutrition/win.htm This site is maintained by the National Institute on Diabetes and Digestive and Kidney Diseases at the National Institutes of Health. It offers publications and videos about medically sound weight loss, as well as information about university-based weight-control programs.

www.shapeup.org This site, founded by the former surgeon general, C. Everett Koop, is the home site of a national program promoting safe, healthy weight loss through increased physical activity. It contains a library of materials related to BMI, weight control, and healthy recipes, as well as evaluations of commercial and noncommercial weight-loss programs.

www.soyfoods.com This is a commercial site sponsored by the Indiana Soybean Board. Although its stated purpose is to promote the consumption of soybeans, it does provide sound scientific information on the benefits of soy as well as guidelines for cooking with soy and links to vendors of commercial soy products.

www.usda.gov/cnpp At this USDA site, consumers can evaluate their diets interactively for fat, saturated fat, cholesterol, and sodium content and can compare them to recommendations from the Food Guide Pyramid. Consumers type in dietary information and receive a nutritional score.

www.veganet.com This site is maintained by the Vegetarian Awareness Network, a nonprofit educational, social service organization that advances public awareness of the benefits of a vegetarian lifestyle and assists consumers in making informed dietary decisions.

www.vrg.org The Vegetarian Resource Group is a non-profit organization dedicated to educating the public on vegetarianism and the interrelated issues of health, nutrition, ecology, ethics, and world hunger.

REFERENCES

Allison, D. B., Fontaine, K. R., Manson, J. E., Stevens, J., & VanItallie, T. B. (1999). Annual deaths attributable to obesity in the United States. *Journal of the American Medical Association, 282*(16), 1530–1538.

Allison, D. B., & Rha, S. S. (1998, July/August). Getting a feel for body mass index (BMI). *The Weight Control Digest,* 740–741.

American Dietetic Association. (1995). Biotechnology and the future of food-position of the American Dietetic Association. *Journal of the American Dietetic Association, 95*(12), 1429–1432.

American Dietetic Association. (2000). Position of the American Dietetic Association: Food irradiation. *Journal of the American Dietetic Association, 100*(2), 246–252.

American Institute for Cancer Research. (Spring 2000). The straight story on soy. Newsletter on Diet, Nutrition and Cancer prevention, p. 5.

Ausman, L. M. (1999). Criteria and recommendations for vitamin C intake. *Nutrition Reviews, 57*(7), 222–224.

Barrette, E. P. (2000). Metabolife 356 for weight loss. *Alternative Medicine Alert, 3*(1), 1–5.

Blackburn, G. L., & He, Y. H. (1999). The changing nature of obesity in the U.S.: How serious is the problem? *Nutrition and the M.D., 25*(6), 1.

Bray, G. A., & James, W. P. T. (Eds.). (1998). *Handbook of obesity.* New York: Marcel Dekker.

Brophy, B., & Schardt, D. (1999, April). Functional foods. *Nutrition Action Newsletter* [On-line]. Available: http://www.cspinet.org/nah/4_99/functional_foods.htm

BT corn pollen from Iowa fields kills Monarch caterpillars [On-line]. (2000, September) Available: http://www.ucsusa.org/

Center for Disease Control (2002). *Patterns of body weight in U.S. adults* [On-line]. Retrieved 8/26/02. Available: http://www.cdc.gov/nchs/releases/02facts/adultweight.htm

Cody, M. (1999, November). *Statement—FDA public meeting; Biotechnology for the year 2000 and beyond* [On-line]. Available: http://www.eatright.org

Cook, J. D., & Monsen, E. R. (1977). Vitamin C, the common cold, and iron absorption. *American Journal of Clinical Nutrition, 30,* 235–241.

Council on Scientific Affairs, American Medical Association. (1991). Biotechnology and the American agricultural industry. *Journal of the American Medical Association, 265*(11), 1429–1436.

CSPI Press Release. (2000, July 18). *FDA urged to halt sale of "functional foods" containing illegal ingredients* [On-line]. Available: http://www.cspinet.org/new/fda_funcfoods.html

DeLorgeril, M., Salen, P., Martin, J. L., Monjaud, I., Delaye, J., & Mamelle, N. (1999). Mediterranean diet, traditional risk factors, and the rate of cardiovascular complications after myocardial infarction; Final report of the Lyon heart study. *Circulation: Journal of the American Heart Association, 99*(6), 779–785.

Dietary supplement health and education act of 1994 (1995). [On-line]. Available: http://vm.cfsan.fda.gov/~dms/dietsupp.html

Douglas, R. M., Chalker, E. B., & Treacy, B. (1999). Vitamin C for preventing and treating the common cold. *The Cochran Library,* Issue 3. Oxford, England: Update Software. Available: http://www.medscape.com/cochran/abstracts/ab000980.html

Eades, M. R., & Eades, M. D. (1996). *Protein power.* New York: Bantam Books.

Eat fat, get thin? (2000). *University of California, Berkeley Wellness Letter, 16*(7), 1–3.

Eaton, B. (1988). *The paleolithic prescription.* London, England: Harper & Row.

Expert Panel of the AICR-WCRF Diet & Cancer Project. (1997, September). *Food, nutrition and the prevention of cancer: A global perspective* (pp. 1–660). Washington, DC: American Institute for Cancer Research.

Expert Panel of the AICR-WCRF Diet & Cancer Project. (1998, July). *Moving towards a plant-based diet: Menus and recipes for cancer prevention* (pp. 1–41). Washington, DC: American Institute for Cancer Research.

Fastats A to Z: Overweight prevalence [On-line]. (1999). Available: http://www.cdc.gov/nchs/fastats/overwt.htm

F-D-C Reports, Inc. (1997). *The Tan Sheet: Dietary supplement sales up 16% to approximately $10.3 bil.* Chevy Chase, MD: Author.

Flegal, K. M., Carroll, M. D., Kuczmarski, R. J., & Johnson, C. L. (1998). Overweight and obesity in the United States. *International Journal of Obesity and Related Metabolic Disorders, 22,* 39–47.

Food and Nutrition Board and Institute of Medicine. (2000). *Dietary reference intakes for vitamin C, vitamin E, selenium and carotenoids, a report of the panel on dietary antioxidants and related compounds.* Washington, DC: National Academy Press.

Fox, N. (1999, September). Another worry: Splicing antibiotic resistance into food. *The Green Guide,* p. 2.

Frost, G., Leeds, A., Trew, G., Margara, R., & Dornhurst, A. (1998). Insulin sensitivity in women at risk of coronary heart disease and the effect of a low glycemic diet. *Metabolism, 47*(10), 1245–51.

Gateway to government food safety information [On-line]. (2000). Available: http://www.FoodSafety.gov

Golub, C. (1999a). Heart-smart advice updated for 2000: More fat, but make it "mono," please. *Environmental Nutrition, 22*(7), 1–4.

Golub, C. (1999b). Making sense of the supplement scene: *EN* picks winners among multis. *Environmental Nutrition, 22*(11), 1, 4–5.

Goodman, M. T., Wilkins, L. R., Hankin, J. H., Lyu, L. C., Wu, A. H., & Kolonel, L. N. (1997). Association of soy and fiber consumption with the risk of endometrial cancer. *American Journal of Epidemiology, 146*(4), 294–306.

Grodner, M., Anderson, S. L., & DeYoung, S. (2000). *Foundations and clinical applications of nutrition, a nursing approach* (2nd ed.). St. Louis: Mosby.

Halaas, J. L., Gajiwala, M., Maffei, K. S., & Cohen, M. (1995). Weight reducing effects of the plasma protein encoded by the obese gene. *Science, 269*(5223), 543–546.

High-protein, low-carb diets: Do they really work? (2000, January). *Women's Health Advocate,* pp. 1–2, 7.

A history of victories over the FDA. (2000, March). *Life Extension,* p. 10.

Ikramuddin, A. (1999, October). Far afield: Biotech propaganda and the truth. *The Green Guide,* pp. 1–3.

Jacobs, R. A. (1999). Vitamin C. In M. E. Shils, J. A. Olson, M. Shike, & A. C. Ross (Eds.), *Modern nutrition in health and disease* (9th ed., pp. 467–483). New York: Williams and Wilkins.

Johnson, R. A., & Kennedy, E. (2000). The 2000 dietary guidelines for Americans: What are the changes and why were they made? *Journal of the American Dietetic Association, 100*(7), 769–774.

Judd, J. T., Clevidence, B. A., Muesing, R. A., Witts, J., Sunkin, M. E., & Podczasy, J. J., (1994). Dietary trans fatty acids: Effect on plasma lipids and lipoproteins of healthy women. *American Journal of Clinical Nutrition, 59*(4), 861–868.

Katan, M. B., Zock, P. L., Mensink, R. P., et al. (1994). Effects of fats and fatty acids on blood lipids in humans: An overview. *American Journal of Clinical Nutrition, 60*(6 suppl), 1017S–1022S.

Korkeila, M., Rissanen, A., Kaprio, J., Sorensen, T. I., & Koskenvuo, M. (1999). Weight-loss attempts and risk of major weight gain: A prospective study in Finnish adults. *American Journal of Clinical Nutrition, 70*(6), 965–975.

Krebs-Smith, S. M., Cook, A., Subar, A. F., Cleveland, L., & Friday, J. (1995). US adults fruit and vegetable intakes, 1989 to 1991: A revised baseline for the Healthy People 2000 objective. *American Journal of Public Health, 85,* 1623–1629.

Kriketos, A. D., Thompson, H. R., Greene, H., & Hill, J. O. (1999). (-)- hydroxycitric acid does not affect energy expenditure and substrate oxidation in adult males in a postabsorptive state. *International Journal of Obesity Related Metabolic Disorders, 23*(8), 867–873.

Lark, S. (2000, July). Boundless energy, part 1. *The Lark Letter,* pp. 1–3.

Lean, M. E., Han, T. S., & Seidell, J. C. (1998). Impairment of health and quality of life in people with large waist circumference. *The Lancet, 351*(9106), 853–856.

Lu, L. J., Anderson, K. E., Grady, J. J., Kohen, F., & Nagamani, M. (2000). Decreased ovarian hormones during a soya diet: Implications for breast cancer prevention. *Cancer Research, 60*(15), 4112–4121.

MacMahon, S. (1999). Blood pressure and the risk of cardiovascular disease. *New England Journal of Medicine, 342*(1), 50–52.

Margolis, S., & Cheskin, L. J. (1999). *Weight control.* New York: Medletter.

Margolis, S., Cheskin, L. J., & Wilder, L. B. (2000). *Nutrition and weight control for longevity.* New York: Medletter.

Marshall, E. (1999). *High-tech harvest: A look at genetically engineered foods.* Danbury, CT: Franklin Watts.

Mellon, M. (1997). Wholesome harvest. *Nucleus* [On-line], *19*(4). Available: http://www.ucsusa.org/Nucleus/97w.harvest.html

Meyer, K. A., Kushi, L. H., Jacobs, D. R., Slavin, J., & Sellers, T. A. (2000). Carbohydrates, dietary fiber and incident type 2 diabetes in older women. *American Journal of Clinical Nutrition, 71*(4), 921–930.

Must, A., Spandano, J., Coakley, E. H., Field, A. E., Colditz, G., & Dietz, W. H. (1999). The disease burden associated with overweight and obesity. *Journal of the American Medical Association, 282*(16), 1523–1529.

National Academy Press Food and Nutrition Board (1989). *Recommended dietary allowances* (10th ed.). Washington, DC: National Academy Press.

National Institutes of Health. (1994). *Optimal calcium intake.* NIH consensus statement. Bethesda, MD: Office of Medical Applications of Research.

Neville, K. (1999). "Worried about pesticides? *EN* offers advice to minimize risk. *Environmental Nutrition, 22*(8), 1, 6.

New study tarnishes chromium. (1999). *University of California, Berkeley Wellness Letter, 15*(9), 1–2.

ORAC of selected fruits and vegetables [On-line]. (2000). Available: http://www.hntc.tufts.edu/researchprograms/USDALabResProgDes/Oracchrt.html.

Ornish, D. (1996). *Dr. Dean Ornish's program for reversing heart disease.* New York: Ivy Books.

Pauling, L. (1980). Vitamin C therapy for advanced cancer [letter to the editor]. *New England Journal of Medicine, 302*(12), 694–695.

Pawling, G. P. (1999, September 18). Here's the skinny on contestants' weights: They are not normal. *Miss America News,* p. 3.

Pennington, J. A. (1998). *Bowes & Church's food values of portions commonly used* (17th ed.). Philadelphia: Lipincott.

Phytoestrogens—Hormones from plants (2000, February 7) [On-line]. Available: http://www.mayohealth.org/mayo/0002/htm/hormones.htm

Pritikin, N. (2000). *The Pritikin principle: The calorie density solution.* New York: Time Life.

Putnam, J. J., & Allshouse, J. E. (1997). Food consumption, prices, and expenditures, 1970–1997. *USDA Statistical Bulletin, 965,* 17–25.

Sears, B. (1995). *Enter the zone.* New York: HarperCollins.

Slavin, J. L., Martini, M. C., Jacobs, D. R., & Marquat, L. (1999). Plausible mechanisms for the protectiveness of whole grains. *American Journal of Clinical Nutrition, 70* (suppl), 463S–495S.

Smith-Warner, S. A., Spiegelman, D., Yuan, S., van den Brandt, P. A., Folsom, A. R., Goldbohm, R. A., Graham, S., Holmberg, L., Howe, G. R., Marshall, J. R., Miller, A. B., Potter, J. D., Speizer, F. E., Willett, W. C., Wolk, A., & Hunter, D. J. (1998). Alcohol and breast cancer in women. *Journal of the American Medical Association, 279*(7), 535–540.

Solfrizzi, V., Panza, F., Torres, F., Mastroanni, F., Del Parigi, A., Venezia, A., & Capruso, A. (1999). High monounsaturated fatty acids intake protects against age-related cognitive decline. *Neurology, 52*(8), 1563–1569.

Vitamin and nutritional supplements [On-line]. (1997). Available: http://www.mayohealth.org/mayo/9707/htm/me_jun97.htm

Washburn, S., Burke, G., & Morgan, T. (1999). Effect of soy protein supplementation on serum lipoproteins, blood pressure, and menopausal symptoms in perimenopausal women. *Menopause: The Journal of the North American Menopausal Society, 6*(1), 7–13.

Webb, D. (1999, February 16). Super foods that act like medicine. *Family Circle*, pp. 54–60.

Welland, D. (1999). Drink to good health, especially water: Here's why and how much. *Environmental Nutrition, 22*(10), 1, 6.

Westman, E. C., Yancy, W. S., Edman, J. S., Tomlin, K. F. & Perkins, C. E. (2002). Low carb diet reduced weight by 10% in 6-month study. *American Journal of Medicine 113*(1), 30–36.

Whitney, E., Cataldo, C., & Rolfes, S. (1998). *Understanding normal and clinical nutrition* (5th ed.). San Francisco, CA: West/Wadsworth.

Yanovski, J. A., & Yanovski, S. Z. (1999). Recent advances in basic obesity research. *Journal of the American Medical Association, 282*(16), 1504–1506.

Zock, P. L., & Katan, M. B. (1997). Butter, margarine, and serum lipoproteins. *Atherosclerosis, 131*(1), 7–16.

4

Substance Abuse and Dependence

Elaine R. Feeney

Objectives

1. Identify seven theories of substance abuse causation.
2. Describe the difference between substance abuse and substance dependence.
3. Identify five risk factors for substance abuse and substance dependence that are specific to females.
4. State three unique ways in which substance abuse/dependence impacts women psychosocially.
5. Compare and contrast physiological and social differences between males and females that lead to differences in reactions to substances of abuse.
6. Describe the treatment for each category of drug and the signs and symptoms of withdrawal.
7. Describe brief intervention and identify one possible variable that may facilitate or restrict the success of this intervention among women.
8. Discuss the need for ongoing support, the appropriateness and availability of such support in the community, and available alternatives.

Introduction

One of the most prevalent myths about substance abuse is that it is primarily a male problem. We are bombarded daily with media images that reinforce this perception, such as images of young men bloodied from bar fights and drug-related shootings or men nodding off in filthy rooms with tourniquets in place and needles in their arms. Images of intoxicated males as perpetrators in vehicular homicide or domestic abuse are also all too common. The public face of drug and alcohol abuse masks the fact that they are common problems for women as well as men, often with even more devastating consequences. The public is generally not aware that women abuse some substances at a higher rate than men and that, although the incidence of cocaine and alcohol abuse is declining in men, it is rising in women. The public is unaware also that women become addicted to alcohol and other drugs more easily than men and develop serious physical consequences more rapidly. Alcohol, tobacco, and other commonly abused drugs act on the physiological mechanisms in all body systems. For example, they affect neurotransmitters and other elements in the central nervous system, cardiovascular system, and respiratory system and impair digestive processes and hormone activity. The social consequences of drug and alcohol abuse are at least as devastating for women as men and are often more so, due to different behavioral expectations for the two genders. The purpose of this chapter is to provide an overview of the problem of addiction in American society, to explore in depth the phenomena related to addiction in women, and to describe strategies for preventing and treating substance abuse in women.

Background

The problems associated with substance abuse and dependence have been a matter of record since biblical times. Historically, drunkenness and, more recently, the abuse of other mind-altering chemicals have been seen as a *moral and legal issue*. Over time, however, this morally judgmental attitude has not proved effective in producing a change in the behavior of substance-abusing individuals, except in very select circumstances. Fortunately, drug and alcohol abuse are now coming to be viewed as *diseases*, rather than evidence of moral degeneracy.

The earliest indication that a change was occurring in the way substance abuse/dependence was being viewed was in the area of alcohol dependence. The change involved conceptualizing alcohol dependence as a disease rather than as a moral issue. The first known reference to alcohol dependence as a disease was made in 1785 by **Benjamin Rush,** a Philadelphia physician. In the same year, **Thomas Trotter,** a British physician, also claimed that alcoholism is a disease (Blum & Payne, 1991). It was not until 1960, though, that the first scientific document describing alcoholism as a disease was written.

Although much research is currently being conducted that involves addictive substances other than alcohol, the preponderance of research is still focused on alcohol. This may be due to the relative ease of studying the abuse/dependence of a substance that is easily obtainable and has no inherent legal problems associated with it. The fact that alcohol is still the most abused substance in the United States (National Institute for Drug Abuse, 1999a) may demand attention that the use of other addictive substances does not demand.

Definition of Terms

Among the terms used in this chapter are *substance dependence, substance abuse, addiction,* and *substance use.* Healthcare providers rely on the *Diagnostic and Statistical Manual of Mental Disorders,* 4th edition (*DSM-IV*) (American Psychiatric Association, 1994) for guidance in diagnosing and treating substance abuse and substance dependence. The criteria for the diagnosis of substance abuse and the diagnosis of substance dependence are different in terms of severity of the consequences of substance use and the degree of control over such use. *Lack of control* over use and the requirement of gradually increasing amounts of the substance to achieve the desired effect (**tolerance**) are the hallmarks of *substance dependence.* Social and other problems related to substance use but not associated with lack of control or tolerance are usually seen as evidence of *substance abuse* (American Psychiatric Association, 1994).

In this chapter, the term *addiction* is used synonymously with the term *substance dependence,* and the term *substance use* is defined as the use of any substance of abuse. The term *substance abuse* is used to represent the *DSM-IV* description of the phenomenon.

The terms *binge* and *heavy* are usually used in conjunction with alcohol use. A binge use of alcohol refers to the ingestion of five or more alcoholic drinks at one occasion during the past 30 days. The "heavy use of alcohol" refers to the ingestion of five or more alcoholic drinks at five or more occasions during the past 30 days. These terms are from the National Household Surveys of 1995 and 1996 (Substance Abuse and Mental Health Services Administration, 2000).

Theories of Causation

In the field of substance abuse/dependence, a number of theories explain the cause of substance abuse/dependence and delineate approaches to the treatment of affected individuals. Brower, Blow, and Beresford (1989) provide a description of the theories of causation as the moral model, learning model, disease model, self-medication model, and social model. Others include the biopsychosocial model (Group for the Advancement of Psychiatry Committee on Alcoholism and the Addictions, 1991), and the public health model (Leavell & Clark, 1965; Westermeyer, 1987).

The Moral Model

The moral model consists of concepts such as moral weakness, lack of willpower, evil character, temptations, religious concepts, punishment, amends, responsibility, and consequences. This model was widely accepted for many years and is still in use today. Several of the **Alcoholics Anonymous (AA)** 12 steps (listed below) reflect these concepts:

- Made a decision to turn our wills and lives over to the care of God, as we understood Him;
- Made a searching and fearless moral inventory of ourselves;
- Admitted to God, to ourselves, and to another human being the exact nature of our wrongs;
- Were entirely ready to have God remove all these defects of character;
- Humbly asked Him to remove our shortcomings;
- Made direct amends to such people, wherever possible, except when to do so would injure them or others;
- Continued to take personal inventory and when we were wrong, promptly admitted it;
- Sought through prayer and meditation to improve our conscious contact with God, as we understood him, praying only for knowledge of his will for us and the power to carry it out. (Alcoholics Anonymous World Services, 1976, p. 59)

For more information on the 12 steps, Alcoholics Anonymous World Services publishes a number of volumes and pamphlets to aid in understanding.

The Learning Model

According to the learning model, substance abuse/ dependence is a consequence of an individual's having learned *maladaptive* habits and attitudes. Therefore, substance abuse can be overcome via *new learning* in the areas of self-control, coping skills, etc. **Moderation management (MM)**, a self-help program, uses many of the concepts included in the learning model and can be viewed as an alternative to Alcoholics Anonymous. However, MM was recently dealt a tremendous blow from which it may not recover; its founder, Audrey Kishline, was sentenced to 4½ years in prison after being convicted of driving while intoxicated and causing the deaths of two individuals in a car crash (Ashton, 2000).

The Disease Model

The disease model, developed by Jellinek (1960), has been embraced by the healthcare community with varying levels of enthusiasm. The "disease" alcoholism has been described as chronic and progressive, as marked by periods of exacerbation and remission, and as having predictable stages. Jellinek (1960) also drew parallels between the physiopathological changes caused by alcohol and those caused by the prolonged use of other drugs, such as morphine, cocaine, and barbiturates. It is important to note that Jellinek conducted his investigations on white males in AA. Females were not represented in any of the early studies of addiction.

The Self-Medication Model

The self-medication model deals with concepts such as coexisting mental disorders, mental functioning, psychotherapy, pharmacotherapy, and diagnosis and treatment. Dependent individuals are assumed to be suffering from an *underlying disorder*, such as, depression or anxiety, and to be using addictive substances as a means of easing their *symptoms*.

The Social Model

The social model involves concepts and constructs such as environment, society, role function, coping, social supports, social skills, and social problems. In a sense, it is similar to the learning model in that coping skills are taught. However, the social model views the surroundings of the individual, or the context in which the substance use occurs, as the major factor contributing to addiction. Poverty, isolation, and social disadvantages are viewed as direct causes of a number of social ills, including addiction.

The Biopsychosocial Model

Since the early 1990s, the biopsychosocial model (Group for the Advancement of Psychiatry Committee, 1991) has received considerable attention. Wallace (1990) used this model in designing a strategy for relapse prevention among cocaine addicts. This model implies the presence of multiple factors contributing to substance abuse. Genetic and other biological factors, psychological factors, and social factors are considered together in the development of substance abuse and dependence. Although the term *biopsychosocial* was first used in the early 1990s, the conceptual basis is as old as the beginnings of the scientific study of alcoholism. In Jellinek's (1946) study of AA members, he identified a number of interacting factors related to the development of alcoholism. These factors involved inherited characteristics, early life experiences and responses, educational level, social experiences (including education and marital experiences), and cultural influences. Later, his view of alcoholism was revised to the disease concept, whereby the cause was seen as physiological (Jellinek, 1960).

The Public Health Model

The original public health model (see Figure 4–1) was developed by Leavell and Clark (1965). It conceptualizes addictions as related to three factors: the *host*, the *agent*, and the *environment*. Westermeyer (1987) refined the model by addressing more fully the interactions among the three factors.

According to Westermeyer's conceptualization, independent factors are associated with each component of the model. **Host** factors include all the attributes of the individual: sex, race, ethnicity, genetic or biological makeup, psychological makeup, and so on. The **agent** is the nature of the substance being ingested: its solubility, half-life, pharmacodynamics (what the drug does to the body, such as action, effects, and addicting power), and pharmacokinetics (what the body does to the drug in terms of metabolism, excretion, detoxification, and so on). The **environment** is the cultural, social, economic, and community context in which the drug use occurs. An example of the application of this model can be seen in the consideration of epidemiology and the risk factors related to addiction. Alcohol, in itself, is not a strongly addictive substance, considering the number of individuals who ingest it without experiencing any of the signs and symptoms of dependence. However, if an individual has a strong genetic or biological predisposition to a dependence on alcohol, the chances of this substance's being addictive to the individual are increased. If environmental factors facilitate the use of alcohol in such an individual, her chances of experiencing alcohol dependence are increased further. With a highly addictive substance such as crack cocaine, minimal genetic predisposition or environmental facilitating factors are required for dependence on this substance to occur.

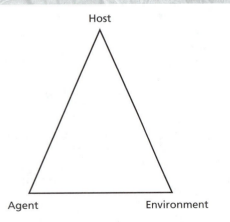

Figure 4–1   Public Health Model

Host

Agent

Environment

Some other theories of causation are the neurobiological theory, genetic theory, personality theory, psychoanalytic theory, systems theory, and economic theory (Allen, 1996), but their concepts and assumptions seem to be based on the models already discussed in this section.

Epidemiology

The study of substance abuse and dependence in women is a recent event in science. The early research and treatment of substance dependence were directed toward men. This may have been in part the result of differences in the socialization of men and women. Two classic works by Naegle (1988) and Gomberg (1989) highlighted the emergence of substance dependence among women into the public consciousness. Both authors indicated that, because of the immediate post–World War II ethic, in which women were seldom seen working outside the home, the economic and social consequences of alcohol dependence were not seen as easily in women as in men. Public drinking by men was accepted, but drinking, especially to excess, by women was stigmatized. As a result, alcohol- and drug-dependent women drank and used their drugs at home, and their substance-abuse problems were overlooked or hidden. This changed, somewhat, with the advent and growth of the **feminist movement.** Women went to work outside of the home, began demanding equality, and became more visible, and the double standard regarding gender-appropriate behavior became less stringent, although it remained.

In reports of the prevalence of substance abuse (see Table 4–1), cocaine use continuously dropped for males each year from 1985 to 1995, with the exception of a 0.5 percent increase from 1990 to 1991 and a 1 percent increase from 1992 to 1993. Although cocaine use by females was reported by 7.9 percent of those interviewed in 1985 and 1995, the use of this substance *increased for females* 0.5 percent each year until 1990, when it remained at 8.7 to 8.9 percent until 1993, when use began to taper off. The use of cocaine by females was reported by 8.4 percent of the respondents in 1993 and 8.2 percent in 1994 (Office of Applied Studies, 1996).

Of particular interest are the statistics regarding binge drinking. For males, there has been a significant decline in binge drinking since 1985, but there is no statistical significance to any change in binge drinking for females over the same period. In 1996, however, both males and females reported a statistically greater risk of having four or five drinks nearly every day, when compared with the responses in 1994. Adding to the confusion is that the percentages of males and females reporting great risk of having five or more drinks once or twice a week were significantly lower in 1996 than in 1994.

It has been known for some time that women use psychotropic drugs at a greater rate than men, but only recently has research been conducted to examine whether this extends

TABLE 4–1 Percentage of people reporting the use of substances by gender and types of substance (among respondents age 12 and older): 1985, 1995, and 1998.

		Lifetime Use		Past Year Use		Past Month Use		Past Month Use
		1985	1995	1985	1995	1985	1995	1998
Any illicit drug	Females	30.1	29.8	13.3	8.7[a]	9.5	4.5[a]	4.5
	Males	39.0	39.1	19.7	12.9[a]	14.9	7.8[a]	8.1
Marijuana	Females	24.5	26.8	10.2	6.5[a]	7.1	3.3[a]	3.5
	Males	34.7	35.6	17.2	10.5[a]	12.6	6.2[a]	6.7
Cocaine	Females	7.9	7.9	3.6	1.2[a]	2.1	0.4[a]	0.5
	Males	14.7	12.8	6.8	2.3[a]	3.9	1.1[a]	1.1
Alcohol	Females	80.7	79.2	68.2	61.1[a]	52.0	45.1[a]	45.1
	Males	89.6	85.8	78.0	70.1[a]	69.2	60.1[a]	58.7
Binge alcohol	Females	——	——	——	——	9.8	8.5	8.6
	Males	——	——	——	——	31.6	23.8[a]	23.2
Heavy alcohol	Females	——	——	——	——	3.2	2.1[a]	2.4
	Males	——	——	——	——	13.8	9.4[a]	9.7
Cigarettes	Females	71.6	66.9	36.2	29.5[a]	34.5	26.8[a]	25.7[b]
	Males	85.1	77.1[a]	45.3	34.6[a]	43.4	31.1[a]	29.7

Source: Adapted from U.S. Department of Health and Human Services, Public Health Service, Substance Abuse and Mental Health Services Administration (SAMHSA), Office of Applied Studies, National Household Survey on Drug Abuse (1995); *National household survey on drug abuse, preliminary data* [On-line]. Available: http://www.samhsa.gov/retrieved June 26, 2000.
[a]Difference between 1985 and 1995 is statistically significant at $p > .05$ level.
[b]Difference between 1995 and 1998 is statistically significant at $p > .05$ level.

to the use of prescription drugs that have the potential for abuse. A recent study by Simoni-Wastila (2000) revealed that women are 48 percent more likely than men to use prescription drugs with the potential for abuse. This study controlled for a number of confounding variables, such as demographics, health status, economic status, and diagnosis. As with any study, a number of questions need to be answered, not the least of which is, how and why is this happening?

Substance Use During Pregnancy

A study of women who delivered children during a 10-month period in 1992–1993 revealed that more than an estimated 5 percent of those pregnant women used illicit drugs during their pregnancy (National Institute for Drug Abuse, 1999b). The consequences of alcohol and other drug use among pregnant women are especially serious, in that they affect not only the health of the woman but fetal

health and development as well. Alcohol and other drug use on the part of a pregnant woman can cause her to develop anemia, thrombocytopenia (a blood disorder), and hypertension (high blood pressure). The consequences to the fetus can be even more severe. Miscarriage (spontaneous abortion), ectopic, or tubal, pregnancy, and stillbirth can occur. The children who survive intrauterine drug exposure can experience low birth weight, immature or poorly developed body systems, small head circumference, and other temporary or permanent impairments (National Institute for Drug Abuse, 1999b). These statistics do not include the most devastating consequence of substance use during pregnancy, the use of alcohol and its relationship to **fetal alcohol syndrome (FAS)** (FAS Community Resource Center, 1999).

Fetal alcohol syndrome (FAS) is a group of physical and mental birth defects that are the direct result of the consumption of alcohol by a woman while pregnant. Alcohol affects the child by crossing the placenta into the child's bloodstream, impairing normal intrauterine development. *Alcohol has more deleterious effects on the developing fetus than any* other known substance, even crack cocaine (FAS Community Resource Center, 1999), and these effects are irreversible. FAS affects nearly 2 infants out of 1,000 born in North America (FAS Community Resource Center, 1999). Infants born with FAS have a small head and body, a characteristic facial appearance, and brain damage. FAS is the leading known cause of **mental retardation.** Care for FAS children is extremely expensive. The cost of caring for one FAS child over her lifetime is $1.4 million (National Organization on Fetal Alcohol Syndrome, 1999).

The impairment of fetal development does not always take the extreme form of FAS, however. **Fetal alcohol effects (FAE)** is a less obvious developmental impairment of the fetus caused by alcohol ingestion by the pregnant mother. FAE usually manifests itself in behavioral and mental problems. Affected individuals are not able to understand the connection between their behavior and related consequences (National Organization on Fetal Alcohol Syndrome, 1999). Attention deficits are also noted in FAE children (FAS Community Resource Center, 1999). In addition, **alcohol-related birth defects (ARBD),** such as heart defects, vision and auditory problems, and joint problems, and **alcohol-related neurological disorders (ARND)** can also include obsessive/compulsive disorder, in addition to the attention and behavior deficits (FAS Community Resource Center, 1999). One out of every 100 babies have some degree of disability related to alcohol ingestion by the mother during her pregnancy (FAS, FAE, ARBD, or ARND) (FAS Community Resource Center, 1999). Perhaps the most alarming fact related to FAS and the associated anomalies is that *there is no agreement on the amount of alcohol needed to cause any of these syndromes* (Bradley, Badrinath, Bush, Boyd-Wickizer, & Anawalt, 1998; National Organization on Fetal Alcohol Syndrome, 1999). In some instances, the consumption of *any* alcohol by a pregnant woman can cause FAS. It seems that the threshold beyond which alcohol brings about impaired fetal development is different for each woman and each pregnancy. It is recommended that pregnant women avoid alcohol altogether; in fact, it is advisable for any woman who plans to get pregnant to begin *avoiding alcohol before attempting to conceive* (Bradley et al., 1998).

Despite public education initiatives regarding the effect of alcohol on a developing fetus, women continue to consume alcohol during pregnancy. In a report by the Substance Abuse and Mental Health Administration (2000), 16.1 percent of the 69.4 percent of women who reported using any alcohol in the past month were pregnant, as were 1.6 percent of the 15 percent who reported binge alcohol use and 0.5 percent of the 3.5 percent who reported heavy alcohol use (defined as drinking five or more drinks per occasion on five or more days in the previous 30 days) (*National Household Survey on Drug Abuse,* 1995; 1996).

Cocaine preparations (especially crack cocaine) used by a pregnant woman cross the placenta and enter the fetus's bloodstream, causing physical and neural problems in the newborn. These **crack babies** are born underdeveloped, with a number of other abnormalities, such as brain hemorrhage, generalized edema (swelling), and congenital anomalies (birth defects). Some are **stillborn** or die shortly after birth. Those who do survive may experience impaired vision, hearing, and language ability, in addition to behavior problems (Church, Crossland, Holmes, Overbeck, & Tilak, 1998). Other researchers have also identified maternal crack cocaine use as a primary factor in negative neonatal outcomes (Datta-Bhutada, Johnson, & Rosen, 1998; Eyler, Behnke, Conlon, Woods, & Wobie, 1998); however, other factors have also been identified such as maternal age, poor relationships on the part of the mother, and marijuana use (Datta-Bhutada et al., 1998; Richardson & Day, 1994). The fact that women who use crack cocaine are often members of the lowest socioeconomic group has led other researchers to suggest that there may be social and economic factors that contribute to the crack baby phenomenon, such as poor or no prenatal care, poor maternal diet, poor parenting skills, and lack of education (Church et al., 1998; Eyler et al., 1998; LaGasse, Seifer, & Lester, 1999; Litt, & McNeil, 1997; Lyons & Ritter, 1998).

When a pregnant woman is dependent on **opiates** (such as heroin), the drug crosses the placenta into the fetus's bloodstream, resulting in retarded intrauterine growth. More important, the *fetus becomes addicted to opiates as well.* **Detoxification** of the neonate must be initiated at birth. The drug phenobarbitone is used to manage withdrawal symptoms (Vance, Chant, Tudehope, Gray, & Hayes, 1997). Despite the initial problems these infants experience at birth, research has shown that, by their first birthday, many have made up their growth deficits (Vance et al., 1997), but they continue to demonstrate mildly impaired psychomotor development (Bunikowski et al., 1998).

Although the risk to the fetus is great and consequences to the parents and child are grave in psychosocial and economic terms, too little is being done to identify the women at risk for having a child affected by substance abuse. A study conducted in Chapel Hill, North Carolina, demonstrated that the rate at which women at risk are identified can be increased through the use of improved *screening tools.* Rather than asking questions about drug use that could be answered with a simple "yes" or "no," Clark, Dawson, & Martin (1999) asked respondents how *frequently* they used tobacco, alcohol, and other drugs. The experimental screening tool increased the identification of pregnant women at risk for a less than optimum outcome of the pregnancy due to smoking and/or alcohol use from 21 percent to 72 percent, any drug use from 12 percent to 18 percent, and alcoholism/drug addiction from 0 percent to 6 percent (Clark et al., 1999). These alarming statistics are only frightening when one considers the lack of attention given to the problem of alcohol, tobacco and other drug use during pregnancy.

Risk Factors for Substance Abuse and Dependence

Risk factors are elements that predispose an individual to the abuse or dependence of alcohol or other drugs. Some risk factors can be controlled; others cannot. The most widely accepted factors that place an individual at risk for substance abuse and dependence are described in the following sections. As with other areas of research involving abuse and dependence, the risk factors for alcohol abuse/dependence have been the most widely studied.

Ethnicity

The National Institute for Drug Abuse (1999a) reports that the tendency toward drinking differs among the various ethnic groups. Fewer African American women (54 percent) than Euro-American women (66 percent) drink alcohol, and, when alcohol abuse/dependence has been studied, it has been found that women of both groups suffer in equal proportions. The types of problems, however, have been found to be different. African American women experience *more physical health problems* related to alcohol intake, whereas Euro-American women experience *more psychosocial problems.* Hispanic women have been described as "infrequent drinkers, or abstainers" (National Institute for Drug Abuse, 1999a). However, age seems to be a confounding factor, in that moderate and/or heavy drinking has been seen in younger, American-born Hispanic women.

Predisposing or Co-Occurring Psychiatric Disorders

The reasons for substance abuse and dependence are more complex for females than for males (National Institute for Drug Abuse, 1999a). Hence, attention to risk factors may play a more important role in prevention and treatment for women. Women usually begin using drugs later in life than men, and their use usually follows a breakdown of *protective factors,* such as family protection, individual coping skills, and environmental controls. There may be an increase in fears, anxiety, and a history of poor interpersonal relationships (National Institute for Drug Abuse, 1999b).

The National Institute for Drug Abuse (1999b) reports that as many as 70 percent of all women in substance-abuse treatment experienced **childhood sexual abuse.** This does not mean that 70 percent were raped or experienced sexual penetration as children, but the fact that these women were still recalling experiences they were unable to consent to (fondling, unwelcome kissing, and sexual intercourse) indicates the potential consequences of any form of sexual abuse.

Gil-Rivas, Fiorentine, and Anglin (1996) found that childhood sexual abuse and other physical abuse are related to symptoms of post-traumatic stress disorder (PTSD). However, they also found that the prognosis for the recovery of women experiencing these symptoms is not worse than for men. Although PTSD is not always linked to childhood sexual abuse, the appearance of PTSD as a co-occurring diagnosis among women seeking substance-abuse treatment is not unusual. The National Institute for Drug Abuse (1999b) reports that women diagnosed with PTSD are 17 times more likely to experience major substance-abuse problems than are women with no PTSD diagnosis. In the same report, the National Institute for Drug Abuse (1999b) indicates there is a strong relationship between eating disorders (particularly binge eating) and substance abuse.

Loss

One significant risk factor for substance abuse, particularly alcohol abuse, is loss of social or cultural role. The loss of the role of wife through divorce or death, the loss of the role of mother due to the death of child or the child's leaving home, and the loss of the role of worker through layoff, dismissal, or retirement are all related to an increased risk for alcohol abuse and resulting alcohol-related problems. The resulting damage to self-esteem and self-worth is more involved than simply the loss of a love object. In many cases, it is the loss of the role offered by the love object that causes the most grief. For example, certainly the loss of a child is devastating to a woman, but the woman is mourning not only the loss of the child but also the loss of her role as mother to that child (National Institute for Drug Abuse, 1999b).

Elective abortion can also be conceptualized as involving a loss of some type, whether loss of role, love object, or self-esteem. Elective abortion has recently been closely associated with subsequent substance abuse; those aborting their first pregnancy are four to five times more likely than the general population to demonstrate substance abuse (Reardon & Ney, 2000).

Other Psychosocial Risk Factors

Women who do not work outside of the home are at greater risk for alcohol problems than women who do. In fact, the multiple roles that pose such a challenge to women seem to constitute a protective factor regarding alcohol abuse. In addition, women who have never married, who are divorced or separated, or who are living with a partner to whom they are not married run a greater risk of developing alcohol abuse or dependence (National Institute for Drug Abuse, 1999a). The risk of other drug use (particularly cocaine) is increased for women who are living with a drug-using male. The attempt to maintain or develop an intimate relationship with a drug-using male seems to mandate that the woman use the drug as well (National Institute for Drug Abuse, 1999b).

Genetic Factors

Until recently, evidence of genetic factors involved in substance use, abuse, and dependence was gathered through the study of twins and the adoption of twins into different families (Cadoret, Troughton, & O'Gorman, 1987; Cloninger, Christiansen, Reich, & Gotteman, 1978). The researchers sought to determine whether the genetic or environmental influences on the development of alcohol dependence could be identified. Because identical twins have an identical genetic makeup, if their alcohol dependence was caused by genetic factors alone, the appearance of alcoholism in one twin would naturally result in the alcoholism in the other twin, whether or not the twins lived together with their biological families or were adopted into different families. These early studies found that genetic influences seemed stronger for males than females for the development of substance abuse and dependence.

More recent research calls into question the methodology of earlier studies and highlights the difficulties of this type of research. Nevertheless, Van den Bree, Johnson, Neale, and Pickens (1998) used more sophisticated statistical procedures but obtained results similar to those of the earlier studies; they found that **men** demonstrate very strong **genetic** influence in the development of substance abuse and dependence, whereas, women are more influenced by environmental factors. **Environmental** factors, such as parental substance abuse, the use of substances of abuse by peers, the availability of such substances, sexual and other abuse, and co-occurring psychiatric diagnoses. Incidentally, the same environmental influences were found to result in substance use by males, but it was the genetic influence that determined whether this recreational use developed into abuse or dependence. A similar study, conducted two years earlier using different methodology, offered an explanation for the gender-based differences in genetic influence. Cadoret, Yates, Troughton, Woodworth, and Stewart (1996) found that **female** twin subjects who were adopted at birth demonstrated a strength of genetic influences similar to that of **males** when the methodology included an examination of **additional variables.** For example, aggressiveness or antisocial personality on the part of the biological parent seem to be linked to female substance abuse and dependence, and these female offspring are usually found to have conduct disorders themselves. This is a new area of study that deserves attention. It may be that the antisocial personality disorder of the biological parents is part of the genetic package for women that predisposes them to substance abuse/dependence. The fact that these women were **adopted** at birth eliminates the possibility that parental aggressiveness and antisocial personality are *environmental* influences.

Another study of female twins suggests that there may be two sets of genetic risk factors that influence substance use: one set influencing the initiation of substance use and the other influencing misuse. This research suggests also that family environment has an impact on the *initiation* of substance use, but not on the development of substance abuse or dependence (Kendler, Dardowski, Corey, Prescott, & Neale, 1999).

With the advent of newer technology, genetic studies are being conducted that are identifying the more complex and specific components of inherited predisposition to substance abuse/dependence. Vanyukov et al. (1998) have discovered that the **DRD5 gene** may be the origin of one sex-related predisposing factor to substance abuse and dependence among women. These are exciting findings and invite future scientists to join in the search for the genetic contribution to addiction.

It is important to bear in mind that a genetic predisposition to addiction does *not* make it inevitable that the individual will become an addict. The public health model of addiction suggests that the environment plays a very important role in determining whether substance abuse or dependence develops. If environmental factors provide protective mechanisms against substance use, then the genetic impact is mediated. If, however, the environment fosters or allows for substance use, the genetic predisposition to addiction may be translated into actual addiction. For example, marriage or a committed, long-term relationship is a strong protective factor that has been found to lessen the impact of a genetic predisposition to alcohol abuse/dependence (National Institute for Drug Abuse, 1999b).

Gateway Drugs

Gateway drugs are drugs that lead to the use of other drugs (Witters, Venturelli, & Hanson, 1992). Inherent in this definition is that the gateway drug is the first substance of abuse to which the individual is exposed. The major gateway drug for females is cigarettes; for males, it is alcohol (National Institute for Drug Abuse, 1999a). It is not known why this difference exists.

Classification of Substances of Abuse

Table 4–2 lists the effects and symptoms of overdose and withdrawal associated with general categories and agents of substances of abuse/dependence. The categories covered are **narcotics, depressants, stimulants, hallucinogens,** and **inhalants.** It is important to note that the signs and symptoms of overdose reflect the effect the agent has on the lower centers of the brain which control respiration, heart action, and autonomic nervous system activity. Logically, the signs and symptoms of withdrawal are almost always the opposite of the effects of the agent.

TABLE 4–2 Substances of abuse/dependence: their effects and symptoms of overdose and withdrawal.

Agent	Effects	Overdose	Withdrawal
Narcotics (morphine, heroin, and other opiates, prescription sleeping pills, and pain relievers)	Euphoria, drowsiness, respiratory depression, constricted pupils, nausea	Slow and shallow breathing, clammy skin, convulsions, coma, death	Watery eyes, runny nose, yawning, loss of appetite, irritability, tremors, panic, abdominal cramps, nausea, chills, excessive sweating
Depressants (alcohol, tranquilizers)	Slurred speech, disorientation, drunken behavior (may be present with or without odor of alcohol)	Shallow respirations, clammy skin, dilated pupils, weak and rapid pulse, coma, death	Anxiety, insomnia, tremors, excitability, delirium, convulsions, death (alcohol)
Stimulants (caffeine, amphetamines, some appetite suppressants, certain nasal decongestants)	Hyperalertness, excitation, euphoria, increased pulse and blood pressure, insomnia, loss of appetite	Agitation, increase in body temperature, hallucinations, convulsions, death	Apathy, long periods of sleep, irritability, depression, disorientation
Hallucinogens (LSD, marijuana and cannabis, peyote mushrooms, other peyote preparations)	Illusions and hallucinations, poor perception of time and distance, euphoria, possible increase in appetite, disorientation	Longer, more intense "trip" episodes; psychosis; paranoia; death	Cannabis—insomnia, hyper-activity, decreased appetite, possible violence; other hallucinogens—no symptoms reported
Inhalants (amyl nitrate, gasoline and other petroleum-based products, nitrous oxide, airplane glue, aerosol propellants)	Euphoria, headaches, nausea, fainting, stupor, rapid heartbeat	Lung, liver, kidney, and/or bone marrow damage; suffocation; choking; anemia; stroke; sudden death	Insomnia, increased appetite, depression, irritability, headache

Sources: Adapted from NIDA web site—http://www.nida.nih.gov; and Witters, W., Venturelli, P., & Hanson, G. *Drugs and society* (3rd ed). Copyright 1992. Jones & Bartlett Publishers, Sudbury, MA. www.jbpub.com. Reprinted with permission.

The Unique Psychosocial Impact of Substance Abuse/ Dependence on Women

When viewed from a psychosocial perspective, women have more frequent and more severe problems associated with substance abuse than men. Female substance abusers have more frequent psychiatric hospitalizations; more of a family history of psychiatric problems, including substance abuse; and more frequent visits to mental health clinics (Davis & DiNitto, 1996). Male substance abuse is often viewed as a factor contributing to the physical abuse of females. Although this is certainly true, Wilson et al. (1996) found an association between the abuse of females and substance abuse on the part of the victim herself. This controversial finding bears further examination, with other contributing factors deserving of further study as well.

Although substance abuse is strongly related to a high risk of divorce for both genders (Fu & Goldman, 2000), the risk of becoming impoverished as a consequence of divorce is greater for women than men. Even when poverty is not a direct consequence, the resulting impact of divorce on children is significant. Children whose parents are divorced are more likely to lack coping and social skills, and to use substances of abuse than children whose parents are not divorced (Hoffmann, 1995; Neher & Short, 1998). Because more mothers are awarded custody of children in divorce proceedings, any problematic behavior on the part of children most directly impacts the female parent. It seems clear that negotiating the demands of everyday life is more of a challenge for female substance abusers than for their male counterparts.

Role of Physiological, Sex-Based Differences in Substance Abuse/Dependence

The characteristics, progression, and impact of drug abuse and addiction differ in the two sexes. For example, women may develop a full-blown addiction to certain illicit drugs more rapidly than men. Heavy alcohol use may also have much more severe consequences for women than for men (National Institute for Drug Abuse, 1999b). Women who consume 2 to 2.9 alcoholic drinks daily have been seen to increase their relative risk of death significantly. In contrast, the relative risk of death does not increase significantly for men until daily consumption reaches 4 standard drinks daily (Bradley et al., 1998). Other consequences of substance abuse in women include an increased risk for reproductive problems; spontaneous abortion; gastrointestinal, cardiovascular, and neurological diseases; and certain cancers (Center on Addiction & Substance Abuse, 1993; National Institute for Drug Abuse, 1999a, National Institute for Drug Abuse, 1999b; Wartenberg & Liepman, 1990).

Bradley et al. (1998) also found an increased risk of injury, fatal injury and bone fractures. Interestingly, the researchers found that heavy alcohol consumption *increases* bone density among postmenopausal women. A related finding was that postmenopausal women who drink heavily and take estrogen replacement therapy have up to three times the serum estrogen levels of women who take estrogen and do not drink heavily. Because estrogen contributes to the maintenance of bone density, it does not appear that the increased fracture rate among postmenopausal women is related to osteoporosis. However, there is some evidence that premenopausal women who drink heavily may be predisposed to develop osteoporosis later in life. Bradley et al. (1998) also reported that women substance abusers have a greater risk of developing HIV/AIDS, as well as infertility (especially tubal disease), ovulatory dysfunction, and endometriosis. Dysmenorrhea (painful menstrual periods), premenstrual disorders, and psychiatric comorbidity (the presence of psychiatric problems in addition to drug abuse) were also found more frequently among heavy drinkers (Bradley et al., 1998). Interestingly, imbibing only one alcoholic drink daily can increase the chance of developing breast cancer, and the risk increases with increased consumption. Of course, because estrogen has been found to contribute to the development of breast cancer, the increase in breast can-

TABLE 4–3   Why women are more affected by drugs than men.

- Lower weight
- Higher percent body fat
- Less efficient alcohol metabolism
- Menstrual cycle

cer may be related to the increased serum estrogen levels among heavy drinkers. There is some disagreement about the relationship between alcohol intake and gynecologic cancers. Some studies have found a relationship, whereas other studies have not found a correlation (Bradley et al., 1998). This conflict may be due to inadequate methodologic techniques used in the research studies.

There are a number of reasons for the differences between men and women regarding the impact of substances of abuse (see Table 4–3). Among the simplest explanations is the difference in *body weight*. As a rule, men weigh more than women and, as a result, are able to manage larger dosages of drugs.

Another explanation lies in men's greater water-to-fat ratio, which means that, all other contributing factors (weight, age, general health, and so on) being equal, women have less water and more fat tissue in their bodies than men. A consequence of this is that a given amount of a water-soluble substance, such as alcohol, will be more concentrated in the bodies of women than in those of men (Lex, 1991). In addition to alcohol, other substances of abuse that fall into the water-soluble category are cocaine and morphine derivatives. Substances that are fat soluble are also more problematic for women than men. Methamphetamines, tetrahydrocannabinol, benzodiazepines, most barbiturates, fentanyl, and other **opiate agonists** (substances that work in a manner similar to opiates) are substances that are stored in fatty tissue. Because females have more fatty tissue than males, more of these substances can be stored in the female body. A possible result is that women may take longer to withdraw from these substances, and, depending on the rate at which the substances are released from the fat in which they are stored, the withdrawal symptoms may be less severe. This has not been documented, but seems logical.

Another factor contributing to women's greater susceptibility to the damaging effects of drugs is the way in which women *metabolize* alcohol. Women produce lower levels of a stomach enzyme called **alcohol dehydrogenase** than men do. This enzyme reduces the amount of ethanol that is absorbed into the bloodstream by converting it to acetaldehyde. Frezza et al. (1990) found lower levels of gastric alcohol dehydrogenase in alcohol-dependent women than in alcohol-dependent men. In some instances, no alcohol dehydrogenase was found in female alcohol-dependent subjects. As a result, more unmetabolized ethanol is absorbed into the bloodstream, resulting in greater toxicity to vital organs and systems. In their classic study, Orford and Keddie (1985) determined that women progress more quickly to more serious consequences of alcoholism than do men. The researchers referred to this phenomenon as "telescoping." The Frezza et al. (1990) finding was not replicated until 1996, when Haber et al. (1996) conducted in vitro studies which indicated that when gastric cells from men were incubated with ethanol, those cells produced more than twice as much **acetate** (a byproduct of ethanol metabolism) than did gastric cells from women. The finding that the gastric cells from women were not as efficient or effective in converting ethanol to acetate supports the finding of the study by Frezza et al. (1990).

More research must be done on the implications of female physiology in drug abuse. There is much that is not known. For example, the menstrual cycle appears to have some impact on the effects of some drugs, particularly cocaine. After intranasal administration of cocaine, average peak levels of cocaine in the blood are higher in the *follicular phase* of the menstrual cycle (the period following the cessation of menstrual flow, when the new egg is developing in the ovary and blood estrogen levels increase) than in the *luteal phase* (Lukas et al., 1996). The luteal phase is the period following ovulation (the release of the egg into the fallopian tubes) and there is an increase in **progesterone** at that time. This difference raises the question of the impact of female sex hormones, on drug metabolism. In comparison with females, males achieve higher peak blood levels of cocaine, experience the cocaine high faster, and report a larger number of good effects (Lukas et al., 1996).

A degree of male-as-norm bias continues in science. Wilke (1994) points out that alcoholism research has been based on the assumption that the disease is the same for both sexes. When judged according to the male standard, women are found to be **sicker** and more **difficult to treat than their male counterparts.** This is beginning to change as more research is being conducted that is specific to substance abuse and dependence among women.

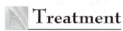 # Treatment

Treatment of drug abuse and dependence involves both primary and secondary prevention, as well as treating established drug abuse.

Prevention

In the treatment of substance dependence, *primary prevention* activities are directed toward *preventing substance use in a population at risk.* These activities are frequently conducted in a school setting, and are begun early in the curriculum. The effectiveness of these activities has been disappointing, however, with a considerable erosion of their impact over time (White & Pitts, 1998). It may be that any attempts to conduct interventions at this level need to be repeated frequently during the school curriculum, and that the method of intervening needs to change.

Secondary Prevention

Secondary prevention activities are directed toward *reducing substance use once it has begun but before true dependence on a given substance has occurred.* Secondary prevention often takes the form of **brief intervention.**

Brief intervention characteristically takes place during a visit to a primary care provider, when the provider becomes aware that a client's ingestion of substances of abuse may be problematic. The client's use of the substance is discussed, and the primary care provider cautions and encourages the client to change the substance-use behavior. Education regarding the rationale for the intervention is offered, and this brief intervention may be repeated during subsequent visits to the provider (Vranas & Allen, 1996).

Studies of brief interventions for alcohol use during pregnancy have resulted in conflicting findings as to its *efficacy.* Chang, Wilkins-Haug, Berman, and Goetz (1999) found that pregnant drinkers who received a brief intervention did *not* decrease their drinking behavior more than those in a control group who received no intervention. However, in a study of a subset of the population used in their 1999 study, Chang, Goetz, Wilkins-Haug, and Berman (2000) reported that, when the subjects' intention was to abstain from drinking during their pregnancy, a significant number did reduce their alcohol intake following the brief intervention. Further refining those studies, Conrod, Stewart, Pihl, Fontaine, and Dongier (2000) found that, when the *style* of the brief intervention was matched to the *personalities* of the subjects and their *reasons* for substance use, there was a significantly reduced frequency and severity of alcohol and drug use for six months after the intervention. The groups receiving the *unmatched* intervention showed no such reduction. In identifying the factors related to the success of brief interventions, more may be required than simply establishing the fact that a brief intervention was conducted. It may be that the type of intervention and how well it fits with personality and other characteristics, should be considered as well.

TREATING ESTABLISHED ADDICTION

Although the American Medical Association classified *alcoholism* as a disease as early as 1954, drug dependence was not so identified until 1962, when the U.S. Supreme Court ruled as unconstitutional the classification of drug dependence (in itself) as a crime. These events paved the way for

TABLE 4–4 Substances of abuse and the medications used in detoxification.

Substance of Abuse	Detoxification Medications
Alcohol	Benzodiazepines (Librium, Klonopin, Tranxene, Valium)
Opioids	Clonidine, Methadone
Benzodiazepines and other sedative-hypnotics	Decreasing doses of problem drug; use of phenobarbital; substitution of another drug from this classification, then withdrawal from all drugs
Stimulants/cocaine	No specific medication for withdrawal; individuals are treated with medications to relieve severe symptoms

Source: Adapted from Feigenbaum, J. C., & Allen, K. M. (1996). Detoxification. In K. M. Allen (Ed.), *Nursing care of the addicted client* (pp. 139–175). Philadelphia: Lippincott Williams-Wilkins.

the treatment of substance dependence in healthcare centers using sound medical practices.

Treatment usually consists of **inpatient medical detoxification** for seriously dependent individuals. Because of the physiological factors impacting their substance dependence, women's detoxification should be individualized. If women are not monitored by a healthcare professional familiar with their specific needs, their withdrawal may be more complicated and unpredictable. Also, because of the higher concentrations of ethanol in women—and women's greater stores of body fat, where many drugs are stored—detoxifying women may take a longer period of time, and the cravings and effects of the drugs may persist (Feigenbaum & Allen, 1996).

Table 4–4 lists the medications used in detoxification from specific substances. In addition to those listed, there are standard detoxification protocols used for individuals who are addicted to more than one drug. For example, when an individual is alcohol-dependent, **benzodiazepines** are the medication of choice, regardless of what the other addictive substances s/he may use. The only exception to this is when the individual is addicted to alcohol *and* benzodiazepines. In that case, **phenobarbital** is the drug used for detoxification.

The detoxification of an opiate-dependent pregnant woman is risky to both the woman and her unborn child. The lack of certainty regarding the dosages of medication needed to control withdrawal symptoms in the fetus, in addition to other factors, is the reason the drug **Methadone** is

frequently used to treat opiate addiction in pregnant women. Methadone is an addictive narcotic sometimes prescribed for addicts so they will not have to obtain drugs illegally in order to satisfy their cravings. Although controversial, the use of Methadone by pregnant opiate addicts has been described as beneficial for many opiate-dependent women and their children (Kandall, Doberczak, Jantunen, & Stein, 1999). However, impaired fetal central nervous system development and changes in fetal behavior related to the use of Methadone have been identified (Anyaegbunam, Tran, Jadali, Randolph, & Mikhail, 1997). Nevertheless, current medical practice is based on the assumption that it is more advisable to have a newborn who was exposed to Methadone in utero than to deal with a newborn who is addicted to heroin and other opiates. It is standard practice that, whenever possible, the opiate-addicted pregnant woman is detoxified with Methadone (American Society of Addictions Medicine, 1998).

Many of the medications used in the detoxification process (review Table 4–3) are addictive in themselves, so a period of *weaning* off them may be required. During detoxification, skilled nursing staff monitor the individual's progress and the effects of the detoxifying medications to assure that the dosages are adequate but not excessive. Following detoxification, patients are usually referred to a tertiary facility for a continuing program of rehabilitation. These programs are of various lengths and configurations; some take place in inpatient facilities, where the length of stay is planned for 28 days or longer.

Eisenstadt (1993) identified nine elements that are important to effective, high-quality rehabilitation for substance-dependent women. These elements have been endorsed by the Center for Substance Dependence Treatment (CSDT) and include the following:

1. *A warm, welcoming atmosphere is provided.*
2. *Initial contact is with experienced clinicians or trained recovering counselors.*
3. *Staff communicates to the substance-dependent woman that she is important as a person.*
4. *Various treatment modalities are including women-only groups.*
5. *Social role problems and conflicts are addressed.*
6. *Staff is culturally competent and able to apply family systems theory.*
7. *Staff refrains from diagnosing substance-dependent women as depressed until a complete assessment can be performed.*
8. *The special needs of lesbian women are addressed.*
9. *HIV/AIDS education integrated into every facet of the program and into all services offered.*

In order to treat addiction in women effectively, a wide range of *therapies* and *services* must be provided. For example, women must be *assessed* and *treated* for certain problems, including malnutrition, physical and psychological trauma resulting from abuse (including sexual abuse), co-existing psychiatric disorders, and sexually transmitted diseases. Women must also be *educated* on a variety of topics, such as breast self-examination, smoking cessation, the consequences of drug use during pregnancy, and parenting skills. Finally, women must know how to access child-care services and obtain legal assistance if necessary (Vranas & Allen, 1996).

The Center for Substance Dependence Treatment (1999) has identified positive associations between *favorable* treatment outcomes and such variables as *length of stay* in treatment facilities and the degree of program *structure* and *intensity*. In addition, the center assumes the position that substance-abuse treatment, welfare reform, and child protection are "intimately related and dependent upon each other for success" (Center for Substance Abuse Treatment, 1999). It suggests that all three issues need to be addressed at the same time or all will fail. On the basis of their meta-analysis of drug-abuse outcome studies, Stanton and Shadish (1997) reported that the availability of family therapy in a treatment program increases the retention rates over programs without this component. Family therapy may be a key factor in tertiary care.

Because of changes in the manner in which healthcare providers are reimbursed for their services, and the growth of managed care, rehabilitation facilities have been forced to demonstrate their effectiveness. For example, many insurance companies require frequent updates on the condition of their clients and demand that certain *outcomes* be documented to justify continued inpatient care. Because few instruments that measure *behavioral* outcomes have been developed, most inpatient rehabilitation centers use *physiological* outcomes, such as stabilized or normalized liver, heart, and kidney function. Once these outcomes have been achieved, many insurance companies refuse to pay for further inpatient care. The patient then has the option of *paying* for a continued stay or being *transferred* to an outpatient facility. The latter option is usually the only one that is feasible.

There are a number of types of outpatient care. Most involve group and individual therapy sessions with professional or semiprofessional staff who have received special training and certification in addictions counseling. Some require attendance at Alcoholics Anonymous (AA) and/or Narcotics Anonymous (NA) meetings, with the expectation that attendance at these meetings will continue throughout the patient's lifetime. Some outpatient rehabilitation programs require patients to have a **sponsor** and **home group** as a condition for discharge. A sponsor is an individual in AA or NA, preferably of the same sex, who has a period of abstinence from drugs and alcohol and who has followed the 12-step program of recovery as outlined by *Alcoholics Anonymous* (Alcoholics Anonymous World Services, 1976). A home group is a regular meeting of AA or NA, in which a member commits to regular attendance and

to contributing to the functioning of the group by acting as coffee maker, secretary, and greeter. Outpatient rehabilitation programs can usually be tailored to the needs of the individual. For example, there are all-day programs which provide intensive interventions as well as evening programs, which are geared toward individuals who are employed. This benefits the individual in that there are strong support and therapy available during the period of reentry into the workplace.

Community Resources

Alcoholics Anonymous and Narcotics Anonymous are the most widely known groups that provide ongoing support for individuals desiring to maintain abstinence from alcohol and other drugs. Although the size of their membership is difficult to estimate because of the anonymity assured to the members, there are approximately 2 million members in Alcoholics Anonymous worldwide, in more than 98,000 local groups (Alcoholics Anonymous World Services, 1999). Narcotics Anonymous acknowledges the problem of collecting these types of data because of the criminality of drug use and the associated criminal behavior engaged in by many members but estimates its membership at 5,000 worldwide (Narcotics Anonymous World Services, 1999).

In addition to Alcoholics Anonymous and Narcotics Anonymous, there are other groups in the community that assist in recovery from substance dependence. These include Rational Recovery Systems, the Resource Center on Substance Abuse Prevention and Disability, Secular Organizations for Sobriety (SOS), Women for Sobriety, Moderation Management, and The Womens Health Network. (See the Resources section at the end of this chapter for further information.) Two groups that offer viewpoints different from those of Alcoholics Anonymous and Narcotics Anonymous are Rational Recovery Systems (Trimpey, 1996) and Moderation Management (Kishline, 1996).

Rational Recovery was started as an *alternative* to the 12-step programs, mainly Alcoholics Anonymous and Narcotics Anonymous. Critics maintain that the 12-step groups are *religious* in nature, and therefore incompatible with the views of some addicted persons. They also object to the focus on *powerlessness* and the requirement that members maintain a *lifelong affiliation* with the groups (Trimpey, 1996). The Rational Recovery program is based on the assumption that addicted persons have the *internal resources* they need to overcome addiction. It stresses personal responsibility and agency and teaches its members to use *logic* to internally dispute denial and other unrealistic thinking patterns that support addiction. It is difficult to know how popular or successful Rational Recovery is, however, as no estimates of its membership, or success rate, have been published. It is also difficult to find Rational Recovery centers or meetings. Trimpey (1996), however, maintains that attending only *a few* training sessions and reading the organization's *literature* prepares substance-dependent individuals for lifelong abstinence.

Kishline (1996), the creator of Moderation Management, describes alcoholism as a *learned* behavior that, as such, can be *unlearned*. She claims that many alcoholics can be taught to drink socially; however, she does acknowledge that some cannot resume social drinking without falling back into alcoholism. Again, it is difficult to locate local groups, so it is difficult to refer individuals for this type of help. Moreover, legal difficulties involving Kishline have raised considerable skepticism regarding this treatment program.

Alternative, or Complementary, Treatment

For centuries, Asian societies have used herbs, touch, stimulation via acupuncture, meditation, and other methods, and techniques to maximize health and treat disease. These techniques have been viewed as outside the acceptable limits of Western medicine and science and, thus, have been termed alternative, or complementary (see Chapter 10). Nevertheless, there is striking anecdotal and empirical evidence that some of these techniques are safe and often quite effective in treating a number of conditions, including substance dependence. As early as 1979, the World Health Organization (WHO) identified acupuncture as an appropriate treatment for addictive disease (World Health Organization, 1979). Early research into the use of auricular (ear) acupuncture for substance dependence treatment indicated that, when acupuncture was used in detoxification from alcohol, subjects did not experience expected alcoholic seizures and recidivism was significantly decreased. When acupuncture was used for heroin and cocaine withdrawal, subjects experienced milder, more manageable withdrawal symptoms and cravings (Brumbaugh, 1992). The **National Acupuncture Detoxification Association (NADA)** has sponsored clinics that incorporate the use of alternative medicine, including the use of herbs, in treating clients. Herbs such as chamomile, hops, catnip, skullcap, peppermint, and yarrow are used in combination to make a hot drink that promotes sleep. This is particularly important for clients who are withdrawing from alcohol and other sedatives, as insomnia is often a problem (Brumbaugh, 1992).

Barriers to Treatment and Hope for Recovery

During the years 1994 and 1995, only 30 percent of the **females** over age 12 who needed substance-abuse/dependence treatment received it. The 70 percent who did not receive treatment were different from **males** who did not receive treat-

ment in a number of ways. When compared with males, the females were *more* likely to be married, white, high school graduates and living with one or more children. They were *less* likely to be employed full-time, less likely to be dependent on alcohol, and less likely to have initiated substance abuse before the age of 15 (Office of Applied Studies, 1996). Women are truly a medically underserved population in terms of substance-dependence treatment. Only recently has this problem been identified and efforts begun to understand it.

A new and growing body of knowledge is pointing to the need for special treatment for addicted women (Allen, 1994; Allen & Dixon, 1994; Office of Applied Studies, 1997). Although no single program will meet the needs of all women, these researchers have identified barriers to addictions treatment for women. Despite the current popularizing of addictions treatment and the public acknowledgment of drug and alcohol problems on the part of celebrities, there is a strong *moral* component to the view of addiction, especially when the addict is a woman with children. Support from a significant other (husband, parent, lover, and so on) seems to be important to women's recovery, and is sometimes difficult for them to obtain (Allen, 1994). The need for childcare is a barrier for many women, in that there are few treatment settings that will take a woman's children as residents. Because women are greatly represented in the poorest of the poor in the United States (U.S. Administration Office on Aging, 2001), a lack of health insurance is a barrier to treatment that may be impossible to overcome. Other barriers identified by Allen (1994) include feelings of hopelessness, fear of the unknown, shame, fear of commitment to a treatment program, family responsibilities, relationships with men, and an unwillingness to ask family members to sacrifice financially or socially.

In order for treatment facilities to be useful to women, then, they must provide services tailored to their specific needs and characteristics. For women with few or no skills or economic advantages, residential treatment is preferable to outpatient treatment. Residential treatment enables a women to leave a setting where recovery from substance dependence may be impossible due to drug use in the home, a lack of social support, and so on. However, the residential facility must accommodate children. School or job skills training is needed by many women, as are half-way house facilities, so that once the most intensive treatment and skills instruction is completed, the women and their children have a protected environment while the woman begins to work, or continues with school. Many women must undergo intensive psychotherapy for the treatment of underlying or co-occurring psychiatric disorders, including post-traumatic stress disorder, if they are to remain abstinent from drugs and alcohol. A supportive and loving environment can assist a woman in developing self-respect and self-esteem.

Field et al. (1998) found that when provided with educational, vocational, and parenting classes, as well as drug and alcohol rehabilitation for six months, teenage, drug-abusing mothers and their children recovered to the point at which they were indistinguishable from a nondrug-using control group. The teen mothers were less apt to continue their drug use, had fewer repeat pregnancies, and improved their parenting skills greatly, when compared with a drug-using group not receiving the intervention. The children thrived in this environment. They showed improved communication skills, increased head circumference, and fewer illnesses and other complications.

Wellness Self-Assessment

Because of the male-as-norm bias, most standard screening and assessment tools are more likely to identify problems in men than in women. There are few assessment guides specifically for women, and they are primarily focused on pregnant women. However, given what is known about the nature of the problems caused by addictions in women, there are some questions that can reveal the need for further assessment or treatment by professionals skilled in addictions treatment. You may wish to consult a professional if you have experienced (to any degree) *any* of the following:

1. *Disagreements or arguments with a husband or significant other about your substance use.*
2. *Expressions of concern about the care of your children or your ability as a mother.*
3. *Physical problems following episodes of substance use.*
4. *Being told by a friend that he or she is concerned about your substance use.*
5. *Hiding the fact of substance use or the amount of substance use, regardless of the reason.*
6. *Feelings of guilt over substance use.*
7. *Loss of control over substance use or changing your mind about how much you will use once the use has begun.*
8. *Awareness of the need to control your substance use.*
9. *Being told you engaged in behavior you don't remember.*
10. *Medical or legal advice to stop substance use.*

New Directions

In 1998, three researchers from Yale University—Margolin, Avants, and Kleber—identified a methodological flaw ubiquitous in the research to date on the value of acupuncture in treating substance dependence; they found that, in many studies, the subjects had not been *randomly assigned* to their groups. Because of the resources recently made available by the National Center for Complementary and Alternative Medicine (part of the National Institutes of Health), Margolin, Avants, and Kleber (1998) are in the process of remedying this situation. They are conducting the largest controlled study of cocaine addiction treatment ever undertaken. Five hundred cocaine-dependent subjects have been assigned randomly to treatment groups. The groups are being treated using various techniques and the results will be analyzed upon completion of the study. Among the topics to be studied are appropriate control conditions, point location for needle insertion, and the efficacy of acupuncture in comparison with more traditional therapies.

In 1997, Schuckit, Tipp, Smith, and Bucholz found that female sex is a predictor of maintained abstinence from alcohol for three months after treatment. The results of this study challenged the previous assumption that alternating periods of abstinence and heavy drinking are common in alcoholics of both sexes. The Schuckit et al. study also contributed to a growing body of knowledge that contradicts earlier findings that female alcoholics are more difficult to treat. More studies specific to substance-abusing and substance-dependent women are needed to expand our knowledge further and to identify the factors that are involved in successful treatment.

Much more needs to be done in order to answer the many perplexing questions raised by the existing research into substance dependence in women. The number of variables contributing to substance abuse and dependence is enormous. Before researchers can determine how these variables interact to bring about substance-use problems, the variables need to be identified. **Naturalistic inquiry** (qualitative) into the experience of women during the addicted state and their experience in treatment may help identify more variables that can be used in quantitative analysis to bring about some valuable answers for these women.

QUESTIONS FOR REFLECTION AND DISCUSSION

1. *What are the physical, emotional, and social implications of substance abuse and dependence in women?*
2. *If you were in a position to contribute to a discussion of policy with regard to substance-dependent women, what sorts of treatment options would you promote? Why?*
3. *Discuss the meaning of the phrase "continuing cycle of addiction."*
4. *What is meant by the phrase "male as norm bias"?*

RESOURCES

Community Organizations

Alcoholics Anonymous
World Service Office
475 Riverside Drive
New York, NY 10115
Phone: 212-870-3400
Web: www.alcoholics-anonymous.org/

National Council on Alcoholism and Drug Dependence, Inc.
Public Information
12 W. 21st Street, 7th Floor
New York, NY 10010
Phone: 212-206-6770
Web: www.ncadd.org

Rational Recovery Systems
P.O. Box 800
Lotus, CA 95651
Phone: 916-621-2667
Web: www.rational.olg/recovery/

Resource Center on Substance Abuse Prevention and Disability
1331 F Street, NW
Suite 800
Washington, DC 20004
Phone: 202-783-2900

Secular Organizations for Sobriety (SOS)
P.O. Box 5
Buffalo, NY 14215
Phone: 716-834-2922

Women for Sobriety
P.O. Box 618
Quakertown, PA 18951
Phone: 1-800-333-1606
Web: www.secularhumanism.org/sos/

Women's Health Network
1325 G Street, NW
Washington, DC 20005
Phone: 202-347-1140

Websites

Narcotics Anonymous World Services
www.na.org/

Hazelden (publishers of addictions-treatment literature and literature for use by recovering individuals)
www.hazelden.org/

Staying Cyber—Alcoholics Anonymous meetings on the World Wide Web
http://stayingcyber.org/

Alcoholics Anonymous—meetings listed by state
www.soberspace.com

Join Together—to decrease substance abuse and gun violence
www.jointogether.org/

National Women's Resource Center for the Prevention and Treatment of Alcoholism, Tobacco, and Other Drug Addiction
www.healthfinder.gov/text/orgs/HR2462.htm

Center for Substance Abuse Prevention
www.samhsa.gov/CSAP/CSAP.htm

Center for Substance Abuse Treatment
www.samhsa.gov/CSAT/CSAT.htm

REFERENCES

Alcoholics Anonymous World Services. *Alcoholics Anonymous,* (1976). (3rd ed.). New York City: Author.

Alcoholics Anonymous World Services. (1999). *Welcome to Alcoholics Anonymous Home page* [On-line]. Available: http://www.alcoholics-anonymous.org/

Allen, K. M. (1994). Development of an instrument to identify barriers to treatment for addicted women, from their perspective. *International Journal of the Addictions, 29*(4), 429–444.

Allen, K. M. (1996). *Nursing care of the addicted client.* Philadelphia: Lippincott-Raven.

Allen, K. M., & Dixon, M. (1994). Psychometric assessment of the Allen barriers to treatment instrument. *The International Journal of the Addictions, 29*(5), 545–563.

American Psychiatric Association. (1994). *Diagnostic and statistical manual of mental disorders* (4th ed.). Washington, D.C.: American Psychiatric Association.

American Society of Addictions Medicine. (1998). *Home page* [On-line]. Available: http://www.asam.org/

Anyaegbunam, A., Tran, T., Jadali, D., Randolph, G., & Mikhail, M. S. (1997). Assessment of fetal well-being in methadone-maintained pregnancies: Abnormal nonstress tests. *Gynecological and Obstetrical Investigation, 43*(1), 25–28.

Ashton, L. (2000, August 11). Alcoholism activist sentenced in drunken-driving accident. Associated Press Release.

Blum, K., & Payne, J. E. (1991). *Alcohol and the addictive brain: New hope for alcoholics from biogenetic research.* New York: Free Press.

Bradley, K. A., Badrinath, S., Bush, K., Boyd-Wickizer, J., & Anawalt, B. (1998). Medical risks for women who drink alcohol. *Journal of General Internal Medicine, 13,* 627–639.

Brower, K. J., Blow, F. C., & Beresford, T. P. (1989). Treatment implications of chemical dependency models: An integrative approach. *Journal of Substance Abuse Treatment, 6*(3), 147–57.

Brumbaugh, A. G. (1992). Acupuncture: New perspectives in chemical dependence treatment. *Journal of Substance Abuse Treatment, 10,* 35–43.

Bunikowski, R., Grimmer, I., Heiser, A., Metze, B., Schafer, A., & Obladen, M. (1998). Neurodevelopmental outcome after prenatal exposure to opiates. *European Journal of Pediatrics, 157*(9), 724–730.

Cadoret, R. J., Troughton, E., & O'Gorman, T. W. (1987). Genetic and environmental factors in alcohol abuse and antisocial personality. *Journal of Studies on Alcohol, 48,* 1–8.

Cadoret, R. J., Yates, W. R., Troughton, E., Woodworth, G., & Stewart, M. A. (1996). An adoption study of drug abuse/dependency in females. *Comprehensive Psychiatry, 37*(2), 88–94.

Center on Addiction and Substance Abuse at Columbia University (CASA). (1993). *The cost of substance abuse to America's health care system.* New York: Author.

Center for Substance Abuse Treatment (CSAT). (1999). *Treatment improvement exchange* [On-line]. Available: http://www.treatment.org/externals/tips.html

Chang, G., Goetz, M. A., Wilkins-Haug, L., & Berman, S. (2000). A brief intervention for prenatal alcohol use: An in-depth look. *Journal of Substance Abuse Treatment, 18*(4), 365–369.

Chang, G., Wilkins-Haug, L., Berman, S., & Goetz, M. A. (1999). Brief intervention for alcohol use in pregnancy: A randomized trial. *Addiction, 94*(10), 1499–1508.

Church, M. W., Crossland, W. J., Holmes, P. A., Overbeck, G. W., & Tilak, J. P. (1998). Effects of prenatal cocaine on hearing, vision, growth, and behavior. *Annals of New York Academy of Science, 846,* 12–28.

Clark, K. A., Dawson, S., & Martin, S. L. (1999). The effect of implementing a more comprehensive screening for substance use among pregnant women in North Carolina. *Maternal and Child Health Journal, 3*(3), 161–166.

Cloninger, C. R., Christiansen, R. C., Reich, T., & Gotteman, I. (1978). Implications of sex differences in the prevalences of antisocial personality, alcoholism and criminality for familial transmission. *Archives of General Psychiatry, 35,* 941–951.

Conrod, P. J., Stewart, S. H., Pihl, R. O., Fontaine, C. S., & Dongier, M. (2000). Efficacy of brief coping skills interventions that match different personality profiles of female substance abusers. *Psychology of Addictive Behaviors, 14*(3), 231–242.

Datta-Bhutada, S., Johnson, H. L., & Rosen, T. S. (1998). Intrauterine cocaine and crack exposure: Neonatal outcome. *Journal of Perinatology, 18*(3), 183–188.

Davis, D. R., & DiNitto, D. M. (1996). Gender differences in social and psychological problems of substance abusers: A comparison to nonsubstance abusers. *Journal of Psychoactive Drugs, 28*(2), 135–145.

Eisenstadt, B. L. (1993, February). Quality treatment for women. *Employee Assistance,* pp. 31–33, 35.

Eyler, F. D., Behnke, M., Conlon, M., Woods, N. S., & Wobie, K. (1998). Birth outcome from a prospective, matched study of prenatal crack/cocaine use: II. Interactive and dose effects on neurobehavioral assessment. *Pediatrics, 101*(2), 237–241.

FAS Community Resource Center. (1999). *Home page* [On-line]. Available: http://come-over.to/FAS/

Feigenbaum, J. C., & Allen, K. M. (1996). Detoxification. In K. M. Allen (Ed.), *Nursing care of the addicted client* (pp. 139–175). Philadelphia: Lippincott.

Field, T. M., Scafid, F., Pickens, J., Prodromidis, M., Pelaez-Negueras, M., Torquati, J., Wilcox, H., Malphuras, J., Shanberg, S., & Kuhn, C. (1998). Effects of interventions for drug-abusing teen age mothers. *Adolescence, 33*(129), 117–43.

Frezza, M., DiPadova, C., Pozzato, G., Terpin, M., Baraona, E., & Lieber, C. S. (1990). High blood alcohol levels in women: The role of decreased gastric alcohol dehydrogenase activity and first-pass metabolism. *New England Journal of Medicine, 322*(2), 95–99.

Fu, H., & Goldman, N. (2000). The association between health-related behaviours and the risk of divorce in the USA. *Journal of Biosocial Science, 32*(1), 63–88.

Gil-Rivas, V., Fiorentine, R., & Anglin, M. D. (1996). Sexual abuse, physical abuse, and post-traumatic stress disorder among women participating in outpatient drug abuse treatment. *Journal of Psychoactive Drugs, 28*(1), 95–102.

Gomberg, E. S. (1989). Alcoholic women in treatment: Early histories and early problem behaviors. *Advances in Alcohol and Substance Abuse, 8*(2), 133–147.

Group for the Advancement of Psychiatry Committee on Alcoholism and the Addictions. (1991). Substance abuse disorders, a psychiatric priority. *American Journal of Psychiatry, 148*(10), 1291–1300.

Haber, P. S., Gentry, R. T., Mak, K. M., Mirmiran-Yazdy, S. A. A., Greenstein, R. J., & Lieber, C. S. (1996). Metabolism of alcohol by human gastric cells: Relation to first-pass metabolism. *Gastroenterology, 111*(4), 863–870.

Hoffmann, J. P. (1995). The effects of family structure and family relations on adolescent marijuana use. *International Journal of the Addictions, 30*(10), 1207–1241.

Jellinek, E. M. (1946). Phases in the drinking history of alcoholics: An analysis of a survey conducted by the official organ of Alcoholics Anonymous. *Quarterly Journal of Studies on Alcohol, 7,* 1–88.

Jellinek, E. M. (1960). *The disease concept of alcoholism.* New Haven, CT: Hillhouse Press.

Kandall, S. R., Doberczak, T. M., Jantunen, M., & Stein, J. (1999). The methadone-maintained pregnancy. *Clinical Perinatology, 26*(1), 173–183.

Kendler, K. S., Dardowski, L. M., Corey, L. A., Prescott, C. A., & Neale, M. C. (1999). Genetic and environmental risk factors in the aetiology of illicit drug initiation and subsequent misuse in women. *British Journal of Psychiatry, 175,* 351–356.

Kishline, A. (1996). *Moderate drinking: The moderation management guide for people who want to reduce their drinking.* New York: Crown.

LaGasse, L. L., Seifer, R., & Lester, B. M. (1999). Interpreting research on prenatal substance exposure in the context of multiple confounding factors. *Clinical Perinatology, 26*(1), 39–54.

Leavell, H. R., & Clark, E. G. (1965). *Preventive medicine for the doctor in your community.* New York: McGraw-Hill.

Lex, B. W. (1991). Some gender differences in alcohol and poly-substance users. *Health Psychology, 10,* 121–132.

Litt, J., & McNeil, M. (1997). Biological markers and social differentiation: Crack babies and the construction of the dangerous mother. *Health Care Women, International, 18*(1), 31–41.

Lukas, S. E., Sholar, M., Lundahl, L. H., Lamas, X., Kouri, E., Wines, J. D., Kragie, L., & Mendelson, J. H. (1996). Sex differences in plasma cocaine levels and subjective effects after acute cocaine administration in human volunteers. *Psychopharmacology, 125*(4), 346–354.

Lyons, P., & Ritter, B. (1998). The construction of the crack babies phenomenon as a social problem. *American Journal of Orthopsychiatry, 68*(2), 313–320.

Margolin, A., Avants, S. K., & Kleber, H. D. (1998). Rationale and design of the Cocaine Alternative Treatments Study (CATS): A randomized, controlled trial of acupuncture. *Journal of Alternative and Complementary Medicine, 4*(4), 405–418.

Naegle, M. A. (1988). Substance abuse among women: Prevalence, patterns, and treatment issues. *Issues in Mental Health Nursing, 9*(2), 127–137.

Narcotics Anonymous World Services. (1999). *Home page* [On-line]. Available: http://www.na.org/

National Household Survey on Drug Abuse (1995). U.S. Department of Health and Human Services, Public Health Service, Substance Abuse and Mental Health Services Administration, Office of Applied Studies. Rockville, MD: Author.

National Household Survey on Drug Abuse (1996). U.S. Department of Health and Human Services, Public Health Service, Substance Abuse and Mental Health Services Administration, Office of Applied Studies. Rockville, MD: Author.

National Institute for Drug Abuse. (1999a). *Home page* [On-line]. Available: http://www.nida.nih.gov/

National Institute for Drug Abuse. (1999b). *Women's Health & Gender Differences (WHGD) home page* [On-line]. Available: http://www.nida.nih.gov/WHGD/WHGDHome.html

National Organization on Fetal Alcohol Syndrome. (1999). *Home page* [On-line]. Available: http://www.nofas.org/

Neher, L. S., & Short, J. L. (1998). Risk and protective factors for children's substance use and antisocial behavior following parental divorce. *American Journal of Orthopsychiatry, 68*(1), 154–161.

Office of Applied Studies. (1996). *National Household Survey on Drug Abuse, 1996.* Rockville MD: U.S. Department of Health and Human Services, Public Health Service, Substance Abuse and Mental Health Services Administration, Office of Applied Studies.

Orford, J., & Keddie, A. (1985). Gender differences in the functions and effects of moderate and excessive drinking. *British Journal of Clinical Psychology, 24,* 265–279.

Reardon, D. C., & Ney, P. G. (2000). Abortion and subsequent substance abuse. *American Journal of Drug and Alcohol Abuse, 26*(1), 61–75.

Richardson, G. A., & Day, N. L. (1994). Detrimental effects of prenatal cocaine exposure: Illusion or reality? *Journal of the American Academy of Child and Adolescent Psychiatry, 33*(1), 28–34.

Schuckit, M. A., Tipp, J. E., Smith, T. L., & Bucholz, K. K. (1997). Periods of abstinence following the onset of alcohol depen-dence in 1,853 men and women. *Journal of Studies on Alcoholism, 58*(6), 581–589.

Simoni-Wastila, L. (2000). The use of abusable prescription drugs: The role of gender. *Journal of Women's Health Gender Based Medicine, 9*(3), 289–297.

Stanton, M. D., & Shadish, W. R. (1997). Outcome, attrition, and family-couples treatment for drug abuse: A meta-analysis and review of the controlled, comparative studies. *Psychology Bulletin, 122*(2), 170–191.

Substance Abuse and Mental Health Administration. (2000). *National household survey* [On-line]. http://samhsa.gov/

Trimpey, J. (1996). *Rational recovery: The new cure for substance addiction.* New York: Pocket Books.

U.S. Administrative Office on Aging (2001). [On-line]. Meeting the needs of older women: A diverse and growing population. Retrieved September 3, 2002. Available: http://www.aoa.dhhs.gov/factsheet/ow.html

Vance, J. C., Chant, D. C., Tudehope, D. I., Gray, P. H., & Hayes, A. J. (1997). Infants born to narcotic dependent mothers: Physical growth patterns in the first 12 months of life. *Journal of Pediatrics and Child Health, 33*(6), 504–508.

Van den Bree, M. B., Johnson, E. O., Neale, M. C., & Pickens, R. W. (1998). Genetic and environmental influences on drug use and abuse/dependence in male and female twins. *Drug and Alcohol Dependence, 52*(3), 231–241.

Vanyukov, M. M., Moss, H. B., Gioio, A. E., Hughes, H. B., Kaplan, B. B., & Tarter, R. E. (1998). An association between a microsatellite polymorphism at the DRD5 gene and the liability to substance abuse: Pilot study. *Behavioral Genetics, 28*(2), 75–82.

Vranas, M., & Allen, K. M. (1996). Interventions and treatment. In K. M. Allen (Ed.), *Nursing care of the addicted client* (pp. 176–194). Philadelphia: Lippincott.

Wallace, B. C. (1990). Treating crack cocaine dependence: The critical role of relapse prevention. *Journal of Psychoactive Drugs, 22*(2), 149–158.

Wartenberg, A. A., & Liepman, M. R. (1990). Medical complications of substance abuse. In W. D. Lerner & M. A. Barr (Eds.), *Handbook of hospital-based substance abuse treatment* (pp. 45–63). New York: Pergamon Press.

Westermeyer, J. (1987). Cultural patterns of drug and alcohol use: An analysis of host and agent in the cultural environment. *Bulletin on Narcotics, 38*(2), 11–27.

White, D., & Pitts, M. (1998). Educating young people about drugs: A systematic review. *Addiction, 93*(10), 1475–1487.

Wilke, D. (1994). Women and alcoholism: How a male-as-norm bias affects research, assessment, and treatment. *Health and Social Work, 19*(1), 29–35.

Wilson, L. M., Reid, A. J., Midmer, D. K., Biringer, A., Carroll, J. C., & Stewart, D. E. (1996). Antenatal psychosocial risk factors associated with adverse postpartum family outcomes. *Canadian Medical Association Journal, 154*(6), 785–799.

Witters, W., Venturelli, P., & Hanson, G. (1992). *Drugs and society* (3rd ed.). Boston: Jones and Bartlett.

World Health Organization. (1979). *Viewpoint on acupuncture* (Revised). New York: United Nations.

5

Environmental Toxins

Karl Kleiner

Objectives

1. *Differentiate between how sexual differences and gender differences affect women's exposure to environmental toxins.*
2. *Differentiate between a toxin and a hazard.*
3. *Discuss the limitations of establishing the cause and effect of environmental toxins.*
4. *Identify the four components of risk assessment.*

Introduction

During the first half of the 1900s, human exposure to chemical toxins was largely unregulated and unsolicited. By 1962, the work of one woman, Rachel Carson (1907–1964), had enlightened the American public to the hazards of one cause of toxic contamination, excessive pesticide use. Carson's book, *Silent Spring,* was prompted by a friend, Olga Huckins, who owned a private bird sanctuary in Massachusetts. Following an unannounced spray program with DDT to control mosquitoes near the sanc-tuary, Huckins witnessed the deaths of several birds and implored Carson to find someone to investigate the effects of pesticides on wildlife. Carson, who was a U.S. Fish and Wildlife Service biologist, undertook the investigation her-self and quickly discovered that research on the environ-mental effects of pesticide use was severely lacking. *Silent Spring* was Carson's metaphor for the long-term conse-quences of extensive and excessive pesticide use, and it al-luded to a spring without the voices of the birds and the drone of honeybees (Hynes, 1989).

Silent Spring was widely read by scientists, politicians, industrialists, and the general public, and it engaged the nation in a public debate about the benefits and hazards of chemical pesticides. It also threatened the booming pesti-cide industry, which was still taking advantage of the "silver bullet" status of dichlorodiphenyltrichoroethane (DDT), an extremely toxic pesticide that seemed virtually harmless to animals, including humans. Carson was la-beled a food-faddist, a nature nut, and a hysterical woman. Her book's validity was attacked by the agricultural and chemistry industries because of the belief that Carson, a woman, could not possibly understand the technical na-ture of her subject matter. Carson, who was battling breast cancer at the time, responded to her critics and defended the validity of her research. The work of Rachel Carson has been credited with tightening the regulations concerning the sale and use of pesticides, spurring the start of the environmental movement as we know it and influencing the creation of the U.S. Environmental Protection Agency (EPA) (Hynes, 1989).

It was the untimely death of wildlife that motivated Rachel Carson to write *Silent Spring*, but ultimately it was the latent danger that uncontrolled exposure to pesticides posed to the human race that spurred members of the public to take interest in their exposure to environmental toxins. The price that people were paying for the temporary destruction of a few insect pests was a slow poisoning. However, not all people respond the same way to environmental toxins. In particular, women may be disproportionately affected by **anthropogenic** (human-made) toxins, as compared with men (National Institute of Environmental Health Sciences, 1997b). Documented cases of toxicity from anthropogenic compounds in the early 1900s were based mostly on the exposure of men in the workplace. However, during the latter half of the 1900s, both the number of women entering the workforce and the amount of chemical substances brought into the household increased. A nationwide survey suggests that women exposed to environmental pollutants are more likely to develop cancer and have diabetes, kidney and liver problems, and urinary tract disorders. Men, on the other hand, do not show an increased incidence of disease with exposure to pollutants (Christensen, 1998).

It is unclear whether the incidence of pollutant-related disease is higher in women because women are exposed more **frequently** to potentially harmful substances or whether they are more **sensitive** to them (Ness & Kuller, 1997). *Sex differences* are based on genetic and physiological differences between women and men and are considered to be biological or **intrinsic** determinants of risk. Factors such as sex steroid hormone metabolism, body size, immunological functioning, and body metabolism can all contribute to gender differences in susceptibility to environmental contaminants (Setlow, Lawson, & Woods, 1998). For example, smoking can increase the risk of coronary heart disease among women who use oral contraceptives (Castelli, 1999) and increase women's risk for osteoporosis (Baron, La Vecchia, & Levi, 1990) and endometrial cancer (Austin, Drews, & Partridge, 1993; Brinton et al., 1993). Another reason for the different responses of women and men to environmental toxins is women's smaller body size. Exposure to the same amount or concentration of a toxin results in a higher dose in women than in men (Christensen, 1998).

Gender differences reflect the interaction of the sociocultural environment, economic status, employment patterns, and family and are regarded as nonbiological or **extrinsic** factors (Ness & Kuller, 1997). Men and women are often exposed to different musculoskeletal and psychological stressors and environmental toxins at work even when employed in the same job sector (Messing, 2000). For example, in the healthcare sector, where 72 percent of the workers are women, they constitute 94 percent of the registered nurses but only 20 percent of the physicians. In the Canadian poultry industry, the higher accident rate among women, compared with men, was explained in large part by the differences in duties and the ergonomics of the work environment (such as the height of workstations). Traditional patterns of job assignment still largely prevail, and men are more likely to do "dirty" industrial work. Women, however, may be exposed to chemicals both on the job and in the home, which can affect their reproductive health (Rosenstock & Lee, 2000). Women who work outside their homes still do 90 percent of the work inside the home and thus are exposed to additional contaminants from household chemicals (Stellman, 1998). Moreover, the combined stress of the workplace environment and domestic responsibilities may make women's immune systems more susceptible to environmental toxins (Stellman, 2000; Swanson, 2000). It is known that stress compromises the immune system, and a study of factory workers at Volvo, the Swedish car manufacturer, indicated that, although both men and women possessed the same level of stress on the job, the similarity vanished when they got home. At the end of the day, the stress level of the men went down, whereas that of the women went up (Frankenhaeuser, 1989). The very determination of how men and women differ in response to occupational hazards, such as exposure to carcinogens is also influenced by gender. Historically, white women have been underrepresented in gender-specific occupational cancer epidemiologic research, compared with white men, by a ratio of 6:1, and nonwhite women have been virtually ignored (a 40:1 discrepancy, compared with white men). Moreover, detailed studies on women have tended to use weaker methodologies, which provide less conclusive data on the occupational cancer risks that women face (Zahm, Pottern, Ward, & White, 1994).

Weight gain and loss can influence susceptibility to toxins and differences in dieting and the natural phenomena of pregnancy lead to more cycles of weight gain and loss in women. Many environmental toxicants stored in adipose tissue may be released during periods of weight loss and this could be a significant factor in the gender differences in response to environmental toxins (Kumanyika, 1998).

Evaluation of Environmental Toxins

Environmental toxins and their potential for causing ill health in humans have been the subject of heated debate in recent years. Understanding what constitutes an environmental toxin, and how its relative danger is estimated, can help the public make informed choices regarding personal behavior and proposed public policy.

What Are Environmental Toxins?

Whereas, synthetic chemicals are commonly seen by the public as the villains of environmental toxicity, chemicals produced in nature are generally regarded as safe. However, over millions of years of evolution, plants and animals have waged an evolutionary war with their predators and competitors (Rosenthal & Janzen, 1979). This escalating "natural" arms race has resulted in a diverse abundance of naturally toxic chemical substances (Rodricks, 1992). Nerve toxins, skin irritants, phototoxic compounds, metabolic disrupters, digestion inhibitors, anesthetics, intoxicants, and sedatives are just some of the categories of toxic compounds produced by plants and animals (Ottoboni, 1997). Ricin, a protein found in castor bean seeds, is one of the most toxic chemicals known. It is so toxic that only 0.3 billionths of a gram supplied intravenously will induce death in a mouse. An aspirin-sized tablet of ricin, divided evenly, could kill 1 million people (Cunningham & Saigo, 1999). On the other hand, some of the toxic substances found in nature, such as lead and mercury, become harmful to humans only when they are excavated and used.

The perception that natural chemicals are good and synthesized chemicals are bad largely stems from the association between human health problems and synthesized substances. It is true, however, that 14 of the top 20 hazardous substances listed by the Agency for Toxic Substances and Disease Registry (1999) are synthetic. The other 6 substances (arsenic, lead, mercury, cadmium, chloroform, and chromium) occur naturally but are released into the environment by human activities. (Chromium III is an essential nutrient that helps maintain the human body's normal metabolism of glucose, cholesterol, and fat. It is dangerous only in extremely high doses.)

The degree of toxicity exhibited by a chemical is not necessarily related to whether it is natural or synthetic, whether it is biodegradable or nonbiodegradable, or whether it has a complex or simple structure. Indeed, approximately half of the known organic chemical compounds either have been isolated in the lab or are synthetic versions of naturally occurring forms. However, chemicals synthesized or exploited by humans generally possess two attributes not necessarily shared by naturally produced substances. The first attribute is that synthetic chemicals and their breakdown products are generally persistent in their environment. The second is that humans are more likely to come into contact with these chemicals than with naturally produced compounds. The length of time a compound persists in the environment is not an essential criterion for toxicity. Many natural substances, such as bones, seashells, and wood, are

slow to biodegrade (Ottoboni, 1997). However, environmental persistence does offer the opportunity for some toxic substances to be transported around the globe, thereby increasing human exposure. The United Nations Environment Programme has identified a dozen chemical compounds (see Box 5–1) that pose a serious threat to the health of both humans and wildlife (Fisher, 1999). All 12 chemicals belong to a class of compounds known as **persistent organic pollutants (POPs).** These are compounds that resist degradation by light, biological compounds, and chemicals. Moreover, many are semivolatile, permitting them to disperse long distances into the atmosphere.

Criteria for Concern

What characteristics make a chemical a toxin? Philippus T.A.B. von Holenheim (1493–1541), better known as Paracelsus, established the essential tenet of toxicology in writing the following: "All substances are poisons; there is none which is not a poison. The right dose differentiates a poison and a remedy." In essence, "the dose makes the poison" (Furst & Fan, 1996). **Toxicology** is the study of toxic properties or adverse health effects due to chemicals or other agents. **Toxicity** is a measure of how harmful a substance is and refers to a chemical's ability to damage organs or disrupt metabolic processes. Frequently, a toxic substance is synonymously referred to as a *hazardous substance,* but there is a distinction between a hazard and a toxin. The term **hazard** implies conditions of use, and its definition has two components: (1) the toxicity of the chemical and (2) the *likelihood of exposure.* For example, the chemical ricin is about 200 times more toxic than dioxin, an industrial by-product, but the likelihood of being exposed to ricin is far less than for dioxin. Dioxin is therefore a more hazardous substance than ricin (Cunningham & Saigo, 1999; Miller, 1998; Ottoboni, 1997).

Two of the most important criteria in ascertaining the toxicity of a chemical are the *size of the dose* (how much chemical is involved) and *duration of exposure.* An **acute exposure** occurs over a very short time period (hours) and generally involves a large single dose, resulting in an **acute response,** during the same time frame, that may be reversible. A **chronic exposure** involves a smaller dose over a longer period of time (months to years) and can generate a **chronic response**—a long-lasting effect that may be permanent. Many chemicals exhibit properties of chronic toxicity, making links between cause and effect difficult. For example, a one-time ingestion of a large amount of metallic mercury (from a broken thermometer) will not cause illness or death. Very little will be absorbed by the intestine, and the remainder will be excreted. However, exposure to a small amount of metallic mercury every day will produce chronic mercury intoxication. Conversely, some chemicals have a high acute toxicity but an extremely low chronic toxicity and, in fact, may be essential to health, in small doses. Vitamin D is such an example. We each need approximately $10\mu g$ (1×10^{-7} g) a day for good health, but an oral dose of 1,000 times that amount (10 mg/kg or 1×10^{-4} g), technically makes vitamin D a **poison** (Ottoboni, 1997).

Difficulties of Establishing Cause and Effect

By definition, the **acute** toxicity of a chemical can be determined fairly readily because it involves investigating a short-term response. Far less is known about the **chronic toxicity** of chemicals because doses may be low, responses may be subtle, and over a long time period other factors may interact to obscure the response of the chemical under investigation. However, chronic responses, such as cancer, are what strike fear in the minds of most people. Although many chemicals are linked with chronic diseases, it can be difficult to determine if and how a particular substance causes harm.

Part of the problem with linking adverse health effects with specific substances lies in the sheer number of chemical compounds that have been produced. The total number of chemical compounds that have been synthesized may be close to 10 million. There are anywhere from 70,000 to 110,000 chemicals currently in use, with approximately

1,000 to 2,000 added annually. The majority of these compounds are produced in small quantities, but nearly 3,000 are produced or imported in quantities at or above 1 million pounds per year. The U.S. Environmental Protection Agency (EPA) (1998) has found that basic toxicity data (human or animal) do not exist for 43 percent of these high-volume chemicals and that a full set of basic information is available for only 7 percent. Studies to establish basic toxicity data (acute toxicity, chronic toxicity, developmental and reproductive toxicity, etc.) take several years and cost over $200,000 per compound. For chemicals in consumer products or to which children might be exposed, more detailed tests, which cost millions of dollars per compound, are needed. As a consequence of these limitations, the National Toxicology Program, the nation's largest toxicology program, can initiate only 10 long-term cancer studies and 10 reproductive studies per year (Lucier & Schecter, 1998). The current regulatory system considers these chemicals innocent until proven guilty on a case-by-case basis—a system that greatly benefits the chemical industry. Surprisingly, to test the nearly 3,000 high-production-volume chemicals would cost the chemical industry only approximately 0.2 percent of the total 1996 annual sales for the top 100 chemical companies (EPA, 1998).

In addition to the volume of tests needed to ascertain the safety of the multitude of individual chemicals, tests on the many chemical mixtures that people are exposed to are critically needed. It is an environmental reality that people experience several chemicals *simultaneously* or *sequentially* via multiple exposure routes. Mixtures of chemicals are ubiquitous in the air we breathe, the water we drink, and the food we eat (Lang, 1995). Exposure to two or more compounds may result in an additive, antagonistic, or even synergistic effect (Carpenter et al., 1998). It is estimated, however, that to conduct studies of two-way interactions with the 500 most widely used industrial chemicals would require 125,000 experiments and that to conduct all of the three-way combinations would require a physically and financially impossible 20.7 million experiments (Miller, 1998).

Because of the dearth of available information, scientists often cannot directly ascertain whether a given chemical is harmful or not. The method used to estimate the safety of chemicals about which not much is known is to extrapolate from other data. This limits scientists' ability to conclude with certainty that a given compound is the cause of a particular health effect. *Anecdotal evidence* and *case reports* from physicians provide the least amount of reliability on the health effects of a given compound. They have limited usefulness because they are few in number, the health status of the individual is generally unknown, and usually the dose and duration of exposure have not been controlled or are unknown. However, such evidence may alert health officials that a particular chemical has potentially adverse health effects and may stimulate more rigorous testing (Miller, 1998; Ottoboni, 1997).

Animal testing is the most commonly used and widely accepted method for assessing the acute and chronic toxicity of various chemicals. These studies are known as **dose-response assessments** because they produce a relationship between the dose of a compound and the incidence of the adverse health effect in the treatment group. These experiments produce reliable results because they consist of treating animals under controlled conditions, which eliminate confounding factors to the greatest degree possible. Moreover, a **test group** is compared with a **control group,** which is not exposed to the chemical. This permits health researchers to account for common diseases that might occur in the test group but that are unrelated to the treatment chemical (Ottoboni, 1997).

The use of animal testing as the methodology for determining the toxicity of substances to humans has been openly challenged. A criticism is that the animals are exposed to much higher doses of whatever material is being tested than humans would ever be. However, using very high doses in animal research is necessary in order to reduce the number of test animals needed to yield valid statistics. With the use of very high doses, only hundreds or thousands of animal subjects are needed, whereas without it, millions or at least hundreds of thousands, would be needed. The results from the high-dose experiment are extrapolated to low doses using mathematical models. Then these low doses are extrapolated to humans to estimate toxicity (National Institute of Environmental Health Sciences [NIEHS], 1998a). This procedure has been highly criticized because any substance when administered at a high enough concentration (such as saccharine) may be carcinogenic (Cohen, Kaufman, Ruttenberg, & Fano, 1998). The use of animals as models for humans has also been criticized on the grounds that animal response does not always predict what will happen in humans (Salsburg, 1983). Historically, the implementation of proper workplace precautions for asbestos were delayed for decades (Enterline, 1988), and the tobacco industry was able to delay government warnings against smoking, because tests on animals produced results that were contradictory to human responses (Barnard & Kaufman, 1997). Unrelated species do react differently to the same compounds. Ninety-five out of 226 chemicals thought to be carcinogenic to both rats and mice produced cancer in one species but not the other (Ames, Magaw, & Gold, 1987). Whereas, more than 400 chemicals have been found to be carcinogenic to rodents, only 20 to 30 have been proven toxic for humans (Lewis, Ioannides, & Parke, 1998).

However, the National Institute of Environmental Health Sciences (1998a) considers that as mammals even as mice are more similar to humans in their biological function, physiology, and biochemistry than bacteria, they are the best surrogate models. The successful development of antibiotic sulfanilamide drugs depended on the screening of the prospective compound, prontosil, in mice, because the same compound had no effect on bacteria in culture. The use of sulfonamide drugs has reduced death from puerperal sepsis (a disease contracted by mothers after childbirth due to hemolytic streptococci) from 200 to 5 of every 100,000 births (Botting & Morrison, 1997). Ironically, relying entirely on test animals could result in the unwarranted labeling of some compounds as unsafe for humans. For example, Tamoxifen, a therapeutic agent used in the treatment of breast cancer, is a known carcinogen to rodents and other test animals but is metabolized differently by humans and is generally regarded as acceptable for use by younger women (Fisher, Powles, & Pritchard, 2000; Gail et al., 1999).

Animal testing is also opposed by animal rights groups, prompting scientists to look for ways to reduce the number of animals used by conducting tests on bacteria, cell and tissue cultures, and chicken egg membranes, and through human biopsies and autopsies (Cohen et al., 1998; NIEHS, 1998b). However, these tests can provide information only about acute toxicity. The best way to obtain information about the chronic toxicity of chemicals is to test them on humans. Considering that this is not an ethically acceptable approach, health scientists rely on epidemiological studies to understand what factors are responsible for causing illness in one group of people but not another.

Although **epidemiology** originally focused on the occurrence and distribution of disease in human populations, it is now widely used to study the health effects of environmental pollutants and food additives. The purpose of epidemiology is to discover the chain of association between diseases and their causative agents in an effort to protect humans by preventing repeated exposure to a harmful substance. Epidemiological studies rely on logical thinking, systematic documentation, and rigorous statistical analysis to compare the health of people who have been exposed to a particular substance or environment with that of people who have not. For example, during the early 1960s, outbreaks of neonatal jaundice in a hospital in the Imperial Valley of California appeared to be associated with the use of cotton defoliants. For several years in a row, cases of neonatal jaundice increased during the late summer months, which was coincidentally about the same time that cotton defoliants were being used in the agricultural area that surrounded the relatively new hospital. It was conjectured that the defoliants were causing liver damage in the newborns, and thus preventing the breakdown of excess bilirubin and leading to jaundice. However, other hospitals that were also situated in the same agricultural area reported no such annual outbreak (Ottoboni, 1997). Independent of these events, a nurse in England observed that newborns placed in cribs near windows were less likely to have jaundice (Fincher, 1985). In retrospect, it was apparent that both defoliant spraying and the increased incidence of jaundice occurred at a time of the year when people of all ages (including newborns) tended to stay indoors to avoid the heat. This, combined with the fact that the new hospital had fewer windows than other area hospitals, suggests that the Imperial Valley jaundice outbreaks were associated with the lack of bright light, rather than exposure to cotton defoliants.

The central limitation of epidemiological studies is that they may make a strong, moderate, weak, or no association between a potentially harmful agent and its health effects, but they cannot establish a cause and effect relationship. A significant contributor to this limitation is that such studies are generally an after-the-fact science. They cannot control the size of the dose, nor can they control for the myriad of potentially interacting substances that individuals may be exposed to during their lifetimes. In fact, establishing the dose often depends on the memory of the subjects (Ottoboni, 1997).

Epidemiological studies are limited in their ability to detect small differences in the rates of common diseases. Such studies may not account for genetic differences, called **polymorphisms,** that may make some people more susceptible to a disease and thus obscure the impact of a chemical (Kaiser, 1997). For example, approximately 5 to 10 percent of breast cancer cases can be linked to inherited breast cancer susceptibility genes (Sakorafas & Tsiotou, 2000). Moreover, genetic polymorphisms will make some individuals more susceptible than others to the harmful effects of a chemical.

Environmental Toxins of Special Concern to Women

Because of the nature of women's reproductive physiology, and the fact that many women bear and nurse infants, certain environmental toxins pose a special danger to them. These include endocrine disruptors, dioxins, lead, mercury, and organic solvents.

Endocrine Disruptors

Endocrine disruptors are synthetic or plant-derived compounds that affect the endocrine systems of animals. Some have been associated with birth defects, sexual abnormalities, and reproductive failure in natural and laboratory animal populations, and there is speculation that they may be generating hormone-related cancers in women and reduced sperm counts in men. An endocrine disruptor is defined as "an exogenous substance or mixture that alters the function of the endocrine system and consequently causes adverse health effects in an intact organism or its progeny or sub-populations" (EPA, 1997b).

The endocrine system is one of the two communication systems of the body (the other is the nervous system) that regulate the response and function of both short-term processes (such as maintaining the body's internal steady state) and long-term processes (such as growth, development, and reproduction). Steroid hormones are the messengers of the endocrine system, and they have specific chemical conformations that match the receptor sites of the target cells in a manner much like a lock and key arrangement (Eubanks, 1997). Scientists at one time thought that the protein receptor site in a cell would accept only a specific hormone and no other, but the discovery of other compounds (endocrine disruptors) that can also unlock receptor sites quickly changed this perception (McLachlan & Arnold, 1996).

The most commonly used synonym for endocrine disruptors is **environmental estrogens.** These are substances that mimic or partly mimic the function of true steroid hormones, such as estrogen and androgens, through their ability to bind to hormone target receptor sites and initiate a sequence of events in the same way that a hormone would. Other synonyms for endocrine disruptors are estrogen mimics, hormone mimics, and xenoestrogens. Not all hormone mimics stimulate the functioning of the endocrine system. Some compounds block the ability of the body's hormones to bind with the hormone receptor site. These compounds are called **anti-estrogens,** or **anti-androgens** (male hormones). The type of environmental disruptors, known as **modulators,** do not bind to the hormone receptor site but can alter how the body's hormones are produced or bind to the receptor. They can indirectly turn on genes and alter cell growth and cell division. Moreover, a single chemical may act on the endocrine system in more than one way (Center for Bioenvironmental Research, 2000).

Phytoestrogens are estrogen-like compounds that are produced naturally by plants. They occur in many plant-derived foods, including many legumes (soybeans and soy products), whole grains, vegetables (beans, carrots, cabbage, and potatoes), fruits (dates, pomegranates, cherries, and apples), and even coffee. Unlike the synthetic xenoestrogens that are generally harmful, phytoestrogens in low doses may have a beneficial effect. Epidemiological studies have indicated that phytoestrogens may offer long-term protection against some cancers, including breast, endometrial, colon, prostate, liver, and leukemia. In addition, the consumption of phytoestrogens may delay the onset of menstruation in young women and reduce the occurrence of hot flashes in menopausal women. Phytoestrogens may also protect against osteoporosis. At very high concentrations, phytoestrogens have reduced the fertility of wildlife and farm animals and have altered sexual cycles in female rats (Barret, 1996).

Compounds that can act as endocrine disruptors span a wide range of artificially produced chemicals (see Table 5–1). The main concern is that, if the human body requires only very small amounts of endogenously produced hormones to function, then exposure to a small amount of environmental estrogen could be harmful. However, many environmental estrogens and phytoestrogens have activities

TABLE 5–1 Some hormone-disrupting chemicals and their most common sources and routes of exposure.

Chemical	Sources	Exposure
Polychlorinated biphenyls (PCBs)	Lubricants and coolants in electrical equipment	Consumption of contaminated fish and shellfish, breathing of contaminated air
Dichlorodiphenyltrichoroethane (DDT)	Pesticides	Consumption of contaminated root and leafy vegetables; meat, fish, and poultry may also contain very low levels of these compounds
Dioxins, furans	Combustion of PVC plastics, chlorine-based solvents and bleaches, pesticides	Consumption of contaminated meat, fish, eggs, and dairy products
Phthalates	Teething toys, plastic wrap	Direct ingestion or through contamination of meats, cheeses, or microwaved food covered with plastic wrap
Bisphenol A	Epoxy resins, polycarbonate plastic	Lining in food cans, plastic dental fillings
Alkyl phenol (nonyl phenols)	Industrial detergents, active ingredient in (nonyl-9) spermicides	Consumption of contaminated drinking water
Fungicides, herbicides, organochlorine pesticides	Pesticides	Consumption of contaminated vegetables and animal products
Lead, mercury, cadmium	Combustion of fossil fuels and municipal waste, cigarette smoke (lead, cadmium)	Consumption of contaminated vegetables (lead, cadmium) and fish (mercury), breathing of contaminated air

Adapted from: "Most Unwanted, Persistent Organic Pollutants," by B. Fisher, 1999, *Environmental Health Perspectives, 107,* A18–A23; "Endocrine Disruption from Environmental Toxicants," by T. Colborn, 1998, in W. N. Rom (Ed.), *Environmental and Occupational Medicine, 3rd ed.,* pp. 398–415, Philadelphia: Lippincott-Raven; "Hormone Disrupting Chemicals," [online], Hormone Disrupting Chemicals Homepage, 2000. Retrieved July 11th, 2000. Available: http://www.website.lineone.net/~mwarhurst/

that are far below that of estradiol, the primary and most potent human estrogen (see Table 5–2). Moreover, humans are exposed to low estrogen doses through the consumption of phytoestrogens in the diet; it is estimated that estrogenic compounds of industrial origin contribute to only 0.0000025 percent of the total daily intake of dietary estrogens (Safe, 1995b). Whether xenoestrogens are metabolized by the body, like phytoestrogens, or are bioaccumulated in adipose tissue remains unclear (American Council on Science and Health [ACSH], 1999; Barret, 1996).

Evidence demonstrating cause and effect between man-made chemicals or their breakdown products and adverse effects on human health via an endocrine-disrupting mechanism is lacking (American Council on Science and Health, 1999; EPA, 1997b; Safe, 1995a, 1995b). However, high doses of estrogenic chemicals have been demonstrated to have endocrine-mediated effects on wildlife species, laboratory colonies of animals, and cell cultures, thus generating cause for concern for humans (ACSH, 1999; Colborn, Dumanoski, & Myers, 1996; Foster, 1998).

TABLE 5–2 Relative potencies of selected estrogenic substances compared with estradiol.

Chemical	Potency Ratio
Estradiol—the most abundant and potent human estrogen	1.00—represents the greatest estrogenic potency and the standard by which estrogen activity is measured
Diethylstilbestrol (DES)—a drug prescribed to prevent miscarriages	0.64—DES is 0.6 times as potent as estradiol.
Coumestrol—a phytoestrogen found in sunflower seeds and alfalfa sprouts	0.01—Coumestrol is 77 times less potent than estradiol.
p-Nonylphenol—a chemical used in some plastics	0.0002—p-Nonylphenol is 5,000 times less potent than estradiol.
Bisphenol A—a chemical used in some plastics	0.00007—Bisphenol A is 15,000 times less potent than estradiol.
β-Sitosterol—a natural plant compound used as an anticholesterol agent	0.000005—β-Sitosterol is 220,000 times less potent than estradiol.
Testosterone—a male sex hormone	0.000004—Testosterone is 226,000 times less potent than estradiol.
Methoxychlor—a pesticide	0.0000002—Methoxychlor is 5 million times less potent than estradiol.
DDT—a pesticide	0.0000001—DDT is 8 million times less potent than estradiol.
DDE—a breakdown product of DDT	0.00000004—DDE is 24 million times less potent than estradiol.

Adapted from "Evaluation of Chemicals with Endocrine Modulating Activity in Yeast-based Steroid Hormone Receptor Gene Transcription Essay," by K. W. Galdo, et al., in *Toxicology and Applied Pharmacology, 143,* 205–212. Copyright 1997, Elsevier Science (USA). Reproduced by permission of the publisher.

Dioxin

Dioxin is the generic name for a group of 75 chlorinated aromatic hydrocarbons, which include the chlorinated dibenzo-p-dioxins (CDDs), chlorinated dibenzofurans (CDFs), and certain polychlorinated biphenyls (PCBs). The most notorious members of this group is 2,3,7,8-TCDD, which first gained notice in 1970 when it was discovered to be a contaminant of the herbicide **Agent Orange** (2,4,5,-T), the defoliant that was sprayed on the forests in Vietnam. TCDD is the most toxic of the CDDs and is the most studied.

The incineration of municipal and medical waste is the largest source of dioxin in the environment, followed by the chlorine bleaching of paper pulp, the chlorination of waste and drinking water, and pesticide manufacturing (Agency for Toxic Substances and Disease Registry, 1999; EPA, 2000b). Dioxins enter the human food chain primarily by atmospheric deposition on plants and soil. Approximately 95 per-

cent of our exposure to dioxins is through the dietary intake of animal fats. Breast-feeding constitutes a significant amount (14 percent) of the cumulative human exposure to dioxin prior to reproductive age, after which 65 to 90 percent of exposure occurs through eating contaminated food, particularly meat, dairy products, and fish. However, the benefits of breast-feeding outweigh the risks of dioxin exposure (EPA, 2000c; Patandin et al., 1999).

Dioxins are emblematic of the difficulty of linking cause and effect with any potentially toxic compound. Prior to the mid 1900s, there was little awareness of the dangers of chemicals; heavy metals, such as lead and mercury, were used freely and without protection. This resulted in a substantial data set documenting the toxicity of these chemicals to humans. During the latter half of the 1900s to the present, workers have been offered greater protection and, for the most part, are not intentionally subjected to chemicals without prior knowledge of their toxicity. However, it is not possible (legally or ethically) to test a putatively toxic chemical on humans in an attempt to obtain toxicity data. We must rely on those few cohorts that have been subject to accidental or occupational exposure at levels greater than background levels, such as the residents of Seveso, Italy who were exposed to dioxin (Bertazzi, Bernucci, Brambilla, Consonni, & Pesatori, 1998), and workers involved in the production of chemicals contaminated with TCDD (Fingerhut et al., 1991). When follow-up studies were conducted on these cohorts, few clinically significant effects were found, even though dioxin is considered to be one of the most toxic substances produced by humans.

One of the most consistently documented health problems linked with dioxin exposure is the acute response of chloracne, a skin condition resembling acne. In addition to chloracne, the long-term consequences of exposure to TCDD include elevated levels of gamma glutamyl transferase (GGT), an enzyme indicative of obstructed bile ducts and associated with liver disease, and alterations in male reproductive hormones. Aside from these effects, no definite cause and effect relationships have been established for reported health effects, such as nerve damage, fatigue, depression, personality changes, hepatitis, enlarged liver, abnormal enzyme levels, and porphyria cutanea tarda—a disorder that involves liver dysfunction and photosensitive dermatitis. Although the rates of many cancers are greater in those cohorts exposed to levels of TCDD greater than background, the magnitude is generally small because of the small sample sizes involved (EPA 2000a; International Agency for Research on Cancer [IARC], 1997). The acute effects of dioxins in animals are better established and include weight loss, liver damage, chloracne, and weakening of the immune system. In female animals, exposure to dioxins can induce miscarriages, generate hormonal irregularities in the estrous cycle, and reduce fertility. Birth defects associated with the transplacental transfer of dioxins from mother to fetus include skeletal deformities, kidney defects, weakened immune responses, lower birth weight, hyperpigmentation of the gums and nails, conjunctivitis, and bronchitis (Agency for Toxic Substances and Disease Registry, 1999; Fisher, 1999; Rogan et al., 1988). Human epidemiological studies alone have not provided unequivocal evidence that dioxins are dangerous to people. Nevertheless, TCDD has been characterized as a "human carcinogen" and other dioxins as "likely human carcinogens" on the basis of human studies coupled with animal studies and the inferences that can be drawn from cellular and biochemicalmechanistic studies (EPA, 2000a; International Agency for Research on Cancer, 1997).

It has been suggested that exposure to dioxin confers a risk of *endometriosis*. Although correlations exist between the incidence of endometriosis and blood serum levels of dioxins or the degree of industrialization in the community, it remains unclear whether dioxins actually cause endometriosis in humans (Koninckx, 1999; Mayani, Barel, Soback, & Almagor, 1997). One preliminary study found no relationship between the severity of endometriosis in women and blood serum levels of dioxins (EPA, 1997b). The strongest evidence for a relationship between dioxins and endometriosis was provided by a long-term study of female rhesus monkeys. After four years of exposure to TCDD, a dose-dependent response in the severity of the disease was noted (Rier, Martin, Bowman, Dmowski, & Becker, 1993). Popular literature (Houppert, 1995; Yannello, 1998) has indicated that the rayon fibers of tampons used to contain dioxins and thus posed an increased risk for endometriosis. Rayon is made from cellulose fiber derived from wood pulp, and in the past, wood pulp was bleached using a process that did produce dioxin. While the U.S. Food and Drug Administration (FDA) (1999) has indicated that the dioxin levels in tampons were far below the EPA's threshold for consumer risk, this assessment was based on the data provided by the tampon manufacturers. Currently, the FDA states that the cellulose used in U.S. tampons is now produced using a process that does not involve dioxin.

Lead

Lead is a naturally occurring mineral, found in the earth's crust, that has been distributed throughout the environment (plants, animals, soil, and water) due to human activities, such as mining, manufacturing, and the burning of fossil fuels. Prior to 1973, auto emissions constituted 90 percent of the lead in the atmosphere but now amount to less than 35 percent. Vegetable foods are the leading sources of exposure to lead. Lead emitted by power plants, industry, and auto emissions is deposited on soil, where it is absorbed by crops. Other sources of exposure to lead include cigarette smoke, contaminated air, and crystal and ceramic containers. Lead-soldered cans and plumbing were significant sources at one time, but both have been banned. However, lead-soldered plumbing still exists in many older homes. Children are more likely to be exposed to lead through the ingestion of lead-containing paint chips (an abnormal eating habit known as *pica*) and soil. In comparison with adults, children who consume food, beverages, or other substances contaminated with lead absorb more of the ingested lead via the gastrointestinal tract. Because of this difference in metabolism, children tend to develop higher blood levels of lead than adults (ATSDR, 1999; Chiras, 1998). Although exposure to lead in the U.S. population has decreased since the late 1970s, some population groups—namely, low-income groups, minorities, and those inhabiting older homes (pre 1946)—remain at significant risk (Pirkle et al., 1998).

Almost every organ system in the body is affected by lead. The most sensitive is the *central nervous system*, but lead also damages the kidneys and the immune system. Although lead acetate and lead phosphate have been demonstrated to be carcinogenic to animals, no cause and effect has been demonstrated for humans. Lead exposure in infants and young children decreases intelligence (I.Q.) scores, slows growth, and causes hearing problems. Unborn children are at particular risk; they may be born prematurely, have a low birth weight, and have decreased mental abilities and learning difficulties.

Lead is an important health issue for women who breast-feed, since the majority of lead in breast milk comes from maternal bone and diet. By adulthood, 90 to 95 percent of the body burden of lead has been stored in the bones, but this may be resorbed into the blood and circulated in the body under two conditions: (1) during pregnancy and lactation and (2) during aging (National Institute of Environmental Health Sciences [NIEHS], 1997a). Studies done on infant subjects during the first 60–90 days postpartum indicated that 36 to 80 percent of the breast-fed infants' blood lead levels had come from breast milk. The blood lead levels in the breast-fed infants, however, were similar to the levels in the infants fed with formula. Breast-fed infants are at risk only if the mother has a history of high lead exposure or is currently exposed to high concentrations from external sources (Gulson et al., 1998; Sinks & Jackson, 1999).

Mercury

Mercury is a chemical element that occurs naturally in the earth's crust, as well as in the environment in several forms due to human and natural processes. Most of the mercury in the atmosphere is in the elemental form, whereas the mercury found in water, soil, plants, and animals is either a form of inorganic mercury or organic mercury (methylmercury). Mercury is persistent in the environment but may change forms when combined with other elements. Microorganisms in the water or soil can combine mercury with carbon to create **methylmercury** (the organic form), the main form that accumulates in the adipose tissue of fish (EPA, 1997a).

The most familiar anthropogenic source of metallic mercury is glass thermometers, but mercury is also found in dental fillings, batteries, fluorescent lamps, and electrical switches, and it is used to produce chlorine gas and caustic soda. Mercury salts are used in skin-lightening creams, antiseptic creams and ointments, and as a preservative in many pharmaceutical products. The dominant pathway of exposure to mercury is through the consumption of contaminated fish and shellfish (methylmercury), and through breathing the vapors during the use of mercury in the workplace (elemental mercury) (ATSDR, 1999). The typical U.S. consumer who eats fish in restaurants and from grocery stores is not in danger of ingesting harmful levels of mercury. However, some demographic groups, such as recreational anglers, and cultural groups that depend heavily on fish as part of their diet, have higher body burdens of mercury.

Both methylmercury and elemental mercury can cross placental and blood-brain barriers. Once across these barriers, the mercury is oxidized, which impedes its return to the general circulatory system. Approximately 80 percent of the mercury vapor continually released by dental amalgams is reabsorbed by the lungs, making dental fillings the greatest source of inorganic mercury; however, the actual amount of mercury released by amalgams and the hazards associated with them are disputed (American Dental Association, 1995; Barret & Gots, 1998; Lorscheider, Vimy, & Summers, 1995). Although all forms of mercury can accumulate in humans and animals, methylmercury is taken up at a faster rate and with greater efficiency, and it is eliminated more slowly than elemental and inorganic mercury. The avenues of elimination from the body vary for the three forms of mercury but include urine, feces, exhaled air, sweat, breast milk, and saliva (EPA, 1997a).

Methylmercury is listed by the International Program of Chemical Safety as one of the six most dangerous chemicals in the environment (Gilbert & Grant-Webster, 1995). However, all three forms of mercury have been associated with adverse human health effects. The nervous system is the most sensitive to mercury exposure, but mercury can also cause renal dysfunction and degenerative changes in the liver, kidney, and other organs. There is currently no evidence that mercury is carcinogenic. Developing embryos and fetuses are at highest risk for toxicity due to mercury exposure. High levels of prenatal exposure through the maternal diet can result in severe mental retardation and cerebral palsy–like behavior (ATSDR 1999; Factor-Litvak, Stein, & Graziano, 1993; Gilbert & Grant-Webster, 1995; Mottet, Shaw, & Burbacher, 1985). A slight increase in neuropsychological dysfunctions (language, attention, memory) has been found for the children of women living in some communities that rely on fish as a source of protein (Grandjean, Weihe, White, & Debes, 1998; Muckle, Dewailly, & Ayotte, 1998; Myer & Davidson, 1998). Breast milk is also a source of methylmercury to infants. Both the frequency of fish consumption and the number of dental amalgams have been correlated with the concentration of methylmercury in breast milk. The amounts of mercury in a mother's breast milk will, of course, depend on her diet and environmental circumstances, but the concentration may be the same as that of infant formula (Drasch, Aigner, Roider, Staiger, & Lipowsky, 1998; Oskarsson et al., 1996). Furthermore, the benefits of breastfeeding on infant development outweigh any potential adverse effects mercury may have (Grandjean, Weihe, & White, 1995). The removal of amalgam fillings during pregnancy can do more harm than good by increasing mercury levels in the blood and breast milk of pregnant and lactating women and subjecting the fetus or infant to unnecessary mercury exposure (Sandborgh-Englund, Elinder, Langworth, Schultz, & Ekstrand, 1998; Vimy, Hooper, King, & Lorscheider, 1997).

Organic Solvents

Exposure to organic solvents is sometimes seen as more of a concern for men, but many women, particularly those of childbearing age, are also exposed to organic solvents, either in an occupational setting or through common household products. Some of the solvents that women are most likely to come into contact with in an occupational setting include trichloroethylene (cleaning solvent), xylene (chemical solvent and paint thinner), vinyl chloride (used to make PVC and plastics), and acetone (chemical solvent). Women-dominated occupations with the potential for exposure to organic solvents include jobs in the clothing and textile industries, laboratory technology and chemistry, art and graphic design, and printing (Khattak, K.-Moghtader, Barrera, Kennedy, & Koren, 1999). Women employed as postal service personnel, healthcare professionals, and hairstylists are also at increased risk for organic solvent exposure (Schenker & Jacobs, 1996; Swanson & Burns, 1997). The consequences of occupational exposure to organic solvents highlights the distinction between *gender differences* and *sex differences* when humans are exposed to environmental toxins. In cohorts with an unexpectedly high incidence of an uncommon salivary gland cancer, the women were more likely to be hair dressers, whereas the men were more likely to be oil and gas salespeople and railroad workers. However, the women's tumors were often characterized as benign, whereas the men's tumors were more often characterized as malignant (Swanson & Burns, 1997). The risks of salivary gland cancer are associated not only with professional hairstylists; the incidence of this cancer is also higher among individuals who apply their own hair dye (Spitz, Fueger, Goepfert, & Newell, 1990).

The consequences of organic solvent exposure are well known and include central nervous system toxicity, liver, renal and dermatologic injury, and irritation of the respiratory pathways. Pregnant women who are exposed to organic solvents put the health of their child at risk; organic solvents are absorbed through women's skin, lungs, and digestive tract; enter the bloodstream; and then cross the placenta to the developing fetus. Children born to women who are exposed to organic solvents at the workplace or at home are more likely to be born with malformations, such as deafness, clubfoot, spina bifida, and central nervous system and cardiovascular abnormalities; as adults, they are more likely to have reduced fertility and an increase in miscarriages (Homlberg, 1979; Khattak et al., 1999; Silberg, Ransom, Lyon, & Anderson, 1979).

Keeping It in Perspective

The majority of environmental toxins are acutely toxic, but, by the same token, most people are able to avoid acute exposure to these compounds. On the other hand, a causative link between most environmental toxins and chronic human health effects has been difficult to establish, even though it is widely accepted that such toxins have an adverse health effect on wildlife. It makes prudent sense that, as individuals, we would wish to reduce our exposure to potentially harmful substances (see Box 5–2). However, even if we know that

---

Box 5–2   Top 10 Ways to Reduce Exposure to Potential Environmental Toxins

1. Buy organic fruits and vegetables.
2. Don't use chemical pesticides, herbicides, and fungicides.
3. Wash fruits and vegetables before eating.
4. Eat lower on the food chain. Reduce your intake of carnivorous fish and other fatty foods.
5. Filter your drinking water.
6. Use nontoxic household cleaners.
7. Microwave in glass or ceramic containers—avoid using plastic wrap.
8. Recycle and compost all the waste that you can.
9. Buy durable goods and avoid excessively packaged goods.
10. Quit smoking.

---

a substance is harmful, it is necessary to make an assessment of the actual risk associated with that substance. There are four components to **risk assessment:** (1) identifying the hazards involved, (2) estimating the probability of exposure (or event), (3) estimating the severity of the exposure, and (4) estimating the degree of damage or harm that may be done (Roberts & Abernathy, 1996). Whether a risk is acceptable depends on two factors: (1) our perception of the harm that it can cause and (2) the perceived benefits associated with the risk. Moreover, we may be more willing to accept a risk if we feel that we are in control of the circumstances that expose us to the risk. For example, we may be willing to accept the risk of dying in an automobile accident, which, in a given year is about 2.4 in 10,000, because we can control whether we take the risk and we derive considerable benefit from taking it. We may also accept the greater risk of dying from smoking a pack of cigarettes per day (3.6 in 1,000) for the same reasons. In contrast, we may resent, and worry a lot about, contaminated drinking water, even though the risk of dying from drinking water with the EPA's limit of trichloroethylene is about 2 in 1 billion (Wilson & Crouch, 1987). These examples provide a perspective from which we might consider which risks we will take for granted and which ones we will avoid.

The effect that a risk has on our lives can be expressed as the **loss of life expectancy,** or **LLE.** The LLE represents the number of years of life that will be lost due to the presence of a risk factor. The LLEs for some common avoidable risk factors are as follows: smoking (3.9 years for females smoking one or more packs a day); being 20 percent overweight (about 2.8 years); drinking alcohol (about 1 year for the average American); drinking contaminated water (1.3 days). The LLE for exposure to cancer-causing pollution is 30 days, and, for exposure to pollution that causes non-cancerous diseases, it is 20 days. For exposure to pesticide residues on food (including more than 200 chemicals), it is 12 days (Cohen, 1992).

Approximately 65 to 70 percent of human cancers can be attributed to smoking, diet, alcohol, and behavior (Henderson, Ross, & Pike, 1991; Higginson, 1993). We can easily avoid or modulate our exposure to those substances that are strongly linked with cancer, but, unfortunately, some of the greatest risks that people face are those they may not be able to avoid. For example, the LLE for people living in an area of poverty in the United States is about 9 years, and the LLE for being of the male gender is 7.5 years. However, there are many risk factors we can avoid by making wise lifestyle choices.

New Directions

Given the paucity of information on the human health effects of the 3,000 chemicals that are produced in volume, the field is wide open for the testing of these chemicals. The Agency for Toxic Substances and Disease Registry maintains and updates its list of the environmental and human health effects of more than 100 hazardous substances. Six federal agencies (the National Center for Toxicological Research, National Institutes of Health, National Institute for Environmental and Health Sciences, Food and Drug Administration, National Institute for Occupational Safety and Health, and Centers for Disease Control and Prevention) participate in the National Toxicology Program, which supports long-term carcinogenesis studies, short-term toxicity studies, immunotoxicity studies, continuous breeding studies, short-term reproductive and developmental toxicity studies, and teratology studies. However, these studies use rats and mice as subjects. Fortunately, the National Institute for Environmental and Health Sciences (NIEHS) recognizes that much of the human data is based on male occupational studies, and therefore the NIEHS is supporting epidemiological studies with women, such as research on the role of the environment in breast carcinoma.

Currently, 50 percent of the cases of breast carcinoma can be accounted for by genes, the number of first-degree relatives with breast carcinoma, age at menstruation, and age at menopause. It is suspected that environmental components are risk factors in the remaining 50 percent of the cases (Johnson-Thompson & Guthrie, 2000). The Sisterhood Study, which follows women who are sisters of breast carcinoma survivors, is currently being conducted. Because these sisters are considered to be at twice the risk for the development of breast carcinoma, they are an ideal cohort for examining the role of suspected environmental toxins. The

NIEHS also recognizes that African American women have the highest mortality rate from breast carcinoma and has placed special emphasis on this demographic in studies examining the roles of diet, lifestyle choices, and endocrine disruptors as risk factors.

No single study, however, can be the basis for definitive conclusions on the hazards of any given substance. Many government agencies, such as the Environmental Protection Agency and The Center for the Evaluation of Risks to Human Reproduction, provide timely, unbiased, scientifically sound assessments of potentially hazardous substances to the public. These summaries are based on numerous animal and human occupational studies, accidental exposure reports, follow-ups, and planned epidemiological studies.

QUESTIONS FOR REFLECTION AND DISCUSSION

1. *Consider the tenet "The dose makes the poison." Using your research skills, find a substance that is not acutely toxic at low doses but is toxic at high doses.*
2. *Because any chemical can potentially be a poison, should we be concerned with occasional exposure to chemical toxins?*
3. *A physician files a case report suggesting that a certain chemical is toxic. What steps should be taken to evaluate this substance? What information would you need before providing safety information to people?*
4. *Should you be more concerned about an acute exposure or a chronic exposure? What factors must be considered in answering this question?*
5. *Should you be more concerned about being exposed to occasional home pesticide use or pumping your own gasoline? Explain.*
6. *Using the four components of risk assessment, assess the avoidable and unavoidable risk factors in your environment. On what basis do you avoid some risks and not others?*
7. *The risk of dying from a shark attack (1 in 300 million) is smaller than the risk of dying while driving to the beach (1 in 5,000), yet which do you fear more? Why?*

RESOURCES

Books

Barret, S. J., & Gots, R. E. (1998). *Chemical sensitivity: The truth about environmental illness.* Amherst, NY: Prometheus Books.

Colborn, T., Dumanoski, D., & Myers, J. P. (1996). *Our stolen future: Are we threatening our fertility, intelligence and survival?—A scientific detective story.* New York: Dutton Books.

Ottoboni, M. A. (1997). *The dose makes the poison: A plain language guide to toxicology.* (2nd ed.). New York: Van Nostrand Reinhold.

Rodricks, J. A. (1992). *Calculated risks: Understanding the toxicity and human health risks of chemicals in our environment.* Cambridge, England: Cambridge University Press.

Websites

Agency for Toxic Substances and Disease Registry. http://www.atsdr.cdc.gov/

Center for Bioenvironmental Research at Tulane and Xavier Universities. http://www.mcl.tulane.edu/ECME/eehome/

Center for the Evaluation of Risks to Human Reproduction (CERHR). http://cerhr.niehs.nih.gov/index.html

Hormone Disrupting Chemicals Home Page. http://website.lineone.net/~mwarhurst/

National Center for Environmental Assessment. http://www.epa.gov/ncea/

National Health and Environmental Effects Research Laboratory. http://www.epa.gov/nheerl/

National Institute of Environmental Health Sciences. http://www.niehs.nih.gov/

TOXNET (Toxicology Data Network). http://www.toxnet.nlm.nih.gov/

REFERENCES

Agency for Toxic Substances and Disease Registry. (1999). *Top 20 hazardous substances. ATSDR/EPA priority list for 1999* [On-line]. Available: http://www.atsdr.cdc.gov/atsdrhome.html

American Council on Science and Health (1999). *Endocrine disruptors: A scientific perspective.* New York: American Council on Science and Health.

American Dental Association. (1995). *Dental amalgam: 150 years of safety and effectiveness. ADA news releases* [On-line]. Available: http://www.ada.org/newsrel/1195/nr-02a.html

Ames, B. N., Magaw, R., & Gold, L. S. (1987). Ranking possible carcinogenic hazards. *Science, 236,* 271–280.

Austin, H., Drews, C., & Partridge, E. E. (1993). A case-control study of endometrial cancer in relation to cigarette smoking, serum estrogen levels, and alcohol use. *American Journal of Obstetrics and Gynecology, 169,* 1086–1091.

Barnard, N. D., & Kaufman, S. R. (1997). Animal research is wasteful and misleading. *American Scientific, 276*(2), 80–82.

Baron, J. A., La Vecchia, C., & Levi, F. (1990). The antiestrogenic effect of cigarette smoking in women. *American Journal of Obstetrics and Gynecology, 162,* 502–514.

Barret, J. (1996). Phytoestrogens: Friends or foes? *Environmental Health Perspectives, 104,* 478–482.

Barret, S. J., & Gots, R. E. (1998). *Chemical sensitivity: The truth about environmental illness.* Amherst, NY: Prometheus Books.

Bertazzi, P. A., Bernucci, I., Brambilla, G., Consonni, D., & Pesatori, A. C. (1998). The Seveso studies on early and long-term effects of dioxin exposure: A review. *Environmental Health Perspectives, 106* (Suppl. 2), 625–633.

Botting, J. H., & Morrison, A. R. (1997). Animal research is vital to medicine. *Scientific American, 276*(2), 83–85.

Brinton, L. A., Barret, R. J., Berman, M. L., Mortel, R., Twiggs, L. B., & Wilbanks, G. D. (1993). Cigarette smoking and the risk of endometrial cancer. *American Journal of Epidemiology, 137,* 281–291.

Carpenter, D. O., Arcaro, K. F., Bush, B., Niemi, W. D., Pang, S., & Vakharia, D. D. (1998). Human health and chemical mixtures: An overview. *Environmental Health Perspectives, 106* (Suppl. 6), 1263–1270.

Carson, R. (1962). *Silent spring.* Boston: Houghton Mifflin.

Castelli, W. P. (1999). Cardiovascular disease: Pathogenesis, epidemiology, and risk among users of oral contraceptives who smoke. *American Journal of Obstetrics and Gynecology, 180,* S349–S356.

Center for Bioenvironmental Research. (2000). *Environmental estrogens and other hormones* [On-line]. http://www.mcl.tulane.edu/ECME/eehome/

Chiras, D. D. (1998). *Environmental science: A systems approach to sustainable development.* Belmont, CA: Wadsworth.

Christensen, D. (1998). Pollutants may pose greater danger to women. *Medical Tribune: Internist and Cardiologist Edition, 39*(17), 6.

Cohen, B. L. (1992, June). How to assess the risks you face. *Consumer's Research,* pp. 11–16.

Cohen, M. J., Kaufman, S. R., Ruttenberg, R., & Fano, A. (1998). *A critical look at animal experimentation* (5th ed.). [On-line]. Shaker Heights, OH: Medical Research Modernization Committee. Available: http://www.mrmcmed.org/critcv.html

Colborn, T., Dumanoski, D., & Myers, J.P. (1996). *Our stolen future: Are we threatening our fertility, intelligence and survival?—A scientific detective story.* New York: Dutton Books.

Cunningham, W. P., & Saigo, B. W. (1999). *Environmental science: A global concern* (5th ed.). New York: WCB/McGraw-Hill.

Drasch, G., Aigner, S., Roider, G., Staiger, F., & Lipowsky, G. (1998). Mercury in human colostrum and early breast milk. Its dependence on dental amalgam and other factors. *Journal of Trace Elements in Medicine and Biology, 12,* 23–27.

Enterline, P. E. (1988). Asbestos and cancer. In L. Gordis (Ed.), *Epidemiology and health risk assessment* (pp. 242–258). New York: Oxford University Press.

Environmental Protection Agency. (1997a). *Mercury Study report to Congress* (EPA-452/R-97-003) [On-line]. Available: http://www.epa.gov/oar/mercury.html

Environmental Protection Agency. (1997b). *Special report on environmental endocrine disruption: An effects assessment and analysis* (NTIS No. PB97-137772INZ) [On-line]. Available: http://www.epa.gov:80/reg5ogis/risk/endocrin.pdf

Environmental Protection Agency. (1998). *Chemical hazard data availability study* [On-line]. Available: http://www.epa.gov/opptintr/chemtest/hazchem.htm

Environmental Protection Agency. (2000a). *Dioxin: Scientific highlights from draft reassessment (2000). Information sheet 2* [On-line]. Available: http://www.epa.gov/nceawww1/pdfs/dioxin/factsheets/dioxin_long.pdf

Environmental Protection Agency. (2000b). *Exposure and human health reassessment of 2,3,7,8-tetrachlorodibenzo-p-dioxin (TCDD) and related compounds, Part I: Estimating exposure to dioxin-like compounds. Volume 2: Sources of dioxin-like compounds in the United States (EPA/600/P-00/001Ab)* [On-line]. http://www.epa.gov/nceawww1/pdfs/dioxin/part1/volume2/volume2.pdf

Environmental Protection Agency (2000c). *Exposure and human health reassessment of 2,3,7,8-tetrachlorodibenzo-p-dioxin (TCDD) and related compounds, Part II: Health assessment for 2,3,7,8-tetrachlorodibenzo-p-dioxin (TCDD) and related compounds (EPA/600/P-00/001Ae)* [On-line]. Available: http://www.epa.gov/nceawww1/pdfs/dioxin/part2/dritoc.pdf

Eubanks, M. W. (1997). Hormones and health. *Environmental Health Perspectives, 105,* 482–487.

Factor-Litvak, P., Stein, Z., & Graziano, J. (1993). Increased risk of proteinuria among a cohort of lead-exposed pregnant women. *Environmental Health Perspectives, 101,* 418–421.

Fincher, J. (1985). Notice: Sunlight may be necessary for your health. *Smithsonian, 16*(3), 71–76.

Fingerhut, M. A., Halperin, W. E., Marlow, D. A., Piacitelli, L. A., Honchar, P. A., Sweeney, M. H., Greife, A. L., Dill, P. A., Steenland, K., & Suruda, A. J. (1991). Cancer mortality in workers exposed to 2,3,7,8-tetrachlorodibenzo-p-dioxin. *New England Journal of Medicine, 324,* 212–218.

Fisher, B. (1999). Most unwanted, persistent organic pollutants. *Environmental Health Perspectives, 107,* A18–A23.

Fisher, B., Powles, T. J., & Pritchard, K. J. (2000). Tamoxifen for the prevention of breast cancer. *European Journal of Cancer, 36,* 142–150.

Foster, W. G. (1998). Endocrine disruptors and development of the reproductive system in the fetus and children: Is there cause for concern? *Canadian Journal of Public Health, 89* (Suppl. 1), S37–S41.

Frankenhaeuser, M. (1989). The physiology of sex differences as related to occupational status. In M. Frankenhaeuser, U. Lundberg, & M. Chesney (Eds.), *Women, work and health* pp. 340–349. New York: Plenum Press.

Furst, A., & Fan, A. M. (1996). Principles and highlights of toxicology. In A. M. Fan & L. W. Chang (Eds.), *Toxicology and risk assessment* (pp. 3–7). New York: Marcel Dekker.

Gail, M. H., Costantino, J. P., Bryant, J., Croyle, R., Freedman, L., Helzlsouer, K., & Vogel, V. (1999). Weighing the risks and benefits of Tamoxifen treatment for preventing breast cancer. *Journal of the National Cancer Institute, 91,* 1829–1846.

Gilbert, S. G., & Grant-Webster, K. S. (1995). Neurobehavioral effects of developmental methylmercury exposure. *Environmental Health Perspectives, 103* (Suppl. 6), 135–142.

Grandjean, P., Weihe, P., & White, R. F. (1995). Milestone developments in infants exposed to methylmercury from human milk. *Neurotoxicology, 16,* 27–33.

Grandjean, P., Weihe, P., White, R. F., & Debes, F. (1998). Cognitive performance of children prenatally exposed to "safe" levels of methylmercury. *Environmental Research, 77,* 165–172.

Gulson, B. L., Jameson, C. W., Mahaffey, K. R., Mizon, K. J., Patison, N., Law, A. J., Korsch, M. J., & Salter, M. A. (1998). Relationships of lead in breast milk to lead in blood, urine, and diet of the infant and mother. *Environmental Health Perspectives, 106,* 667–674.

Henderson, B. E., Ross, R. K., & Pike, M. C. (1991). Toward the primary prevention of cancer. *Science, 254,* 1131–1138.

Higginson, J. (1993). Environmental carcinogenesis. *Cancer, 72* (Suppl. 3), 971–977.

Holmberg, P. C. (1979). Central nervous system defects in children born to mothers exposed to organic solvents during pregnancy. *The Lancet, 2,* 177–179.

Houppert, K. (1995, February 7). Pulling the plug on the sanitary protection industry. *The Village Voice,* pp. 24–27.

Hynes, P. H. (1989). *The recurring silent spring.* Elmsford, NY: Pergamon Press.

International Agency for Research on Cancer. (1997). Polychlorinated dibenzo-para-dioxins and polychlorinated dibenzofurans. *IARC Monographs on the Evaluation of Carcinogenic Risks to Humans* 69 [On-line]. Available: http://193.51.164.11/htdocs/Indexes/Vol69Index.html

Johnson-Thompson, M. C., & Guthrie, J. (2000). Ongoing research to identify environmental risk factors in breast carcinoma. *Cancer, 88* (Suppl. 5), 1224–1229.

Kaiser, J. (1997). Environment Institute lays plan for gene hunt. *Science, 278,* 569–570.

Khattak, S., K.-Moghtader, G., Barrera, M., Kennedy, D., & Koren, G. (1999). Pregnancy outcome following gestational exposure to organic solvents. *Journal of the American Medical Association, 281,* 1106–1109.

Koninckx, P. R. (1999). The physiopathology of endometriosis: Pollution and dioxin. *Gynecologic and Obstetric Investigation, 47* (Suppl. 1), 47–50.

Kumanyika, S. (1998). Environmental exposure and nutrition. In V. P. Setlow, C. E. Lawson, & N. F. Woods (Eds.), *Gender differences in susceptibility to environmental factors: A priority assessment: Workshop report* [On-line]. (pp. 38–43). Washington, DC: National Academy Press. Available: http://books.nap.edu/books/0309064236/html/R1.html

Lang, L. (1995). Strange brew: Assessing risk of chemical mixtures. *Environmental Health Perspectives, 103,* 142–145.

Lewis, D. F. V., Ioannides, C., & Parke, D. P. (1998). Cytochrome P450 and species differences in xenobiotic metabolish and activation of carcinogen. *Environmental Health Perspectives, 106,* 633–641.

Lorscheider, F. L., Vimy, M. J., & Summers, A. O. (1995). Mercury exposure from "silver" tooth fillings: Emerging evidence questions a traditional dental paradigm. *The FASEB Journal, 9,* 504–508.

Lucier, G. W., & Schecter, A. (1998). Human exposure assessment and the National Toxicology Program. *Environmental Health Perspectives, 106,* 623–627.

Mayani, A., Barel, S., Soback, S., & Almagor, M. (1997). Dioxin concentrations in women with endometriosis. *Human Reproduction, 12,* 373–375.

McLachlan, J. A., & Arnold, S. F. (1996). Environmental estrogens. *American Scientist, 84,* 452–461.

Messing, K. (2000). Ergonomic studies provide information about occupational exposure differences between men and women. *Journal of the American Medical Women's Association, 55,* 72–75.

Miller, T. G. (1998). *Living in the environment: Principles, connections and solutions.* (10th ed.). Belmont, CA: Wadsworth.

Mottet, N. K., Shaw, C. M., & Burbacher, T. M. (1985). Health risks from increases in methylmercury exposure. *Environmental Health Perspectives, 63,* 133–140.

Muckle, G., Dewailly, E., & Ayotte, P. (1998). Prenatal exposure of Canadian children to polychlorinated biphenyls and mercury. *Canadian Journal of Public Health, 89* (Suppl. 1), S20–S25.

Myer, G. J., & Davidson, P. W. (1998). Prenatal methylmercury exposure and children: Neurologic, developmental, and behavioral research. *Environmental Health Perspectives, 106* (Suppl. 3), 841–847.

National Institute of Environmental Health Sciences. (1997a). *Annual report for fiscal year 1997* [On-line]. Available: http://www.niehs.nih.gov/dert/annrpt.htm

National Institute of Environmental Health Sciences. (1997b). *Women's health and the environment. National Institutes of Health fact sheet #10* [On-line]. Available: http://www.niehs.nih.gov/oc/factsheets/womens.htm

National Institute of Environmental Health Sciences. (1998a). *Medicine for the layman—environment and disease* [On-line]. Available: http://www.niehs.nih.gov/oc/factsheets/ead/ead.htm

National Institute of Environmental Health Sciences. (1998b). *NIEHS and the use of alternative methods in toxicological research and testing* [On-line]. Available: http://www.niehs.nih.gov/oc/factsheets/analt.htm

Ness, R. B., Kuller, L. H. (1997). Women's health as a paradigm for understanding factors that mediate disease. *Journal of Women's Health, 6,* 329–336.

Oskarsson, A., Schultz, A., Skerfving, S., Hallen, I. P., Ohlin, B., & Lagerkvist, B. J. (1996). Total and inorganic mercury in breast milk in relation to fish consumption and amalgam in lactating women. *Archives of Environmental Health, 51,* 234–241.

Ottoboni, M. A. (1997). *The dose makes the poison: A plain language guide to toxicology* (2nd ed.). New York: Van Nostrand Reinhold.

Patandin, S., Dagnelie, P. C., Mulder, P. G. H., deCoul, E. O., van der Veen, J. E., Weisglas-Kuperus, N., & Sauer, P. J. J. (1999). Dietary exposure to polychlorinated biphenyls and dioxins from infancy until adulthood: A comparison between breast-feeding, toddler, and long-term exposure. *Environmental Health Perspectives, 107,* 45–51.

Pirkle, J. L., Kaufmann, R. B., Brody, D. J., Hickman, T., Gunter, E. W., & Paschal, D. C. (1998). Exposure of the U.S. population to lead, 1991–1994. *Environmental Health Perspectives, 106,* 745–750.

Rier, S. E., Martin, D. C., Bowman, R. E., Dmowski, W. P., & Becker, J. L. (1993). Endometriosis in rhesus monkeys (*Macaca mulatta*) following chronic exposure to 2,3,7,8-tetrachlorodibenzo-*p*-dioxin. *Fundamentals of Applied Toxicology, 21,* 433–441.

Roberts, W. C., & Abernathy, C. O. (1996). Risk assessment: Principles and methodologies. In A. M. Fan & L. W. Chang (Eds.), *Toxicology and risk assessment* (pp. 245–270). New York: Marcel Dekker.

Rodricks, J. A. (1992). *Calculated risks: Understanding the toxicity and human health risks of chemicals in our environment.* Cambridge, England: Cambridge University Press.

Rogan, W. J., Gladen, B. C., Hung, K.-L., Koong, S.-L., Shih, L.-Y., Taylor, J. S., Wu, Y.-C., Yang, D., Ragan, N. B., & Hsu, C.-C. (1988). Congenital poisoning by polychlorinated biphenyls and their contaminants in Taiwan. *Science, 241,* 334–336.

Rosenstock, L., & Lee, L. J. (2000). Caution: Women at work. *Journal of the American Medical Women's Association, 55,* 67–68.

Rosenthal, G. A., & Janzen, D. H. (1979). *Herbivores: Their interaction with secondary plant metabolites.* New York: Academic Press.

Safe, S. H. (1995a). Do environmental estrogens play a role in development of breast cancer in women and male reproductive problems? *Human and Ecological Risk Assessment, 1,* 17–23.

Safe, S. H. (1995b). Environmental and dietary estrogens and human health: Is there a problem? *Environmental Health Perspectives, 103,* 346–351.

Sakorafas, G. H., & Tsiotou, A. G. (2000). Genetic predisposition to breast cancer: A surgical perspective. *British Journal of Surgery, 87,* 149–162.

Salsburg, D. (1983). The lifetime feeding study in mice and rats—An examination of its validity as a bioassay for human carcinogens. *Fundamental and Applied Toxicology, 3,* 63–67.

Sandborgh-Englund, G., Elinder, C. G., Langworth, S., Schultz, A., & Ekstrand, J. (1998). Mercury in biological fluids after amalgam removal. *Journal of Dental Research, 77,* 615–624.

Schenker, M. B., & Jacobs, J. A. (1996). Respiratory effects of organic solvent exposure. *Tubercle and Lung Disease, 77,* P4–P18.

Setlow, V. P., Lawson, C. E., & Woods, N. F. (1998). *Gender differences in susceptibility to environmental factors: A Priority assessment: Workshop report* [On-line]. Washington DC: National Academy Press. Available: http://books.nap.edu/books/0309064236/html/R1.html

Silberg, S. L., Ransom, D. R., Lyon, J. A., & Anderson, P. S. (1979). Relationship between spray adhesives and congenital malformations. *Southern Medical Journal, 72,* 1170–1173.

Sinks, T., & Jackson, R. J. (1999). International study finds breast milk free of significant lead contamination. *Environmental Health Perspectives, 107,* A58–A59, A60–A61.

Spitz, M. R., Fueger, J. J., Goepfert, H., & Newell, G. R. (1990). Salivary gland cancer: A case-control investigation of risk factors. *Archives of Otolaryngology and Head and Neck Surgery, 116,* 1163–1166.

Stellman, J. (1998). Environmental exposure in the workplace. Environmental exposure and nutrition. In V. P. Setlow, C. E. Lawson, & N. F. Woods (Eds.), *Gender differences in susceptibility to environmental factors: A priority assessment: workshop report* [On-line]. (pp. 34–38). Washington, DC: National Academy Press. Available: http://books.nap.edu/books/0309064236/html/R1.html

Stellman, J. M. (2000). Perspectives on women's occupational health. *Journal of the American Medical Women's Association, 55,* 69–71.

Swanson, G. M., & Burns, P. B. (1997). Cancers of the salivary gland: Workplace risks among women and men. *Annals of Epidemiology, 7,* 369–374.

Swanson, N. G. (2000). Working women and stress. *Journal of the American Medical Women's Association, 55,* 76–79.

U.S. Food and Drug Administration. (1999). *Tampons and asbestos, dioxin, and toxic shock syndrome.* [On-line] . Available: http://www.fda.gov/cdrh/ocd/tamponsabs.html

Vimy, M. J., Hooper, D. E., King, W. W., & Lorscheider, F. L. (1997). Mercury from maternal "silver" tooth fillings in sheep and human breast milk. A source of neonatal exposure. *Biological Trace Element Research, 56,* 143–152.

Wilson, R., & Crouch, E. A. C. (1987). Risk assessments and comparisons: An introduction. *Science, 236,* 267–270.

Yannello, A. (1998, May 20). Medical field "unaware" of tampon-dioxin link. *The Press-Tribune* [On-line]. p. 3. Available: http://frontiernet.net/~ruthb/page3.html

Zahm, S. H., Pottern, L. M., Ward, M. H., & White, D. W. (1994). Inclusion of women and minorities in occupational cancer epidemiologic research. *Journal of Occupational Medicine, 36,* 842–847.

6

Rest and Exercise

Susan Sponsler and Marian C. Condon

CHAPTER OUTLINE

Objectives

1. *Describe the nature and hallmarks of restful sleep.*
2. *List the signs and symptoms of sleep deprivation.*
3. *Identify strategies for preventing insomnia.*
4. *List the health benefits associated with cardiorespiratory fitness.*
5. *List the health benefits associated with flexibility and muscle strength.*
6. *Describe methods of safely improving fitness, flexibility, and strength.*

Introduction

The new national health goals described in the document *Healthy People 2010: National Health Promotion and Disease Prevention Objectives* (U.S. Department of Health and Human Services, 1998) outline a realistic standard of well-being for Americans to achieve by the year 2010. In addition to focusing on disease prevention and health promotion, the goals emphasize physical, mental, and spiritual well-being; quality of life, and functional capacity. The overall goal is that people adopt a healthy lifestyle that will allow them to achieve a lifetime of wellness. **Rest** and **exercise** are both essential components of such a lifestyle.

Women who wish to improve their lifestyles in terms of rest and exercise must have a basic understanding of both. Although rest and exercise could be viewed as opposite components of a healthy lifestyle, each supports the other in significant ways. For example, a study done by Higdon (1997) at the Sleep and Aging Research Laboratory at the University of Washington in Seattle, demonstrated that exercise improves sleep. Participants who ran or walked regularly for six weeks lengthened the period they spent in deep sleep by 33 percent. A number of other studies have shown that a program of regular exercise increases total time spent in sleep and that exercise-induced *increases in lean body mass* and *maximal oxygen consumption* promote sleep (Kubitz, Landers, Petruzzello, & Han, 1996; O'Connor & Youngstedt 1995). Conversely, getting an adequate amount of sleep or rest is essential to a successful fitness program. Rest supports energy level and propensity to exercise, and it is during periods of rest following exercise that muscle fibers and bone are strengthened. Rest also allows our bodies to heal when ill or injured. Exercise and rest are interdependent and essential for good health.

Rest

Sleep is an essential part of our existence. Human beings spend approximately *one-third* of their lives (on average, 24 years) sleeping. We cannot achieve maximum wellness without sufficient amounts of quality sleep. Individuals who suffer from chronic insomnia have been found to be more likely to develop psychoemotional problems and to make more frequent use of healthcare services (Dement, 1999). Although everyone sleeps, not everyone sleeps similarly; sleep is as varied in character and quality as other aspects of our lives.

The Sleep Cycle

Our daily pattern of sleep and wakefulness is one of our **circadian rhythms,** the daily patterns that regulate every function in the body from alertness and appetite to heartbeat and hair growth. These fluctuations are controlled by the **hypothalamus,** the portion of the brain that acts as the body's internal pacemaker. Normal sleep also involves **cycles**—90-minute sequences comprising several stages of sleep, which occur in a predictable order. In the first two stages, sleep is relatively *light*. In stage 1, the muscles relax and brain waves are rapid and irregular. In stage 2, brain waves become more pronounced, reflecting bursts of electrical activity. Stages 3 and 4 are stages of *deep sleep,* in which individuals are more difficult to awaken than during the lighter stages of sleep. Deep sleep is followed in turn by what is known as **REM (rapid eye movement) sleep.** The REM phase is an *active* phase, in which heart rate, respiratory rate, and blood pressure are about the same as in the waking state, and it is during REM sleep that *dreams* occur. After one cycle of sleep has been completed, another begins. About 25 percent of each night's sleep is spent in REM sleep. Interestingly, REM sleep causes a temporary *paralysis,* perhaps so that individuals do not act out their dreams, regardless of how active or frightening. Although the exact functions of the REM and non-REM phases of sleep are not fully understood, it is known that frequent awakening, with consequent failure to complete the normal cycles, is damaging to physical and mental health (Dement, 1999).

Sleep needs and patterns are individualized—within certain parameters. Whereas most people are thought to need about eight hours of sleep per night for optimal well-being and performance, some individuals do very well with less. Similarly, some people are morning people, and others are more productive later in the day. However, almost everyone's internal clock is set for sleep at **night,** especially the hours between **midnight and dawn.** Most people also get a bit sleepy in the middle of the day between 1 P.M. and 4 P.M.—the so-called **siesta zone.** We sleep best when we heed the rhythm of our internal clocks. Individuals who are *out of synchrony* with their clocks, such as shift workers who never fully adjust to nighttime work and daytime sleep, underperform both physically and mentally (Dement, 1999). Women who rotate shifts at work are more likely to suffer irregular menstrual cycles, to have difficulty becoming pregnant, miscarry a pregnancy, or to have a low birth weight baby (Sleep Foundation, 2001m).

Sleep patterns change as we age: Newborns and children spend more time than adults in deep sleep. As we grow older, sleep becomes more fragmented; we spend more time in the lighter stages and tend to retire and get up earlier. Senior citizens tend to sleep for shorter periods than younger people, but, because they still need the same overall *amount* of sleep, they need more *episodes* of sleep. They may wake in the middle of the night, engage in some activity for a while, and then go back to sleep. *Naps* are another way for older individuals to ensure that they get enough sleep (Sleep Foundation, 2001i).

Whether we are getting enough sleep to satisfy our unique needs is reflected not in the absolute number of hours we spend in sleep, but in how we feel and function. People who are getting enough sleep wake up feeling refreshed and do not find themselves nodding off in meetings or while driving.

Sleep Deprivation

The term *sleep deprivation* refers to a pattern of not getting as much sleep as the body requires for optimum functioning. Sleep deprivation is epidemic in our fast-paced, work-obsessed society: A poll of more than 1,000 adults conducted by the National Sleep Foundation (Sleep Foundation, 2001g) suggested that almost two-thirds of Americans fail to get 8 hours of sleep a night and that about one-third fail to get even 7. Many respondents also reported struggling to stay awake on their jobs and experiencing drowsiness while driving (Sleep Foundation, 2001k). The average woman age 30 to 60 years averages only 6 hours and 41 minutes of sleep per night during the workweek. The Sleep Foundation survey suggests that the more time individuals spend at *work,* the less sleep they tend to get. People who work 60 hours a week habitually get only 6 hours of sleep a night, and even people who work 40 hours get only 7.1 hours. *Having children* also shortens hours spent in sleep. Adults with children average only 6.7 hours per night, whereas those without children average 7.2 hours (Sleep Foundation, 2001i).

The signs and symptoms of sleep deprivation include fatigue, irritability, depression, decreased attention span, lack of concentration, lapses in memory, frequent illnesses, and loss of productivity. The accumulated number of hours of sleep needed but not obtained is called the **sleep debt.** The larger the sleep debt, the more pronounced and potentially serious the symptoms of sleep deprivation will be. Unfortunately, people often ignore signs that they are not getting enough sleep. Sleep debt is like monetary debt; it must be paid back, and, until proven otherwise, it is reasonable and safer to assume that accumulated lost sleep must be paid back hour for hour (Dement, 1999).

One of the most serious consequences of sleep deprivation is *drowsy driving.* In a poll conducted by the U.S. National Highway Traffic Safety Administration, 62 percent of all the adult respondents said they had driven a car or another vehicle while drowsy during the previous year, and 27 percent reported having dozed off while driving. Drivers who are sleep deprived are at risk for accidents, as are those who drive long distances without stopping to rest and those who drive during hours they are normally asleep. Sleep-related accidents are most common among *young* drivers, who tend to stay up late, sleep too little, and drive at night. Another at-risk group is *shift workers,* particularly those who are driving home from the night shift (Sleep Foundation, 2001c).

Insomnia

The term *insomnia* refers to difficulty in falling asleep or remaining asleep. Chronic or frequent insomnia can seriously interfere with quality of life and productivity. There are many causes of insomnia, including stress, worry, excitement, general anxiety, depression, and chronic illness. A number of *medications* can contribute to insomnia as well.

Insomnia can be transient, short-term, or chronic. **Transient insomnia** lasts only a few nights and is usually related to stress, excitement, or a change in one's usual sleeping environment. **Short-term insomnia** lasts two or three weeks and is often related to a stressful situation or a medical or emotional problem that will be resolved relatively quickly. **Chronic insomnia** persists for more than a month and is usually related to an underlying medical or emotional problem; depression and anxiety are frequent causes.

Chronic insomnia may also be related to the consumption of beverages and foods that interfere with sleep. For example, drinking coffee, tea, or soda that contains *caffeine* within four to six hours of bedtime may stimulate the body and mind enough to prevent sleep. Even foods and drinks high in *sugar* can have a stimulating effect. Drinking *alcoholic* beverages in the evening can also cause insomnia; although alcohol is sedating initially, it is notorious for causing people to wake up after a few hours and be unable to get back to sleep (Sleep Foundation, 2001a). *Sleeping pills and tranquilizers* can also disrupt the normal sleep cycle. Over-the-counter sleeping aids should be used only for a short time, to cope with transient stressors. Professional help should be sought for persistent sleep problems. *Exercising* too close to bedtime can stimulate the sympathetic nervous system and prevent sleep. A study done at the Mayo Clinic suggests that late afternoon is the best time for persons prone to insomnia to exercise (Dement, 1999). Also, both *going to bed hungry* and *trying to sleep on a full stomach* can interfere with rest, and having a source of *light* in a room can prevent the release of the hormone *melatonin,* which promotes sleep. Even the small amount of light from a VCR display can do this (Dement, 1999). Opaque window shades can be used to block the light from streetlights, traffic signals, and so on. *Noise* from traffic, barking dogs, a partner who snores, and other sources can cause insomnia. Sources of "white noise," such as fans and machines especially designed for that purpose, can be used to block disturbing sounds. *Temperature* can also be a factor in insomnia; a room that is too hot or too cold can interfere with sleep. Temperatures below 54 and above 75 will awaken many people (Sleep Foundation, 2001k).

Developing consistent sleep habits can help ward off insomnia. It is a good idea to go to bed and get up at the same times, even on weekends and during vacations. It is also a good idea to use one's bed only for sleeping, not for reading, watching TV, or paying bills. This trains the body and mind to associate lying in bed with sleep. Box 6–1 lists some behavioral strategies for preventing insomnia.

Box 6–1 Strategies for Preventing Insomnia

- Avoid alcohol, caffeine, and sugar in the evening.
- Use sleeping and antianxiety medications only briefly.
- Exercise regularly, but not within four hours of bedtime.
- Manage stress.
- Remember that both feelings of hunger and a full stomach can interfere with sleep; allow at least three hours to digest a big meal.
- Sleep in a dark room.
- Provide "white noise," if necessary.
- Go to bed and wake up at the same time each day; continue the pattern on weekends and vacations.
- Use your bed only for sleeping.
- Maintain a comfortable room temperature.
- Ease into bedtime. Choose end-of-day activities that are calming.
- Do relaxation deep breathing or progressive relaxation exercises, or meditate, at bedtime.

Box 6–2 Dealing with Insomnia

- Don't toss and turn. Get up, go to another room, and do some light reading or something else calming.
- Drink a glass of warm milk.
- Don't do housework or pay bills.
- Don't keep checking the clock; it can actually make you more stressed.
- Once you feel sleepy, go back to bed.

Women may be especially prone to insomnia if they suffer from PMS (premenstrual syndrome) (see Chapter 17). Some women with PMS report difficulty falling asleep and staying asleep. Women with PMS have also been found to experience shortened periods of deep sleep all month long (Sleep Foundation, 2001m). Pregnant women may also have difficulty sleeping. During the first and third trimesters of pregnancy, the need to urinate may wake them during the night (Sleep Foundation, 2001m). Hot flashes associated with menopause (see Chapter 24) can also interfere with women's sleep.

Almost everyone occasionally has the experience of waking up in the middle of the night and not being able to get back to sleep. Should this happen, the best strategy is to get up and engage in a *nonstimulating* activity, such as reading. Lying in bed, staring at the clock only increases anxiety and delays sleep. Box 6–2 lists some strategies for dealing with insomnia once it has occurred.

If insomnia persists, it is important to contact a healthcare provider. She can rule out medical, psychological, or emotional causes. Keeping a *sleep diary* may provide information that can help identify the underlying problem. A sleep diary can be downloaded from the National Sleep Foundation website listed at the end of this chapter.

Sleep Disorders

A number of conditions, characterized as **sleep disorders,** can interfere with normal sleep and give rise to sleep deprivation and its attendant symptoms. The sleep disorders typically cause a symptom known as **excessive daytime sleepiness (EDS).** When EDS is present, the individual feels very drowsy during the day, even after having gotten enough sleep the night before. People with this problem fall asleep in situations in which they need to be fully alert, such as during work and when driving a car. Chronic EDS can have serious social consequences; individuals afflicted with it may be seen by others as lazy, unmotivated, or unintelligent and are often frustrated and angry.

SLEEP APNEA

Apnea means absence of breath. **Sleep apnea** is a disorder in which breathing is periodically interrupted during sleep. Although considered more common in men, sleep apnea afflicts *one in four women over the age of 65* (Sleep Foundation, 2001m) and may be underdiagnosed in women. Persons most at risk for sleep apnea include those who are overweight, who snore loudly, or who have a physical abnormality in the upper airway. Sleep apnea occurs in some people because the muscles in the throat and tongue relax during sleep and block the airway. The presence of excessive amounts of tissue in the airway can also cause it to become blocked during sleep. Sleep apnea is known to contribute to high blood pressure. Sleep apnea tends to run in families and may have a genetic cause. Episodes of apnea during sleep cause low levels of oxygen and high levels of carbon dioxide in the blood. These chemical changes alert the brain to danger and the person wakes up. Frequent arousals prevent a person from getting enough deep, restorative sleep (Sleep Foundation, 2001j).

People who have sleep apnea may not realize it. Although they are tired during the day, and may fall asleep at inopportune moments, they are unaware of what befalls them during sleep. It may be a partner, friend, or relative who recognizes the nighttime pattern of *snoring heavily* and periodically *gasping for breath* as a symptom of sleep apnea. A tentative diagnosis of sleep apnea can be confirmed through specific tests usually carried out in the patient's home or in sleep disorder centers. A variety of behavioral, mechanical, and even surgical interventions are used to treat it. Drug therapy is usually not effective.

RESTLESS LEG SYNDROME

Restless leg syndrome (RLS) is said to be present when the individual experiences uncomfortable sensations in the legs, with a need to move or rub them. The sensations are usually described as a creeping or crawling, tingling, cramping, or burning. Sometimes, only the perceived need to move is present. The sensations are most likely to emerge when the person is sitting or lying down.

Restless leg syndrome is thought to afflict 28 percent of women overall and up to 15 percent of pregnant women. Its cause is unknown; it may be inherited, and some cases have been related to nerve damage in the legs subsequent to diabetes, kidney problems, or alcoholism. RLS tends to worsen over time and is most severe in middle to old age. Fortunately, it responds well to treatment with medications from a number of classes (Sleep Foundation, 2001e). A related disorder, **periodic limb movements in sleep (PLMS),** involves twitching or jerking the limbs during sleep. Whereas some individuals are undisturbed by PLMS, others are awakened by the movement. Thirty-five percent of people over the age of 65 experience it, and women and men are affected in equal numbers. The cause of PLMS is unknown. If it interferes with sleep, it is treated in the same way as RLS (Sleep Foundation, 2001d).

JET LAG

Jet lag is a very common, temporary sleep disorder. Jet lag arises from an upset in the body's natural clock caused by travel to different time zones, as the body's circadian rhythms are influenced by exposure to natural light (Sleep Foundation, 2001f). When we travel to a different time zone, our circadian rhythms are slow to adjust and remain on their original schedule for several days. They tell us it is time to sleep in the middle of the afternoon and tell us to stay awake during the night. Behavioral adjustments made before, during, and after travel can minimize some of the unpleasant effects of jet lag:

- Anticipate the time change by getting up and going to bed earlier several days in advance of an eastward trip and later for a westward trip.
- Select a flight that arrives in the early evening and stay up until at least 10 P.M. local time. Avoid napping earlier in the day, or nap no longer than two hours.
- Maximize your chances of sleeping well after you reach your destination by not eating heavily before bed and by avoiding alcohol and caffeine.
- Get out into the sunshine as much as possible the next day to reset your biological clock.

NARCOLEPSY

Narcolepsy is a chronic central nervous system (brain and spinal cord) disorder that causes people to fall asleep at times when they would normally be awake (Sleep Foundation, 2001h). It is a genetic disorder; therefore, it runs in families, but its exact cause is unknown. About 1 in every 2,000 people suffer from narcolepsy. It affects women and men in equal numbers and typically manifests around puberty. Although excessive daytime sleepiness is usually the first symptom to appear, and the most troubling overall, a phenomenon known as *cataplexy* can also occur. A narcoleptic person having a cataplexic episode experiences a sudden partial or total loss of muscle control; she might become very weak or collapse entirely. Cataplexy typically occurs in the context of a strong emotion, such as anger, or during a fit of laughter. Persons with narcolepsy also experience *sleep paralysis,* the inability to move or talk for a brief period when falling asleep or awakening, and *automatic behavior*—performing routine or familiar tasks while in a sleeplike state.

If narcoleptic individuals do not seek treatment, the periods of daytime sleep they experience can seriously impede their ability to get a good night's sleep. Fortunately, a variety of drug and behavioral treatments are available. Like other people at risk for insomnia, narcoleptics are advised to avoid caffeine, alcohol, and exercise too close to bedtime and to establish a routine time for going to sleep and getting up. Stimulant drugs may be prescribed to decrease daytime sleepiness, and antidepressants are used to control cataplexy and sleep paralysis.

Exercise

Exercise is a vital component of a healthy lifestyle. Its numerous benefits in terms of physical and emotional well-being have been exhaustively documented. Nevertheless, many women are unused to exercise; it has been estimated that 60 percent of adults do not get the recommended 30 minutes per day of physical activity and that 25 percent of adults are almost completely sedentary (*How Much Exercise is Enough,* 1999). Getting and staying *motivated* to work out regularly is problematic for many, but, without motivation, lifelong fitness will remain an elusive goal. Another key to achieving fitness is embarking on a realistic program—one that is appropriate to the individual's existing level of aerobic endurance, strength, and flexibility and that allows for any medical limitations. A comprehensive program addresses the three main components of fitness: cardiorespiratory (aerobic) endurance, muscular strength and endurance, and flexibility. Each plays a vital role in a woman's health and well-being.

Why Bother? The Benefits of Exercise

Women who are knowledgeable about the many benefits of fitness are more likely to choose to make regular exercise a part of their lives. Aerobic exercise, exercise that builds muscle strength, and exercise that enhances flexibility all benefit us physically and mentally. Overall fitness is associated with a lower incidence of many diseases and has been found to support self-esteem and mental health.

BENEFITS OF AEROBIC CONDITIONING

Aerobic exercise contributes substantially to health. First and foremost, aerobic exercise decreases women's risk of coronary heart disease. This is an extremely important benefit for women, as coronary heart disease (discussed in detail in Chapter 12), poses the single greatest risk to women's health overall (Schnirring, 1997). The heart is a muscle with a staggering workload; it contracts an estimated 2.5 billion times during an average lifetime and it never rests. Aerobic exercise can strengthen the heart muscle itself (Huelskamp, 1999) while lowering blood pressure (Kelly, 1989) and assisting in weight control (*How Much Exercise Do You Need?,* 1999). A number of studies have documented that even a modest level of aerobic exercise decreases women's risk of coronary heart disease. Data from the health histories of the more than 72,000 women who participated in the Nurses' Study, a longitudinal study of women's health, suggest that women who walked briskly for five hours a week had a 50 percent reduction in their risk of having a heart attack (Manson et al., 1999). Schnirring (1997) found that women who walked as few as three hours per week have a 40 percent lower risk of heart attack and stroke than more sedentary women.

Aerobic exercise also decreases the risk for diabetes and breast cancer (Van Dam, 1988). Analysis of data from the Nurses' Study suggests a direct correlation between frequent moderate to vigorous exercise and a reduced risk of breast cancer. Women who exercised for 7 or more hours/wk lowered their breast cancer risk by 20 percent (Rockhill et al., 1999). Exercise is also an effective antidote to depression, which occurs frequently in women. Both modest and significant fitness gains have been associated with a decrease in depressive symptoms (Moore et al., 1996).

BENEFITS OF INCREASED FLEXIBILITY

Increasing flexibility through stretching exercises or disciplines such as yoga is also very important for women. *Flexibility* refers to the ability of a joint to move easily and fully through its range of motion. Although women tend to be more flexible than men, because men tend to have greater muscle mass and less pliable ligaments, women cannot afford to take their flexibility for granted. If they do not take steps to maintain their flexibility, it will gradually decrease. Muscles will become shorter and tighter; tendons, ligaments, and joint capsules will become less pliable, and more stress will be placed on the joints. Eventually, stiffness and joint injury may result. Back pain, a common complaint, can also be caused by a lack of flexibility in the hamstrings (located in the back of the thigh), together with weak abdominal muscles. Muscle strains and ligament sprains are often caused solely by lack of flexibility, and poor flexibility can interfere with even simple, everyday tasks that require the ability to bend and stretch. Unfortunately, despite its importance, the flexibility component of fitness is one that is often ignored or minimally addressed.

BENEFITS OF MUSCLE STRENGTH AND ENDURANCE

Women can derive many benefits from becoming stronger through strength training. They can enhance their autonomy by not requiring assistance with tasks such as carrying groceries and lifting substantial objects at home and at work. Women can decrease their susceptibility to joint injuries, osteoporosis, and the overall disability that too often accompany aging. Women who maintain a good muscle mass can also more easily maintain a healthy weight. Increased self-confidence and self-esteem naturally arise from these benefits.

Strengthening muscles decreases the risk of soft tissue injury by providing greater stability to joints. Resistance training strengthens antigravity muscles, thus improving posture, reducing wear and tear on the back, and preventing lower back pain (Nieman, 1999). Strengthening the muscles adjacent to joints can also decrease the symptoms of osteoarthritis, as a substantial muscle mass can absorb physical stress, which would otherwise be transferred to the joint (Harvard University, 1998). Improving leg strength can lead to better balance thereby decreasing the chance that a fall

that could result in a fracture will occur (Bryant, Peterson, & Franklin, 1998). Bone density is increased, and the incidence of osteoporosis decreased, when strength training is performed over an extended period of time (Nelson, Fiatrone & Morganti, 1994). Building muscle mass contributes to the maintenance of a healthy weight because muscle has a higher resting metabolic rate than fat, so an abundance of muscle tissue causes more calories to be burned at rest. Unfortunately, inactive women can expect to lose 50 percent of their muscle mass between the ages of 20 and 90 (American College of Sports Medicine, 1998a). Too often, weight also increases with age, as high metabolic rate muscle is replaced by low metabolic rate fat. Women who are physically strong tend to have higher self-esteem and self-confidence than weaker women (Bryant et al., 1998). Strength training has also been found to enhance both the quality and quantity of sleep (Bryant et al., 1998).

One of the greatest benefits strength training can confer on women is enhanced self-sufficiency in old age. Improved musculature is invaluable in helping senior citizens maintain independence and self-esteem. Americans, especially women, are living longer, and many live with physical and functional limitations. Women outnumber men in nursing homes by three to one (see Chapter 2). Experts attribute at least 50 percent of the physical problems that render older people unable to live on their own to muscle atrophy caused by lack of use (U.S. Department of Health and Human Services, 1996). Data gathered from a large ongoing study of health in Framingham, MA shows that over 40 percent of women age 55 and older cannot lift 10 pounds (Butler, Davis, Lewis, Nelson, & Strauss, 1998). It is muscle strength that makes rising from a chair, getting into and out of a car or a bathtub, and going up and down stairs possible. An ongoing program of strength training can enable a woman to continue to carry out these activities of daily living as she ages. Women who maintain good muscle strength do not experience the physical deterioration observed in women who are not physically active, regardless of their age (Nelson, 1997). Fortunately, it is never too late to increase one's strength; Nelson et al. (1994), demonstrated that even octogenarians can increase muscle strength and functional ability through a program of weight training. The benefits of exercise are summarized in Box 6–3.

Following a program that emphasizes aerobic fitness, flexibility, and muscular strength, preferably in conjunction with other aspects of a healthy lifestyle, can reduce a woman's risk of developing many health problems. Developing and maintaining motivation is one of the keys to taking full advantage of exercise, in order to gain a significant amount of control over one's health.

Motivation Whether an individual will have the motivation to begin and stick with an exercise program depends on factors such as desires, expectations, activity preferences, and special interests. Attention to these factors can make the dif-

Box 6-3   Health Benefits of Exercise

Exercise Increases	Exercise Decreases
Size and strength of the heart muscle	Work load of the heart
Function and efficiency of the heart	Resting pulse
Blood volume	Electrical irritability
Amount of blood pumped per minute	Blood pressure
Oxygen supplied to the heart	Triglycerides
Electrical stability	Total cholesterol
Blood vessel size and strength	Low-density lipoproteins
Number of red blood cells	Stickiness of platelets
Blood flow regulation	Coronary heart disease progression
High-density lipoproteins	Glucose intolerance
Blood sugar regulation	Body fat and obesity
Insulin sensitivity	Muscle loss during dieting
Self-esteem	Bone loss
Emotional outlook	Stress hormone secretion
Energy regulation and efficiency in cells	Psychological depression
Growth hormone	Harmful effects of psychic stress
Lean body mass	
Efficiency of thyroid gland	
Tolerance for stress	
Strength in skeletal muscles	
Joint range of motion	
Density and strength of bones	
Strength of ligaments and tendons	

ference between a program that is soon abandoned and one that becomes a permanent part of lifestyle.

Because American society places such a premium on women's *appearance,* many women's motivation to exercise comes not from a desire to improve their health but from a desire to improve the way their body looks. However, any motivation is better than no motivation. The desire to change body image can be positive, but realistic goals must be established. The gaunt, willowy standard of beauty endorsed by the media is attainable only by a minority of women who were born with that body type. Women who are very concerned with body image are encouraged to consult a professional trainer, who can help them set realistic goals and a safe, healthy program.

Once the decision has been made to begin an exercise program, it is important to identify potential activities that are relatively appealing. Although some women truly enjoy exercise, for most it is drudgery undertaken only for the sake of appearance, and few have the discipline to persist long in activities they absolutely detest. Preferences regarding the location (indoor, outdoor, a gym, at home), the type of equipment, and whether a partner or professional trainer is desired should be explored. Women should also take into consideration any special interests or goals they have, such as developing a certain skill, pursuing a particular activity, or achieving a specific accomplishment.

The information in the following sections can serve as a guide to setting up a basic personal exercise program. Although fitness experts are excellent resources, much of what they do is founded on the basics presented in this chapter.

Getting Off to a Good Start   The American College of Sports Medicine (ACSM) has established guidelines for determining whether an individual needs to get a physical exam or stress test before beginning an exercise program. An apparently healthy woman, with no signs or symptoms of coronary heart disease and no more than one risk factor for coronary heart disease (see Chapter 12) may exercise at a moderate level (30 minutes per day, most days of the week) without a prior exam. Individuals who have two or more major risk factors, but no symptoms, can also engage in a moderate program, provided they see a physician first for testing and clearance. The ACSM also recommends that women over 50 have a stress test (see Chapter 12) before engaging in a more vigorous program. Individuals with existing cardiac, pulmonary, or metabolic disease should also be tested and cleared by a physician. Women can generally exercise safely during pregnancy if they limit cardiovascular workouts to 30 minutes of moderate-intensity exercise and avoid increases in core temperature, extreme exhaustion, and dehydration (Schnirring 1997). The Physical Activity Readiness Questionnaire (PARQ) is a tool widely used by medical professionals and exercise specialists to assist people in determining whether they should have a physical examination before embarking on an exercise program. It can be found at the Canadian Society of Exercise Physiology website (see the Resources section at the end of this chapter).

Becoming Fit

All well-designed fitness programs include guidelines as to how often one should carry out an activity (*frequency*), how difficult the activity should be (*intensity*), how long the activity should be done (*time or duration*), and what *type* of activity will help achieve the goal. The acronym for this is *FITT*. The minimum amount of activity necessary to produce benefits in each area of FITT is called the **threshold of training.** The American College of Sports Medicine has established FITT guidelines for each area of fitness: cardiovascular endurance, flexibility, and muscular strength and endurance.

Developing Cardiovascular Endurance Safely

Activities that build cardiovascular endurance, also known as aerobic fitness, have the following attributes: large muscles in the body are used, activities can be maintained for a long period of time, movements are rhythmic, and the activities stimulate the heart, lungs, and muscles.

Almost any activity can be made into an aerobic activity if it fits into the exercise prescription guidelines established by the ACSM. Whether a team or an individual sport is considered aerobic often depends on the skill level of the individual involved. If the activity requires the person to use major muscle groups and keep moving for substantial periods of time, it probably meets the ACSM criteria. However, if the activity does not raise the heart rate and keep it elevated, it is not considered an aerobic activity.

A few of the common aerobic activities are walking, jogging, running, biking, swimming, stair climbing, treadmill walking or running, rowing, elliptical training, dance aerobics, step aerobics, stationary bicycling, cycle spin aerobics, in-line skating, one-on-one basketball, tennis and Frisbee, cardio-boxing, and cross-country skiing. Bench steps and jump ropes are affordable pieces of exercise equipment that can be used in the home. In order to carry out activities that develop cardiovascular health and fitness safely, the following FITT guidelines should be followed:

1. *Frequency—three to seven times days per week*
2. *Intensity—40 to 85 percent of maximal heart rate*
3. *Time—15 to 60 minutes*

Intensity is the most important factor in improving cardiovascular endurance. The ACSM's recommendations regarding minimum intensity were higher at one time than they are now. They have been systematically lowered over the past two decades because research has shown that individuals are more likely to stick with lower-level cardiovascular exercise regimens and that health benefits can be realized at lower intensities if they are also done for longer periods of time (*How Much Exercise is Enough?*, 1999). Intensity should be tailored to a woman's current fitness and activity levels; women whose level of fitness is *low* initially should begin exercising at a relatively low level of intensity, which can be increased as fitness develops.

There are several simple methods that can be used to gauge the intensity of aerobic exercise and ensure that one is safely within the exercise guidelines. These include establishing a target heart rate, gauging the rate of perceived exertion, and the using talk test.

Establishing the Target Heart Rate The heart rate, or pulse, can be used as a measure of the intensity of an aerobic activity because it is easy to calculate and correlates well with the amount of oxygen consumed. Heart rate is the number of times the heart beats per minute. It is found by feeling the pulse through the skin at one of several locations on the body and counting it for one minute. As the heart rate slows rapidly when one stops an exercise, however, it is best to count the pulse for only 10 seconds instead of a full minute. Multiplying the 10-second count by six will yield the equivalent of a one-minute count. The two pulse sites easiest to use to monitor the heart rate are the *carotid pulse* and the *radial pulse*. The carotid pulse is located on either side of the trachea, or windpipe, just under the jaw. The radial pulse is located at the bend of the wrist, just below the thumb, on the palm side. The pulse is found and counted by applying gentle pressure with the first and second fingers of the hand. Using the thumb should be avoided, as it has its own pulse, which may confuse matters. Regardless of which pulse site is used, it is important to practice finding the proper spot ahead of time, so that it can be done quickly and easily. Pulse monitoring is used to keep the heart rate within a certain target range, or zone—for example, between 120 and 150 beats per minute.

The terms *training zone* and *target heart rate* are used interchangeably to refer to the zone within which an individual will reap cardiovascular benefits from exercise without exceeding safe limits. The method that the authors recommend for determining one's target heart rate (THR) or training zone is the **Karvonen method** (Donatelle, Snow, & Wilcox, 1999). This method takes into consideration the individual's age, her resting heart rate, and the desired intensity level of the exercise. The intensity level is expressed as a percentage and is chosen on the basis of one's age, medical condition, and existing fitness level. It can range from low (40 to 50 percent), to moderate (60 to 70 percent), to high (75 to 85 percent). In the Karvonen method, the target heart rate (THR) is determined according to a formula that includes the maximum heart rate (MAR), resting heart rate (RHR), and level of intensity desired. The Karvonen formula is THR = (MHR−RHR) × (intensity %) + RHR. The maximum heart rate equals 220 minus one's age. The resting heart rate is the pulse rate when the body is at rest.

The first step in using the Karvonen formula is determining one's resting heart rate (resting pulse). The best time to count the pulse for this purpose is first thing in the morning before arising and before any stimulants, such as caffeine or nicotine, have been ingested. The resting heart rate is counted on 3 consecutive mornings and recorded. Then, the 3 numbers are added together, and an average is determined by dividing by 3. An example of this is as follows: Mary has taken her pulse on three consecutive mornings and has recorded resting heart rates of 78, 80, and 82. She adds them up for a total of 240. She divides 240 by 3 to get an average resting heart rate of 80. That number is the resting heart rate to be used in the Karvonen formula.

The second step in using the Karvonen formula is determining one's maximal heart rate. This is very easy to determine, as MHR equals 220 minus one's age. The third step, deciding the intensity at which one wishes to exercise, is one of the most important aspects of designing a safe but effective program. People who are out of shape should start at a low level of intensity and plug 40 or 50 percent (.40 or .50) into the formula. The less intense an activity is, the longer it needs to be sustained to be effective. Conversely, more intense activities need be sustained for relatively shorter periods of time.

A sedentary person one who engages in very little physical activity would start at the lower end of the guidelines. A program for such a person might consist of taking a brisk walk for 15 minutes, three times a week, within an intensity of 40 to 50 percent. If this person were 45 years old with a resting heart rate of 72 and a maximum heart rate of 175 (220 − her age), her Karvonen target heart rate calculation for the *low end* of her target heart range (40 percent) would be as follows:

THR = MHR (175) − RHR (72) × (intensity .40) + RHR (72)

THR = 103 × .40 + 72

THR = 113

Her *high-end* (50 percent) calculation would be as follows:

THR = MHR (175) − RHR (72) × (intensity .50) + RHR (72)

THR = 103 × .50 + 72

THR = 123

Thus, this relatively sedentary woman would want to keep her heart rate in the target zone between 113 and 123 in order to exercise safely while still deriving a conditioning benefit.

In contrast, a somewhat more fit women who does a lot of walking during the course of a day, takes the stairs instead of the elevator, and does all of her own gardening and housework would need a more challenging program. She would need to work out at a moderate level of intensity, 60 to 70 percent, for 20 to 30 minutes, in order to improve her cardiorespiratory endurance. Finally, a woman who is already in pretty good shape, and exercises consistently, would need to

Box 6–4 Karvonen Method of Determining Training Zone/Target Heart Rates

THR (target heart rate)

MHR (maximum heart rate) = 220 − your age

RHR (resting heart rate) = Average of three consecutive morning pulse rates

Low-Intensity Zone Formulas

Minimum target heart rate: THR = (MHR − RHR) × .40 + RHR =

Maximum target heart rate: THR = (MHR − RHR) × .50 + RHR =

Intermediate-Intensity Zone Formulas

Minimum target heart rate: THR = (MHR − RHR) × .60 + RHR =

Maximum target heart rate: THR = (MHR − RHR) × .70 + RHR =

High-Intensity Zone Formulas

Minimum target heart rate: THR = (MHR − RHR) × .75 + RHR =

Maximum target heart rate: THR = (MHR − RHR) × .85 + RHR =

train at the upper ranges of the guidelines—that is, for 40 to 60 minutes, five to seven times per week, at an intensity level of 75 *to* 85 percent in order to improve her fitness. The formulas for computing target heart rates for low, moderate, and high levels of intensity are shown in Box 6–4.

The Karvonen formula is an invaluable tool for establishing a safe heart rate range during exercise. People who are in good health often choose to work in the middle range—60 to 70 percent of their maximal heart rate. Working below the 40 percent level will not promote a significant change in the body, and exercisers should take care not to work at intensities beyond the upper (85 percent) limit of their maximal heart rate for more than a few seconds. Doing so can cause fatigue, discomfort, possible disturbances in heart rhythm, and other problems. The pulse should be counted approximately every 10 minutes during exercise. This will decrease the possibility that a person will unknowingly exercise at an intensity that is too low or too high. Paying attention to the body and using common sense are the keys to exercising safely. A feeling of extreme fatigue is a signal to slow down.

The heart rate decreases when exercise is discontinued. When the heart rate decreases to fewer than 100 beats per minute, the heart is said to have recovered from exercise. How quickly the recovery heart rate is achieved after a workout is an indicator of how aerobically conditioned a person is; the more rapid the recovery, the better the conditioning. The pulse should be taken 2 to 5 minutes after exercising, and, ideally, the heart rate should be below 100 beats per minute. If the heart rate fails to return to its pre-exercise level within 10 minutes after the workout, the exerciser probably overexerted.

Individuals who adhere to an aerobic training program consistently for six to eight weeks should notice that their resting pulse is slower and that their heart rate decreases more rapidly after exercise. This is an indication that it is time to retake the resting heart rate in the morning and recalculate the target heart rate zone. After this initial recalculation, it should be necessary to recalculate only once or twice a year if exercise is continued consistently.

A phrase for everyone interested in fitness to keep in mind is "Use it or lose it." This phrase refers to what is known as the **principle of reversibility.** This principle states that improvement gained through an exercise program will be lost when the training is discontinued (Donatelle et al., 1999). If a program of exercise is interrupted for longer than several weeks, some of the endurance that was built up will be lost. In that event, when the program is resumed, a downward adjustment will need to be made, so that the program is not excessively intense. The longer an individual goes without exercise, the more conditioning she will lose.

The rate of perceived exertion and the talk test are two other methods a person can use to determine whether she is exercising in a safe and effective zone of exertion.

Gauging the Rate of Perceived Exertion   This method, originated by Gunnar Borg (1970), a noted exercise physiologist, requires that the exercisers get in touch with how they feel during a workout. By noting how their bodies feel at different heart rates, individuals can learn to estimate the level of intensity at which they are exercising. In the Borg method, activity is classified on a continuum from extremely light to extremely hard. A level of exertion classified as *extremely light* is at the lowest end of the intensity level, whereas exertion classified as *extremely hard* is at the maximal end, and an exerciser would not want to continue at that level for long. An activity classified as moderately hard falls somewhere in the middle (60 to 70 percent) of the intensity range.

Using the Talk Test   This simple approach does not require a person to wear a watch or memorize numbers. The objective is for the person to exercise at a level of intensity that allows her to *talk comfortably.* As long as she can do that, she has not exceeded the upper limit of her training zone. Working at very high intensities increases the body's demand for oxygen. A person exercising at a high level must breathe deeply and rapidly and cannot talk comfortably. This un-complicated method also allows a person to exercise with a *partner,* which can be an effective motivator.

Putting It All Together   The FITT acronym can be used to put together a personalized cardiorespiratory endurance exercise program:

1. Frequency. *Get a calendar and block out days and times that are convenient for your workout. Try to do the workout at about the same time each day, as this will help you establish a routine and make exercise a permanent part of your lifestyle. Remember that, in order to receive optimal benefit from your program, you must work out at least three times a week but no more than seven times per week. At least one day off per week is needed for recovery and rest.*
2. Intensity. *Calculate your maximal heart rate and your resting heart rate and put them into the Karvonen formula at your desired minimal and maximal intensity levels. The two numbers delineate your personal training zone. Plan to exercise at the lower or higher limits of your zone, depending on your present level of fitness.*
3. Type. *Determine the type of aerobic activity or activities you will engage in. Variety is important and helps prevent boredom. If you choose outdoor activities, keep environmental conditions in mind and plan accordingly. Drink plenty of fluids before, during, and after exercise, especially on warm days. The rule of thumb is 8 ounces every 20 minutes. Wear lightweight and light-colored clothing on warmer days and layered clothing on cold days.*
4. Time. *Determine the number of minutes you will spend exercising. Less intense activities should be done for a longer period of time in order to be beneficial. More intense activities may be done for shorter periods of time but no less than 15 minutes.*

As your level of fitness improves, you will want to increase either the number of days you work out or the length of time you devote to each workout, in order to continue to challenge your heart. This is called the **overload principle** (Donatelle et al., 1999). In general, cardiovascular benefits increase with the length and intensity of workouts; however, exercising more than 60 minutes per day confers no additional health benefits and may pose some risks (*How Much Exercise Is Enough?* 1999).

ENHANCING FLEXIBILITY SAFELY

Stretching exercises are generally used to promote flexibility. Proper stretching will improve performance, prevent injury, and increase mobility. The American College of Sports Medicine (ACSM, 2000) has prepared guidelines for stretching exercises that stipulate frequency, intensity, and duration:

1. *Frequency—three to five repetitions of each stretch, done at least three days a week*

Figure 6-1   Flexibility Exercises

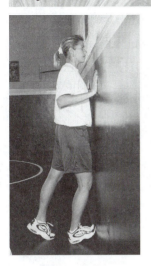

Calf Stretch. Stand facing the wall. Place hands shoulder width apart on the wall. Extend one leg behind you, fully extended. Place the forefoot of the other leg against the wall, with the knee extended. You will feel the stretch of the muscle in the belly of the calf. Hold the stretch for a 15- to 30-second count. Switch to the other leg. (If you bend your knee and keep the heel flat on the floor, you will stretch the achilles tendon.)

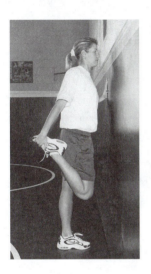

Quadriceps Stretch. Stand with feet shoulder distance apart. Grab one foot and bend it toward the buttocks until you feel a pull or slight stretch. Balance on the other leg, with the knee slightly bent. Hold for 15 to 30 seconds. Switch to the other leg.

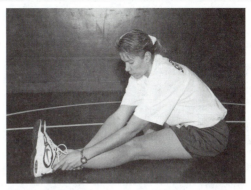

Hamstring Stretch. Sit on the floor. The leg you want to stretch should be extended out in front of you, with the back of the knee touching the floor. The other leg should be bent, with the foot flat on the floor. (Do not grab your foot and bend the leg toward the buttocks while you stretch; this will damage the knee ligaments.) Lean forward, reaching toward the toes. Go to the point of pull or slight stretch and hold for 15 to 30 seconds. Switch to the other leg.

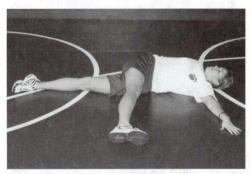

Hip Stretch. Lie flat on the floor on your back, with arms extended at shoulder level against the floor. Left leg should be extended and right leg will rotate across your body with leg extended. The goal is to try to lay it on the floor. Hold for 15 to 30 seconds. Switch to the other leg.

2. *Intensity—using proper form, stretch only to the point of "pull" or mild discomfort*

3. *Duration—10 to 60 seconds; the longer the stretch is held, the greater the gains in range of motion; a reasonable duration is 15 to 30 seconds*

4. *Type—specific stretches designed for specific muscles. Figure 6-1 illustrates stretching exercises for each major area of the body.*

Stretching is most beneficial if done *after* the body has warmed up. Five to 10 minutes of activities, such as slow running and biking, will raise body temperature sufficiently. A good stretching routine should take no less than 10 to 15 min-utes. Stretching each of the major muscles in the body three times, each with a 15- to 30-second hold, will take at least 15 to 20 minutes. Boredom often leads to noncompliance in this area of fitness. Listening to music, watching television, or talking to a training partner can prevent monotony from sabotaging the stretching phase of the fitness program.

DEVELOPING A MUSCLE-STRENGTHENING PROGRAM SAFELY

The muscle-strengthening component of fitness is one that many women tend to shy away from. This is unfortunate, as muscle strengthening is tremendously beneficial for women.

Figure 6–1   Flexibility Exercises (Continued)

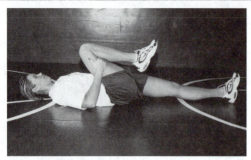

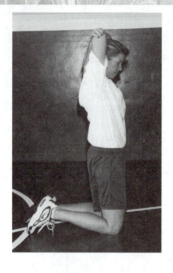

Triceps Stretch. Take elbow overhead in a bent position. With the other hand, grab at the elbow and push backwards. Hold for a 15- to 30-second count. Switch to the other arm.

Low Back Stretch. Lie supine on your back, with left leg extended. Place right hand behind the knee at the hamstring muscles and bend the knee; pull it up toward the chest and head. Hold for 15 to 30 seconds. Switch to the other leg.

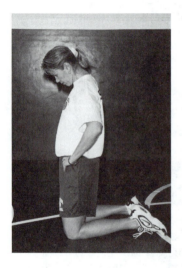

Trapezius Stretch. Bend the chin toward the chest until you feel mild discomfort. Hold for a 15- to 30-second count. Relax and repeat.

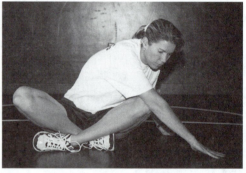

Latissimus Dorsi Stretch. Sit with legs in a crossed position. Lean slightly forward and twist to the left and hold when you feel the stretch. Hold for a 15- to 30-second count. Then switch to the other side.

The following are a few commonly held misconceptions about the ways in which strength training affects women:

1. *"I will look like a man." A belief that keeps many women from developing their muscles is that a woman will become masculine if she lifts weights. This is not true. Women do not have the genetic potential to develop large, bulky muscles because their bodies do not make enough of the hormone testosterone. It is men's high testosterone levels that allow them to develop large, bulging muscles if they work hard enough. Women who train with weights develop only toned, shapely muscles. In order to develop large, bulging muscles, women must use steroids or other artificial and potentially harmful substances.*

2. *"Intensive strength training will rid the body of fat." This is only partially true. Strength training does create more lean body mass by firming and toning muscles, and with increased lean body mass there is an increase in the resting metabolic rate (the rate at which calories are burned at rest). However, many believe that strength training can remove fat from specific areas of the body, and that is not true; unfortunately, there is no such thing as spot reducing. Stored fat is removed from the body only when the body's expenditure of energy exceeds its intake of energy in the form of food. The areas from which fat is most readily removed are genetically determined (Bryant & Peterson, 1998).*

3. *"Muscles turn to fat when you stop training." Muscles do not have the ability to change from one type of tissue to another. However, if muscles are not used, they will atrophy (become smaller), and, if the same number of calories are consumed in the absence of the energy expenditure associated with training, fat will be stored in the body.*

4. *"Weight lifting makes you muscle bound." Properly done, strength training does not decrease flexibility; it increases it. If each muscle is put through its full range of motion during strength training, flexibility will be enhanced. If, however, muscles strain against weight in a limited range of motion, they will shorten. A strength/resistance program should always be done in conjunction with a flexibility program.*

5. *"Long, hard sessions are better." On the contrary, the quality of a workout is more important than performing it for an extensive amount of time. Following the ACSM guidelines assures that weight training is performed safely.*

6. *"No pain, no gain." This is a very common misconception. Workouts should not be painful; the presence of pain indicates injury to muscular tissue. Workouts may involve mild discomfort, but they should never cause pain.*

7. *"You have to take protein supplements to build muscle." The average diet contains more than sufficient protein to support muscle building. Taking in excess protein does no good and actually is counterproductive. The body does not have the ability to store protein; excess protein is dismantled and its components used to synthesize fat, which is stored. Moreover, taking in excess protein can lead to both dehydration and loss of calcium. Chronic calcium loss from an excessive protein intake increases a woman's risk of osteoporosis.*

8. *"Strength training is for young people." A higher level of muscular fitness will improve women's quality of life and can extend their functional life span. A woman is never too old to improve her level of muscular fitness; women in their eighties and nineties have demonstrated the ability to increase their muscular strength and balance through resistance training (Nelson, 1997).*

The ACSM guidelines for muscle resistance training for healthy adults stipulate the frequency, intensity, and duration with which resistance training should be carried out. In order to determine the optimum intensity for a resistance program, an individual must first determine the maximum amount of weight she can lift. This can be done through trial and error. That amount is used to calculate the amount that will actually be lifted during each exercise session. The duration of the training program is determined by the total number of times the weight is lifted or moved. Each lift or move is called a **repetition,** and a certain number of repetitions make up a **set.** For example, a strength-training program might call for three sets of eight repetitions each. A beginning program should consist of a

minimum of one set of five to seven repetitions of each exercise. The goal is to work each targeted muscle group to near fatigue. Two goals are addressed in the ACSM guidelines: increasing muscle strength and increasing muscle endurance. Increasing muscular endurance strengthens the body for repetitive activities. Most women should participate in a muscular strength program unless they are engaging in endurance activities, such as bicycling, running, or walking long distances, or have a job that requires repetitive motions as well as strength. The ACSM guidelines are as follows:

1. *Frequency—two to three times per week on nonconsecutive days*
2. *Intensity—for strength, 60 to 80 percent of the maximum weight; for endurance, 50 percent of the maximum weight*
3. *Duration—for strength, 3 sets of 5 to 7 repetitions with 60 to 80 percent of the maximum weight; for endurance, 3 sets of 12 to 15 repetitions with 50 percent of the maximum weight*
4. *Rest—for strength, 1 to 5 minutes between sets; for endurance, 15 to 60 seconds between sets*

A muscle-strengthening program should be done a minimum of twice a week and should consist of a minimum of 8 to 10 exercises that work the major muscle groups of the body. Following the ACSM guidelines can help women who are new to strength training to develop a solid foundation. They can then progress to more specific advanced programs if they so desire. There are many excellent weight-training resources available through bookstores and libraries. Professional trainers may also be enlisted to help in developing sound strength programs.

Figure 6–2 illustrates isotonic exercises for all major areas of the body using free weights and machines. **Isotonic** exercise training uses both *concentric* muscle contractions (muscle shortens about the joint) and *eccentric* muscle contractions (muscle lengthens about the joint). Both types of contractions contribute to the development of muscular strength.

Preventing Exercise-Related Problems

Certain problems, such as joint pain, muscle pain, and breathlessness may arise when an individual incorporates exercise into her lifestyle. Some of these are more common to the novice exerciser, whereas others plague more experienced exercise adherents. The following suggestions may prevent these problems and allow individuals to maintain a consistent and comfortable exercise program.

Choosing an exercise that is appropriate for an individual's unique characteristics can make all the difference. Weight-bearing exercises such as walking and jogging can be excellent choices for some but may be too demanding for those who are overweight or who have arthritis. Alternatives

Figure 6–2   Strength Exercises

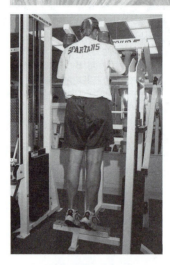

Calf Raises—Muscle Developed Is the Calf. Stand flat-footed, feet shoulder width apart. Holding a barbell on the shoulders or standing in the calf machine, rise up on toes as high as possible. Hold for a two-second count and then return to the starting position.

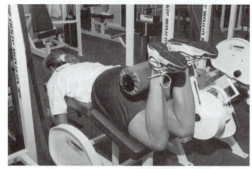

Leg Curls—Muscle Developed Is the Hamstring Group. Lie prone on the bench. Place the roller at the achilles tendon just below the calf muscle. Flex the knee and curl the lower leg toward the buttocks. Hold for a two-second count and then return slowly to the starting position.

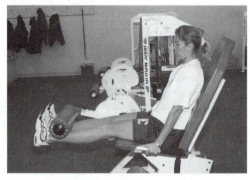

Leg Extensions—Muscle Developed Is the Quadriceps Group. Sit on the bench, with legs hanging over the bench. Place the roller on the lower legs just above the bend of the ankle. Straighten legs to extension, slowly. Hold for a two-second count and then slowly return to the starting position.

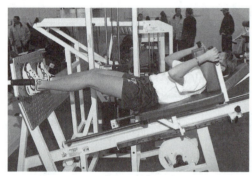

Leg Press—Muscles Developed Are the Gluteus, Quadriceps, Hamstrings, and Calf. Lie supine, with knees bent at a 90° angle. Extend legs slowly and do not snap legs into a locked position. This will injure the knee. Hold for a two-second count and then slowly return to the starting position.

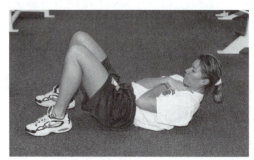

Crunches—Muscles Developed Are the Abdominals. Lie supine, with arms by the side or bent across the chest. Bend the chin toward the chest. Contract abdominal muscles and curl up until the shoulder blades are about 10 to 12 inches off the ground. Hold for a two-second count and then return to the starting position.

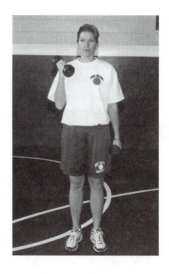

Arm Curls—Muscle Developed Is the Biceps. With feet shoulder width apart, hold dumbbell in hand, with arm straight down by the side. Slowly bend the elbow and curl the weight toward the shoulder. Hold for a two-second count and then slowly return to the starting position. Alternate arms.

Figure 6–2   Strength Exercises (Continued)

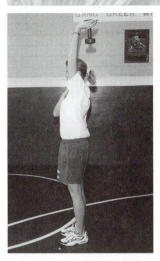

Overhead Extensions— Muscle Developed Is the Triceps. Stand with feet shoulder width apart. Hold the weight behind the head, with the elbow flexed. Slowly extend the weight straight upward. Hold for a two-second count and then slowly return to the starting position.

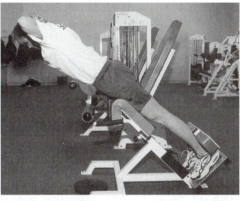

Back Extensions—Muscles Developed Are the Erector Spinae. Lie prone on the extension bench (you can use a flat bench if someone holds your feet) and then lean forward as far as you can. Tighten the buttocks and move your body up into an extended and level position. Hold for a two-second count and then return to bent position.

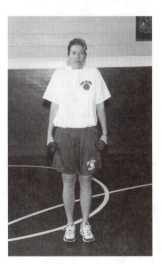

Shoulder Shrugs—Muscle Developed Is the Trapezius. Stand with feet shoulder width apart. Hold dumbbells in both hands. Arms are extended. Shrug shoulders upward as high as possible. Hold for a two-second count and then slowly return to the starting position.

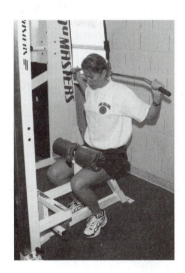

Lateral Pulldown— Muscle Developed Is the Latissimus Dorsi. Sit on the bench, with feet flat on the floor. Reach above the head and place hands on the bar a little wider than shoulder distance apart. Pull bar down behind the head. Hold for a two-second count and then slowly extend the arms and return to the starting position.

include nonweight-bearing exercises in which the body is supported. These include bicycling and exercising in water.

Because the upper body is a relatively weak area in many women, exercises involving barbells or dumbbells can be stressful to joints, especially the elbows and shoulders. Women can minimize stress on their joints by using weight machines instead of free weights. If free weights are used, it is important to move the weight slowly, so as to maintain control and prevent potential problems. Other frequent errors that occur with the use of free weights include failing to lift through the entire range of motion, locking the knees while lifting, and lifting with back muscles rather than the stronger muscles in the legs.

The manner in which an exercise is done can be critical, even in the case of such simple exercises as walking. Improper technique can overstress joints and other areas of the body. For example, when a woman who has embarked on a walking program wishes to increase her pace, it may seem natural to take longer strides. However, doing so can place excessive stress on the shins. A preferable technique is to walk more rapidly, without increasing the length of the stride.

The way in which an exerciser breathes is extremely important. Novice aerobic exercisers tend to breathe more shallowly and more rapidly as their bodies demand more oxygen. However, this type of breathing causes a feeling of breathlessness to develop because it does not allow oxygen to make its way to the depths of the lungs, where it is needed. A better approach is to take in slower, deeper breaths. Breathing technique is also important during weight training. It is a mistake to take a deep breath and hold it just before lifting or moving weight. Doing so strains the body and can trigger a reflex that can slow the heart rate or cause an abnormal rhythm to develop. Lifting or pulling should be done on exhalation, and the next breath should be taken during relaxation or while returning the weight to its original position.

Another pitfall for exercisers is the temptation to do too much, too soon. Most people make rapid gains in the beginning stages of an exercise program, and the temptation to rush toward one's ultimate goals can be strong. However, accelerating the rate at which additional demands are placed on the body must be resisted, as pushing too hard can easily lead to injury. Even veteran exercisers can fall into this trap, particularly if they have had to interrupt their program because of illness or another circumstance; they tend to push themselves too hard in an attempt to regain their former level of fitness quickly.

Although exercise is one of the most important elements of a healthy lifestyle, it must be remembered that vigorous exercise places a great deal of stress on the body. Whereas a healthy body will adjust to the demands of exercise by becoming more fit, an unhealthy one can be overwhelmed. The American College of Sports Medicine recommends that persons who have coronary heart disease, or are at risk for it, see their physicians to make sure that an exercise program is appropriate for them.

Rest and Exercise Wellness Self-Assessment

Use the following questions to evaluate your degree of wellness related to rest and exercise:

1. *I get at least seven to eight hours of sleep most nights.*
2. *I usually awaken feeling fresh and rested in the morning.*
3. *If I awaken during the night, I am usually able to get back to sleep.*
4. *I seldom nod off in meetings or when I would prefer to be wide awake.*
5. *Feeling sleepy while driving is a rare occurrence for me.*
6. *I can bend over and touch my toes from a standing position.*
7. *I perform general stretching exercises or do yoga in order to maintain or increase my flexibility.*
8. *I can easily lift grocery bags, small children, and so on.*
9. *I can walk up two flights of stairs without becoming short of breath.*
10. *I perform some type of aerobic exercise for a minimum of 20 minutes three times a week.*

QUESTIONS FOR REFLECTION AND DISCUSSION

1. *Do you feel your daily routines and habits promote healthy sleep? Why or why not?*
2. *What changes, if any, do you need to make in your sleep hygiene?*
3. *Do you believe your current level of cardiovascular conditioning and strength is adequate to meet your health, work, and leisure-time needs? Why or why not?*
4. *Do you now, or do you plan to someday, incorporate aerobic and muscular strength conditioning into your lifestyle? Why or why not?*
5. *What factors motivate or would motivate you to embark on, and stick with, a fitness program?*

RESOURCES

Books

Nelson, M.E. (2000). *Strong women stay young.* New York: Bantam Books.

Peterson, J.A., Bryant, C.X., & Peterson, S.L. (1995). *Strength training for women.* Champaign, IL: Human Kinetics.

Websites

Canadian Society of Exercise Physiology—contains guidelines for exercise and a readiness to exercise self-assessment tool www.paguide.com.

Fitness Partner Connection Jumpsite—a comprehensive resource for fitness information; includes a calorie counter and a searchable library http://www.primusweb.com/fitnesspartner/

National Sleep Council—information on sleep and sleep disorders; provides information gleaned from a poll on the sleep habits and problems of Americans http://www.sleepfoundation.org/publications/sleepdiary.html

President's Council on Physical Fitness and Sports—workout schedules and basics of fitness programs http://www.hoptechno.com/book11.htm

The Internet's Fitness Resource—offers information on fitness planning, specific sports, and special topics http://www.netsweat.com/

The Sleep Well—an excellent resource for information on sleep and sleep disorders http://www.stanford.edu/~dement/~

REFERENCES

American College of Sports Medicine. (1998a). Exercise and physical activity for older adults. *Medicine and Science in Sports and Exercise, 30*(6), 992.

American College of Sports Medicine. (1998b). The recommended quantity and quality of exercise for developing and maintaining cardiorespiratory and muscular fitness, and flexibility in healthy adults. *Medicine and Science in Sports and Exercise, 30*(6), 975.

American College of Sports Medicine. (2000). *Guidelines for exercise testing and prescription* (6th ed.). Philadelphia: Lea and Febiger.

American Heart Association. (1997). *Heart and stroke facts. Statistical supplement.* Dallas, TX: American Heart Association.

Borg, G. A. V. (1970). Perceived exertion as an indication of somatic stress. *Scandinavian Journal of Rehabilitation Medicine, 2,* 92–98.

Bryant, C. X., & Peterson, J. A. (1998). Strength for women through the stages of life. *Fitness Management, 14*(7), 36.

Bryant, C. X., Peterson, J. A., & Franklin, B. A. (1998). Fountain of youth. *Fitness Management, 14*(10), 44.

Butler, R. N. Davis, R., Lewis, C. B., Nelson, M. E., & Strauss, E. (1998). Exercise prescription for older women. *Geriatrics, 53*(11), 45–46.

Canadian Society for Exercise Physiology. (1996). The Canadian activity, fitness, and lifestyle appraisal: CSEP's plan for healthy active living. Ottawa, Canada: Author.

Cooper, K. H. (1995). *Faith based fitness.* Atlanta, GA: Thomas Nelson.

Dement, W. C. (1999). *The promise of sleep.* New York: Dell.

Donatelle, R., Snow, C., & Wilcox, A. (1999). *Wellness choices for health and fitness.* Belmont, CA: Wadsworth.

Griffen, J. C. (1998). *Client-centered exercise prescription.* Champaign, IL: Human Kinetics.

Harvard University. (1998). Stay stronger longer with weight training. *Harvard Health Letter, 23*(12), 1.

Hastings, M. (1998). The brain, circadian rhythms, and clock genes. *British Medical Journal, 317,* 17404–17408.

Higdon, H. (1997, October). Rest assured: We can help you sleep better, reduce fatigue and improve performance. *Runner's World,* pp. 102–108.

How much exercise do you need? (1999, April). *University of California, Berkeley Wellness Letter,* p. 6.

How much exercise is enough? (1999, April). *Women's Health Advisor,* pp. 4–5.

Huelskamp, S. (1999, October). Broken hearts. *Advance for Directors in Rehabilitation,* pp. 26–32, 56.

Kelly, G. A. (1989). Aerobic exercise and resting blood pressure among women: A meta-analysis. *Preventive Medicine, 28*(3), 264–275.

Kubitz, K. A., Landers, D. M., Petruzzello, S. J., & Han, M. (1996). The effects of acute and chronic exercise on sleep: A meta-analytic review. *Sports Medicine, 21,* 227–291.

Manson, J. E., Hu, F. B., Rich-Edwards, J. W., Colditz, G. A., Stampfer, M. J., Willett, W. C., Speizer, F. E., & Hennekens, C. H. (1999). A prospective study of walking as compared with vigorous exercise in the prevention of coronary heart disease in women. *New England Journal of Medicine, 341*(9), 650–658.

Modifica, M. (1998). Exercise and aging. *Fitness Management, 14*(10), 48.

Moore, K. A. (1996). A review of recent studies linking exercise and improved mental health. *Primary Psychiatry, 3*(1), 75–91.

Motluk, A. (1997, May). Emotions need forty winks. *New Scientist,* 20–21.

Nelson, M., Fiatrone, M., & Morganti, C. (1994). Effects of high intensity strength training on multiple risk factors for osteoporosis fractures: A randomized, controlled trial. *Journal of the American Medical Association, 272,* 1904–1914.

Nelson, M. E. (1997). *Strong women stay young.* New York: Bantam Books.

Nieman, D. C. (1999). *Exercise testing and prescription: A health-related approach.* Mountain View, CA: Mayfield.

Novitt-Moreno, A. (1998, October). Why sleep? Getting a good night's sleep is important to your health and also to your success in life. *Current Health, 2,* 6–13.

O'Connor, P. J., & Youngstedt, S. D. (1995). Influence of exercise on human sleep. *Exercise Sports Science Review, 23,* 105–134.

Rockhill, B., Willett, W. C., Hunter, D. J., Manson, J. E., Hankerson, S. E., & Colditz, C. A. (1999). A Prospective Study of Recreational Physical Activity and Breast Cancer Risk. *Archives of Internal Medicine, 159*(19), 2290–2296.

Schnirring, L. (1997). What's new in treating active women? *The Physician and Sportsmedicine, 25*(7), 34–36.

Sleep Foundation. (2001a). *Don't go to bed yet* [On-line]. Available: http//www://sleepfoundation.org/publications/ travel.html

Sleep Foundation. (2001b). *Excessive daytime sleepiness* [On-line]. Available: http//www://sleepfoundation.org/epworth/ quizfaq.html

Sleep Foundation. (2001c). *Facts about drowsy driving* [On-line]. Available: http//www://sleepfoundation.org/publications/ travel.html

Sleep Foundation. (2001d). *Facts about PLMS* [On-line]. Available: http://www.sleepfoundation.org/ publications/fact_plms.html

Sleep Foundation. (2001e). *Facts about restless legs* [On-line]. Available: http://www.sleepfoundation.org/ publications/fact_rls.html

Sleep Foundation. (2001f). *Jet lag: The traveling sleep disorder* [On-line]. Available: http//www://sleepfoundation.org/ publications/travel.html

Sleep Foundation. (2001g). *Less fun, less sleep, more work: An American portrait.* Available: http://wwwsleepfoundation. org/PressArchives/lessfun_lesssleep.htm

Sleep Foundation. (2001h). *Living with narcolepsy* [On-line]. Available: http//www://sleepfoundation.org/publications/ livingnarcolepsy.html

Sleep Foundation. (2001i). *The nature of sleep* [On-line]. Available: http//www://sleepfoundation.org/publications/ nos.html

Sleep Foundation. (2001j). *Sleep apnea* [On-line]. Available: http//www://sleepfoundation.org/publications/sleepap.html

Sleep Foundation. (2001k). *Sleep and the traveler* [On-line]. Available: http://www.sleepfoundation.org/publications/ travel.html

Sleep Foundation. (2001l). *Women and sleep* [On-line]. Available: http://www.sleepfoundation.org/publications/women.html

Sleep Foundation. (2001m). Rotating shifts [On-line]. Available: http://www.sleepfoundation.org/publications/shifts.html

Stuhr, R. M. (1998). Strategies for beating the barriers to exercise for women. *ACSM's Health and Fitness Journal, 2*(5), 20.

U.S. Department of Health and Human Services. (1996). *Physical activity and health: A report of the surgeon general.* Atlanta, GA: Author.

U.S. Department of Health and Human Services. (1998). *Healthy People 2010 objectives: Draft for comments.* Washington, DC: Author.

Van Dam, S. M. (1988). Effect of exercise on glucose metabolism in post-menopausal women. *American Journal of Obstetrics and Gynecology, 159,* 82–86.

7

Women and Stress

Normandie Gaitley

Objectives

1. *Identify common stressors for women.*
2. *Discuss the relationship among stress, coping, and well-being.*
3. *Identify personal characteristics that confer resistance to stress.*
4. *Identify sociocultural factors related to the greater role strain experienced by women.*
5. *Identify techniques for minimizing and coping with stress.*

Introduction

A Fable of Two Frogs

Two frogs fell into a can of cream, or so I've heard it told.
The sides of the can were shiny and steep, the cream was deep and cold.

"Oh what's the use?" said number one, " 'Tis fate, no help's around."
"Good bye, my friend, Good bye sad world!" and weeping still, he drowned.

But number two, of sterner stuff, dog paddled in surprise.
For awhile she wiped her creamy face and dried her creamy eyes.

Poem *A Fable of Two Frogs:* A Fable of Two Frogs [Internet]. A Gift of Poetry, Wombarra, NSW, Australia. Allen Jesson, owner. [Modified 2001, Aug., cited 2001, Aug.]. Available: http://www.agiftofpoetry.com/Work/Workfunny_two_frogs.htm

"I'll swim awhile, at least," she said, or so it has been said.
"It wouldn't really help the world if one more frog were
    dead."

An hour or two she kicked and swam, not once she
    stopped to mutter.
But kicked and swam and swam and kicked, then hopped
    out via butter.

Author unknown

*T*his fable highlights a reality often observable in human behavior. Individuals respond to stress differently. For some, life stressors induce *paralysis* and *inactivity;* for others, they precipitate *creativity* and *growth.* In the general stress literature, the linkage between exposure to stress and the effect of stress on personal well-being is not clear. However, it is likely that the effects of a given stressor are related to how it is perceived.

The accelerated and hectic pace of modern lifestyles subjects individuals to frequent and intense stress. Rapid and abrupt cultural and technological changes are stressful for many people. In addition, environmental pollution, random crime, fear about AIDS, nuclear accidents, and terrorism are growing concerns. The turbulence of modern life suggests that managing stress will continue to be a significant part of life in the second millennium. Every individual is challenged to accept this reality and to learn to develop the skills needed to live happily and productively. Failure to cope positively with stress can have dire health consequences: Stress is known to contribute to a host of disease states, including high blood pressure, coronary heart disease, and depression, and is believed to be implicated in some instances of cancer (see Chapter 26). It has been reported that stress-related illnesses and symptoms cost industry over $150 billion a year in lost productivity, medical expenses, and absenteeism (Hafen, Karren, Frandsen, & Smith, 1996).

This chapter will begin with a brief exploration of modern theories of stress and coping. It will consider the personal qualities that are thought to make individuals stress-resistant and will examine the environmental stressors at home and at work that create special stress for women. The chapter will conclude with a review of the practices that are known to help individuals reduce or cope with stress.

Stress and Coping

Stress is a subjective concept; what is perceived as stressful by one individual may be experienced as merely stimulating by another. The ability to cope with stressful phenomena also varies from individual to individual.

Stress

For the purpose of this chapter, *stress* is defined as the belief that a given situation is both *threatening* and *demanding* and that one does not have the ability to cope with it (Cohen & Wills, 1985). Contemporary definitions of stress include two important processes: appraisal and demand. The term **appraisal** refers to the process of making a judgment as to whether a situation, an occurrence, or a circumstance constitutes a *threat.* Whether a threat is perceived depends on variables such as learning, memory, judgment, and thought (Lazarus, 1966), as well as on factors related to both the perceiver and the circumstance, such as the individual's past experiences, beliefs, and personality and the characteristics of the situation. For example, if a boss asks an employee to work late, the request may be viewed as a threat, because the boss has the power to hire and fire. The threat is increased if the employee is fearful about retaining her job and if other employment opportunities are few. The developmental level of the person involved, and the cultural setting in which the stress is experienced, also influence the degree to which a given situation is perceived as threatening (Lazarus, 1966).

The term **demand** refers to an environmental situation that prompts changes in an individual's physiological or psychological functioning. Such situations might involve changes in task, technology, workload, time constraints, or authority.

The coping strategies that stressed individuals choose influence the overall, ultimate effects stressful situations have on well-being. This is illustrated by one model of the relationship between stress and coping, the mediated effects model (see Figure 7–1). According to this model, the degree to which a given stressor affects an individual's well being is determined by how well s/he is able to cope with it. A person who can cope well with a given stressor will suffer few or no ill effects; a person who cannot may experience serious consequences. Various methods of managing the symptoms of stress, such as relaxation and exercise, will be discussed later in this chapter.

Coping

Coping has been defined as a constantly changing cognitive and behavioral process used to manage specific external or internal demands that are appraised as taxing or exceeding

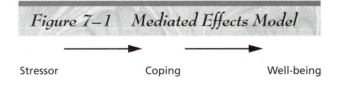

Figure 7–1   Mediated Effects Model

Stressor   Coping   Well-being

the resources of a person (Lazarus & Folkman, 1984). As this definition suggests, coping necessitates taking action or changing one's thinking patterns in order to deal with a stressor. There are generally thought to be two basic ways of coping with a stressful situation: one, known as **instrumental coping,** is to take some form of action; the other, known as **emotional coping,** is to change one's thoughts about, or attitudes toward, the stressor (Lazarus & Folkman, 1984).

An important feature of effective coping is that it involves more than just problem solving; it also involves managing or altering the problem causing distress, as well as regulating the emotional response to the problem (Dewe, 1992). According to Latack (1986), attempts at coping have one of three goals: control, escape, or symptom management. Based on their analysis of the existing literature on both human and animal methods of coping with stress, researchers from the University of California at Berkeley (Taylor et al., 2000) theorize that there may be a prototypically "female" method of coping with stress, which differs in some important ways from male coping. Taylor and her colleagues note that, unlike males, the females of many species tend to initiate social contact with others when stressed. They may seek the company of other females or nurture their young. Differing hormone activity in the two sexes may explain this behavior: Oxytocin, a hormone that promotes calmer, more social behavior and encourages maternal behavior, such as nurturing and comforting, is present in the systems of both males and females of many species. However, oxytocin's effects are enhanced by estrogen and mitigated by testosterone. Taylor has dubbed the female response to stress the **tend-and-befriend** response and theorizes that it may explain why women are less vulnerable than men to stress-related diseases, such as alcoholism and hypertension. More studies are needed to confirm Taylor's hypotheses, however, because most stress research (and research on other topics as well) has been done on male subjects (see Chapter 1).

A number of personality characteristics are associated with **resilience,** or the ability to withstand stress. These characteristics are self-efficacy, hardiness, internal locus of control, and Type B personality.

SELF-EFFICACY

Self-efficacy is defined as a person's belief that she can successfully accomplish a specific task. Efficacy expectations are different from outcome expectations. Efficacy expectations are the conviction that one is *capable* of executing a necessary or desired new behavior, whereas outcome expectations are the person's estimate of whether the new behavior will achieve the desired outcome.

Expectations regarding efficacy and outcome influence both the initiation and the persistence of coping behavior. An individual's beliefs regarding efficacy will determine, at least in part, whether she will even try to cope with a given situation. Self-efficacy has been shown to be an even better predictor of behavior toward unfamiliar threats than is past performance (Bandura, 1977).

An important dimension of self-efficacy is that it is not a stable characteristic; it can change over time. People's beliefs regarding self-efficacy and the controllability of the environment are based on their experience. Success breeds confidence because it validates personal efficacy and environmental controllability. Failure, on the other hand, particularly repeated failure, can erode confidence and the sense of efficacy (Wood & Bandura, 1989).

HARDINESS

The term **hardiness** refers to the capacity to withstand stress without becoming ill. Kobasa (1979), who also wrote under the name Oulette, examined hardiness as a personality trait and found that it is comprised of three general characteristics: control, commitment, and challenge. Hardy individuals possess the following characteristics:

- The belief that they can control or influence the events related to themselves
- A deep feeling of being involved in or committed to the activities of their lives
- The ability to see change as an exciting challenge for further development

In a study of more than 800 executives, Kobasa (1979) found that executives who had high levels of stress but low levels of illness could be distinguished from high-stress, high-illness executives on the basis of *personality*. The high-stress, low-illness executives were, at least in some ways, more in control, more committed, and more oriented to challenge than the high-stress, high-illness executives. The high-stress, low-illness executives possessed commitment to the self, a sense of vigorousness about life, a sense of meaningfulness, and an internal locus of control (discussed in the next section). In a prospective study that measured hardiness, social support, exercise, and other variables in 73 pregnant women, hardier women were found to have fewer problems during labor and more positive perceptions about their infants than less hardy women. Of the variables hardiness, social support, and exercise, hardiness was found to be the most powerful predictor of health a year later (Priel, Gonik, & Rabinowitz, 1993).

Interestingly, in the Priel et al. study, when hardiness was low, family support *increased* the risk of illness. This counterintuitive interaction appeared to be the result of the differing types of family support that the hardy and less hardy individuals received. For the hardy individuals, family support seemed to consist of nurturing, engaging kinds of interactions, whereas, for the less hardy, family support was characterized by an absence of mutuality and nonengaging "yes person" types of interactions. The connection between hardiness and health is likely due to the positive effect hardiness has on immune functioning (see Chapter 27).

INTERNAL LOCUS OF CONTROL

Locus of control is a personality dimension that reflects whether individuals believe their fate lies primarily in their own hands or in the hands of others. *Locus* means locality. Individuals with an **internal** locus believe that much of what happens to them is *controlled by them;* individuals with an **external** locus believe that their fate depends on *forces outside themselves* (Parasuraman, 1977). Persons with an internal locus of control consider their successes to be the result of their own persistence, intelligence, and efforts, whereas persons with an external locus of control consider their successes to be the result of good luck. In the fable recounted at the beginning of this chapter, the first frog, who has an internal locus, sees the outcome of his situation as already determined: " 'tis fate, no help's around." The second frog, who has an internal locus, assumes she can influence the outcome of her situation. Locus of control is a function of relatively stable beliefs about self-efficacy, and it involves the appraisal of events (Newton & Keenan, 1990). Locus of control often underlies consistent styles of coping behavior.

Persons with an internal locus of control and persons with an external locus of control tend to be affected differently by certain types of job-related stress (Newton & Keenan, 1990). For example, uncertainties about job responsibilities and frustrations with the work environment were found to increase the stress experienced by persons with an external locus of control but to have little effect on persons with an internal locus. However, an excessive workload or simultaneous demands from home and work increased the degree of strain experienced by persons with an internal locus of control. Although these findings suggest that internals report less stress *overall,* they also suggest that internality may lead to more stress under certain job-related conditions (Newton & Keenan, 1990).

Actual or perceived control over events in one's life is important to well-being, and acquiring the ability to control even mundane things can dramatically affect an individual's life. In a landmark study of nursing home patients, Rodin and Langer (1977) found that the residents who were given the right to make decisions concerning their day-to-day activities were more active, happier, healthier, and more likely to be alive 18 months later than were those who were not given this right.

TYPE B PERSONALITY

Two different constellations of behavioral characteristics have been labeled Type A and Type B. Both types involve characteristic styles of responding to and coping with environmental stressors. A **Type A** personality orientation is characterized by impatience, perfectionism, and a desire for achievement. Some Type A individuals display free-floating or nonsituational hostility and cynicism as well. People with a **Type B** orientation are more easygoing and less competi-

tive and display lower levels of hostility (Parasuraman, 1977). Although it was once assumed that the hurried, competitive, and possibly hostile behavior of Type A individuals would lead to greater career success, research suggests that this is only true to a point. Type As advance more rapidly than Type Bs in the early and middle stages of their careers, but they do not make it to the top more often. It has been suggested that the reason for this is that Type A persons sometimes do not take the time to form the *relationships* that help individuals advance within an organization. Alternatively, some studies suggest it is only the hostile Type A individuals who are ultimately hampered in their careers.

It is not clear whether Type A individuals always experience more *stress* than Type Bs. Some studies suggest that they do, but Newton and Keenan (1990) found, surprisingly, that persons with Type A personalities seem to experience *less* psychological strain than Type Bs. This may, however, be true only in situations in which action may be taken, as Type A individuals are known to favor *instrumental* coping strategies (Edwards, Baglioni, & Cooper, 1990). Type As may experience equal or greater stress than Type Bs in situations in which *emotional* coping is called for. Type A individuals who display hostility and cynicism have definitely been found to suffer more coronary heart disease than Type Bs do. Ornish (1998) has suggested that the key to this association is the problems that hostile Type A individuals tend to have with intimacy and personal relationships. An instrument that you can use to assess your hostility level can be found at the end of this chapter.

Stressors at Home and at Work

The range of roles women play in American society has been increasing steadily over the last century. One result of this change is that most women must now contend with stressors encountered both at home and in the course of paid employment.

The Changing Roles of Women

Throughout much of our history, the concept of work has generally had a masculine connotation, and the concept of family has had a feminine one (Singer, 1991). In the past, women were more likely to be socialized to fill *expressive roles,* emphasizing nurturance and emotional sustenance, whereas men were more likely to be socialized to fill *instrumental roles,* emphasizing achievement and accomplishment (Vanfossen, 1981). Traditionally, women worked within their own homes or on their own farms. At the turn of the twentieth century, however, about 20 percent of all the women in America were working outside their homes. This percentage continued to increase, from 19.7 percent in 1900 to 66.9% in 1988 (Matthews & Rodin, 1989). Today, almost *three out of every four* women work outside their homes, and it has been estimated that 99 percent of all U.S. women will work for pay at some point in their lives (Hales, 1999). Moreover, more women than ever before are opting for careers, as opposed to jobs. This change may be related to women's increasing interest in the money, power, and prestige that accompany high-status careers (Regan & Roland, 1985).

Only 20 years ago, a Yankelovitch Poll found that a solid majority of those queried defined *masculinity* in terms of *the ability to provide for a family* (Hales, 1999). In contemporary society, however, the traditional family model in which the husband is breadwinner and the wife homemaker, is fast becoming a vestige of the past. In most contemporary heterosexual American families, both the woman and the man work; in one out of four families, the woman earns more than the man. Moreover, *women are the sole breadwinners in two of every five families* (Hales, 1999).

A source of stress for the many women who work outside their homes is conflict between their domestic and employment-related responsibilities. Figure 7–2 illustrates the variety of relationship and responsibility patterns that can characterize women's lives. Some of the possible role combinations illustrated in Figure 7–2 are employee/mother; employee/wife; employee/wife/mother; and employee/single woman. Many women also take on the role of caretaker for aging parents and relatives.

Workplace Stress

Since the dawn of the industrial age, women and men have experienced workplace stress. Common stressors they have faced include work overload; ineffective, hostile, and incompetent bosses; lack of personal fit with a job; lack of recognition; job ambiguity, and uncertainty about career progress. The 1990s ushered in new business stressors, such as global competition and reorganization, technological change, an increasingly diverse workforce, teamwork, employee empowerment, and violence in the workplace.

It is sobering that, even today, working women face additional stressors related to gender. For one thing, women still make less money then men in *comparable* jobs; overall, women earn only about 74 percent of what men do. The gap is narrowing in certain sectors, however. Young women in entry-level positions in science and technology now earn

about *98 percent* of what their male colleagues earn. Elsewhere, unfortunately, salary discrepancies persist, even as women and men are promoted (Hales, 1999). Despite their increasing participation in the workforce, women are still generally found in low-skill, low-pay jobs *within occupational groupings* such as construction. Women in such low-level jobs often lack the technical and mechanical skills or the physical strength and stamina needed to gain recognition and advancement. Women attempting to make the transition from job to career or from entry level to middle or upper management often face barriers as well, including gender discrimination, conflicts between work and home, and poorly articulated career goals. It is particularly difficult for women in traditionally male-dominated fields to advance, as they are sometimes excluded from *informal social networks* and held to higher standards then men are. Authorities (Hales, 1999) in the field of gender equity believe the following:

- A given occupation must be comprised of at least *40 percent women* before women can have the same opportunities for promotion and advancement as men.
- Gender bias works against women applying for a given position unless at least *25 percent* of the applicants are female.

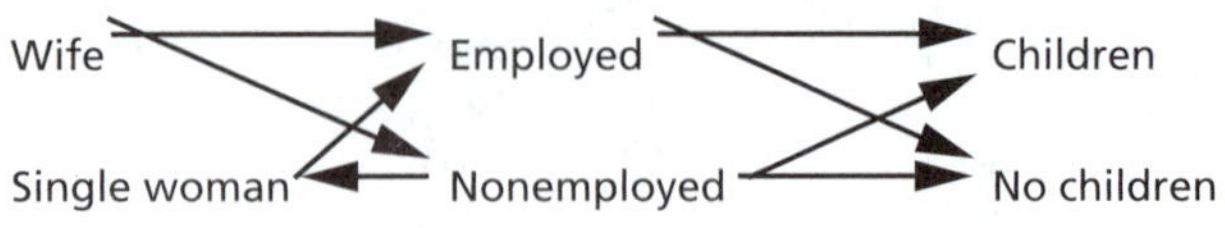

Some fields, such as law, seem to pose particular difficulties for women. A 1996 report by the American Bar Association found that women lawyers earn less than men at every level of experience and are less likely to advance to the rank of partner or judge (Hales, 1999). Almost as many women as men are now attending law school, however, and, when women constitute almost half the profession, those patterns may change (Guinier, Fine, & Balm, 1997). Women workers are making excellent gains in some areas. Women fill 48 percent of the managerial and professional positions in corporations and 33 percent of government positions at the decision-making level. Women are joining the ranks of *entrepeneurs* at an astonishing rate—they are going into business for themselves at twice the rate of men. The number of businesses owned by women increased by 78 percent between 1987 and 1996 (Hales, 1999).

Women pioneers in the male-dominated world of work found it difficult to reconcile female gender role characteristics with the male traits that seemed essential for career success. Carolyn Duff captured this dilemma in her essay *We Were Damned Whatever We Did:*

> *If we acted like men, men often felt threatened by our directness and competitiveness, and many women found us alienating and difficult to work with. On the other hand, if we acted like women—seeming reluctant to play power politics and insisting on bringing relationship-based values into an objective, competitive "male" workplace—men found our feminine behavior a sign of weakness. (Duff, 1993, p. 244)*

Figure 7–2   Relationship/ Responsibility Patterns

Wife → Employed → Children
Single woman → Nonemployed → No children

As women's presence alongside men in the world of work has become more commonplace and accepted, women have developed a distinctive managerial and leadership style that is being increasingly valued and copied by men. Contemporary women in positions of authority and responsibility often emphasize *flexibility, cooperation,* and *team building* and are more likely than men to make decisions by consensus and to encourage individual growth in employees (Hales, 1999).

Role Conflict

Role conflict occurs when the roles associated with different environments create simultaneous, irreconcilable demands on one person (Barnett, 1995). Roles are aspects of *identity,* which is generally defined as persons' perceptions of themselves as they relate to their environment. Many women have multiple roles, such as spouse, parent, and employee. A role is made up of three components: the structurally determined demands, the individual's personal role conception, and the individual's personal role behavior. **Structurally determined demands** are responsibilities that flow from a particular role, due to its intrinsic nature and societal or organizational norms. An example is the work-related tasks associated with the role of employee. **Role conception** is an individual's beliefs about what a given role entails. **Role behavior** refers to what an individual actually does to carry out a particular role; it is a function of both personal role conception and structurally determined demands (Hall, 1972).

Women's increased participation in the workplace has caused role conflict to emerge as a significant problem for them. **Work-family conflict** occurs when the demands of work and family roles are incompatible in some respect, so that participation in either the work or the family role is more difficult because of participation in the other role. Research findings indicate that work role characteristics and family structure demands contribute independently and additively to work-family conflict (Voydanoff, 1988). Research done on dual-career families in the early 1980s indicates that conflicts between professional and parental roles are especially stressful for the female spouse (Gilbert, Holahan, & Manning, 1981). Sekaran (1985) reported results indicating that multiple role pressures and the number of children in the family have direct adverse consequences on the mental health of the women, but not of the men, in dual-career families. The stress that women experience so acutely tends to emanate from the role of *mother,* rather than that of employee (Barnett & Baruch, 1985). The situation in which many women who juggle the roles of spouse/mother/employee find themselves is illustrated by Perlow's (1997) description of the research participant "Laura":

> Laura does not feel she has the option to make an open-ended commitment to work. Her husband works at the same company, in a different division, at a level equivalent to her boss, the software manager. Laura explained that her husband is the one who oversees the details around the house: "He organizes the lawn service; he hires the maid; he pays the bills; he calls the dentist; he does the weekly shopping. He is the administrator. I take care of the children; I do the cleaning beyond the maid; I pick up; I cook; I do laundry, gardening, ironing and the shopping, besides the weekly grocery shopping." Laura said her husband works longer hours than she does. If he does get involved in transporting the children to day care, he prefers to drop them off in the morning, so he has the flexibility at night. He usually comes home between six-thirty and seven, just as Laura is serving dinner. She says they quibble a lot over whose work meetings are more important and who should have to skip out to care for the kids, but ultimately her husband says, "If there is ever a real question, my work wins out."
>
> When one of the children is sick, it is Laura who usually stays home. Her mother who is recovering from a serious illness also lives with them. According to Laura, her mother is not much help around the house or with the children. (Perlow, 1997, p. 28)

Laura's situation includes the three factors identified by Beehr and Bhagat (1985) as stress-producing: *importance, uncertainty,* and *duration.* Although employed full-time, Laura's husband does not see her work responsibilities as equal in importance to his. In addition to her full-time job, Laura has the primary responsibility for the home and children. She is the primary provider of the care of sick children—an unpredictable, and therefore uncertain, occurrence. Finally, Laura's situation is of long duration, with no immediate relief in sight. Hers is a classic case of work-family conflict.

Sociologists have traditionally seen the assumption of multiple roles as a drain on an individual's scarce energy resources. More recently, sociologists with an expansionist view have suggested that human activity generates energy as well as depletes it and that the benefits of role accumulation, such as role-related privileges and status, security, personality enrichment, and ego gratification, may *outweigh* the generated stress—at least in certain circumstances (Sieber, 1974). Indeed, some investigators have found that multiple roles do not always equal more perceived stress. In a study of faculty women, Yogev (1982) found that women with children felt no more overworked than single women who worked significantly fewer hours. *Control* and *support* are two variables that seem to influence the degree to which women experience multiple roles as stressful. In one study, women who occupied a greater number of roles but perceived a higher level of personal control and social support reported fewer stress-related symptoms than those who occupied fewer roles but had less control and support (Amatea

& Fong, 1991). In a study of Mexican American families, spousal support and effective social networks were found to promote affinity toward both family and work and to reduce role conflict (Holtzman & Gilbert, 1987).

A pressing issue for employers and society is to identify and support workplace and domestic arrangements that foster maximal emotional, social, and cognitive development of employees' children while promoting employees' own personal and marital/domestic satisfaction. The value an organization places on its human resources is reflected by the degree to which its personnel policies are *family-friendly*. Fortunately, family-friendly policies seem to be in organizations' best interests, as well as employees'. In one study, 88 percent of the 58 employers surveyed indicated that work/family programs increased their ability to attract employees (Dewe & Guest, 1990). In another study of 204 companies with childcare programs, employers ranked an improved ability to recruit and improved morale among the top benefits of such programs (Galinsky & Stein, 1990). Indeed, the need to attract top employees seems to provide strong motivation for companies to establish family-friendly policies. In a study that looked at a sampling of companies from across the nation, Kammerman and Kahn (1987) found that the ability to attract a talented and stable workforce was the primary motivation for companies to establish family support services. Support in life was found to moderate the relationship between work stress and burnout for women (Etzion, 1984). Although women were found to experience more stress than men (Etzion, 1984), they also reported more social support in their lives (Shinn, Rosario, Morch, & Chestnut, 1984).

Flexible schedules, parental leave, and childcare assistance are just some of the new policies that have been adopted in the private and public sectors to ease the strain between work and family roles. Issues related to the effectiveness of these policies, who should pay for them, and whether they should be mandated through legislation are intensely debated (Matthews & Rodin, 1989).

At least some of the stress in our lives is unavoidable, and can cause symptoms such as feeling tense and irritable, as well as a host of physical problems, including headache, stomach problems, back pain, and many more. In the remainder of this chapter, practices that can be used to relieve these symptoms are described. The major responsibility for implementing effective measures for relieving stress rests with the individual, who is primarily responsible for her own well-being.

Strategies for Relieving Stress and Promoting Well-Being

A number of techniques from the Eastern and Western traditions have been found effective in stress management. A brief overview of some of them will be provided in this section (and see Chapter 11).

The Relaxation Response

The term **relaxation response** was coined in 1971 by Herbert Benson, a cardiologist interested in stress and the mind/body connection (Roush, 1997). The relaxation response is the opposite of the stress response. When we are fully relaxed and free of stress, heart rate, respiratory rate, blood pressure, and muscle tension all decrease, as does the level of stress hormones circulating in the body. The relaxation response has been used to ameliorate many physical and emotional problems. It has been used therapeutically as part of the treatment of disorders of heart rate and rhythm, hypertension, asthma, insomnia, headache, epilepsy, menstrual disorders, depression, anxiety, and sexual dysfunction. It has also been used to halt premature labor (Gregerson, 1998). Many methods of diverting the mind from stressful thoughts and allowing the relaxation response to occur have been documented, including imaging, biofeedback, breathing techniques, music therapy, progressive muscle relaxation, prayer, and various forms of meditation. Although some might disagree, prayer has been described as the most effective method of eliciting the relaxation response (Hafen et al., 1996).

As scientists learn more about the hormones and neurotransmitters that brain cells use to communicate with each other and with the rest of the body, they are gaining insight into the physiological changes that occur when we are under stress and how to minimize them. Although mind/body research is still evolving, and new techniques for controlling stress will likely be developed, individuals can use current insights into phenomena such as the relaxation response to improve their quality of life and, likely, their health as well (Benson, 1993).

Progressive muscle relaxation is an easily learned, effective way of eliciting the relaxation response. Progressive muscle relaxation involves consciously relaxing each part of the body, one after the other, beginning at the feet and slowly working one's way up to the head. The relaxation response can also be elicited while engaging in rhythmic, repetitive exercises, such as walking, jogging, or swimming, even though the body is not fully relaxed; freeing the mind of stressful preoccupations and thoughts is enough. Research suggests that focusing on a sound, word, phrase, or prayer and passively disregarding other thoughts when they come to mind decrease the metabolic rate of persons who are performing simple, repetitive exercises, such as walking, jogging, and swimming (Benson, 1993). Summoning the relaxation response during workouts could yield important benefits to many stress-ridden exercisers. Regularly eliciting the relaxation response can both decrease the amount of stress perceived and protect the body from the negative effects of unavoidable stress. An additional bonus is that those

Box 7–1   Progressive Muscle Relaxation

You can do this exercise by yourself, or you can have a partner read the following steps. Be sure you focus on and relax each part of the body in turn and spend approximately 1 full minute on each. Allow 15–20 minutes for your session.

1. Begin by sitting or lying quietly with no distractions. Close your eyes.
2. Take a deep breath, allowing your belly to rise, and release it fully, through the mouth, with an audible sound, such as a-a-h-h. Repeat four or five times.
3. Breathe naturally. Imagine tension leaving the body with each exhalation.
4. Focus your attention on your toes and feet, and imagine them becoming soft and warm. Let your toes and feet become completely relaxed (30 seconds).
5. Feel all tension flowing away from your calves. Let them become soft, relaxed, and warm. Remember to let your belly rise with each breath (one minute).
6. Allow your thighs to just let go. Notice how warm and relaxed they feel. Imagine any tension in your legs just flowing down your thighs and calves and out of your body through your feet and toes (one minute).
7. Relax your buttocks. Just let those muscles go limp. Just let them sink right into the (chair, bed, floor). Allow any tension to just flow right down your legs and out of your body (one minute).
8. Notice your belly rising with each breath. Just release all tension there. Let it rise and fall, and let all tension flow down through your fingertips and out of your body (one minute).

9. Relax your arms, forearms, and upper arms. Allow them to become heavy and warm and to just sink into the (chair, bed, floor). Notice whether your palms are beginning to feel warmer (one minute).
10. Let go of all tension in your shoulders. Just feel them drop a little. As you exhale, let them sink more deeply into the (chair, bed, floor). Allow any tension to flow down your arms and out of your body through your fingers (one minute).
11. Now, relax the muscles in your chest. Notice any tightness there, and let it go. Notice that your breathing is becoming just a bit slower as you relax more and more deeply (one minute).
12. Bring your attention to your neck and head. Allow them to relax completely. Let them sink deeply into the (chair, bed, floor). Notice your jaw. Let all the muscles that hold it in place relax. If your mouth wants to open, let it.
13. Release all tension from your cheeks, eyes, and forehead. Allow your face to become a bit warmer as you relax all the muscles around your mouth and nose (one minute).

After you have relaxed all parts of your body, lie still for a few moments and enjoy the feeling. When you are ready to conclude the exercise, start moving your fingers and toes gradually. Open your eyes and slowly return to your normal state. With practice, you will notice that it becomes easier to relax fully. You may notice that your breathing slows automatically and that you develop a feeling of warmth or tingling in the palms of your hands. If you choose to incorporate progressive muscle relaxation into your lifestyle, you will realize maximum benefit by engaging in two sessions per day.

---

who regularly achieve the relaxation response during exercise tend to experience mild euphoria in a relatively short time. Box 7–1 contains guidelines for doing progressive muscle relaxation.

Box 7–2 outlines the steps in eliciting the relaxation response during repetitive exercises, such as walking, jogging, or swimming. Persons who are over 40 years old, have a health problem, or are not in sufficiently good condition that that they can exercise without becoming excessively short of breath should consult a healthcare provider before beginning an exercise program.

The Practice of Mindfulness

The central goal of **mindfulness** is to become more *aware,* aware of one's thoughts, feelings, and behaviors. Awareness is the quality of being in touch with life and with whatever is happening in one's own mind and body at the time it is happening. The practice of mindfulness involves reserving a portion of one's attention for self-monitoring. Mindfulness leads to *insight* and is invaluable in the identification of subtle stressors. It is also a necessary part of learning positive new habits and unlearning negative ones. Everyday sounds, such as those made by car horns, watch alarms, beepers, and telephones, can be used as reminders to pause and ask ourselves how we are feeling, what thoughts we were just having, and whether our behavior is in accord with our values. With much practice, mindfulness can be maintained during almost all activities. Choosing a commonplace activity and carrying it out in a highly mindful way can be a good introduction to mindfulness practice and its revelations (Kabat-Zinn, 1993).

Box 7–2   *Eliciting the Relaxation Response During Physical Exercise*

- Do your usual warm-up exercises.
- As you begin to exercise, keep your eyes fully open, but attend to your breathing.
- After you fall into a regular pattern of breathing, focus in particular on its in-and-out rhythm.
- As you breathe in, say to yourself silently, "In"; when you exhale, say, "Out." In effect, the words *in* and *out* are mental devices that help you concentrate.
- After you complete your exercise, return to your normal after-exercise routine. If the in/out rhythm is uncomfortable for you (you might feel that your breathing is too fast or too slow), you can focus on something else. For example, you can become aware of your feet hitting the ground, silently repeating, "One, two, one, two," or "Left, right, left, right."

There is nothing wrong with focusing on a faith-oriented word or phrase during exercise; in fact, it could make your exercise more satisfying. Remember to form a passive attitude, simply disregarding disruptive thoughts. When they occur, think to yourself, "Oh, well," and return to your repetitive focus word or phrase.

Adapted from Benson, H. (1993). The Relaxation Response. In Goleman, D., & Gurin, J. (Eds.) *Mind, body, medicine* (pp. 233–259). Yonkers, NY: Consumer Reports Books.

Box 7–3   *Eating Mindfully*

- Take a few breaths and direct your attention inwardly, to yourself. Note your feeling state in the moments before your begin to eat. Notice whether you are feeling relaxed, stressed, calm, anxious, happy or depressed.
- Now bring your full attention to the food you intend to eat. Observe it. Carefully note its characteristics; what is its shape, color, texture? Think about the origin of this food: What plant or animal did it come from? Who prepared it?
- Tune into your feelings as you prepare to eat this food: Are you experiencing anticipation, eagerness, reluctance, worry, fear, or a sense of hurry? If you notice a feeling that surprises you, take a moment to reflect on its origin.
- Now place your attention on the physical sensations in your body. How does the anticipation of eating this food affect your body? Notice any sensations in your nose, mouth, throat, stomach, or abdominal area. Notice your breathing: Has its pattern changed since you started focusing on the food?
- Bring the food, or a portion of it, close to your nose and mouth. Inhale its aroma. Note any thoughts, feelings, or physical sensations that arise.
- Slowly place the food in your mouth. Note any thoughts, feelings, or physical sensations.
- Begin to chew the food. Go slowly, and allow yourself to fully experience the food's taste and texture. Notice any desire to swallow the food more quickly, or to hasten your eating. Notice whether willing yourself not to eat more quickly brings up any fear, anger, impatience, etc.
- Prepare to swallow your food mindfully. Be aware of your intention to swallow, and focus on the actual process of swallowing. Note any feelings that arise, and the sensations you feel in your body.
- Notice that you can prolong the pleasure of eating by taking longer to chew and swallow each mouthful. Small portions can be as satisfying as larger ones.
- Finish your meal, following process outlined above with each mouthful.
- At the conclusion of the meal, review any relationships you've noted between eating and stress, or eating and feelings such as anxiety or depression.

Eating is an example of an everyday activity that can be done mindfully. In mindful eating, one focuses one's attention fully on the food and on the actions and sensations involved in eating. When eating mindfully, there is no conversation, no television, no reading, and no gazing about the room. Attention is focused only on the appearance of the food, its aroma, and the acts of taking it in and chewing, tasting, and swallowing it. This exercise can be used with any meal, a part of a meal, or even with one mouthful. The idea is to eat with awareness, focusing moment by moment on seeing the food, taking it in, chewing it, tasting it, and swallowing. It is easier to practice mindful eating if one eats in silence, rather than while conversing with other people. However, even in a group, one can eat mindfully simply by concentrating on doing so. Box 7–3 outlines the steps to be followed in mindful eating.

The term *mindfulness meditation* refers to an adaptation of traditional Buddhist meditation practice (see Chapter 11) developed by Jon Kabat-Zinn, director of the Stress Reduction Program at the University of Massachusetts Medical Center (Kabat-Zinn, 1993). In mindfulness meditation, one focuses the mind on a phrase, an image, or simply on the breath, in order to cultivate calmness and stability. As in most other forms of meditation, one simply notes the inevitable thoughts as they occur and observes them nonjudgmentally. Thoughts, feelings, and reactions that might go unnoticed often come into conscious awareness during meditation. By dispassionately observing them, rather than becoming caught up in them, individuals can achieve *clarity of thought* and *insight* into problems, circumstances, fears, and aspirations (Kabat-Zinn, 1993).

The adoption of a mindfulness meditation practice constitutes a major change in lifestyle for most people. It requires a commitment of 45 minutes a day, at least six days a week. The cultivation of mindfulness involves facing, accepting, and even welcoming tension, stress, fear, anger, frustration, disappointment, and feelings of insecurity and unworthiness. It may also involve accepting physical pain. According to the theory that underlies mindfulness meditation practice, acknowledging present-moment reality, as it actually is, whether pleasant or unpleasant, is the first step toward transforming that reality and the individual's relationship to it. Facing and inquiring into reality, rather than suppressing or fleeing from it, fosters inner strength and balance. Such traits allow individuals to face and respond to all life situations with greater stability, clarity, dignity, and effectiveness.

Biofeedback

Biofeedback is a therapeutic process in which individuals attempt to exert control over unhealthy voluntary or involuntary processes in the body and receive information as to how they are doing. Many negative physiological or mental conditions are caused or exacerbated by stress and respond well to interventions that short-circuit the stress response. For example, stress triggers the release of chemicals that can cause arteries to constrict and blood pressure to rise. People with high blood pressure can use biofeedback to learn to dilate their blood vessels and lower their blood pressure.

When receiving biofeedback, the individual is hooked up to devices that continuously measure one of several *involuntary* physiological variables—notably, muscle tension, skin temperature, brain activity, blood pressure, or pulse. A meter, light, computer display, or tone provides *feedback,* which tells the individual whether the variable is increasing or decreasing. Individuals experiment with a variety of techniques for inducing the relaxation response and thereby changing the target variable. Such techniques include deep breathing, visualization, or focusing on certain sensations, thoughts, or feelings. The feedback confirms that the desired response, which might otherwise be hard to detect, is occurring. Learning to control physiological processes takes time and effort. Individuals are instructed and coached by skilled therapists until they master a technique that will con-

trol the target variable; then they continue to use the technique at home. Through biofeedback, individuals have learned to do the following (Schwartz & Schwartz, 1993):

- Tighten muscles at the neck of the bladder to control impaired bladder function
- Abort migraine headaches
- Decrease blood pressure
- Decrease pain and spasms in irritable bowel syndrome
- Reuse muscles of the legs and arms after an operation
- Use alternate muscles to move a limb if the primary ones can no longer do the job

Biofeedback is sometimes described as a "mirror" that lets individuals see processes within their body that they aren't aware of and cannot presently control. When biofeedback is successful, it helps people recognize their bodies' habitual responses to stress and learn to control them. It can replace feelings of helplessness with a sense of control (Schwartz & Schwartz, 1993).

Exercise

Stress is recognized as a major contributor to coronary heart disease, and researchers recognize that one of the most profound influences of stress is its effect on the cardiovascular system (Hafen et al., 1996). Studies suggest that people who exercise regularly respond in a healthier way to emotional stress than do sedentary people (Keller, Manning, Newhouse, Sloss, & Wasserman, 1989). Exercise triggers the release of morphinelike substances, which have a positive effect on mood. Such effects include the well-known *runner's high,* as well as antidepressant and antianxiety effects. Almost everyone who exercises experiences an increased sense of well-being.

Long-Term Planning

We can be certain that the future holds two things in store for us—change and stress. The information revolution has shrunk the globe and spawns technological advances daily. Our modern world is fast-paced and fluid. A long-term strategy for handling stress is to develop a personal philosophy and outlook that are in step with the spirit of this new age, which many hope will be one of mutuality and integration. Traditional dichotomies, such as body/spirit, masculine/feminine, us/them, work/family, and personal/professional, which have often been sources of stress, are beginning to blur and may one day disappear. In society at large, differences are beginning to be seen as *complementary,* with each informing the other. Personally adopting such a perspective will certainly improve our ability to cope with differences and change and will improve our health as well.

Reducing, or learning to better cope with, the amount of stress in our lives usually involves several or all of the following: setting goals and priorities, getting organized, exercising self-discipline, assertively refusing to overcommit ourselves, getting along with people, being patient, and maintaining a sense of humor through it all. An optimistic outlook, together with a sense of our own efficacy and hardiness, helps us put life's occurrences in perspective and use the inevitable frustrations of life as opportunities for *growth*. The information in this chapter can be reduced to three prescriptions:

- Assume personal responsibility for your well-being.
- Know yourself and your limits.
- Live with some degree of intentionality and self-regulation.

Research efforts and clinical experiments suggest that the dichotomy between mind and body long taken for granted in Western philosophy is *illusory*. Scientists have begun to outline plausible ways in which the mind and emotions can affect physical health. They have deepened our understanding of the effects of stress on the body and are accumulating convincing evidence that virtually all the organs and systems in the body can be influenced by the mind. Chapter 27 contains more information about mind/spirit/body communication mechanisms.

 # Wellness Self-Assessment

There are two parts to this wellness self-assessment: determining your stress style, or the way in which you typically respond to stress, and determining your average level of hostility. Guidelines on how to go about reducing your hostility, if necessary, are provided.

Determining Your *Stress Style*

People experience stress in different ways, and those differences sometimes determine which relaxation techniques are most effective for specific individuals. Some people react to stress mostly in their bodies, whereas others have primarily mental reactions, and about a third of people experience stress both mentally and physically. The following short quiz can give you a rough idea of your tendency. When you're feeling anxious, what do you typically experience? Check all that apply.

1. _____ My heart beats fast.
2. _____ I find it difficult to concentrate because of distracting thoughts.
3. _____ I worry too much about things that don't really matter.
4. _____ I feel jittery.
5. _____ I get diarrhea.
6. _____ I imagine terrifying scenes.
7. _____ I can't keep anxiety-provoking pictures and images out of my mind.
8. _____ My stomach gets tense.

9. _____ I pace up and down nervously.
10. _____ I'm bothered by unimportant thoughts running through my head.
11. _____ I become immobilized.
12. _____ I feel I'm losing out on things because I can't make decisions fast enough.
13. _____ I perspire.
14. _____ I can't keep worrisome thoughts out of my mind.

Scoring: Give yourself a "body" point for each of the following: 1, 4, 5, 8, 9, 11, 13.

Give yourself a "mind" point for each of the following: 2, 3, 6, 7, 10, 12, 14.

Developed by Michael Sachs, professor of psychiatry, Weil Medical College. Used with permission.

If you have more mind than body points, you tend to have mental reactions to stress. If you have more body points than mind points, your stress reaction style tends to be physical. If you have about the same number of each, you're a mixed reactor; you experience stress both mentally and physically.

These are rough guidelines only, but, if you are seeking a way to handle stress, they may help you find an approach suited to your stress style. Those who experience stress mainly mentally, through worrisome thoughts and the like, often find relaxation in activities that engage the mind completely—such as meditating, reading an absorbing book, or playing a challenging game, such as chess. Those who experience stress in a mostly physical manner often benefit from vigorous exercise, such as jogging or swimming. Methods of deep muscle relaxation or yoga, which also break up the physical stress response pattern, may also be helpful. Those who experience stress both mentally and physically do well with physically involving activities that also demand full mental engagement: competitive sports like tennis, racquetball, or volleyball. Engaging in mindfulness meditation while exercising may also be helpful.

How Hostile Are You?

Hostility is made up of three components: cynicism, anger, and aggression. Hostility has been associated with increased risk for coronary heart disease. To get a sense of your general level of hostility, answer the following questions related to the three components of hostility.

Cynicism

1. *When in the express checkout line at the supermarket, do you often count the items in the baskets of the people ahead of you to be sure they aren't over the limit?*
2. *When an elevator doesn't come as quickly as you think it should, do your thoughts quickly focus on the inconsid-*

erate behavior of the person on another floor who's holding it up?

3. Do you frequently check up on family members or co-workers to make sure they haven't made a mistake in some task?

Anger

1. When you are held up in a slow line in traffic, at the bank, or at the supermarket, do you quickly sense your heart pounding and your breath quickening?

2. When little things go wrong, do you often feel like lashing out at the world?

3. When someone criticizes you, do you quickly begin to feel annoyed?

Aggression

1. If an elevator stops too long on a floor above you, are you likely to pound on the door?

2. If people mistreat you, do you look for an opportunity to pay them back, just for the principle of the thing?

3. Do you frequently find yourself muttering at the television during a news broadcast?

If you answered yes to at least one question in each area or to four or more questions overall, your hostility level is probably high.

Adapted from Williams, R. & Williams, V. (1999). *Lifeskills* (pp. 212–213). New York: Random House. Used with permission.

Reducing Your Level of Hostility

1. Admit to a friend that your hostility level is too high and let her know you are trying to reduce it.

2. When cynical thoughts come into your head, yell, "Stop!" (Silently, if you are in public.)

3. Try to talk yourself out of being angry. Reason with yourself.

4. Distract yourself when you're getting angry. For example, pick up a magazine from the rack if you're kept waiting in a supermarket checkout line.

5. Force yourself to be quiet and listen when other people are talking.

6. Learn how to meditate, and use this skill whenever you become aware of cynical thoughts or angry feelings.

7. Try to become more empathetic to the plight of others.

8. When someone is truly mistreating you, learn how to be effectively assertive, rather than aggressively lashing out.

9. Take steps to make more connections with others, thereby countering the tendency of hostile people to ward off social support.

10. When people do you wrong, forgive them.

11. Cultivate friendships. Seek out compatible people where you work, worship, or relax.

12. Volunteer to help others less fortunate than yourself.

13. Learn to laugh at your hostile tendencies.

14. Engage in regular exercise.

15. Get a pet. People who have pets live longer and are healthier overall. Pets who are well treated provide unconditional love.

16. Learn more about the core teachings of your chosen faith or belief system: A central principle of all spiritual teachings is that we must treat others as we would have them treat us.

17. Pretend that this day is your last. That will help you bring minor annoyances into perspective.

Adapted from Williams, R. & Williams, V. (1999). *Lifeskills* (pp. 212–213). New York: Random House. Used with permission.

New Directions

Recent research (Wolkowitz, 1999) suggests that stress may play a prominent role in the development of depressive states. Although it was assumed in the past that depression is caused by low levels of the neurotransmitter serotonin (Sapolsky, 1996), scientists have found that stress hormones, such as cortisol, act on serotonin and other neurotransmitters in ways that set the stage for depression. Drug companies are in the process of developing a new class of antidepressants (Evans, 2000) that will, if they prove effective, reduce the output of stress hormones and break the link between stress and depression. This may be of great consequence to women, as women suffer from both stress and depression more than men. It will not suffice, however, to merely devise new methods of lessening the negative effects of stress. We must work also to address the *underlying factors* that create the stress we all face in our changing society.

Traditionally, stress, particularly in the form of work-family role conflicts, has been perceived to be the result of personal decisions made by individuals, and they were expected to cope with it, using whatever resources they had. Although employees must still make wise choices based on their values and manage their time effectively, it is unrealistic to expect that all problems related to work-family stress can be solved solely by workers' efforts. In contemporary society, the informal and formal community systems that once eased the family-related burdens of workers have eroded; neighborhoods are virtually empty during working hours.

Enlightened organizations are becoming increasingly aware that family support programs have been empirically shown to increase employees' perception of organizational support and family support, as well as their commitment to their jobs (Orthnew & Pittman, 1986). Organizations serious about reducing employee stress would do well to adopt Leavy's (1983) suggestion that support be conceptualized in terms of structure, content, and process. Building flexibility into employee scheduling and career paths would address the structural aspect, whereas educational programs would address the content dimension. The process dimension could be addressed via managerial training focused on enhancing managers' understanding of work-family issues and the adoption of a work-family culture within the organization (Regan, 1994).

Work stress, however, is experienced by so many people at different socioeconomic levels, and with different employment relationships, that it is unrealistic to expect the corporate world to solve all of the problems by itself. As there will always be variability in the extent to which private sector employers are willing and able to address employees' family needs, it is imperative that both communities and the government play a role in supporting family life in a manner that reduces work-family role stress. The government, the nonprofit sector, and local communities are also major stakeholders in this area, and each of these must do more. Relevant issues must be brought before the public in order to foster awareness and debate and to stimulate other segments of society to plan and implement stress-reducing initiatives. Finding solutions to work-related problems will require a cooperative effort among employees, employers, communities, and government agencies.

QUESTIONS FOR REFLECTION AND DISCUSSION

1. *To what degree does stress influence overall health?*
2. *Is it more likely that stress increases, decreases, or remains the same as a person grows older? What factors might influence this?*
3. *Can individuals with little control over their environment decrease their stress?*
4. *What stresses people the most?*
5. *Do women and men experience stress differently? If so, in what way?*

RESOURCES

Books

Benson, H., & Stuart, E. (1993). *The wellness book: The comprehensive guide to treating stress-related illnesses.* Delta.

Byron, W. (2000). *Answers from within: Spiritual guidelines for managing setbacks in work and life.* Books Worldwide.

Carlson, R. (1999). *Don't sweat the small stuff.* Hyperion.

Domar, A. (1999). *Self-nurture: Learning to care for yourself as effectively as you care for everyone else.* Viking Penguin.

Kabat-Zinn, J. (1990). *Full catastrophe living.* Delta.

Kremen Bolton, M. (2000). *The 3rd shift: Managing hard choices in our careers, homes and lives as women.* Jossey-Bass.

Lazarous, J. (2000). *Stress relief and relaxation techniques.* Contemporary.

Sachs, J. (1997). *Break the stress cycle! 10 steps to reducing stress for women.* Adams Media Corp.

Smallen, D. (2000). *7 simple steps to unclutter your life.* Storey Books.

Research Institutes

Center on Work and Family
Boston University
232 Bay State Rd.
Boston, MA 02215
Phone: 617-353-7225

Families and Work Institute
330 7th Ave.
New York, NY 10001

Work/Family Directions
930 Commonwealth Ave.
West Boston, MA 02215-1274
Phone: 508-256-8783
Web: http://www.wfd.com

Work & Family Issues Research Team
George Mason University
Psychology Department
David King Hall
Fairfax, VA 22030-4444
Phone: 703-993-1363

Work and Family Research Group
Drexel University
Department of Management
College of Business and Administration
Philadelphia, PA 19104
Phone: 215-895-1796

Websites

The Livelihood Journey:
http://www.pbs.org/livelihood/index6.html

The Mind-Body Institute: http://www.mindbody.harvard.edu

REFERENCES

Amatea, W., & Fong, M. (1991). The impact of role stressor and personal resources on the stress experience of professional women. *Psychology of Women, 15,* 419–431.

Bandura, A. (1977). Self-efficacy: Toward a unifying theory of behavioral change. *Psychological Review, 84,* 191–215.

Barnett, R. (1995). Change in job and marital experience and change in psychological distress: A longitudinal study of dual-earner couples. *Journal of Personality and Social Psychology, 69,* 839.

Barnett, R., & Baruch, G. K. (1985). Women's involvement in multiple roles and psychological distress. *Journal of Personality and Social Psychology, 49,* 135–144.

Beehr, T. A., & Bhagat, R. S. (1985). *Human stress and cognition in organizations: An integrated perspective.* Ottawa, Canada: John Wiley & Sons.

Benson, H. (1993). The relaxation response. In Goleman, D., & Gurin, J. (Eds.), *Mind, body, medicine* (pp. 233–259). Yonkers, NY: Consumer Reports Books.

Cohen, S., & Wills, T. A. (1985). Stress, social support, and the buffering hypothesis. *Psychological Bulletin, 98,* 310–357.

Dewe, P. J. (1992). Applying the concept of appraisal to work stressors: Some exploratory analysis. *Human Relations, 45,* 143–165.

Dewe, P. J., & Guest, D. E. (1990). Methods of coping with stress at work: A conceptual analysis and empirical study of measurement issues. *Journal of Organizational Behavior, 11,* 135–150.

Duff, C. (1993). We were damned whatever we did. In C. Duff & B. Cohen (Eds.), *When women work together: Using our strengths to overcome our challenges* (pp. 10–20). Berkeley, CA: Conari Press.

Edwards, J. R., Baglioni, A. J., & Cooper, C. L. (1990). Stress, Type-A, coping, and psychological and physical symptoms: A multi-sample test of alternative models. *Human Relations, 43,* 919–957.

Etzion, D. (1984). Moderating effect of social support on the stress-burnout relationship. *Journal of Applied Psychology, 69,* 615–622.

Evans, K. (2000, April). Is stress wrecking your health? *Health,* 119–124.

Galinsky, E., & Stein, P. J. (1990). The impact of human resources policies on employees. *Journal of Family Issues, 11,* 285–290.

Gilbert, L. A., Holahan, C. K., & Manning, L. (1981). Coping with conflict between professional and maternal roles. *Family Relations, 30,* 419–427.

Gregerson, M. (1998). Relaxation. In E. Blechman & K. Brownell. *Behavioral medicine and women* (pp. 279–283). New York: Guilford Press.

Guinier, L., Fine, M., & Balm, J. (1997). *Becoming gentlemen. Women, law school and institutional change.* Boston: Beacon Press.

Hafen, B., Karren, K., Frandsen, K., & Smith, N. L. (1996). *Mind/body health.* Needham Heights, MA: Simon & Schuster.

Hales, D. (1999). *Just like a woman.* New York: Bantam Books.

Hall, D. T. (1972). A model of coping with role conflict: The role of behavior of college educated women. *Administrative Science Quarterly,* 471–486.

Holtzman, W., & Gilbert, L. A. (1987). Social support networks for parenting and psychological well-being among dual-earner Mexican-American families. *Journal of Community Psychology, 15,* 176–184.

Kabat-Zinn, J. (1993). Mindfulness meditation: Health benefits of an ancient buddhist practice. In D. Goleman & J. Gurin (Eds.), *Mind, body, medicine* (pp. 259–276). Yonkers, NY: Consumer Reports Books.

Kammerman, S. B., & Kahn, A. J. (1987). *The responsive workplace: Employers and a changing labor force.* New York: Columbia University Press.

Keller, E., Manning, W., Newhouse, J., Sloss, E., & Wasserman, J. (1989). The external costs of a sedentary life-style. *American Journal of Public Health, 79,* 975–981.

Kobasa, S. C. (1979). Stressful life events, personality, and health: An inquiry into hardiness. *Journal of Personality and Social Psychology, 37,* 1–11.

Latack, J. C. (1986). Coping with job stress: Measures and future directions for scale development. *Journal of Applied Psychology, 71,* 377–385.

Lazarus, R. S. (1966). *Psychological stress and the coping process.* New York: McGraw-Hill.

Lazarus, R. S., & Folkman, S. (1984). *Stress, appraisal and coping.* New York: Springer.

Leavy, R. A. (1983). Social support and psychological disorder: A review. *Journal of Community Psychology, 11,* 3–21.

Matthews, K. A., & Rodin, J. (1989). Women's changing work roles. *American Psychologist, 44,* 1389–1393.

Newton, T. J., & Keenan, A. (1990). The moderating effect of the Type A behavior pattern and locus of control upon the relationship between change in job demands and change in psychological strain. *Human Relations, 43,* 1229–1255.

Ornish, D. (1998). *Love and survival.* New York: Harper Perennial.

Orthnew, D. K., & Pittman, J. F. (1986). Family contributions to work commitment. *Journal of Marriage and the Family, 48,* 573–581.

Parasuraman, S. (1977). *Sources and outcomes of organizational stress: A multidimensional study of the antecedents and attitudinal and behavioral indices of job stress.* Unpublished doctoral dissertation, State University of New York.

Perlow, L. (1997). *Finding time: How corporations, individuals and families can benefit from new work practices.* Ithaca, NY: Cornell University Press.

Priel, B., Gonik, N., & Rabinowitz, B. (1993). Appraisals of childbirth experience and newborn characteristics: The role of hardiness and affect. *Journal of Personality,* 299–315.

Regan, M. C., & Roland, H. E. (1985). Rearranging family and career priorities: Professional women and men of the eighties. *Journal of Marriage and the Family, 47,* 985–992.

Rodin, J., & Langer, E. J. (1977). Long term effects of control relevant intervention with the uninstitutionalized aged. *Journal of Personality and Social Psychology, 35,* 897–902.

Roush, W. (1997). Herbert Benson: Mind-body maverick pushes the envelope. *Science, 276,* 357–359.

Sapolsky, R. (1996). Why zebras don't get ulcers. New York: Scribner.

Schwartz, M., & Schwartz, N. (1993). Biofeedback: Using the body's signals. In D. Goleman & J. Gurin (Eds.), *Mind, body, medicine* (pp. 40–52). Yonkers, NY: Consumer Reports Books.

Sekaran, U. (1985). The paths to mental health: An exploratory study of husbands and wives in dual-career families. *Journal of Occupational Psychology, 58,* 129–137.

Shinn, M., Rosario, M., Morch, I., & Chestnut, D. E. (1984). Coping with job stress and burnout in the human services. *Journal of Personality and Social Psychology, 46,* 864–878.

Sieber, S. D. (1974). Toward a theory of role accumulation. *American Sociological Review,* 567–578.

Singer, J. (1991). Women's work. *Report from the Institute for Philosophy and Public Policy, 11,* 1–5.

Taylor, S. E., Klein, L. C., Lewis, B. P., Gruenwand, T. L., Gurung, R. A., & Updegraff, J. A. (2000). Biobehavioral responses to stress in females: Tend and befriend, not flight or fight. *Psychology Review, 107*(3), 411–429.

Vanfossen, B. E. (1981). Sex differences in the mental health effects of spouse support and equity. *Journal of Health and Social Behavior, 22,* 130–143.

Voydanoff, P. (1988). Work role characteristics, family structure demands, and work/family conflict. *Journal of Marriage and the Family, 50,* 749–761.

Wolkowitz, O. (1999). Treatment of depression with anti-glucocorticoid drugs. *Psychosomatic Medicine, 6*(5), 698–711.

Wood, R., & Bandura, A. (1989). Social cognitive theory of organizational management. *Academy of Management Review, 14,* 361–383.

Yogev, S. (1982). Are professional women overworked? Objective versus subjective perception of role loads. *Journal of Occupational Psychology,* 165–169.

8

Relationships

Barbara Barski-Carrow and Marian C. Condon

CHAPTER OUTLINE

Objectives

1. *Discuss the theory of women as relational beings.*
2. *Identify ways in which the quality and nature of relationships influence health.*
3. *List the characteristics of healthy relationships.*
4. *Identify the limiting factors in relationships.*
5. *Discuss the importance of the following in maintaining healthy relationships: skillful communication and conflict management, boundaries, intimacy, and assertiveness.*
6. *Identify differences in the ways in which women and men sometimes approach communication, conflict management, and the like.*

Introduction

In this chapter, the meaning and importance of relationships in women's lives is addressed, and information about what women value in friendships and sexual/romantic relationships is provided. The connection between women's relationships with friends, family members, and romantic partners and women's health is also explored. Healthy elements in relationships are contrasted with unhealthy ones, and communication and conflict-management strategies for building and maintaining positive relationships are presented. Theories regarding differences in the ways in which men and women approach communication, intimacy, conflict, and negotiation are also presented.

Women and Relationships

Research on the historical and current patterns of women's relationships with friends and spouses in Western culture suggests that the nature of female friendships, and spousal relationships, has shifted over time. Relationship patterns, like other cultural phenomena, are greatly influenced by factors that affect society as a whole. Age, life circumstances, and ethnicity also determine, at least partially, the ways in which women relate to each other as friends. The nature of spousal relationships has evolved in concert with the ways in which gender is constructed in the overall society (see Chapter 1).

Women as Relational Beings

A connection to others is seen by some (e.g., Miller, 1976) as the central organizing feature of women's development. Theorists who see women as inherently *relational beings* argue that women are socialized, and possibly genetically inclined, to value and seek close, intimate relationships with others and that women's development takes place in a context of *connection to others*. According to relational theory, women's sense of self and self-worth are grounded in their ability to make and maintain the relationships that shape not only their families but society as well. An extensive literature supports the contention that women desire emotionally intimate relationships with others and tend to share feelings and problems, and otherwise *reveal themselves,* in the context of relationships. The literature also suggests that men, in contrast, are relatively less concerned with establishing intimate relationships and are relatively more concerned with achieving *autonomy* and establishing their place in a *hierarchy* through *competition* (Connell, 1995). Men also have been found to tend to *resist personal disclosure* in the context of relationships and prefer to discuss sports, politics, and other external topics instead (Tannen, 1994). Although there is general agreement that American women have tended to desire emotional intimacy in relationships more than men, the reasons that this should be so are debatable.

One theory, summarized in a book on women's nature (Blaffer-Hrdy, 1999) is that women's relational tendencies are a product of *natural selection* over the course of human evolution. According to this theory, in the past, women who tended to be more inclined to make and maintain relationships with others had a better chance of passing on their genes to future generations through successful childrearing than were women who were less so inclined. Relationally oriented women would be more likely to have friends who might assist them in finding food and caring for their children and perhaps even to bond emotionally with males who could aid in protecting offspring. A corollary to this theory is that, although natural selection promotes a relational inclination in women, it promotes a more *competitive* inclination in men. Men who were successful at hunting, and/or relatively more dominant in their societies, would have been more likely to pass on their genes. A successful hunter could provide sufficient food to sustain his mate and offspring through harsh winters, and a dominant male could deny other men access to fertile women. According to this theory, successful hunters and dominant males reproduced more successfully than other males, and they passed certain sex role–related traits to their descendants. One such trait is a tendency to form primarily *instrumental* alliances with each other. An instrumental alliance is an alliance made for the purpose of reaching some goal or achieving a desired end. This arose because men were more successful in killing large animals when they banded together in hunting groups. Because hunting activities must be conducted in relative silence, men developed the trait of working alongside each other with a minimum of verbal interaction. Therefore, according to the biological theory of how gender-related differences came to be, it is natural selection that causes men to tend to be more oriented toward competition and hierarchy and to form practical alliances, rather than alliances based on emotional bonding.

More psychodynamically oriented theorists have a somewhat different explanation for women's greater affinity for relationship in comparison with men. They argue that women's orientation toward relationship and men's toward autonomy and competition are functions of their differing *developmental tasks.* For example, according to Nancy Chodorow (1974), girls do not have to differentiate themselves from their mothers (who are the same sex) in order to develop an individual identity, whereas boys do. Females need never sever the mother-child link to the degree that males must and are therefore forever more comfortable than males with deep connection and sharing.

A rather large popular literature on male-female relations is based on the purported "innate" differences between men and women. John Gray's highly successful "Venus and Mars" series (2000) is an example. Gray's books seek to educate readers on the nature of problematic gender differences and to promote understanding and accommodation. An objection to the uncritical acceptance of biological and developmental gender difference theories, however, is that they provide men and women with an *excuse* for failing to change patterns of behavior that may be limiting in both professional and domestic relationships. After all, it can seem rather hopeless to attempt to change an inborn tendency, or one developed very early in life. What is often overlooked, however, is the fact that human beings are marvelously adaptable organisms, and the plentiful evidence that whatever genetic and developmentally based tendencies may exist can be both fostered and blunted by environment—that is, by the culture. Critics of innate difference theories point out that the patterns of female and male friendships cannot be unalterably "hardwired" because they are not the same in all cultures. For example, Derlega and Stepian (1977) found that the male Polish university students in their study believed that intimate self-disclosure is *equally appropriate* for men and women. Other studies have found that intimate relationships between men have long existed in Asian and Native American cultures (Williams, 1992). *Cultural mores* and *gender socialization,* rather than genetic or developmental predisposition, may explain the gender differences in orientation to relationship and competition observed in American men and women. Women have historically been barred from competing with men in the world of commerce and, so, have been relatively more in need of the assistance that a web of relationship can provide. Men, in contrast, have been socialized to repress their emotions and deny weakness and any need for assistance (see Chapter 1). These patterns are changing rapidly in the developed world, however, and it will be interesting to see whether gender differences in the ways in which women and men value relationships and autonomy will persist or will eventually fade away.

Relationships and Women's Health

Social support is recognized as a powerful influence on human health. People who have friends to whom they can turn for affirmation, empathy, and affection are more likely to survive health challenges, such as heart attacks and major surgery (Hafen & Frandsen, 1987). Kenneth Pelletier, a researcher in disease prevention at Stanford University, characterizes a sense of connection to other people as *a basic human need*—as important to health in the long term as food and shelter (Pelletier, 1994). A 10-year study focusing on the connection between relationships and health that involved 3,000 adults found that those who were socially involved had the best health. The individuals for whom social ties were broken for some reason developed higher rates of certain diseases, such as coronary heart disease, cancer, arthritis, and mental illness (Hafen & Frandsen, 1987). Although married people of both genders seem to have better health overall than single people (Berkman & Syme, 1979), women seem to derive the greatest health benefit from relationships *with other women*. A study involving 900 elderly people found that the women with the most friends enjoyed the best health (Preston & Grimes, 1987). In that study, whereas the main source of social support for the married men was their wives, the married women relied more heavily on family members and friends than on their spouses. In their book *The Healing Connection,* Miller and Stiver (1998) assert that women are more oriented toward empathy and the needs of others than are men and that,

in heterosexual relationships, it is the women who are most active in keeping the relationship alive and fostering its growth. Whereas men are empowered by women's empathy, even though they may be oblivious to it, women do not usually receive sufficient empathy from their male partners to be similarly empowered by the relationship. The theme of unequal contribution is familiar to many women and is frequently developed in popular women's magazines. For these reasons, women would do well to cultivate nourishing relationships with other women. Another factor worth considering is that women typically live almost 10 years longer than men, and 6 out of 10 elderly women spend the last decade or so of their lives without a spouse (Sheehy, 2000). Therefore, women who do not value and cultivate friendships with other women risk dying alone.

Miller and Stiver (1998) report that women believe that *both the giver and the receiver* benefit from a caring or nurturing exchange. Consider an example illustrating this point: Lora, who had just lost her father to lung cancer, took time away from her office duties to tend to family responsibilities relating to the funeral, the estate, and her mother's health. Lora's boss, Linda, was very empathetic to her situation, since Linda herself had recently lost her mother a few months ago. Linda allowed Lora ample time away from the office and was very empathetic to her needs when she returned to work. Both women felt they had benefited from the situation, and both were able to engage their work with more energy and enthusiasm.

Relationships also promote emotional and psychological *growth.* Daphne Rose Kingma (1998) maintains that relationships are one of the most important vehicles by which we create our *identities,* come to a better understanding of ourselves, and define ourselves. How we relate to someone we care for provides an extremely clear and accurate mirror of how we relate to ourselves, and our friends act as mirrors that reflect back to us the messages we send (Welwood, 1996). Women often rely on their friends to provide a safe person to whom to vent angry or hostile feelings about a third person. This allows them to express their anger without creating or escalating conflict or taking actions they might later regret. The *intimacy* women experience with their very close friends allows them to share their darkest secrets and otherwise reveal themselves as they truly are. Having the acceptance of a friend who really knows you is one of life's more *ego-affirming* experiences.

Friendship

Patterns of friendship among women in Western culture have changed over time. Whereas, accounts of friendships between women recorded prior to the seventeenth century are relatively rare, literacy among women was more common in the seventeenth and eighteenth centuries, and middle- and upper-class women left many records of their friendships in *diaries and letters*. Like their forebears, seventeenth- and eighteenth-century women (at least middle- and upper-class women) were not allowed to interact with unrelated men without a chaperone, and women's friendships were made primarily with other women. Although *marriage* may have involved loyalty and tenderness, at least for fortunate women, it is only recently that spouses have expected to share friendship—that is, interests and confidences—with each other.

Many women in the seventeenth and eighteenth centuries seem to have formed deep, intimate bonds with other women. The words of Katherine Phillips, an English poet, to her friend are quite typical of the era: "Oh, my Lucasia, let us speak our Love. . . . I've all the world in thee" (Sheehy, 2000, p. 5). These committed attachments were known as **romantic friendships.** They were recognized and accepted in American culture, and both married and unmarried women participated in them freely, apparently with no objections from husbands and family members. Women known to share close bonds were commonly invited to social gatherings as a couple. Scholars differ in their opinions as to the true nature of such relationships (Sheehy, 2000). Some argue that intense expressions of ardor merely reflected the Victorian penchant for *idealizing* relationships and that sexual expression was generally not involved. Others maintain that societal tolerance for such bonds between women was a naïve function of the Victorian assumption that women are devoid of sexual feelings. However, it is hard to believe that *all* the seventeenth- and eighteenth-century women involved in such relationships were lesbian in orientation, as homosexuality is currently estimated to occur in only 1 to 10 percent of the population (D'Milio & Freedman, 1988). Moreover, the contemporary popular literature contains many references to platonic love as an element of deep friendships between women. In an article in Oprah Winfrey's extremely popular magazine, *O,* Elizabeth Young-Bruehl and Faith Bethelard (2001) adapted the exquisite seventeenth-century word *cherishment* to describe the essence of deep friendship between women. *Cherishment* means loving someone "sweetly and indulgently," as well as spontaneously, generously, and playfully (p. 131).

The dawn of the twentieth century brought the first of a series of changes that marked the end of the golden age of women's friendships. In 1897, the word *lesbian* was used by Havelock Ellis in the first of his multivolume work, *Studies in the Psychology of Sex.* Shortly thereafter, Freud contended that unconscious urges can influence behavior. These two developments caused overt demonstrations of affection between women to be increasingly viewed with suspicion. It was also during this time that women were (belatedly) given the right to vote and began to become educated and employed in larger numbers. Rigidly patriarchal Victorian marriages gradually gave way to **companionate marriages,** in which wives and husbands were considered equal partners—even though their roles were still defined by gender. This shift negatively affected female friendships also, as women in companionate marriages were expected to put all their emotional energy into their relationships with their husbands (Sheehy, 2000).

In the 1950s, women were expected to find not only financial security and sexual gratification in their marriages but validation and support as well (Sheehy, 2000). Middle-class women were encouraged in the popular media to be friendly and cordial to each other but to reserve true intimacy for the marital relationship. Girls in the 1950s and 1960s grew up believing that all their emotional needs would be fulfilled in marriage and that forming close relationships with other women was unnecessary. Interviews with women born before 1940 (Sheehy, 2000) reveal that they did *not* discuss personal problems with each other and that married women prioritized the needs of spouses and children over those of friends. Among single women, relationships with each other ran a distant second to the all-important relationship with a man; it was understood that a woman would cancel any plans she had made with another woman if a man were to ask her out. Ironically, women's increasing freedom to venture outside the domestic sphere also undermined female friendships, as women who worked outside their homes had less time for socializing with others. By the early 1960s, the tide had begun to turn once again. Increasing numbers of women began to voice a sense of emotional isolation and dissatisfaction with the quality of their lives. They banded together to demand more equal rights in society and gave birth to the **feminist movement.**

One of the greatest accomplishments of the early feminists was to get women to connect intimately with each other once again. So successful were they that interviews conducted with women born after 1950 (Sheehy, 2000) found that the priorities and values of these younger women differ significantly from those of the previous generation. Younger women reported that they freely confide dissatisfactions and problems to close friends, and they prioritize the needs of intimate female friends equally, or almost equally, with those of spouses and family members. Among today's middle-aged women, canceling a social commitment with another female to accommodate a male is considered not only bad manners but an act of disloyalty as well.

Not all the friendships that modern women make are deep and intimate. Women also make peripheral friendships, based on a liking for the same activity, proximity, and the like. To be regarded as a friendship rather than a mere acquaintanceship, however, the relationship must include certain ingredients (Sheehy, 2000). **Mutuality** is one such ingredient; both parties must regard the other as a friend. The most fundamental requirement of friendship is that both individuals **value** each other; they must find something of *worth* in the other's unique set of characteristics and traits. **Reciprocity** is another vital ingredient of friendship; both participants must contribute approximately equal amounts of time and attention, and, of course, **comfort** is essential in a friendship. Each participant must feel *at ease* and find more pleasure than pain in the relationship. **Trust** is extremely important in friendship.

We must be able to trust that a friend will not habitually wound us, through malicious criticism or betrayal of confidences. Optional, but important ingredients of friendship include empathy, tactful honesty, and dependability. Friends demonstrate their empathy for each other by listening attentively and helping each other feel understood and validated. Being tactfully honest involves sharing one's truth with a friend while still protecting her ego. For example, one friend might suggest that the other reject a garment in a store without going into excessive detail about the figure flaws it reveals. Dependability means that friends can generally count on each other to be there—whether to provide emotional support or to supply a ride to the airport.

IMPLICATIONS OF CLASS AND ETHNICITY FOR WOMEN'S FRIENDSHIPS

Sheehy (2000) found that working-class women make as many friends as wealthier women but for somewhat different reasons. Whereas wealthier women see friends as a source of leisure companionship and emotional support, poorer women value friends for the emotional and material support they can provide. Material support includes baby-sitting, providing transportation, and helping with projects.

Sheehy also found that meaningful friendships exist between women with different ethnic backgrounds. Some Euro-American women had African American friends, Latina friends, and so on and vice versa. However, most women, particularly women who were nonwhite, expressed a strong need to also have friends who share their ethnic and cultural background. They felt that only women who shared more or less the same domestic and public life experiences could offer true empathy and understanding. African American women reported that one topic they seek to avoid in the context of relationships with Euro-American women was race. Discussing racial issues with a white friend was seen as too risky and potentially damaging to the relationship.

FRIENDSHIPS WITH MEN

The literature on friendships between men and women is sparse in comparison with the vast literature on heterosexual romance, as it is only recently that women have had the freedom to associate with men to whom they are not related or married. For example, the key issue in the popular movie *When Harry Met Sally* is whether it is even possible for heterosexual men and women to share a platonic (nonsexual) friendship. Although in that film the friendship between Harry and Sally turned into romantic love, there is evidence that it is indeed possible, and beneficial, for both women and men to have a real friend of the opposite gender.

In her research on women's friendships, Sheehy (2000) found that having a male friend can provide a woman with an "interpreter," who can help her understand and negotiate the male culture. Women who have friendships with both men and women report that, although they do not typically enjoy the same level of deep intimacy with male friends, they often get more *instrumental* assistance from men. A male friend, for instance, may be more likely to be able to help a woman with her car than a female friend. Interestingly, men who have friendships with both other men and women, report benefiting from the greater intimacy they are able to enjoy with female friends.

Sexual/Romantic Relationships

Before World War II, the expectations that women had for their male spouses were primarily instrumental. Most women married for reasons related to social expectation, financial support, sexual/romantic attachment, and legitimate procreation but did not generally expect their partners to be their major source of emotional support and companionship (Sheehy, 2000). As the ideals of companionate marriage and equality between the sexes became more widespread, however, women came to expect more from men. Research on heterosexual couples suggests that contemporary women tend to expect to share emotional intimacy with men and to be valued and respected as well. Ball (2000) found that the women in her small, qualitative study wanted to feel cherished by their husbands. For these women, being cherished meant knowing that their husbands valued them highly and were emotionally available to them. In a six-year study of the factors that ultimately predict divorce, it was found that the likelihood of eventual divorce was high in couples in which the husbands systematically rejected their wives' suggestions and wishes (Gottman, 1994).

Romantic love has been characterized in many ways. It has been described as power, light, and the energy of life; it is said to be mysterious, beautiful, and productive of happiness and hope. It cannot be bought or forced, and, when we are in love, no one can talk us out of it (Kingma, 1998).

Whereas **sexual attraction** is based largely on appearance and surface characteristics, **compatibility** is based on a deep emotional connection and moral interests (Crenshaw, 1996). Opposites may attract, but it is likes who pair up most successfully. We link up to someone who *fits;* we look for our romantic twin. This person is usually a mirror image of us, or we have so much in common with him or her that an automatic bond forms. **Attraction** seems to work somewhat differently for men than for women. Men are initially attracted to a woman's *physical appearance,* whereas women are initially attracted more by *personality and status* (Gray, 1995). Eventually, as both people get to know each other, the man learns to love the inner woman and the woman becomes attracted to the man's body.

Five stages of romantic relationships have been identified (Campbell, 1999): (1) romance, (2) power struggle, (3) stability, (4) commitment, and (5) co-creation. Stage 1, the *romance stage,* is filled with positive feelings, and the partners often feel that they must keep each other happy. They ignore or deny any differences they observe in each other. The positive energy that characterizes this stage helps the partners develop the emotional bond and the trust they will need to sustain the relationship later, when differences become more noticeable. The danger, however, is that each can become so enamored with the other that they both deny any awareness about the negative elements in the relationship. The hormone **phenylethylamine (PEA),** known as the "molecule of love" (Crenshaw, 1996, p. 55), seems to play a large role in romantic infatuation. PEA is produced in the body and is a natural form of amphetamine. It has an antidepressant, stimulating effect in both sexes, and it causes feelings of giddiness and excitement. An individual's PEA levels soar when s/he is in romantic love. Conversely, when romance ends abruptly, PEA levels drop precipitously, and the painful feelings of lovesickness ensue. Interestingly, the intensity or even the presence of romantic love does not play an important role in predicting the success of a marriage. **Marital success** is based on many important factors, including similarity of values, realistic expectations, and how happy the childhoods of the two participants were (Larson, 2000).

Stage 2, the *power struggle,* begins when infatuation wears off and the couple begin to notice differences between them. Couples in which one or both partners are having difficulty in establishing boundaries and negotiating the terms of the relationship may experience considerable conflict during this stage. One person may try to dominate the other, or both may feel the other is being too assertive and demanding. Many marriages and other forms of committed relationships do not make it beyond this stage, because it is during this period that each partner's true personality emerges.

In stage 3, *stability,* the couple starts to put the power struggle into perspective. They realize that, although unresolved issues remain, addressing them can be a growth experience for both. They begin to communicate more effectively about their differences and gain an even more enhanced perspective. It is in this stage that the couple begin to see a larger picture of what they can create together.

Stage 4 is the *commitment* stage. Commitment is defined as a subjective state that represents a long-term orientation to the relationship. It is characterized by *psychological attachment* to a partner and the *desire to maintain the relationship* through good and bad times (Banfield & McCabe, 2001). In this stage, the couple begins to perceive their interdependence. Each person appreciates the uniqueness of his or her own personality and that of the other. They begin to see that together they can build a true partnership. They understand that grappling with the disappointments and surprises that arise in the context of the relationship can foster the growth of both individuals.

In stage 5, the *co-creation* stage, both partners are able to love the other unconditionally. They begin to accept the uncertainty of life as well as its preciousness, and they allow each other to stretch beyond old limits to new challenges and possibilities. Both partners shift their focus from security and control to growth and discovery.

Markers of Healthy Relationships

Relationships that can be considered basically healthy are those in which the growth of both participants is fostered (Hendricks & Hendricks, 1992). Such relationships have a number of features, or markers, in common. Although the literature on relationships has focused more on sexual/romantic relationships, the markers discussed in this section—self-awareness, understanding, acceptance, sharing and support, nurturing, and intimacy—can be applied to close friendships as well.

Self-Awareness

The first marker of a healthy relationship is a reasonable level of *self-awareness* on the part of both participants. Being self-aware means being in touch with who we are and valuing ourselves. Self-awareness encompasses self-esteem and self-confidence; it is difficult to love someone else if we cannot love ourselves. Each person has a past during which s/he may have acquired certain beliefs and assumptions, which may not support continued growth. It is our responsibility to let go of negative messages that could be destructive to our continued growth and participation in society. Self-awareness also involves having *insight* into the ways in which we interact with ourselves and with others. Is the internal dialogue we have with ourselves positive or negative? Do we have a pleasant and happy demeanor that will attract people to us? Do we manage our anger or allow it to control us? Do we trust ourselves? When we trust, we are able to give in abundance (Zukav, 1989). Those who radiate love and compassion toward others generally receive it back. Trust also allows us to be playful and light-hearted, which is important if we are to gaze clearly and unflinchingly at ourselves.

Understanding

The second marker of a healthy relationship is *understanding.* Both partners in the relationship must put in the effort required to come to truly understand the other person. Understanding can be gained through both verbal communication and observations of a friend or partner's behavior. Behavior is a language in itself, and people often reveal themselves more by what they *do* than by what they *say.* It is important that messages transmitted behaviorally be understood and affirmed. For example, if one of a pair of friends or partners does something that pleases the other, it is important that the other both acknowledge the behavior and express appreciation. For example, if one partner demonstrates caring by clearing snow off the other's car, it is important for the recipient of the gesture to comment on it, express appreciation, and perhaps perform some service or favor for the other in return.

Acceptance

The third marker of a healthy relationship is *acceptance*. Although it is not necessary to like everything about a friend or lover, it is necessary to accept the person *in spite of* the characteristics or behaviors we could do without (Gilmer & Neumeyer, 1992). Liking or loving friends and partners unconditionally gives them the gift of freedom to grow, whereas manipulating them, and restricting them from being who they really are, causes resistance, the shutting down of communication, and likely the demise of the relationship. Being required to remold one's personality to meet another person's needs inhibits and distorts personal development (Sheehy, 2000). We wish to be loved for who we are now—we don't want our friends, lovers, or spouses to try to change us. Many women mistakenly believe they can change a romantic partner after they get married. This is almost always a delusion, and women who take that position can count on having many marital problems. Maintaining a successful relationship, whether a friendship or a romance, requires a considerable amount of acceptance and compromise on the part of both participants.

Sharing and Support

The fourth marker is the combined presence of the related elements *sharing* and *support*. It is painful to go through life without being able to share one's experiences, great and small, with another, and it is equally painful to have to do without the support and caring of loved ones. We all need someone to listen to us and give us feedback if we are to flourish, rather than just exist. Providing sharing and support, however, requires effort.

Sharing means that each partner is open to being told what is going on in the other's life and shares the details, including joys and disappointments, of his or her own life. Sharing provides the circumstance under which support can be offered. We cannot support a friend or partner in a circumstance we do not know of. Sharing can also involve participating in mutually enjoyable activities with each other. Sharing can pose a challenge for friends and couples in the busy world of today. Although the demands imposed by career and family can seem overwhelming, it is important to make the effort to keep in touch with our friends and partners if we are unable to see them on a daily basis.

Providing friends and romantic partners with emotional, and sometimes tangible, support is key to maintaining successful relationships (Goulton, 2001). Providing adequate support can overcome myriad difficulties that may exist in a relationship; there are many relationships in which the partners seem to have great rapport, even though they seem to be complete opposites in personality. One of the secrets to making sure a friend or partner feels supported is applying active listening skills in the relationship. Active listening involves focusing our attention on our partner when the partner is speaking, and asking for clarification if necessary, so that the partner knows we are truly interested in what he or she is saying. This is particularly important if significant personality differences exist (Mackay & Paleg, 1994). Paying attention and listening are the keys to understanding, and understanding frees one to offer support. Most differences in perspective can be accepted if both friends or partners truly understand where the other is coming from. Paying attention is essential if empathy, a component of support that is particularly important to women, is to be provided. The primary way in which women express empathy for the other person in a relationship is by listening attentively and then using body language and/or words to convey understanding (Sheehy, 2000).

Nurturing

The fifth marker of a healthy relationship is *nurturing*. Although the following description of a nurturing relationship refers to a romantic one, it really applies to all close relationships:

> *Nurturing means appreciating your partner, keeping it current, warm and juicy, sparking with gratitude, burnished with respect. Nurturing your love means you give it the same attention you give your career, your children, and your commitment to your community. It is the act of creating an environment in which the relationship and each person can flourish.* (Louden, 1994, p. 201)

Merely caring about a friend or partner and wishing that person the best does not constitute nurturing. Nurturing is an *active process* that involves both *promoting* the person's well-being and *restraining oneself from inflicting harm* in a moment of anger or frustration. Conveying affection for a friend or partner is an important part of promoting a friend or partner's well-being (Hooks, 2000). Trust, an absolutely essential component in healthy relationships, develops only in a nurturing relationship in which hurtful behaviors occur only infrequently (Sheehy, 2000). It is important to recognize that as humans we all need caring to grow and that nurturing is a *reciprocal* process (Louden, 1994).

An important part of nurturing is providing affirmation. *Affirmation* means conveying one's respect and affection *for* another person *to* that person. Affirmation is food for the soul, and every person needs it. It is very important to recognize a friend's or lover's value and to let that person know it in a loving and appreciative way. Each person in a relationship should have a repertoire of affirmation cues—terms or gestures of endearment, such as a wink, a smile, a pet name, a squeeze of the hand, or a hug. Bestowed liberally, affirmations are part of the glue that holds a relationship together (McGraw, 2000).

Intimacy

The sixth marker of a healthy relationship is *intimacy*. The word *intimacy* can be used in several ways, but it always connotes a deep connection in which both friends or partners feel safe enough to reveal a personal vulnerability because they trust the other person to respond in an accepting, nonjudgmental, nonpunitive manner. In research done on married couples, intimacy has been found to correlate with both individual well-being and satisfaction with the relationship (Gottman & Notarius, 2000). In romantic relationships, there is a sexual component to intimacy as well. The quality of the sexual relationship is often, but not always, a barometer of the degree of genuine intimacy and trust that exists in the relationship overall. Good sex (see Chapter 22) revitalizes both partners and consistently brings them closer as a couple. Over a long period of time, the meaning of sexual intimacy changes as the relationship changes.

Common Limiting Factors in Relationships

If a relationship is to be a healthy one, it is important that the personal growth and development of each participant is supported, not suppressed. However, a number of factors can limit personal growth and negatively affect the relationship itself. These include relational dynamics, such as fusion, codependence, and entanglement; personal characteristics, such as low self-esteem and inadequate boundaries; and behaviors, such as concealing old wounds and issues.

Fusion and Codependence

For a relationship to be considered a healthy one, both people involved must have a reasonable degree of self-knowledge regarding unresolved past issues. If they do not, they may unconsciously choose a friend or partner who resembles the person—often a parent—who was the *source* of pain experienced earlier in their lives. This is done in the usually vain hope of receiving that which was withheld by the person who was the original source of the pain (Turndorf, 1999). A story concerning a 30-year-old woman we will call Kate illustrates this principle.

While in her late teens, Kate moved away from her parents' home in order to build her own life and career in a metropolitan area. Kate eventually met a man she came to love, and she married him. Shortly after the marriage, however, Kate began accusing her husband of not meeting her needs. She complained that he failed to thank her for small favors, discounted her suggestions, and was not empathetic regarding her work-related problems. Although Kate's husband did not react angrily to her accusations, he seemed very surprised. Later that month, Kate's father became ill, and she went to visit him for several uneasy, tension-filled days. As she was driving back home after the visit, Kate was struck by the realization that she had been accusing her husband of doing what her father had done to her during that visit—and her entire childhood as well. When Kate arrived home, she explained her insight to her husband and apologized to him. Her newfound awareness allowed Kate to become more conscious of her feelings and behavior.

When one or both partners are operating on the basis of repressed needs and issues, fusion, rather than true closeness, develops in the relationship. The term **fusion** means that the participants have no independent selves to bring to the relationship; they feel alive and whole only when they are with a partner (Gilbert, 1992). A related problem exists when one or both participants in a relationship sacrifice their own development in order to preserve the friendship or, more likely, the partnership. When both participants exhibit this pattern, the relationship is said to be **codependent.** Individuals who have a strong sense of self and feel whole within themselves, do not look to another to provide them with a sense of completion. Fusion and codependence cause anxiety in relationships and inhibit the personal development of both participants.

Relationships in which fusion and codependence are present are characterized by a lack of acceptance and respect, and one or both partners generally attempts to control the other. Entangled relationships involve many conflicts, in which one or both participants believe themselves to be right and the other wrong. One or both always want to remake the other person to fit their image of what the other should be and try to change the other person's beliefs, opinions, values, desires, and so on. Usually, one or both are trying to get something from the other person that they did not get from their parents. This seldom works, because no other person can give an adult what was needed as a child. Adults must find ways to provide for themselves whatever was missing. A hallmark of an entangled relationship is the feeling on the part of one or both partners that they cannot speak the truth to the other.

Most of the fusion and codependence literature addresses sexual/romantic relationships. The goals for each person in healthy relationships of all types, however, is to actively work on themselves and to be committed to their *own* growth. Doing so will strengthen the two participants, as well as the relationship itself.

A strategy women can use to get in touch with the deep wishes, fears, and strong emotions that may be conjured by the challenge of a close relationship is to **journal** their feelings and thoughts after they have spent time with the other person. When we write in a journal, we create a dialogue with ourselves, which can be very therapeutic. The process of writing freely and honestly often puts us in touch with our deepest thoughts and can help us become more cognizant of our focus and desired direction in life.

Low Self-Esteem

A *low self-esteem* on the part of one or both participants in a relationship can lead to problems. Self-esteem has two interrelated components (Branden, 2001): **self-efficacy,** a sense of basic self-confidence in the face of life's challenges, and **self-respect,** the sense of being worthy of happiness. The stronger one's self-esteem, the higher one's goals and ambitions are likely to be. In contrast, individuals with low self-esteem tend to question what they want to say or do, and their insecurity may prevent them from acting. High self-esteem is one of the most important predictors of a person's ability to form satisfying and lasting friendships and sexual/romantic relationships (Branden, 1998). If one or both participants in a friendship or romantic relationship lack a self that is mature and able to grow both psychologically and emotionally, the relationship may suffer. Individuals who seem incapable of maintaining close, companionable relationships often have self-esteem issues that are getting in the way. People who do not feel loveable may attract others that will reflect their poor self-image back to them by treating them badly. People who feel fundamentally unworthy of love and respect may become unjustifiably suspicious of their friend's or partner's motives and behaviors. Such behavior does not promote a good relationship and can wreak havoc in a friendship or romantic relationship.

Inadequate Boundaries

Another common unhealthy dynamic in close relationships is a lack of adequate boundaries on the part of one or both participants. **Boundaries** are limits that define a person as separate from others (Katherine, 1991). It is our boundaries that give us a clear sense of ourselves and allow us to resist other people who may try to invade us psychologically or physically. Part of defining our boundaries is deciding how we wish to be treated by other people and what limits we will set as to the ways in which we will allow them to interact with us. To be a good friend or partner in a relationship, a person must have sufficient boundaries to clearly define him or her as an individual. People with poorly defined boundaries often believe they are responsible for the choices of others and that others are responsible for the choices they themselves make. They may offer unwanted advice to another person and feel frustrated and angry when it is not taken (Sheehy, 2001). Individuals who allow others to control them, or to abuse them emotionally, physically or sexually, may have been raised in homes in which they were not allowed to establish appropriate boundaries. An important issue that couples need to understand when establishing boundaries is that each partner requires a certain amount of privacy. Each partner must respect the other's need for his or her own time and space. Relationships are harmed when one or both partners become too focused on always being with the other. Both

must be allowed to develop interests and friends of their own (Page, 1994).

Old Wounds and Issues

A related unhealthy dynamic exists when one or both participants *deliberately* conceal certain past experiences or difficulties from the other. In healthy relationships, both persons have a good level of understanding regarding the life experiences, beliefs, values, desires, fears, and aspirations of the other. If a participant has undisclosed issues related to something in the past, such as a history of psychological or physical abuse, the relationship is likely to be stressed severely. Consider the example of a woman named Daria, whose story illustrates the value of being straightforward about past experiences. Prior to her marriage, Daria and her fiancé, Glenn, had visited a therapist for premarital counseling. One of the things the therapist had invited Daria and Glenn to do was to tell each other about their respective wounds and issues. Daria had said she was very susceptible to feelings of abandonment ever since her father had left her mother and the family when Daria was very young. When Daria had elaborated on her feelings around this issue, Glenn had listened with empathy and had appreciated her honesty. Glenn had shared some of his insecurities as well, and both partners felt that the experience had been extremely beneficial in that it had allowed them to enter into their marriage with a better sense of each other's vulnerabilities.

Strategies for Maintaining Healthy Relationships

A relationship is a *process,* not a destination; it is not necessarily the final emotional resting place of the persons who enter into it, rather, but is a vital, growing entity that has a life and a lifetime of its own (Kingma, 1998). A relationship can be thought of as a *third organism,* a new living entity beyond the two people in it. If this new organism is to thrive, it must have adequate protection and nourishment; ongoing, thoughtful attention is required. A person who wishes to maximize the likelihood that an important relationship will survive the tests of time and human nature must make the relationship the most important thing in her life (McGraw, 2000). A relationship can be compared to a flowering plant. If we want it to produce a beautiful bloom, we need to water it, prune its leaves, provide it with sunshine, and in all other ways take care it. Relationships need a similar quality of care.

A healthy relationship is a partnership. Partners cooperate, support each other, and depend on one another; they do not compete, and no one "keeps score" (McGraw, 2000). When both partners possess good communication skills, such as substituting *I* statements for *you* statements, listening actively, asking for what they want, and decoding gendered communication, the chances that the relationship will flourish and deepen are greatly increased. Having good conflict-management skills, such as coping with differences and expressing feelings constructively, is also very important.

Cultivating Communication Skills

Communicating with other people in a manner that maximizes understanding and minimizes misperception and the potential for conflict is not easy. The quality of communication in a relationship, however, is a decisive factor in whether it is able to thrive (Page, 1994). Mastering and implementing four relatively simple strategies can enhance communication in relationships and thereby strengthen them. The four strategies are (1) substituting *I* statements for *you* statements, (2) listening actively, (3) asking for what you want, and (4) decoding gendered communication.

SUBSTITUTING *I* STATEMENTS FOR *YOU* STATEMENTS

Substituting *I* statements for *you* statements is a way of taking the assignment of blame out of a discussion or an argument. The following is an example of a *you* statement: "*You* betrayed me by telling your mother about our fight." *You* statements are inherently blaming. Most people have a tendency to blame others when things go wrong—especially when they get angry. Accusing people, however, usually causes them to become angry in return, and the result is often a highly negative confrontation instead of a reasoned discussion. Substituting a more informative and less accusatory *I* statement, such as, "I felt betrayed when you told your mother about our fight," provides the other person involved with relevant, but much less highly charged, information. Using *you* statements to express anger or annoyance to people is essentially accusing them of having done something wrong, before having heard the facts of their side of the story. The following exchange illustrates the likely effect of an accusation made in the form of a *you* statement:

Liza: You are so insensitive to my needs; you never ask me what I would like to do. You just go ahead and make plans that suit your interests.

Seth: You are never satisfied! Whatever I do or choose, you criticize me. It makes me so mad!

Had Liza brought up her concern by using an *I* statement, the results would likely have been more positive:

Liza: Seth, I would like it if we made decisions together about what shows we see on weekends. When you decide on your own, it feels as if you don't care what I want.

Seth: Oh, sure, we can do that. I guess I just assumed you'd like what I like. Of course, I care what you want.

In the second example, Liza does not sound angry; rather, she is telling Seth what she wants and why she wants it. Our friends and partners will be more accepting of our suggestions if we use *I*, rather than *you*, statements to let them know how we feel.

LISTENING ACTIVELY

Listening actively means giving our full attention to a person who is speaking. It means being present and available (Powell, 1985). Being present and available refers not just to physical presence and availability but also to personal presence and availability. It means focusing our full attention on what people are saying and how they are saying it, without drifting into unrelated thoughts. Listening actively also involves giving other people time to express themselves without trying to hurry them. Making eye contact, if culturally appropriate, enhances active listening, as does mentally putting yourself in the other person's position before responding. Listening actively tells other people that we respect and care about them (Wetzler, 1998). People want to be heard and affirmed, and active listening contributes to both.

The following short anecdote about Jim and Kathy illustrates the problems that can arise in a relationship when one partner is not a good listener.

Jim and Kathy have been married for three years. Kathy is the type of person who can carry out several tasks at the same time, and she has a lot of friends with whom she keeps in contact. It was Kathy's extroverted, high-energy personality that had really made her attractive to Jim, whose personality is quite the opposite. Jim is an introverted individual, who rarely talks about his everyday thoughts and keeps his own counsel about what goes on at work. Jim is the type of person who does one thing at a time and focuses on it until it is completed. Kathy recently received a new position at work, which is exciting and stimulating to her. When she gets home in the evening, she typically chats animatedly about her day. However, Kathy has begun to notice some changes in Jim's behavior. He seems not to want to converse with her and does not want to listen when she talks about her job. Kathy has decided to ask Jim what was wrong. He responds by telling her that, when they talk, she seems to assume that he knows what she is talking about, even though she often jumps from one subject to another. On the contrary, though, he says he is seldom sure which topic she is on and feels unable to keep up with her. Jim also tells Kathy that, whenever he tries to say something, she interrupts him. Jim finds Kathy's conversational behavior frustrating and does not know how to respond to it, so he has decided to just keep quiet.

Had Kathy been listening more actively to Jim, she might have noticed his inability to keep up with her conversation sooner. Had Jim been willing to ask for what he wanted, he would have told Kathy of the difficulties he was having and asked her to slow down and clarify what she was saying. Communication problems such as this are not unusual in relationships. Friends and partners often assume that their friends think and feel the same as they do and wonder why they seem to be communicating at cross-purposes.

ASKING FOR WHAT YOU WANT

Asking for what you want is another key to effective communication. Although it may sound easy, it can be difficult for many women to do. There are a number of reasons that a woman might have difficulty expressing wants and needs. One factor is that many women have been socialized to behave in a relatively passive manner, rather than risk seeming too pushy or forward. Another factor is that women are often socialized to focus on the needs of others, rather than on their own, and some are not even fully in touch with their own wants and desires. A third factor is the common belief that, if a person (particularly a man) really loves a woman, he will *know* what she wants. This is a falsehood, and the opposite is more often true; due to their differing socialization (see Chapter 1) and life experiences, men and women may have considerable difficulty anticipating and divining each other's thoughts and feelings. Even friends of the same gender cannot always know each other's mind. It is very important that friends and partners communicate their wants and needs clearly to each other.

Consider the case of Susan and Amy, who had decided to rent a beach house on weekends over the summer months. Unbeknown to Susan, Amy's intention in renting the beach house had been to spend more intimate time with Susan in hopes that they could become a committed couple and live together as sexual partners. Although Susan cared for Amy, her primary intention in renting the beach house had been to have a place to which she and Amy could invite friends for swimming and cookouts. After two frustrating weekends during which the beach house was full of friends, Amy shared with Susan her original motivation in renting the beach house and expressed her wishes and hopes for their summer together. Once Susan understood Amy's intention, she agreed to compromise. Susan and Amy decided that they would keep most of the remaining weekends for themselves but still share some with friends.

Another key to constructive assertiveness is *asking* for what one wants, rather than *demanding* it. People who have difficulty in making their needs and wants known directly sometimes delay doing so until they have become highly frustrated and then angrily demand an action or a response from their friend or partner. A polite request delivered in a pleasant tone of voice is much more likely to be well received than a belligerent demand. Polite requests can be repeated, after a suitable interval, if necessary. Many partners who would only dig in their heels when con-

fronted with force or an ultimatum eventually respond to this tactic (Schnebly, 1994).

DECODING GENDERED COMMUNICATION

Decoding gendered communication means being aware of and alert for ways of talking that are common in men but frequently misinterpreted by women, and vice versa. In her research on men and women in communication, linguist Deborah Tannen (1990) found that men and women tend to express themselves somewhat differently in conversation, due to gender differences that may be genetic, developmental, social, or a combination of all three. Tannen found that, from early childhood, men use language to *protect their independence* and to achieve and *maintain a one-up position* in relation to others. Women, on the other hand, use language to *seek affirmation* and *reinforce intimacy*. These tendencies are related to men's greater orientation toward autonomy, hierarchy, and competition and women's greater orientation toward affiliation and egalitarianism.

According to Tannen, men tend to be more direct, and women more indirect, in conversation. Men tend to *state clearly* what they want, whereas women are more likely to *hint* at what they want. An example of this similar to one contained in Tannen's (1990) book *You Just Don't Understand: Men and Women in Conversation* is the following exchange between a married couple driving together in a car:

Mary: John, would you like to stop for ice cream?

John: No, I'm not hungry.

Mary (thinking to herself): He's so inconsiderate.

Mary was actually hinting that *she* would like to stop for ice cream but had phrased her desire in a subtle, indirect way that felt appropriately restrained to her. John, in contrast was used to expressing himself directly, took Mary's statement as a straightforward question, and answered it.

Another communication-related gender difference discussed by Tannen is the differing ways in which men and women typically approach decision making and negotiation. Men who must make a decision are less likely to invite input from other people initially. They typically announce a unilateral decision but then expect others to challenge it if they disagree. Men expect to have to negotiate. Women, on the other hand, are more likely to ask other people for input first and then come to a decision. When men make a decision unilaterally, women often see them as egotistical and inconsiderate, hear the decision as final, and fail to attempt to negotiate it. When women ask for input before making decisions, men may interpret that as a sign of weakness and indecisiveness.

A related difference that has tremendous implications for men and women in close relationships is the way in which men and women handle problems and difficulties. Women are more likely than men to confide problems to friends and partners and do so in considerable detail. When they do, they expect the other person to listen closely to them and to empathize. When women confide problems to other women, they generally get the response they want. When they confide problems to men, however, they are likely to get a less satisfactory response. Because men do not typically use talking as a way of getting closer to another person, as women do, they tend to hear a disclosure that a problem exists as a request for assistance. They do not realize that the woman only wants to be heard, and they tend to cut her off as soon as they think they understand the nature of the problem, so that they can offer her a solution. Women typically interpret this as a rejection of their intimate disclosure and as a sign that the man does not care about them.

Sharing and support are handled differently in male culture. Men tend to be much less verbal than women when they confide in and support each other. When a man shares a problem with a male friend, he is likely to do it quickly and rather sketchily; men tend not to engage in the lengthy analyses typical of women. Another major difference is that men support each other primarily by their presence, rather than by verbal commiseration. A man can experience intimacy with a male friend by working alongside him, even though relatively few words are exchanged (Goodman & O'Brian, 2001).

According to Tannen, men and women also tend to have different patterns of talking at home. Women are usually eager to converse with their partner at the end of the workday, in order to connect and reinforce the bonds between them. Unlike men, women tend to use talking as a way of establishing intimacy, as well as in instrumental ways. In contrast, men who return home after a day of work often desire a respite from the need to talk, at least for a while. This is because most of men's conversation during the workday is instrumental—they are trying to "win" and move up in the hierarchy. To them, simply sharing space with their partner or spouse at the end of the day feels intimate and comforting. This difference causes many women to complain that their male partners will not talk to them as much as they would like and to interpret men's relative silence as lack of interest.

Women in close relationships with men often complain that men do not readily share their feelings. Although it is true that many men do not share feelings as readily as women, the sharing they do allow themselves with the women in their lives may be very important to them. Because the emphasis on competition in male culture causes many men to be reluctant to share problems with other men (lest they be perceived as weak), a man's female friend or partner is often the only person to whom he can fully reveal himself. Warren Farrell (1999), who writes about masculinity and the male experience, suggests that, paradoxically, men's very need for closeness with women can inhibit men's emotional expression. It can be difficult and frightening for a man to communicate certain feelings to his partner or spouse, because, if she withdraws, it feels to him as if his entire emotional support system has collapsed.

When men and women attempt to communicate with each other, the result is often misunderstanding and hurt feelings. It is important to remember how differently men and women may view the sharing of feelings and how culture and tradition still play a large role in the behavior of the sexes.

Managing Conflict

People often fall out of love and friendship because of their differences. The two people in any sort of close relationship are bound to have somewhat different backgrounds and life experiences, which means that their needs, wants, viewpoints, preferences, and priorities will not always be the same. Differences may emerge around any subject, small or large, and can lead to overt conflict and fighting. Conflict, therefore, is likely to occur in *all* close relationships; there is no way to avoid it. It is not, however, conflict itself that causes difficulties in relationships but, rather, unskillful ways of *handling* it (Paul & Paul, 1990). A conflict is merely the catalyst that precipitates an often-predictable chain reaction of responses and consequences. Trying to avoid conflict in a relationship is usually counterproductive and undermines honesty and genuineness (Fisher & Brown, 1994). Similarly, hurried and poorly thought-out measures designed to end conflict are likely to cause more problems than they prevent. Two keys to managing conflict are coping with differences in a skillful manner and expressing feelings constructively.

COPING WITH DIFFERENCES

Learning to *cope* well with differences is key to minimizing conflict in a relationship (Fisher & Brown, 1994). The following strategies can help friends or partners cope with their differences in a positive manner:

1. Set clear boundaries around the topic of discussion. *It is imperative that the participants stick to the topic at hand and not bring up other areas of disagreement or attack each other personally. Doing so can result in a vitriolic free-for-all (McGraw, 2000).*
2. Maintain a balance between reason and emotion. *Logical arguments should be accompanied by an acknowledgment of the feelings that accompany them. Conversely, neither partner should rely solely on emotion to make his or her case. Nor should one partner attempt to restrict the other from either using reason or expressing emotion.*
3. Make every effort to understand each other's position and point of view. *To achieve an outcome that is satisfactory to both parties, each must fully explore and take into consideration the other's feelings, interests, and perceptions; it follows that both must be willing to reveal them.*
4. Use persuasion rather than coercion. *Force never works. People perceive force as manipulation, and no one wants to be manipulated. Both partners should ask for what they want, rather than demanding it. Neither friend or partner should engage in emotional outbursts, sulk, or attempt to make the other feel guilty.*

5. Be reliable. *Each partner must keep whatever agreement is made. Compromise becomes difficult when one or both participants in a relationship have learned that the other cannot be trusted to keep his or her word.*

EXPRESSING FEELINGS CONSTRUCTIVELY

Sometimes, expressing feelings is difficult. We may be reluctant to express certain feelings or are temporarily out of touch with them. It is common to ask people about their feelings only to hear a response such as, "Nothing is wrong," "I didn't mean to say that," or "The comment was not meant for you." Our feelings are often too complex to discuss, and many times we try to disguise them. Nevertheless, it is important to try to describe the feelings that *are* accessible during an interaction. Framing feelings in relation to the problem and sharing feelings without evaluating them are two strategies that may help (Stone, Patton, Heen, & Fisher, 2000).

Framing feelings in relation to the problem means prefacing a description of one's feelings with a statement regarding the discomfort that is associated with them. For example, a person who is uncomfortable with her own feelings of anger or resentment toward another person might begin by saying, "It's hard for me to say this to you . . ." and then proceed to share what is on her mind. *Sharing feelings without evaluating them* means not subjecting our feelings to our own censorship. Although it is often prudent to refrain from expressing certain feelings in superficial relationships, it is generally not appropriate to do so in intimate ones. It's important to share our feelings without making a judgment about them. Feelings are what they are, and "stuffing" them, or feeling that it is not safe to express them, is one of the hallmarks of an unhealthy relationship. The mandate to express feelings, however, should not be taken as a license to be abusive or manipulative while doing so. A degree of tact, together with a concern for the feelings of one's friend or partner and for the welfare of the relationship itself, is always appropriate. When engaged in a dialogue that involves disagreement or anger, we would do well to consider the following question: If I say what I am thinking of saying to my partner, will I be promoting the relationship, or will I be undermining it? Being insensitive to a partner's needs and feelings is destructive to a relationship.

Because some feelings around a certain topic may not be immediately accessible, the topic may need to be readdressed at a later time, after feelings have had a chance to surface. Multiple conversations about an area of conflict are often necessary in order to resolve it.

Learning from Broken Relationships

Although the dissolution of a close friendship or marriage is usually a painful experience for both persons involved, it can also be a profound learning experience, which will make success in future relationships more likely. The key is to reflect on the breakup and on the part that one's own attitudes, beliefs, and behaviors played in it.

Broken Friendships

In the course of doing research on women's friendships, Sandy Sheehy (2001) catalogued the reasons that the women in her study had lost friends. A few of the major ones included (1) leftover baggage from earlier relationships with mothers and sisters, (2) a tendency to withdraw in the face of conflict rather than staying to work things out, (3) competition, (4) judgment, (5) self-absorption, (6) an inability to keep confidences, (7) envy and jealousy, (8) poor social skills, and (9) life transitions.

Unresolved issues with mothers and sisters can be played out in close female friendships. A woman who had a mother who was unpredictably moody is likely to find that characteristic hard to tolerate in a friend. Women who were young when their mothers died, or who had mothers who were emotionally unavailable to them, may have difficulties relating to other women because of abandonment issues. Women who were constantly embroiled in conflict with sisters are likely to assume a wary and defensive stance in their relationships with other women. The positive aspect of women's tendency to unconsciously identify other women with their mothers and sisters is that friendship can provide a space in which old issues can be confronted and overcome, provided both participants are willing to remain in the relationship.

Unfortunately, many women have been socialized to be very uncomfortable with **conflict,** especially conflict with another woman. Women are generally expected to be society's peacemakers—to cooperate and smooth over differences. Because they are unwilling to bring an element of conflict into a friendship, many women choose not to express a difference of opinion or a dissatisfaction to another woman. If the burden of unspoken grievances becomes too great, a friendship may simply collapse. Women are much more likely to vent their dissatisfaction with a friend or coworker to a third party than to the person herself. Although venting to another person can be a safety valve if done occasionally, a policy of *never* directly confronting one's friends derails personal growth and the possibility of working out longstanding issues in the arena of friendship.

Competition is another friendship killer among women. Whereas men are socialized to see competition as a desirable mechanism for establishing the hierarchy with which they are comfortable, women often see competition as antithetical to *loyalty, trust,* and *support,* the premier female friendship values. Although the presence of underlying competition is one factor that distinguishes superficial office collegiality from true friendship, even women who merely work together may feel betrayed when female colleagues oppose a plan they have suggested, or fail to support it. Many find it exceedingly difficult to deal with feelings of competitiveness toward a personal friend, whether in the context of sports, academic achievement, homemaking ability, or some other area.

Judgment is a limiting factor in all forms of relationships. Personal disclosure is the hallmark of friendship among women, and, when a friend reacts to a confided belief, attitude, feeling, or behavior with judgment instead of acceptance and understanding, a friendship can be badly fractured. Judgment can also arise out of differences in lifestyle. For example, a woman who works outside her home may fail to accept a friend's choice to be a full-time wife and mother, or vice versa. Sheehy (2001) notes that, in such a case, the friendship can be salvaged, and even made stronger, if both parties honestly divulge the *feelings* that underlie their inability to accept the other's choice. For example, an employed woman might admit that her friend's choice to stay home with her children makes her feel guilty for having gone back to work.

Self-absorption kills friendships by unbalancing the give and take of confiding and supporting. Self-absorbed people are fundamentally interested only in themselves and betray that by wanting to discuss only *their* experiences and problems. Although most women are willing to do most of the listening while a friend is going through a particularly rough patch, they begin to feel used if consistently denied the opportunity to confide their own concerns.

The inability to treat sensitive information shared by friends as **confidential** is a major barrier to sustained friendship. One of the basic criteria for true friendship is that both parties feel safe in revealing their darkest secrets; there is no surer way to lose a friend than by betraying a confidence.

Sheehy (2001) describes **envy** and **jealousy** as the "twin enemies of friendship." Although there are similarities between the two attributes, they are not the same. *Envy* involves resenting a friend because of something she possesses—her social status, financial position, job, lover, and so on. *Jealousy* is the feeling that a third person is getting more love, attention, or special treatment from someone we care about than we are. For example, if Mary's friend, Teresa, starts spending a lot of time with a new friend, Sue, Mary may feel both jealous of Sue and angry with Teresa for "deserting" her. This scenario is particularly likely to arise if one participant in a friendship puts a higher value on it than the other does. Contrary to what is portrayed in the media, sexual jealously does not seem to be a major reason for the dissolution of friendships among women (Sheehy, 2001). Women who are envious of a friend for some reason often feel guilty enough to end the relationship, because they know that friends ideally rejoice in each other's good fortune. The person who is the object of envy may also end the relationship if she feels she cannot freely share her successes and triumphs.

Limited social skills are another reason friendships between women break down. A woman who repeatedly fails to show up for engagements, who is chronically late, or who does not recognize the value of "please" and "thank you" will find it hard to maintain relationships with other women.

Finally, a significant **change** in the life of one partner in a friendship can spell the end of the relationship. For example, whereas some friendships survive the geographic relocation of one of the participants, others do not. Getting married (or embarking on a serious romantic relationship), getting divorced, or becoming a mother can change the relational dynamic between a woman and her friend in any number of ways. The woman who married or gave birth may have less time to spend with her friend; there is a tacit understanding among women that time spent with friends cannot impinge on time spent with family. Another possibility is that the friend may not care for the woman's partner or spouse. When two friends are both married, the divorce of one can conjure so much fear in the other that the relationship crumbles. A similar sundering can occur if one of a pair of friends becomes seriously ill or suffers a great misfortune, such as the death of a husband or child. Whereas some friends will remain staunchly loyal in the face of such circumstances, others will be too uncomfortable to remain in the relationship.

Broken Sexual/Romantic Relationships

Over the past decade, some very enlightening research has been done on the factors that contribute to the dissolution of initially committed sexual/romantic relationships. Gottman and Notarious (2000) reviewed this research, including studies done by Gottman himself with various other collaborators. Gottman studied married couples over periods of up to six years, videotaping them repeatedly as they addressed various sources of conflict in their relationships. He and his colleagues noted the ways in which the spouses interacted with each other and were able to identify patterns that correlated with eventual divorce. The couples who eventually divorced interacted more *negatively* with each other, right from the beginning of the research, than couples who did not. Four specific patterns of negative interaction were ultimately found to be highly predictive of divorce: **criticism, defensiveness, contempt,** and **stonewalling.** The couples who eventually divorced also tended to **escalate the degree of negativity** in their interactions. For example, if a husband criticized his wife, she might not only counter his criticism with criticism of her own but also display contempt for him. In contrast, the couples who stayed together generally reciprocated each other's criticism but did not escalate the negativity into contempt or stonewalling. Another factor found to be predictive of divorce was the husband's tendency to routinely **reject** influence from his wife. The husbands who demonstrated this pattern generally ignored their wives' viewpoints and preferences and paid little attention to their complaints. Interestingly, a pattern of wifely rejection of the husband's influence did *not* predict divorce.

When a serious relationship or marriage ends, it is common for one or both partners to enter a new relationship, or marry again, relatively soon. Often, however, this is a mistake. When people part, it is important that both learn something from the experience. Each should take the time to reflect on the relationship and the part that he or she played in its demise. It is also important that the former partners take enough time to get to know themselves as single people before coupling again (Kingma, 1987). The following story illustrates this principle.

Ed married his first wife, Lana, because the timing had been right. He had just graduated from medical school and wanted to start a family. After the birth of Ed and Lana's first child, Ed's medical practice started to grow. As Ed became more successful, however, he and Lana rarely spent any time together. Finally, after 10 years of marriage and three children, they separated and divorced. Within 2 years of his divorce from Lana, Ed entered into a second marriage, which he later came to see as a *rebound relationship*. This second marriage lasted 12 years. After his second divorce, Ed vowed never to marry again, thinking that he did not know who he was, what he wanted, or how to choose a partner. Ed then changed his lifestyle dramatically; he gave up his medical practice and entered the academic community. During this university period, he spent time with his children and dated women he met through his university friends. At a dinner party for friends, Ed met Tara, a woman who had her own professional career and who would become his third wife. After a 6-year relationship, they married. Ed says he is happier now than he has ever been and attributes this to having taken the time to find out more about himself and what he wanted in a relationship before marrying for the third time. Ed feels that he is growing as a person in his present relationship. Because Ed and his partner are emotionally mature, they give each other the freedom to pursue various interests—something that had been missing in their previous relationships. Ed feels that working on projects he has long been interested in has stimulated him intellectually; he is writing and making a contribution to the community. Ed admits that, previously, he had done little reflecting on his relationships and did not perceive or understand the patterns that had been present in them. He has learned that being committed to a relationship or marriage requires a willingness to assess previous behavioral patterns and to learn new communication and negotiating skills.

Success Is Possible

Today, we are fortunate in that a variety of assistance is available to individuals and couples who desire help in forming or negotiating relationships. Individuals can see a therapist, make use of commercial relationship assessment/enhancement materials, or attend one of the many workshops and retreats that focus on many forms of relationships (Larson, 2000). Another way that couples can better understand their own and their partner's behavior is by becoming familiar with the various scales on the Myers-Briggs Type Inventory (MBTI). The MBTI reflects the degree to which an individual possesses various personality characteristics, such as introversion and extroversion, which are organized into 16 basic types. Many organizations use the MBTI to help employees understand the differences in personality and preferences among co-workers with whom they must work closely. It is also widely used to facilitate understanding and communication between couples who are in counseling. A slim volume, *People Types and Tiger Stripes* (Lawrence, 1987), serves as a good introduction to "type."

Cultivating successful relationships takes time and effort. In order to hold up our end of a friendship or romantic liaison, we must be willing to reflect on our own motivations and actions, strengthen our communication and conflict-resolution skills, and provide our partner with ongoing empathy and support. We must prioritize our important relationships, not neglect them on account of conflicting demands on our time. The rewards of doing so far outweigh the costs; healthy relationships feed the body, mind, and spirit; even those that ultimately fade provide us with an opportunity for growth and personal development.

Relational Wellness Self-Assessment

Respond to the following statements honestly. The more statements you agree with, the more likely it is that your relationships are supporting your physical, mental, and spiritual health.

1. *I have at least one close female friend in whom I can safely confide.*
2. *I make a conscious effort to provide my friends and romantic partners with support without judgment.*
3. *I am strict with myself about keeping friends' confidences confidential.*
4. *I do not allow friends and romantic partners to dictate my attitudes, beliefs, and behaviors.*
5. *I allow my friends and romantic partners to be themselves, without trying to control them.*
6. *I do not expect any one friend or romantic partner to meet all my needs for companionship and support.*
7. *I can and do apologize to friends and romantic partners when I know I have spoken or acted inappropriately.*
8. *I do not refuse to address issues that are important to my friends and partners.*
9. *I raise important issues with my friends and partners, even though some degree of conflict may result.*
10. *When involved in a conflict with a friend or partner, I stick to the subject and do not bring up old or unrelated issues.*
11. *I value close relationships with others and prioritize them accordingly.*

New Directions

Recent discoveries regarding the importance of relationships to women's physical, emotional, and spiritual health have resulted in a resurgence of interest in women's relational patterns and new research on women's friendship and sexual/romantic relationships. For example, scholars at the Wellesley Centers for Women are currently conducting ongoing investigations into the ways in which women reconcile their orientation toward connection with the competition that is inherent in many of the roles they now occupy in society. They are also mapping out patterns of friendship among women of various ages and ethnic backgrounds and attempting to find out whether men would benefit from adopting more "feminine" relational patterns.

Researchers who study committed sexual/romantic relationships are continuing to identify the factors associated with both enduring and broken relationships in order to find ways of helping couples withstand the stressors that doom so many marriages and other forms of committed relationships. The factors currently being investigated include gender role orientation, ethnicity, employment patterns, socioeconomic status, social support, domestic task allocation, conflict-resolution style, communication patterns, and various aspects of personality.

QUESTIONS FOR REFLECTION AND DISCUSSION

1. *Are women's and men's relational patterns likely to become more or less similar? In what ways? Why?*
2. *Which aspects of women's typical relational orientation do you see as positive? negative? Why?*
3. *The divorce rate is now over 50 percent. Do you expect that to improve or to worsen over time? Why?*
4. *What are your strengths and weaknesses as a friend?*

RESOURCES

Organizations

Wellesley Centers for Women
Wellesley College
106 Central Street
Wesley, MA 02481
Phone: 781-283-2484
Web: www.wcwonline.org

Books

Goodman, E., & O'Brian, P. (2001). *I know just what you mean: The power of friendship in women's lives.* Fireside.

Lerner, H. (2001). *The dance of connection: How to talk to someone when you are mad, hurt, scared, frustrated, insulted, betrayed or desperate.* New York: HarperCollins.

McGraw, P. (2000). *Relationship rescue: A seven step strategy for reconnecting with your partner.* New York: Hyperion.

Ryan, M. J. (2002). *Attitudes of gratitude in love: Creating more joy in your relationships.* New York: Conari Press.

Schwartz, P. (1994). *Love between equals: How peer marriage really works.* New York: Macmillan.

Sheehy, S. (2000). *Connecting: The enduring power of female friendships.* Morrow.

Websites

Ask Alice About Relationships—Columbia University's question-and-answer Internet service
www.goaskalice.columbia.edu/Cat8.html

The Coalition for Marriage, Family and Couples—A nondenominational, nonprofit organization dedicated to disseminating information that helps couples remain in relationship
www.smartmarriages.com

International Society for the Study of Personal Relationships—A nonprofit organization of professionals interested in all aspects of relationships
www.isspr.org

REFERENCES

Ball, L.J. (2000). How gender differences contribute to divorce: A restrospective, qualitative study. *Dissertation Abstracts International, 60*(9-B), 4874.

Banfield, S., & McCabe, M. P. (2001). Extra relationship involvement among women: Are they different from men? *Archives of Sexual Behavior, 30*(2), 119–142.

Berkman, L. E., & Syme, S. L. (1979). Social networks, host resistance, and mortality: A nine-year follow up study of Alameda County residents. *American Journal of Epidemiology, 109,* 186–204.

Blaffer-Hrdy, S. (1999). *Mother nature.* New York: Pantheon.

Branden, N. (1998). *A woman's self-esteem: Struggles and triumphs in the search for identity.* San Francisco: Jossey-Bass.

Branden, N. (2001). *The psychology of self-esteem: A revolutionary approach to self-understanding that launched a new era in modern psychology.* San Francisco: Jossey-Bass.

Campbell, S. M. (1999). *The couple's journey: Intimacy as a path to wholeness.* New York: HarperCollins.

Chodorow, N. (1974). Family structure and feminine personality. In Rosaldo, M., & Lamphere, L. (Eds.), *Women, culture and society* (pp. 42–66). Palo Alto, CA: Stanford University Press.

Connell, R. W. (1995). *Masculinities.* Berkeley: University of California Press.

Crenshaw, T. (1996). *The alchemy of love and lust.* New York: Pocket Books.

Derlega, V., & Stepian, E. (1977). Norms regulating self-disclosure among Polish university students. *Journal of Cross-Cultural Psychology, 8*(3), 369–376.

D'Milio, J., & Freedman, E. (1988). *Intimate matters: A history of sexuality in America.* New York: Harper & Row.

Farrell, W. (1999). *Women can't hear what men don't say: Destroying myths, creating love.* New York: Tarcher/Putnam.

Fisher, R. (1994). *Getting together: Building a relationship that gets to yes.* Boston: Harvard Negotiation Project/Houghton Mifflin.

Gilbert, R. (1992). *Extraordinary relationships: A new way of thinking about human interactions.* Minneapolis: Chronimed.

Gilmer, T., & Neumeyer, J. (1992). *Redefining Mr. Right: A career woman's guide in choosing a mate.* Oakland, CA: New Harbinger & Marin.

Goodman, E., & O'Brian, P. (2001). *I know just what you mean: The power of friendship in women's lives.* New York: Fireside.

Gottman, J. M. (1994). *What predicts divorce: The relationship between marital processes and marital outcomes.* Hillsdale, NJ: Erlsbaum.

Gottman, J. M., & Notarius, C. I. (2000). Decade review: Observing marital interaction. *Journal of marriage and the family, 62*(4), 927–947.

Goulton, M. (2001). *The 6 secrets of a lasting relationship: How to fall in love again and stay there.* New York: Putnam's & Sons.

Gray, J. (1995). *Mars and venus in the bedroom: A guide to lasting romance and passion.* New York: HarperCollins.

Gray, J. (2000). *Mars and venus in touch: Enhancing the passion with great communication.* New York: HarperCollins.

Hafen, B., & Frandsen, K. (1987). *People who need people are the healthiest people: The importance of relationships.* Provo, UT: Behavioral Health Associates.

Hendricks, G., & Hendricks, K. (1992). *Conscious loving: The journey to co-commitment.* New York: Bantam Books.

Hooks, B. (2000). *All about love: New visions.* New York: William Morrow.

Katherine, A. (1991). *Boundaries: Where you end and I begin.* New York: MJF Books.

Kingma, D. R. (1987). *Coming apart: Why relationships end and how to live through the ending of yours.* New York: Fawcett Crest.

Kingma, D. R. (1998). *The future of love: The power of the soul in intimate relationships.* New York: Doubleday.

Larson, J. (2000). *Should we stay together? A scientifically proven method for evaluating your relationship and its chances for long-term success.* San Francisco: Jossey-Bass.

Lawrence, L. (1987). *People types and tiger stripes* (2nd ed.). Gainesville, FL: Center for the Application of Psychological Type.

Louden, J. (1994). *The couple's comfort book: A creative guide for renewing passion and pleasure.* San Francisco: Harper & Co.

Mackay, F., & Paleg, K. (1994). *Couple skills: Making your relationship work.* Oakland, CA: New Harbinger.

McGraw, P. (2000). *Relationship rescue: A seven step strategy for reconnecting with your partner.* New York: Hyperion.

Miller, J. B. (1976). *Toward a new psychology of women.* Boston, MA: Beacon Press.

Miller, J. B., & Stiver, I. P. (1998). *The healing connection: How women form relationships in therapy and in life.* Boston: Beacon Press.

Page, S. (1994). *The 8 essential traits of couples who thrive.* New York: Dell.

Paul, J., & Paul, M. (1990). *Do I have to give up me to be loved by you?* Minneapolis: Compcare.

Pelletier, K. (1994). *Sound mind, sound body: A new model for lifelong health.* New York: Simon & Schuster.

Powell, J. (1985). *Will the real me please stand up? So we can all get to know you: 25 guidelines for good communication.* Allen, TX: Argus.

Preston, D., & Grimes, J. (1987). A study of differences in social support. *Journal of Gerontological Nursing, 13*(2), 36–40.

Schnebly, L. (1994). *I do? Being happy being married.* Tucson, AZ: Fisher Books.

Schwartz, P. (1994). *Love between equals: How peer marriage really works.* New York: Macmillan.

Sheehy, S. (2001). *Connecting: The enduring power of female friendships.* New York: HarperCollins.

Stone, D., Patton, B., Heen, S., & Fisher, R. (2000). *Difficult conversations: How to discuss what matters most.* New York: Penguin.

Tannen, D. (1994). *Talking from 9 to 5.* New York: William Morrow & Co.

Tannen, D. (1990). *You just don't understand: Women and men in conversation.* New York: Ballantine Books.

Turndorf, J. (1999). *Till death do us part (unless I kill you first): A step-by-step guide for resolving marital conflict.* New York: Henry Holt.

Welwood, J. (1996). *Journey from the heart: Intimate relationships and the path to life.* New York: Harper Perennial.

Wetzler, S. (1998). *Is it you or is it me? Why couples play the blame game.* New York: Harper Perennial.

Williams, W. (1992). Relationship between male-male friendship and male-female marriage: American Indian and Asian comparisons. In P. Itardi (Ed.), *Men's friendships: Research on men and masculinities* (Vol. 2., pp. 250–261). Newbury Park, CA: Sage.

Young-Bruehl, E., & Bethelard, F. (2001, August). Cherishment. *O Magazine,* pp. 131–133, 176.

Zukav, G. (1989). *The seat of the soul.* New York: Fireside Books/Simon & Schuster.

SECTION III

The Emerging Healthcare Delivery System

9

Traditional Healthcare

Jacquelin H. Harrington and Deborah Lessard

Objectives

1. *Compare and contrast fee-for-service insurance plans with managed care.*
2. *List the factors that should be taken into consideration in choosing a health insurance plan.*
3. *Describe the credentials of, and services provided by, selected healthcare professionals and nonprofessionals.*
4. *Identify the strategies by which consumers can maximize their likelihood of obtaining safe, effective healthcare.*
5. *Discuss healthcare consumers' rights regarding information, treatment, and privacy.*

Introduction

The days when healthcare consumers had only to consult the healthcare provider of choice and rely on their insurance to cover most of the medical bills are gone or on their way out for many Americans. Today, selecting an insurance plan that will ensure good medical care requires careful preparation. This chapter will address the changes that have occurred in the healthcare delivery system, the realities of the present managed care environment, and strategies that consumers can use to obtain the best healthcare. Information about the educational preparation and scope of practice of physicians, nurses, and other categories of licensed and unlicensed healthcare providers will also be presented, as will information about healthcare consumers' legal and generally agreed-upon rights.

Knowing the System

Paying for Healthcare

Relatively few people who live in modern societies pay for the bulk of their healthcare by making payments directly to providers. Instead, they make payments, known as **premiums** to **third-party payers,** who actually reimburse the providers. Third-party payers may be insurance companies, managed care companies, government agencies, or a combination. In the past, persons who had health insurance were most often covered by what is known as **fee-for-service,** or **private,** insurance plans. Today, in an effort to keep healthcare costs down, **managed care** is rapidly supplanting private insurance. For most people, health insurance is linked with employment as a benefit. Employees pay a portion of the premium, and the employer pays the rest as a tax-deductible business expense. Employees are not taxed on the cash value of their insurance premium benefit.

PRIVATE INSURANCE

Under private, or fee-for-service, insurance plans, physicians, hospitals, and so on are reimbursed on the basis of the **services** they provide. Private plans are based on the principle of pooling both risk and money, and they operate under the law of large numbers. Although it is difficult to predict what health problems a given individual will develop over a period of time, it is relatively easy to estimate (on the basis of known statistical likelihood) the problems that will arise in a *pool* (group) of people and the costs of treating them. Simply put, insurance companies who offer fee-for-service plans adjust their premiums in such a way that the total estimated healthcare costs, plus a margin of profit, are distributed equally (according to level of coverage) among the pool of insurance customers. Some people wind up paying more in premiums than the insurance company spends on them, whereas others pay less. Because of a number of factors, such as the development of sophisticated medical technology and the increasing numbers of people who live into old age, however, the *cost* of medical care has been skyrocketing over recent decades. Fee-for-service plans that place few or no restrictions on the services that will be provided once an illness or injury occurs are becoming extremely expensive and increasingly unattractive to employers who must assume part of the cost of employees' healthcare.

Even though fee-for-service insurance plans are still available, they are rapidly being replaced by what is known as managed care. In 1992, a survey of workers in settings that had more than 200 employees found that only 4 percent still had traditional private insurance plans that involved no precertification or other form of managed care. Another 43 percent had traditional plans that used recertification or other controls on use of the plan. The remaining 53 percent provided benefits through managed care programs (Potter & Perry, 1997).

MANAGED CARE

The term *managed care* refers to the practice of monitoring and adjusting healthcare benefits for the purpose of managing costs. The end result is the placing of limits on coverage and access to healthcare services. Managed care affects insurance companies, employers, providers, and clients. Most enrollees in managed care plans are employees of businesses that contract for health insurance as a benefit; many managed care plans, especially the plans that enroll Medicare beneficiaries, do not accept individual enrollees. Although certain managed care arrangements have been around for some time, the number of people employed in the private sector who are enrolled in managed care plans through their employers has increased dramatically in recent years.

Under managed care, providers are paid on the basis of **capitation.** Under capitation, the insurance plan pays the primary provider (usually a physician) a flat fee for each patient, instead of reimbursing the provider for discrete units of care provided. Managed care organizations are healthcare organizations that are responsible for both the *provision* of care and the *financing* of care. Managed care organizations assume responsibility for enrollees' healthcare, including hospitalization and outpatient care, at a fixed cost per client, regardless of the amount of care given. If a given enrollee does not need care, the provider keeps all of the allotted capitation monies, anyway. On the other hand, if the enrollee needs to be seen by a specialist or to receive expensive, high-tech care, the primary provider must pay for that out of the capitation funds. This arrangement is meant to provide an incentive for physicians and other providers to keep their patients healthy.

There are three common types of managed care organizations: health maintenance organizations (HMOs), preferred provider organizations (PPOs), and point-of-service (POS) organizations.

HMOs The health maintenance organization (HMO) is the most prevalent type of managed care organization. HMOs provide the *least expensive* type of managed care. Premiums are 8 to 10 percent lower than traditional plans, there are no deductibles or coinsurance payments, and copayments are only $5 to $10 per visit (*Is an HMO Right for You?*, 1996). Whereas the fee-for-service (or *indemnity*) insurers, such as Blue Cross/Blue Shield, were responsible only for paying for the treatment patients received, HMOs are responsible for actually providing care to their enrollees. Because of this, HMOs must seek to balance the need to provide appropriate, high-quality care with the need to reduce costs. Therefore, although HMOs are the most inexpensive type of managed care provider, they are also the most *restrictive*.

HMOs keep costs down by requiring all patients to have a **primary care physician (PCP),** who becomes the gatekeeper to all services. HMO enrollees must get the approval of their primary care physician in order to access all healthcare services. Referrals to specialists and approval for emergency room care, X rays, surgery, and so on must all come from the PCP. This provision reduces the demand for costly medical services.

HMOs contract with providers, such as hospitals, laboratories, radiologists, physician specialists, and druggists, for discounted prices. The aggregate of all the providers that have contracted with an HMO is called the *network*. Participants in HMOs must use the providers that have contracted with the HMO; they cannot go outside of the network for services. HMOs are usually the best choice for people (particularly those who have children) who are new to a community and have no established ties to certain providers or hospitals. HMOs also work well for people whose current provider and hospital are part of the HMO network (Pyenson & O'Connor, 2000).

PPOs   Preferred provider organizations (PPOs) are similar to group or network HMOs in that the insurance company contracts with physicians and hospitals to provide care to their enrollees. PPOs are usually more expensive than HMOs because they offer more *choices*. The physicians and hospitals with which the insurance company contracts are called **preferred providers.** Participants who use preferred providers are rewarded with low deductibles and copayments. Usually, 80 percent of claims are covered. If an enrollee wishes to see someone besides a preferred provider, or go to a hospital outside the network, she pays a higher deductible and copayment, and usually only 60 to 70 percent of the claim is covered. Therefore, although enrollees are not required to see a preferred provider, there is a considerable financial incentive to do so. PPOs also differ from HMOs in that they do not require enrollees to get permission from a gatekeeper before receiving care. PPOs are usually most satisfactory for people who want more choice about providers and whose provider is already part of the network (Pyenson & O'Connor, 2000).

POS Plans   A point-of-service (POS) plan is a hybrid cross between a traditional indemnity policy and a PPO. Point-of-service (POS) organizations represent attempts by insurance companies to better meet patient demands for choice and quality of care. Basically, a POS plan functions the same as an HMO, except that the enrollee has the option of receiving medical care from any provider. As long as the enrollee stays "in network"—that is, the enrollee receives care through the traditional HMO network—she pays only a small copayment (typically less than $25). However, if an employee elects to receive care "out of network," there is a financial penalty. Usually, the enrollee must pay a deductible, such as $500, and then the plan reimburses the enrollee for only 80 percent of "rea-

sonable and customary" charges. This means that the enrollee may have to pay the deductible plus a percentage of reasonable and customary charges. Moreover, unlike enrollers in PPOs, POS enrollers must pay 100 percent of charges not deemed "reasonable and customary" by the POS organization. Although it can be very expensive to go outside of the network, the option is available in POS plans (Lancaster, 1999).

Watchdog Agencies   There are public and private agencies and organizations that seek to ensure that managed care organizations provide quality care and respond to consumer concerns. The **National Committee on Quality Assurance (NCQA)** is a nonprofit organization that evaluates HMOs according to 50 standards related to a plan's ability to provide good healthcare. The **Joint Commission on the Accreditation of Healthcare Organizations (JCAHO),** which evaluates hospitals, nursing homes, and other health facilities, has also begun to evaluate managed care plans. Recently, the book *Making a Killing: HMOs and the Threat to Your Health,* by Jamie Court and Frank Smith, has been made available, at no charge, on the Internet. Consumers can read the book, and communicate their own stories to the authors, at http://makingakilling.org.

Acute care facilities, such as hospitals, have been dramatically affected by managed care. Hospitals have variously been forced to close, merge, change their bed capacity, and develop integrated healthcare systems. **Integrated systems** combine all three components of healthcare delivery (medical care providers, hospitals, and insurance companies) in one system. They represent the latest organizational model to evolve as a result of economic environmental forces. Integrated systems sometimes merge with one another to form large health care networks, or systems.

Choosing a Managed Care Plan   All facets of healthcare delivery have been affected by the economic changes in healthcare. Both private and public healthcare delivery systems have changed. Managed care plans vary widely in services, cost, and quality of care. Many are excellent; some are not. It is vital that consumers choose the most appropriate plan for their families and themselves. Because the current healthcare delivery system is characterized by ongoing dramatic shifts in terms of financing, method of care delivery, and nature of providers, consumers of healthcare need current information in order to make intelligent decisions.

Prior to choosing a plan, consumers must take stock of their healthcare needs and preferences, both present and future. Information should be collected about plans of interest, including their rules and provisions, and the satisfaction level of their enrollees. Consumers would be well advised to ask themselves the following questions before choosing a plan:

• Do I have a pre-existing condition that I need care for?
• Do I have a family history of a serious disease that may require special treatment?

- Do I want alternative therapies, such as acupuncture or massage?
- Is staying with my current physician an important consideration?
- What can I afford to pay for my medical care?
- Are the healthcare facilities in the HMO network located conveniently for me?
- Am I concerned about a limited choice of doctors and having less control over treatment decisions? (If so, a POS or PPO may be a better choice than an HMO.)
- Is the plan accredited by the NCQA or JCAHO?
- Does the plan have a good review process? Is it approved by the NCQA?
- Does the plan provide for consumer feedback, and is there a way to evaluate patient satisfaction and quality of care?
- Are the plan's findings regarding enrollees' satisfaction verified by outside sources?
- How many enrollees decided to leave the HMO the previous year? Did they join another HMO or return to a fee-for-service plan?
- What is the procedure for registering consumer complaints? Is there a grievance process if the plan denies care?
- Are the plan's physicians and other providers board certified?
- Does the plan review the providers' performance? If so, how often?
- Are providers paid on a salaried or per-enrollee basis?
- Do providers earn bonuses if they limit referrals to specialists and avoid expensive tests and procedures?
- How many physicians and other providers leave the plan each year?
- How long does it take to get an appointment with a primary care provider or specialist?
- How flexible is the plan? Can enrollees keep their current physicians, or will they be assigned to new ones they may not like?
- Does the plan have a "gag" clause? Some plans discourage their providers from giving enrollees information concerning treatment options. Currently, 15 states have outlawed this practice (*Is an HMO Right for You?*, 1996). Consumers should know whether their own state prohibits gag clauses.
- What prescription drugs are covered? Physicians may be limited as to which drugs they may prescribe. Often, the HMO will issue a drug formulary, which lists medications that will be paid for. If the physician feels an unlisted drug is needed, the patient must pay for that drug out-of-pocket. Potential enrollees should also inquire about whether a plan has a cap on the amount it will spend on drugs in one year.
- Does the plan allow enrollees to see a specialist without additional cost?
- If enrollees need hospitalization, which hospitals may they use? What conditions are considered serious enough to warrant hospitalization and what services need to be authorized in advance?
- How does the plan define medical emergencies? Are there certain conditions under which the plan can refuse to pay for emergency-room care?
- Will the plan cover out-of-town care? Although all plans cover emergencies, most will not reimburse for routine care received outside of the plan's network.
- What is the contraceptive coverage? The American College of Obstetricians and Gynecologists says 49 percent of traditional insurers and almost half of managed care plans do not routinely pay for birth control that requires a prescription.
- What are the plan benefits for mental health? According to Assistant Surgeon General Susan Blumenthal, twice as many women as men will experience depression or panic. Nine times as many women as men will experience depression.

Strengths and Weaknesses of Managed Care   Managed care has both strengths and weaknesses. Its major strength is related to cost containment, and its major weaknesses are related to access and inclusion.

Thus far, managed care has been successful at exerting some control over skyrocketing medical costs. Although the rate at which the cost of medical care rises (inflation) went up in 1997 to pay for two years of rollback and sagging profits, the current rate is the lowest since 1973. Managed care, with its emphasis on health maintenance, also has the potential to increase societal health through patient education, screening, and the provision of optimal healthcare (Swansburg & Swansburg, 1999). Consumer satisfaction, however, will not be improved until some of the weaknesses of managed care are addressed.

Managed care's critics point to such practices as recruiting only patients who are healthy, refusing to care for genuinely ill patients, promoting the use of less skilled healthcare workers, and forcing physicians to withhold costly treatments—thus undermining patients' trust in their physicians' motives. Researchers and individuals working in the healthcare field have also expressed concern that cost controls are being implemented at the expense of appropriate care (Clancy & Brody, 1995).

Managed care's emphasis on cost reduction and competition has its most negative effect on the poor and underinsured. Many Americans have no way to pay for insurance. Sixty percent of insured Americans do not have adequate insurance, and 33 million have no insurance at all (Potter & Perry, 1997).

Access to health care has been decreased overall under managed care because coverage is usually tied to employment. As small businesses find their healthcare benefit costs escalating, they often begin to eliminate healthcare-related benefits. Self-employed individuals with marginal incomes may be unable to purchase insurance because of the high costs of individual policies. Moreover, the practice of raising deductibles and copayments in order to encourage people to use services wisely sometimes causes families to delay or avoid timely care. *Geographic* access to healthcare is becoming even more of a concern than in the past. Many small rural hospitals have had to close their doors, thus denying convenient diagnostic and treatment services to local residents. When a hospital closes, healthcare providers often leave the area, causing residents to lose their source of primary care as well. People in economically depressed urban areas have always had problems with access to healthcare and continue to do so in the age of managed care. Relatively few healthcare workers choose to practice in poor neighborhoods, and residents are forced to travel long distances to receive care. Public transportation is frequently inadequate and inconvenient. *Sociocultural factors* also affect access to healthcare. Many people have historically been excluded from both high-quality care and entry to the health professions because of their ethnicity, gender, or economic status (see Chapters 1 and 2). Currently, ethnic-minority and poor persons are still often made to feel uncomfortable in the healthcare system. This may cause them to fail to seek both preventive healthcare and treatment.

The practice of excluding people from insurance coverage because of pre-existing conditions or the potential for serious health problems is also a concern. Genetic testing has become more extensive, and some insurance companies have been using the results as a reason to deny coverage to healthy individuals. The importance of this issue will increase as more genetic tests become available.

Appealing Managed Care and Insurance Plan Decisions
HMOs and other insurance plans are often quick to refuse to authorize (agree to pay for) tests and procedures. Authorization requests and claims are often processed by persons who are not licensed healthcare providers. Even those who are licensed providers are expected to base their decisions on a set of arbitrary criteria. Some critics of managed care have even accused certain HMOs of routinely denying coverage in the hope the consumer will simply accept the decision. It is imperative that consumers *challenge decisions with which they disagree*. Sometimes resubmitting the claim along with a provider's statement that the test or procedure is medically necessary (written on a prescription pad or letterhead stationary) is all that is necessary. Most HMOs have an appeals system and will expedite a consumer's case if time is of the essence. Information about appeal procedures should be included in the policy booklet or the **certificate of coverage,** which is the contract between the consumer and the insurer. A written complaint may have to be filed and the process may be long and cumbersome. Nevertheless, it is imperative that the consumer follow through. In the event that an appeal is turned down, consumers may contact their state insurance commissioner's office for assistance. The National Association of Insurance Commissioners maintains a website at www.naic.org/consumer/state/usamap.htm. Some states now allow patients to *sue* HMOs that deny necessary coverage. Similar federal legislation is currently pending. The threat of lawsuits may help HMOs become more responsive to patients' needs. Many consumers obtain their health insurance through their place of employment. Dissatisfaction with an employment-related plan should also be communicated to the department of human resources, as complaints from employees may motivate employers to reconsider the plan they have chosen.

Who's Who in Traditional Healthcare

Today's healthcare consumers encounter many different providers—some familiar and some not so familiar. Physicians and nurses remain as fixtures in the healthcare delivery system, but the nurse's role has been expanded. Relatively new providers, such as physician's assistants, paramedics, emergency medical technicians, and a variety of unlicensed assistive personnel (UAP), have expanded the services provided to the public and have assumed responsibilities once reserved for physicians and nurses.

PRIMARY CARE PROVIDERS

The term **primary care** refers to the routine medical care needed by most people. It includes treatment for minor illness, periodic immunizations, and health screening via physical examinations and laboratory tests. In managed care systems, primary care providers also serve as gatekeepers to more complex medical care. At one time, only physicians provided primary care; however, as demands on the healthcare system increased, other professionals joined the ranks of primary care providers. Primary care providers now include advanced practice nurses and physician's assistants, as well as doctors of medicine and doctors of osteopathy (Ellis & Hartley, 1998). The types of physicians currently classified by the federal government as primary care providers are general practitioners, pediatricians, obstetricians, and physicians certified in family practice or internal medicine. There is a shortage of primary care physicians and a surplus of specialists. Therefore, it is currently being recommended that advanced practice nurses (APNs) and physician's assistants (PAs) be used more extensively in providing primary care.

Doctors of Medicine   A doctor of medicine (M.D.) is a physician who has earned her degree by completing an approved course of study at an accredited medical school and by passing the National Board Examination. An M.D. usually enters a hospital internship or residency program for one year of postgraduate training before beginning practice or further training in a specialty. To practice medicine, an M.D. is required to obtain a license from the state in which professional services will be performed.

Doctors of Osteopathy   Six percent of all U.S. physicians are doctors of osteopathy (D.O.). D.O.s have essentially the same qualifications in terms of medical education, internship, licensure, and requirements for recognition as specialists as M.D.s. They are equal with M.D.s under the laws of all 50 states and are recognized as physicians by the American Medical Association (AMA). Central to traditional osteopathic medical theory is the importance of the human body's musculoskeletal system (bones, muscles, tendons, tissues, nerves, and spinal column) to the person's well-being. Traditional osteopathic physicians, who are very much in the minority today, use the manipulation of muscular and skeletal structures as all or part of their treatment regimen. Although many osteopathic physicians have abandoned traditional methods of treatment in favor of conventional ones indistinguishable from those provided by M.D.s, there is currently a resurgence of interest in traditional osteopathic medicine (see Chapter 11).

Advanced Practice Nurses Advanced practice nurses (APNs) are registered nurses (RNs) whose formal education and clinical preparation extend beyond the basic requirements for nursing licensure. Advanced practice nurses hold either certificates or master's degrees, with master's degrees (in addition to the prerequisite baccalaureate degree) being more common. Most categories of APNs, with the exception of clinical nurse specialists, are dually licensed by their states as registered nurses and APNs.

The educational background of physicians and advanced practice nurses is similar in some ways and different in others. Both types of practitioners typically have four years of basic healthcare education—nursing school or medical school—and then additional education in a field of specialization. Physicians receive more training in the basic sciences than nurses, but nurses receive more education than physicians in the areas of health education and promotion, disease prevention, community and home-based care, and the facilitation of clients' access to community health services (Mundinger & Kane, 2000). The categories of advanced practice nurses include the following:

1. Clinical nurse specialist (CNS). *A clinical nurse specialist holds both a baccalaureate and a master's degree in nursing and has expertise in a specialized area of practice. Areas in which a CNS may work include primary care, acute care, restorative care, and community-based settings. In addition, the CNS may specialize in specific diseases, such as diabetes mellitus, cancer, or congestive heart failure, or in a specific field, such as obstetrics or acute care. A CNS may provide direct care as an expert clinician or may function as an educator, a case manager, a consultant, or a researcher (Potter & Perry, 1997).*
2. Nurse practitioner (NP). *A nurse practitioner is a registered nurse who has advanced education in nursing and clinical experience in a specialized area of nursing practice. NPs obtain certification in their area of practice by passing an examination administered by a professional organization, such as the American Nurse Credentialing Center. They are also licensed in the state in which they practice. NPs usually provide primary care to patients with common acute or stable medical conditions, often in an outpatient, ambulatory care, or community-based setting. A study published in the* Journal of the American Medical Association *found that nurse practitioners and physicians gave equally effective care to the patients in the study (Mundinger & Kane, 2000). It has been noted that, "one particularly strong element in the practice of the NP is the provision of patient education regarding lifestyles, health care options, and maintenance of normal function, no matter what the client's objective health status may be". (Schwirian & Moloney, 1998, p. 146).*
3. Certified registered nurse anesthetist (CRNA). *A nurse anesthetist is an RN who has received advanced training in an accredited program in anesthesiology. Most CRNA master's degree programs require two to three years of full-time study (Schwirian & Moloney, 1998). CRNAs provide all aspects of anesthesia care. Most CRNAs practice in hospital operating rooms, but they also provide service wherever patients require anesthesia, such as in physician's offices, outpatient surgery centers, labor and delivery rooms, and dentists' offices.*
4. Certified nurse-midwife (CNM). *A certified nurse-midwife is an RN who is also educated in midwifery and is certified by the American College of Nurse-Midwives. Most nurse-midwives hold master's degrees. The definition of nurse-midwifery today is "the independent management of women's health care, focusing particularly on pregnancy, childbirth, the post-partum period, care of the newborn, and family planning and gynecological needs of women" (Romaine-Davis, 1997, p. 132).*

Supporters of APNs suggest that the increased use of nurse practitioners as primary care providers is key to providing quality care to all consumers while holding down costs. Research has shown that the care provided by APNs is both *comparable in quality with* and *less expensive than* that provided by physicians (Safriet, 1993).

Physician's Assistants Another primary care giver is the physician's assistant (PA). Physician's assistants must complete a course of study ranging from one to four years in a university. Many persons who enroll in university physician assistant programs have prior medical or emergency training acquired in the military or previous healthcare occupations. PAs have no licensure of their own and must always work under the direction of a physician (Ellis & Hartley, 1998). In some states, PAs may prescribe medications. PAs provide routine primary care in hospitals, clinics, and private physicians' offices.

OTHER HEALTHCARE PROVIDERS

Many different kinds of healthcare workers provide professional and non-professional care in settings such as hospitals, clinics, external care facilities, and patients homes. These include professional nurses, licensed practical nurses, unlicensed assistive personnel, physical therapists, occupational therapists, respiratory therapists, paramedics, and emergency medical technicians.

Registered Nurses Registered nurses (RNs), otherwise known as *professional nurses,* are familiar providers of healthcare. Currently in the United States, an individual can become eligible to take the RN licensing examination by completing any one of three types of preparatory programs: a three-year hospital diploma program, a two-year associate degree program in a college, or a four-year baccalaureate degree program in a college or university. RNs work in a wide variety of settings, including physicians' offices, hospitals, clinics, schools, and home health agencies. Whereas many RNs provide direct care to patients and clients, others work in supervisory or other administrative capacities.

RNs who deal directly with consumers assess the healthcare needs of individuals and families and provide appropriate teaching, counseling, or care. RNs can initiate many of the services they provide independently but require a physician's order to administer medications and carry out certain procedures. The main focus of professional nursing is assisting individuals and families to achieve and maintain optimal health.

Licensed Practical Nurses A licensed practical nurse (LPN), or licensed vocational nurse (LVN), is trained in basic nursing techniques and provides direct patient care. LPNs and LVNs generally receive one year of education and training in a technical program, after which they are eligible to take the LPN/LVN licensing examination. LPNs and LVNs who work in hospitals and other healthcare agencies do so under the supervision of a registered nurse. LPNs and LVNs are also frequently employed in physicians' offices.

Unlicensed Assistive Personnel Unlicensed assistive personnel (UAP) are individuals who assist nurses in healthcare agencies. Also, many are employed in physicians' offices or the offices of other primary care providers. Such unlicensed healthcare workers as patient care technicians, certified medical technicians, and nursing assistants fall into the UAP category. Short, freestanding training programs leading to certification, or employee programs in agencies, provide the preparation for these occupations. UAP in healthcare agencies function under the direct supervision of an RN.

Physical Therapists Physical therapists (PTs) are licensed to assist physicians in examining, testing, and treating patients with physical disabilities. PTs usually receive their training in a six-year college program, which leads to a Master of Science degree in physical therapy (Potter & Perry, 1997). Treatment modalities used by physical therapists include the prescription and supervision of specific exercises and devices, the application of heat and cold, the use of sonar waves, and other treatment procedures. PTs practice in hospitals, clinics, rehabilitation centers, and home healthcare agencies.

Occupational Therapists Occupational therapists (OTs) work with patients who have physical limitations. They are licensed or certified to develop and use adaptive devices to assist such patients in performing the activities of daily living, such as bathing and feeding. OTs receive their education in four-year college programs in occupational therapy (Potter & Perry, 1997). Like PTs, OTs work in a variety of settings.

Respiratory Therapists Respiratory therapists (RTs) are licensed to deliver respiratory treatments to patients with respiratory problems or diseases. RTs can receive their basic education and training in six-month technical programs, two-year associate degree programs, or four-year baccalaureate programs (Potter & Perry, 1997). RTs are usually employed in healthcare institutions.

Social Workers Social workers provide certain kinds of counseling and services. Social workers who are employed in the mental health field provide psychotherapy to clients. Nonmental health social workers provide information about, and make arrangements for, community resources. They work with a variety of individuals and families: those facing severe or terminal illness, the elderly, the poor, and children. Social workers generally hold both a baccalaureate and a master's degree in social work (Potter & Perry, 1997).

Paramedics Paramedics provide advanced emergency medical care in *prehospital* settings, such as at the scene of accidents and in emergency transportation vehicles (ambulances). They receive extensive training in the identification, assessment, and treatment of a variety of sudden, life-threatening injuries and illnesses in certificate, associate degree, and, increasingly, baccalaureate degree programs. Paramedics work under the supervision of a physician through written standing orders or radio communication and are required to maintain current certification in their field.

Emergency Medical Technicians Emergency medical technicians (EMTs) also provide prehospital care. They receive approximately 128 hours of initial training in the administration of basic emergency care and the transportation of victims of acute illness or injury to a medical facility. EMTs receive ongoing training in new procedures and must qualify for national recertification every two years. EMTs often work as volunteers on community ambulances. Paid positions are available to them in healthcare institutions.

Getting the Best from Providers

In the managed care environment, healthcare priorities have been redefined. Emphasis has been shifted away from the treatment of illness and toward wellness and health (Grohar-Murray & DiCroce, 1997). The fact that consumers, especially among the middle class, are no longer content with only illness care and are demanding care to maximize wellness constitutes a major transformation in American culture. Easy access to health information, a growing recognition of their own rights, and dissatisfaction with the paternalistic attitude of some providers have caused many consumers to take a more active role in their own care. Consumers who feel personally invested in health promotion and health maintenance expect a higher level of response from healthcare providers and are often unwilling to blindly accept providers' recommendations. They wish to be both informed about their options and empowered to collaborate with providers.

A reality of the current managed care environment is that the need to keep costs down sometimes takes precedence over the need to provide high-quality care. Because of this, healthcare consumers must, more than ever, take charge of their health and healthcare.

CHOOSING A PROVIDER

Many consumers enrolled in managed care plans no longer have an unlimited choice as to who their primary care provider will be. Nevertheless, there is usually some element of choice. Most HMOs, PPOs, and other third-party providers give enrollees a list of primary care providers from which to choose. Individuals whose choice of provider is not restricted can obtain lists of providers from the local medical association or nearby hospitals. One strategy for choosing a primary care provider is to ask relatives, friends, and business associates for the names of providers in whom they trust and with whom they feel comfortable.

The provider-patient relationship is a very important one. Consumers must consider what characteristics they desire in a provider and then actively and assertively seek out providers who have those characteristics. For example, some consumers prefer providers who will collaborate with them in making decisions about care. Others, however, prefer providers who are more authoritarian. It is entirely appropriate for consumers to schedule appointments for the sole purpose of *interviewing* providers in whom they are interested. The following points should be considered when choosing a provider:

- Is the provider licensed by the state in which she practices and board certified in the specialty in which she practices?
- Is the provider taking new patients? A call to the health plan or provider's office will yield this information.
- Is the office open at a convenient time? Is it well staffed? How long must patients typically wait before

they can schedule an appointment? How many patients does the provider typically see in one hour?

- What is the office policy regarding payment? Must patients pay a certain amount for each visit or are they billed later?
- Who substitutes for the primary care provider when she is away?
- What provisions have been made for urgent care outside of office hours?
- Does the provider practice at a hospital covered by your insurance plan?

FOSTERING OPTIMAL PROVIDER-PATIENT COMMUNICATION

Provider-patient communication has suffered under managed care. HMOs often place restrictions on the amount of time providers can spend with individual patients. In order to obtain good care, consumers must make every minute count. Consumers who are seeing a provider for the first time must be prepared to answer questions about their medical history, including diseases and surgical procedures. Often, they will be given a checksheet to fill out in the waiting room. Providers will want to know about any diseases, such as diabetes, coronary heart disease, and breast cancer, that run in the family.

It is an excellent idea for consumers to write their most important symptoms and questions on a piece of paper and refer to it while conversing with the provider, and it is important to be as *specific* as possible. The more specific information the provider has, the more able she will be to assist the consumer.

It is important to be *open* and *frank* with providers. Many serious medical conditions could be treated early if patients were more willing to disclose problems and details that may be somewhat embarrassing. For example, many people are reluctant to discuss sexual problems or problems related to bowel or bladder function. If these problems are not addressed, however, successful treatment cannot occur.

Consumers who desire information about their illness, tests, or treatment should not hesitate to ask for it. Requesting printed material, which can be reviewed later, is always a good idea. Patients who are pressed for time can write down any medical terms they don't understand and look them up later. If the provider wishes to order a test, it is imperative that the consumer understands what the provider hopes to learn from the test and what, if any, risks are involved.

Consumers must not hesitate to be *assertive* with providers if the situation calls for it. For example, if a provider is standing with her hand on the doorknob and the consumer still has unanswered questions or is confused, the consumer must speak up and let the provider know that she has more questions. There is no reason for a consumer to leave a provider's office with unanswered questions. Being assertive with providers, especially traditionally minded physicians, is difficult for many. In the past, patients were not encouraged to question physicians' decisions or otherwise think for themselves. The paternalism of the past was harmful to patients then, and it has even more potential for being so now. In today's healthcare environment, consumers can ill afford to take a "doctor knows best" approach to their healthcare.

TAKING MEDICATIONS SAFELY

Medications, whether purchased over-the-counter (OTC) or by prescription, can be ineffective, or actually harmful, if not properly prescribed and used. Consumers must do everything they can to see that the appropriate medications are recommended or prescribed by healthcare providers and dispensed by pharmacists. Consumers must also learn about their medications in order to take them properly and be alert for complications.

Consumers can take steps that will greatly increase the likelihood that providers will prescribe or recommend drugs appropriately. Providers need certain information in order to make good decisions regarding drugs and other treatments. They need to know about any *allergic reactions* consumers have had; whether they are pregnant or breast-feeding; whether another doctor is treating them; whether they use alcohol, tobacco, or "street drugs"; and whether they have diabetes, kidney disease, or liver disease. Providers also need to be aware of all medications patients are already taking. This includes over-the-counter items, such as vitamins, herbs, aspirins, and laxatives, as well as prescription drugs.

Consumers sometimes fail to carry out providers' written instructions as to how a drug should be taken because they cannot read the instructions. Patients who cannot read what the provider has written must insist on clarification. Consumers can also ask the pharmacist who fills the prescription to review the manner in which the drug should be taken. A way of avoiding the possibility of taking harmful combinations of medications is to purchase all OTC drugs and have all prescriptions filled *at the same pharmacy.* Computer records of past purchases are kept, and pharmacists can warn customers who are about to add an incompatible drug to their regimen. This is especially important if the consumer has been getting prescriptions from more than one provider.

It is imperative that consumers take responsibility for learning about the drugs they are taking. Consumers can find out about side effects, contraindications, potential interactions with other drugs, and so on by asking their pharmacist or by consulting drug references, such as the *Physician's Desk Reference (PDR),* which can be found in libraries. The PDR provides information about almost every FDA-approved drug available. It is updated yearly, and consumers must be sure they are consulting the latest edition. Every prescription drug comes with a package insert, which contains extensive information about it. These inserts are not typically given to consumers, but consumers have a right to ask for and receive them. Pharmacists are excellent resources for the public. Pharmacists are healthcare professionals who have completed five to six years of postsecondary education in a college or university pro-

gram in pharmacology. Pharmacists are licensed by the states in which they practice. They provide information about drug reactions and side effects, whether drugs should be taken with food, and so on. Websites (see those listed in the Resources section at the end of this chapter) also provide reliable information about drugs. Consumers should know the following about every drug they are taking:

- The name of the drug, why they are taking it, and what it's supposed to do
- When and for how long the drug should be taken
- What the most likely side effects are and what should be done if they occur
- Whether any food, drink, activities, dietary supplements, or other drugs should be avoided while the drug is being taken

USING GENERIC VERSUS BRAND-NAME DRUGS

The difference between generic drugs and brand-name drugs is important for consumers to understand. A **generic name** is a name assigned to a chemical substance, such as the drug *acetominophin.* A **brand name** is the proprietary name a pharmaceutical company gives to the generic drug it markets. For example, the McNeil Pharmaceutical Company markets the drug *acetominophin* under the brand name *Tylenol.* Some companies, particularly pharmacy and grocery store chains, market their own line of generic drugs, which are less expensive than their brand-name twins. For example, the Weiss chain of grocery stores sells a generic acetominophin that is considerably less expensive than Tylenol. The label on the bottle reads Weiss Quality Pain Reliever with the word *acetominophin* written below.

Brand-name drugs are more expensive than generics, in part because they are heavily advertised; companies must charge more in order to offset advertising costs. Not all drugs are available in generic form, however. When a pharmaceutical company develops and patents a new drug, it may market that drug under a brand name for several years before other companies are allowed to do so, either generically or under their own brand names. Most established drugs, though, are available in generic form. In the case of prescription drugs, pharmacists are allowed to *substitute* generic drugs for brand-name versions with the approval of the patient who will purchase the drug. Consumers can keep medication costs down by choosing generic over brand-name drugs.

SEEKING HEALTH AND DRUG INFORMATION ON THE INTERNET

There is a vast amount of information about medications to be found on the Internet. Internet sites also contain information on diseases and treatments. Currently, there are more than 15,000 health sites that offer detailed information on hundreds of diseases and drugs. Consumers must be careful, however, because the information on the Internet is not always accurate and is often biased. It is best to use only websites associated with reputable healthcare agencies, organizations, and authorities. Organizations such as the American Medical Association, the American Heart Association, and the American Diabetes Association all maintain websites containing consumer information. A site specifically dedicated to pharmaceuticals, http://www.rxlist.com, contains lengthy articles about hundreds of prescription drugs. A wide range of information, including information about costs, is provided. The site also assists consumers in identifying unknown medications by matching the code imprinted on the tablet or capsule with information in an extensive database. Dr. Everett Koop (1999), former surgeon general of the United States, has a web page, www.drkoop.com, which rates about 1,500 sites for credibility and content and gives the public an opportunity to provide feedback. Commercial sites, the addresses of which end in *.com,* often contain useful and, in some cases, well-documented information. The information may, however, be biased in favor of products or services sold. Another thing about which consumers should be concerned is whether the information presented on a website is *current*. The date on which an article was posted on a website should be displayed. If it is not, it is unwise to assume that the information is current, as healthcare changes very rapidly. (The addresses of a sampling of reliable websites can be found in the Resources section at the end of this chapter.)

Dealing with Hospitalization

Patients who are acutely ill and in need of nursing and medical care are admitted to hospitals. Sometimes, patients have a choice as to which hospital they will be admitted; at other times, where they go is dictated by their health plan or the nature of their condition. There are two kinds of hospitals in which patients may find themselves: *teaching* hospitals and *nonteaching* hospitals. The two differ in some respects as regards medical care and medical staffing, as well as the experiences patients admitted to them are likely to have. Nursing care is generally organized in the same way in teaching and community (nonteaching) hospitals.

TEACHING HOSPITALS

Teaching hospitals generally have state-of-the-art equipment and, because of their *emphasis on research,* may offer innovative diagnostic and treatment procedures. Teaching hospitals also tend to attract top physician specialists who are involved in research along with their teaching and patient-care duties. Teaching hospitals are also usually affiliated with a *medical school,* which means that patients may interact with medical students, who are not yet licensed physicians, as well as with other types of students enrolled in programs in the health professions. Some examinations and procedures may be performed on patients by students who need to practice doing them, rather than by more experienced personnel.

In teaching hospitals, patients will likely receive at least some of their care from *resident physicians.* Resident physicians are licensed physicians who act as employees of the hospital while they undergo the training they need to become certified in their specialty. They are paid a modest salary to care for patients and may have anywhere from one month to several years of experience as practicing physicians. They may have limited or extensive experience with a given patient's particular problem. In some hospitals, residents in their first year of training are known as *interns*. If a patient's own physician is primarily responsible for the patient's care, she is referred to as the *attending* physician. On occasions when the attending physician is not available, or if there is no attending physician, resident physicians provide the patient's medical care.

NONTEACHING HOSPITALS

Hospitals not affiliated with medical schools do not have resident physicians who are completing a training program. Patients are cared for by their own private physicians or by physicians who have completed their training and have been hired by the hospital. Physicians in private practice who have the right to admit patients to the hospital and treat them there are said to have *privileges* in that hospital. Attending physicians may invite other physicians, usually specialists, to participate in their cases as *consultants,* both in nonteaching and teaching hospitals. If a patient in a nonteaching hospital develops a problem that does not constitute an emergency, the nursing staff generally contacts the patient's private physician. If she is not available, a designated substitute, or *covering* physician (who will not have previous knowledge of the patient's case), will be contacted. Hospitalized patients have certain rights, regardless of what type of hospital they are in. These rights are spelled out in The Patient's Bill of Rights, a document put out by the American Hospital Association, (see Box 9–1).

ACCREDITATION OF HOSPITALS

The Joint Commission on the Accreditation of Healthcare Organizations (JCAHO) is an independent organization that makes regular inspections of healthcare facilities and certifies that an institution's services and procedures meet predetermined high standards. Consumers may check on the accreditation of any hospital by calling the Joint Commission on the Accreditation of Healthcare Organizations at 630-792-5600. The commission's reports on individual hospital performances in 50 areas of activity are available to the public.

NURSING CARE

Patients are admitted to hospitals because they need nursing care in addition to medical treatment. If they did not need nursing care, their medical treatment would likely be provided on an outpatient basis (Mundinger, 1996). Nurses provide a wide range of services to patients. Some provide direct patient care, whereas others work in supervisory positions, or as coordinators of care.

One of the most important aspects of nursing care is ongoing patient *observation and assessment*. Professional nurses (RNs), assisted by LPNs and UAP, assess their patients' physical, emotional, and mental status frequently in order to gauge the effectiveness of medical treatment and to detect developing complications early. It is nurses who contact or summon physicians in the event of an emergency or a turn for the worse. Nurses also assess and meet patients' and family members' needs for education, emotional support, and assistance with coping. Nurses also administer most of the medications and treatments patients receive.

In addition to providing direct care to patients, registered nurses *supervise* patient care on all hospital units. The RN who bears 24-hour responsibility for the nursing care on a given hospital unit is referred to in most hospitals as the *nurse manager*. The RN who is in charge of the unit on a given shift (most RNs, LPNs and UAP work either 8- or 12-hour shifts) is the *charge nurse*. On some hospital units, RNs known as *team leaders* are responsible for the team of RNs, LPNs, and UAP who care for patients on *wings, halls,* or other subsets of larger hospital units. Patients who have concerns about the care they are receiving should not hesitate to ask to speak with the charge nurse or the nurse manager.

Most patients in hospitals are also assigned a *case manager,* an RN who has expertise regarding managed care. The patient's case manager coordinates the various aspects of the patient's care to ensure that the care provided is both cost-effective and high-quality. The case manager apprises patients and physicians of any impending problems regarding insurance coverage and may work to obtain authorization for additional care. Case managers also anticipate the care patients will need after discharge, and they expedite the needed paperwork and authorizations.

As hospitals are under tremendous pressure to keep costs down, RNs who provide direct care to patients are increasingly being replaced by LPNs, technicians, and aides (Blegen & Vaughn, 1998; Hall, 1997). Although these individuals may be highly conscientious and concerned about patient welfare, they have not had the same education as a professional nurse and do not have equal competencies. Indeed, research has shown that adequate staffing with professional nurses is linked with better patient outcomes. A study done by the Agency for Healthcare Research revealed that one additional hour of care by a registered nurse cuts a patient's risk of pneumonia by 8 percent and the risk of contracting a urinary tract infection by 10 percent (Kovner & Gergan, 1998). In another study (McCloskey, 1998), an inverse relationship was found between the number of hours of care patients received from RNs and rates of medication errors, bedsores, and patient complaints. Regrettably, presumably in an effort to disguise the scarcity of RNs, some hospitals forbid staff to place their titles (such as RN, LPN, or Technician) on their name tags. Patients have the right to know the credentials of the staff members who are caring for them and should not hesitate to ask. If credentials are not plainly visible on name tags, a complaint should be lodged with the hospital administrator.

Surgery

Although many medical procedures can be quite daunting for patients, perhaps none is as feared as surgery. Surgery can be performed in hospitals or in free-standing surgical centers if the patient is to go home afterward. Although some surgical procedures are more inherently risky than others, there is no such thing as *minor surgery*. Any surgical procedure requires special training and skill and involves risk. Patients who are told they need surgery should be sure to get a *second opinion*. Most health insurance programs now pay for second opinions concerning surgical procedures. Experience has shown that there are often alternatives to a given operation considered necessary by a particular physician. Some health plans actually *require* that a second opinion be obtained before they will pay for nonemergency surgeries.

There is no reason for consumers to feel embarrassed or uncomfortable about telling a surgeon they want to get another opinion. No reputable physician is threatened by this request. Consumers should immediately flee any physician who says something along the lines of, "I'm the best and, if you want another opinion, you don't want me." Any physician who displays that level of arrogance and disregard for her patient's concerns will likely be an unsatisfactory provider in other ways as well. Consumers should go *outside the practice* for a second opinion, rather than consulting one of the original physician's partners. Physicians in partnership are sometimes reluctant to disagree with each other and have an equal interest in the financial health of the practice.

Consumers who are scheduled for surgery must be sure to tell both the *surgeon* and the *anesthesiologist* of any pre-existing medical conditions or problems. A number of potent drugs are used to induce and maintain anesthesia, and the anesthesiologist bears a large part of the responsibility for the patient's welfare during surgery. It is never wise to assume that your surgeon or anesthesiologist is familiar with your medical history. Both the surgeon and the anesthesiologist should also be made aware of all medications patients are taking. This includes herbal preparations, as well as over-the-counter and prescribed medications. Aspirin, nonsteroidal anti-inflammatory drugs (such as ibuprofen), and high doses of blood-thinning herbs (see Chapter 11) should be avoided starting at least two weeks prior to surgery (Eliopoulous, 1999).

Because of the wide range of drugs that may be administered to surgical patients, it is imperative that medical and nursing personnel be aware of any allergies patients have. Allergies should be clearly marked on patients' charts and on their wrist bands. Wrist bands are put on when patients are admitted to hospitals, surgical clinics, and other medical facilities. The wrist band is an identifier of tremendous importance in medical environments. It lists the name of the patient and any substances to which she is allergic. Patients should make sure the information displayed on their wrist band is correct. This becomes critical if the patient becomes unconscious or otherwise unable to answer questions and supply information.

Although such occurrences are very uncommon, surgeons do sometimes make errors, such as mistaking one patient for another, performing the wrong operation, or operating on the wrong extremity (Blau, 1998). In order to obviate these possibilities, patients should confirm with the operating room staff the nature of the operation and which extremity is to be operated on. They may even use a felt-tipped pen to mark the area of the body to be operated on.

Surgical patients are usually told to *fast* for a certain period prior to surgery. Usually, they are instructed not to eat anything after midnight and not to drink for several hours before surgery. Patients must clarify with the surgeon or anesthesiologist whether they should take prescription medications on schedule prior to surgery. The purpose of making sure that the stomach is empty prior to surgery is to avoid the possibility that patients will vomit during or after surgery and **aspirate** (inhale stomach contents into their lungs). Aspiration is a serious complication, which can cause lung injury, pneumonia, and even death.

One of the things surgical patients are most worried about is *postoperative pain*. Patients should confer with their surgeon and anesthesiologist about what therapies will be used to decrease postoperative pain and should be assured that everything possible will be done to control pain. Studies show that pain is often inadequately treated in hospitals (Dufault & Sullivan, 2000) and in patients who have same-day surgery (Beauregard, Pomp, & Choiniere, 1998). Patients whose physicians do not seem to take preoperative concerns about pain seriously may be well advised to seek medical or surgical care elsewhere. Pain control is of more than subjective importance to patients. Pain stresses most systems in the body. Patients in pain often have higher blood pressure and heart rates than patients whose pain is controlled. Pain can also cause patients to breathe shallowly and not take in enough oxygen. After surgery, patients should not take a stoic attitude toward pain. They must report the presence of pain to the nurses and be prepared to describe its location and intensity. Patients must demand that adequate pain relief be provided.

Patients' Legal Rights

All patients who are receiving medical and/or nursing care, whether in their homes or in healthcare institutions, have certain legal rights. Patients have rights to knowledge about the nature of proposed treatments, rights to privacy regarding medical records, the right to refuse treatment, and the right to prepare documents about their care.

Informed Consent

Every consumer of medical care should be aware of a concept known as **informed consent,** an ethical standard in medicine that mandates that patients be given an explanation of their treatment that they fully understand. Patients who are mentally competent should be able to explain, in their own words, the reason for and nature of their treatment. They should know the statistical likelihood that the proposed procedure will accomplish what it's supposed to accomplish. Both the potential benefits and the accompanying risks must be identified clearly, and patients about to undergo treatment that is experimental must be informed of that fact. Consumers also have the right to expect that physicians will review with them all the feasible alternatives to the recommended treatment. Although there are no guaranteed outcomes in medicine, informed consent enables consumers to make rational decisions about their treatment.

Medical Records

The Joint Commission on the Accreditation of Healthcare Organizations (JCAHO) requires that all facilities treating patients maintain adequate medical records to serve as a basis for the planning of patient care and for continuity in the evaluation of the patient's condition and treatment. The medical record is where clinical information about the patient is recorded; it is a repository of information and a means for communication among healthcare providers involved in a patient's care.

The medical record serves other purposes as well. It is used as a *business record* of the hospital and is accessed by departments and personnel not involved in direct patient care, including administrative staff, quality-assurance and risk-management departments, finance departments, and peer review committees. External organizations, such as governmental organizations and accreditation bodies, monitor hospital and individual provider performance by reviewing medical records; third-party payers review medical records for reimbursement; and, in multiple types of litigation, the record serves as the principle source of evidence.

The owner of medical records is generally recognized to be the *healthcare facility* that made the record. Ownership does not prohibit access by the patient, but, in certain instances, such as when the patient is not competent to manage her affairs, the patient's requests for access may not be immediately be satisfied. In such instances, as with a request for medical records from a minor, the request will not be granted unless the legal guardian makes the request. Similarly, mental health records may not be immediately released to patients. The request may be circuited to the treating provider, who will issue an opinion as to whether the request should be honored.

Certain kinds of information contained in medical records will be disclosed to third parties, such as government agencies, because of *mandatory reporting requirements* stipulated in state health and public welfare statutes and by federal and government organizations. Information about certain infectious diseases, as well as suspected child abuse, suicides, and traumatic injury by gunshot or knife, must be released to the appropriate agency or body. Agencies and individual professionals who do not comply with mandatory reporting requirements may incur civil consequences (including fines, disciplinary proceedings, and licensure suspensions or revocations) and criminal penalties.

There is both an ethical and a legal basis for the confidentiality of medical information. The *ethical* principle of confidentiality, which is incorporated into the standards of all health professions, originates from the idea that an assurance of confidentiality encourages patients to seek needed medical care and to be candid about their conditions. People receiving medical care are entitled, both by case law and statute, to privacy regarding their conditions and the care received. The *legal* basis for confidentiality derives from the physician-patient privilege, which is a statutorial privilege. The physician-patient relationship is one of several relationships recognized by the law. The other recognized relationships are attorney-client, husband-wife, and priest-penitent. The preservation of confidentiality is deemed essential to the maintenance of these relationships. The need for confidentiality in the physician-patient relationship gives rise to a legal *privilege*, which means that, absent a patient authorization or waiver or an overriding law or public policy, physicians cannot be compelled to disclose medical information about a patient. Some states have extended the physician-patient privilege to other healthcare professionals. In the absence of a statute, however, there is no privilege between *nurses* who have acted independently and patients. If a nurse, a physician assistant, or another healthcare professional is employed by a physician, however, physician privilege generally extends to them as well.

Once privilege is determined to exist, it is considered to extend beyond oral communications and covers written entries in the medical record as well as lab results, X rays, and so on. For patient information to be privileged, it must satisfy certain criteria:

- It must have been communicated in the context of the physician-patient relationship.
- It must have been given with the expectation that it remain confidential.
- It must be necessary for the diagnosis and treatment of the patient.

These requirements mean that, although the patient is legally entitled to confidentiality with respect to her medical records concerning diagnosis and treatment, other information, such as a patient's name and address and the fact that she is receiving medical treatment, is not privileged.

An issue related to confidentiality is the need to balance the principle that patient information is private with the legitimate needs of individuals who require access to a medical record, even though they are not involved in a patient's care.

The privilege of confidentiality belongs to the patient, because that is the person for whose benefit it exists. In some cases, however, the patient does not even know that the release of confidential information about her medical care has been requested. For example, the attorneys for patient A, who is alleging negligence on the part of a provider or an institution, may request patient B's records to strengthen their case. In such instances, privilege on patient B's behalf is asserted by the physician or the healthcare institution. Frequently, the court will allow an in camera inspection, meaning that only the judge will view the records, to determine which materials are relevant. Identifying information may be deleted from the materials found to be relevant. Although privilege can be *asserted* by someone other than the patient on the patient's behalf, only the patient or the patient's legal representative can *waive* privilege.

Patients who bring a personal injury lawsuit concerning a medical condition for which they were treated or who otherwise disclose, or consent to the disclosure of, a significant part of the communications previously made to a treating physician lose the privacy privilege. The reason for the implicit waiver is that the patient has placed information about her medical condition in issue and is no longer entitled to privilege.

According to standards set by the JCAHO, patient information may be used in both internal and external reviews of the performance of healthcare organizations without patients' consent. Committees and organizations created to conduct peer review or quality of care reviews have access to patient records. Committee members must carefully balance their dual responsibilities to protect patients and to be fair to those under review.

The Health Care Quality Improvement Act (HCQIA) of 1986—intended to further protect the public from unqualified, incompetent, or criminal healthcare providers—was passed by Congress in October 1986 and signed by President Reagan on November 14, 1986. It requires that certain disciplinary actions taken against providers, as well as licensure sanctions and malpractice convictions, be reported to the National Practitioner Data Bank.

The HCQIA applies to organizations that are "healthcare entities," including hospitals, HMOs, group medical practices, professional societies, and other entities that provide healthcare services and follow a formal peer review process. It does not apply to POSs, PPOs and similar "broker" organizations because they do not actually provide care.

The storage and transfer of medical records via computers has created new challenges to patient privacy. State departments of health and departments of public welfare, which set forth the regulations that govern electronic recordkeeping and electronic communication are hard put to produce guidelines that are specific enough to provide direction and protection yet are broad enough to encompass rapid technology growth. States are in varying stages of regulation development; some are drafting their first electronic regulatory language that provides direction and protections beyond the written medical record, whereas others have this basic language and are in the process of refining it.

Issues related to the protection of computerized and electronic records become even more complicated as *interstate transmission* of patient records and information from one healthcare provider or institution to another become more commonplace, because laws regarding confidentiality, privilege, and disclosure laws may differ from state to state.

Patient information related to substance abuse, mental health treatment, and HIV/AIDS diagnosis and treatment is managed and treated in a special manner. Mandates for the special protection of privacy in these highly sensitive areas can be found in a variety of statutes and regulations.

SUBSTANCE ABUSE

Some states require healthcare providers to report or keep records of the names of persons for whom addictive drugs are prescribed. When the constitutionality of such a statute was challenged in *Whalen v. Roe*, the U.S. Supreme Court upheld the state statute, finding that it was a reasonable exercise of the state's broad police powers and did not unduly infringe on the patient's right of privacy.

States have statutes that regulate the accessibility and confidentiality of alcohol and other drug-abuse records. Most state's acts provide that alcohol and other drug-abuse patient records are confidential and may be disclosed (in a nonemergency situation) only with the patient's consent and then only to medical personnel for the treatment of the patient or to government and other officials who are privy to such information. Most regulations prohibit treatment facilities from disclosing whether an identified individual is or has been diagnosed or treated for substance abuse; however, under certain circumstances, they may disclose that a given individual has never been treated in the facility. Substance-abuse record regulations also contain guidelines for the disclosure of the records of minor, incompetent, and deceased patients.

As with other types of patient records, hospitals and other drug-treatment facilities may release confidential information without the patient's written consent for such purposes as data processing, bill collecting, and audit and evaluation activites. They may also release patient information to entities having direct administrative control over the program, as well as to elements of the criminal justice system that referred the patient to the program. Information may also be released in certain circumstances involving crimes committed on the program's premises or against program personnel and involving suspected child abuse and neglect.

Confidential substance-abuse records will be released in response to a court order. Federal regulations mandate court orders and a subpoena must be issued to compel disclosure. Under the federal regulations, a court order authorizing disclosure may only be issued if patient information related to drug treatment meets one of the following criteria:

1. *Disclosure of the information is necessary in order to protect against an existing threat to life or serious bodily injury.*
2. *Disclosure of the information is necessary in connection with the investigation or prosecution of an extremely serious crime, such as the purchase of a firearm by a person addicted to controlled substances.*
3. *Disclosure of the information is necessary in connection with a legal proceeding in which the patient will offer evidence regarding confidential information.*

Most regulations require that programs notify their patients regarding the federal confidentiality requirements at the time of admission. The notification usually provides the patient a written summary, which includes the following information:

1. *A general description of the exceptions to the confidentiality protections*
2. *A statement that violation of the confidentiality statute and regulations is a crime and that suspected violations may be reported in accordance with the regulations*
3. *A statement that the regulations do not protect information relating to patient crimes on the program premises*
4. *A statement that reports of suspected child abuse and neglect required under the state law are not protected*
5. *Copies of pertinent statutes and regulations*

In the event that federal drug and alcohol abuse confidentiality laws and regulations conflict with state laws, the law that imposes the more *strict* control on disclosure of confidential information obtains.

MENTAL HEALTH

Psychiatric records also have special protection. All state regulations pertaining to privacy include an act that is specific to psychiatric records. A fundamental issue in the area of mental health is the determination of **competency.** Generally, people who lack the capacity to know and understand the effect of their actions are not competent to give valid authorization for the disclosure of their medical record information. If a mentally incompetent patient consents to the release of confidential information, a valid later claim may be asserted that the consent was invalid by reason of incompetency.

As a general rule, confidential patient information is not released to law enforcement officials without patient consent or statutory authority for release. In some states, however, a healthcare provider may be able to disclose information to law enforcement officers on the basis of **qualified privilege.** Qualified privilege is a common-law concept that provides immunity from civil liability for the communication of information by a person who has an interest in making the communication to someone acting in an official capacity who has a duty or an interest in receiving the information. Clear guidelines as to the circumstances under which a healthcare provider must or should release information do not exist. The duty not to disclose confidential information may be outweighed by a duty to take reasonable steps to protect third parties from foreseeable harm.

HIV/AIDS

Most states have enacted statutes designed to protect the confidentiality of patient information relating to testing for the human immunodefiency virus (HIV), which causes acquired immune deficiency syndrome (AIDS) and AIDS-related complex (ARC). Such regulations are designed to balance the privacy interests of a person against the need for information that will assist in controlling the spread of AIDS and protect people who are at risk for infection by the infected person. Most statutes have clear language regarding consent to testing, confidentiality requirements, and the penalties for unauthorized testing and disclosure of confidential information.

The information generally covered by HIV confidentiality statutes and regulations includes:

1. *Any information that is likely to identify someone as having been tested for or actually having HIV infection, antibodies to HIV, AIDS, or related infections or illnesses or someone suspected of having HIV as a result of high-risk activities*
2. *Any information pertaining to an application for or recipient of treatment, services, or benefits*
3. *Information about an individual's family or partner(s)*

Information is generally covered regardless of the source—that is, the client and the client's family or partner—and regardless of whether it was obtained from oral, written, or electronic communication and regardless of whether the information was obtained intentionally or unintentionally. In states that lack specific AIDS confidentiality legislation, HIV/AIDS-related records are protected by general public health record confidentiality laws.

State and federal law may conflict in certain situations. For example, a state statute may permit the disclosure of confidential HIV-related information for the purpose of warning the spouse or sexual partner of an infected patient or for warning healthcare workers. This type of disclosure would be permitted under the federal regulations only in situations constituting a medical emergency or after obtaining a court order.

National Practitioner Data Bank

The **National Practitioner Data Bank** is a mandatory reporting agency to which some healthcare professionals must report lawsuits brought against them and the outcome. Access to information in the data bank is limited to hospitals and other healthcare entities, state medical and dental licensing boards, plaintiffs' attorneys in very limited circumstances, and individual physicians and dentists. Many consumer groups are lobbying for this information to become public. At the same time, many large and powerful organizations, such as medical and hospital associations, are lobbying to retain limited access.

Refusing Treatment

The competent patient at all times has the right to refuse treatment and to leave a healthcare facility. The hospital staff will document that the patient is refusing a treatment, or the staff will document that a patient has left the hospital *against medical advice (AMA)*.

Competency, Incompetency, Advance Directives, and Living Wills

Under most circumstances, adults are considered competent to make decisions regarding their healthcare and otherwise to manage their own affairs unless they have been declared incompetent by a judge in a court of law. All too often, however, unforeseen illnesses and accidents render an individual incapable of making decisions. In the absence of legal documents called **advance directives,** family members or even institutions will have to petition the court to grant them the right to make decisions on behalf of the incapacitated person. Such petitions are time-consuming and expensive and are avoidable if individuals plan ahead for the possibility that they may become incapacitated. Advance directives include legal documents, such as living wills and durable powers of attorney for healthcare. In a durable power of attorney for healthcare, one or more individuals are designated as guardians, who are able to make decisions related to healthcare on behalf of another person who has become incapacitated. It is highly advantageous to have such a document in place before the need arises.

The following scenario illustrates the consequences an unforeseen incapacitation in a person who has prepared no advance directives:

Sue is a healthy, athletic, 25-year-old single woman. However, she begins to have low back pain, which persists for several days. On the third day, the pain is so severe that Sue cannot get out of bed. She calls her parents, who live nearby, and they take her to the hospital. In the Emergency Department, Sue's condition is diagnosed as appendicitis, and she undergoes abdominal surgery.

The surgeon observes that Sue's problem is not related to her appendix. Infectious disease physicians are consulted because Sue's temperature and white blood cell count are rising out of control. Sue's condition deteriorates over the two days following surgery and she becomes unconscious. Sue has no documents in place that allow her family to pay her bills, otherwise manage her affairs, or have a say in her medical treatment. Sue now needs to have a guardian appointed by the court.

Sue's family has to hire an attorney to petition the court to appoint them as Sue's guardians. This process requires that two physicians testify that Sue is indeed incompetent. The two physicians and the attorney each submit a bill in excess of $500 for their services, but this is not the end of the expenses involved. The guardianship was granted on an emergency basis and is time-limited. After 72 hours, the attorney and two

physicians are required to go back into court, so that the nature of the guardianship can be changed. The attorney and the physicians submit additional bills— again each in excess of $500.

Had Sue prepared a durable medical power of attorney naming her parents as guardians in the event she became incapacitated, much distress and expense would have been avoided.

Living wills are a means by which individuals can convey to healthcare providers and family members their wishes as to what should and should not be done in the event that they suffer a life-threatening illness or accident. Some people, for example, would not want treatment to prolong their lives if they were to suffer irreversible brain damage. Also, many persons suffering from terminal diseases, or who are extremely elderly, do not want to be resuscitated should their heart function or breathing stop. Living wills can be quite specific; for example, an individual could stipulate that, in the event pneumonia develops, she does not wish to receive antibiotics but does wish to be hydrated via intravenous therapy if necessary. Living wills are legal in some states, but not all. Individuals may prepare their own documents or use standard forms (see Chapter 28). It is best, however, to have an attorney review the document—especially to confirm that it is signed properly. Some states require the signatures of two witnesses and that all signatures be *notarized*. It is difficult to prepare a living will comprehensive enough to cover all possible circumstances; some interpretation is usually necessary. For that reason, it is imperative that individuals discuss their living wills with family members and review their exact wishes regarding possible scenarios. Family members who truly understand a loved one's values and desires are more likely to see that they are heeded. Copies of the living will should be given to family members and the family physician.

New Directions

A need has been recognized for more research on the ways and means of enhancing the quality and effectiveness of health services in this age of managed care and acute shortages of nurses and other healthcare personnel (Clark, 2001). For example, downsizing in healthcare facilities has resulted in a staff mix that includes fewer registered nurses and licensed practical nurses and more unlicensed assistive personnel (Clark, 2001). Some have suggested that this trend has led to a decreased quality of care, as reflected in morbidity and mortality rates, and corrective legislation has been proposed to mandate certain RN-to-patient ratios (Jacobson, 2001). However, the exact mix of RNs, LPNs, and UAP needed to provide quality care to high, low, and intermediate acuity (relative amount of care needed) patient populations is not known. Additional research in this area is needed to provide policymakers with the information they need to improve the healthcare system's ability to deliver high-quality, accessible healthcare at a reasonable cost.

QUESTIONS FOR REFLECTION AND DISCUSSION

1. *In what ways has managed care affected American's Health?*
2. *What changes in the healthcare system do you, as a consumer, advocate?*
3. *What steps could you take to obtain better healthcare for yourself?*
4. *Would you consider becoming politically active in healthcare legislation? Why or why not?*
5. *Do you have a living will? Why or why not?*
6. *What are the developing threats to privacy regarding medical information and the possible consequences?*

RESOURCES

Books

Blau, S. P. (1998). *How to get out of the hospital alive.* New York: Macmillan.

Websites

Adam.com—A San Francisco–based commercial provider of high-quality health information. Has a distinguished health advisory panel. www.adam.com

CancerNet—A service of the National Cancer Institute. Provides information on various types of cancer, clinical trials, treatment options, support groups, and other support services. www.cancernet.nci.nih.gov

Centers for Disease Control and Prevention—Provides consumer information on health news and a variety of subjects related to health and lifestyle, health and travel, and so on. www.cdc.gov

C. Everett Koop—Headed by the former surgeon general, this commercial site offers news, feature articles on health, and links to on-line support communities for a variety of illnesses. www.drkoop.com

Healthfinder—Maintained by the U.S. Department of Health and Human Services. Provides basic self-care information, information about government health projects, and links to other health sites. www.healthfinder.gov

InteliHealth—Maintained by the Aetna U.S. Healthcare Company and Johns Hopkins University. Provides user-friendly physician-reviewed articles on many topics, an Ask the Doc feature, and a medical dictionary. www.intelihealth.com

Mayo Clinic Health Oasis—Maintained by the Mayo Clinic. Provides physician-reviewed articles that are easy for consumers to understand. Also allows users to e-mail questions to physicians at the clinic. www.mayohealth.org

OncoLink—This cancer-oriented site is maintained by the University of Pennsylvania Cancer Center. Offers news; information on treatment and available clinical trials; a list of useful institutions, organizations, and support groups; and an on-line support community. www.oncolink.upenn.edu

United States National Library of Medicine—Consumer access to the world's largest medical library is available at www.nlm.nih.gov. General health information can be found at www.nlm.nih.gov/medlineplus.

The book *Making a killing: HMOs and the threat to your health,* by Jamie Court and Frank Smith, has been made available, at no charge, on the internet at http://makingakilling.org.

REFERENCES

Beauregard, L., Pomp, A., & Choiniere, M. (1998). Severity and impact of pain after day-surgery. *Canadian Journal of Anesthesia, 45*(4), 304–311.

Blau, S. P. (1998). *How to get out of the hospital alive.* New York: Macmillan.

Blegen, M. A., & Vaughn, T. (1998). A multisite study of nurse staffing and patient occurrences. *Nursing Economics, 16*(4), 196–203.

Clancy, C. M., & Brody, H. (1995). Managed care: Jekyll or Hyde? *Journal of the American Medical Association, 273,* 338–339.

Clark, M. (2001, April 9). The impact of downsizing on nurses and patients. *Advance for Nurses,* p. 29.

Dufault, M. A., & Sullivan, M. (2000). A collaborative research utilization approach to evaluate the effects of pain management standards on patient outcomes. *Journal of Professional Nursing, 16*(4), 240–250.

Eliopoulos, C. (1999). *Integrating conventional and alternative therapies.* St. Louis: Mosby.

Ellis, R. J., & Hartley, C. L. (1998). *Nursing in today's world.* New York: Lippincott.

Grohar-Murry, M., & DiCroce, H. (1997). *Leadership and management in nursing.* Stanford, CT: Appleton & Lange.

Hall, L. M. (1997). Staff mix models: Complementary or substitution roles for nurses. *Nursing Administration Quarterly, 21*(2), 31–39.

Is an HMO Right for You? (1996, November). *AARP Bulletin, 37*(10), 2.

Jacobson, N. (2001, April 9). Nursing advocates tackle the nursing shortage. *Advance for Nurses,* p. 22.

Koop, C. E. (1999, May). Dr. Koop's guide to managed care. *Reader's Digest,* 39–41.

Kovner, C., & Gergen, P. J. (1998). Nurse staffing levels and adverse events following surgery in U.S. hospitals. *Image: Journal of Nursing Scholarship, 30*(4), 304–311.

Lancaster, J. (1999). *Nursing issues.* Philadelphia: Mosby.

McCloskey, J. M. (1998). Nurse staffing and patient outcomes. *Nursing Outlook, 46*(5), 199–200.

Mundinger, M. O. (1996). New alliances: Nursing's bright future. *Nursing Administration Quarterly, 20*(3), 50–53.

Mundinger, M. O., & Kane, R. L. (2000). Health outcomes among patients treated by nurse practitioners or physicians. *Journal of the American Medical Association, 28*(1), 59–68, 106–108.

Potter, P. A., & Perry, A. (1997). *Fundamentals of nursing.* Philadelphia: Mosby.

Pyenson, B., & O'Connor, J. (2000, March). 1.5 million Americans must buy their own health insurance. How to choose wisely. *Bottom Line Personal, 1*(3), 1–16.

Romaine-Davis, A. (1997). *Advanced practice nurses: Education, roles, trends.* Sudbury, MA: Jones & Bartlett.

Safriet, B. J. (1993, March). Health care dollars and regulatory sense: The role of the advanced practice nurse. *Issue Bulletin,* p. 3.

Schwirian, D., & Moloney, M. (1998). *The professionalization of nursing.* St. Louis, MO: Mosby.

Swansburg, R. C., & Swansburg, R. J. (1999). *Introductory management and leadership for nurses.* Sudbury, MA: Jones & Bartlett.

10

Nontraditional Healthcare: Emerging into Integrative Healthcare

Valerie Lincoln

CHAPTER OUTLINE

Objectives

1. *Compare and contrast the traditional Western healthcare model with the holistic healthcare model.*
2. *Demonstrate an understanding of how the traditional bioscience model of healthcare is evolving into an integrated model, which includes elements of the traditional model and the holistic model.*
3. *Identify the philosophical and cultural influences associated with the emergence of the integrative healthcare model.*
4. *Discuss ways in which people's cultural, familial, and social backgrounds influence their healthcare choices.*
5. *Describe the major characteristics and foundational constructs of selected complementary and alternative therapies used in integrated healthcare.*

Introduction

Recent decades have seen a dramatic and controversial shift in the healthcare delivery system in this country. The model of healthcare considered traditional in Western culture has been, and continues to be, challenged by what has become known as the holistic health care model. DiLama and Painter (1998) characterize the holistic healthcare model as one that embraces "a more encompassing perspective of what comprises health, what causes illness and how successful outcomes should be defined" (p. vii). The nature of this model will be addressed more fully in the section on the holistic healthcare paradigm.

Definition and Clarification of Terms

Various terms have been used to describe both the model of healthcare that has been dominant in Western culture (the traditional Western healthcare model), and the newer model that is challenging its primacy (the holistic healthcare model). It is important to understand what is meant by the terms traditional Western healthcare and holistic healthcare. It is also important to understand terms such as alternative, complementary, and integrative, that have arisen as the relationship between the traditional Western healthcare model and the holistic healthcare model continues to evolve.

The Traditional Western Healthcare Model

The traditional Western healthcare model has as its goals the control and eradication of disease and the treatment of disease, particularly acute disease, and injury. It is foundationally supported by **bioscience**—that is, the basic and technological sciences, including pharmaceutics and others. Although the tremendous contributions and advances of this system, known as **traditional healthcare,** are undeniable, its limitations are becoming increasingly obvious. For example, the sometimes inappropriate use of technology conflicts with some of the values and ethics of our society, as when life and suffering are prolonged artificially and unnecessarily. The focus on *acute* diseases and conditions has been at the cost of a decreased emphasis on health promotion, the treatment of chronic disease, and support for psychospiritual health. The insistence on using only those techniques focused on by medical schools allows us to advance only along narrow, bioscience-focused parameters (DiLama & Painter, 1998).

The Holistic Healthcare Model

The holistic healthcare model was first colloquially known as **alternative medicine.** However, it was clear that the term *alternative* connotes an either-or approach to medical care and placed alternative medicine in opposition to the traditional healthcare model. Over time, alternative medicine became known as **complementary medicine** to denote the supportive attributes of the treatments, philosophy, and modalities of this system of healthcare. Even that term, however, suggests subservience to the traditional healthcare model. The label *complementary* has since been conjoined with the label *alternative* to create **complementary and alternative medicine (CAM).** The latest permutation of labeling this model of emergent healthcare is *integrative* healthcare. **Integrative healthcare** is a blend of the best of both traditional healthcare and CAM. This term more accurately reflects reality, in that nontraditional practices and treatments are usually used along with, rather than in place of, traditional interventions (Eisenberg et al., 1993).

The labeling of the dominant system as *traditional healthcare* is highly specific to western culture. What we in America consider new and nontraditional is both familiar and traditional in many other cultures. For instance, in China, medical practitioners often study primarily traditional Chinese medicine (TCM) and augment their healthcare with the techniques, drugs, and technology of Western medicine. The Chinese healthcare system is founded on the tools, techniques, and practices that we in the Western world consider to be CAM.

The Emergence of Holistic Healthcare

The holistic healthcare model has emerged as a serious challenge to the traditional Western model because of a number of factors. These factors include sanction by reputable medical professionals with mainstream credentials, official government recognition, consumer demand, globalization and knowledge expansion, and shifts in our cultural paradigms.

Governmental and Organizational Recognition

The holistic/integrative healthcare movement gained substantial credibility by the establishment of the Office of Complementary and Alternative Medicine by the National Institutes of Health. The office was later more appropriately named the **National Center for Complementary and Alternative Medicine (NCCAM).** The U.S. Congress created this center in 1992 to facilitate the formal evaluation of CAM and to support the integration of effective treatments into mainstream care. To address the issue nationally, a 1996 conference cosponsored by the NCCAM was convened. A panel recommended that complementary care content be integrated into the curricula of medical and nursing schools. Moreover, the NCCAM has recommended that national centers of excellence be developed to foster collaboration among complementary practitioners, nurses, and physicians and to promote synergy among education, research, and clinical practice.

Currently, hundreds of American schools, colleges, and universities are actively involved in teaching, research, and practice that supports the credibility of holistic healthcare. Two examples of this are Western Michigan University in Kalamazoo and the University of Minnesota in Minneapolis. In fact, Western Michigan University has offered a graduate certificate program in holistic healthcare since the mid 1970s. In 1997, the University of Minnesota established the Center for Excellence in Complementary Care in its Academic Health Center.

As a reflection of the emergence of holism into professional practice, several professional organizations have evolved. Three of the most prominent professional organizations are the **American Holistic Medical Association (AHMA),** the **American Holistic Nurses Association (AHNA),** and the **American Holistic Health Association (AHHA).** There are currently several jurried alternative and complementary professional healthcare journals, which are dedicated to the analysis and integration of these therapies. Subspecialty journals often focus on integrative therapy as it relates to their own specialties.

Consumer Demand

There are many divergent influences operational in all evolutionary processes. Consumer demand has been the most pivotal influence related to access to the increasing availability of CAM services in the United States. The public's interest in nonconventional healthcare has risen dramatically in recent years. Eisenberg et al. (1993) at Harvard Medical School demonstrated that one of every three adults in the United States uses a complementary treatment for a health problem. From 1990 to 1997, Americans made more visits to alternative practitioners than they did to traditional practitioners, spending $13.7 billion; $10.5 billion were paid out of-pocket (Eisenberg et al., 1998). Ornish, Brown, and Scherwitz (1990) caught the attention of cardiologists all over the world when they published research that indicated that lifestyle change could not only improve clinical outcomes in persons with coronary heart disease but actually reverse the atherosclerotic process as well.

It has long been recognized that women direct the spending of the vast majority of healthcare dollars. Women dominate the healthcare market and have demonstrated they can be a very powerful force for change. For example, in the 1970s and 1980s, women consumers demanded a more harmonious, healing, and conducive atmosphere in which to experience childbirth. At that time, healthcare providers unilaterally managed deliveries, and women had little say as to the circumstances under which they gave birth. Women demanded change, and the result was no less than a revolution in childbearing.

Financial reimbursement is a very potent influence on the integration of systems. Clearly, the public's willingness to financially support integrative healthcare by spending billions of dollars has encouraged the conventional healthcare system to take notice and to look very closely at the integration of holistic services. An obstacle for many who desire CAM services is a lack of financial reimbursement by third-party payers. Both holistic service providers and consumers have actively pursued this issue. In 1996, Washington was the first state to legally require all insurers and managed care organizations to ensure that subscribers have access to the services of licensed alternative healthcare providers. Since 1996, other states, healthcare systems, and third-party payers have begun to cover the costs of select holistic services.

Globalization and Knowledge Expansion

Another influence on the introduction of integrative healthcare is the incredible rate at which knowledge increases. It has been estimated that humanity had doubled its collective knowledge by A.D. 1500 and had doubled that by 1750—a span of only 150 years. Projections suggest that from now on, the collective knowledge of human civilizations will double every year (Russell, 1992). The advent of the Internet has extraordinarily influenced the proliferation of and access to information related to holistic healthcare.

Globalization has also eased the assimilation of Eastern healing systems into mainstream and holistic healthcare structures. The cultural exchange between the West and China began in the 1960s, with a toast by then President Nixon to Chairman Mao of China. Since then, the fruits of thousands of years of clinical and practical experience with Eastern healing modalities have become available to other cultures around the globe.

Evolving Cultural Paradigms

Transitions such as the integration of healthcare take place because of a variety of influences, of which one is cultural. Sociocultural researcher Ray (1996) has identified a subset within American culture that is comprised of individuals who have interest and investment in holistic healthcare. Ray classifies this subset as the **integral culture.** No longer marginalized, this group consists of nearly 44 million Americans, or 25 percent of the general population. Individuals in this subset, many of whom are women, are concerned with issues such as alternative healthcare, psychology, self-expression, spirituality, self-actualization, social welfare, and the environment.

The individuals who comprise the integral culture subscribe to a different world view, or **paradigm,** than those who do not. A paradigm is the lens through which we compare and contrast all of our experiences in the world. Achterberg (1998) characterizes paradigms as myths that codify beliefs, enforce morality, dictate rituals of healing and politics, and influence culture through the acts of everyday life.

There are five evolving cultural paradigm shifts that continue to influence the integration of holistic healthcare into mainstream culture. The paradigm transitions that are most influential to the integration of holistic healthcare are human centeredness to ecocentrism, time focus to timelessness, mechanism to integration, patriarchy to balance, and designed to natural (Andrus et al., 1999; Lincoln, 1998).

HUMAN CENTEREDNESS TO ECOCENTRISM

Human centeredness, or **anthropocentrism,** is the view that human concerns and needs are primary over all other concerns in creation. An anthropocentric perspective is one in which concerns related to individual humans and human society take precedence over concerns related to other species, the environment, and so on. An **ecocentric perspective,** in contrast, is grounded in the recognition that all of nature, and the entire cosmos, is sacred. All of creation is valued equally, and this value is seen as intrinsic rather than bestowed by humankind. The spiritual insight that human beings are a part of creation rather than the point of creation leads naturally to a greater concern for the integrity of the environment. Holistic health care practitioners are united in their contention that individuals must have access to pure food, water, and air in order to be well, and this point of view is supported by a growing body of evidence that links the health of humankind and the health of the environment.

TIME FOCUS TO TIMELESSNESS

Time focus refers to the phenomenon of great social importance being placed on time. For example, in the United States, which is an exceedingly time-focused culture, watches and clocks are everywhere and deadlines are an important source of stress. There are, however, vast intercultural differences regarding the importance placed on time. For example, many cultures base their time perspective not on days, hours, and seconds but on the dawning day, shifting moon, and changing seasons.

The subjective experience of time is not constant. In some circumstances, five minutes can feel like five hours; in others, like five seconds. Furthermore, we have all experienced moments in which time seems to stand still and we become **timeless.** Time is not objectively constant, either. In his theory of relativity, Einstein demonstrated that velocity and the rate at which time passes are inversely related. For example, Einstein maintained that, if one twin went space traveling at the speed of light and returned after 20 years, she would appear younger than her sister who had remained on earth (Hawking, 1998). Although few would wish to do away entirely with time as a concept, decreasing its exaggerated importance in many societies would reduce overall stress and allow for more *being* as opposed to *doing.* The term *being* refers to a state in which one is fully in touch with one's inner experience in the present moment—one is fully aware of feelings and physical sensations. *Doing,* in contrast, involves focusing on a task and its future consequences. Doing takes the focus away from the self. Excessive doing at the expense of being can result in constant time pressure and stress. Doing is often used as a method of distracting oneself from painful thoughts and emotions. Holistic practitioners typically recommend meditation, yoga, and other practices that direct attention to the present moment, to individuals suffering from a wide range of physical and emotional problems. The benefits of such practices are addressed in Chapters 7 and 11.

MECHANISM TO INTEGRATION

The **mechanistic paradigm** is the view that any whole is no more than the sum of its parts and that the parts operate in isolation from one another. The mind/body separation articulated by French scientist and philosopher René Descartes inaugurated a mechanistic view of human beings, which has persisted unchallenged until recently. Einstein, however, brought us a science of *relationship* via his theory of relativity, and Bohm's (1998) theories of quantum physics guide us toward a science of **inseparability and integration.** These concepts have several implications for the holistic healthcare model. One of the most important is that macrosystems (such as the environment) and the microsystems they contain (such as human beings) influence one another. Another is that the three major domains of personhood, the physical, the mental, and the spiritual, are interrelated and inseparable. Consequently, holistically inclined healthcare practitioners assess the physical, mental, and spiritual health of those who consult them, regardless of the nature of the symptom that has motivated a patient to seek care.

PATRIARCHY TO BALANCE

Patriarchy is the male-centeredness and male dominance pervasive in most societies today. Values traditionally perceived to be masculine, such as science, technology, and defense, are often seen as more important than values traditionally perceived to be *feminine,* such as the arts, human services, environmental issues, and efforts for peace and cooperation (Elkins, 1995). Both masculine and feminine energies are associated with the core values of our culture. However, the masculine influence has been predominant. A shift toward **balance** would integrate so-called feminine values equally with so-called male values. Persons with a holistic worldview often work on behalf of the environment, world peace, and social justice. Holistic health practitioners generally see personal authenticity as an important component of health, and encourage individuals of both genders to free themselves from the influence of gender role stereotypes and get in touch with their true talents, inclinations, desires, passions, and so on.

DESIGNED TO NATURAL

The speed with which technology has become pervasive in our culture is impressive, and there is no doubt that it has brought many benefits. It has also, however, challenged our natural environment to a degree that has alarmed many. Consequently, Americans are beginning to accept the notion that an ecological, organic, sustainable cultural framework is essential to our very survival. The fact that we are beginning to shift from overvaluing that which is *artificial* to revaluing that which is *natural* is evident in many aspects of our culture. For example, the superiority of natural foods over highly processed foods is now evident to many. Natural fibers, such as cotton, flax, silk, and wool, are often preferred over synthetics. Indeed, the most popular synthetics are those that appear most natural. The cultural metaphors of clockwork and machines are transitioning toward metaphors that reflect an organic and ecological worldview (Petzinger, 1999). Though few would wish to return to a pre-industrial way of life, many yearn for a more balanced existence in which human beings are more in tune with the natural world. A major tenet of the holistic paradigm is that it is essential that our society devise ways of living that do not ultimately deplete our natural resources and pollute our environment, and it is essential that we reacquaint ourselves with our spiritual connection to all of creation.

Foundational Concepts of the Holistic Healthcare Paradigm

The holistic healthcare paradigm as a philosophy and model is being increasingly embraced by a wide range of healthcare providers, including physicians and nurses. Several foundational concepts, healing whole person care, challenge and opportunity, and reciprocity and right relationship, underlie the holistic philosophy (Johnson, 1990). Additional important concepts/premises include belief as a catalyst of healing, transpersonality, alignment and congruence, consciousness, energy, connectedness, coherence, and entrainment.

Healing

In holistic philosophy as it relates to healthcare, healing, rather than mere curing, is the ultimate goal of all care rendered. **Healing** is the reestablishment of a sense of harmony, well-being, and peace, even in the face of objective physical illness or impending death (Quinn, 1997). Healing is always possible, even if curing is not. The holistic paradigm recognizes the healing properties inherent in our body systems and supports the view that conscious access to these inherent healing properties can be beneficial. It also recognizes that there are many ways to heal and that there is meaning in all actions and circumstances. **Curing** differs from healing in that, although it may involve eliminating the symptoms of disease, it does not necessarily remove the innate pattern of responses that causes the disease pattern to be present (Quinn, 1997). Curing acknowledges and focuses on only those physical parts of human beings that can be objectively perceived by practitioners themselves or with commonly used technology. Curing is not always possible, and curing can occur in the absence of healing.

Holistic healing involves an emerging way of being in, seeing, and experiencing the world. The process is intentional, not incidental. Holistic healing is not so much about *what* one does but *how* one goes about it. A holistic philosophy of healing embraces conscious awareness, intuition, and intent, as well as critical, logical, and linear thinking. The practitioner's way of being in the world and of being in relationships with patients and clients are seen as crucial aspects of the healing environment.

The metaphors and categorizations used in the traditional *curing* healthcare model reflect its values and assumptions and, so, differ from those used in the holistic healing model. The metaphors of the traditional model reflect its inherent categorization, hierarchy, objectification, either/or thinking, future time orientation, and violence. For example, negative feeling states, such as shame and fear, are considered relevant to emotional, but not physical, problems. Patients, who are categorized and depersonalized by providers in the hierarchy, are often referred to in terms of their illness, as in "the gallbladder in Room 303." Metaphors of control and dominance, such as "the war on cancer" are common. *Patients* (the word contains a message in itself) are also thought of as either *ill* or *cured*; healing is not an operative concept.

Whole Person Care

The second characteristic of the holistic healthcare paradigm is that it focuses on the **whole person**—the integrated aspects of body, mind, and spirit. That these three facets of each person are inseparable is a major assumption in holistic philosophy. (Research that supports this assumption is discussed in Chapter 27.) In holistic philosophy, every person is seen as having an inherent capacity for *wholeness*—that is, unimpeded communication and harmony among the three aspects of the self. Therefore, all individuals have the seeds of change and healing within them. Holistic philosophy also sees each person as constantly *changing,* or having the capacity to change, in every moment. Therefore, no situation is regarded as hopeless, and no effort on the part of a provider is seen as wasted, regardless of the apparent outcome.

Challenge and Opportunity

The third characteristic of the holistic healthcare paradigm is that it views challenges, such as illness and crisis, as *opportunities for multidimensional growth*—physical, mental, spiritual, emotional, and behavioral. Recognizing synchronous events, such as the onset of an illness coincidentally with a particular internal state (such as fear or shame), provides an opportunity to access inner wisdom and to gain insight into positive and negative aspects of our lives. Living an examined life characterized by the holistic processes of **introspection** and **access of deep inner wisdom** supports personal growth and adds dimension and clarity to the search for personal meaning and purpose in life. Challenges such as illness may stimulate individuals to become aware of the more subtle aspects of their consciousness and to access their innate healing capabilities.

Reciprocity and Right Relationship

The fourth characteristic of the holistic healthcare paradigm is that it acknowledges the **reciprocal nature of healing** (between that which is healed and that which heals). To say that healing is reciprocal means that, in an interaction between a healthcare provider and a patient, for example, both the provider and the patient benefit from the healing interaction. Reciprocal healing depends on **right relationship,** a connection between two or more entities that increases energy, supports coherence and creativity, and allows the function of the entities taken as a whole to be greater than the sum of their individual functioning (Quinn, 1997). A person can be in right relationship with another person or group or with an animal, a career, personal choices, and so on. The holistic healing worldview maintains that right relationship on all levels (cellular, organ, body systems, self, other, and planet) is conducive to the health of all participating entities. Right relationships confer a sense of harmony and wellness, regardless of one's objective physical status.

The holistic paradigm also recognizes the importance of a **well-developed sense of self** in relation to one's life's choices and subsequent physical, mental, emotional, and spiritual outcomes. According to the holistic worldview, everything (rocks, animals, plants, people, the stars, the universe) is continuously evolving within itself and is in a dynamic relationship with its environment (Schaef, 1998).

Belief as a Catalyst of Healing

Another important principle of the holistic paradigm is the recognition that all organisms have an ability to heal themselves; practitioner interventions simply remove obstacles to the process. If an individual suffers a severe fracture, for example, a healthcare provider can align the bone and provide immobilization, but it is *nature*—that is, the individual's intrinsic healing ability—that causes fractured bones to knit, or become whole again (Weil, 1983). Although physicians and other caregivers can often remove the factors that delay or block the healing process, such as an infection or malnutrition, they cannot cause wounds to close, tissues to regenerate, and so on. It is well known and understood that factors such as immune competence and adequacy of circulation in-

fluence the healing of the physical body. What is less widely understood, however, is that another factor, **belief,** seems to have an equally powerful effect.

There have been many documented instances in which beliefs seem to have caused physical changes to occur in the body. Some fall into the category of what is known as **voodoo death.** In voodoo death, a shaman believed to possess magical power places a curse on an individual, who then sickens and dies. Others fall into a fascinating and very well-documented category known as **placebo response.** A placebo (Latin for "it shall please") is an inert substance presented to a patient as an active substance or drug. If a patient *believes* the inert substance to be a drug, her body will respond to the substance as though it were a drug. The power of the placebo effect is universally acknowledged by scientists and is controlled in the testing of drugs and other substances. In blinded studies, subjects are not told the nature of the drugs they are receiving, lest their beliefs alter the actual physiological response to the substance. The placebo response is believed to be a function of the unconscious mind and is an exquisite example of the interconnected and inseparable nature of the mind and body (Weil, 1983).

Belief plays a role in patients' response to actual drugs and treatments as well. An enhanced belief in a medicine or a procedure tends to augment its effects (Lavin, 1992). Patients tend to respond faster and better to therapeutic interventions when they are told to expect a rapid, positive result. The degree to which belief is responsible for the effects of substances, such as drugs, and interventions, such as surgery, is not known, but sham (simulated) surgery was shown in one famous study to reduce anginal pain as much as real surgery on the coronary arteries (Diamond, Kittle, & Crockett, 1958).

The *beliefs of the practitioner,* as well as those of the patient, affect the healing process. As Weil (1983) states, "the true art of medicine is the ability of a practitioner to select and present to individual patients those treatments most likely to elicit healing from within" (p. 218). Providers' beliefs regarding the outcome of a disease or treatment are conveyed to patients verbally and through body language and expression (Weil, 1983). Holistic practitioners are acutely aware of the power of their beliefs and consciously monitor their beliefs and attitudes. They also regard belief as a therapeutic ally that can facilitate healing.

Alignment and Congruence

The holistic healing paradigm holds that individuals are more likely to access their inner wisdom and the cosmic energy source when their behavior and lifestyle choices are in *alignment* with their sacred purpose and meaning in life. In the truly healthy individual, thoughts, words, and deeds are *congruent*. A fundamental premise of holistic therapies is that the integration of the body, mind, and spirit is a fundamental mechanism supporting health and healing.

Transpersonality

Another concept foundational to the holistic healing paradigm is **transpersonality.** That which is transpersonal transcends the limits and boundaries of the physical body and allows for cosmic possibilities. The term *transpersonal* may refer to experiences of *connection* with people, the environment, the cosmos, and the spirit. Quinn (1997) characterizes transpersonal healing as that which promotes the flow and coherence of biological processes. Transpersonal healing may occur without curing and is supported by optimism, a sense of hope, and multisensory awareness. Transpersonal healing cannot be coerced, controlled, or scheduled. A transpersonal system of healing looks beyond the development and expression of the self to the greater, more cosmic global and spiritual concerns of the human community. The transpersonal nature of the holistic healing paradigm views dreams, visions, images, and prayer as healing tools (Achterberg, Dossey, & Kalkmeier, 1994).

Dossey (1999) refers to transpersonality as **nonlocality.** He maintains that nonlocal events, such as distant healing, intercessory prayer, precognitive and shared dreams, and intuitive or distant diagnosis, are worthy of recognition by physicians and other providers. Some remarkable research findings relevant to one transpersonal intervention, *prayer,* have come out of Duke University's Monitoring and Actualization of Noetic Training (MANTRA) Study. In that study, 150 subjects who had been diagnosed as having unstable angina or acute myocardial infarction (heart attack) and who were scheduled for an invasive procedure that would disclose blockages in their coronary arteries were randomly divided into five groups, each of which received a different treatment. The control group received standard therapy. The other groups received guided imagery, prayer, touch therapy, or relaxation. Off-site individuals who had volunteered to participate in the study prayed for the participants in the prayer group, and the participants in the control and prayer treatment groups did not know which of the two groups they had been placed in. The subjects in the guided imagery, touch therapy, and stress-relaxation groups experienced 30 percent fewer adverse outcomes overall, in comparison with the subjects in the control group. The subjects in the prayer group, however, experienced 50 to 100 percent fewer adverse outcomes than did the subjects in the control group (Horrigan, 1999).

Consciousness

Another important concept in the holistic paradigm is **consciousness.** A phrase often heard in CAM circles, "Consciousness counts," reflects the paramount importance assigned to consciousness in the holistic paradigm. Although there is considerable debate about the specific nature of consciousness, holistic philosophy holds that consciousness is the infrastructure, or building block, of energy and matter

(Horrigan & Schlitz, 1998). According to Candice Pert, a prominent scientist, "Consciousness exists prior to the physical realm" (1997, p. 257). Consciousness is thought to be a universal, integral, patterning form of *information* that can circumvent and penetrate the barriers of space and time and that may play a part in transpersonal, or nonlocal, phenomena. In holistic healthcare, consciousness is seen as foundational to human experience in the world: "Consciousness is fundamental, a pervasive, implicit field of all existence, both seen and unseen" (Burch, 1994, p. 101). Some theorists see consciousness as the basic *stuff* of which humans are made: "The person does not possess consciousness, the person is consciousness" (Newman, 1986, p. 33).

Well-known consciousness researcher Marilyn Schlitz (Schlitz & Braud, 1997) offers an integral model of consciousness as extending beyond physical modulators, such as the brain and central nervous system. Schlitz suggests that it is consciousness that lends humankind its uniqueness and makes human relationships with all sentient beings and potentially the cosmos as a whole, possible. Many holistic practitioners hold that humans are spiritual beings who are having a temporary physical experience. Indeed, it has been suggested that, if consciousness were universally accepted as a concept relevant to health, healthcare would be greatly improved: "Models including consciousness as a determinant of health will open up possibilities for the prevention and management of disease by methods less dangerous, less costly, and more effective than many in favor today" (Weil, 1983, p. 273).

The dominant view, in contrast to that of the holistic paradigm, is that the term *consciousness* is merely a euphemism for measurable, quantifiable **electrochemical processes** in the body that can be controlled in the process of scientific research. From the perspective of mainstream medical scientists, the world is overwhelmingly physical. Indeed, many hold the view that humans are physical beings and that there are physiological explanations for all spiritual experiences.

These differing views relative to the role and the very existence of consciousness constitute a major barrier to the full integration of complementary and alternative medicine (CAM) with conventional medicine. A continued dialogue and empirical research are necessary to reduce the philosophical barriers between these two worldviews.

Energy

One of the tenets of the holistic paradigm is that all created and existing life is suffused with a universal life force known as **energy.** This energy is considered to be intrinsic and connected with all life. Energy is the *force* that supports transpersonal healing (Schwartz, 1997). Hundreds of cultures recognize this phenomenon and have variously named it ch'i, prana, ki, life force, and so on. The holistic healthcare paradigm considers this life force energy to be as important to human function as the heart.

The existence of this pervasive and fundamental energy is, for the most part, not recognized by Western medicine, although there is a sizable cohort of researchers and physicians who do research in what is known as **subtle energies.** In other parts of the world, however, the existence of life force energy is unquestioned. For example, after hundreds of years of experience with acupuncture, the Chinese mapped out a system of the energy channels, called meridians, that traverse the body. Many CAM modalities are based on the manipulation of energy (see Chapter 11).

Connectedness

Connectedness is a pivotal construct of the holistic model. Andrews (1996) reported that multiple studies have been conducted to determine the value and extent of the effect of connectedness. He summarized that individual and global health could depend on the degree to which we individually and collectively share a sense of connectedness and *belonging* with others and with nature. Ornish et al. (1990) have written that developing a sense of connection with others can promote health and well-being, and even one's chances for survival. This sense of connectedness can also extend to the immediate natural environment, *soul and soil,* and to the larger environment, *person and planet* (Lincoln, 1999). Wilderness psychologists, who take troubled persons out into nature, list many positive manifestations of this connection: feeling renewed, invigorated, or self-actualized; being more mindful and focused; and having a sense of transcendence (Cumes, 1999). **Social connectedness,** one measure of the amount of love in one's life, has been found to be positively related to health, whereas social isolation has been found to be positively related to illness (Green & Shellenberger, 1996). In a 17-year follow-up health risk survey, Reynolds and Kaplan (1990) found social isolation to be an illness risk factor for women as evidenced by an increase in cancer incidence and mortality. Thus, the capacity to fully experience relationships may underlie health and wholeness.

Coherence

Coherence has been defined as "the ordered, harmonious function between systems" (Institute of HeartMath, 1997, p. 6). The holistic worldview holds that all aspects of the body, mind, and spirit influence each other. Research conducted at the Institute of HeartMath in Colorado has demonstrated that states of mind and emotions have a direct and measurable influence on the autonomic nervous system and that the status of the autonomic nervous system (ANS) affects heart rate and rhythm. The HearthMath researchers have also found that the heart communicates with and influences the brain through neurological mechanisms, biochemical mechanisms, pressure waves, and perhaps energy.

The ANS controls the body's vital functions, one of which is the beating of the heart. The ANS is divided into two branches: the sympathetic and the parasympathetic. Sympathetic stimulation increases the heart rate, whereas parasympathetic stimulation decreases it. It is the momentary balance between the relative activity of the sympathetic and parasympathetic systems that determines heart rate in a given moment. Numerous studies have demonstrated that mental or emotional stress causes an increase in sympathetic activity, which over time can compromise the function of the heart and the immune and hormonal systems as well. Conversely, a decrease in the level of stress experienced causes an increase in parasympathetic activity and a reduction of the demands placed on the cardiovascular and other systems.

The HeartMath research suggests that negative emotions, such an anger, stimulate the sympathetic system, whereas positive ones, such as feelings of love, caring, or appreciation, stimulate the parasympathetic system (Institute of HeartMath, 1997). The variable the institute uses to reflect sympathetic and parasympathetic stimulation is **heart rate variability (HRV).** HRV, reflected in waveforms, is a measurement of the subtle, beat-to-beat changes in heart rate that constitute the heart's response to changing levels of sympathetic and parasympathetic stimulation. The presence of a synchronous heart rhythm that displays little variability in beat-to-beat intervals is termed **cardiac coherence.** Positive emotions have been found to increase calming (parasympathetic) activity and decrease HRV, whereas anger has been found to increase the activity of stress (sympathetic) mechanisms and increase HRV. Tiller, McCraty, and Atkinson (1996) asked a group of subjects to focus their attention on stimuli designed to evoke negative emotions. When the subjects did so, their HRV increased, which means that their cardiac coherence decreased. When the subjects were asked to stop paying attention to the negative stimulus and to focus on their hearts in a meditative way, however, their thoughts and emotions became more positive and their HRV decreased—meaning that their cardiac coherence improved. The HeartMath scientists believe that the heart is, in fact, as much the center of feeling, wisdom, and intuitive knowing in actuality as it is in folklore. They maintain that it is no accident that such words and phrases as *heartbroken* and "I knew it *in my heart*" are commonly used in our culture. The HeartMath scientists also regard the heart as the locus of positive feeling—qualities such as love, caring, understanding, appreciation, and a sense of security. Focusing on the heart evoked positive emotions in the subjects in the Tiller et al. study, as well as in a similar study done by McCraty, Atkinson, Tiller, Rein, and Watkins (1995).

Focusing on the heart seems to result not only in changes in emotional state and degree of cardiac coherence but also in objectively measurable changes in the brain. Song, Schwartz, and Russek (1998) found that heart-centered activities seemed to stimulate direct electromagnetic interactions between the heart and brain, which synchronized the subjects' electrocardiogram activity with their electroencephalogram activity, possibly by the mechanism of entrainment, discussed below. Electrocardiograms reflect the pattern and rhythmicity of the electrical activity in the heart, and electroencephalograms reflect similar characteristics of electrical activity in the brain. These findings support the holistic principle of mind/body connection via physiological, and perhaps energetic, mechanisms.

Entrainment

Entrainment, an essential concept in the holistic paradigm, is the tendency of organisms to come into alignment, or *synchrony,* with each other. McPartland and Mein (1997) define *entrainment* as the integration or harmonization of oscillators. Entrainment was developed as a scientific hypothesis when the inventor of the pendulum clock noted that clocks with similarly sized pendulums began to swing synchronously. This synergy of oscillators also occurs in living organisms. Stogatz and Stewart (1993) found that heart cells located in separate petri dishes (round, shallow glass containers) emit a synchronous electrical charge. The heart generates the body's most powerful electromagnetic field, and it entrains other energy fields into alignment.

Entrainment can involve cells and organisms, including people. Entrainment may explain why people often begin to feel depressed while in the company of another who is depressed. It may also explain the tendency of individuals gathered in large groups to behave in a similar manner—the "crowd phenomenon." For example, fireflies tend to flash synchronously with other, nearby fireflies. Women who work or live together tend to experience their menstrual cycles at the same time (McClintock, 1998). Healthcare practitioners can consciously use the entrainment principle to align body, mind, and spirit in order to carry out a healing intention (McCraty et al., 1995). McPartland and Mein (1997) propose that entrainment and synchrony within a person's body/mind/spirit can be enhanced by the centering techniques used by many complementary therapy practitioners. In the process of centering, one intentionally turns one's attention inward to consciously serve others by intending and embodying a healing presence.

Provider-Client Equality

Holistic practitioners speak of valuing the patient's *individuality* and *subjective experience.* They value *cooperation* and *partnership* and work to maintain *egalitarian* relationships and to *personalize* their care (Dossey, 1997). Holistic practitioners also attempt to use *both/and thinking,* as opposed to either/or thinking, and to be as concerned with the present as they are with the future. The holistic healing paradigm encourages caregivers to shed the cloak of authority and use

TABLE 10–1	Traditional curing and integrative healing Healthcare Models.

Curing Model	Integrative Healing Model
Categorizing process	Individualizing process
Objectification	Personification
Either/or thinking	Both/and thinking
Hierarchical approach	Cooperative approach
Future-time orientation	Present-time orientation
Seeing is believing	Believing is seeing
War metaphor	Lesson metaphor
Treatment of parts	Treatment of relationships
Body and mind	Body, mind, and spirit
Problems to be solved	Challenges to be met
Cure	Heal
Practitioner as authority	Patient-practitioner partnership
Patient as recipient	Patient as responsible

their wisdom and experience to help patients make wise choices (see Table 10–1).

In no way are these broad generalizations intended to imply that there is nothing of merit in the traditional healthcare model. Overall, medical science has been a great boon to humanity. It is both foolish and inaccurate to argue otherwise. Nor are the generalizations meant to imply that CAM practitioners always support healing and that traditional practitioners never do. Having training in an alternative modality does not automatically imbue a given practitioner with a healing persona. Conversely, many practitioners trained in traditional health disciplines are true healers by virtue of their personalities and ways of being.

The paradigm that has informed healthcare over the course of human history has evolved over time and is continuing to do so. The integration of holistic insights, experiences, and approaches with the best features of the traditional model represents an important phase of the evolution of healthcare. The only absolute requirement for integrative healthcare is that it facilitate movement toward wholeness within the self, others, and the planet.

Women and Integrative Healthcare

As an emerging domain within healthcare, CAM modalities are in the beginning stages of validation by evidence-based methodologies of inquiry. Perhaps to avoid repeating the history of the noninclusive nature of medical research practices in the past, the integrative healthcare community in the West has, from the beginning, included and focused research on integrative healthcare as it relates specifically to women's health. For example, The National Institutes of Health (NIH) and its subunit, the National Center for Complementary and Alternative Medicine (NCCAM), established the **Specialty Center for Complementary and Alternative Medicine Research in Women's Health,** hosted by Columbia University. This specialty arm of the NCCAM was established to implement a research agenda for CAM practices specifically related to women's health. The center's functions include providing comprehensive literature reviews on such integrative topics as pregnancy care, prelabor and labor management, menstruation-related disorders, menopausal problems, and breast cancer, to name only a few. From this comprehensive literature review, an evidence-based research agenda will be enhanced by collaborative research in high-priority areas. Networks of researchers, clinicians, and others interested in women's health are being formed to assist in the achievement of the center's goals regarding research, collaboration, and the provision of technical assistance.

Research Methodologies and Integrative Healthcare

The successful integration of CAM will depend on its ability to produce research the results of which will be accepted by the traditional medical establishment. Evidence-based theoretical frameworks that address the *efficacy* and *mechanisms* of alternative interventions must be developed (Schwartz & Russek, 1997). There is, however, considerable philosophical disagreement between orthodox-traditional (OT) medical science and complementary and alternative medicine (CAM) concerning methodology.

One of the most important and controversial issues confronting the credibility and integration of CAM therapies is how these CAM therapies should be evaluated. Gatchel and Maddrey (1998) state that the gold standard in medical research has been the *randomized, double-blind, controlled clinical trial (RCT)* in which subjects are randomly divided into treatment and control groups and neither the subjects nor the investigators know which subjects are in which group. In addition, extraneous variables are removed to the greatest degree possible.

From the perspective of many CAM therapy practitioners (Dossey, 1995), the RCT is not always the investigative tool of choice for a number of reasons. First, CAM recognizes the existence and relevance of variables, such as consciousness, that cannot be *controlled*. In CAM philosophy, all elements of consciousness—beliefs, attitudes, degree of connection, and so on—influence the processes of body/mind/spirit. Thus, it would be difficult to set up an exquisitely controlled research study, because the consciousness of the subjects would differ

and evolve significantly. Another challenge with the RCT model is its inherent presumption that any change noted would be due conclusively to the research intervention. This worldview assumes that subjects will not spontaneously change or evolve during the trial. CAM researchers do not accept this assumption, as they view human beings as constantly evolving and view health and illness as a multicausal, complex spectrum of processes (Green & Shellenberger, 1996). Myers and Benson (1992) suggest that a hallmark of scientific inquiry does not rest alone on the clarity associated with the independent variable but, rather, on whether the observed outcomes are measurable, reliable, and reproducible.

Congruent with **systems theory,** which holds that, in a system composed of parts, all parts mutually and reciprocally affect and are affected by each other, CAM philosophy views the internal landscape of a human being to be in a state of constant flux and influenced by a multitude of inter- and intrarelated factors. Thus, from a holistic perspective, it is virtually impossible to determine the impact of a *single* independent variable. In the perspective of orthodox-traditional (OT) scientists, however, the overall effect of such internal variables as mood, beliefs, and intention is insignificant. This disagreement between OT and CAM scientists about the significance of internal states has forestalled an agreement about what constitutes good science and good research.

CAM scientists point out that, although OT scientists criticize CAM research for a paucity of RCTs, OT scientists themselves do not always use RCT methodology. Sheldrake (1998) and colleagues surveyed representative mainstream scientific literature done over a two-year period; only 24 percent of the medical research and 0.2 percent of the biological research surveyed was done using RCT methodology. Sheldrake surmised that, even in conventional medical and other sciences, blind techniques are not always deemed appropriate or applicable.

CAM researchers do not totally disavow the usefulness of RCTs. Many CAM therapies appear to be highly physical, and, for them, the RCT is seen as an appropriate research methodology. It is important to understand that not all CAM therapies are homogeneously aligned. CAM therapies cover a wide spectrum; some are highly physical, while others involve consciousness, subtle energies, and the effect of intention, love, and support. For example, many CAM therapies and processes focus on and support the quality and meaning of life as a whole, rather than a particular isolated aspect of function (Guzzetta, 1997). Such processes and therapies are not suitable to RCT analysis, and other methodologies would be more appropriate. "All that counts cannot be counted" is a well-known rubric in CAM.

Qualitative research is a systematic, subjective form of research that is used to discover ways in which people experience certain events and situations (Guzzetta, 1997). Qualitative research probes subjective human experience and the meaning ascribed to the experience. Qualitative research has been used to explore subjective human responses to experiences such as having breast cancer and states such as health, loneliness, pain, and comfort. Qualitative research focuses on understanding the *whole* of something, which is consistent with the holistic philosophy that is an essential component of integrative healthcare. Qualitative CAM studies often stimulate further quantitative research, deepen our knowledge of lived experience, and support theory development—adding dimension and richness to our understanding.

Case study is another research methodology that often lends itself to CAM investigations (Lukoff, Edwards, & Miller, 1998). In case studies, investigators look at all aspects of an occurrence or a situation, sometimes by using a combination of quantitative and qualitative methodology. An example of a case study would be intensely studying one woman who is in treatment for breast cancer as a means of investigating the nature of the experience of having breast cancer. *Qualitative inquiry* would be used to elicit the woman's *subjective* experience—her perceptions, feelings, beliefs, and attitudes, as well as those of her friends and family. *Quantitative methods* might be used to analyze her diet and various health parameters, as well as her physical response to treatment. The data aggregate would yield rich information about what it is like to experience the breadth of breast cancer.

Science is an inferential process. RCT and other designs must be used where appropriate to assess both the quantitative value of CAM therapies and the qualitative outcomes. The important issue is not only the methodological process used but the methodological integrity as well. The use of sound research methodologies in CAM supports the credibility and efficacy of CAM research and the cost-effective use of CAM healthcare dollars.

The full integration of traditional healthcare and CAM will not occur overnight, but it is inevitable. Jean Achterberg (1998) has identified four principles that apply to the transition that is in progress:

1. *Science does not change by evolution, but by revolution.*
2. *Paradigm shifts are caused by crises.*
3. *Major shifts will emanate from a multidisciplinary vision.*
4. *All pending revolutions threaten the proponents' current body of knowledge and belief systems.*

As Dossey (1999) has noted, "Science changes funeral by funeral" (p. 14).

The integration of holistic healthcare into mainstream American healthcare is similar to the diffusion of all innovations into the culture at large. In the early 1900s, noted philosopher and psychologist William James (1955) wrote:

> When a thing was new, people said, "It's not true."
> Later, when its truth became obvious, people said,
> "Anyway, it is not important." And when its
> importance could not be denied, people said, "Anyway,
> it is not new." (p. 204)

More and more consumers and providers of contemporary healthcare are acknowledging the validity and importance of

at least some elements of the holistic paradigm. The day may not be far off when healthcare will be comprised of an integrated array of effective services representing the collected wisdom of many traditions.

New Directions

Proponents of integrative healthcare argue that true integration of the traditional Western healthcare model and the Holistic healthcare model has yet to occur. They observe that Western medicine still emphasizes heroic treatment of advanced disease at the expense of wellness and disease prevention, and generally fails to address the mental, emotional, and spiritual concerns of people with illnesses that manifest in the physical realm. A prime reason for this continuing imbalance is that healthcare professionals typically lack education regarding the crucial importance of lifestyle and the environment to health, and the importance of holistic care to healing. Fortunately, this problem is being addressed. A number of professional development programs in CAM are springing up around the country. An example of such a program for physicians is the Program in Integrative Medicine at the University of Arizona Health Sciences Center, in Arizona, U.S.A. Founded by Andrew Weil, M.D., a respected proponent of integrative medicine and graduate of Harvard Medical School, the program provides 2-year residential fellowships to licensed physicians, and month-long rotations to medical students. The program's Integrative Medicine Clinic provides its patients with comprehensive treatment, which includes recommendations regarding diet and dietary supplements, strategies for reducing environmental toxins, mind-body techniques, and assistance in choosing alternative therapies that may prove beneficial (Weil, 2001).

Programs of professional education in Nursing are increasingly incorporating holistic concepts and principles into their curricula. An example is the Rush University College of Nursing at Rush Presbyterian–St. Luke's Medical Center in Chicago (Sierpina, 2001). The undergraduate program at Rush offers a course on issues in holistic health, and graduate students may choose among several holistically oriented courses. A faculty member at Rush, Janice Zeller, RN, PhD, has conducted published research on a number of alternative therapies and interventions.

QUESTIONS FOR REFLECTION AND DISCUSSION

1. *Would you consider consulting a CAM practitioner? Why or why not?*
2. *If you have consulted a CAM practitioner, was that experience different from your encounters with traditional practitioners? In what ways?*

3. *What potential positives and negatives do you foresee as consequences of the increasing integration of traditional Western medicine and CAM? Explain your answers.*

4. *Do you have difficulty accepting any of the concepts that underlie the holistic healthcare model? Which ones? Why?*

5. *What barriers exist to the establishment of a truly integrated system of healthcare?*

RESOURCES

Books

Davis-Floyd, R., & St. John, G. (1998). *From Doctor to Healer: The Transformative Journey.* New Brunswick, NJ: Rutgers University Press.

Sierpina, V. S., M.D., (2001). *Integrative Health Care: Complementary and Alternative Therapies for the Whole Person.* Philadelphia: F. A. Davis.

CD

Weil, A. (2000). *Integrative Medicine.* Boulder, CO: Sounds True. Three CDs. Running time: 3.5 hours.

Organizations

American College for Advancement in Medicine
2312 Verdugo Drive, Suite 204
Laguna Hills, CA 92653
Phone: 800-532-3688 ext. 3.
Web: *http://www.acam.org*

American Holistic Medical Association
6728 Old McLean Village Drive
McLean, VA 22101
Phone: 703-556-9245
Web: *http://www.holisticmedicine.org*

American Holistic Nurses Association
P.O. Box 3130
Flagstaff, AZ 86003-3130
Phone: 800-278-2463
Web: *http://www.ahna.org*

REFERENCES

Achterberg, J. (1998). Between lightning and thunder: The pause before the shifting paradigm. *Alternative Therapies in Health and Medicine, 4*(3), 62–65.

Achterberg, J., Dossey, B. M., & Kalkmeier, L. (1994). *Rituals of healing: Using imagery for health and wellness.* New York: Bantam Books.

Andrews, S. (1996). Promoting a sense of connectedness among individuals by scientifically demonstrating the existence of a planetary consciousness. *Alternative Therapies, 2*(3), 39–45.

Andrus, V., Gold, J., Johnson, M., Lincoln, V., Thornton, L., & Yetter Lunt, J. (1999). *Phase 1: The Certificate Program in Holistic Nursing.* Shutesbury, MA: Seeds and Bridges.

Bohm, D. (1998). *Quantum theory.* Mineola, NY: Dover.

Burch, S. (1994). Consciousness: How does it relate to health? *Journal of Holistic Nursing, 12*(1), 101–116.

Cumes, D. (1999). Nature as medicine: The healing power of the wilderness. *Alternative Therapies in Health and Medicine, 4*(2), 79–85.

Diamond, E., Kittle, C., & Crockett, A. (1958). Evaluation of internal mammary artery ligation and sham procedure in angina pectoris. *Circulation, 18,* 712–713.

DiLama, S. N., & Painter, S. B. (Eds.). (1998). *Holistic health promotion and complementary therapies: A resource for integrated practice.* Gaithersburg, MD: Aspen.

Dossey, B. M. (1997). Holistic nursing practice. In B. M. Dossey (Ed.), *Core curriculum for holistic nursing* (pp. 4–12). Gaithersburg, MD: Aspen.

Dossey, L. (1995). How should alternative therapies be evaluated: An examination of fundamentals. *Alternative Therapies in Health and Medicine, 1*(2), 6–10, 79–85.

Dossey, L. (1999). Healing and modern physics: Exploring consciousness and the small-is-beautiful assumption. *Alternative Therapies in Health and Medicine, 5*(4), 12–17, 102–108.

Eisenberg, D., Davis, R., Ettner, S., Appel, S., Wilkey, S., Rompay, M., & Kessler, R. (1998). Trends in alternative medicine use in the United States, 1990–1997. *Journal of the American Medical Association, 280*(18), 1569–1576.

Eisenberg, D. M., Kessler, R. C., Foster, C., Norlock, F. E., Calkins, D. R., & Delbanco, T. L. (1993). Unconventional medicine in the United States: Prevalence, costs, and patterns of use. *New England Journal of Medicine, 328*(4), 252–265.

Elkins, D. N. (1995). Psychotherapy and spirituality: Toward a theory of the soul. *Journal of Humanistic Psychology, 35*(2), 78–98.

Gatchel, R. J., & Maddrey, A. M. (1998). Clinical outcome research in complementary and alternative medicine: An overview of experimental design and analysis. *Alternative Therapies in Health and Medicine, 4*(5), 36–42.

Green, J., & Shellenberger, R. (1996). The healing energy of love. *Alternative Therapies in Health and Medicine, 3*(3), 46–56.

Guzzetta, C. (1997). Holistic nursing and related research. In B. M. Dossey (Ed.), *Core curriculum in holistic nursing* (pp. 74–80). Gaithersburg, MD: Aspen.

Hawking, S. (1998). *A brief history of time.* New York: Bantam Books.

Horrigan, B. (1999). Mitchell W. Krucoff, M.D.: The MANTRA study project. *Alternative Therapies in Health and Medicine, 5*(3), 75–82.

Horrigan, B., & Schlitz, M. (1998). On consciousness, causation, and evolution. *Alternative Therapies in Health and Medicine, 4*(4), 82–90.

Institute of HeartMath. (1997). *Research overview: Exploring the role of the heart in human performance.* Boulder Creek, CA: Author.

James, W. (1955). *Principles of psychology, 1.* London: Dover Publications.

Johnson, M. (1990). The holistic paradigm in nursing: The diffusion of an innovation. *Research in Nursing and Health, 13,* 129–139.

Lavin, M. (1992). A second look at the placebo response. *American Journal of Psychiatry, 149*(12), 1760.

Lincoln, V. (1998). *Healing healthcare.* Seminar presentation at Abbot Northwest Medical Center, Minneapolis, MN.

Lincoln, V. (1999). Accessing an ecospiritual consciousness. *Creative Nurse Journal, 2,* 11–12.

Lukoff, D., Edwards, D., & Miller, M. (1998). The case study as a scientific method for researching alternative therapies. *Alternative Therapies in Health and Medicine, 4*(2), 44–52.

McClintock, M. K. (1998). Whither menstrual synchrony? *Annual Review of Sex Research, 9,* 77–95.

McCraty, R., Atkinson, M., Tiller, W. A., Rein, G., & Watkins, A. D. (1995). The effects of emotions on short-term power spectral analysis of heart rate variability. *American Journal of Cardiology, 76*(14), 1089–1093.

McPartland, J. M., & Mein, E. A. (1997). Entrainment and the cranial rhythmic impulse. *Alternative Therapies in Health and Medicine, 3*(1), 40–45.

Myers, S. S., & Benson, H. (1992). Methodological and conceptual issues in research on social support. *Hospital Community Psychiatry, 16,* 5–11.

Newman, M. A. (1986). *Health as expanding consciousness.* New York: Mosby.

Ornish, D., Brown, S. E., & Scherwitz, L. W. (1990). Can lifestyle changes reverse coronary heart disease? *Lancet, 336,* 129–133.

Pert, C. (1997). *Molecules of emotion.* New York: Touchstone.

Petzinger, T. (1999). *The new pioneers: Men and women who are transforming the workplace and marketplace.* New York: Simon & Schuster.

Quinn, J. F. (1997). Transpersonal human caring and healing. In B. M. Dossey (Ed.), *Core curriculum for holistic nursing* (pp. 13–16). Gaithersburg, MD: Aspen.

Ray, P. H. (1996). The rise of the integral culture. *Noetic Sciences Review, 37,* 4–15.

Reynolds, P., & Kaplan, G. (1990, Fall). Social connections and risk for cancer: Prospective evidence from the Almeda County study. *Behavioral Medicine,* 101–110.

Russell, P. (1992). *The white hole in time.* San Francisco: Harper.

Schaef, A. (1998). *Living in process: Basic truths for living the path of the soul.* New York: Ballentine Wellspring.

Schlitz, M., & Braud, W. (1997). Distant intentionality and healing: Assessing the evidence. *Alternative Therapies in Health and Medicine, 3*(6), 62–73.

Schwartz, G. E. (1997). Information and energy: The soul and spirit of mind-body medicine. *Advances, 13*(1), 75–77.

Schwartz, G. E., & Russek, L. G. (1997). Dynamical energy systems and modern physics: Fostering the science and spirit of complementary and alternative medicine. *Alternative Therapies in Health and Medicine, 3*(3), 46–56.

Sheldrake, R. (1998). Experimenter efforts in scientific research: How widely are they neglected? *Journal of Scientific Exploration, 12*(1), 73–78.

Sierpino, V. (2001). Progress notes: Rush University College of Nursing. *Alternative Therapies, 7*(3), 141.

Song, L. Z. Y., Schwartz, G. E., & Russek, L. S. (1998). Heart-focused attention and heart-brain synchronization: Energetic and physiological mechanisms. *Alternative Therapies in Health and Medicine, 4*(5), 44–62.

Stogatz, S. H., & Stewart, I. (1993, December). Coupled oscillators and biological synchronization. *Scientific American,* pp. 102–109.

Tiller, W. A., McCraty, R., & Atkinson, M. (1996). Cardiac coherence: A new invasive measure of autonomic nervous system order. *Alternative Therapies in Health and Medicine, 2*(1), 52–65.

Weil, A. (1983). *Health and healing.* Boston: Houghton Mifflin.

Weil, A. (2001). CAM and continuing education: the future is now. *Alternative Therapies, 7*(3), 32.

11

Holistic Health: Complementary Therapeutic Disciplines and Remedies

Valerie Lincoln and Karl Kleiner

Objectives

1. *Identify reasons for the increasing popularity of alternative remedies and therapies.*
2. *Identify four major categories of alternative interventions.*
3. *Discuss the ontological assumptions that underlie the use of energy therapies.*
4. *Compare and contrast traditional Chinese medicine and Ayurveda in terms of underlying assumptions and treatment modalities.*
5. *Discuss the historical role of herbs in healing and medicine.*
6. *Compare and contrast food supplements and drugs in terms of physical characteristics and laws pertaining to advertising and marketing.*
7. *Discuss selected herbs in terms of indications for use, therapeutic efficacy, side effects, and potential interactions with other herbs and drugs.*

Introduction

As we enter the new millennium, women and their families can choose from among an array of nontraditional therapies in addition to therapies and procedures associated with the traditional Western healthcare model. This chapter will provide an overview of what is known about the nature and efficacy of selected therapies that are currently regarded as alternative, or complementary.

The nontraditional healing modalities commonly used in holistic healthcare have a wide range of geographic, philosophical, and cultural origins. Many are rooted in one or more of the following: Eastern wisdom traditions, European traditions, Native American medicine traditions, and the medicine of primal peoples from all over the globe. In most cases, these modalities are intended to stimulate or unblock the intrinsic healing capacity of the body.

In a landmark research study done by Eisenberg et al. (1993), one in three people interviewed reported having used an alternative therapy in the previous year. This statistic suggests that more visits are being made to alternative practitioners than to traditional medical practitioners. In a 1997 follow-up survey, Eisenberg and his colleagues (1998) found that this trend had grown exponentially. The 1997 survey estimated the proportion of Complementary and Alternative Medicine (CAM) use among Americans to have increased to 42.1 percent (83 million people). This increase was due primarily to the proportion of the population seeking alternative therapies, rather than increased visits per client. The extrapolated data revealed a 47 percent increase in total visits to CAM practitioners—more visits than to all U.S. primary care physicians combined. Alternative therapies were sought for the treatment of existing medical conditions (42 percent) as well as for health promotion (58 per-

cent) (Eisenberg et al., 1998). As many alternative therapies are not covered by insurance, those numbers also suggest that more out-of-pocket dollars are being spent on nontraditional than traditional therapies. Participants in the Eisenberg study reported a variety of reasons for their decision to seek alternative therapies. Their reasons included the following: a focus on wellness rather than disease prevention; the expectation of taking fewer medications with reduced side effects and lower costs; an increasing awareness of alternative healthcare practices; frustrations with the current medical system; a sense of disconnection with traditional practitioners; increasing scientific support for many alternative therapies; and increasing support on the part of traditional healthcare providers for nontraditional therapies.

The alternative therapies used most commonly in America are vitamin, herbal, and mineral supplements, chiropractic care, relaxation and stress-reduction techniques, massage and bodywork, and acupuncture (Pelletier, Marie, Krasner, & Haskell, 1997). The complaints that most often motivate people to seek alternative treatments are back problems, allergies, arthritis, insomnia, sprains or strains, headache, high blood pressure, digestive problems, anxiety, and depression (Eisenberg et al., 1993). Many people who seek out holistically oriented providers have a *holistic worldview* themselves and believe that all aspects of their lives influence their health. Holistic healthcare providers generally share that view and subscribe to a partnership model of care, wherein consumers are actively involved in their healthcare.

Diet, Nutrition, and Lifestyle Choices

A much discussed scientific study by Dean Ornish (Ornish et al., 1998), a cardiologist and proponent of mind/body awareness, made clear the dramatic role that diet, nutrition, exercise, and stress control can play not only in health promotion but in the reversal of disease processes as well. In Ornish's study, 28 subjects with documented atherosclerotic heart disease actually reversed their disease process by making significant lifestyle changes. The participants in Ornish's study embarked on a yearlong program of lifestyle modification after having attended a weeklong seminar in which the importance of a **low-fat diet**, **smoking cessation**, **exercise** was stressed, and techniques and skills for **stress management** were taught. The prescribed diet was comprised of 10 percent fat, 15 percent protein, and 75 percent carbohydrates. The participants also exercised a minimum of 30 minutes daily and performed centered meditation exercises for one hour each day. They also attended a facilitator-led support group twice weekly. After yearlong participation in the Ornish program, statistically significant improvement was seen in all parameters of the subjects' heart health. Chest pain, body weight, and blood lipid and stress hormone levels were markedly reduced. Repeat cardiac catheterization procedures indicated that the amount of plaque present in the coronary arteries was lessened.

Holistically oriented practitioners stress the importance of a good diet to health. Although a healthy diet should include a variety of foods that provide optimal amounts of protein, carbohydrate, and fat (see Chapter 3), the *quality* of the food is also very important. Many women choose organically produced foods to reduce their exposure to pesticides, herbicides, hormones, steroids, antibiotics, and genetically engineered foods. Avoiding processed foods and refined sugars in favor of whole grains, vegetables, and fruits also minimizes exposure to toxins and maximizes nutrition. Consuming only small amounts of meat, and choosing meats from animals raised organically without prophylactic antibiotics and hormones, is advised, as is abstaining from or moderating intake of alcohol and caffeine. How foods are prepared also has implications for health. Eating whole foods either raw or lightly cooked (except for meats) results in retention of vitamins, minerals, and general micronutrients.

Specific approaches to diet often recommended by holistic practitioners include the Ayurvedic, macrobiotic, and strict vegan diets. In the **Ayurvedic approach,** foods appropriate to one's *dosha,* or body/mind type, are chosen. Ayurvedic practitioners recommend that food be chewed slowly and completely and that one never eat while standing up. Ice cold drinks are not to be taken with meals, as they diminish the digestive fire. Ayurvedic practitioners also advise against overeating; they recommend eating smaller portions of food more frequently and terminating meals while the stomach is still not quite full (Chopra, 1991). Many people turn to a **macrobiotic diet** in order to maintain health or when they experience a health crisis, such as a cancer diagnosis. A macrobiotic diet is comprised primarily of whole grain and raw food sources in prescribed combinations. A **vegan diet** is a strict vegetarian diet that is exclusively vegetable-based and free from animal and animal-derived products. Vegetarians who consume milk and milk products are known as **lacto-vegetarians,** and vegetarians who use both milk products and eggs are known as **lacto-ovo vegetarians** (Sizer & Whitney, 1991). See Chapter 3 for further information regarding the pros and cons of vegetarian diets.

Modalities That Promote Relaxation and Enhance Self-Regulation and Insight

Physical and mental relaxation has proven to be beneficial for persons with a variety of physical and emotional problems. Interventions that assist individuals in gaining some degree of control over involuntary physiological functions, such as blood pressure and bowel activity, have proven useful, as have modalities that promote insight into specific patterns and problems.

Relaxation

There are several methods of eliciting what Herbert Benson, M.D., has called the **relaxation response** (see Chapter 7). The results of regularly inducing the relaxation response include decreased heart and respiratory rates, reduced blood pressure and oxygen consumption rates, lowered metabolism, and reduced muscle tension. Relaxation techniques have been used in the control of high blood pressure, tension headaches, and other such problems. The methods of inducing the relaxation response include progressive muscle relaxation and various breathing techniques and forms of meditation. The relaxation response is either a necessary prelude to, or a beneficial side effect of, many other practices and therapies, such as breathing techniques, biofeedback, imagery, meditation, yoga, and hypnotherapy.

Breathing Exercises

Proper breathing is considered essential to good health. Breathing is a function that is *both voluntary and involuntary.* That is, we can control our breathing if we choose to, but breathing will also occur whether we think about it or not. The breath is a conduit to the *involuntary nervous system,* which regulates our circulation, digestion, and other vital functions. By manipulating the breath, we can influence many systems of the body. In this country, breathing techniques were first used to promote relaxation and control stress by women who desired natural childbirth. Specific patterns of deep breathing, along with deep concentration, are part of the La Maze and Bradley techniques for relaxation and focus during childbirth.

Breathing and the breath are also used in other settings for other purposes. Following the breath in meditation, for example, is a way of both relaxing and developing concentration. Breathing techniques have been used to control blood pressure, improve digestion, decrease anxiety, and improve sleep (Weil, 1995). Andrew Weil, M.D., recommends the following breathing exercise for regaining control and centeredness in moments of anxiety or anger:

- Breathe in through the nose briskly over a count of four.
- Hold the breath (without straining) for a count of seven if possible.
- Exhale audibly through the mouth slowly over a count of eight.
- Repeat the cycle four times.

The main goal is to have exhalation take twice as long as inhalation—a reversal of the usual ratio (Weil, 1995).

Biofeedback

Biofeedback is the information that is presented to an individual about whether she is achieving a desired change in the body at a given moment in time. There are five common types of biofeedback (Schwartz & Schwartz, 1993). **Electromagnetic (EMG) biofeedback** measures muscle tension and is useful for tension headaches, chronic muscle pain, and general relaxation. **Thermal biofeedback** measures skin temperature as a reflection of blood flow and is used for relaxation and the treatment of anxiety and hypertension. **Electrodermal activity (EDA) biofeedback** measures sweat production and is often used to control anxiety and overactive sweat glands. The fourth type of biofeedback, **finger pulse biofeedback,** measures pulse rate and force and is used to treat hypertension, anxiety, and some cardiac arrhythmias. Finally, there is a type of biofeedback (respiratory biofeedback) used to assess *breathing* in terms of rate, volume, rhythm, and locus (chest or abdominal). This type of biofeedback is often useful in the treatment of asthma, hyperventilation, and anxiety, and it is used to promote support relaxation (Schwartz & Schwartz, 1993).

The elicitation of the relaxation response is an essential part of biofeedback, as relaxation is the mechanism by which the autonomic nervous system is influenced and the physiology is changed. Therefore, at the beginning of each session, clients using biofeedback set an intention to relax the mind and body and engage in a breathing or progressive muscle relaxation exercise. Once they are relaxed, clients *visualize* the desired physiological response—the arteries widening, the heart beating regularly, and so on. Electromechanical measuring devices that detect various physical responses and relay them to the patient via visual or auditory cues provide feedback as to whether the desired response is occurring.

Imagery

In **imagery therapy,** individuals use mental images, in conjunction with other self-created sensory experiences, to promote relaxation and to access their inner wisdom to gain insight into problems and circumstances. Imagery can involve all the sensory modalities: visual, olfactory, tactile, auditory, and kinesthetic. The images used include visualizations of real people or situations, fantasies, memories, and dreams. Such images are seen as bridges connecting the mind, body, and spirit (Dossey, 1997). Imagery is a holistic modality that can be done by oneself or under the guidance of a trained facilitator. Imagery is useful for decreasing anxiety, pain, and reactions to stressful states and is used to support healing as well. There are many types of imagery, each using a specialized form of imagery to achieve a specific goal (Achterberg, Dossey, & Kolkmeier, 1994). Rossman (1993) reports that researchers using sophisticated technology, such as positron emission tomography (PET), have documented the physiological activation of specific brain centers during visual im-

aging sessions. The three major outcomes in imagery therapy are physiological shifts, psychological insights, and enhanced awareness of emotions (Rossman, 1993).

Meditation

The term *meditation* refers to a number of techniques used to quiet the mind for a period of time. Meditation involves disengaging the mind from the myriad concerns and goals of the moment and moving into a state of *being* rather than *doing*. There are many reasons that a person might want to engage in a meditation practice. Some meditate primarily to relieve stress and tension. Others wish to get to the bottom of suffering and unhappiness—when the mind is no longer distracted by the mundane, profound insights can arise. Many use meditation as part of a broader spiritual practice. Meditation is a significant aspect of many spiritual traditions, such as Hinduism, Islam, Buddhism, and Christianity.

All of the various techniques of meditation involve both relaxation and focused attention. In **mindfulness meditation,** for example, one sits quietly and simply observes the thoughts that flow through the mind without becoming caught up in them; one simply notices them and allows them to pass. In **transcendental meditation,** one of the most popular forms of meditation in the West, attention is focused on a *mantra*, or sacred word or phrase. Meditation need not be done while sitting. In *walking meditation,* one focuses attention on each slow, deliberate step while setting an intention to create space for personal illumination. One can also meditate while carrying out mundane activities. For example, while washing dishes, one can immerse oneself fully in the activity of the present moment—noticing the feel of the water, the scent of the detergent, and so on. When thoughts of the past or future come up, attention is gently redirected to the present moment.

Meditation plays a prominent role in several well-known therapeutic programs. At the Stress Reduction Clinic at the University of Massachusetts Medical Center, meditation has benefited thousands of people with such disparate problems as chronic pain, anxiety, depression, and coronary heart disease (Kabat-Zinn, 1990). Similar results have been obtained at the Mind/Body Medical Institute in Boston, Massachusetts (Benson, 1996).

Yoga

Yoga is an ancient Hindu spiritual practice. The aim of yoga practice is to link the body, mind, and spirit in a balanced life; the word *yoga* is derived from a Sanskrit word meaning "to bind" or "to yoke." The foundations of yoga include moral precepts and prescribed rules for daily conduct, as well as meditation and physical practices. The physical aspect of yoga involves postures called **asanas,** as well as special breathing techniques. A high level of accomplishment in yoga requires a mastery of the senses, mental concentration, and discipline, as well as access to transpersonal consciousness. In the West, yoga is often seen as merely a physical discipline—a means of acquiring strength and flexibility. Although a superficial, physically focused practice can certainly confer those benefits, much more is to be gained from a more comprehensive practice.

A number of approaches to yoga are taught in the West. The term **hatha yoga** is a nonspecific term that refers to the physical aspect of yoga practice.

There has been some research done on yoga as therapy. Garfinkel et al. (1998) found that a yoga-based regimen including postures and relaxation was more effective than wrist splinting (a common conventional treatment) in relieving some signs and symptoms of carpal tunnel syndrome. Benson (1996) indicated that the physiological changes observed in yoga therapy include decreased oxygen consumption, decreases in respiratory and heart rate, and blood pressure (in patients with high blood pressure), and an increase in alpha waves, which indicates the promotion of relaxation.

Hypnotherapy

The term *hypnotherapy* refers to the use of *hypnosis* in reaching a therapeutic goal. In classical hypnosis, one becomes deeply relaxed and enters a *trancelike state* in order to render one's subconscious mind more susceptible to positive suggestions. People who shift easily into the hypnotic state can influence involuntary physical mechanisms, such as blood pressure, bowel motility, and the inflammatory response (Weil, 1988). *Hypnosis* is defined functionally by Kohen and Olness (1996) as an "alternative state of awareness and alertness in which an individual is selectively focussed, absorbed, and concentrating upon a particular idea or image with the specific purpose of achieving some goal or realizing some potential" (p. 45). Some forms of hypnosis incorporate the relaxation response and some do not.

Contrary to popular opinion, the hypnotic state is *voluntary*. No one can force another person into it. Neither can a hypnotist force anyone to do something contrary to her values (Olness, 1993). Persons in hypnotic trance can see, hear, and move if they choose to and can end the trance at any time. All hypnosis is, in fact, *self-hypnosis*. Subjects consciously decide to accept the suggestions that lead to the trance state and can learn to induce it in themselves without the guidance of a hypnotherapist. Another fallacy about hypnosis is that hypnotic susceptibility correlates with a lack of intelligence or sophistication. This is not true; varying levels of ability to enter trances are found in persons from all levels of education and lifestyles (Kohen & Olness, 1996).

There are three distinct levels of hypnotic trance: light, middle, and deep. Subjects need only achieve the first or second level in order to be able to take suggestions regarding behavioral or attitudinal changes. Deep trance states can be achieved by only about a third of the population, but those individuals are able to anesthetize body tissues and actually undergo surgical procedures with no anesthesia except their hypnotic state (Olness, 1993). The degree of response to hypnosis is positively related to an individual's ability to enter trance, and it is inversely related to the fear of negative outcome or loss of control (Olness, 1993). Hypnotherapy is accepted by many traditional healthcare providers because its efficacy is supported in the scientific literature. For example, hypnotherapy has been found to lessen the inflammatory response to burn injuries and to reduce the healing time of bone fractures (Ginades & Rosenthal, 1999). Hypnotherapy has also proven helpful in the amelioration of acute, chronic, and cancer-related pain. Hypnosis is thought to prevent the entry of pain impulses into consciousness by inhibiting the transmission of pain impulses from thalamic to cortical structures in the brain (Pinnell & Covino, 2000). However, the antics of stage hypnotists and inaccurate depictions of hypnosis in books and films have tainted the reputation of this useful therapy.

Hypnotherapy falls within the scope of the practice of licensed professionals, such as physicians, psychotherapists, dentists, and professional nurses (RNs), and is provided by laypeople with various kinds of preparation. The American Board of Clinical Hypnosis grants certification in hypnotherapy to professionally trained and licensed practitioners.

Humor Therapy

In the past decade, a good deal of research has focused on the healing properties and effects of humor. Humor is a cognitive skill that links *logical left-brain function* with *creative right-brain function*. Laughter stimulates increases in respiratory rate, pulse rate, and muscle tension and increases oxygen consumption. Laughter also stimulates the release of catecholamines, hormones, and endorphins, all of which are important to the healing process. Buxman (1996) reported that the positive outcomes of humor stimulate and strengthen the immune system by increasing the level of natural killer cells (cells that release a tumor-destroying substance) and decreasing serum cortisol levels. Humor is also said to increase levels of T-lymphocytes and salivary IgA, which can protect against upper respiratory infections such as colds and flu (Buxman, 1996). Humor also diminishes anxiety, fear, and tension and can help release anger and frustration, all of which facilitate right relationship and healing.

Art, Dance, Music, and Drama Therapies

Art, dance, music, and drama therapies all involve creative expression, and they are becoming accepted and used as healing modalities. Well-established graduate programs in each of these therapies are found across the country. The participation in creative endeavors addresses the cognitive, physical, social, and spiritual aspects of the self in ways that other modalities may not. Art, dance, music, and drama therapies are evocative and engaging modalities that are intimate and soulful. Immersion into these therapies allows the individual's unconscious to express itself in symbolic and metaphoric language. Such therapies combine behavioral science with art to produce relaxation and achieve desired changes in physiology, emotions, and behavior. Each domain has national professional organizations and credentialing processes.

Transpersonal Therapies

Transpersonal therapies are based on the assumption that all beings are connected in such a way that they can communicate with and influence each other via subtle energies and other nonlocal phenomena (see Chapter 10). Transpersonal therapies include intercessory prayer and various energy-based interventions.

Intercessory Prayer

Many cultures subscribe to the healing power of prayer. Intercessory, or *remote* (nonlocal), prayer has been defined as "an effort to mediate on behalf of someone else" (Dossey, 1997, p. 11). Intercessory prayer is referred to as remote because of the distant location of the person for whom the prayer is intended. Randolph Byrd, a cardiologist, completed the first scientific inquiry into the effectiveness of intercessory prayer in 1988. Byrd (1988) studied 393 consecutive patients who had been admitted to coronary care units. All the patients in the study received standard medical treatment for their condition, but half the patients were prayed for from afar by volunteers from religious groups. The volunteers were given the patients' first names and were given updates on the conditions of the patients for whom they were praying. Both the patients and the medical and nursing staff knew that a study on the effects of prayer was being conducted because the patients who were included in the study were required to sign consent to be prayed for forms. The study was blinded, however, in that neither the patients themselves nor the staff who cared for them knew which patients had been assigned to the prayer group. Byrd used an instrument he devised, called the Hospital Course Score, to quantify complications and untoward events, such as the onset of fever or congestive heart failure. The lengths of stay in the coronary unit and elsewhere were also recorded. Byrd found that the prayed-for patients did somewhat better than the patients who were not prayed for on several measures. For example, the prayed-for patients were less likely to require endotracheal intubation (the placement of a tube in the windpipe in order to provide mechanical assistance with breathing). They also required fewer potent drugs, experienced a lower incidence of pulmonary edema, and required cardiopulmonary resuscitation (CPR) less often. The differ-

ences however, were not statistically significant, except in the case of endotrachial intubation. The Byrd study was criticized on the basis of its small sample size and the modest degree of difference in outcome between the two groups (Posner, 1998). It was also pointed out that the patients in the control group (not prayed for) may have been prayed for by friends and relatives.

The Byrd study led to another, similar study (Harris et al., 1999). The Harris study involved a total of 990 consecutive cardiac patients, who, at the time of their admission to the coronary care unit, were randomly assigned to either the treatment (prayer) group or the control (usual care) group. As in the Byrd study, the first names of the patients in the prayer group were given to a group of multidenominational Christian volunteers outside the hospital, who prayed for the patients daily for four weeks. In the Harris study, however, the volunteers were given no additional information or updates on the patients' conditions. The Harris study was randomized, as was the Byrd study; however, in the Harris study, the patients and staff did not even know that a prayer study was being conducted. The Harris research team received permission from the hospital's research review board to proceed with the study without informed consent from the patients. The instrument used in the Harris study to keep track of patient outcomes (the Coronary Care Unit course, or CCU course) was developed by a team of physicians and tracked essentially the same variables as the instrument used in the Byrd study. The results of the Harris study were similar in terms of magnitude (modest) to the results of the Byrd study. The mean coronary care unit and hospital lengths of stay were not different for the two groups, and there were no statistically significant differences between the groups' scores on any individual component of the CCU score. There was, however, an 11 percent reduction in the prayer group's overall score, in comparison with the usual care group. According to the researchers' calculations, the odds that the 11 percent reduction was due to chance were 1 in 25.

The results of both the Byrd and Harris studies, although modest, suggest that further studies into remote interventions that may benefit those suffering from illness are warranted. Dossey (1997) theorizes that it is the nonlocal, fundamental, omniscient, and causal qualities of consciousness that explain the beneficial effects of prayer, which have thus far been only weakly demonstrated in the scientific literature.

Energy-Based Modalities

Foundational to the theory that underlies energy-based treatment modalities, such as Therapeutic Touch, Healing Touch, and Reiki, is the assumption that all living things are made up of **energy fields.** As well-known nurse-theorist Martha Rogers (1990, p. 7) has stated, "we don't *have* energy fields, we *are* energy fields." The meaning of the term *energy field* can be explained only in terms of rather difficult concepts from the discipline of physics:

> *Energy is one of the most mundane, yet mysterious concepts in modern physics. . . . Although the measurement of energy may be defined precisely, the interpretation of energy is abstract and difficult to comprehend, even by seasoned physicists. The inherent difficulty in understanding energy cannot be overstated. (Schwartz & Russek, 1997, p. 48)*

A comprehensive discussion of the nature of energy will not be attempted here. It suffices to say that the energy field of which human beings and other life forms are comprised is akin to other energy fields, such as electric fields and magnetic fields. The various concepts of energy are really attempts to describe how things *move* in space. Energy influences the motion, and therefore the functioning, of atoms, molecules, cellular processes, and physiological functioning, as well as consciousness and behavior (Schwartz & Russek, 1997).

According to the proponents of energy medicine and healing, the human energy field can be sensed by the self and others, and it can be influenced by conscious means. Health problems cause detectable *alterations* in the field. The practitioners of energy therapies, such as Therapeutic Touch, Reiki, and Healing Touch, use their hands to access, scan, and evaluate the external parts of the human energy field. A systematic assessment of the field surrounding specific body areas is done, after which practitioners use a combination of conscious intention and hand motion to modulate and direct energy in order to restore *balance* to the patient's energy field.

As energy-based therapies are relatively new additions to the CAM modality in this country, a more sophisticated research base regarding their efficacy is needed. Many of the studies suggesting that energy-based touch modalities are helpful in reducing anxiety, tension, and pain have been criticized on methodological grounds. Winstead-Fry and Kijek (1999) recently reviewed 38 formal studies of Therapeutic Touch (TT) (one of the energy-based therapies) and concluded that the outcomes regarding the efficacy of Therapeutic Touch were mixed. While some studies indicated that TT was effective, others did not. Clearly, more research into this and other energy-based modalities is needed.

Bodyways: Body-Based Therapies

Knaster (1996) coined the term **bodyways** to characterize the many holistic therapies that involve the manipulation of the body in some way. Bodyways (sometimes referred to as **bodywork**) therapies are based in both Eastern and Western traditions. Although some are better suited to particular problems and conditions than others, all body-based therapies generally can be used for preventive or corrective purposes. The benefits attributed to them include stress reduction, pain relief, improved posture, increased sensory awareness, better-defined personal boundaries, and improved access to memories and body wisdom (Knaster, 1996). There are many bodyways; only a few of the most available and commonly used will be addressed in this section.

Structural Approaches

Structural approaches to bodywork focus on improving individuals' posture and body mechanics through the manipulation of connective tissue and muscle and by teaching new patterns of movement and posture. The focus of the structural approaches is to enhance structural integrity. Three popular structural approaches are Chiropractic, Craniosacral Therapy and various massage therapies. Structural bodyways offer a wide range of benefits, which include pain reduction, better health, greater range of motion, flexibility, and coordination (Knaster, 1996).

CHIROPRACTIC

David Palmer of Iowa founded chiropractic in 1895. Chiropractic care is based on the philosophy that one's state of health is determined by the *structural integrity* of the spinal column and the emerging nerves. Chiropractic views structure and function as co-existent. Shifts in the structure of the spine (subluxations) lead to abnormalities in function, such as pain and limping. Chiropractic treatment primarily involves the manipulation of the spine in an effort to correct structural and functional imbalances.

Chiropractic therapy is often supported by massage, and chiropractors often make dietary recommendations to their patients as well. According to the Eisenberg et al. (1993) study, chiropractic is the most frequently used CAM therapy in the United States. Mainstream scientific literature supports the efficacy of chiropractic care only for low back pain (Cherkin & MacCornack, 1989).

CRANIOSACRAL THERAPY

Craniosacral Therapy (CST) is derived from the practice of *traditional osteopathy*. Traditional osteopathic medicine concerns the restoration of the body's structural integrity in order to promote balance and health. Traditional osteopathic medicine is distinct from modern osteopathic medicine (see Chapter 9), which has achieved mainstream acceptance; the training of modern osteopaths (D.O.s) is virtually indistinguishable from that undergone by M.D.s. Traditional osteopathy, however, is enjoying a resurgence. Today, a variety of healthcare practitioners use CST to reduce stress and relieve headaches, neck and back pain, and many other disorders (Knaster, 1996). CST training workshops are available and certification can be achieved.

MASSAGE

Therapeutic massage is both an art and a science. It involves the systematic assessment of the skin and body, followed by the selective application of touch, stroking, friction, vibration, percussion, kneading, stretching, compression, and passive or active range of motion (Fritz, 1995). The two basic techniques used in massage have different effects on the body. **Mechanical techniques** are directed toward soft tissue or areas in which fluid has accumulated. **Reflexive techniques** are applied to specific points on the body to stimulate specific biochemical, endocrine, and nervous system changes. Both approaches, however, affect the *autonomic nervous system* and the *endocrine system*. It has been well documented that massage therapies also foster increased blood flow, which improves oxygenation and general cellular nourishment. Massage also decreases edema, relieves muscle spasms, and aids in pain control or reduction (Fritz, 1995).

There are many types of massage available—ranging from fairly light, gentle modalities, such as Swedish massage, to deep, intense forms, such as neuromuscular massage and deep tissue massage. Massage is usually experienced as highly enjoyable and extremely relaxing, although the more intense forms may involve some discomfort as well. A study by Eisenberg (Eisenberg et al., 1998) indicated that massage therapy is the third most frequently used CAM therapy in America. The National Institutes of Health and the National Center for Complementary and Alternative Medicine (NCCAM) have funded research that focuses on therapeutic massage.

Some states require massage therapists to be licensed. Certification in massage therapy is conferred by the National Certification Board for Therapeutic Massage and Bodywork (NCBTMB). The American Massage Therapy Association (AMTA) accredits training programs that meet its 50-hour standard. There are several professional organizations for massage therapists, of which the AMTA is the most prestigious. There are also the American Massage Therapy Association, the International Massage Association, and the Associated Bodywork & Massage Professionals.

REFLEXOLOGY

Reflexology traces its origins to ancient Egypt, with its modern practice having originated in the 1900s in this country. Reflexology is based on the notion that the hands, the feet, and even the ears are mirrors of the entire body and have specific points, or *zones,* that correspond to body function and structure. Applying pressure to specific zones is thought to affect the body structures to which they are connected. Reflexology can also be considered an energy-based therapy, as therapists believe that reflexology detects and relieves energy blockages in targeted areas of the body. Reflexology treatments may also increase blood circulation and endorphin production. Like other massage and touch therapies, reflexology is said to enhance a sense of well-being and promote

relaxation and may thereby support the immune system. The most common type of reflexology is foot reflexology.

The research literature on the efficacy of reflexology treatment is limited and has been criticized on methodological grounds. The NIH via the NCCAM has funded new studies specifically to add to the credibility of findings. A related field, **iridology,** involves diagnosing illness or incipient illness by examining the iris, the colored part of the eye. Iridology is more widely accepted in Europe than in this country, and there is as yet little empirical support for its effectiveness (Collinge, 1997).

Functional Approaches

Functional approaches to bodyways are concerned with remedies for habitual tendencies. Functional therapies focus on bodily awareness skills. Two well-known functional techniques are the **Alexander Technique** and the **Feldenkrais Method.** Both are quite gentle, involving minimal physical manipulation of the body by the therapist and the exploration of new movement patterns by the client. **Rolfing,** however, can be quite vigorous, involving deep tissue work designed to release adhesions in the fascia. Knaster (1996) reports that the outcomes of functional approaches include rejuvenation, enhanced coordination, greater flexibility, improved range of motion, and a reduction in aches, pains, and illnesses, as well as many behavioral and attitudinal improvements.

Ethnomedical Systems

An ethnomedical system of healthcare is a system of healthcare associated with a particular culture. Two such ethnomedical systems, Traditional Chinese Medicine and Ayurveda, have stimulated much interest in the West. Philosophical elements from both have been incorporated into the holistic model of healthcare, and diagnostic and treatment modalities from both are becoming increasingly popular.

Traditional Chinese Medicine

Traditional Chinese Medicine (TCM) is at least 3,000 years old and is rooted in **Taoism,** an ancient Chinese system of philosophy and religion. According to the Taoist worldview, a universal energy flows through the entire natural world, linking humans to the universe and all creation. TCM refers to this universal energy as **ch'i** or **qi** (pronounced chee). In TCM, health is the manifestation of balance and harmony in the flow of ch'i to cells, organs, and systems. TCM is primarily focused on evaluating and manipulating the flow of ch'i energy and on balancing **yin** and **yang.** In TCM, all things have either yin characteristics or yang characteristics. Yin and yang are considered energetically linked opposites that must be present in equal quantities if balance is to be maintained. When the body is in an optimum state of being, ch'i flows without encumbrance, and organ systems are balanced. The five main therapeutic modalities, or "pillars," of TCM include acupressure and acupuncture, the use of traditional Chinese herbs, diet and nutrition counseling, massage, and exercise. Acupressure and acupuncture have become popular CAM therapies in the United States, and two movement practices, Qi Gong and Tai Ch'i, are being used increasingly by Westerners who wish to improve their health.

ACUPRESSURE AND ACUPUNCTURE

Acupressure and acupuncture are two related techniques based on one of the most important concepts in traditional Chinese medicine—the existence of ch'i. In the body, ch'i is thought to flow through distinct pathways called *meridians,* which are patterned, vertical circuits that culminate in the hands and feet. All health problems are thought to reflect imbalances or blockages in the flow of ch'i through the meridian circuits, and both acupressure and acupuncture are methods of evaluating and influencing that flow. In **acupressure,** pressure is applied with the thumbs or fingers to specific points along the meridians. In **acupuncture,** very fine needles are inserted into the skin and underlying tissues to stimulate the points. Modern acupuncturists use sterile, disposable needles. Sometimes the needles are attached to a weak electric current. Alternatively, heat may be applied to the points via a process called **moxibustion.** Once the energy is flowing freely, it is assumed that the body's innate healing mechanisms will come into play.

Acupuncturists must be licensed in some states but are not required to be licensed in others. Licensed acupuncturists, or acupuncturists who hold diplomas from foreign schools, may display the initials LAc or LicAc. The National Commission for Certification of Acupuncturists (NCCA) confers certification and the accompanying title Dipl.Ac—Diplomate in Acupuncture. The National Accreditation Commission for Schools and Colleges of Acupuncture and Oriental Medicine (NACSCAOM) accredits schools of acupuncture. There are a number of professional organizations for acupuncturists. The American Academy of Medical Acupuncture (AAMA) accepts into membership only medical doctors and doctors of osteopathy who have undergone formal training in a program accredited by NACSCAOM as well as a period of apprenticeship in acupuncture. Members have the title MAc—Medical Acupuncturist.

There is a large pool of evidence-based outcomes related to acupuncture. There is less outcome research evaluating the efficacy of acupressure. Like much of the research on alternative therapies, many of the acupuncture studies have been poorly designed, at least in the opinions of orthodox Western scientists. Worldwide, however, the scientific literature suggests that acupuncture can be effective in such problems as tension headache, nausea, osteoarthritis, dys-

menorrhea, high blood pressure, depression and anxiety, back pain, and substance abuse (Knaster, 1996). Westerners who do not accept the existence of ch'i have suggested other mechanisms by which acupuncture may work, such as the stimulation of endorphin production (Collinge, 1997).

QI GONG

Qi Gong is an ancient Chinese movement practice used to promote wellness and self-healing. Its purpose is to improve the flow of Qi (ch'i) throughout the body. One practices the highly orchestrated, deliberate movements of Qi Gong daily for about a half-hour. Qi Gong also includes breathing techniques, which are used in conjunction with the movements. Holding in one's mind the *intention* to balance Qi while engaging in Qi Gong practice is also thought to be important.

TAI CHI

Also known as Tai Chi Chuan, Tai Ch'i is similar to Qi Gong. The goal of both is to balance vital energy, or ch'i. Tai Chi is a blend of *mental exercises* and a series of slow, choreographed, fluid *movements*. An increasing body of evidence suggests that Tai Ch'i practice supports wellness by improving flexibility, balance, and breathing patterns and by decreasing blood pressure and perceived stress (Knaster, 1996). Qi Gong and Tai Chi are as popular in Eastern cultures, such as China, as jogging and aerobics are in the West.

Ayurveda

Ayurveda is the ancient healing system of India. As TCM is an aspect of Taoism, Aruvedic medicine is an integral part of the larger Hindu spiritual tradition. The "pillars" of Aruvedic medicine are a variant of massage known as marma therapy, yoga, breathing exercises known as pranayama, meditation, a diet appropriate to one's **dosha** (body/personality type), and a detoxification regimen known as panchakarma. As with TCM, several universal principles underlie Ayurveda as a system of living and medicine. The first is the universality of the living energy, referred to as ch'i in Taoism and **prana** in Ayurveda. Prana flows through a meridian-like system known as the **nadis** and through energy centers known as **chakras.** The second universal principle is that the universe is made up of intelligent energy—the basic "stuff" of which everything is made. The particular form that this energy takes—mountains, lakes, people, prana, and so on—depends on the rate at which it is *vibrating.* Ayurveda assumes that everything is interconnected and interrelated. In Ayurvedic tradition, there is an immutable relationship between person and universe, which can be perceived via spiritual awareness. Similarly, there is a relationship among the body, mind, and spirit. In Ayurveda, the key to wellness is balance within and among all three spheres. Deepak Chopra, M.D., popularized Ayurveda in his 1991 book *Perfect Health.*

Other Healing Disciplines

A number of therapeutic disciplines not associated with any particular culture have been developed. Three of the better-known ones are naturopathy, homeopathy, and aromatherapy.

Naturopathy

Naturopathy is a system of natural health promotion and care that was brought to this country in the early 1900s, when a German named Benedict Lust founded a school in New York City. Naturopathic physicians take a holistic (whole person) approach to their patients and focus primarily on health maintenance and illness prevention. Naturopaths teach the principles of a healthy diet and the importance of exercise and stress reduction. The goal of naturopathic therapy is to find the *root causes* of ailments, rather than merely to suppress symptoms. Once the root causes have been eliminated, it is assumed that the body's innate healing ability will take over. Naturopaths use herbal therapy, and many are trained in acupuncture, acupressure, and homeopathy (discussed in the next section) as well. A recent resurgence of interest in the more natural healing modalities has shifted naturopathy's sphere of influence to the Pacific Northwest. The accredited schools of naturopathy in North America are located in Seattle, Scottsdale, Portland, Bridgeport, and Toronto. The educational program is a four-year postgraduate program in the health sciences, with admission requirements similar to those of conventional medical schools. The credential is N.D., doctor of naturopathic medicine.

Homeopathy

Homeopathy is a system of healing founded in the 1700s by Samuel Hahnemann. Hahnemann developed homeopathy as an alternative to the so-called **heroic medicine** of the time, which included such therapies as surgery, bloodletting, and the use of toxic, mercury-based purgatives. The American Medical Association was formed largely to suppress homeopaths and other practitioners who competed with physicians.

Homeopathy is based on assumptions that are very difficult for Western scientists and physicians to accept. It is basically an *energy therapy* that relies on curative essences that are not discernible by extant technology. Homeopathic remedies are thought to stimulate the vital energy of the persons who ingest them. Homeopathic remedies consist of extremely dilute preparations of natural substances. A minute amount of a particular substance is ground up and diluted with water—sometimes to the point that not a single molecule of the original substance can be detected. However, in homeopathy, the more *dilute* a remedy is, the more *potent* it is considered to be. The rationale for choosing a specific remedy is also foreign to Western medical thought; the assumption is that "like cures like." Therefore, the remedy for a skin rash might be a dilute preparation of something known to *cause* a rash. Remedies are matched to symptoms, and the ideal remedy is that which would cause the *same* symptoms in a healthy person.

The literature on the efficacy of homeopathic remedies is mixed. Although a carefully conducted meta-analysis of the homeopathic literature (Linde, Clausius, & Ramirez, 1997) failed to identify a single illness for which homeopathy has been demonstrated to be unequivocally effective, the authors did conclude that, overall, homeopathy had an effect that could not be explained by the placebo response. Also, Albrecht and Schutte (1999) found that pigs given homeopathic preparations for the prevention of respiratory ailments had fewer respiratory problems than the swine in a control group given a placebo, and the difference was statistically significant.

The aim of homeopathy is to stimulate the body to heal itself. Homeopaths generally attempt to treat any condition the body is deemed fundamentally capable of resisting or overcoming and seem to do best with acute and chronic diseases in the earlier stages, before too much damage has been done to the body. Homeopathy is not used to treat advanced cancer, physical trauma, and strokes. It may be used, however, to hasten the healing of broken bones. Access to education in homeopathy is widespread across the United States, Canada, and Europe. Information is available through the American Association of Homeopathic Pharmacists and the National Center for Homeopathy. The Council on Homeopathic Education accredits training programs in classical homeopathy.

Aromatherapy

Aromatherapy is a derivative of herbal therapy. The active chemicals of herbs and other plants are concentrated in their oils, and, in aromatherapy, distilled oils (known as **essential oils**) from the leaves, bark, roots, seeds, resins, or rinds of specific plants are used for healing. The aroma, or scent, of the oil is perceived when diffused molecules in the air are inhaled through the nose and reach specialized receptors in the brain. The term *aromatherapy* is a bit misleading, as inhaling the scent of essential oils is not the only method of benefiting from them—essential oils can also be massaged into the skin or added to the bath, and a few can be taken internally. (The internal use of oils, however, is considered herbology rather than aromatherapy.) As essential oils are highly concentrated, they are usually diluted with a carrier oil before being applied to the skin. True essential oils are **steam distillates,** (products recovered from distilled plant extracts) and their production is an exacting and expensive process. **Plant extracts,** although considerably less expensive, usually contain remnants of petrochemical solvents and are therefore not used in clinical aromatherapy.

Aromatherapy is an ancient healing practice that is becoming popular once again. There are hundreds of essential oils available, and each is said to have specific healing properties. There is an extensive quasi-scientific and anecdotal literature on the efficacy of aromatherapy. The number of studies that can be considered truly well designed by prevailing standards is very limited, however, because it is difficult to conduct blinded studies on odoriferous substances (Buckle, 1999). Nevertheless, the evidence for the effectiveness of some oils is persuasive. For example, essential oil of lavender decreased pain and heart rate in a majority of subjects who were patients in an intensive care unit (Woolfson & Hewitt, 1992). Several continuing education opportunities are available for those who wish to learn more about aromatherapy. More information is available through the National Association for Holistic Aromatherapy.

Herbal Remedies

Using herbal remedies to treat illness and disease is one of the most widespread practices in CAM. **Herbs** are plants that elicit pharmacological effects on the body. **Herbal medicinals** consist of intact, unadultered plant parts, or crude preparations made from whole plants. Treating illness or disease with plant extracts is called **herbalism** or **phytotherapy.** The term **phytopharmaceuticals** refers to medicines that contain a standardized amount of an isolated, pharmacologically active constituent of a plant. The term is more commonly used in Europe, where herbs are considered to be drugs. In the United States, however, herbs are classified not as drugs but as *dietary supplements,* and the official term for them is **botanicals** (Barrett, Vohmann, & Calabrese, 1999; Hoffman & Leaders, 1996; L. G. Miller, 1998). Still another term, **nutraceuticals,** describes plants that are used as either food or medicine (Houghton, 1995). An example is garlic *(Allium sativa).* Garlic is a well-known flavoring agent for foods and sauces that also has antibacterial and antioxidant properties, along with the putative ability to lower cholesterol levels and blood pressure, as well as to reduce the amount of plaque in arteries (Berthold, Sudhop, & von Bergmann, 1998; Jungnickel, 1998).

Consumer Demographics

The proportion of the U.S. population that uses herbal medicine is estimated to be between 15 and 37 percent (Barrett, Kiefer, & Rabago, 1999) and continues to increase. In a 1997 follow-up to their original survey in 1991, Eisenberg et al. (1998) reported a 380 percent increase in the number of individuals reporting to use herbal remedies. The annual growth rate of the retail market is estimated to be between 18 and 40 percent (Brody, 1999; PR Newswire, 1999; Williamson & Wyandt, 1998).

Individuals who avail themselves of herbal remedies tend to be well educated and prosperous. The typical consumer is likely to be a college graduate between 35 and 49 years old, with an annual income above $50,000 (Eisenberg et al., 1998). As women constitute two-thirds of the healthcare consumers and make three out of four of the household healthcare decisions (Greenberger, 1998), it is not surprising that the majority of those purchasing and using herbal remedies and supplements are female (Eisenberg et al., 1998; Jacob, 1998). Information gleaned from phone interviews conducted in the United States with English-speaking respondents suggests that African Americans are less likely than members of other ethnic groups to use herbal remedies.

Three theories have been put forth as to why people turn to herbal remedies when there are so many more conventional medicines available. One theory holds that consumers are *dissatisfied* with conventional medicines, which they view as ineffective, impersonal, or too technologically oriented. Another theory maintains that the use of herbal remedies provides individuals with a sense of *personal control* over their healthcare. According to the third theory, the use of herbals, as well as other alternative therapies, is congruent with the spiritual and religious *philosophy* and *beliefs* of the individual. This last theory has been found to be most applicable; research suggests that most of those who use alternative therapies do so because they have a holistic philosophy of health and healthcare. Only those individuals who have a *primary reliance* on alternative healthcare (4 to 17 percent of surveyed alternative healthcare users) do so because of a distrust of and dissatisfaction with conventional medical care (Astin, 1996). Most of those who use alternative therapies use them *in addition to,* rather than in place of, conventional therapies.

In comparison with the rest of the world, the United States still relies heavily on traditional pharmaceuticals for medical relief. In contrast, it is estimated that 80 percent of the nonindustrialized world, or approximately 64 percent of the total world population, relies on plant-derived products to meet their primary medicinal needs (Farnsworth, Akerele, Bingle, Soejarto, & Guo, 1985; Farnsworth & Soejarto, 1991). In South Australia, half of the population uses alternative medicine (McLennan, Wilson, & Taylor, 1996), and, in Germany, the proportion is 62 percent (Robbers & Tyler, 1998).

A Brief History of Herbal Medicine

The contemporary use of herbal remedies in the industrialized West represents not a new phenomenon but, rather, a return to historical perspectives on, and approaches to, treating illness. Whereas mainstream medicine views disease as the malfunction of one specific system and targets only that system for treatment (Houghton, 1995), the much older herbal medical tradition views the body holistically as an assemblage of interacting systems. Disease is seen as causing an imbalance, and herbal preparations are taken to prevent or correct it.

The use of plants to treat illness and disease has a history that extends back at least 60,000 years. Quantities of pollen from eight species of plants were found surrounding the corpse of a Neanderthal man discovered in a burial cave in northern Iraq. Of those eight species, seven are still used in herbal medicine (Solecki & Shanidar, 1975). As early as 4000 B.C.E., the Sumerians were referring to the poppy *(Papaver somniferum)* as the "joy plant" (Lewis & Elvin-Lewis, 1977). The earliest example (circa 3000 B.C.E.) of a written prescription was found at a Sumerian archeological site. Around 1550 B.C.E., the Egyptians were using castor oil as a laxative and opium for pain. Plants have also been a part of traditional medicine in China and India for over 2,000 years. During the medieval period (A.D. 400 to 1580), Christian monks used the plants and herbs they grew in their gardens to treat the sick and maintained records of their medicine in their monasteries. Around A.D. 1240, the Arabs enhanced the empirical use of herbs by developing what is now known as the **apothecary system**—the first known set of drug standards and measurements (Kee & Hayes, 1997; McKenry & Salerno, 1998).

The use of herbs in orthodox Western medicine peaked during the sixteenth and seventeenth centuries and then began to decline (Bateman, Chapman, & Simpson, 1998; Leaders, 1998; Shad, Chinn, & Brann, 1999). The first edition of the *United States Pharmacopoeia* (the written authority for drug standards) was published in 1820 and listed 425 botanical remedies, which constituted 67 percent of the total number (633) of entries. In the twenty-second edition of the *Pharmacopoeia*, published in 1990, however, only 58 of the 2,894 entries (2 percent) were for botanical substances (Williamson & Wyandt, 1998). Some of the decline after 1820 in the rate at which physicians used medications containing plant-derived compounds is attributable to the fact that marketing drugs is more *profitable* for pharmaceutical companies than is marketing herbs.

Pharmaceutical companies, like other companies, are more likely to promote the products from which they can derive the greatest profit. In order to derive profit from the sale of a therapeutic substance, a drug company must be able to sell the substance for more than it costs to develop it. Pharmaceutical companies face a long (10–15 years) and formidable process to bring any drug or therapeutic compound to the market. Developmental costs typically run between $50 and $100 million (Tyler, 1986). Whereas drug companies stand a good chance of realizing a profit on synthetic drugs, it is more difficult to do so in the case of plant-derived substances.

There are two main obstacles to bringing plant-derived drugs to the marketplace. One, there is the tedious, difficult, costly, and largely unrewarding process of *screening plants* and isolating the pharmacologically active ingredients. The second obstacle is the fact that, if the newly isolated compound cannot be synthesized, the company must secure a *raw supply* of material. Often, the raw material is available only from a country that is unwilling to provide it, possibly because it, too, needs the resource (Akerele, Heywood, & Synge, 1991; Taylor, 1996). Also, many countries are increasing the degree of protection and control they exert over their natural resources, thus making it even more difficult for pharmaceutical houses to secure a steady supply of raw materials (Houghton, 1995).

Another impediment to pharmaceutical companies' ability to profit from plant-derived substances has to do with *patents*. Being able to patent drugs they have developed for a period of time protects companies from competition and gives them time to realize a profit. A patent may not be issued for a plant-derived substance, however, if information about its use already exists in the literature. This is frequently problematic, as many medicinal plants have a long history in folk medicine. Consequently, many pharmaceutical companies use plant-derived compounds only as the basis for modified or newly synthesized drugs (Farnsworth & Soejarto, 1991). An example is the derivation of ibuprofen (in 1964) from willow bark, via aspirin (Robbers & Tyler, 1998).

The greater availability of synthetic drugs, together with the empirical evidence of their efficacy provided by drug companies, gradually caused herbal medicinals to go into eclipse. Until very recently, most research on therapeutic substances was funded by drug companies, which had little incentive to fund research on herbals. In the 1900s, however, a resurgence of interest in herbal remedies arose in the United States (Eisenberg et al., 1998) and is continuing unabated. The rise in the popular use of herbal remedies has been attributed to the creation of the National Institutes of Health's Office of Alternative Medicine in 1992 (now the National Center for Complementary and Alternative Medicine—NCCAM). Established by Congress to examine alternative healthcare practices, the work of the NIH began to attract media attention, followed by public interest and increased sales of dietary supplements (*Herbal Rx: The Promise and Pitfalls,* 1999; Neldner, 2000). The NCCAM is currently funding studies of herbs as well as other alternative therapies.

Federal Regulation of Herbal Substances

Throughout the long history of herbal medications, the precise actions that many botanicals have on the body were ill defined and the dosages given inconsistent. The *active ingredient* in most herbs was unknown, and the *potency* varied greatly within and among plants. Moreover, some herbal medicines contained **adulterants**—harmful extraneous ingredients. The methods of chemical analysis were relatively unrefined, compared with today's standards, and the results of testing botanicals on living organisms (bioassays) were variable due to the failure to control for differences among treatment subjects (Leaders, 1998). Because of these circumstances, some early herbal remedies failed to work, were harmful, or caused death (Angell & Kassirer, 1998). Laws intended to protect American consumers from impure, toxic, ineffective, or untested medicines were eventually passed.

The Federal Pure Food and Drug Act of 1906 stipulated that a drug be free of a list of 11 adulterants, including opium, morphine, and heroin—all plant-derived substances. In 1912, the Sherley Amendment, which prohibited fraudulent therapeutic claims, was passed. Another law intended to increase the safety of drugs, the Food, Drug, and Cosmetic Act of 1938, required that all drugs be evaluated for toxicity. In addition, the act required the Food and Drug Administration (FDA) to review all drugs brought to market to ensure that their labels contained accurate information and that literature detailing adverse effects was enclosed. In 1952, the Durham-Humphrey Amendment to the 1938 act was passed. It distinguished between drugs that can be sold with or without a prescription and established a new class of drugs, known as over-the-counter drugs. Prior to 1962, the FDA had lumped herbs and drugs together as pharmaceuticals and had subjected both types of products to the same scrutiny. However, that changed in 1962 with the passage of the Kefauver-Harris Amendment, which required that, in order to be considered a **drug,** a medicinal substance has to be both safe and effective, as demonstrated by specific methods of evaluation (McKenry & Salerno, 1998). After 1962, herbs whose efficacy could not be satisfactorily demonstrated were exempt from regulations that applied to drugs. To date, only nine herbs have met these criteria and have been recognized as drugs by the FDA (Youngkin & Israel, 1996).

In 1993, the FDA proposed controversial regulations that would have required the manufacturers of nondrug medicinals to provide proof of any claim as to their products' ability to treat or alleviate a health-related condition. A grassroots coalition of manufacturers and consumers protested, saying that, due to the inherent difficulties of empirically testing herbal products, such legislation would effectively prohibit the marketing of herbal remedies (*Herbal Rx: The Promise and Pitfalls,* 1999). There was also the suspicion that the increasingly powerful drug companies were pushing the legislation in an effort to have competing botanical products removed from the market. The legislation was defeated, and compromise legislation, the Dietary Supplement Health Education Act (DSHEA), was passed in 1994. The DSHEA placed herbs (along with vitamins, minerals, and amino acids) in a new class of products, now known as **dietary supplements.** Manufacturers are free to market their dietary supplements but are limited as to the claims they can make on the labels. Only documented information about how the herb can affect the structure and function of the human body and how it *may* help a particular condition can be displayed. Manufacturers *cannot* make direct claims that their products can be used to treat, cure, or prevent human *diseases.* Moreover, these dietary supplements are required to carry a disclaimer that they have not been tested or evaluated by the FDA (U.S. Food and Drug Administration, 1995, 1999).

The classification of herbals as dietary supplements means that they undergo less rigorous testing, and less supervision during manufacturing, than prescription or over-the-counter drugs (Leaders, 1998). As a consequence, an herbal product may not contain a pharmacologically active ingredient and may even contain a toxic one (McCarthy, 1998). That said, it is important to keep the relative safety of drugs and food supplements in perspective. There is no doubt that many drugs, particularly prescription medications, are inherently dangerous and can cause serious injury or even death. On average, drugs the FDA has deemed safe cause 125,000 deaths each year, even when appropriately prescribed and administered (Faloon, 1999). When inappropriately prescribed or administered, drugs are even more dangerous; medication errors resulting in adverse drug reactions or death have been on the increase and are estimated to affect as many as 35 percent of hospital patients (Bates et al., 1995; Leape et al., 1991; Phillips, Christenfeld, & Glynn, 1998). In general, herbal remedies that can serve as substitutes for synthetic drugs have been demonstrated to have comparatively fewer adverse effects, such as St. John's wort for mild to moderate depression (Ernst, 1998). When considered on a per capita user basis, the number of fatalities and other serious events in the United States associated with herbal medicines is only in the dozens per year (Barrett et al., 1999). It has been suggested, however, that adverse reactions to botanicals may be *underreported.* People may be more likely to report the serious adverse effects associated with prescription drugs than the moderate or mild effects typically caused by herbals (Alvarez-Requejo, Carvajal, Begaud, Vega, & Arias, 1998; Barnes, Mills, Abbot, Willoughby, & Ernst, 1998).

The oversight of herbal remedies is more stringent in Canada and Germany. In Canada, 57 herbs were banned due to safety concerns and 5 others were given warning labels indicating that they could be harmful to women during pregnancy (Snider, 1991; Youngkin & Isreal, 1996). Shortly after World War II, the pharmaceutical industry in Germany supported projects that optimized the uniformity and efficacy of herbal drugs (Wagner, 1999). More recently (1970–1985), the first phase of an herbal drug investigation was conducted in that country to demonstrate the quality and to determine the active principles of existing phytopreparations. This was followed by clinical trials on 10 phytopreparations that were already on the market (Wagner, 1999). In 1988, a government-designated panel (Commission E) reviewed the literature, clinical trials, and case reports on more than 1,400 herbal drugs, which resulted in a compilation of 300 monographs on herbs and phytomedicines (Youngkin & Isreal, 1996). The **German Commission E Monographs** are considered by some to be the most complete and accurate source of information in the world on the safety and efficacy of herbs. However, because the monographs do not reference the sources of information used to assess the herbs, their credibility has been questioned by many U.S. researchers (NIEHS News, 1998).

TABLE 11–1 Comparison of pharmaceutical medicines with botanical remedies.

Characteristic	Pharmaceutical Medicines	Botanical Remedies
Method of production	Synthesis	Extraction
Outcome of production	Uniform	Variable
Character of product	Homogeneous	Heterogeneous
Structure of active ingredient	Known	Sometimes unknown
Number of active ingredients	One	Sometimes multiple
Product quality	Pure	Compared with a standard

Source: Adapted from "Incorporating Botanical Products into MCO Formularies," by Floyd E. Leaders, JR., RPh, PhD, which appeared in the March 1998 Drug Benefit Trends issue on pp. 34, 36–39, 43.

Phytochemicals in Mainstream Medicine

Despite the decline in the use of herbal remedies in Western medicine during the latter half of the twentieth century, phytochemicals still play an important role in pharmaceutical-based medicine. There are approximately 121 chemicals of known structure that are still extracted from plants for their medicinal value (Farnsworth & Soejarto, 1991), and many of the botanically derived medicinals discovered during the seventeenth and eighteenth centuries are still in use today. For example, purple foxglove *(Digitalis purpurea)* was found through trial and error in 1785 to cure "dropsy" (congestive heart failure) by slowing and strengthening the heartbeat (Ashcroft & Po, 1999). Approximately 25 percent of the drugs dispensed through pharmacies in the United States contain at least one ingredient obtained from a plant (Farnsworth & Soejarto, 1991), and, in Eastern Europe, over 60 percent of prescriptions are for plant-derived drugs (Husain, 1991).

The differences between traditional botanical remedies and pharmaceutical medicines (drugs) lie in their *chemical content* and the different *manufacturing processes* used to produce them (see Table 11–1). Drugs are *synthesized* in laboratories and are *uniform* in terms of chemical composition and potency. The first drug was synthesized in 1899 from salicylic acid, a substance extracted from willow bark *(Salix spp.)*. Teas made from willow bark had long been used to treat headache and pain. Because concentrated salicylic acid was too strong to be administered orally, it was chemically modified into *aspirin,* one of the most widely used medicines in the world (Robbers & Tyler, 1998). Botanical remedies are produced by the process of *extracting* the active ingredient from the plant, and they *vary* in terms of chemical composition and potency. The amount of active ingredient contained in an individual plant is a function of soil conditions, rain, and so on. Other problems with extracted active ingredients are that they may also be unstable or may be effective only if consumed in large quantities. Also, the plants from which the active ingredient is isolated may have limited availability and may not lend themselves to cultivation. For example, the availability of natural taxol for the treatment of breast cancer is limited because it is isolated from the bark of the northwestern yew *(Taxus brevifolia)*. To derive enough taxol for the treatment of one patient would require extracting the bark from six 100-year-old trees (Research Triant Institute, 2000). Because of these difficulties, taxol is now synthesized from a compound extracted from the bark of the much more common English yew *(Taxus baccata)*. Although synthesizing taxol without the use of plant material is possible, it is complicated and not economically feasible (McDonley, 2001; Sanganee & Harrison, 2001).

Only a relatively *small* percentage of the available pharmacologically active plant material is packaged into botanical remedies. Most is used in the process of *synthesizing related drugs*. Nevertheless, some widely sold drugs are still extracted from plants because chemists sometimes find it very difficult to duplicate the complicated chemical structure of a certain plant. In such cases, it is much more cost effective to extract the active ingredients than to synthesize them. An example is the plant steroid diogenin, which is extracted from the yam species *Disocoria* (spp). Nearly all of the *oral contraceptives* used by women are derived from modified diogenin. More recently, oral contraceptives have also been derived from stigmasterol, which comes from soybean oil (Husain, 1991; Plotkin, 1991; Principe, 1991).

Safety of Herbal Remedies

Poisons and medicines are oftentimes the same substance given with different intents.
Peter Mere Latham (1789–1875)

Herbal remedies are often perceived as natural alternatives to traditional pharmaceuticals. Many consumers see herbals as more cost effective, less toxic, and less likely to cause side effects (Leaders, 1998). However, although herbals generally are considerably less toxic than many prescription drugs, they are not without risks, particularly when taken *in conjunction with drugs* (*Adverse Effects to Herbal Medicines,* 1998; Portyansky, 1998). Adverse effects from the use of botanical substances have been reported, both in the United States and in other countries that have a longer history of using herbals. Over one 10-month period, herbal medicine ranked third among the medicines responsible for causing adverse effects in Taiwan and, in Hong Kong, 0.2 percent of all patient admissions were due to adverse reactions to Chinese herbal drugs (Ernst, 1998). In Western cultures, such as Great Britain, approximately 5 to 8 percent of poisonings and adverse drug reactions can be attributed to herbal remedies (Abbot, White, & Ernst, 1996; Perharic et al., 1994).

Whether associated with a synthetic pharmaceutical or a naturally grown herbal remedy, the leading cause of adverse effects and poisonings is *human error.* Thus, most drug- or herb-related complications are preventable. Technical errors, such as miscalculating drug dosages, placing decimal points incorrectly, and using incorrect abbreviations, along with negligence, are often the cause of the adverse events associated with traditional prescription medicines (Leape et al., 1991; Lesar, Briceland, & Stein, 1997). Many adverse reactions to herbal preparations are due to adulteration, accidental overdose, an incorrect prescription or formulation (Bateman et al., 1998), or the false identification of living plants—particularly when common names are used instead of Latin names (Ernst 1998; Frasca, Brett, & Yoo, 1997). For example, one woman drank a tea made from poisonous oleander leaves because she believed she had picked eucalyptus leaves (Snider, 1991). Another cause of adverse reactions to herbal products is inaccurate or inappropriate advice or recommendations made by poorly informed personnel in health-food stores (Vickers, Rees, & Robin, 1998).

A *drug* is any substance that is used to treat a disease or condition (either to cure or mitigate) or used to improve an individual's health through diagnosis or prevention. Although herbal remedies are not considered drugs under current law, they conform to the definition based on the intent of their use (Robbers & Tyler, 1998). If herbs are ingested with the understanding that they will in some way affect the physiology of the body, then it should come as no surprise that herbal remedies can also have adverse or even toxic effects. That herbs are *natural substances* does *not* mean that they cannot cause physiological harm to the human body. See Table 11–2 for a list of potentially toxic herbs.

The active ingredients in plants evolved as part of their *defense mechanisms.* The presence of unpalatable or even toxic chemicals discourages herbivores from eating the plants (Fraenkel, 1959). In response, animals, including humans, have developed an array of enzymes capable of breaking down toxic plant compounds. Unfortunately, however, this breakdown often leads to the formation of toxic intermediates. Because the *liver* is the chemical-processing plant of the body, it is the organ most susceptible to these powerful plant defense compounds and their catabolic intermediates. For example, comfrey *(Symphytum officinale)* contains pyrrolizidine-type alkaloids, which are converted in the liver to toxic pyrrole metabolites. Although the risk of experiencing an adverse reaction to a botanical remedy is relatively low, certain groups of traditional remedies have been associated with some serious adverse side effects (Shad et al., 1999; Shaw, Leon, Kolev, & Murray, 1997). Of the 150 plant species that are used for herbal medicine in China (out of nearly 7,000 species), 10 are considered toxic. Among these are plants from the genus *Aconitum,* which contain highly toxic, aconitine alkaloids that have analgesic, antipyretic, and anesthetic properties and are used to treat arthritic, rheumatic, and musculoskeletal pain. Because of their toxicity, there is a narrow margin of safety between therapeutic and toxic dosages, and there is no antidote for aconitine poisoning (Bateman et al., 1998).

One of the more significant risks associated with the use of herbal remedies lies not in the nature of the herbal remedies themselves but in the *self-diagnosis* that usually precedes their use. Most consumers do not possess the expertise required to accurately diagnose their own illnesses. Many signs and symptoms of serious diseases can be mistaken for those associated with minor illnesses (Robbers & Tyler, 1998). In the United States, the risk for this seems to be high: While 42 percent of respondents in a 1997 survey reported having used some sort of alternative therapy, only 46 percent of those people had consulted either a medical doctor or a practitioner of alternative therapy (Eisenberg et al., 1998). Individuals who self-prescribe herbals also sometimes experience adverse effects related to the pharmacological actions of the active ingredients. This can occur because the herb is inherently dangerous, because the product was ingested in excessive amounts, or because it interacted with a prescription medication. A case that involved both the first and second reasons is that of a woman who drank as many as 10 cups of comfrey tea a day for a year to ease stomach pains and later developed liver disease (Snider, 1991).

It has been estimated that one out of every five people taking prescription medicines is also taking herbals; therefore, approximately 15 million adults are at risk for potential adverse interactions—particularly because nearly 75 percent of these individuals do not tell their providers about the herbals they are taking. Individuals who are at particular risk include those with chronic medical illness, such as liver, kidney, or heart abnormalities (Eisenberg et al., 1993; Greiger, 2000). Many individuals lack the background information required to keep track of the many potential interactions between herbs and prescription drugs. CVS, the largest drug store chain in the country, has provided a safety net for its customers; each time a drug prescription is filled, an automatic printout lists

TABLE 11–2 Some herbs to avoid because of known toxicity.

Herb	Adverse Effects
Borage *(Borago officinalis)*	Hepatic cancer *(oil not harmful)*
Broom *(Cytisus scoparius)*	Strong sedation, tachycardia, cardiac depression
Calamus *(Acorus calamus)*	Cancer
Chaparrel *(Larrea tridentata)*	Liver damage
Coltsfoot *(Tussilago farfar)*	Hepatic cancer
Comfrey *(Symphytum species)*	Hepatic cancer (not harmful when applied externally)
Germander *(Teucrium chamaedrys)*	Liver damage
Life root *(Senecio aureus)*	Liver damage, hepatic cancer
Licorice *(Glycyrrhiza glabra)*	Headache, lethargy, sodium and water retention, hypokalemia, muscle paralysis, hypertension, heart failure, cardiac arrest
Ma huang *(Ephedra sinica)*	Hallucinations, paranoia, stimulation, hypertension, myocardial infarction
Monkshood *(Aconitum napellus)*	Deadly poison: palpitations, arrhythmias, nausea, abdominal pain, diarrhea, heart failure, asphyxiation
Pennyroyal *(Mentha pulegium)*	Liver damage
Sassafras *(Sassafras albidum)*	Cancer
Yohimbe *(Pausinystalia yohimbe)*	Hypertension, tachycardia, paralysis, death

Source: Adapted from "Possible Toxicity of Herbal Remedies, by J. Bateman, R. D. Chapman, and D. Simpson, 1998), *Scottish Medical Journal, 43*, 7–15; "Harmless Herbs? A Review of the Recent Literature," by E. Ernst, 1998, *American Journal of Medicine, 104,* 170–178; *PDR for Herbal Medicines,* (2nd Ed.), by J. Gruenwald, T. Bendler, & C. Jaenicke, 2000, Montvale, NJ: Medical Economics; "Unsafe and Potentially Safe Herbal Therapies," by T. B. Klepser, and M. E. Klepser, 1999. *American Journal of Health-System Pharmacists, 56,* 125–138; "Preoperative Considerations with Herbal Medicines," by J. M. Murphy, 1999. *AORN Journal, 69,* 183–193; "An Herbal Update," by J. S. Williamson, and C. M. Wyandt, 1998, June 1st. *Drug Topics,* pp. 66–75.

potential interactions between the drug and any herbs or vitamins the customer is taking (Business Wire, 2000).

Quality Control in Herbals

Users of herbal remedies are susceptible to another type of toxic poisoning that is related to the lack of stringent rules regarding labeling and general oversight of these products: **adulteration.** Dietary supplements may contain toxic components that are not listed on the label. For example, two individuals taking an herbal dietary supplement that listed plantain (*Plantago spp)* on the label were hospitalized with cardiac symptoms. It was subsequently discovered that the supplement was contaminated with *Digitalis lanata,* a plant that contains cardiac glycosides (Slifman et al., 1998). Chinese herbal remedies may contain steroids or even arsenic, yet these ingredients may not be listed on the label (Anderson, 1996; Graham-Brown, Bourke, & Bumphrey, 1994; Shaw et al., 1997). Herbal reme-

dies used in Ayurvedic medicine may contain high concentrations of lead, arsenic, and mercury as active ingredients, and cases of heavy metal poisoning have been traced to their use (Bateman et al., 1998; Dunbabin, Tallis, Popplewell, & Lee, 1992; Keen, Deacon, Delves, Moreton, & Frost, 1994).

Another problem sometimes encountered with herbals is that packaged remedies may not actually contain the ingredients listed on the label, and, if they do, the label may not reflect the *true concentration*. For example, one brand of yohimbe tablets for erectile dysfunction were found to contain caffeine, but no yohimbe, the active ingredient (De Smet, 1997). In another analysis, the amount of ginseng per pill from 10 brands was found to vary by a factor of 10, although each brand claimed to contain the same amount (*Herbal Roulette,* 1995). Moreover, the amount of the active ingredient (ginsenosides) in each capsule varied by more than 20-fold among the brands. In another analysis underwritten by the *Los Angeles Times,* 10 brands of St. John's wort were analyzed and 3 were found to have less than half the potency claimed on the label (Monmaney, 1998).

Much of the variation in the potency of herbal remedies' active ingredients is natural; potency is affected by a variety of factors. One is that flowers, leaves, roots, seeds, and bark can all contain different concentrations of an active ingredient, representing a substantial source of variation when crude preparations are used. Even a manufacturer that uses only one part of the plant may still produce a product with a wide range of concentrations because the growing conditions experienced by the plant also strongly influence the concentration of active ingredients (Herms & Mattson, 1992). Another factor is that plants may produce more or less of an active ingredient because of *genetic variation*. Many manufacturers standardize the potency of the herbal products they sell by manipulating the amount of active ingredient present. The issue of whether all herbals should be standardized highlights the different philosophies that underlie alternative and conventional medicine. Conventional medicine generally focuses on *isolated substances* with known pharmacological properties. In contrast, many traditional herbal medicines contain a *mixture of compounds,* which may act in different ways on various parts of the body. Some holistically inclined providers maintain that the efficacy of a therapeutic plant lies in the *synergistic balance* among all the chemicals present and that, to focus on only one, and distort its proper proportion in relation to the others, may negatively alter the remedy's effect on the body (Dossey, 2001). The natural variation in the structure of the active compounds may also contribute to herbals' generally longer duration of effect, as each related chemical structure in the plant has a different period of activation in the body. Another point frequently made by herbalists is that fresh herbs are always of better quality than processed ones because harvesting, storage, and processing can degrade the integrity of plant cells and adversely affect the chemical structure of the active ingredients (Krest & Keusgen, 1999; Lindroth & Koss, 1996). Processing can make herbs less effective or more toxic (Chan, Tomlinson, & Critchley, 1993).

The natural variation in the active ingredients of herbals makes the standardization of herbal medicines problematic and controversial and a barrier to quality control for conscientious and responsible companies. The dearth of published standards for the analysis of active constituents also makes it difficult for manufacturers to demonstrate consistency in their products (Houghton, 1995; Matthews, Lucier, & Fisher, 1999).

Popular Herbal Remedies of Importance to Women

Many herbal remedies are safe if used wisely; guidelines are presented in Table 11–3. Women who are or might become pregnant or are nursing should not take any pharmacologically

---

TABLE 11–3 Safety guidelines for women using herbals.

1. Do not take a large quantity of any one herbal preparation.
2. Do not take any herbal remedy on a daily basis for a prolonged period of time.
3. Purchase only herbal products that have been standardized and tested. Look for expiration dates and lot numbers when buying.
4. Buy only preparations that list ingredients and quantities on the package.
5. Do not take herbs if pregnant or attempting to become pregnant.
6. Do not take herbal remedies if you are breast-feeding.
7. Do not use herbals to treat illness in your baby or young children.

Source: Shaw, Leon, Kolev & Murray, 1997; Williamson & Wyandt, 1998; Youngkin and Israel, 1996.

---

active substance except on the advice of a healthcare provider. Most drugs, and the active constituents of herbal remedies, have the ability to cross the placental barrier. Compounds that may be safe for an adult could adversely impact a fetus, particularly during the *first trimester,* when the risk for anatomical malformations is greatest. Lactating mothers may also pass the active constituents of herbal remedies to nursing young. Nursing infants are at risk because their body composition (such as water content, lipids, and proteins) differs from that of adults, and their detoxifying enzyme systems may not be fully developed (Robbers & Tyler, 1998).

BLACK COHOSH *(CIMICIFUGA RACEMOSA)*

Black cohosh, also known as black snake root, rattleroot, rattleweed, bugbane, and bugwort, is reported to have been introduced by Native Americans as a tonic for "female complaints." Black cohosh was one of the main ingredients in Lydia Pinkham's Vegetable Compound, which was marketed successfully to women for 50 years (1875–1925). Black cohosh has been used to treat a wide variety of illnesses and maladies that befall both men and women, including fever, bronchitis, snakebite, lumbago (pain in the lumbar region), malaria, sore throats, and relief from pain. Women have used it historically, and use it currently, to relieve symptoms of both PMS and dysmenorrhea (see Chapter 17). It has also been used to relieve depression, sleeplessness, and hypertension during the female climacteric (menopause) (Crawford, 1997; Gruenwald, Brendler, & Jaenicke, 2000; Hardy, 2000; Miller & Kazal, 1998; Robbers & Tyler, 1998).

How It Works   The known active ingredients in the root of black cohosh include the triterpine glycoside cimifugoside, actein, and 27-deoxyactein. However, it is the isoflavone for-mononetin that is thought to be the active estrogenic compound. During the course of menopause, the secretion of luteinizing hormone (LH) increases as estrogen levels decrease. The active ingredients of black cohosh bind to the estrogen receptors and suppress the release of LH, thus providing an estrogen-like effect. However, recent studies suggest that neither extracts of black cohosh or Remifemin demonstrate hormonelike activity, leaving the mode of action of this plant in question. Black cohosh also contains salicylates, a component of aspirin, which aids in pain relief (Duker, Kopanski, Jarry, & Wuttke, 1991; Einer-Jensen, Zhao, Andersen, & Kristtersen, 1996; Gruenwald et al., 2000; Hardy, 2000; Liske, 1998; Robbers & Tyler, 1998).

Clinical Studies   Most clinical studies of black cohosh use a proprietary formula, called Remifemin, which is standardized with regard to the active ingredients, triterpene glycosides. Remifemin has been demonstrated to be better than placebo at relieving menopausal symptoms (hot flashes, night sweats, changes in the vaginal lining, menstrual cramps, and depression), and in one German study it was found to be superior to both conjugated estrogens and Valium for relieving depression and anxiety. Black cohosh is approved by the German Commission E for climacteric complaints and PMS.

Possible Side Effects   No health hazards or side effects, aside from mild stomach complaints, are associated with the proper administration of therapeutic dosages. However, an overdose of black cohosh can result in vomiting, headaches, dizziness, limb pains, lowered blood pressure, or elevated blood pressure (Israel & Youngkin, 1997). Because of its estrogenic effects in humans and its affinity for estrogen receptors in animal models, its potential for increasing the risk of breast cancer has been suggested but not demonstrated. Although the German Commission E recommended that black cohosh not be taken for longer than six months, recent studies have challenged this precaution (Blumenthal, Goldberg, & Brinckmann, 2000; Gruenwald et al., 2000; Hardy, 2000; Murray & Pizzorno, 1999; U.S. Food and Drug Administration, 1998).

Interactions   Black cohosh may cause a synergistic effect with antihypertensive medications, resulting in hypotension (Gruenwald et al., 2000).

Who Should Not Take It   Because of the potential to induce spontaneous abortion, women who are pregnant should not take black cohosh.

CHASTEBERRY (*VITEX AGNUS-CASTUS*)

Chasteberry is also known as vitex agnus-castus, chaste tree, and monk's pepper. The name chasteberry is derived from the belief that the plant can suppress the libido of women and men (specifically, monks). Chasteberry has been used since the time of the ancient Greeks. Hippocrates wrote of its usefulness in treating injuries, inflammation, swelling of the spleen, and hemorrhages, as well as in encouraging "passing of afterbirth." Decoctions were used as sitz baths for women with uterine diseases. Chasteberry was also used to increase the flow of milk in lactating women, to reduce flatulence, to suppress the appetite, to induce sleep, and to treat impotency and swelling of the testes and ovaries (Brown, 1994; Hardy, 2000).

How It Works   Unlike other herbs used to treat menstrual disorders, extracts of the chasteberry fruit do not contain any plant equivalents of estrogen or progesterone. Rather, Vitex exerts its effects through its dopaminergic properties on the *anterior pituitary*, which secretes prolactin. It increases the production of luteinizing hormone (LH), which causes the release of the ovum and the production of progesterone, and inhibits the release of follicle-stimulating hormone (FSH), which is responsible for the maturation of the follicles into fertile ova and the production of estrogen. Vitex *increases the ratio of progesterone to estrogen*, thereby reducing the symptoms of PMS. Vitex also reduces the secretion of prolactin from the pituitary. It is critical that, in nonlactating women, prolactin be in balance with FSH and LH. Too much prolactin secretion can inhibit the maturation of the follicles in the ovaries and induce menstrual abnormalities and sterility.

Clinical Studies   The German Commission E has approved Vitex for the treatment of menopausal complaints and a number of menstrual disorders, including symptomatic PMS (breast tenderness, cramping, anxiety, craving, headaches, and fluid retention), hypermenorrhea, secondary amenorrhea and polymenorrhea (heavy periods and missed or irregular menstrual cycles), anovulatory cycles (no ovulation), infertility, and hyperprolactinemia (increased prolactin production). Vitex's effects regarding the production of milk are paradoxical; although Vitex has been used to increase milk production and has been clinically proven to do so, it is also known to suppress prolactin, which is responsible for the production of milk after birth (Brown, 1994; Halaska, Raus, Beles, Martan, & Paithner, 1998; Hardy, 2000; Loch, Selle, & Boblitz, 2000).

Possible Side Effects   In one study involving 4,500 women, less than 2 percent reported minor symptoms, such as gastrointestinal upset, itching, mild rash, headaches, and increased menstrual flow (Hardy, 2000).

Interactions   Preparations containing Vitex may weaken the effect of dopamine-receptor agonists drugs used in the management of Parkinson's Disease, such as Bromo-scriptine and Pergolide (Gruenwald et al., 2000).

Who Should Not Take It Women who are pregnant should not take Vitex.

DONG QUAI (*ANGELICA SINENSIS*)

Dong quai, which is not known by other names, is marketed as an all-purpose woman's herb. It has been recommended for menstrual cramps, dysmenorrhea, PMS, hot flashes, and bowel irregularity. Dong quai is purported to possess anti-spasmodic and vasodilating properties and is used to treat constipation, high blood pressure, and insomnia. As a common component of Chinese medical formulas, dong quai is considered a blood tonic as well as a general tonifier that restores function to such organs as the heart, spleen, liver, and kidneys (Alternative Diabetes.com, 2000; Hardy, 2000; Williamson & Wyandt, 1998; Yim et al., 2000).

How It Works The chemical constituents contained in the root of *Angelica sinensis* may explain whatever effects it actually has on the body. An abundance of vitamin B-12, folic acid, and nicotinic acid could explain its purported efficacy in anemia, and the presence of ferulic acid may lend it anti-inflammatory and analgesic properties. The water-soluble fraction is reported to stimulate the uterus, whereas the oil-soluble constituents may promote relaxation, but the active compounds have not been identified (Hardy, 2000).

Clinical Studies The scientific evidence supporting the efficacy of dong quai is weak, consisting primarily of in vitro (test tube) and animal testing. In a double-blind, placebo-controlled clinical study with women, dong quai did not increase endometrial thickness or the maturation of vaginal cells—two expected responses from estrogen therapy for menopause. In traditional Chinese medicine, dong quai is rarely used alone, and its anecdotal effectiveness in treating menopausal symptoms, fibrocystic breast disease, abnormal fetal movements, and pelvic inflammatory disease may be due to the activity of other ingredients (Alternative Diabetes.com, 2000; Hardy, 2000; Hirata, Swiersz, Zell, Small, & Ettinger, 1997; Kotani et al., 1997; Shaw et al., 1997; Williamson & Wyandt, 1998).

Possible Side Effects No evidence exists that dong quai is toxic, but traditional beliefs suggest that this herb be avoided by women during the first three months of pregnancy or by those with extremely heavy menstruation (Alternative Diabetes.com, 2000).

Interactions Dong quai contains coumarins, which act as **photosensitizers** (via the skin) and **blood thinners.** Individuals taking dong quai in conjunction with anticoagulant drugs, such as warfarin (Coumadin), heparin, pentoxifylline (Trental), and aspirin, or with other blood-thinning dietary supplements, such as garlic, ginkgo, and high-dose vitamin E, may be at increased risk for bleeding. Traditional Chinese texts advise against taking dong quai if one is sick with the cold or flu or if one has an acute infection. Because of the interaction with blood thinners and the lack of clinical evidence, the use of this herb is discouraged by some sources (Alternative Diabetes.com, 2000; Bensky, Gamble, & Kaptchuk, 1986; Page & Lawrence, 1999).

ECHINACEA (*ECHINACEA PURPUREA, ECHINACEA ANGUSTIFOLIA, ECHINACEA PALLIDA*)

Echinacea is also known as rudbeckia, Kansas snake root, narrow-leaved echinacea, narrow-leaved purple coneflower, Sampson root, black Sampson, black Susan, pale purple coneflower, and American coneflower. The root of *Echinacea angustifolia* was recommended by the Eclectics, a group of physicians who were prominent during the late nineteenth and early twentieth centuries, as a remedy for cancer, chronic mastitis, chronic ulceration, tubercular abscesses, chronic glandular indurations, and syphilis. Both the root and the herb of *Echinacea angustifolia* have been used externally by the Native Americans of the Great Plains for the treatment of burns, swelling of the lymph nodes, and insect and rattlesnake bites. Echinacea tinctures have been taken by mouth for headaches, stomachaches, measles, coughs, and gonorrhea. The effectiveness of *Echinacea purpurea* root has not been definitively demonstrated for acute and chronic respiratory tract infections and for decreasing susceptibility to infections during periods of temporarily lowered resistance (Alternative Diabetes.com, 2000; Gruenwald et al., 2000; Parnham, 1996).

How It Works The immunostimulating, antibacterial, and antiviral properties of echinacea are derived from alkamides, glycoproteins, caffeic acid derivatives, and polysaccharides. Of these, the polysaccharides seem to play the major role—that is inducing the production of interleukin and interferon. The alkamides exert anti-inflammatory properties. Studies show that extracts of *E. purpurea* increase both the number and the phagocytic (bacteria-engulfing) activity of white blood cells (Blumenthal et al., 2000; Giles, Palat, Vhien, Chang, & Kennedy, 2000; Gruenwald et al., 2000).

Clinical Studies The many misunderstandings that exist as to the proper use of the various available forms of echinacea illustrate the degree to which herbology can be a complicated discipline. There are three species of echinacea (*E. angustifolia, E. purpurea,* and *E. pallida*). The Native Americans and the pioneers in North America primarily used *E. angustifolia,* but the seeds that were taken back to Europe for the development of the drug there happened to be those of *E. purpurea.* Consequently, many of the clinical trials use extracts from this species. To complicate matters further, each part of the plant, (leaves, flowers, seeds, and roots) may be used in remedies, and all four parts may be mixed for use in the same remedy, but not all of the parts are equally effective. Moreover, the active constituents may be readily degraded by processing, resulting in an additional source of variation in the final product. To date, sufficient data have been amassed for the German Commission E to support the use of the *aerial parts* (leaves, flowers, and seeds) of *E. purpurea* to treat the common cold, coughs, bronchitis, infections of the urinary tract, and inflammation of the mouth and pharynx, as well as to decrease the likelihood that infection will develop in wounds and burns. Extracts of the *roots* of *E. pallida* have been approved only to treat fevers and colds.

Echinacea is popularly used both to prevent and to reduce the symptoms of the common cold, but results from clinical trials are mixed (Melchart et al., 1995). In general, research suggests that the juice or extracts of *E. purpurea* aerial parts and extracts of *E. pallida* roots may be effective in reducing the severity and duration of the common cold, as well as bacterial infections of the upper respiratory tract, when taken at the onset of symptoms (Grimm & Muller, 1999). It must be noted, however, that the immunostimulatory properties of echinacea may *decline over time* and that taking preparations on a daily basis as a means of preventing upper respiratory tract infections has not been found to be effective (Melchart, Walther, Linde, Brandmaier & Lersch, 1998). The juice expressed from *E. purpurea* leaves may be useful as a supporting therapy for yeast *(Candida albicans)* vaginal infections (Giles et al., 2000; Melchart, Linde, Fischer, & Kaesmayr, 2000; Turner, Riker, & Gangemi, 2000).

Possible Side Effects   There are few safety issues to consider with the oral administration of echinacea. Aside from potential allergic reactions (echinacea is a member of the daisy family), echinacea has not been found to cause toxicity, even at extremely high doses. The few reported side effects are limited to minor gastrointestinal symptoms and increased urination. *Injections* of echinacea extracts may cause short-term nausea, vomiting, shivering, headache, and fever (Blumenthal et al., 2000; Gruenwald et al., 2000) and are no longer approved by the German Commission E. Because echinacea can stimulate the body's immune system, it has been theorized that echinacea may exacerbate autoimmune diseases, such as rheumatoid arthritis and multiple sclerosis. There is no clinical evidence, however, to support this concern.

Interactions   Although there are no known interactions with prescription or nonprescription drugs, there is an uncertainty as to whether the immune-stimulating effects of echinacea interferes with immunosuppressant drugs.

Who Should Not Take It   There are no known restrictions, but it is recommended that pregnant women avoid taking echinacea by injection.

EVENING PRIMROSE OIL (*OENOTHERIA BIENNSIS*)

Evening primrose oil is also known as fever plant, scabish, scurvish, willow-herb, king's cureall, and sun drop. The oil expressed from the plant's small dark seeds has been used historically as an astringent, an antibiotic, an expectorant, an antitussive, and a digestive stimulant. Currently, it is used to treat the symptoms associated with the menstrual cycle, as well as a host of other problems and diseases.

How It Works   Nearly 80 percent of the oil from evening primrose seeds contain gamma-linolenic acid (GLA), an essential fatty acid that is converted in the body to prostaglandin E1 (PGE1). This hormonelike substance has anti-inflammatory and cell membrane–stabilizing properties (Gruenwald et al., 2000).

Clinical Studies   Evening primrose oil has been shown to provide relief from cyclic mastalgia (breast pain that cycles with the menstrual period). Evening primrose oil has also been clinically tested in patients with eczema and PMS symptoms—both with mixed results. Oral doses of evening primrose oil have not been found to shorten gestation or decrease the overall length of labor. Other diseases and problems for which evening primrose oil has *not* been found to be clinically effective include diabetic neuropathy, rheumatoid arthritis, overweight, asthma, osteoporosis, Raynaud's phenomenon, ulcerative colitis, kidney stones, multiple sclerosis, chronic fatigue syndrome, irritable bowel syndrome, and itching due to kidney failure (Budeiri, Li Wan Po, & Dornan, 1996; Dove & Johnson, 1999; Gateley, Miers, Mansel, & Hughes, 1992; Gruenwald et al., 2000; Hardy, 2000; McFayden, Forrest, Chetty, & Raab, 1992; Morse et al., 1989; Pye, Mansel, & Hughes, 1985; Robbers & Tyler, 1998; Whitaker, Cilliers, & de Beers, 1996).

Possible Side Effects   A small percentage (less than 2 percent, in one study) of people who use evening primrose oil experience side effects, such as mild bloating, nausea, headache, and gastrointestinal distress. However, the seizure threshold may be lowered in patients with seizure disorders (Alternative Diabetes.com, 2000; Gruenwald et al., 2000).

Interactions   There are no known interactions.

GARLIC (*ALLIUM SATIVUM*)

Garlic has been used as a general cure-all for more than 5,000 years and has been used in folk medicine as a treatment for many kinds of ailments. Taken *orally*, garlic has been used to treat inflammatory respiratory conditions, whooping cough, bronchitis, gastrointestinal ailments, menstrual pains, and diabetes. Garlic has also been used *topically* as an antibiotic and as a treatment for corns, warts, calluses, ear infections, muscle pain, neuralgia, arthritis, and sciatica.

More recently, garlic has been proposed as a treatment for asthma, candida, and vaginal infections, but evidence of clinical effectiveness is lacking (Muller & Clauson, 1998). In both Western Europe and the United States, garlic has been widely used to prevent many conditions associated with cardiovascular disease. The German Commission E recommends it for the treatment of high cholesterol, high blood lipid levels, and high blood pressure and as a preventative for arteriosclerosis (Alternative Diabetes.com, 2000; Blumenthal et al., 2000; Gruenwald et al., 2000).

How It Works The thiosulfinate compound allicin is the essential component that is responsible for the antimicrobial, antifungal, and cholesterol-lowering effects of garlic. The putative anticancer effects are due to both allicin and other unidentified compounds. Allicin is formulated when a clove of garlic is cut or damaged, and the allicin-precursor, alliin, is acted on by the enzyme alliinase. The preparation of garlic by drying it can lower the amount of allinase, but enough remains to convert alliin to allicin. Differences in the efficacy of various brands may be related to content, as well as to the method of preparation (Krest & Keusgen, 1999).

Pharmacological research has shown that allicin and other thiosulfinates inhibit blood platelet aggregation and stimulate fibrinolysis (the breakdown of fibrin threads), which leads to increased blood-clotting times (Lamm & Riggs, 2000). There is also evidence that the antioxidative capacity of allicin from aged garlic extracts (but not raw garlic) may reduce the oxidation of LDL cholesterol, a causal factor in arteriosclerosis (Munday, James, Fray, Kirkwood, & Thompson, 1999; Phelps & Harris, 1993). Garlic tablets enhance natural killer cells, which are an important part of the anticancer, antimicrobial, and antifungal properties of garlic (Lawson, 1998).

Clinical Studies Approximately 2,000 clinical studies investigating the potential benefits of garlic have been conducted, and quite a few have assessed its ability to decrease risk factors for coronary heart disease. Clinical studies using dried, powdered garlic standardized to 1.3 percent allicin (either the Kwai® or Sapec® brand) in an amount equivalent to ingesting one-half to one clove of garlic per day, have demonstrated that garlic can lower blood lipid levels. Allicin is the ingredient believed to be responsible for garlic's therapeutic effects. In one study, total blood cholesterol levels dropped by about 9 to 12 percent, and serum triglyceride levels were lowered by 13.4 percent on average. Moreover, the ratio of high-density lipoprotein (HDL) cholesterol to low-density lipoprotein (LDL) cholesterol was increased, primarily through the lowering of LDL cholesterol levels (Silagy & Neil, 1994a). A 4.6 percent reduction in arterial plaque build-up has also been demonstrated in women who were given garlic, in comparison with women who were given a placebo, as has a two-fold decrease in systolic and diastolic blood pressure (Silagy & Neil, 1994b). Garlic is also known

to have blood-thinning properties. The overall cardiovascular benefits of garlic have been reported to reduce the risk of myocardial infarction and stroke by more than 50 percent. The studies that have found garlic to be ineffective in decreasing the risk for cardiovascular disease have generally used garlic oil or garlic tablets that released only one-third as much allicin as the tablets used in studies with more positive results (Berthold et al., 1998). A recent meta-analysis (Stevenson, Pitler, & Ernst, 2000) of 13 methodologically sound clinical trials suggests, however, that garlic's anticholesterol effects are quite modest and that garlic alone is not an adequate treatment for hypercholesterolemia.

Over 200 studies have investigated garlic's potential for reducing the risk of developing cancer. The majority have been *epidemiological studies,* which have found a correlation between decreased cancer rates and the consumption of garlic. *In vitro (laboratory) studies* using garlic have demonstrated its ability to inhibit the growth of some kinds of cancer cells (Siegers, Steffen, Robke, & Pentz, 1999).

Garlic applied topically has been found to have antimicrobial and antifungal properties. One of the oils derived from the fermentation of dried garlic, ajoene, is effective against athlete's foot (Ankri & Mirelman, 1999; Arora & Kaur, 1999; Ledezema et al., 2000). Clinical trials have not, however, found garlic to be effective against the stomach bacterium *Helicobacter pylori,* which causes ulcers (Graham, Anderson, & Lang, 1999).

Possible Side Effects Some individuals on therapeutic doses of garlic have reported such side effects as headaches, myalgia, fatigue, vertigo, abdominal discomfort, and increased body odor. The consumption of raw garlic in excessive amounts will likely result in upset stomach, heartburn, nausea, vomiting, diarrhea, flatulence, facial flushing, rapid pulse, and insomnia. Topical exposure can cause allergic dermatitis (skin irritation, blistering, and even third-degree burns) and some individuals have developed an asthmatic reaction from either the inhalation or the ingestion of garlic (Alternative Diabetes.com, 2000; Gruenwald et al., 2000).

Interactions It is recommended that individuals about to undergo surgery not ingest substantial amounts of garlic, due to its blood-thinning properties. Garlic can also cause excessive bleeding if taken with blood-thinning drugs, such as Warfarin, Heparin, aspirin, or pentoxifylline. Taking garlic with ginkgo or vitamin E may also increase the risk of bleeding problems (Alternative Diabetes.com, 2000; Burnham, 1995; Gruenwald et al., 2000).

Who Should Not Take It Patients about to undergo surgery should not take garlic. Some sources also recommend that nursing mothers should not take garlic, although there is no evidence that the practice is deleterious (Blumenthal et al., 2000; Gruenwald et al., 2000).

Ginkgo Biloba (*Ginkgo Biloba*)

Ginkgo is also known as maidenhair tree, duck foot tree, and silver apricot. In contrast to the current method of using extracts prepared from ginkgo *leaves,* the Chinese have historically made a tea from ginkgo *seeds.* Ginkgo has been used historically for the treatment of asthma, tinnitus, hypertonia, and agina pectoris, as well as for improving brain function (Gaby, 1996; Gruenwald et al., 2000). Today, ginkgo biloba is the most widely prescribed herb in Germany. It is recommended by the Commission E for four main purposes: (1) the symptomatic relief of brain dysfunction typical of *dementia syndromes,* including memory deficits, disturbances in concentration, depressive emotional states, dizziness, tinnitus, and headache; (2) the relief of *intermittent claudication,* a condition in which reduced blood circulation to the legs due to hardening of the arteries causes pain while walking; (3) the relief of *vertigo* (dizziness); and (4) the relief of *tinnitus* (ringing in the ear).

How It Works   Ginkgo extracts improve blood circulation, but it is not precisely known which of the active ingredients are involved or how they operate. At one time, it was believed that the circulation-enhancing properties of ginkgo were responsible for its positive effects on dementia. However, the link between blood circulation to the brain and brain functioning is no longer considered the primary factor; it is now believed that ginkgo improves cognition by protecting nerve cells and their activity more directly (Logani, Chen, Tran, Le, & Raffia, 2000).

The known active constituents of ginkgo are standardized for maximum efficacy at 22 to 27 percent ginkgo flavonol glycosides (kaempferol, quercetin, and isorhamnetin) and 5 to 7 percent terpene lactones (ginkgolides and bilobalide). Ginkolide B is a potent inhibitor of platelet-activating factor (PAF), which can cause bronchoconstriction and lead to a reduced oxygen supply to the brain. The flavonol glycosides are known to be free radical scavenging antioxidants, which can increase the brain's tolerance for being short of oxygen and prevent lipids from being damaged by free radicals which may lead to dementia through tissue and vascular damage and neuronal loss (Alternative Diabetes.com, 2000; Gruenwald et al., 2000; Logani, Chen, Tran, Le, & Raffa, 2000).

Clinical Studies   Clinical studies have demonstrated ginkgo's effectiveness in relieving the symptoms of cerebral insufficiency (poor blood circulation to the brain) due to aging, which include confusion, memory lapses, tinnitus, and headaches. Ginkgo has also been found to be effective for slowing the onset of the symptoms of Alzheimer's disease and, in some cases, has produced small improvements in patients' cognitive abilities, daily living skills, and social behavior (Ernst & Pittler, 1999). Ginkgo's ability to relieve the symptoms of intermittent claudication are also well documented (Blumenthal et al., 2000). Other putative effects of ginkgo have not been sufficiently demonstrated. There is not yet sufficient evidence to support ginkgo as an effective remedy for PMS, macular degeneration, sexual dysfunction, altitude sickness, depression, cyclic edema, acute cochlear deafness, Raynaud's phenomenon, and complications of diabetes (Gruenwald et al., 2000).

Possible Side Effects   Ginkgo has few known side effects. Of the 10,000 participants in clinical trials conducted up to 1991, only .20 percent noted gastrointestinal discomfort, and fewer still reported cases of headaches, dizziness, or allergic skin reactions. The chronic ingestion of excessive amounts of ginkgo has resulted in spontaneous bleeding and the formation of hematomas in the tissue surrounding the brain and in the iris chamber (Alternative Diabetes.com, 2000; Gruenwald et al., 2000).

Interactions   Ginkgo is a potent inhibitor of platelet-activating factor (PAF) and may cause spontaneous bleeding when taken with blood-thinning drugs, such as Coumadin (warfarin), heparin, aspirin, and Trental (pentoxifylline) or with other blood-thinning herbs, such as garlic.

Who Should Not Take It   No restrictions have been established.

St. John's Wort (*Hypericum Perforatum*)

St. John's wort is also known as klamath weed, goat weed, and hypericum. It has been administered both orally and topically since the first century, as an anti-inflammatory, a sedative, an analgesic, a diuretic, an antimalarial, and a **vulnerary** (a substance that enhances healing). It has been widely used in cases of trauma, burns, rheumatism, hemorrhoids, neuralgia, gastroenteritis, snakebite, ulcers, contusions, sprains, diarrhea, menorrhagia, hysteria, bed-wetting, and depression (Gruenwald et al., 2000). The German Commission E has approved St. John's wort for anxiety and depression, as well as inflammation of the skin, blunt injuries, wounds, and burns (Gulick et al., 1999; Lavie et al., 1990; Mukherjee & Suresh, 2000; Schempp, Pelz, Wittmer, Schöpf, & Simon, 1999).

How It Works   Although hypericin has long been considered the ingredient responsible for alleviating the symptoms of depression, a compound known as hyperforin has recently been found to have greater activity and to be naturally more abundant in the plant (Wonnemann, Singer, & Muller, 2000). Consequently, hyperforin is now the **marker compound** for the standardization of extracts. Marker compounds are pharmacologically active plant ingredients that are used to determine whether potency is consistent among batches of herbal products. If the same amount of the marker ingredient is found in all capsules, tablets, and so on, consistency of dosage is assumed. It remains uncertain, however, whether either hypericin or hyperforin alone is responsible for the therapeutic effects of St. John's wort. Although the exact mechanism by which St. John's wort relieves depression remains to be determined, current models are based on the biogenic amine theory of depression (Laakmann, Schule, Baghai, & Kieser, 1998). According to this theory, levels of the neurotransmitters serotonin and norepinephrine are related to mood; adequate levels are related to feelings of well-being, and low levels are associated with depression. Research suggests that St. John's wort inhibits the recycling of serotonin and other neurotransmitters, thus increasing their levels in the brain (Bennett, Phun, & Polk, 1998; Cuccinelli, 1999; Miller, A. L., 1998).

Clinical Studies   Extracts of St. John's wort have been demonstrated to perform better than a placebo and as well as some standard antidepressants, such as fluoxetine and imipramine, in relieving the symptoms of mild to moderate depression (Laakman et al., 1998), but not severe depression, including the symptoms associated with PMS and menopause (Grube, Walper, & Wheatley, 1999; Linde et al., 1996; Maidment, 2000; Stevenson & Ernst, 1999, 2000; Stevenson, Pittler, & Ernst, 2000; Woelk, 2000). Methanol extracts of St. John's wort *(Hypericum hookerianum)*, formulated as an ointment, have been found to stimulate wound healing in rats. The flavonoids in St. John's wort exhibit anti-inflammatory action, and hyperforin has been demonstrated to inhibit the growth of gram-positive bacteria. Studies on the in vitro use of hypericin as an antiretroviral agent have not been supported by a clinical trial with HIV-infected patients.

Possible Side Effects   Compared with synthetic antidepressants, St. John's wort has been demonstrated to be safe, with allergic reactions, gastrointestinal upset, and fatigue each being reported by less than 1 percent of the members of one study group (De Smet & Nolen, 1996). Hypericum can be *phototoxic* to animals, causing burns or blisters on the unpigmented, nonhairy portions of the body. Phototoxicity in humans is unlikely with therapeutic levels but can occur at higher doses, particularly in fair-skinned individuals (Miller, A. L., 1998; Gruenwald et al., 2000). Because patients taking extracts of hypericum have few adverse effects, it has been recommended as a primary treatment for mild to moderate depression (Woelk, 2000).

Interactions   St. John's wort has the potential to interact with many pharmaceutical drugs. Because it increases the levels of serotonin and noradrenaline in the central nervous system, St. John's wort may cause "serotonin syndrome"—sweating, tremors, flushing, confusion, and agitation—when administered with similar antidepressant drugs, such as sertraline or nefazodone. Concomitant use with monoamine oxidase inhibitors (MAOI) should also be avoided (Maid-

ment, 2000). St. John's wort can depress the blood levels of some medications, such as cyclosporin (an organ rejection preventative), digoxin (a heart medication), indinavir (an HIV medication), theophylline (an asthma drug), and warfarin (a blood thinner) (Piscitelli, Burstein, Chaitt, Alfaro, & Falloon, 2000; Ruschitzka, Meier, Turina, Lüscher, & Noll, 2000). Of particular interest to women is the fact that St. John's wort can render *oral contraceptives* containing ethinyloestradiol and desogestrel ineffective (Fugh-Berman, 2000). Extracts of hypericum may also alter the duration of narcotic-induced sleeping times (Gruenwald et al., 2000).

Who Should Not Take It   No current restrictions exist, even for pregnant or lactating women; however, studies have not been conducted with this cohort (Cuccinelli, 1999; McGuffin, Hobbs, Upton, & Golberg, 1997).

New Directions

The NCCAM continues to serve as the seat of government-sponsored scientific research into the efficacy and integration of CAM therapies (see Chapter 10). The NCCAM supports the scientific advancement of CAM therapies by a number of means. It provides grants for training and career development and the establishment of research centers and cooperative agreements, as well as for individual research projects. This broad approach fosters research at all levels of inquiry and encourages communication between individual scientists and centers. Moreover, it facilitates consumer access to the latest scientific findings related to CAM therapies.

NCCAM funding has been provided for research in a wide variety of CAM interventions, such as yoga, herbal therapies, support groups, music therapy, spirituality, and substances which enhance immune functioning. No doubt due to its promising outcomes to date and widespread clinical implications, acupuncture is being evaluated in more than eight studies. As evidenced by the increasing reports found in subspecialty journals, many other privately supported CAM-related studies involving qualitative and quantitative methodology are also in progress across the country.

There is also a definite, although controversial, movement toward greater regulation and standardization of herbal products, and a number of public and private programs have been initiated to scrutinize herbals more closely. For example, the **National Toxicology Program (NTP)** is initiating studies to identify possible adverse health effects associated with the prolonged use of herbals (NIEHS News, 1999). A privately held company, **ConsumerLab.com,** has begun to test herbal products independently and provides a seal of certification to those products that pass its testing program (McDermott & Motyka, 2000). The **National Nutritional Foods Association (NNFA),** which is the largest and oldest nonprofit trade association for the dietary supplement industry, has established a **Good Manufacturing Practices (GMPs) Certification Program** for its members. Manufacturers that pass third-party inspections of their products, facilities, and recordkeeping are allowed to display a seal of approval on their products. Participation in this program will be mandatory for all NNFA members by the year 2002 (McDermott & Motyka, 2000).

The lack of standardization in botanical products has prompted the founding of the **Institute for Nutraceutical Advancement (INA).** The institute represents an international effort among 29 companies to develop standard analytical tests and marker compounds that will serve as indicators for consistency. Via its Methods Validation Program (MVP), the INA selects the marker compounds that will be used as indicators of consistency among specific types of herbal medicines. The establishment of precise analytical methodologies will permit studies to be carried out on the variability and stability of active compounds and will provide a basis by which manufacturers can provide uniformly effective products (Institute for Nutraceutical Advancement [INA], 2000).

Standardization of the chemical constituents of herbals will also allow clinical trials to be conducted in which both the safety and the efficacy of herbal remedies can be evaluated. Clinical trials are needed because the assumptions derived from in vitro (in glass—done on isolated tissues, cells, and so on) studies (chemical analyses, cellular assays, and receptor assays) cannot be completely extrapolated to predict the results of an in vivo (in life—done on living animals) trial (Chang, 1999). For example, in a clinical trial in which the bioavailability of two similar extracts of *Ginkgo biloba* was evaluated, one extract was found to yield ginkgolide blood levels that remained steady for 12 hours, whereas the other produced blood levels that were erratic (Li & Wong, 1997).

If basic pharmacological principles are used in developing herbal medicines, consumers can be confident that they will obtain safe and reliable results from them. Although this approach may be an anathema to individuals who wish to avoid synthetic drugs and the regulations that accompany them, it is the route taken by progressive countries such as Germany, in which most single-ingredient herbal medicines, and many mixtures, are registered as conventional drugs (Wagner, 1999).

QUESTIONS FOR REFLECTION AND DISCUSSION

1. Which assumptions foundational to the various cam systems, therapies and disciplines are best supported by empirical evidence?

2. What are some strengths and weaknesses of holistic healthcare?

3. Which CAM modalities would you personally use? Which would you not use?

4. What are some positive and negative implications of the placebo response?

5. Should herbals be standardized as to the amount of active ingredient present?

6. Should some herbals be available only by prescription?

7. How do food supplements and drugs compare in terms of benefits and risks?

8. What safety precautions should women take before using herbal preparations?

RESOURCES

Books

Benson, H. (1996). *Timeless healing: The power and biology of belief.* New York: Fireside.

Blumenthal, M., Goldberg, A., & Brinckmann, J. (2000). *Herbal medicine: Expanded Commission E monographs.* Boston: Integrative Medicine Communications; Austin, TX: American Botanical Council.

Collinge, W. (1997). *The American Holistic Health Association complete guide to alternative medicine.* New York: Warner Books.

Foster, S. (1999). *Tyler's honest herbal: A sensible guide to the use of herbs and related remedies* (4th ed.). New York: Haworth Herbal Press.

Gerber, R. (2000). *Vibrational Medicine for the 21st Century.* New York: Morrow and Company.

Goleman, D., & Guinn, J. (Eds.). (1996). *Mind-body medicine: How to use your mind for better health.* New York: Consumer Reports Books.

Gruenwald, J., Brendler, T., & Jaenicke, C. (2000). *PDR for herbal medicines* (2nd ed.). Montvale, NJ: Medical Economics.

Hornyak, L., & Green, J. (2000). *Healing from Within: The Use of Hypnosis in Women's Health.* Washington, DC: American Psychological Association.

Knaster, M. (1996). *Discovering the body's wisdom.* New York: Bantam Books.

Robbers, J. E., & Tyler, V. E. (1998). *Tyler's herbs of choice.* Binghamton, NY: Hawthorn Herbal Press.

Weil, A. (1995). *Health and healing.* Boston: Houghton Mifflin.

Journals

Advances: The Journal of Mind-Body Health, John E. Fetzer Institute, Kalamazoo, MI. Phone: 616-375-2000.

Alternative Therapies in Health and Medicine, InnoVision Communications, Aliso Viejo, CA. Phone: 1-800-899-1712.

Brain, Behavior and Immunity, Academic Press Inc., San Diego, CA. Phone: 619-230-1840.

Mind-Body Medicine, Decker Periodicals, Hamilton, Ontario, Canada. Phone: 1-800-568-7281.

Websites

National Institutes of Health Office of Dietary Supplements (ODS) International Bibliographic Information on Dietary Supplements (IBIDS). http://odp.od.nih.gov/ods/databases/ibids.html

Herb Research Foundation. http://www.herbs.org/index

Southwest School of Botanical Medicine. http://chili.rt66.com/hrbmoore/HOMEPAGE/HomePage.html

U.S. Food and Drug Administration. The Special Nutritionals Adverse Event Monitoring System (SN/AEMS). http://vm.cfsan.fda.gov/~tear/aems.html

Organizations

Ayurvedic Institute
P.O. Box 23435
Albuquerque, NM 87192
Phone: 505-291-9698
Web: www.ayurveda.com

Center for Attitudinal Healing
33 Buchanan St.
Sausalito, CA 94965
Phone: 415-331-6161
Web: www.healingcenter.org

Center for Mind-Body Medicine
5225 Connecticut Ave. NW
Suite 414
Washington, DC 17436
Phone: 202-966-2589
E-mail: cmbm@mindspring.com
Web: www.healthy.net/cmbm

Center for Mindfulness
University of Massachusetts Medical Center
419 Belmont Ave.
Worcester, MA 01604
Phone: 508-856-2656
Web: www.mindfulnesstapes.com/email.html

Mind/Body Medical Institute Division of Behavioral Medicine
Beth Israel Deaconess Medical Center
Boston, MA 24823
Phone: 617-632-9530
Web: www.mindbody.harvard.edu

Professional Organizations

Acupressure

American Oriental Bodywork Therapy Association
Laurel Oak Corporate Center, Suite 408
1010 Haddonfield-Berlin Rd.
Voorhees, NJ 08043
Phone: 609-782-1616
Web: www.healthy.net/aobta

Acupuncture

The American Association of Acupuncture and Oriental Medicine
9100 Park West Dr.
Houston, TX 77063
Phone: 1-800-729-4456
Web: www.acaom.edu

American Academy of Medical Acupuncture
5820 Wilshire Blvd., Suite 500
Los Angeles, CA 90036
Phone: 1-800-521-2262

Alexander Technique

Alexander Technique International
1692 Massachusetts Ave.
Cambridge, MA 02138
Phone: 617-497-2242
Web: www.ati-net.com

Aromatherapy

National Association for Holistic Aromatherapy
219 Carl St.
San Francisco, CA 94117-3804
Phone: 415-564-6785

Biofeedback

Biofeedback Certification Institute of America
10200 W. 44th Ave., Suite 304
Wheatridge, CO 80033
Phone: 303-420-2902
Web: www.bcia.org/

Chiropractic

American Chiropractic Association
1701 Clarendon Blvd.
Arlington, VA 22209
Phone: 1-800-986-4636
Web: www.amerchiro.org/index.html

Energy Medicine

International Society for the Study of Subtle Energies and Energy Medicine
356 Goldco Circle
Golden, CO 80403
Phone: 303-425-4625

Environmental Medicine

American Academy of Environmental Medicine
10 Randolph St.
New Hope, PA 18938
Phone: 215-862-4544
Web: www.aaem.com

Feldenkrais Method

The Feldenkrais Guild
P.O. Box 489
Albany, OR 97321
Phone: 541-926-0981 or 1-800-775-2118
Web: www.feldenkrais.com

Guided Imagery

The Academy for Guided Imagery
P.O. Box 2070
Mill Valley, CA 94942
Phone: 1-800-726-2070
Web: www.healthy.net/univ/profess/schools/edu/imagery/index_net.html

Holistic Medicine

American Holistic Medical Association
6728 Old McLean Village Dr.
McLean, VA 22101
Web: www.holisticmedicine.org

Holistic Nursing

American Holistic Nurses' Association
P.O. Box 2130
Flagstaff, AZ 86003-2130
Phone: 1-800-278-2462
Web: www.ahna.org

Homeopathy

American Association of Homeopathic Pharmacists
1441 West Smith Rd.
Ferndale, WA 98248
Phone: 1-800-478-0421

National Center for Homeopathy

801 N. Fairfax St., #306
Alexandria, VA 22314
Phone: 703-548-7790
Web: www.healthy.net/nch

Hypnosis

American Society of Clinical Hypnosis
33 W. Grand Ave., Suite 402
Chicago, IL 60610
Phone: 312-645-9810
E-mail: info@asch.net
Web: www.asch.net

Massage

American Massage Therapy Association
820 Davis St., Suite 100
Evanston, IL 60201
Phone: 708-864-0123
Web: www.amtamassage.org

Music Therapy

American Music Therapy Association
8455 Colesville Rd., Suite 1000
Silver Spring, MD 20910
Phone: 301-589-3300
Web: www.musictherapy.org

Naturopathy

The American Association of Neuropathic Physicians
601 Valley St., Suite 105
Seattle, WA 98109
Phone: 206-298-0126
Web: http://aanp.net

American Naturopathic Medical Association

P.O. Box 96273
Las Vegas, NV 89193
Phone: 702-897-7053
Web: www.anma.com

Homeopathic Academy of Naturopathic Physicians

12132 SE Foster Place
Portland, OR 97266
Phone: 503-761-3298

Osteopathy

American Osteopathic Association
142 East Ontario St.
Chicago, IL 60611
Phone: 1-800-621-1773
Web: www.aoa-net.org

Reflexology

International Institute of Reflexology
5650 First Ave., North
P.O. Box 12642
St. Petersburg, FL 33733-2642
E-mail: ftreflex@concentric.net
Web: www.reflexology-usa.net

Reiki

The Reiki Alliance
P.O. Box 41
Cataldo, ID 83810
Phone: 208-682-3535

Rolfing

The Rolf Institute
205 Canyon Blvd.
Boulder, CO 80302
Phone: 303-449-5903

Therapeutic Touch

Nurse Healers-Professional Associates International
1211 Locust St.
Philadelphia, PA 19107
Phone: 215-545-8079
Web: www.therapeutic-touch.org

Yoga

B. K. S. Iyengar Yoga National Association of the United
    States
Phone: 1-800-889-YOGA
International Association of Yoga Therapists
20 Sunnyside Ave., Suite A-243
Mill Valley, CA 94941
Phone: 415-332-2478

REFERENCES

Abbot, N. C., White, A. R., & Ernst, E. (1996). Complementary medicine. [Letter to the editor]. *Nature, 381,* 361.

Achterberg, J., Dossey, B., & Kolkmeier, L. (1994). *Rituals of healing: Using imagery for health and wellness.* New York: Bantam Books.

Adverse effects to herbal medicines: An increasing problem? (1998). *Drug and Theraputics Perspective, 11,* 14–16.

Akerele, O., Heywood, V., & Synge, H. (1991). *Conservation of medicinal plants.* Cambridge: Cambridge University Press.

Albrecht, H., & Schutte, A. (1999). Homeopathy versus antibiotics in metaphylaxis of infectious diseases: A clinical study in pig fattening and its significance to consumers. *Alternative Therapies, 5*(5), 64–68.

Alternative Diabetes.com. (2000). *Herbs and supplements: GLA (gamma-linolenic acid)* [On-line]. Available: http://alternativediabetes.com/altdiab/pg000002.html

Alvarez-Requejo, A., Carvajal, A., Begaud, B., Vega, T., & Arias, L. H. (1998). Under-reporting of adverse drug reactions. Etimate based on a spontaneous reporting scheme and a sentinal system. *European Journal of Clinical Pharmacology, 54,* 483–488.

Anderson, L. A. (1996). Concern regarding herbal toxicities: Case reports and counseling tips. *Annals of Pharmacotherapy, 30,* 79–80.

Angell, M., & Kassirer, J. P. (1998). Alternative medicine—The risks of untested and unregulated remedies. *New England Journal of Medicine, 339,* 839–841.

Ankri, S., & Mirelman, D. (1999). Antimicrobial properties of allicin from garlic. *Microbes and Infection, 1,* 125–129.

Arora, D. S., & Kaur, J. (1999). Antimicrobial activity of spices. *International Journal Antimicrobial Agents, 12,* 257–262.

Ashcroft, D. M., & Po, A. L. W. (1999). Herbal remedies: Issues in licensing and economic evaluation. *Pharmacoeconomics, 16,* 321–328.

Astin, J. A. (1996). Why patients use alternative medicine: Results of a national study. *Journal of the American Medical Association, 279,* 1548–1553.

Barnes, J., Mills, S. Y., Abbot, N. C., Willoughby, M., & Ernst, E. (1998). Different standards for reporting ADRs to herbal remedies and conventional OTC medicines: Face-to-face interviews with 515 users of herbal remedies. *British Journal of Clinical Pharmacology, 45,* 496–500.

Barrett, B., Kiefer, D., & Rabago, D. (1999). Assessing the risks and benefits of herbal medicine: An overview of scientific evidence. *Alternative Therapies, 5*(4), 40–49.

Barrett, B., Vohmann, M., & Calabrese, C. (1999). Echinacea for upper respiratory infection. *Journal of Family Practice, 48,* 628–635.

Bateman, J., Chapman, R. D., & Simpson, D. (1998). Possible toxicity of herbal remedies. *Scottish Medical Journal, 43,* 7–15.

Bates, D. W., Cullen, D. J., Laird, N., Petersen, L. A., Small, S. D., Servi, D., Laffel, G., Sweitzer, B. J., Shea, B. F., Hallisey, R., Vliet, M. V., Nemeskal, R., & Leape, L. L. (1995). Incidence of adverse drug events and potential adverse drug events. *Journal of the American Medical Association, 274,* 29–34.

Bennett, D. A., Phun, L., & Polk, J. F. (1998). Neuropharmacology of St. John's wort (hypericum). *Annals of Pharmacotherapy, 32,* 1201–1208.

Bensky, D., Gamble, A., & Kaptchuk, T. (1986). *Chinese herbal medicine: Materia medica.* Seattle: Eastland Press.

Benson, H. (1996). *Timeless Healing.* New York: Fireside.

Berthold, H. K., Sudhop, T., & von Bergmann, K. (1998). Effect of a garlic oil preparation on serum lipoproteins and cholesterol metabolism. *Journal of the American Medical Association, 279,* 1900–1902.

Blumenthal, M., Goldberg, A., & Brinckmann, J. (2000). *Herbal medicine: Expanded commission E Monographs.* Boston: Integrative Medicine Communications, Austin, TX: American Botanical Council.

Brody, J. E. (1999, February 9). Americans gamble on herbs as medicine. *New York Times,* pp. D1, D7.

Brown, D. J. (Summer 1994). Vitex agnus castus *Clinical Monograph. Quarterly Review of Natural Medicine* [On-line]. Available: http://www.thorne.com/townsend/oct/herbal.html

Buckle, J. (1999). Use of aromatherapy as a complementary treatment for chronic pain. *Alternative Therapies in Health and Medicine, 5*(5), 42–51.

Budeiri, D., Li Wan Po, A., & Dornan, J. C. (1996). Is evening primrose oil of value in the treatment of premenstrual syndrome? *Controlled Clinical Trials, 17,* 60–68.

Burnham, B. E. (1995). Garlic as a possible risk for postoperative bleeding. *Plastic and Reconstructive Surgery, 95,* 213.

Business Wire. (2000, January 20). *CVS becomes first pharmacy to implement program about potential herb-drug interactions* [On-line]. Available: http://www.herbs.org/current.botest.html

Buxman, K. (1996). A look at PNI through the eyes of Drs. Lee Berk and Stanley Tan. *Therapeutic Humor: The Newsletter of the American Association for Therapeutic Humor: IX,* (5–6), 1.

Byrd, R. (1988). Positive therapeutic effects of intercessory prayer in a coronary care unit population. *Southern Medical Journal, 81*(7), 820–826.

Chan, T. Y. K., Chan, J. C. N., Tomlinson, B., & Critchley, J. A. H. (1993). Chinese herbal medicines revisited: A Hong Kong perspective. *Lancet, 342,* 1532–1534.

Chang, J. (1999). Scientific evaluation of traditional Chinese medicine under DSHEA: A conundrum. *Journal of Alternative and Complementary Medicine, 5,* 181–189.

Cherkin, D., & MacCornack, F. (1989). Patient evaluations of low back pain care from family physicians and chiropractors. *Western Journal of Medicine, 150*(3), 351–355.

Chopra, D. (1991). *Perfect Health.* New York: Harmony Books.

Collinge, W. (1997). The American Health Association complete guide to alternative medicine. New York: Warner Books.

Crawford, A. M. (1997). *Herbal remedies for women: Discover nature's wonderful secrets just for women.* Rocklin, CA: Prima.

Cuccinelli, J. H. (1999). Saint-John's-wort *(Hypericum perforatum). Clinician Reviews, 9,* 102–105.

De Smet, P. A., & Nolen, W. A. (1996). St. John's wort as an antidepressant. *British Medical Journal, 313,* 241–242.

De Smet, P. A. G. M. (1997, April). Adverse effects of herbal remedies. *Adverse Drug Reaction Bulletin, No. 183,* 695–698.

Dossey, L. (1997). The return of prayer. *Alternative Therapies in Health and Medicine, 3*(6), 10–17, 113–119.

Dossey, L. (2001). Being green: On the relationship between people and plants. *Alternative Therapies in Health and Medicine, 7*(3), 12–16, 132–139.

Dove, D., & Johnson, P. (1999). Oral evening primrose oil: Its effect on length of pregnancy and selected intrapartum outcomes in low-risk nulliparous women. *Journal of Nurse Midwifery, 44,* 320–324.

Duker, E. M., Kopanski, L., Jarry, H., & Wuttke, W. (1991). Effects of extracts from *Cimicifuga racemosa* on gonadotropin release in menopausal women and ovariectomized rats. *Planta Medica, 57,* 420–424.

Dunbabin, D. W., Tallis, G. A., Popplewell, P. Y., & Lee, R. A. (1992). Lead poisoning from Indian herbal medicine (Ayurveda). *Medical Journal of Australia, 157,* 835–836.

Einer-Jensen, N., Zhao, J., Andersen, K. P., & Kristtersen, K. (1996). *Cimicifuga* and *Melbrosia* lack oestrogenic effects in mice and rats. *Maturitas, 25,* 149–153.

Eisenberg, D. M., Davis, R. B., Ettner, S. L., Appel, S., Wilkey, S., Rompay, M. V., & Kessler, R. C. (1998). Trends in alternative medicine use in the United States, 1990–1997: Results of a follow-up national survey. *Journal of the American Medical Association, 280,* 1569–1575.

Eisenberg, D. M., Kessler, R. C., Foster, C., Norlock, F. E., Calkins, D. R., & Delbanco, T. L. (1993). Unconventional medicine in the United States: Prevalence, costs, and patterns of use. *New England Journal of Medicine, 328,* 246–252.

Ernst, E. (1998). Harmless herbs? A review of the recent literature. *American Journal of Medicine, 104,* 170–178.

Ernst, E., & Pittler, M. H. (1999). *Ginkgo biloba* for dementia. A systematic review of double-blind, placebo-controlled trials. *Clinical Drug Investigations, 17,* 301–308.

Faloon, W. (1999, May). The plague of RDA regulation. *Life Extension,* p. 7.

Farnsworth, N. R., Akerele, O., Bingle, A. S., Soejarto, D. D., & Guo, Z. G. (1985). Medicinal plants in therapy. *Bulletin of the World Health Organization, 63,* 965–981.

Farnsworth, N. R., & Soejarto, D. D. (1991). Global importance of medicinal plants. In O. Akerele, V. Heywood, & H. Synge (Eds.), *Conservation of medicinal plants* (pp. 25–51). Cambridge: Cambridge University Press.

Fraenkel, G. S. (1959). The raison d'etre of secondary plant substances. *Science, 129,* 1466–1470.

Frasca, T., Brett, A. S., & Yoo, S. D. (1997). Mandrake toxicity: A case of mistaken identity. *Archives of Internal Medicine, 157,* 2007–2009.

Fritz, G. (1995). *Fundamentals of therapeutic massage.* New York: Mosby-Year Book.

Fugh-Berman, A. (2000). Herb-drug interactions. *Lancet, 355,* 134–138.

Gaby, A. R. (1996). Ginkgo biloba extract: A review. *Alternative Medicine Review, 1,* 236–242.

Garfinkel, M., Singhal, A., Katz, W., Allan, D., Reshetar, R., & Schumacher, H. (1998). Yoga-based intervention for carpal tunnel syndrome. *Journal of the American Medical Association, 280,* 1601–1603.

Gateley, C. A., Miers, M., Mansel, R. E., & Hughes, L. E. (1992). Drug treatments for mastalgia: 17 years experience in the Cardiff Mastalgia Clinic. *Journal of the Royal Society of Medicine, 85,* 12–15.

Giles, J. T., Palat, C. T., Vhien, S. H., Chang, Z. G., & Kennedy, D. T. (2000). Evaluation of echinacea for treatment of the common cold. *Pharmacotherapy, 20,* 690–697.

Ginades, C., & Rosenthal, D. (1999). Using hypnosis to accelerate the healing of bone fractures: A randomized controlled pilot study. *Alternative Therapies in Health and Medicine, 5*(2), 67–70.

Graham, D. Y., Anderson, S. Y., & Lang, T. (1999). Garlic or jalapeno peppers for treatment of *Helicobacter pylori* infection. *American Journal of Gastroenterology, 94,* 1200–1202.

Graham-Brown, R. A., Bourke, J. F., & Bumphrey, G. (1994). Chinese herbal remedies may contain steroids. [Letter to the editor]. *British Medical Journal, 308,* 473.

Greenberger, P. (1998). Herbal medicines: Are supplements safe? *Journal of Women's Health, 7,* 1077–1079.

Greiger, L. (2000). *Herb-drug interactions* [On-line]. Available: http://www.heartinfo.org/nutrition/herbdrug062499.htm

Grimm, W., & Muller, H. H. (1999). A randomized controlled trial of the effect of fluid extract of *Echinacea purpurea* on the incidence and severity of colds and respiratory infections. *American Journal of Medicine, 106,* 138–143.

Grube, B., Walper, A., & Wheatley, D. (1999). St. John's wort extract: Efficacy for menopausal symptoms of psychological origin. *Advances in Therapy, 16,* 177–186.

Gruenwald, J., Brendler, T., & Jaenicke, C. (2000). *PDR for herbal medicines* (2nd ed.). Montvale, NJ: Medical Economics.

Gulick, R. M., McAuliffe, V., Holden-Wiltse, J., Crumpacker, C., Liebes, L., Stein, D. S., Meehan, P., Hussey, S., Forcht, J., & Valentine, F. T. (1999). Phase I studies of hypericin, the active compound in St. John's wort, as an antiretroviral agent in HIV-infected adults. AIDS clinical trials group protocols 150 and 258. *Annals of Internal Medicine, 130,* 510–514.

Halaska, M., Raus, K., Beles, P., Martan, A., & Paithner, K. G. (1998). Treatment of cyclical mastodynia using an extract of *Vitex agnus castus:* Results of a double-blind comparison with a placebo. *Ceska Gynekologie, 63,* 388–392.

Hardy, M. L. (2000). Women's health series: Herbs of special interest to women. *Journal of the American Pharmacy Association, 40,* 234–242.

Harris, W. S., Gawda, M., Kolb, J. W., Strychacz, G. P., Vacek, J. L., Jones, P. G., Forker, A., O'Keefe, J. H., & McCallister, B. D. (1999). A randomized, controlled trial of the effects of remote, intercessory prayer on outcomes in patients admitted to the coronary care unit. *Archives of Internal Medicine, 159* (19), 2273–2278.

Herbal roulette. (1995, November). *Consumer Reports,* p. 698.

Herbal Rx: The promise and the pitfalls. (1999, March). *Consumer Reports,* pp. 44–48.

Herms, D. A., & Mattson, W. J. (1992). The dilemma of plants: To grow or defend. *Quarterly Review of Biology, 67,* 283–335.

Hirata, J. D., Swiersz, L. M., Zell, B., Small, R., & Ettinger, B. (1997). Does dong quai have estrogenic effects in postmenopausal women? A double-blind, placebo-controlled trial. *Fertility and Sterility, 68,* 981–986.

Hoffman, F. A., & Leaders, F. E. (1996). Botanical (herbal) medicine in health care: A review from a regulatory perspective. *Pharm News, 3,* 23–35.

Houghton, P. J. (1995). The role of plants in traditional medicine and current therapy. *Journal of Alternative and Complementary Medicine, 1,* 131–143.

Husain, A. (1991). Economic aspects of exploitation of medicinal plants. In O. Akerele, V. Heywood, & H. Synge (Eds.), *Conservation of medicinal plants* (pp. 125–140). Cambridge, England: Cambridge University Press.

Institute for Nutraceutical Advancement. (2000, February 6). [On-line]. Available: http://www.nutracueticalinstitute.com/whoweare/index.html

Israel, D., & Youngkin, E. Q. (1997). Herbal therapies for perimenopausal and menopausal complaints. *Pharmacotherapy, 17,* 970–984.

Jacob, J. (1998, August 17). Untended garden. *AMA News,* p. 28.

Jungnickel, P. W. (1998). Nutraceuticals for management of dyslipidemia and atheroclerosis. In L. G. Miller & W. J. Murray (Eds.), *Herbal medicines: A clinicians guide* (pp. 163–187). Binghamton, NY: Pharmaceutical Products Press.

Kabat-Zinn, J. (1990). *Full catastrophe living.* New York: Delta.

Kee, J. L., & Hayes, E. R. (1997). *Pharmacology: A nursing approach* (2nd ed.). Philadelphia: W. B. Saunders.

Keen, R. W., Deacon, A. C., Delves, H. T., Moreton, J. A., & Frost, P. G. (1994). Indian herbal remedies for diabetes as a cause of lead poisoning. *Postgraduate Medical Journal, 70,* 113–114.

Knaster, M. (1996). *Discovering the body's wisdom.* New York: Bantam Books.

Kohen, D. P., & Olness, K. N. (1996). Self-regulation therapy: Helping children help themselves. *Ambulatory Child Health, 2,* 43–58.

Koscielny, J., Klussendorf, D., Latza, R., Schmitt, R., Radtke, H., Siegel, G., & Keisewetter, H. (1999). The antiatherosclerotic effect of *Allium sativum. Atherosclerosis, 144,* 237–249.

Kotani, N., Oyama, T., Sakai, I., Hashimoto, H., Muraoka, M., Ogawa, Y., & Matsuki, A. (1997). Analgesic effect of a herbal medicine for treatment of primary dysmenorrhea—A double-blind study. *American Journal of Chinese Medicine, 25,* 205–212.

Krest, I., & Keusgen, M. (1999). Quality of herbal remedies from *Allium sativum:* Differences between alliinase from garlic powder and fresh garlic. *Planta Medica, 65,* 139–143.

Laakmann, G., Schule, C., Baghai, T., & Kieser, M. (1998). St. John's wort in mild to moderate depression: The relevance of hyperforin for the clinical efficacy. *Pharmacopsychiatry, 31* (suppl. 1), 54–59.

Lamm, D. L., & Riggs, D. R. (2000). The potential application of *Allium sativum* (garlic) for the treatment of bladder cancer. *Urological Clinics of North America, 27,* 157–162.

Lavie, G., Mazur, Y., Lavie, D., Levin, B., Ittah, Y., & Meruelo, D. (1990). Hypericin as an antiretroviral agent. *Annals New York Academy of Science, 616,* 556–562.

Lawson, L. D. (1998). Garlic: A review of its medicinal effects and indicated active compounds. In L. D. Lawson & R. Bauer (Eds.), *Phytomedicines of Europe: Chemistry and biological activity.* (pp. 176–209). Washington, DC: American Chemical Society.

Leaders, F. E. (1998). Incorporating botanical products into MCO formularies. *Drug Benefit Trends, 10*(34), 36–39, 43.

Leape, L. L., Brennan, T. A., Laird, N., Lawthers, A. G., Localio, A. R., Barnes, B. A., Hebert, L., Newhouse, J. P., Weiler, P. C., & Hiatt, H. (1991). The nature of adverse events in hospitalized patients: Results of the Harvard medical practice study II. *New England Journal of Medicine, 324,* 377–384.

Ledezma, E., Marcano, K., Jorquera, A., De Sousa, L., Padilla, M., Pulgar, M., & Aptiz-Castro, R. (2000). Efficacy of ajoene in the treatment of tinea pedis: A double-blind and comparative study with terbinafine. *Journal of the American Academy of Dermatology, 43,* 829–832.

Lesar, T. S., Briceland, L., & Stein, D. S. (1997). Factors related to errors in medication prescribing. *Journal of the American Medical Association, 277,* 312–317.

Lewis, W. H., & Elvin-Lewis, M. P. F. (1977). *Medical botany: Plants affecting man's health.* New York: John Wiley & Sons.

Li, C. L., & Wong, Y. Y. (1997). The bioavailability of ginkgolides in *Ginko biloba* extracts. *Planta Medica, 63,* 487–584.

Linde, K., Clausius, N., & Ramirez, G. (1997). Are the clinical effects of homeopathy placebo effects? A meta-analysis of placebo-controlled trials. *Lancet, 350,* 838–843.

Linde, K., Ramirez, G., Mulrow, C., Pauls, A., Weidenhammer, W., & Melchart, D. (1996). St John's wort for depression—An overview and meta-analysis of randomized clinical trials. *British Medical Journal, 313,* 253–258.

Lindroth, R. L., & Koss, P. A. (1996). Preservation of salicaceae leaves for phytochemical analysis: Further assessment. *Journal of Chemical Ecology, 22,* 765–771.

Liske, E. (1998). Therapeutic efficacy and safety of *Cimicifuga racemosa* for gynecologic disorders. *Advances in Therapy, 15,* 45–53.

Loch, E. G., Selle, H., & Boblitz, N. (2000). Treatment of premenstrual syndrome with a phytopharmaceutical formulation containing *Vitex agnus castus. Journal of Women's Health and Gender-Based Medicine, 9,* 315–320.

Logani, S., Chen, M. C., Tran, T., Le, T., & Raffa, R. B. (2000). Actions of *Ginko biloba* related to potential utility for the treatment of conditions involving cerebral hypoxia. *Life Sciences, 67,* 1389–1396.

Maidment, I. (2000). The use of St John's wort in the treatment of depression. *Psychiatric Bulletin, 24,* 232–234.

Matthews, H. B., Lucier, G. W., & Fisher, K. D. (1999). Medicinal herbs in the United States: Research needs. *Environmental Health Perspectives, 107,* 773–778.

McCarthy, M. W. (1998). Alternative therapy: Focus on herbal products. *Pediatric Pharmacotherapy, 4,* 1–4. (Available on-line at http://www.hsc.virginia.edu/cmc/pedpharm/v4n5.htm)

McDermott, J. H., & Motyka, T. M. (2000). Expert column—Assessing the quality of botanical preparations [On-line]. Available: http://www.medscape.com/Medscape/pharmacology/journal/2000/v02.no1/mp0128.mcde/mp0128.mcde-0

McDonley, D. (2001). *Taxus sp. and the ethnobotanical and chemical origins of taxol* [On-line]. Available: http://glider/yage.net/taxol.htm

McFayden, I. J., Forrest, A. P., Chetty, U., & Raab, G. (1992). Cyclical breast pain—Some observations and the difficulties in treatment. *British Journal of Clinical Practice, 46,* 161–164.

McGuffin, M., Hobbs, C., Upton, A., & Golberg, A. (1997). *American Herbal Product Association's botanical safety handbook.* Boca Raton, LA: CRC Press.

McKenry, L. M., & Salerno, E. (1998). *Pharmacology in nursing* (20th ed.). St. Louis: Mosby.

McLennan, A. H., Wilson, D. H., & Taylor, A. W. (1996). Prevalence and cost of alternative medicine in Australia. *Lancet, 347,* 569–573.

Melchart, D., Linde, K., Fischer, P., & Kaesmayr, J. (2000). Echinacea for preventing and treating the common cold. *The Cochrane Database of Systematic Reviews (Computer File), 2,* CD000530.

Melchart, D., Linde, K., Worku, F., Sarkady, L., Holzmann, M., Jurcic, K., & Wagner, H. (1995). Results of five randomized studies on the immunomodulatory activity of preparations of echinacea. *Journal of Alternative and Complementary Medicine, 1,* 145–160.

Melchart, D., Walther, E., Linde, K., Brandmaier, R., & Lersch, C. (1998). Echinacea root extracts for the prevention of upper respiratory tract infections: A double-blind, placebo-controlled randomized trial. *Archives of Family Medicine, 7,* 541–545.

Miller, A. L. (1998). St. John's wort *(Hypericum perforatum)*: Clinical effects on depression and other conditions. *Alternative Medicine Review, 3,* 18–26.

Miller, L. G. (1998). Herbal medications interface with conventional medicine: An overview. In L. G. Miller & W. J. Murray (Eds.), *Herbal medicinals: A clinician's guide*. Binghamton, NY: Hawthorn Press.

Miller, L. G., & Kazal, L. A. (1998). Herbal medications, nutraceuticals, and hypertension. In L. G. Miller & W. J. Murray (Eds.), *Herbal medicinals: A clinician's guide*. Binghamton, NY: Hawthorn Press.

Monmaney, T. (1998, September 1). Labels' potency claims often inaccurate, analysis finds. *Los Angeles Times,* p. A6.

Morse, P. F., Horrobin, D. F., Manku, M. S., Stewart, J. C., Allen, R., Littlewood, S., Wright, S., Burton, J., and Gould, D. J., et al. (1989). Meta-analysis of placebo-controlled studies of the efficacy of Epogam in the treatment of atopic eczema. Relationship between plasma essential fatty acid changes and clinical response. *British Journal of Dermatology, 121,* 75–90.

Mukherjee, P. K., & Suresh, B. (2000). The evaluation of wound-healing potential of *Hypericum hookerianum* leaf and stem extracts. *Journal of Alternative and Complementary Medicine, 6,* 61–69.

Muller, J. L., & Clauson, K. A. (1998). Top herbal products encountered in drug information requests (Part 1). *Drug Benefit Trends, 10,* 43–50.

Munday, J. S., James, K. A., Fray, L. M., Kirkwood, S. W., & Thompson, K. G. (1999). Daily supplementation with aged garlic extract, but not raw garlic, protects low density lipoprotein against in vitro oxidation. *Atherosclerosis, 143,* 399–404.

Murray, M., & Pizzorno, J. (1999). *Encyclopedia of natural medicine* (2nd ed.). Rocklin, CA: Prima.

Neldner, K. H. (2000). Complementary and alternative medicine. *Dermatologic Clinics, 18,* 189–193.

NIEHS News. (1998). Herbal health. *Environmental Health Perspectives* [On-line]. 106. Available: http://ehpnet1.niehs.nih.gov/docs/1998/106-12/niehsnews.html

NIEHS News. (1999). Medicinal herbs: NTP extracts the facts. *Environmental Health Perspectives* [On-line]. 107. Available: http://ehpnet1.niehs.nih.gov/docs/1999/107-12/niehsnews.html

Olness, K. (1993). Hypnosis: The power of attention. In D. Goleman & J. Gurin (Eds.), *Mindbody medicine: How to use your mind for better health* (pp. 277–290). New York: Consumer Reports Books.

Ornish, D., Scherwitz, L. W., Billings, J. H., Gould, K., Merritt, T. A., et al. (1998). Intensive lifestyle changes for reversal of coronary heart disease. *Journal of the American Medical Association, 280* (23), 2001–2007.

Page, R. L., & Lawrence, J. D. (1999). Potentiation of warfarin by dong quai. *Pharmacotherapy, 19,* 870–876.

Parnham, M. J. (1996). Benefit-risk assessment of the squeezed sap of the purple coneflower *(Echinacea purpurea)* for long-term oral immunostimulation. *Phytomedicine, 3,* 95–102.

Pelletier, K. R., Marie, A., Krasner, M., & Haskell, W. L. (1997). Current trends in the integration and reimbursement of complementary and alternative medicine by managed care, insurance carriers, and hospital providers. *American Journal of Health Promotion, 12*(2), 112–123.

Perharic, L., Shaw, D., Colbridge, M., House, L., Leon, C., & Murray, V. (1994). Toxicological problems resulting from exposure to traditional remedies and food supplements. *Drug Safety, 11,* 284–294.

Phelps, S., & Harris, W. S. (1993). Garlic supplementation and lipoprotein oxidation susceptibility. *Lipids, 28,* 475–477.

Phillips, D. P., Christenfeld, N., & Glynn, L. M. (1998). Increase in US medication-error deaths between 1983 and 1993. *Lancet, 351,* 643–644.

Pinnell, C. M. & Covino, N. A. (2000). Empirical findings on the use of hypnosis in medicine-a critical review. *International Journal of Experimental Hypnosis, 45*(2), 70–94.

Piscitelli, S. C., Burstein, A. H., Chaitt, D., Alfaro, R. M., & Falloon, J. (2000). Indinavir concentrations and St John's wort. *Lancet, 355,* 547–548.

Plotkin, M. J. (1991). Traditional knowledge of medicinal plants—The search for new jungle medicines. In O. Akerele, V. Heywood, & H. Synge (Eds.), *Conservation of medicinal plants* (pp. 59–63). Cambridge, England: Cambridge University Press.

Portyansky, E. (1998). Alternative medicine. *Drug Topics, 142,* 44–50.

Posner, G. (1998). An examination of the media coverage of a prayer study in progress. *The scientific review of alternative medicine, 2*(2), 34–37.

Price, D. D., & Barrell, J. J. (2000). Mechanisms of analgesia produced by hypnosis and placebo suggestion. *Progress in brain research, 1222,* 255–271.

PR Newswire. (1999, September 29). *US herbal market nearing saturation* [On-line]. Available: http://www.herbs.org/current/saturation.html

Principe, P. P. (1991). Valuing the biodiversity of medicinal plants. In O. Akerele, V. Heywood, & H. Synge (Eds.), *Conservation of medicinal plants* (pp. 79–124). Cambridge, England: Cambridge University Press.

Pye J. K., Mansel, R. E., & Hughes, L. E. (1985). Clinical experience of drug treatments for mastalgia. *Lancet, 2,* 373–377.

Research Triant Institute. (2000). *Fact sheet: RTI's discovery of taxol* [On-line]. Available: http://www.rti.org/patents/taxol.cfm

Robbers, J. E., & Tyler, V. E. (1998). *Tyler's herbs of choice*. Binghamton, NY: Hawthorn Press.

Rogers, M. E. (1990). Nursing: Science of unitary man. In E. A. M. Barrett (Ed.), *Vision of Rogers' science-based nursing* (pp. 5–11). New York: National League for Nursing.

Rossman, M. L. (1993). Imagery: Learning to use the mind's eye. In D. Goleman & J. Gurin (Eds.), *Mind-body medicine: How to use your mind for better health* (pp. 291–300). New York: Consumer Reports Books.

Ruschitzka, F., Meier, P. J., Turina, M., Lüscher, T. F., & Noll, G. (2000). Acute heart transplant rejection due to Saint John's wort. *Lancet, 355,* 548–549.

Sanganee, H. J., & Harrison, K. (2001). *Taxol—Molecule of the month* [On-line]. Available: http://www.ncl.ox.ac.uk/mom/taxol/taxol.htm

Schempp, C. M., Pelz, K., Wittmer, A., Schöpf, E., & Simon, J. C. (1999). Antibacterial activity of hyperforin from St John's wort, against multiresistant *Staphylococcus aureus* and gram-positive bacteria. *Lancet, 353,* 21–29.

Schwartz, G., & Russek, L. (1997). Dynamical energy systems and modern physics: Fostering the science and spirit of complementary and alternative medicine. *Alternative Therapies in Health and Medicine, 3*(3), 46–56.

Schwartz, M. S., & Schwartz, N. M. (1993). Biofeedback: Using the body's signals. In D. Goleman & J. Gurin (Eds.), *Mindbody medicine: How to use your mind for better health* (pp. 301–314). New York: Consumer Reports Books.

Shad, J. A., Chinn, C. G., & Brann, O. S. (1999). Acute hepatitis after ingestion of herbs. *Southern Medical Journal, 92,* 1095–1097.

Shaw, D., Leon, C., Kolev, S., & Murray, V. (1997). Traditional remedies and food supplements. A 5-year toxicological study (1991–1995). *Drug Safety, 17,* 342–356.

Siegers, C. P., Steffen, B., Robke, A., & Pentz, R. (1999). The effects of garlic preparation against human tumor cell proliferation. *Phytomedicine, 6,* 7–11.

Silagy, C., & Neil, A. (1994a). Garlic as a lipid lowering agent—A meta-analysis. *Journal of the Royal College of Physicians of London, 28,* 39–45.

Silagy, C., & Neil, A. (1994b). A meta-analysis of the effect of garlic on blood pressure. *Journal of Hypertension, 12,* 463–468.

Sizer, F., & Whitney, E. (1991). *Nutrition: Concepts and controversies*. St. Paul: West.

Slifman, N. R., Obermeyer, W. R., Musser, S. M., Correll, W. A., Cichowicz, S. M., Betz, J. M., & Love, L. A. (1998). Contamination of botanical dietary supplements by *Digitalis lanata*. *New England Journal of Medicine, 339,* 806–811.

Snider, S. (1991). *Herbal teas and toxicity*. FDA consumer. (DHHS Publication No. FDA 92-1185). Washington, DC: U.S. Government Printing Office.

Solecki, R. S., & Shanidar, I. V. (1975). A Neanderthal flower burial in northern Iraq. *Science, 190,* 188.

Stevenson, C., & Ernst, E. (1999). Hypericum for depression. An update of the clinical evidence. *European Neuropsychopharmacology, 9,* 501–505.

Stevenson, C., & Ernst, E. (2000). A pilot study of *Hypericum perforatum* for the treatment of premenstrual syndrome. *British Journal of Obstetrics and Gynecology, 107,* 870–876.

Stevenson, C., Pittler, M. H., & Ernst, E. (2000). Garlic for treating hypercholesterolemia. A meta-analysis of randomized clinical trials. *Annals of Internal Medicine, 133,* 420–429.

Taylor, D. (1996). Herbal medicine at a crossroads. *Environmental Health Perspectives, 104,* 924–928.

Turner, R. B., Riker, D. K., & Gangemi, J. D. (2000). Ineffectiveness of echinacea for prevention of experimental rhinovirus colds. *Antimicrobial Agents and Chemotherapy, 44,* 1708–1709.

Tyler, V. E. (1986). Plant drugs in the twenty-first century. *Economic Botany, 40,* 279–288.

U.S. Food and Drug Administration. (1995). *Dietary Supplement Health Education Act of 1994* [On-line]. Available: http://vm.cfsan.fda.gov/~dms.dietsupp.html

U.S. Food and Drug Administration. (1998). *The Special Nutritionals Adverse Event Monitoring System (SN/AEMS)* [On-line]. Available: http://vm.cfsan.fda.gov/~tear/aems.html

U.S. Food and Drug Administration. (1999). *An FDA guide to dietary supplements*. Publication No. (FDA) 99-2323 [On-line]. Available: http://vm.cfsan.fda.gov/~dms.fdsupp.html

Vickers, A. J., Rees, R. W., & Robin, A. (1998). Advice given by health food shops: Is it clinically safe? *Journal of the Royal College of Physicians of London, 32,* 426–428.

Wagner, H. (1999). Phytomedicine research in Germany. *Environmental Health Perspectives, 107,* 779–781.

Weil, A. (1988). *Health and healing*. Boston: Houghton Mifflin.

Weil, A. (1995). *Spontaneous Healing*. New York: Alfred A. Knopf.

Whitaker, D. K., Cilliers, J., & de Beers, C. (1996). Evening primrose oil (Epogam) in the treatment of chronic hand dermatitis: Disappointing therapeutic results. *Dermatology, 193,* 115–120.

Williamson, J. S., & Wyandt, C. M. (1998, June 1). An herbal update. *Drug Topics*, pp. 66–75.

Winstead-Fry, P., & Kijek, J. (1999). An integrative review and meta-analysis of therapeutic touch. *Alternative Therapies in Health and Medicine, 5*(6), 58–67.

Woelk, H. (2000). Comparison of St John's wort and imipramine for treating depression: Randomized controlled trial. *British Medical Journal, 321,* 536–539.

Wonnemann, M., Singer, A., & Muller, W. E. (2000). Inhibition of synaptosomal uptake of 3H-L-glutamate and 3H-GABA by hyperforin, a major constituent of St. John's wort: The role of amiloride-sensitive sodium conductive pathways. *Neuropsychopharmacology, 23,* 188–197.

Woolfson, A., & Hewitt, D. (1992). Intensive aromacare. *International Journal of Aroma, 4*(2), 12–14.

Yim, T. K., Wu, W. K., Pak, W. F., Mak, D. H., Liang, S. M., & Ko, K. M. (2000). Myocardial protection against ischaemia-reperfusion injury by a *Polygonum multiflorum* extract supplemented 'dang-gui decoction for enriching blood,' a compound formulation, ex vivo. *Phytotherapy Research, 14,* 195–199.

Youngkin, E. Q., & Israel, D. S. (1996). A review and critique of common herbal alternative therapies. *Nurse Practitioner, 21,* 39, 43–45, 49–52, 54–56, 59–60, 62.

SECTION IV

Physical Health

12

Cardiovascular Wellness and Illness

Oma Riley-Giomariso

CHAPTER OUTLINE

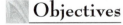 Objectives

1. *List five risk factors for coronary heart disease and ways to minimize them.*
2. *Identify the normal limits for blood pressure readings and blood lipid levels.*
3. *Identify the symptoms of angina and myocardial infarction often seen in women.*
4. *Identify the reasons that coronary heart disease is sometimes misdiagnosed in women.*
5. *Describe the symptoms of stroke.*

Introduction

One in five women between the ages of 45 and 65 have some form of heart or blood vessel disease. Women are at greater risk of dying from heart disease than from any other disease, including breast cancer. Although there has been an overall reduction in the death rate from heart disease in recent years, the rate of decline is less for women than for men. It is of the utmost importance that women be knowledgeable about their cardiovascular system, its basic anatomy and physiology, and the indicators that either reassure that it is healthy or warn that it is not. For many years, one of the most dangerous forms of heart disease, coronary artery disease (CAD) also known as coronary heart disease (CHD), has been thought of incorrectly as a disease that primarily afflicts men. A majority of women polled in 1997 still viewed coronary heart disease as primarily a man's problem (Legato, Padus, & Slaughter, 1997). In a similar study done in 1999, most women identified breast cancer as the greatest risk to their health and were not aware that coronary heart disease is the leading cause of death among women. Additionally, although 80 percent of the women reported that they would be comfortable discussing CHD with their physicians, less than 33 percent had done so (Mosca et al., 2000). Women who do not perceive cardiovascular disease as a substantial health concern may do nothing to reduce their risk, and thus jeopardize their lives.

In this chapter, the hallmarks, or markers, of cardiovascular wellness are identified and explained. Some guidelines for promoting cardiovascular wellness through the elimination or control of risk factors, and the use of appropriate screening tests and examinations, are provided. The mechanisms by which risk factors such as smoking, poor diet, overweight, and a sedentary lifestyle are thought to harm the heart and blood vessels, and the controversies regarding them, are discussed. Three serious cardiovascular conditions that afflict large numbers of women (coronary heart disease, hypertension, and stroke) are addressed in terms of their basic pathophysiology, their symptoms in women, and their diagnosis and treatment. Mitral valve prolapse, a heart valve abnormality, once thought to be more common in women, is not discussed in this chapter, as it is now known to be distributed equally between the genders and not particularly consequential.

Markers of Cardiovascular Wellness

The cardiovascular system consists primarily of the heart and blood vessels. Women, on average, have smaller, lighter hearts than men, and their coronary arteries (the arteries that provide the heart with oxygen-rich blood) are smaller (Wingate, 1997). When the cardiovascular system is functioning optimally, it is able to deliver adequate amounts of oxygen and nutrients to all the body's organs and tissues. A healthy heart beats strongly and regularly, pumping oxygenated blood throughout the body. Healthy arteries and veins are supple, have smooth inner surfaces, and can dilate and contract appropriately. When the cardiovascular system is structurally healthy and functioning well, the resting heart rate (the heart rate while the body is at rest) and blood pressure are within normal limits. The sounds heard when listening to the heart with a stethoscope reflect the appropriate opening and closing of the heart valves. Healthy arteries are free of the fatty deposits known as plaque, so exertion, such as walking or running, does not bring on pain in the chest or calf area. Blood also flows reliably to the brain; no circulation-related alterations in consciousness or cognition occur. The intact electrical system of a healthy heart is reflected on a normal resting electrocardiogram (EKG) as a heart rate that is mostly regular and without signs of disease. An EKG is a recording of the electrical impulses that cause the heart to beat rhythmically.

Normal Heart Rate

The term *heart rate,* or *pulse,* refers to the number of times the heart beats in one minute. A healthy person's heart rate can vary tremendously, depending on the circumstances. Women tend to have a higher resting heart rate, and greater fluctuations in their heart rate, than men. The normal pulse rate in a healthy individual varies from a low of 50 (for athletic adults) to rates exceeding 100 during exercise. Generally speaking, a person who has been sitting or lying quietly for five minutes (resting), and who is not excited or fearful, should have a heart rate of between 60 and 85 beats per minute. People who exercise aerobically and are in good physical condition tend to have lower resting heart rates than those who do not. The pulse should also be regular; the beat-to-beat interval should be consistent, and there should be no skipped beats or flurries of beats. Occasional extra beats, or **palpitations,** are normal and may be related to caffeine or nicotine intake. Frequent palpitations may be a sign of illness, and a healthcare provider should be consulted.

Normal Blood Pressure

A person's blood pressure is comprised of two numbers, as in 120/80. The top number is the systolic blood pressure, and the bottom number is the diastolic blood pressure. The **systolic blood pressure** is the internal pressure that the blood volume exerts within the arteries when the heart is contracting, or beating. The **diastolic blood pressure** is the internal pressure that the blood volume exerts within the arteries when the heart is relaxed and in the process of filling with blood. The systolic pressure is always stated first, the diastolic second. Simply stated, the higher (systolic) number is the pressure when the heart is beating, and the lower (diastolic) number represents the pressure when the heart is resting between beats.

The Sixth Report of the Joint National Committee on Prevention, Detection, Evaluation, and Treatment of High Blood Pressure (JNC VI) (1997) set the most recent parameters for optimal, normal, and high blood pressure. The *optimal* resting blood pressure with respect to cardiovascular risk is between 120/80 and 100/60. *Normal* blood pressure should not be greater than 130/85; a blood pressure that is higher than 135/85 is associated with an increased risk of cardiovascular disease, stroke, and death. *High–normal* blood pressure is a systolic number between 130 and 139 *or* a diastolic number between 85 and 89. Individuals with blood pressure within this range should begin to lower their blood pressure through lifestyle changes, such as exercise, diet, and, if indicated, weight loss. *High* blood pressure is a systolic blood pressure ranging from 140–159 *or* a diastolic pressure ranging from 90–99. When systolic and diastolic pressures fall into different categories, the higher category classifies the individual's blood pressure. A single elevated blood pressure reading is not sufficient proof that the blood pressure is consistently elevated, but it is a sign to seek evaluation from a healthcare professional, according to the JNC VI. Many individuals have blood pressure that is consistently too high for years, known as hypertension, without knowing it, because they usually do not experience symptoms. That is why hypertension is called the "silent killer."

A form of hypertension known as **isolated systolic hypertension** is the most common type of high blood pressure for women and individuals older than 50. This occurs when the systolic blood pressure rises to 140 or greater and the diastolic blood pressure remains less than 90. A recent study concluded that isolated systolic hypertension alone justifies a diagnosis of hypertension among this age group (Lloyd-Jones, Evans, & Larson, 1999). At one time, it was thought that it was normal for blood pressure to increase with aging, but this is no longer considered the case. Among the elderly, systolic blood pressure is a better predictor than diastolic pressure of coronary heart disease, stroke, heart failure, and renal disease. *Low* blood pressure is a far less common problem than high blood pressure. In most instances, blood pressure that runs on the low side is not considered problematic unless it produces symptoms such as lightheadedness and fainting.

The **pulse pressure** is the difference between the systolic blood pressure and the diastolic blood pressure. Among middle-aged and older people, there is a strong correlation between abnormal pulse pressure and the development of coronary heart disease and hypertension (Franklin, Khan, & Wong, 1999). A pulse pressure of 40 (the difference between 120 and 80) is considered average. Pulse pressures of more than 40 points reflect an arterial wall stiffness.

Adults should be screened for hypertension at every healthcare visit or a minimum of once yearly. If a person's blood pressure seems high on one occasion, it is rechecked after at least five minutes have passed. If it is still high, it should be checked again on at least one other occasion. The diagnosis of hypertension is based on the average of *two or more readings,* taken at each of two or more visits to a healthcare provider following an initial screening. JNC IV recommendations are that blood pressure readings be obtained with the individual in three different positions: lying down, seated, and after standing for two minutes. Many people take and keep track of their own blood pressure, using devices specifically designed for that purpose. Blood pressure measuring devices are also available in drugstores and shopping malls. However, if calibrated improperly, these devices can provide incorrect information. Everyone should have her blood pressure evaluated by a healthcare provider on a regular basis.

Several factors can elevate blood pressure temporarily. People who are going to have their blood pressure taken should refrain from smoking and drinking caffeinated beverages for at least 30 minutes prior to the measurement, because these activities are known to increase blood pressure. They should also sit quietly for approximately 5 minutes before a blood pressure measurement, because talking is known to raise blood pressure. Repeated blood pressure measurements should be taken at least 2 minutes apart and in different arms in order to yield accurate results. The use of an upper arm blood pressure cuff that is too large or too small will also result in an inaccurate reading. A blood pressure cuff that is *too small* for the person's arm will give a falsely *elevated* reading; conversely, a cuff that is *too large* will give a falsely *low* reading. The blood pressure cuff should be wide enough to cover about 80 percent of the upper arm.

Some individuals develop elevated blood pressure, termed *white coat hypertension,* while in the presence of healthcare providers. Presumably, such individuals find visits to providers stressful. Although some clinicians see white coat hypertension as benign, others argue that increased blood pressure in response to such a stressor is in itself diagnostic of hypertension.

Screening for hypertension should be a part of every routine healthcare visit. A blood pressure that is consistently 135/85 or higher requires treatment. The initial therapy is lifestyle modification, including losing weight and restricting the amount of sodium in the diet. If, after three months of lifestyle modification, the blood pressure remains elevated (Mosca et al., 1999), treatment with medication is initiated. The treatment of hypertension is discussed in more depth in the Cardiovascular Illnesses section of this chapter.

Normal Heart and Vascular Sounds

The heart produces sounds that can be heard through a stethoscope. The term **auscultation** means listening to heart sounds (or lung or other sounds) with the aid of a stetho-

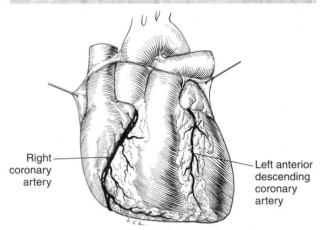
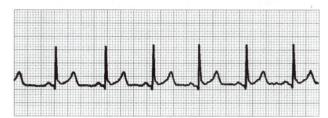
scope. Heart sounds provide information about heart rate, heart rhythm, and abnormalities of the heart valves or chamber walls. Characteristic normal sounds are made as the heart valves close during **systole** (contraction of the heart) or **diastole** (relaxation of the heart). The first heart sound is labeled S1 (lub), and the second heart sound is labeled S2 (dub). Abnormal heart sounds indicate potential problems with the heart valves or chamber walls. For example, if there is a problem with one of the valves in the heart, it may produce a sound called a **murmur.** Other sounds, called **bruits,** may be heard over major arteries in the body if plaque has narrowed the artery and partially obstructed the flow of blood. For example, a **carotid bruit** is a swishing sound heard over the carotid artery located in the neck. The American Heart Association lists asymptomatic carotid bruit as a risk factor for stroke, which is discussed in the Cardiovascular Illnesses section of this chapter.

Adequate Tissue Perfusion

Perfusion is the ability of the arteries to carry oxygen-rich blood to all areas of the body under all normal conditions, including exercise. Organs and other tissues that are inadequately perfused will be oxygen-deficient; they will malfunction, and symptoms will arise. For example, an individual whose heart is not receiving enough blood through the coronary arteries (see Figure 12–1) may experience chest pain and/or a progressive weakening of the heart muscle. The extremities (hands and feet) of individuals with normal perfusion are warm and normal in color. People who tend to have chilly hands and feet probably have

adequate perfusion, as long as the skin color in those areas is normal. The presence of pale, cool, lower extremities and/or calf or thigh pain with exercise suggests compromised blood flow, most likely due to atherosclerosis—the buildup of plaque in the walls of arteries. When plaque in the arteries that feed the legs interferes with blood flow to the point that symptoms develop, **arterial peripheral vascular disease** is said to be present.

Normal Electrical Functioning

An electrocardiogram EKG (see Figure 12–2) provides information about heart rate and rhythm, as well as the effects of various drugs and substances on the heart. Abnormalities on the EKG can also indicate the presence of certain types of coronary heart disease. The impulses that stimulate the heart to beat travel by way of specialized tissue, and any alteration in those tissues can be detected on an EKG. Heart muscle cells that are **ischemic** (short of oxygen) or dead conduct electrical impulses differently than healthy cardiac tissue. Therefore, EKGs can be used to detect and follow the various stages of a heart attack (McCance & Heuther, 1998). An EKG cannot *predict* a heart attack, however, and some individuals have heart attacks without having an abnormal EKG.

Women have a less pronounced wave amplitude (height) on a resting EKG than men. The differences between the size of the EKG waves in men and women, and their anatomical and physiological differences, make the accurate diagnosis of various kinds of coronary heart disease more difficult in women (Laurienzo, 1997). However, every woman should consider having a baseline EKG. This examination is important, even when there is no diagnosis of coronary heart disease, because it establishes baseline information about the electrical function of the heart. Should a heart attack occur, the baseline EKG is useful for comparison with the most recent EKG to determine abnormal changes in electrical conduction.

Promoting Cardiovascular Wellness

Promoting cardiovascular wellness is a matter of pursuing a healthy lifestyle and taking advantage of screening tests that reveal the presence of risk factors or coronary heart disease in its early stages. It is important to both *avoid behaviors* that increase the risk of CHD and to *choose behaviors* that are known to reduce it. Actively promoting cardiovascular wellness may compensate for any predisposing genetic factors.

The risk factors for cardiovascular disease are the circumstances, characteristics, and behaviors that increase the likelihood that an individual will develop hypertension, coronary heart disease, and stroke (see Box 12–1). The risk factors involve the processes, behaviors, and circumstances that ultimately cause injuries to the inner lining of the blood vessels that supply the heart and brain with oxygen and nutrition. Long-standing injury can lead to atherosclerosis, commonly known as *hardening of the arteries*. Atherosclerosis involves the gradual accumulation of plaque within and on the inside surface of the arterial walls (see Figure 12–3). Plaque is made up of cholesterol, calcium, scar tissue, and fat. As plaque deposits enlarge, they can gradually or suddenly occlude the arteries in the brain and heart, as well as elsewhere in the body. When the arteries that feed an area of the heart are blocked and heart tissue dies, a heart attack occurs; when the arteries that feed the brain are blocked, brain cells die and a stroke occurs. **Plaque burden** is said to exist in the coronary arteries when an atherosclerotic plaque reaches the stage of development at which it is in danger of rupturing or eroding. Either a rupture or an erosion can cause a heart attack. The more extensive the coronary atherosclerosis, the greater the chance of plaque rupture (Grundy, 1999).

The American Heart Association (2000) has identified the major risk factors for coronary heart disease: increasing

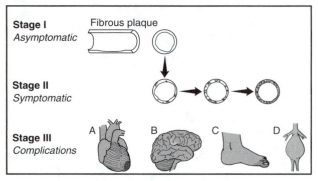

Figure 12–3   Arterial Plaque

Stages I and II. Side views and cross sections of artery illustrating progression of atherosclerosis (described in the text). *Stage III.* Complications produced by atherosclerosis: **A.** Myocardial infarction. **B.** Brain infarction. **C.** Gangrene. **D.** Aneurysm.

Source: ADULT NURSING: ACUTE AND COMMUNITY CARE 2e by Burrell/Gerlach/Pless © 1997. Reprinted by permission of Pearson Education, Inc., Upper Saddle River, NJ.

age, male sex, heredity (including ethnicity), smoking, high blood cholesterol, high blood pressure, physical inactivity, obesity or overweight, and diabetes. Some additional risk factors are elevated levels of LDL cholesterol, low HDL cholesterol, and high blood glucose levels (Grundy, 1999). Cholesterol is discussed in detail in the section on modifiable risk factors. Other factors thought to confer the risk for cardiovascular disease, but not yet officially recognized by the American Heart Association, are elevated homocysteine, fibrinogen, iron, and c-reactive protein levels, and hypothyroidism (Sinatra, 2000). Recently, researchers (Wilson et al., 1998) have defined low-risk individuals as nonsmoking, nondiabetic persons who have a total cholesterol of 160 to 199, an LDL cholesterol level between 100 and 129, an optimal blood pressure of 120/80 or less, and an HDL cholesterol of at least 45 for men and 55 for women. Even individuals in this low-risk group may need attention as they age and their risk status changes. The general notion is that, the more risk factors an individual has, the more aggressive the intervention should be (Grundy, 1999). Whereas some risk factors can be avoided, others are genetic to varying degrees and can only be minimized.

There are three levels of prevention in healthcare: primary, secondary, and tertiary. The most optimal, **primary prevention,** involves reducing the risk factors that could lead to the development of cardiovascular disease. **Secondary prevention** involves detecting and managing cardiovascular disease in an early stage. **Tertiary prevention** involves maximizing health by taking measures to prevent an existing condition from worsening and complications from developing in persons who have established cardiovascular disease.

Box 12–1   Cardiovascular Risk Factors for Women

- ♦ Increasing Age
- ♦ Heredity
- ♦ Smoking
- ♦ High blood cholesterol level
- ♦ High blood pressure
- ♦ Physical inactivity
- ♦ Obesity or overweight
- ♦ Diabetes
- ♦ Previous heart attack, stroke, or TIA

Source: Adapted from Health risk awareness [On-line]. *American Heart Association.* Retrieved August 23, 2001. Available: http://www.americanheart.org.

Circumstances such as male sex, and coronary heart disease in one's family, are considered *nonmodifiable risk factors,* because nothing can be done about them. Other characteristics, however—such as having diabetes, hypertension, an undesirable lipid profile, or a high fibrinogen, iron, or homocysteine level, or being menopausal or hypothyroid—are *modifiable,* or *controllable,* to varying degrees. Still other risk factors, such as smoking, being overweight, leading a sedentary lifestyle, and having high levels of life stress, are, for most people, completely *avoidable* or at least highly modifiable. Taking all measures to obviate modifiable risk factors and to control the physical problems that contribute to coronary heart disease can greatly mitigate the influence of a nonmodifiable factor, such as family history.

Nonmodifiable Risk Factors

Nonmodifiable risk factors include increasing age, male sex, a family history of coronary heart disease, and diabetes.

INCREASING AGE

Most people who die of cardiovascular disease are age 65 or older. As women age, their chances of developing coronary heart disease increases. When women approach menopause, their risk of CHD and stroke begins to increase, and it keeps increasing as they age (see Chapter 24).

MALE GENDER

Cardiovascular disease is the number one killer of both men and women. Men, however, have a greater risk of heart attack than women. African American males have a higher incidence of coronary heart disease than Euro-American males do.

FAMILY HISTORY

A family history of CHD is a strong risk factor for developing it. This is especially true if the family member is a close relative, such as a parent or sibling, and if any family member developed CAD at an early age (Assmann et al., 1999). Having a mother who had a heart attack before age 65 and/or a father who had a heart attack before age 55 puts a woman at risk for cardiovascular disease. A family history of CHD confers risk because a genetic predisposition for characteristics such as central obesity (excess weight carried mainly in the abdomen), abnormal lipid metabolism, or high blood pressure may be present and because people tend to adopt family lifestyle patterns related to food choice and physical activity, smoking, and so on. If a woman with a strong family history has any symptoms that she is concerned about, she should seek immediate medical attention.

A related factor, ethnicity, can also confer a risk of developing CHD. African American women have a greater risk of coronary heart disease and stroke than Euro-American women. African Americans as a group have more severe high blood pressure than Euro-Americans and are therefore at higher risk for coronary heart disease. The incidence of coronary heart disease is also higher among Mexican Americans, American Indians, native Hawaiians, and some Asian Americans. This is partially due to higher rates of obesity and diabetes within these cultures (American Heart Association, 2000; Carter, Pugh, & Monterrosa, 1996).

DIABETES

Ten million Americans have a diagnosis of diabetes, and another 5 million are estimated to have undiagnosed diabetes. Diabetes is an independent risk factor for cardiovascular disease in both men and women (Grundy, Benjamin, et al., 1999). However, diabetes is a more serious risk factor in women than in men. Diabetic women are three to seven times more likely to develop cardiovascular disease than are nondiabetic women, whereas diabetic men are only two to three times more likely to develop the disease than are men who do not have diabetes. This difference may be due to the strong negative effect diabetes has on lipid levels and blood pressure in women. Detecting cardiovascular disease is also more difficult in individuals with diabetes because they have decreased pain perception and may not feel chest pain. Consequently, multivessel coronary heart disease may be present before the symptoms appear (Grundy, Benjamin, et al., 1999).

Sixty-five percent of all diabetic persons who die prematurely fall victim to cardiovascular disease. Diabetes also increases the risk of stroke, heart failure, renal disease, and carotid atherosclerosis (Grundy, Benjamin, et al., 1999). Even impaired glucose tolerance or slightly elevated blood sugars can increase the risk of high cholesterol and hypertension (Assmann et al., 1999). Insulin resistance, considered a precursor to adult onset diabetes, is increasingly being seen as a risk factor for CHD. Insulin resistance is said to exist when the cells become resistant to insulin, causing blood insulin and glucose levels to increase gradually. Insulin resistance has recently been classified as a multisystem disorder that is caused by genetics, obesity, physical inactivity, and advancing age. Over time, insulin resistance leads to high blood pressure, weight gain, and atherosclerosis (Grundy, Benjamin, et al., 1999).

Women with insulin resistance or actual diabetes need to be vigilant to protect themselves from cardiovascular disease. Smoking cessation is a primary goal, because nicotine constricts blood vessels and increases abnormal plaque formation on the walls of the vessels. Women with diabetes can reduce their risk of coronary heart disease by controlling the risk factors to a degree greater than that recommended for the general population. They should strive to lower their LDL cholesterol level to less than 100, increase their HDL level to greater than 50, and maintain a blood pressure of less than 135/85. In many instances, taking lipid-lowering drugs and antihypertensive medications will help them meet these goals. Additionally, the current recommendation of the Expert Committee of the Diagnosis and Classification of Diabetes Mellitus is for individuals with diabetes to consistently control their blood sugars so they are near normal or less than 126.

Modifiable Risk Factors

The modifiable risk factors include hypertension, an undesirable lipid profile, a high fibrinogen level, a high c-reactive protein level, postmenopausal status, and hypothyroidisim.

HYPERTENSION

Hypertension is a significant risk factor for women over 45. Approximately 60 percent of Euro-American women and almost 80 percent of African American women in this age group are hypertensive. A woman with high blood pressure has 2 to 10 times the CHD risk of a woman who does not. Even moderate elevations of blood pressure raise women's risk; hypertension causes blood vessel walls to become irritated by the increased pressure, and the irritation makes them vulnerable to plaque formation.

Unfortunately, a large portion of the population with hypertension is inadequately treated (Whelton & Appel, 1996), and often the disease is not recognized until it is in the later stages. The treatment of hypertension reduces the risk for coronary heart disease in both sexes. Meeting target blood pressures, such as those outlined by the Joint National Committee on the Prevention, Detection, Evaluation, and Treatment of High Blood Pressure is important for preventing stroke and reducing the progression of CHD. A blood pressure of 135/85 or less is the target for all persons. Hypertension is further discussed in the Cardiovascular Illnesses section of this chapter.

UNDESIRABLE LIPID PROFILE

The lipid substances found in the blood include cholesterol and triglycerides. Although both substances are needed for the proper functioning of the body, excessive amounts are believed to contribute to coronary heart disease.

The lipid most closely associated with coronary heart disease in the minds of most people is cholesterol. Cholesterol is actually a wax the body uses to form cell membranes and other tissues. The body's supply of cholesterol comes from two sources: from the cholesterol it manufactures itself and from foods, such as meats and dairy products. Foods from plants, such as fruits, vegetables, and grains, do not contain cholesterol. The dietary consumption of cholesterol itself has less of an effect on blood cholesterol levels than does one's overall intake of *fat*. High-fat diets stimulate the body to manufacture more cholesterol than it ordinarily would. Fat from food first undergoes digestion in the body and is then taken to the liver, where it is processed into cholesterol. Unfortunately, some individuals suffer from **familial hypercholesterolemia** (high levels of cholesterol) and are genetically predisposed to make large amounts of cholesterol, regardless of how much fat they consume. This trait, particularly in combination with a high-fat diet, increases a person's risk of developing cardiovascular disease. Familial hypercholesterolemia can be diagnosed at birth through blood tests.

Excessive levels of cholesterol in the blood, particularly certain kinds of cholesterol, can lead to atherosclerosis in the arteries throughout the body. Just as atherosclerosis in the coronary arteries causes CHD, atherosclerosis in the arteries of the legs causes peripheral vascular disease and atherosclerosis in brain arteries causes stroke (discussed in the Cardiovascular Illnesses section of this chapter). Atherosclerosis is also implicated in hypertension; as arteries become infiltrated with plaque, they become less flexible and distensible, a condition called **arteriosclerosis.** Atherosclerosis is thought to be the primary contributor to the development of arteriosclerosis, which, in turn, causes the most common form of hypertension.

Cholesterol is transported in the bloodstream by large carrier molecules called **lipoproteins.** Several types of lipoprotein molecules exist and are classified according to their density. All lipoproteins contain triglycerides (a type of lipid), and protein, in addition to cholesterol. The higher the percentage of lipid in relation to protein, the lower the density of the lipoproteins will be. The classes of lipoproteins currently thought to be most influential in the development of atherosclerosis are low-density lipoprotein (LDL), high-density lipoprotein (HDL), and Lipoprotein a, known as Lp (a). Triglyceride, another blood lipid, is also thought to play a significant role in the development of atherosclerosis (McCance & Heuther, 1998).

Among the lipoproteins, it is LDL, the so-called bad cholesterol, that contributes most significantly to the development of arteriosclerosis and constitutes an independent risk factor for cardiovascular disease in men and women. LDL carries large amounts of cholesterol from the liver to the cells, where it is used to make hormones. Unfortunately, LDL also carries cholesterol to the walls of the arteries—particularly, the walls of medium-sized and large arteries. Cholesterol is one component of atherosclerosis plaque. An excessively high level of LDL in the blood, therefore, is a risk factor for cardiovascular disease.

Making appropriate lifestyle choices can lower blood LDL levels. A diet that limits total fat intake to less than 35 grams per day, and saturated fat intake to 7 grams per day (NIH News Release, 2001), will decrease the amount of LDL in the blood. Increasing the amount of fiber in the diet will also lower LDL levels. Controlling stress and quitting smoking will also reduce LDL levels. Some individuals, however, may not be able to reduce the amount of LDL in their blood through lifestyle-related efforts alone. Fortunately, recent studies indicate that lipid-lowering medications can be used effectively to treat these individuals.

Conversely, high-density lipoprotein (HDL), also known as good cholesterol, has a *protective* effect against atherosclerosis. HDL carries cholesterol away from the cells and away from the walls of the blood vessels. It also picks up LDL molecules in the blood and carries them back to the liver, where they are dismantled. A *decreased* level of HDL is a risk factor for cardiovascular disease. High-density lipoprotein levels increase with exercise and estrogen replacement and as a result of a diet low in fat. Simply stated, whereas LDL carries cholesterol *to* the arterial walls, HDL carries cholesterol *from* the arterial walls.

Lp(a) is essentially an LDL particle with a somewhat different protein structure. It is currently the topic of much research and investigation. Lp(a) is thought to promote clot formation, because it is structurally similar to plasminogen, a protein invalued in clotting. Blood levels of Lp(a) are at least partially genetically determined, and elevated levels are a risk factor for atherosclerosis. Lp(a) may contribute to cardiovascular disease by interfering with the breakup of blood clots, which often play a role in heart attacks. Lp(a) has also been found in plaques in the arteries. This finding may be significant for understanding plaque development. The presence of Lp(a) in women 65 years old or younger increases the risk for coronary heart disease (Pay, Ozcan, & Tokgozoglu, 1997). The statin class of lipid-lowering drugs does not bring Lp(a) levels down and may even increase them. Estrogen replacement therapy has been shown to decrease Lp(a) levels, as has niacin therapy (Sinatra, 2000). More research is needed to determine whether measuring Lp(a) in women's blood is an appropriate screening measure. Research that may demonstrate that lowering Lp(a) results in a reduction in coronary heart disease risk has not been completed.

Another blood lipid of some importance is **triglyceride.** Excessive levels of triglyceride put *women* at risk for coronary heart disease, but not their male counterparts. Increased triglyceride levels in women seem to make LDL more likely to cause coronary artery lesions. Trigylceride levels increase with diets in which almost all calories are derived from carbohydrates, diabetes, increased fat intake, alcohol consumption, obesity, and menopause. Individuals with a high triglyceride level and a low HDL level are likely to have an inherited syndrome known as *familial hypertriglyceridemia.* These individuals are also at very high risk for early heart attack and diabetes. Most heart attacks in women younger than 40 occur in individuals with either familial hypercholesterolemia or hypertriglyceridemia (Castelli, 1988).

Lipid screening is an important part of preventive healthcare for women and men. By the age of 30, every woman should have had a complete blood lipid profile, which should consist of total cholesterol, LDL cholesterol, HDL cholesterol, LDL:HDL cholesterol ratio, and triglyceride level. A person must fast for approximately 12 hours before a blood sample is taken; however, it is permissible to drink water and take most medications during the fasting period. The National Cholesterol Education Panel provides uniform standards for the treatment of hyperlipidemia. The currently recommended therapeutic goals for individuals with no cardiovascular risk factors, or fewer than two risk factors, are to reduce LDL to less than 160; to increase HDL to greater than 35 and, if possible, 45; and to decrease total cholesterol

to less than 200. In an individual with two or more risk factors, the goal is to keep LDL below 130. Individuals with known CHD or diabetes should decrease their LDL to less than 100 (*Looking Beyond LDL Cholesterol,* 2001).

Newly diagnosed individuals with **mild** hyperlipidemia (excessively high blood lipid levels) are generally advised to try to reduce their lipid levels through diet modification (see Chapter 3) and exercise (see Chapter 6) for three to six months. If no significant results have occurred after that time, medications are usually prescribed. Although the combination of exercise and a diet low in saturated and trans fat and high in whole grains, vegetables, and fruit works for a large number of individuals, recent studies have shown that diet changes alone may not achieve the desired results. This seems to be especially true for postmenopausal women.

If making lifestyle changes is not sufficient to bring blood lipid levels down to desirable levels (see Box 12–2), lipid-lowering medications can be used. Lipid-lowering therapy for patients with established coronary artery disease can prevent acute coronary events and cardiac death. In individuals who have high lipid levels without established coronary artery disease, the correction of abnormal lipid levels may deter the development of atherosclerosis. Lipid-altering drugs also improve coronary **endothelial** (vessel wall) function. Unfortunately, whereas 26 million adults have high blood lipid levels significant enough to warrant treatment, only 5.3 million are receiving drug therapy. Specific types of lipid altering-agents are used to treat specific abnormal blood lipid patterns (Yu, Pasternak, & Ginsburg, 2000).

There are currently five classes of lipid-lowering medications: statins, bile acid binding resins, niacin, fibric acid derivatives, and estrogen. Statins and bile acid binding resins are highly effective for the reduction of low-density lipoprotein levels. The drugs in these classes have have also been shown to be effective in the prevention of CAD. Clinical trials have shown a regression of CAD, improvement in endothelial function, a reduction in the incidence of coronary events, and a decrease in CAD-related mortality (Lenfant, 1986; Rossouw, Lewis, & Rifkind, 1990).

Statins work in a variety of ways, but primarily by inhibiting an enzyme (HMG-CoA reductase) that is necessary for cholesterol synthesis. This results in a decreased LDL level, because more of the LDL in the body is taken up by the liver and removed from the circulation. Statins profoundly reduce LDL levels and improve HDL and triglyceride levels as well. Currently, they are the drugs of choice for individuals with hyperlipidemia, particularly individuals with increased LDL levels. Individuals taking these medications can expect LDL to decrease by approximately 20 to 40 percent, triglyceride to decrease by approximately 10 to 30 percent, and HDL to increase by 5 to 10 percent. The trade names of the statins are Mevacor, Zocor, Pravacol, Lescol,

Box 12-2 Lipid Levels and Associated Risk of Coronary Heart Disease

Total Cholesterol	Degree of Risk
Less than 200 mg/dl	Desirable—minimal risk
200–239 mg/dl	Borderline high—increases risk
240 mg/dl and above	High—doubles the risk in comparison with a person whose level is < 200

LDL Cholesterol	
Less than 100 mg/dl	Optimal—minimal risk
100–129 mg/dl	Desirable—low risk
130–159 mg/dl	Borderline high—increases risk
160–189 mg/dl	High—increases risk substantially
190 mg/dl and above	Very high—CHD risk is high

HDL Cholesterol	
60 mg/dl and above	Optimal—minimal risk
40–59 mg/dl	Good—low risk
< 40 mg/dl	Too low—a major risk factor

Triglyceride	
< 150	Normal—low risk
150–199	Borderline high—increases risk
200–499	High—increases risk substantially
500 and above	Very high—high risk

Source: Reproduced from the National Heart, Lung, and Blood Institute publication titled *Cholesterol-Heart Disease Connection: Measuring Your Blood Cholesterol.*

and Lipitor. Currently, Lescol is the least potent, and Lipitor is probably the most potent on the market. Some of the side effects of these medications are diffuse abdominal pain, constipation, mild fatigue, flatulence, dyspepsia, headache, sleep disturbances, and muscle aches. Most patients find that the side effects subside within the first two weeks. It takes approximately three months for statin drugs to begin to improve lipid levels. Because of the effect of these drugs on the liver, healthcare providers order liver function tests before beginning statin therapy. The tests are repeated after six weeks and are then done approximately every six months thereafter. Adjustments in medication dosage may require more frequent testing. Overall, the statins have reduced the need for combination drug therapy. Nevertheless, certain in-

dividuals still require treatment with more than one drug to achieve a healthy lipid profile.

The **bile acid binding resins** include drugs such as Questran and Cholested. These medications have local, rather than systemic, effects and are therefore the safest of all the lipid-lowering drugs. They remain in the gastrointestinal tract and are not absorbed into the blood. They work by binding with bile acids in the intestine and causing them to be excreted in stool, rather than returned to the liver. The liver is forced to synthesize more bile acids to make up for this loss, and, because cholesterol is used in this process, blood cholesterol levels go down. Bile acid binding resins are prescribed for individuals who need moderate LDL lowering or a slight increase in HDL. They typically lower LDL by 15 to 30 percent, slightly increase HDL, and have no effect on triglyceride. The combination of a low-fat diet and the use of bile acid binding resins can also decrease the **vasoconstriction** (narrowing) associated with hypercholesterolemia in persons with normal coronary arteries and enhance the regression of atherosclerosis in persons with CAD. The most common side effects of these medications are bloating, abdominal pain, constipation, and nausea. Individuals taking them need to maintain a high water intake. Liver function tests are also required before and during therapy with resins. Also, this class of drugs may interfere with the absorption of other medications, such as digoxin and Coumadin.

Niacin, or nicotinic acid, is also used to lower cholesterol levels. Although niacin is a water-soluable B complex vitamin, its function as a lipid-lowering agent has nothing to do with its role as a vitamin. Niacin was the first lipid-altering agent shown to reduce mortality in the secondary prevention of coronary artery disease. Its primary effect appears to be on very low-density lipoprotein (VLDL) synthesis and secretion and apolipoprotein B synthesis. VLDL is a precursor of LDL, and apolipoprotein B is another small particle thought to be implicated in CAD. Niacin also increases HDL levels, but the mechanism for this is unclear. Niacin improves HDL levels by 15 to 30 percent and lowers LDL levels by approximately 15 to 25 percent. Niacin also lowers triglyceride levels in some individuals by 20 to 50 percent. In addition, niacin decreases lipoprotein Lp(a) levels; niacin and estrogens are the only agents known to do so. Niacin and Niaspan are common trades names for niacin. The side effects reported most often are flushing and itching; taking aspirin or ibuprofen before the niacin dose may prevent these effects. Liver function tests are also necessary when taking this agent, and individuals with diabetes who take it may have increased insulin requirements. Niacin is contraindicated for individuals who have liver disease or peptic ulcer disease.

Fibric acid derivatives, such as gemfibrozil (Lopid) and fenofibrate, are agents most known for their ability to lower triglyceride levels. They can also be used to increase HDL. They lower triglyceride by about 20 to 50 percent and improve HDL by 10 to 15 percent. They are believed to work by enhancing VLDL clearance. However, fibric acid derivatives may raise LDL levels, so it is unclear whether they should be used as a single agent in the primary prevention of CAD. These agents have also been associated with the development of pancreatitis, gallbladder disease, and muscle inflammation. Therefore, fibric acid derivatives should be used judiciously to treat severe hypertriglyceridemia.

The use of *estrogen* as a hyperlipidemic agent is controversial. Some studies have suggested that postmenopausal estrogen use can significantly reduce the incidence of cardiac events (Grodstein, Stampfer, & Colditz, 1997). Estrogen works by increasing serum levels of VLDL and HDL and decreasing LDL levels. However, another study (Hulley, Grady, & Bush, 1998) raised the possibility that estrogen is associated with an increased clotting effect, which could lead to a heart attack or death in some groups of women. Currently, many practitioners recommend estrogen for postmenopausal women with hypercholesterolemia only after other lipid-lowering therapies have been considered or if the woman had been on estrogen before coronary heart disease was diagnosed. Pre-existing breast cancer and a history of blot clots are contraindications to estrogen use. **Hormone replacement therapy (HRT)** with both synthetic estrogen and progestins has been associated with a higher morbidity and mortality rate in women with pre-existing CHD. However, estradiol (a form of estrogen) that is identical to that produced in women's bodies, has been associated with plaque regression (*Hormone Replacement and Your Heart,* 2001). The issues related to hormone replacement and CHD are explored more fully in Chapter 24.

Garlic, although once touted as a cholesterol-lowering substance, has not lived up to its promise. A meta-analysis of randomized, double-blind, placebo-controlled trials found that, although garlic was superior to placebo in lowering total cholesterol levels, the size of the effect was too modest to be of clinical significance (Stevenson, Pitler, & Earnst, 2000). Although the evidence as to whether the *isoflavones* (beneficial micronutrients in *soy products*) decrease cholesterol levels is contradictory, the American Heart Association recommends that persons who have elevated cholesterol levels consume 25 to 50 grams per day of soy protein (*Hormone Replacement and Your Heart,* 2001).

HIGH FIBRINOGEN LEVEL

Fibrinogen is a blood component that is involved with the formation of clots. Elevated levels of fibrinogen have been linked with an increased risk of stroke and heart attack. Fibrinogen levels tend to rise in women after menopause, as estrogen levels fall (Sinatra, 2000), and some women inherit a tendency toward high levels. The normal range for blood fibrinogen is 185–360 (Sinatra, 2000). Women who have high fibrinogen levels, and who also smoke or take birth control pills, are at a higher risk of developing a blood clot, which may lead to a heart attack or stroke. Many providers are now advising their middle-aged patients to take *aspirin* daily as a primary or secondary preventative against heart attack and stroke, providing

that their blood pressure is not elevated, there is no history of a bleeding disorder, and they are taking no other blood-thinning substances. Aspirin makes the blood slightly less likely to form a clot that could obstruct a coronary artery. Preventive aspirin therapy in a dose of 75–150 mg/day has been shown to decrease the incidence of heart attack in women (*Another Angle on Aspirin,* 2000).

HIGH C-REACTIVE PROTEIN LEVEL

C-reactive protein is a marker for inflammation, the process by which the body responds to injury. Although inflammation is a desirable and protective process in the short term, chronic inflammatory processes within the blood vessel walls are thought to contribute to atherosclerosis and may make plaques in the coronary vessels unstable and at risk for rupture. Chronic inflammation also increases the risk that blood clots will form within the blood vessels.

An elevated c-reactive protein (CRP) level may constitute a risk factor for cardiovascular disease. It has been demonstrated that levels can be elevated for many years before a first heart attack or stroke occurs (Packard et al., 2000), and an elevated CRP level has been shown to predict heart attacks independent of lipid levels, Lp(a), fibrinogen, body mass index, diabetes, hypertension, and a number of other risk factors (Grundy, 1999). A recent study of patients with unstable coronary artery disease (Lindahl, Henrik, Siegbahn, Venge, & Wallentin, 2000) suggests that elevated levels of c-reactive protein and elevated levels of troponin T (a marker for myocardial damage) may signal the likelihood of death from cardiovascular causes. Sinatra (2000) suggests using the **high sensitivity c-reactive protein test (HS-CRP)** to detect low levels of inflammation in the body. The normal range for this test is 0.1–2.0. A value of 1.8 or greater has been associated with myocardial infarction; however, larger studies are needed to demonstrate definitively that an elevated CRP level is a cause and not merely an effect of infarction (Sinatra, 2000).

HIGH HOMOCYSTEINE LEVEL

Homocysteine is one of several new variables whose role in developing cardiovascular disease is under investigation. **Homocysteine** is an amino acid that is formed when **methionine,** another amino acid, which is found in red meat, poultry, ricotta cheese, avocado, and some other foods, is improperly metabolized. Adequate levels of vitamin B-6, folate, and vitamin B-12 are required for the proper metabolism of methionine. In their absence, the dangerous protein homocysteine is formed (Sinatra, 2000). At elevated levels, homocysteine can make the blood vessels less pliable and allow atherosclerosis to build up. Elevated levels are referred to as **hyperhomocysteinemia.** Hyperhomocysteinemia is considered a prevalent and independent risk factor for acute myocardial infarction (MI), stroke, peripheral vascular disease, and thrombosis (blood clot) (Ridker et al., 1999). Insufficient blood levels of folate and vitamin B-6 have been similarly linked with heart attack risk, and an increased intake of these substances has been shown to lower homocysteine levels. Normal blood concentrations of homocysteine are considered to be between 5 and 15 umol/L. Levels between 16 and 30 umol/L are considered to be moderately elevated. Levels higher than 100 umol/L are considered severely elevated.

High homocysteine levels can often be brought down by a diet that provides the currently recommended daily allowances of 400 µg of folate, 2 mg of vitamin B-6, and 6 µg of vitamin B-12. This can be accomplished by eating vegetables, fruits, fish, and fortified grains and cereals. In cases in which diet alone does not control homocysteine levels, two food supplements, betaine and trimethylglycine (TMG), at dosages of 500 to 1,000 mg/day have been reported to lower homocysteine levels (Sinatra, 2000). Smokers should be aware that they may be prone to elevated homocysteine (Mosca et al., 1999).

POSTMENOPAUSAL STATUS

Menopause is caused by the lowering of endogenous estrogen levels in women's bodies which occurs as women age. The term *endogenous* means produced by the body. Because it is associated with declining estrogen levels, menopause doubles or triples women's risk of developing CHD (Wilson et al., 1998). The risk is even higher in menopausal women who have coexisting **hypertension** and an **increased fibrinogen level** (Ernst & Resch, 1993). Endogenous estrogen is known to confer a protective effect against cardiovascular disease. Younger women are much less likely to develop CHD than women who are 10 to 15 years postmenopause. Prior to menopause, a women's risk of a cardiovascular event is considerably less than that of a man; but after menopause, the risk that a significant cardiovascular event will occur becomes equal in both sexes (Dennerstein, 2000; McCance & Heuther, 1998). Endogenous estrogen is known to reduce many of the *risk factors* for coronary heart disease. For example, premenopausal women have lower LDLs and Lp(a)s and higher HDLs than men. However, after natural or surgical menopause HDL decreases and LDL and Lp(a) gradually rise until they exceed the average level in men (Matthews, Kuller, Sutton-Tyrrell, & Chang, 2001). Estrogen also promotes optimal functioning of the inside (endothelium) of the vessel wall, even in coronary arteries that contain plaque. Estrogen may also stabilize plaque, making it less vulnerable to rupture and allowing blood vessel walls to *dilate*, rather than *constrict*, in response to stress. Vasoconstriction in response to stress occurs more often in postmenopausal women who are not taking estrogen (Tikkanen, 1993).

Although unavoidable, menopause is not necessarily a non-modifiable risk factor. **Hormone replacement therapy (HRT)** has been seen as a way of decreasing the likelihood that older women will develop CHD, and a number of studies have suggested that this is the case. HRT has been found to return LDL, HDL, and Lp(a) values to premenopausal levels and to normalize endothelial vasodilation (Guetta & Cannon, 1996; Tikkanen, 1993). Walsh et al. (2000) demonstrated that taking ERT or HRT reduces homocysteine levels. The results of the Postmenopausal Estrogen/Progestin Interventions

(PEPI) trial, which involved over 800 women, provided convincing evidence that both estrogen replacement therapy (ERT) and estrogen/progestin combination therapy (HRT) reduce most of the risk factors for coronary heart disease (Wenger, 2000). Estrogen replacement therapy has also been shown to lower the risk for *stroke* by about 20 percent (Update on Estrogen and the Heart, 1999).

However, more recent studies, such as the HERS study, the ERA study, and a new study undertaken as part of the Women's Health Initiative (all addressed in Chapter 24), have cast doubt on the ability of HRT (but not necessarily ERT) to prevent or ameliorate coronary artery disease in postmenopausal women. The American Heart Association is now advising *against* using HRT to prevent coronary artery disease and second heart attacks (News, 2002). It is not yet known whether postmenopausal women who have undergone hysterectomy, and can therefore safely take ERT, will derive benefit from estrogen replacement alone.

HYPOTHYROIDISM

The thyroid gland helps control the rate of body function. It does this through the production of thyroid hormone, which helps regulate the body's metabolism. **Hypothyroidism** is said to be present when the thyroid fails to produce sufficient thyroid hormone (see Chapter 21). Hypothyroidism commonly affects middle-aged women and is a risk factor for coronary heart disease. It contributes to high lipid levels and also decreases the heart's rate and ability to pump efficiently. Treatment for hypothyroidism must be approached cautiously, however; if coronary artery disease is present, the sudden introduction of excessive amounts of thyroid hormones into the body can stress the heart and cause angina, heart attack, or sudden death.

Avoidable Risk Factors

Avoidable risk factors for CHD (smoking, excess body weight, stress, and a sedentary lifestyle) exert a negative effect on the health of the cardiovascular system through mechanisms that are well understood, in some cases, but still under investigation in others. Making informed and wise lifestyle choices is extremely important in promoting cardiovascular health. Psychological, emotional, and spiritual factors can also increase the risk for CHD.

SMOKING

The single most important thing women can do to protect their health is to avoid smoking. Smoking greatly increases one's chance of developing coronary artery disease; two out of every five smoking-related deaths result from it. A woman who smokes only one to four cigarettes per day is twice as likely to have cardiovascular disease as a woman who does not smoke. Heavy smokers are twice as likely to suffer a heart attack as nonsmoking women are. Women who do smoke must **quit.** Quitting smoking reduces the risk for coronary events by 50 percent and is the most effective means of preventing coronary disease (Schenck-Gustafsson, 1996). Quitting also improves morbidity and mortality in patients with existing coronary artery disease (Wenger, 1996a).

Smoking has a number of negative effects on the cardiovascular system. Smoking increases the release into the blood of substances called **catecholamines.** Catecholamines cause the blood vessels to constrict and thereby contribute to hypertension. Smoking lowers estrogen levels, which causes levels of undesirable low-density lipoprotein (LDL) to increase in the blood, while the levels of heart-protective high-density lipoprotein (HDL) decrease. Nicotine, the addicting ingredient in cigarettes, masks chest pain, which can result in a smoker's unknowingly having a heart attack. It also irritates the lining of the coronary arteries, causing them to constrict and even go into spasm—which can trigger a heart attack. Smoking further contributes to the likelihood of having a heart attack by inducing increased **platelet aggregation,** which causes blood cells to clump together in the coronary arteries. The carbon monoxide in cigarette smoke causes lowered oxygen levels in the blood, increasing the possibility of a coronary event in women who may already have narrowed or diseased coronary arteries (McCance & Heuther, 1998). Women who use nicotine patches must not smoke while wearing the patch, because the cumulative effects of the nicotine in cigarettes and the nicotine from the patch increase the risk for heart attack. Smoking and smoking cessation are addressed in more detail in Chapter 13.

Excess Body Weight

Most women with coronary artery disease are overweight (American Heart Association, 2000). Heart attack risks double if women are 15 to 30 percent overweight. Obesity increases a women's risk for high blood pressure, diabetes, high cholesterol, and high triglyceride levels, and weight gain is associated with increased LDL, increased total cholesterol, and decreased HDL. The pattern of weight gain is also important. Central obesity is associated with the greatest risk (Rexrode et al., 1998). Central obesity is present if one's waist measurement divided by one's hip measurement is greater than 0.9. A more general rule of thumb is that a person whose waist measures more than 35 inches has central obesity (*Hormone Replacement and Your Heart*, 2001). In people under age 50, obesity poses a greater risk for coronary artery disease than any other risk factor. See Chapter 3 for a discussion of the problem of overweight and ways of addressing it.

Sedentary Lifestyle

Exercise is very important to good cardiovascular health. Unfortunately, women tend to get less exercise than men (see Chapter 6). High-demand multiple roles and depression have been identified as some of the reasons women have sedentary lifestyles and tire easily when they are involved in physical activity (McGrath, 1998).

The most recent information on the benefit women can derive from exercise comes from the Nurses' Health Study.

The Nurse's Health Study has been in progress for many years, and thousands of female nurses have taken or are taking part. Thus far, data from the Nurses' Health Study suggest that brisk walking reduces the risk of MI in women (Manson & Lee, 1996). The women in the study who walked at a rate of 30 mph or more for at least three hours per week had a 30 to 40 percent lower risk of suffering a heart attack than the women who did not. However, spending even *more* time exercising appears to confer an even greater benefit; the women who walked briskly for five hours per week had a 50 percent lower risk of coronary heart disease. Interestingly, the women who engaged in vigorous exercises, such as aerobics or jogging, had the same time-related reduction in risk. These results are important because they demonstrate that even *moderate* levels of exercise exert a protective effect against cardiovascular disease.

In the Nurses' Study, even the women who smoked, were overweight, or had other risk factors for CHD significantly reduced their risk of developing cardiovascular disease by exercising. Aerobic exercise lowers LDL, raises HDL, lowers resting heart rate and blood pressure, decreases body fat, increases muscle mass, and reduces stress. The benefits of exercise are further discussed in Chapter 6.

Stress

Stress is a term used to describe the conditions that result from a person's response to physical, chemical, emotional, and environmental factors. Stress can refer to physical effort as well as mental tension. A body of evidence points to a relationship between the risk for cardiovascular disease and environmental and psychosocial factors, such as job strain, social isolation, and stress-prone personality. Lack of social support, depression, and low socioeconomic status are also associated with an increased risk for cardiovascular disease (Assmann et al., 1999; Uchino, Cacioppo, & Keicolt-Glaser, 1996). Chronic stress may affect other coronary risk factors, such as high blood pressure and cholesterol levels, and contribute to behaviors such as smoking, physical inactivity, and overeating. Denollet and Brutsaert (1998) found that people who are distressed— that is, people with Type D personalities, are four times more likely to suffer a second heart attack than are non-D types. Characteristics of distressed persons include ongoing worry and anxiety, insecurity, and nonassertiveness.

There are several physiological mechanisms by which stress may promote atherosclerosis. One of these mechanisms involves blood clotting. When we are stressed physically or psychologically, the body exhibits what is known as the *fight-or-flight response*. As a part of that response, chemicals that make the blood stickier and more likely to form a clot are released into the circulation. Over time, this continual, stress-induced hypercoagulability may contribute to plaque buildup in the arteries. A second way in which stress contributes to coronary heart disease is by triggering chemical changes in the body that increase *free radical damage* to the coronary arteries. Finally, under stressful conditions, catecholamines, such as *norepinephrine*, are produced in greater than usual amounts. High levels of norepinephrine in the blood can trigger spasms in the walls of the coronary arteries (McCance & Heuther, 1998).

There is evidence that stress affects the cardiovascular system negatively even before we are born. Babies who have a low birth weight for their length are at risk for CHD in adulthood. Dr. Janet Rich-Edwards of Harvard reported in 1997 that, of 70,297 American women studied, those born weighing less than 5.5 pounds had a 23 percent higher incidence of cardiovascular disease (Rich-Edwards et al., 1997). According to Rich-Edwards, if a pregnant woman is under stress, certain conditions in her body may both stunt her baby's growth and make the baby more vulnerable to stress later in life. Under stressful conditions, the mother's body produces *cortisol,* one of the stress hormones. If this cortisol reaches the fetal brain, the child is likely to be especially susceptible to stress in adulthood. Under optimal circumstances, an enzyme in the placenta deactivates the cortisol, but, if the mother is not well nourished, her body may not produce the enzyme. Scientists also suspect that suboptimal maternal nutrition during gestation raises the fetus's risk of developing hypertension and high cholesterol levels as an adult (Barker, 1995).

The highly successful Dr. Dean Ornish Program for Reversing Heart Disease emphasizes the importance of stress management. Patients learn meditation, yoga, and other techniques for inducing what is known as the relaxation response, which is an antidote to stress (see Chapter 7). The Ornish program also includes a very low-fat diet, an exercise program, and group support sessions in which patients meet to learn more about their problems and act to express them. The health insurer Hallmark both pays for and provides the Ornish program. In the state of Pennsylvania, there have been no deaths, heart attacks, strokes, or bypass surgeries among program participants since its inception in 1997 (Brekke, 2001).

PSYCHOLOGICAL, EMOTIONAL, AND SPIRITUAL FACTORS

Hostility, antagonistic behavior, depression, social isolation, and low or absent religious involvement have all been associated with atherosclerotic cardiovascular disease (Everson, Kauhanen, & Kaplan, 1997; Siegman, Townsend, Civelek, & Blumenthal, 2000). Conversely, optimism, social support, and religiosity have been associated with superior levels of cardiovascular health and superior health in general (see Chapter 27).

Hostility as a component of personality has been associated with cardiovascular risk and has a demonstrated correlation with coronary artery calcification, which is a marker of subclinical atherosclerosis (Iribarren et al., 2000). A number of theories explaining this relationship have been put forward. Some studies suggest that hostile people are more likely to have risk factors, such as smoking, alcohol use, and physical inactivity (Iribarren et al., 2000). However, in a study involving 1,950 women with a family history of coro-

nary atherosclerosis, Knox et al. (2000) found that hostility correlated positively to the presence of plaque in the carotid arteries, even when the researchers controlled smoking, alcohol use, and physical inactivity. Cardiologist Dean Ornish (1998) believes hostility to be a barrier to intimacy and love, which he sees as crucial to cardiovascular health.

Social isolation is also a risk factor for CHD. An analysis of pooled data from six studies involving more than 20,000 participants suggests that people who are socially isolated have a rate of premature death two to four times higher than that of individuals with supportive friends and family (Linden, Stossel, & Maurice, 1996).

Depression has also been associated with an increased risk for CHD. In a large study involving over 3,000 young adults with normal blood pressure, participants who scored high on screening tests for depression were *twice as likely* as their happier peers to develop high blood pressure within five years (Davidson, Jonas, Dixon, & Markovitz, 2000). In another large study, Penninx et al. (2001) found that among over 2,000 elderly subjects who started out free of coronary artery disease, those suffering from major depression were nearly *four times more likely* to eventually die of a heart attack than those who were not. In the same study, individuals with major depression who already had CHD were *three times as likely* to die as those who also had CHD but were not depressed. In their meta-analysis of the literature on depression and coronary heart disease, Linden et al. (1996) concluded that, after statistical adjustment for risk factors such as poor diet, smoking, and lack of exercise, depression increases the risk of developing coronary artery disease by 60 percent and the risk of having a heart attack by 50 percent. Depressed patients are also known to exhibit higher mortality rates, compared with nondepressed patients after myocardial infarction (Kubzansky & Kawachi, 2000). Dr. Thomas Pickering, a cardiologist at Mount Sinai Medical center is quoted in *Health Magazine* (Chen, 2001) as saying that depression "is probably as important as blood pressure and physical inactivity as a risk factor for developing heart disease" (p. 109).

Anxiety has also been implicated as a factor that contributes to the development of coronary heart disease. Men who suffer from anxiety related to phobias such as fear of flying, and individuals with panic disorder, an extreme form of anxiety, have higher rates of sudden cardiac death and coronary artery disease than less anxiety-prone individuals (Kubzansky & Kawachi, 2000). Worry, a component of anxiety, can also contribute to the development of heart disease. The relationship between worry and coronary events was studied in a cohort of older men over a period of 20 years. The investigators (Kubzansky et al., 1997) found that subjects who worried the most, particularly about social conditions, were about *twice as likely* to suffer a fatal or nonfatal heart attack as subjects who worried less.

Several mechanisms have been identified by which negative emotions may contribute to morbidity and mortality related to coronary artery disease. One is **increased platelet**

aggregation (clumping), which makes the blood more likely to form a clot that can occlude a coronary artery. Lederbogen et al. (2001) found that major depression increases platelet aggregation. Another mechanism is loss of what is known as **heart rate variability.** Normally, the nervous system signals the heart to quickly speed up or slow down in response to the body's demands. The loss of this flexibility is an important risk factor for adverse cardiovascular events. For example, after myocardial infarction, a reduction in beat-to-beat heart rate variability is a strong predictor of death. Individuals with high hostility scores, and patients with anxiety or depressive disorders, have low heart rate variability (Gorman & Sloan, 2000) and may be at increased risk for cardiovascular death associated with coronary heart disease and abnormal electrical activity in the heart. A weakened immune response may also be a factor. Depression is known to affect the immune system adversely, and a decrease in the body's ability to heal injured arterial walls may foster inflammation and the build up of plaque in coronary arteries (Chen, 2001).

Many women simultaneously occupy high-demand occupational and homemaking roles. This often causes them to give priority to providing service and care to others and neglect their own well-being. Taking time to care for themselves physically, psychologically, emotionally, and spiritually, however, is important to women's cardiovascular health.

Cardiovascular Illnesses

Hypertension, coronary artery disease, congestive heart failure (the inability of the heart to pump adequately), and stroke are serious health problems that afflict women in significant numbers. Women do not always experience coronary heart disease the same way men do, and healthcare providers may not respond in the same way to CHD in men and women. The reasons for these differences are varied and have to do with anatomy, physiology, and gender roles, among other factors. It is important that women be familiar with the early signs of cardiovascular disease, and with relevant diagnostic procedures and treatment.

Hypertension

Hypertension is defined as a systolic blood pressure > 139 and a diastolic pressure > 89, and even moderate elevations of blood pressure pose serious risks for women (Grundy et al., 1998). High blood pressure increases the risks for heart attacks, strokes, kidney failure, damage to the eyes, congestive heart failure, and atherosclerosis. Hypertension causes the heart to work harder than normal and renders both the heart and the arteries more prone to injury. When high blood pressure exists with obesity, smoking, high cholesterol levels, or diabetes, the risk for heart attack or stroke increases

several times. Many hypertensive individuals are asymptomatic but may have a degree of target organ disease, which may not appear until 10–20 years of disease progression. The target organs of hypertension are the **heart, kidneys, brain,** and **eyes.**

Higher levels of both systolic and diastolic blood pressure cause an increased risk for morbidity, disability, and mortality. In the past, it was thought that an elevated diastolic blood pressure posed more risk than an elevated systolic blood pressure. It is now known, however, that an elevated systolic blood pressure is a risk factor for CHD, stroke, heart failure, and peripheral artery disease, whether the diastolic blood pressure is elevated or not. The evaluation and treatment of systolic hypertension are particularly important for reducing risk in women and the elderly (Kannel, 1999).

Approximately 50 million Americans have hypertension. African-Americans, the elderly, those with less education, and those from a lower socioeconomic group are at increased risk of developing hypertension. More women than men have the disease, but men, particularly African-American men, have greater **morbidity** and **mortality** related to hypertension. This disease typically appears between ages 30 and 55. The major risk factors that pertain to women are smoking, elevated cholesterol levels, diabetes, age greater than 60 or postmenopausal status, and a family history of premature CHD. Additional factors are obesity, stress, high fat and sodium intakes, oral contraceptive use, and a significant alcohol intake.

Blood vessels can constrict for a variety of reasons, including emotional states and physical demands placed on the body. Constriction causes an increase in **peripheral arterial resistance,** or the pressure the heart must overcome in order to pump blood into the arteries. Increased peripheral arterial resistance is the basic cause of hypertension (McCance & Huether, 1998). When there is increased constriction in the vessels, the heart has to work harder to force the blood to flow through the constricted arterial system. If hypertension is not treated, the heart must work harder and harder to pump enough blood and oxygen to the tissues of the body, and it may become enlarged and weakened because of its increased workload.

The mechanism that controls the constriction and relaxation of blood vessels is located in the brain. In response to physical and emotional stress, the brain initiates the fight-or-flight response, which is mediated by the sympathetic branch of the nervous system. This response causes blood vessels to constrict in order to shunt blood to vital organs. For reasons that are not clearly understood, the blood vessels of hypertensive individuals are easily stimulated; they are very sensitive to norepinephrine, one of the powerful vasoconstrictors released when the sympathetic nervous system is stimulated. When vasoconstriction occurs, the kidneys do not receive their normal blood supply. This causes them to retain salt and water, which increases blood volume and contributes to the hypertension. The kidneys also release chemicals which cause even more powerful vasoconstriction of blood vessels. Some hypertensive individuals are highly sensitive to the sodium in table salt (and other food substances) and increase their blood volume when they consume too much.

The first step in the treatment of hypertension is lifestyle modification. Quitting smoking, losing weight, exercising, decreasing sodium intake, reducing stress, and decreasing alcohol intake are all ways to begin to manage hypertension. A reduction in weight of just 10 pounds will reduce blood pressure an average of 3 mm (American Heart Association, 2000). Women who exercise for 30 minutes three times a week reduce their cardiovascular risk by 50 percent (Folsom et al., 1993; Manson & Lee, 1996).

Decreasing sodium intake will also decrease blood pressure in many hypertensive individuals. Sodium promotes the retention of water, resulting in an increase in blood volume. Sodium, along with chloride, is a component of table salt, so keeping the ingestion of salt to no more than 2,400 mg a day is recommended by the American Heart Association. This is about 1 1/4 teaspoons of salt. Sodium is an ingredient in many prepared foods (see Chapter 3), and hypertensive individuals should limit their intake of it. An awareness of both natural and added sodium content is important when trying to control one's salt intake. It is important to read labels when buying prepared and packaged foods. The words *soda* and *sodium* and the symbol *Na* on labels signal the presence of sodium in products. Fresh or frozen foods (without added salt) will likely contain less sodium than prepared foods sold in boxes or cans. Using salt/sodium-free or low-sodium products, and using spices and herbs in place of table salt, can result in a significant decrease in sodium intake. Older individuals, and individuals of African or Asian ancestry, tend to be particularly sensitive to sodium. Damage to the arteries by the excessive consumption of dietary fat, oil, and cholesterol also fosters hypertension, as does a diet too low in potassium (Sinatra, 2000). Reducing and managing stress (see Chapter 7) is also important in the treatment of hypertension.

Numerous medications are available for treating hypertension when lifestyle modification alone does not suffice. There are several major classes of medications used to treat hypertension. **Beta-blockers** reduce or block the action of chemicals in the body that stimulate blood pressure and heart rate. Beta-blockers are also prescribed for some patients with cardiovascular disease because they decrease the heart's workload by lowering blood pressure and heart rate. Common side effects are fatigue, constipation, depression, decreased libido, and difficulty reaching orgasm during sexual activities. The trade names of commonly prescribed beta-blocking drugs include Inderal, Lopressor, and Tenormin.

Calcium channel blockers also reduce blood pressure, as well as heart rate and the overall workload of the heart. They block the movement of calcium into the muscle cells in the artery walls, thus limiting the vessels' ability to contract. Common side effects are swelling of the ankles due to fluid retention, constipation, dizziness, and either a fast or slow heartbeat. The trade names of two commonly prescribed calcium channel blocking drugs are Verapamil and Diltiazem.

Angiotensin converting enzyme (ACE) inhibitors lower blood pressure and reduce the work of the heart. They decrease blood pressure by inhibiting an enzyme that leads to the formation of the vasoconstricting hormone **angiotensin**. Prinivil and Zestril are brand names for the ACE-inhibiting drug lisinopril. Vasotec is a brand name for another commonly prescribed ACE inhibitor, enalapril. ACE inhibitors are contraindicated during pregnancy, as they can injure the developing fetus. Some individuals, particularly women, develop a dry, irritating cough while on ACE inhibitor therapy, but this side effect typically disappears within a week or 10 days

Diuretics act on the kidneys and foster the removal of excess sodium and fluid from the body, reducing blood volume and, consequently, blood pressure. Most diuretics also remove potassium from the body, and it is important that potassium stores be replenished through a diet that includes potassium-containing foods, such as raisins and other dried fruits, potatoes, and citrus fruits and juices. Some individuals on diuretic therapy may need potassium supplements to maintain optimum potassium blood levels. Commonly prescribed diuretics include Lasix, Diuril, Esidrix, and Oretic.

Coronary Artery Disease

Coronary artery disease, which is also referred to as coronary heart disease, exists when plaque partially blocks sections of one or more coronary arteries, which supply the heart muscle with oxygen-containing blood. Coronary artery disease is the *single largest killer of women;* more than 500,000 women die annually from it. The age-adjusted mortality rate for coronary artery disease is four times higher in Euro-American women, and six times higher in African-American women, than the mortality rate for breast cancer. Whereas, statistically, one in every two women will eventually die of coronary artery disease, only one in nine will die of breast cancer. Contemporary women are developing coronary artery disease at a younger age than their forebears did; more than one-fourth of the women who die from cardiovascular disease are under the age of 50. Coronary artery disease is also the leading cause of death and disability in women over 40. CAD is associated with aging in both sexes, but women typically develop it 10 years later than men do, because women are protected by estrogen when they are younger. The downside of this apparent blessing is that women with coronary artery disease, being older, typically do not fare as well as men (American Heart Association, 2000).

The heart receives its blood supply from the coronary arteries. The heart has a high need for an uninterrupted supply of blood, as it has a great deal of work to do. A normal heart beats approximately 60–80 times and pumps out approximately five quarts of blood every minute. The heart rate increases and decreases automatically in response to the body's varying demand for the oxygen and glucose carried by the blood. If coronary artery disease is present, the heart has difficulty getting the blood supply it needs to function optimally. In coronary artery disease, also known as **coronary atherosclerosis,** the lumen (interior) of the coronary artery becomes narrowed, usually from a buildup of plaque. Although there are a number of theories as to how coronary artery disease develops, the exact mechanism by which plaque forms in arteries is unknown. Factors such as hypertension, injury, hyperlipidemia, and oxidation have all been implicated (Danesh et al., 2000). Some studies suggest that atherosclerosis may be precipitated by an ongoing inflammation within arterial walls (Danesh et al., 2000).

Research indicates that there are two broad types of plaque development in arteries (Davies, 1990; Libby, 1995). One type involves the gradual formation of dense, stable plaque on the *inner surface* of the artery where the blood flows. When the arterial narrowing from this form of plaque becomes severe, coronary blood flow decreases, producing **angina,** the pain experienced when the heart muscle becomes deprived of sufficient oxygen. The second type of plaque development is the formation of unstable plaque that is hidden *within the walls* of the arteries. This form of plaque consists of soft fat, or even a dense liquid, held in place by thin, fibrous tissue. This type of plaque is considered unstable because it is prone to rupture or erosion (abrasion). If plaque, which is a living substance, ruptures or is abraded, the injury will activate the clotting process. A blood clot, which will likely obstruct the artery partially or completely, will form at the site of injury. This is known as an **acute thrombotic event,** and it usually leads to a heart attack. These hidden plaques often go undetected by conventional diagnostic procedures, such as **coronary angiography,** an invasive test in which dye is instilled into the coronary arteries in order to determine whether plaque is present. This pattern of plaque development may explain why some individuals who die from a heart attack without warning (sudden death) are found on autopsy to have no narrowing of their coronary arteries. Women tend to have single-vessel coronary artery disease, whereas men tend to have multiple-vessel disease (Douglas & Ginsberg, 1996).

Prior to the late 1980s, when the National Institutes of Health began funding research on women and CAD, most CAD research had been done on *men*. Because of this, the incidence and severity of CAD in women went unrecognized, as did differences in the ways in which coronary artery disease typically manifests in the two genders.

ANGINA

Whereas in men an actual heart attack (the death of muscle cells due to lack of oxygen in an area of the heart) is often the first symptom of coronary artery disease, women are more often warned by the pain of angina (Lerner & Kannel, 1986). Once coronary atherosclerosis has progressed be-

yond a certain point, the arteries become so narrowed that, under certain circumstances, they cannot supply the heart with enough oxygen. When the heart muscle needs more oxygen than the coronary arteries can supply, it becomes ischemic (short of oxygen), and anginal pain results. Angina in women often manifests differently than it typically does in men. Although women *may* experience the burning or squeezing chest pain typical of angina in men, they are more likely to experience a dull, aching discomfort under the breastbone. Women may also experience angina as pain in the jaw or in the upper abdomen (Danesh et al., 2000). Many women mistake angina for heartburn (Philpott, Boynton, Feder, & Hemingway, 2001). Both men and women may also experience angina as pain down their arms, especially the left arm, with or without accompanying chest pain. In men, angina typically develops during exercise or other exertion and goes away with rest; however, in women, it can arise and subside for no obvious reason (Sinatra, 2000). Angina is categorized according to the circumstances under which it occurs and the rapidity with which it becomes more severe. An individual can have classical, or typical angina; variant angina; or unstable angina.

Classical angina (referred to simply as *angina*) develops during physical exercise or under conditions involving emotional stress. A typical example is angina experienced while shoveling snow or during a bout of anger. If the CAD is severe, classical angina may occur with even mild physical activity. Classical angina is relatively stable; it worsens slowly, over time. As the atherosclerotic coronary artery becomes more and more occluded, however, individuals with classical angina become more at risk of having a heart attack. This progression tends to occur more rapidly in men than women. Women often experience repeated anginal episodes for months or years before they finally have a heart attack. Eighty percent of anginal episodes in women eventually subside and do not culminate in a heart attack; in men, however, 43 percent of anginal episodes evolve into an MI (Lerner & Kannel, 1986).

Variant angina, also called Prinzmetal's angina, occurs when a person is at rest and is caused by a coronary artery spasm. Approximately two-thirds of the people who experience such spasms have severe coronary atherosclerosis in at least one major vessel, and the spasm usually occurs very close to areas where partial blockage exists (American Heart Association, 2000). Variant angina is a serious symptom, because people who have it also tend to experience heart attacks; severe cardiac dysrhythmias, such as ventricular tachycardia and fibrillation; and sudden cardiac death (American Heart Association, 2000). **Ventricular tachycardia** is an abnormal rhythm caused by an abnormality in the heart's electrical system. The heart beats rapidly, and dangerously low blood pressure usually results. The appearance of ventricular tachycardia is considered a medical emergency. **Ventricular fibrillation** is a life-threatening dysrhythmia in which a catastrophic electrical disturbance in the heart causes it to quiver rather than contract. No blood is circulated, and death will result unless a more normal rhythm is established quickly. The term **sudden cardiac death** refers to an unexpected and almost immediate death that is almost always due to ventricular fibrillation.

Unstable angina is a very serious form of angina caused by plaque damage and subsequent blood clotting. Six to 8 percent of those with unstable angina die or have a heart attack within the following year (*What Is Unstable Angina?* 2000). As its name suggests, unstable angina is not predictable. Plaque can sustain damage and initiate the clotting process and inadequate blood flow to the heart at any time, even during sleep or rest. The only difference between an attack of unstable angina and a heart attack is that, in unstable angina, the body dissolves the clot before heart muscle is damaged. When it fails to do so, unstable angina evolves into true myocardial infarction.

Diagnosis   CAD is suspected on the basis of symptoms and is confirmed via various testing modalities. Because CAD was seen as a man's disease for so long, the male pattern of symptoms remains uppermost in the minds of some clinicians. Consequently, women's chest pain is sometimes dismissed as related to anxiety or a gastrointestinal problem (Wenger, 1996b). It is important for women who believe they may be experiencing symptoms of CAD to demand appropriate testing, if it is not offered to them. Because of differences between female and male physiology, some testing modalities have been found to be more accurate in women than men and vice versa.

One of the most common procedures performed when a woman complains of symptoms that *may* suggest the presence of CAD is exercise stress testing, also referred to as treadmill testing. An electrocardiogram is taken while the individual exercises on a treadmill. One problem with this common diagnostic test is that it can yield a *false positive* result in women. A false positive result is a result that suggests the presence of CAD when it does not actually exist. Hormone replacement therapy can cause a false positive result, as can breast tissue that distorts the EKG tracing. Women are also more likely than men to have **repolarization abnormalities** in the heart's electrical system (Mosca et al., 1997), which cause atypical patterns on EKG. A second problem with stress testing in women is that stress tests are more likely to pick up triple-vessel disease, which is more common in men, than single-vessel disease, which is more often seen in women. A third problem with stress testing is that some older women are unable to exercise at a high enough level to stress their hearts sufficiently (Sinatra, 2000). The use of an imaging agent, such as thallium, which provides actual pictures of blood flow to the heart during the stress test, improves the accuracy of stress tests in women.

Tests that are considered more accurate in women include the echocardiogram, ultrafast electron beam computed tomography (UFCT), positron emission tomogra-

phy (PET), and cardiac angiography. An **echocardiogram** is a noninvasive test that provides three-dimensional ultrasound images of the heart. It reveals the motion of the heart's muscular walls as they expand and contract. Areas that are receiving insufficient oxygen display abnormal motion on the echocardiogram (Sinatra, 2000). Echocardiography can be performed in combination with a stress test to provide accurate information about the status of women's coronary arteries (Cerqueira, 1995; Marwick et al., 1995).

UFCT is a simple, noninvasive, 10-minute test that can detect the presence of plaque in its early stages, before it significantly obstructs coronary arteries (Sinatra, 2000). UFCT (also called electron beam computerized tomography, or EBCT) is successful in detecting the calcium deposits that mark the beginning of plaque deposit 85 to 95 percent of the time. A grade called the **calcium score** reflects the amount of calcium deposited in arterial walls. UFCT is also useful for tracking the progression of plaque formation in persons with known CAD. The test is relatively inexpensive at about $400. A limitation of UFCT is that is does not detect the presence of soft plaque. Therefore, a negative UFCT test does not absolutely rule out the presence of coronary artery disease.

Positron emission tomography (PET) scanning has been dubbed "the woman's test for coronary heart disease" (Sinatra, 2000, p. 349). PET scanning reflects **myocardial perfusion**—that is, the amount of blood being taken up by the heart muscle. Coronary arteries free of plaque permit excellent perfusion of all areas of the myocardium, whereas the presence of plaque partially blocks the arteries and causes areas of the heart musculature to be underperfused. In PET scanning, a harmless radioactive substance that causes glucose, nitrogen and other metabolites present in blood to become visible is injected intravenously. When the radioactive blood reaches the heart muscle, areas that are well perfused "light up" on the scan, whereas areas that are not as well perfused do not. Although more expensive and invasive than UFCT, PET scanning is highly accurate in detecting CAD in women (Sinatra, 2000).

Cardiac arteriography, or cardiac catherization, is an invasive diagnostic test that is considered the gold standard in the diagnosis of CAD. It provides a direct visual picture of the coronary arteries, heart chambers, and valves on X ray. A cardiologist places a thin plastic tube, called a catheter, in a peripheral artery or vein (or both) and slowly guides it upward until it reaches the coronary arteries. A liquid dye, which makes the blood flowing through the heart and arteries visible on X ray, is injected through the catheter, and high-speed X-ray moving pictures are taken. The flow of blood through the arteries is seen to narrow in areas that are partially obstructed by plaque. If this test reveals the presence of a dangerous amount of plaque in one or more coronary arteries, an aggressive intervention, such as coronary artery bypass surgery, can be undertaken immediately. Unfortunately, because women's complaints of chest pain are not always taken seriously, women with chest pain are less likely than men to have coronary angiography (Kudenchuk, Maynard, Martin, Wirkus, & Weaver, 1996).

Treatment   There are various treatments for coronary artery disease. The type of treatment available depends on personal choice and the type, extent, and location of the plaque. If the CAD is causing angina, but has not progressed to the point where it is threatening life, it can be treated with drugs that improve the supply of blood to the heart and drugs that help decrease the heart's demand for oxygen. Nitrates (nitroglycerine preparations) dilate coronary and peripheral arteries and provide the heart with more oxygen while decreasing its workload. Beta-blockers can also be used to control angina. Calcium channel blockers are effective in preventing the coronary spasms that cause variant angina. Invasive therapies are also available for the treatment of angina. They include angioplasty with stenting and coronary artery bypass surgery.

Angioplasty   *Angioplasty,* also known as percutaneous transluminal coronary angioplasty (PTCA) and balloon angioplasty, is a procedure used to dilate narrowed coronary arteries. It is an established treatment for coronary artery disease and a less traumatic and less expensive alternative to bypass surgery. In PTCA, a cardiologist inserts a catheter, with a deflated balloon at its tip, into a peripheral artery and threads it upward until it reaches the coronary arteries. The balloon is positioned in the narrowed part of the artery and is inflated, compressing the plaque and enlarging the inner diameter of the blood vessel, so that blood can flow more easily (see Figure 12–4). Women are three times as likely as men to die or suffer a complication during the angioplasty procedure (Mosca et al., 1997). This is probably due to the fact that women's arteries are smaller, and women with coronary artery disease tend to be older and to have more comorbidities than men. Women whose procedures go smoothly, however, have the same excellent long-term prognosis as men (Mosca et al., 1997).

A variant of angioplasty is **laser angioplasty,** in which a catheter with a laser at the tip is positioned near the plaque. The laser emits pulsating beams of light, which vaporize the plaque. This procedure can be used alone or with balloon angioplasty. The first laser device was approved in 1992, and laser angioplasty is now available at many major medical centers. Whether the laser can be used depends on the location, degree, and extent of the blockage.

In some patients who undergo angioplasty, the dilated segment of the artery renarrows within six months after the procedure, a process known as **restenosis.** If restenosis occurs, another PTCA procedure, or even coronary artery by-

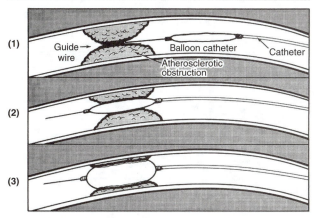

Source: *Meltzers Intensive Coronary Care* by Dracup. Copyright 1995. Reprinted by permission of Pearson Education, Inc., Upper Saddle River, NJ.

pass surgery, may then be required. In a very small percentage of patients, the angioplasty procedure fails to open the artery, and emergency coronary artery bypass surgery is needed. For this reason, the American College of Cardiology and the American Heart Association recommend that angioplasty be done only in institutions that have an experienced cardiovascular surgical team available as backup in case the patient needs emergency surgery (American Heart Association, 2000).

Stents   A *stent* (see Figure 12–5) is a short mesh tube made of wire or another material. Increasingly, stents are being used to prop open coronary arteries after angioplasty: The stent is collapsed to a small diameter, placed over a balloon catheter, and positioned in the area of the blockage. When the balloon is inflated, the stent expands, locks in place, and holds the artery open, improving blood flow and relieving the symptoms of chest pain. Stents also reduce the incidence of restenosis. Stent technology is ongoing, and newer stents have been developed that are coated with drugs, and even radioactive material, which help prevent the blood vessel from re-stenosing (*How Well Do Stents Work?* 2000). Currently, individuals who have a stent in one or more of their coronary arteries must take blood-thinning agents, such as aspirin, Ticlid, or Plavix, to discourage clot formation within the lumen of the stent. Periodic clotting tests are done to make sure the drug therapy does not cause bleeding (American Heart Association, 2000). There is insufficient information to say whether stents work better or less well in either gender.

Figure 12–5 Coronary Stent

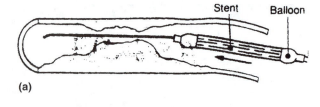

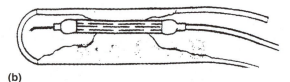

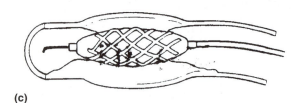

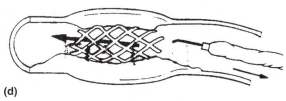

Insertion of a coronary stent. **(a)** Catheter in narrowed coronary artery. **(b)** Catheter is positioned so that the stent is within the narrowed region of the coronary artery. **(c)** Balloon is inflated, causing the stent to expand and stretch the coronary artery. **(d)** Balloon catheter is withdrawn, leaving the stent behind to keep the vessel open.

Source: *Meltzers Intensive Coronary Care* by Dracup. Copyright 1995. Reprinted by permission of Pearson Education, Inc., Upper Saddle River, NJ.

Atherectomy The term *atherectomy* refers to a procedure by which plaque is removed from an artery. In coronary atherectomy, either a laser or a rotating device is used to remove plaque from the lumen. Lasers vaporize plaque and rotating devices shave it off. As in angioplasty, a catheter, with the device at its tip, is inserted into a peripheral artery and threaded into the coronary arteries. Balloon angioplasty or stenting can be done after the atherectomy to increase the likelihood that the artery will remain **patent** (open). To date, there is not sufficient data to indicate whether women and men benefit similarly from atherectomy procedures.

Figure 12–6 Coronary Artery Bypass Graft

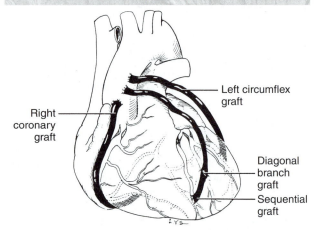

Source: Way, L. W. (ed): *Current Surgical Diagnosis & Treatment*, ed. 9. Norwalk, CT, Appleton & Lange, 1991. Reprinted with permission of The McGraw-Hill Companies.

Coronary Artery Bypass Surgery Coronary artery bypass surgery, also known as coronary artery bypass grafting, is sometimes referred to as CABG, or "cabbage," and involves open-heart surgery. Sections of veins or arteries taken from elsewhere in the patient's body are used to bypass clogged or blocked coronary arteries (see Figure 12–6). This procedure improves the supply of blood and oxygen to the heart, thereby improving angina and helping prevent a heart attack. Women are slightly more likely than men to die during this procedure, but overall intra-operative mortality is low in both sexes. The 15-year survival rate is the same (50 percent) in women and men (Mosca et al., 1997). The traditional way of accessing the heart was through an incision in the breastbone, or **sternum.** A newer approach, called **minimally invasive heart surgery,** involves accessing the heart through one or more smaller incisions. Whether this approach can be used depends on the location and severity of the plaque deposits. After a bypass operation, patients are advised to reduce their risk factors by controlling their diet, stopping smoking, slowly increasing physical activity to regain their strength, and, for some, taking medication. In most cases, recovery usually takes four to six weeks.

Whether balloon angioplasty, stents, atherectomy, or coronary artery bypass surgery is used to treat coronary artery disease depends on such factors as the location, extent, and number of blockages, as well as the risk of complications, the likely effect on quality of life, and personal choice.

Individuals who require invasive treatment for CAD should indicate to their physicians their desire to be apprised of all treatment options appropriate for them, as well as the potential benefits and risks of each.

HEART ATTACK

The most serious consequence of coronary artery disease is a myocardial infarction (MI) known as a "heart attack." An MI occurs when an area of the heart muscle becomes so deficient in oxygen that it cannot live; it becomes increasingly ischemic and finally dies. Women who have heart attacks tend to be older than their male counterparts and are more likely to have diabetes and high blood pressure. Women who have heart attacks also develop more complications, such as cardiac arrest, than men do, and their mortality rates are higher. The mortality rate among women who have an MI is 44 percent, compared with a 27 percent mortality rate in men (Mosca et al., 1997). African American women have an additional 22 to 40 percent chance of dying after an MI (American Heart Association, 2000). Women who have heart attacks also do poorly over the long term; during the first six years following an MI, 33 percent of women have a second heart attack, whereas only 21 percent of men do.

Two studies reported in the July 1999 *New England Journal of Medicine* examined gender differences in heart attack–related morbidity and mortality. In the first study (Vaccarino, Parsons, Every, Barron, & Krumholz, 1999), the death rate during hospitalization was 16.7 percent for women and 11.5 percent for men. In the second study (Hochman et al., 1999), it was reported that, at the 30-day post-MI mark, the rates of both complications and death were higher for the women in the study than for the men.

There are factors in addition to age and its attendant health problems that may influence the morbidity and mortality experienced by women who have M.I.s. For one thing, women often fail to seek prompt treatment when they experience symptoms. In a number of studies (Becker et al., 1994; Dracup & Bryan-Brown, 1997; Jenkins et al., 1994) among a population of women and men who had symptoms of heart attack, the women waited hours longer than the men before going to the hospital. A likely reason for this is that women tend to experience less painful heart attack symptoms than men. Women may not realize the serious nature of such symptoms and delay treatment, thus making extensive damage to the heart more likely. Additionally, women may feel that their family responsibilities overshadow their need for healthcare, so they minimize their symptoms and take a watch-and-wait approach to their illness.

Relatively few premenopausal women have heart attacks; however, when they do, they also have a greater risk of death than men do. In the Vaccarino et al. (1999) study, the rate of death among the female subjects less than 50 years of age was almost double that of the male subjects. The high mortality rates among younger women who have heart attacks may be due, at least in part, to differences in medical treatment. However, in these studies, treatment differences and the women's poorer overall health explained only one-third of the MI-related mortality difference between the men and women (Vaccarino et al., 1999). Some researchers (Burke et al., 1998) have speculated that young women who have MIs may lack the protective effect of estrogen because their bodies may use the hormone differently. Others suggest that such women may have an as yet unknown additional potent risk factor, or lack an unknown protective factor that is normally present in women (Vaccarino et al., 1999). Nevertheless, a consensus panel statement from the American Heart Association and American College of Cardiology (Mosca et al., 1999) indicates that there are alarming trends in the prevalence and management of risk factors in women. Some authors indicate that there is clear evidence that women often do not receive aggressive therapies to prevent and treat coronary artery disease (Heim & Brunsell, 2000; Roger et al., 2000). This disparity is due to a form of gender bias: CAD has long been considered a disease of men, and the symptoms considered classic are those typically experienced by men, but not necessarily by women.

Overall, the MI-related mortality gap is most prominent in women younger than 50, who are *twice* as likely as men to die if they have a heart attack. Women have a 7 percent higher risk of dying for each five years below age 75. However, the gap narrows with time and eventually disappears later in life; by age 80, men who have heart attacks have a slightly higher risk of dying than women (Vaccarino et. al., 1999).

Symptoms Women who are having a heart attack often experience symptoms that are different from the symptoms typically experienced by men. Women may have mild chest pain, or pain only in the arm or jaw. When women do get chest pain, it is often a feeling of pressure or burning, rather than the crushing, unmistakable pain typically experienced by men. Women may experience only abdominal pain that resembles indigestion with or without nausea, vomiting and shortness of breath (Wenger, 1996a). Many women experience extreme fatigue before a heart attack. The term *chest discomfort* is a better descriptor of a potential heart attack, because not all individuals, particularly women and diabetics, present with chest *pain*. The following is a list of the most common, or classic, warning signals of a heart attack (American Heart Association, 2000):

- Uncomfortable pressure, fullness, squeezing, or pain in the center of the chest that lasts more than a few minutes or that goes away and comes back
- Pain that spreads to the shoulders, neck, or arms
- Chest discomfort with lightheadedness, fainting, sweating, nausea, or shortness of breath

The following are some less common warning signs of heart attack:

- Atypical chest, stomach, or abdominal pain
- Nausea or dizziness (without chest pain)

- Shortness of breath and difficulty breathing (without chest pain)
- Unexplained anxiety, weakness, or fatigue
- Palpitations, cold sweat, or paleness

Any delay in the treatment of a developing heart attack increases the risk of serious complications and death. *The early detection, diagnosis, and treatment of a heart attack is imperative.* Approximately two-thirds of all sudden deaths due to cardiovascular disease occur out of the hospital, and most occur within two hours of the onset of symptoms (American Heart Association, 1997). The American Heart Association has developed a series of critical interventions to prevent death from cardiovascular disease. These critical interventions are called the "chain of survival." The components of the chain are early access, early CPR, early defibrillation, and early advanced care. Early access starts with the early recognition of chest discomfort and then progresses to activation of the 911 system. The statement "Time is muscle!" draws attention to the importance of early recognition in preventing damage to the heart muscle. Women may not feel as weak and sick as men often do and may not realize that a serious and potentially fatal event is taking place.

Diagnosis The diagnosis of heart attack is based on the symptoms that the patient is experiencing, together with a review of existing risk factors for cardiovascular disease, a through physical examination, an electrocardiogram (EKG), and blood tests. Some studies suggest that some women can be having a heart attack and still have a normal EKG (Roger et al., 2000). Wexler (1999) suggests that younger women are less likely than younger men to be diagnosed correctly, because they often do not present with the "classic" EKG findings that are common in men. This is one of several reasons that diagnosing heart attacks in women can be more difficult than diagnosing them in men.

The development of new blood tests has made the early detection of heart attack possible. These tests detect the presence of **cardiac enzymes,** which are chemicals released into the blood by damaged heart muscle cells. The enzyme most commonly used to confirm the existence of heart muscle damage is **creatine kinase myocardial band,** or **CK-MB.** This enzyme can be detected in the blood about six hours after the onset of a heart attack. Another, more recently discovered marker for cardiac damage is **troponin,** a protein released from damaged heart cells. Measuring blood troponin levels allows for even earlier and more sensitive detection of heart muscle injury. Troponin levels increase within several hours of the onset of muscle damage and remain in the blood for a week or more after damage has occurred (McCance & Heuther, 1998).

In women, heart attacks, as well as angina, are sometimes misdiagnosed as heartburn or a physical manifestation of anxiety. This is due, in part, to the fact that women are less likely to present with the symptoms experienced by men and

expected by physicians (Roger et al., 2000). However, this phenomenon is almost certainly also related to the societal view that women are more prone than men to anxiety and other emotional problems (see Chapter 1). Because the prompt diagnosis of myocardial infarction is so crucial to survival, women who think they may be having a heart attack must insist on aggressive diagnosis and treatment.

Treatment When a coronary artery becomes blocked, the area of heart muscle fed by that artery does not die instantly; it becomes ischemic first and then injured. The injury becomes progressively more severe if the artery remains blocked. The actual death of cardiac tissue, however, typically takes place over a period of hours and can be interrupted if appropriate therapy is begun in time. This means that *delaying treatment increases the damage to the heart and reduces the chance of survival.* Anyone experiencing the warning signals of a heart attack should call 911 and be taken by ambulance to the nearest hospital. It is not a good idea to have a family member or friend drive the person to the hospital if ambulance service is available. Ambulance crews are equipped to perform life-saving interventions in the ambulance during transport, should they become necessary. Nor should a person drive herself to the hospital, as this endangers the general public as well as the individual involved. Most communities have hospitals that are equipped to treat heart attacks.

The goal of treatment for the person experiencing a heart attack is the early reperfusion of the heart and the prevention of additional heart damage. *Reperfusion* means that the blockage in the coronary artery is removed, and an adequate supply of blood is restored to the heart muscle. If an individual with chest discomfort gets to an emergency department soon enough, reperfusion techniques can be used to increase the blood supply to the heart muscle. This can be accomplished in several ways. The least invasive method is the administration of drugs known technically as **thrombolytics** and colloquially as *clot busters.* Clot busters are administered intravenously to dissolve the clot that has blocked the artery. Other reperfusion techniques include angioplasty and coronary artery bypass surgery. Many healthcare providers now advise their patients to chew an aspirin tablet if they believe they are having a heart attack, in order to lessen the likelihood that the clot will enlarge on the way to the hospital. Chewing, rather than swallowing the tablet whole, speeds the action of the aspirin.

Unfortunately, women who suffer heart attacks may not receive aggressive treatment for their condition. Because the ways in which men experience myocardial infarction have been accepted as the norm, women are less likely to be diagnosed correctly and placed under the care of a cardiologist. They are also less likely to undergo cardiac catheterization, to receive reperfusion therapies, and to be admitted to an intensive care unit (Roger et al., 2000). Another problem related to the treatment of heart attack is the recent findings of researchers concerning the indecision and undertreatment of patients by healthcare providers and specialists, such as cardiologists (Berger, Schulman, & Gersh, 1999; Francis, Go, & Dauterman, 1999).

Another important aspect of the treatment of myocardial infarction is **cardiac rehabilitation.** Cardiac rehabilitation programs help individuals who are recovering from a heart attack minimize disability and develop a healthier lifestyle, which lessens the likelihood that another heart attack or another cardiac disorder will develop. After the acute period of illness is over, patients are taught to reduce their risk factors through healthy eating, stress management, and exercise. Cardiac rehabilitation programs are usually located in outpatient centers and staffed by registered nurses, exercise physiologists, nutritionists, and a medical director. Each patient is placed on an individualized program after being assessed for such problems as smoking, overweight, hypertension, diabetes, depression, and other psychosocial problems. Patients and their spouses or companions attend classes on nutrition, weight reduction, stress management, and risk-factor management. Patients also receive what is known as an **exercise prescription,** which stipulates the type and intensity of the exercise the patient will do at the center under the supervision of the nursing staff. During exercise sessions, the patient's EKG, heart rate, and blood pressure can be monitored continuously if indicated. Cardiac rehabilitation programs also provide avenues to social support; patients and their families meet other individuals who are coping with similar challenges. Studies of the efficacy of cardiac rehabilitation programs suggest that women benefit from them as much as men (Mosca et al., 1997). Because not all physicians are diligent about referring patients, however, women who are recovering from a heart attack should not hesitate to inquire about whether cardiac rehabilitation would be of benefit to them. Cardiac rehabilitation programs can also be very helpful to patients with angina and heart failure and patients who have had cardiac surgery.

Congestive Heart Failure

Approximately 1 million American women suffer from *congestive heart failure (CHF).* CHF is the only major cardiovascular disorder that is increasing in incidence, rather than decreasing (Packer et al., 1999). In the most common form of congestive heart failure, the left ventricle of the heart (the chamber that pumps freshly oxygenated blood throughout the body) has been weakened by untreated high blood pressure, a heart attack, diabetes, valvular disease, alcoholism, or another cause and can no longer pump a sufficient amount of blood to the tissues and organs of the body.

A number of factors can contribute to the development of CHF. Sustained high blood pressure and diabetes both cause the peripheral arteries to narrow, and the heart has to work very hard to pump blood through them. Over time, the left ventricle **hypertrophies,** or thickens, in an attempt

to manage its heavy workload, but eventually it becomes too weak to pump out a sufficient amount of blood with each contraction (Packer et al., 1999). Coronary artery disease can also cause CHF; if the heart is chronically malnourished, its muscular wall can become thin, dilated, and too weak to contract strongly. A heart attack can also cause CHF, because the dead heart muscle cells are replaced by scar tissue, which cannot contract and assist with pumping. The various forms of valvular heart disease can also cause heart failure (Chavey, 2000). Overall, women are more at risk for CHF than men. The left ventricle is smaller in women but contracts at a higher velocity. This pattern of extra work, plus the eventual loss of estrogen, may explain women's greater tendency to develop an abnormally enlarged left ventricle and congestive heart failure as they age.

SYMPTOMS

Congestive heart failure causes symptoms such as edema (swelling) in the legs, difficulty breathing at night if the head is not propped up on pillows, and shortness of breath on exertion. These symptoms are caused indirectly by the heart's inability to pump enough blood to the kidneys. When the kidneys fail to receive enough blood, they incorrectly assume that there is insufficient fluid in the blood vessels. In an attempt to remedy this, they release chemicals into the bloodstream that are designed to raise blood pressure and improve perfusion. Unfortunately, over the long term, the resulting vasoconstriction and retention of salt and water only make it more difficult for the straining heart to pump enough blood to sustain life. The retained water increases blood volume to the point at which plasma seeps out of the walls of the blood vessels and into surrounding tissues, where it is visible as edema. A similar edema-producing process in the lungs interferes with gas exchange and causes shortness of breath on exertion and, in extreme situations, at rest.

DIAGNOSIS

The diagnosis of CHF is based on the patient's medical history, a physical examination, X-ray and laboratory findings, and the results of tests that evaluate the heart's ability to pump. The clinician uses a stethoscope to listen for abnormal heart and lung sounds. An EKG is done and evaluated for evidence of a prior heart attack and/or an enlarged left ventricle. A chest X ray is taken, as it will reveal the presence of edematous fluid in lung tissues. However, the single most important test in the evaluation of CHF is the **echocardiogram with doppler.** This test can detect abnormal wall movement in specific areas of the heart and provides information about the overall ability of the heart to pump (Packer et al., 1999). In addition, the New York Heart Association (NYHA) classification system is commonly used to assess the functional status of individuals with CHF. Under this system, the presenting symptoms and the patient's activity tolerance are used to quantify the degree of heart failure.

It is extremely important to *prevent* CHF by intervening early in the conditions that can give rise to it. Screening for and effectively managing hypertension prevents many cases of CHF, as does treating heart attacks promptly, before tissue death occurs (Packer et al., 1999).

TREATMENT

The treatment of CHF involves both the use of medication, and lifestyle changes. The medical management of heart failure consists of finding the underlying cause and treating it with the appropriate drugs. The choice of drug or drugs depends on the symptoms experienced by the patient and the cause and stage of the disease. The medications most commonly used in the treatment of CHF are angiotensin converting enzyme inhibitors, diuretics, beta-blockers, and digoxin.

Angiotensin converting enzyme (ACE) inhibitors are an important advance in the management of CHF. These medications work by preventing the conversion of the enzyme **angiotensin** to **angiotensin II.** Angiotensin II is a powerful vasoconstrictor, which narrows the blood vessels and reduces blood flow to the kidneys, causing sodium and water to be retained in the body. When the conversion of this enzyme is blocked by a drug, the vessels dilate, and the heart is able to pump more efficiently. An added benefit of ACE inhibitor therapy is that it prevents the body from retaining extra sodium and fluid. ACE inhibitors are used to treat many patients with CHF; however, improvement may not be seen for several weeks after therapy has begun.

Diuretic medications help relieve the fluid retention and edema that many patients with heart failure experience. The diuretic Aldactone has been shown to reduce mortality when added to standard therapy for the treatment of heart failure (Packer et al., 1999).

Beta-blockers work by blocking adrenalin and other stress hormones, which, if unopposed, would constrict blood vessels and cause the heart to beat faster. Intended to assist in the fight-or-flight response, these hormones are produced inappropriately in response to the stress of heart failure. Beta-blocking drugs are used to protect the compromised heart from the extra workload imposed by these hormones. In the Beta-Blocker Evaluation Survival Trial, patients with heart failure who were given beta-blockers in addition to ACE inhibitors, diuretics, and the drug digoxin demonstrated significantly improved mortality rates (Domanski, 1999).

Digoxin is an older drug that has been a standard treatment for CHF. It is used to improve the heart's pumping ability and to control an abnormal cardiac rhythm—atrial fibrillation, which sometimes arises in heart failure patients.

Lifestyle modification is extremely important in the management of CHF. Smoking must be stopped, because it robs the body—particularly the heart—of oxygen. Alcohol, which is toxic to the heart in large doses, should be limited or discontinued. Activity and exercise should be part of the treatment whenever possible, and cardiac rehabilitation helps improve exercise capacity. Some individuals may require temporary or ongoing oxygen therapy to reduce fatigue.

Diet is another important factor in the management of CHF. Sodium intake is generally limited to 2 gm/day. Exceeding that level of sodium intake causes fluid retention, edema, and hypertension, which strain the heart. It is important to read food labels to determine the sodium content of foods, particularly packaged foods. In some cases, fluid intake must be limited. Nonsteroidal anti-inflammatory drugs (NSAID), such as ibuprofen, should not be taken, because they can cause fluid retention (McCance & Heuther, 1998). Consuming a diet that is low in fat and high in vegetables, fruits, and whole grains is also necessary to slow the progression of atherosclerosis.

The daily *monitoring* of the signs and symptoms of heart failure is also important. When the body begins to retain fluid, weight gain results. A pint of fluid weighs approximately 1 pound. Individuals with CHF may need to keep a daily weight log. They should report a weight gain of 3 pounds in one day or 5 pounds in one week to the primary physician and/or cardiologist, so that medication dosages can be adjusted. It is important to have an accurate scale and to weigh at the same time each day. Swollen ankles, a bloated abdomen, and tight rings or tight clothing may also be signs of fluid retention and worsening CHF.

It may be particularly difficult for low-income women with CHF to care for themselves well. Low-sodium foods cost more, and many women may need assistance with transportation to a cardiac rehabilitation program (Halm & Penque, 2000). Congestive heart failure support groups can be helpful to all women and are available in some communities. They provide additional education on managing CHF and an opportunity to meet other individuals facing similar concerns.

Stroke

A stroke, known technically as a **cerebrovascular accident (CVA)** or **brain attack,** is a neurological emergency that can occur suddenly or over a period of a few hours. In a stroke, the flow of blood through an artery that supplies oxygen and nutrients to an area of the brain is blocked. Although most strokes are similar to heart attacks in that a blood clot is usually the precipitating factor, a stroke can also be caused by a blood vessel that has burst. When part of the brain is deprived of the blood that it needs, death soon follows if rapid treatment is not begun, and often even if it is. Stroke is the leading cause of brain injury in adults and the third largest cause of death. Each year, approximately 100,000 women die of stroke, and, at all ages, more women than men die of it. Although the elderly account for the majority of stroke fatalities, they do not account for all of them; stroke ranks third as a cause of death among middle-aged individuals. The mortality rate from stroke is higher in African-American women and men; African-Americans are more than twice as likely as Euro-Americans to suffer death and disability from stroke. The higher number of risk factors present among African-Americans may partially explain these statistics. Stroke is the leading cause of serious, long-term disability in the United States. In 1998, 553,000 women were discharged from the hospital after having had a stroke (American Heart Association, 2000).

CLASSIFICATIONS OF STROKE

Strokes can be classified into two major categories: (1) **ischemic strokes,** which occur when a blood vessel supplying the brain is occluded, and (2) **hemorrhagic strokes,** which occur because a cerebral artery ruptures. Ischemic stoke accounts for approximately 75 percent of all strokes. In ischemic stroke, the occlusion is caused by a blood clot that either develops within the brain or is carried to the brain from elsewhere in the body via the circulation. If the clot developed in the brain, it is referred to as a **thrombus.** If it originated in another location and was carried to the brain, it is referred to as an **embolus.** Thrombi most often form in arteries that have been injured by arteriosclerosis and/or hypertension. Emboli most often originate in the heart and can form because of an irregular heart rhythm, an abnormal heart valve, or a heart attack. Ischemic strokes rarely cause immediate death, whereas hemorrhagic strokes are usually fatal at the onset. In a hemorrhagic stroke, a defective artery in the brain bursts, covering the surrounding tissue with blood and depriving the tissue it was meant to nourish of oxygen and glucose. Trauma can also cause damage to blood vessels in the head, as can cocaine use. Overall, the most common cause of stroke is hypertension.

Reducing stroke risk factors is the best way to prevent a stroke. Whereas genetic predisposition, increasing age, male gender, African-American ethnicity, and a prior stroke are risk factors that are not preventable, hypertension, diabetes, and an abnormal heart rhythm called atrial fibrillation are stroke risk factors that can often be controlled. After the age of 50, women develop high blood pressure, the most important risk factor for stroke, twice as often as men do. Diabetes significantly increases a woman's risk of having a stroke and is associated with severity and mortality (Mosca et al., 1999). Atrial fibrillation, an abnormal condition in which the upper chambers of the heart contract erratically, can cause blood clots to form in the heart, and, if such a clot is swept up to the brain by the circulation, an embolism will result.

Elevated blood lipid levels contribute to atherosclerosis and, therefore, to stroke. Obesity contributes to increased blood pressure, because every pound of fat contains miles of tiny blood vessels through which the heart must pump blood. Cigarette smoking increases blood pressure, reduces the amount of oxygen available in the blood, and causes the blood to thicken, thus making the formation of blood clots more likely. Imbibing more than two alcoholic drinks a day raises blood pressure, and an episode of binge drinking can trigger a stroke (American Heart Association, 2000).

SYMPTOMS

The symptoms of stroke depend on the area of the brain affected. The symptoms of a major stroke commonly include motor, sensory, and cognitive deficits. It is crucial to heed the early warning signs that a stroke is occurring and obtain medical assistance. The early warning signs are as follows: feelings of unsteadiness; dizziness; loss of speech (or difficulty in talking or understanding speech); loss of vision, especially in one eye; and any unexplained numbness or weakness in the face, in the extremities, or on one side of the body (American Heart Association, 2000). If treatment is obtained in time, these symptoms can be temporary; if not, individuals who have suffered a stroke can be left with permanent muscle paralysis, as well as speech and visual problems. They can also lose their ability to understand what another person is saying or to recognize common objects. Unfortunately, research indicates that most stroke victims and their families are not educated about the symptoms of stroke and wait too long to seek care (American Heart Association, 2000).

Transient ischemic attacks (TIAs) are commonly known as mini-strokes. They differ from classic strokes in that the symptoms last from minutes to hours and then subside spontaneously. A person who is having TIAs is in great danger of having a classic stroke, which can cause permanent neurological deficits.

DIAGNOSIS AND TREATMENT

The diagnosis of a stroke is made by a CAT scan or an MRI scan, both of which provide a picture of the area of the brain that is affected. How quickly therapy is initiated is a major determinant of whether the victim will survive and the degree of recovery that will be possible. If the stroke was caused by a blood clot, a thrombolytic agent, such as those used in the case of heart attack, can be used to dissolve it before the death of brain tissue occurs. An intravenous clot buster with the brand name Tissue Plasminogen Activator (TPA) was the first drug approved by the Food and Drug Administration for the treatment of stroke. Other treatments after the acute stage of stroke include the use of of antiplatelet aggregating and antithrombotic drugs, such as aspirin, ticlopidine, or Coumadin. Aspirin given within 48 hours of stroke onset has been shown to be effective in both women and men; however, the use of aspirin for primary stroke prevention in women has not been determined (Mosca et al., 1997).

The treatment of hemorrhagic stroke consists of measures to curtail bleeding through the administration of blood pressure–lowering drugs and drugs that speed clot formation. The dramatic curtailing of the stroke process that is possible with ischemic strokes is not, unfortunately, possible in hemorrhagic stroke.

Cardiovascular Wellness Self-Assessment

Responding to the following statements can help you estimate your degree of cardiovascular wellness. The more of the statements you are able to agree with, the better your cardiovascular health is likely to be.

1. *I am aware that coronary heart disease is a major killer of women.*
2. *I know the risk factors for coronary heart disease and stroke.*
3. *I know the symptoms of angina and heart attack in women.*
4. *My blood pressure, lipid profile, weight, and thyroid hormone levels are all within normal limits.*
5. *I do not experience weakness, nausea, or discomfort in my chest, jaw, back, arm, or abdominal area when I exert myself.*
6. *I do not experience pain in my calves when I walk.*
7. *I have never experienced any of the following: sudden, transient weakness in an arm or leg; transient, unexplained visual abnormalities; or transient difficulty in speaking or understanding words.*
8. *I do not smoke.*
9. *I consume fruits and vegetables frequently, and I usually eat fish twice a week.*
10. *I minimize my consumption of full-fat dairy products, stick margarines, fried foods, and fatty meats.*
11. *I get regular aerobic exercise.*

New Directions

Advances in the treatment of cardiovascular disease are being made almost daily. The overall goal is to develop new treatments that are more effective, faster, and less invasive than the old. There have been several innovations in the battle against cornary artery disease. For example, off-pump coronary artery bypass (OPCAB) has made open heart surgery safer for the patient. The old procedure required the surgeon to stop the heart and put the patient on a heart-lung machine, which put the patient at risk for a number of complications. When OPCAB is used, the heart is not stopped, and no heart-lung machine is required. The surgeon operates on a beating heart with the help of newly developed instruments, which help hold parts of the heart steady.

Another advancement in the treatment of coronary artery disease is the implantation of tiny capsules, which contain growth factor, in the wall of the heart. This innovation stimulates the growth of new or collateral vessels and improves the blood supply to the heart. In a related technique, called **percutaneous myocardial revascularization (PMR)**, a laser-tipped catheter is used to drill tiny holes in ischemic areas of the heart. This stimulates the growth of new blood vessels.

The procedure known as balloon catheter or angioplasty has also been improved to lessen catheter-induced scar formation within the coronary artery wall. In the new technique, tiny radioactive pellets are introduced into the plaque via the catheter and left in place for several minutes. The radiation reduces the scar tissue formation that could trigger the development of new blockages.

A new technique for detecting the presence of plaque in arteries has also been developed. It involves a refined use of magnetic resonance imaging (MRI) in a procedure known as intravascular ultrasonography (IVUS). IVUS is an invasive procedure in which a catheter probe and sonic waves are used to distinguish between hard plaques, which form in the interior lumen of coronary arteries, and soft plaques, which form within their walls. This is an important advance, because soft plaques have previously been difficult to detect and are believed to cause 70 percent of all MIs. Individuals found to be at high risk can be placed on medications, such as statin drugs, that stop the growth of artery wall plaque, or even shrink it.

Isolating the genes that control plaque formation in the arteries is another area of investigation. Researchers hope to identify the genetic roots of plaque formation. This work may eventually help prevent cardiovascular disease (Hunter, 2001).

In recent years, the American Heart Association, clinicians, and researchers have recognized the need to improve the system of cardiovascular care to optimize patient survival. The use of early cardiac defibrillation improves survival rates for victims of heart attack and sudden cardiac death. The placement of automated external defibrillators (AEDs) in the community is now recognized as an important part of early cardiac care. Many nonmedical professionals have been educated on the use of this equipment (American Heart Association, 1997). As the price of the automated external defibrillator becomes more affordable, it may become a standard part of safety equipment in the home.

QUESTIONS FOR REFLECTION AND DISCUSSION

1. *What percentage of funding related to cardiovascular disease should go toward educating the population about risk factors and what percentage toward developing new treatment technology?*
2. *To what degree were you surprised to learn of the danger cardiovascular disease poses for women? To what do you attribute your surprise or lack of it?*
3. *What strategies would be most effective in convincing people in your age group to take steps to minimize their risk factors for cardiovascular disease?*
4. *What are some of the barriers in your life that prevent you from achieving good cardiovascular health?*
5. *How will you begin to develop a heart-healthy lifestyle?*

RESOURCES

Books

Heart Sense for Women by Steven T. Sinatra, M.D., Jan Sinatra, RN, MSN & Roberta Jo Lieberman. Lifeline Press. 2000.

Love & Survival: The Scientific Basis for the Healing Power of Intimacy by Dean Ornish, M.D. Harper Collins. 1998.

Lifeskills, by Redford Williams, M.D., and Virginia Williams, Ph.D. Times Books. 1999.

Newsletters

Heart Advisor. Published monthly by the Cleveland Clinic. $39.00/yr. P.O. Box 420235, Palm Coast, FL 32142-0235. Phone: 1-800-829-2506.

Organizations

American Association of Cardiovascular and Pulmonary Rehabilitation
7611 Elmwood Ave., Suite 201
Middleton, WI 53562
Phone: 608-831-6989
Web: www.aacvpr.org

American Heart Association National Center
7272 Greenville Ave.
Dallas, TX 75231-4596
Phone: 214-373-6300
Web: www.americanheart.org

National Heart, Lung, and Blood Institute Information Center
P.O. Box 30105
Bethesda, MD 20824-0105
Phone: 301-592-8573
Web: www.nhlbi.nih.gov

WomenHeart—The National Coalition for Women with Heart Disease
818 18th St., N.W., Suite 730
Washington, D.C. 20006
Phone: 202-728-7199
Web: www.womenheart.org

National Stroke Association
96 Inverness Dr. E, Suite I
Englewood, CO 80111-5112
Phone: 303-649-9299
Web: www.stroke.org

REFERENCES

American Heart Association. (1997). *Basic life support for health-care providers.* Dallas, TX: American Heart Assocation.

American Heart Association. (2000). *Heart and stroke: Statistical update.* Dallas, TX: Author.

Another angle on aspirin. (2000). *Heart Watch, 4*(2), 1–2.

Assmann, G., Carmena, R., Cullen, P., Fruchart, J., Jossa, F., Lewis, B., Mancini, M., & Paoletti, R. (1999). Coronary heart disease: Reducing the risk, a worldwide view. *Circulation, 100,* 1930–1938.

Barker, D. J. P. (1995). Fetal origins of coronary heart disease. *British Medical Journal, 311,* 171–174.

Becker, R. C., Terrin, M., Ross, R., Knatterud, G. L., Desvigne-Nickens, P., Gore, J. M., & Braunwald, E. (1994). Comparison of clinical outcomes for women and men after acute myocardial infarction. The Thrombolysis in Myocardial Infarction Investigators. *Annals of Internal Medicine, 120*(8), 638–645.

Berger, A. K., Schulman, K. A., & Gersh, B. J. (1999). Primary angioplasty versus thrombolysis for the management of acute myocardial infarction in elderly patients. *Journal of the American Medical Association, 282,* 341–348.

Brekke, M. (2001, January/February). Outcome-based research: Part 11. *Beginnings,* p. 30.

Burke, A. P., Farb, A., Malcom, G. T., Liang, Y., Smialek, J., & Virmant, R. (1998). Effect of risk factors on the mechanism of acute thrombosis and sudden coronary death in women. *Circulation, 97,* 2110–2116.

Carter, J. S., Pugh, J. A., & Monterrosa, A. (1996). Non-insulin-dependent diabetes mellitus in minorities in the United States. *Annals of Internal Medicine, 125,* 221–232.

Castelli, W. P. (1988). Cardiovascular disease in women. *American Journal of Obstetrics and Gynecology, 6*(2), 1553–1560.

Cerqueira, M. D. (1995). Diagnostic testing strategies for coronary artery disease: Special issues related to gender. *American Journal of Cardiology, 75,* 52D–60D.

Chavey, W. E. (2000). The importance of beta-blockers in the treatment of heart failure. *American Family Physician, 62*(11), 2453–2465.

Chen, I. (2001, September). Can your moods affect your heart? *Health,* 109–116.

Danesh, J., Whincup, P., Walker, M., Lennon, L., Thompson, A., Appleby, P., Gallimore, J. R., & Pepys, M. B. (2000). *British Medical Journal, 321*(7255), 199–204.

Davidson, N. K., Jonas, B. S., Dixon, K. E., & Markovitz, J. H. (2000). Do depression symptoms predict early hypertension incidence in young adults in the CARDIA study? Coronary artery risk development in young adults. *Archives of General Psychiatry, 160*(10), 1495–1500.

Dennerstein, L. (2000). 5th European Congress on Menopause. *Medscape Women's Health 5*(4), 2000 Medscape, Inc. Retrieved 8/1/2000 from the World Wide Web. Available: http://womenshealth.medscape.com/Medscap . . . v05.n04.wh0719.denn/pnt-wh0719.denn.html.

Dracup, K., & Bryan-Brown, C. W. (1997). Reducing patient delay in seeking treatment. *American Journal of Critical Care, 6*(6), 415–417.

Davies, M. J. (1990). A macro and micro view of coronary vascular insult in ischemic heart disease. *Circulation, 82,* 38–46.

Denollet, J., & Brutsaert, D. L. (1998). Personality, disease severity, and the risk of long-term cardiac events in patients with a decreased ejection fraction after myocardial infarction. *Circulation, 97,* 167–173.

Domanski, M. (1999). *B-blocker evaluation survival (BEST) trial.* Paper presented at the 72nd Scientific Sessions of the American Heart Association, Atlanta, GA.

Douglas, P. S., & Ginsberg, G. S. (1996). The evaluation of chest pain in women. *New England Journal of Medicine, 344,* 1311–1315.

Eaker, E. D. (1998). Psychosocial risk factors for coronary heart disease in women. *Cardiology Clinics, 16,* 103–111.

Ernst, E., & Resch, K. L. (1993). Fibrinogen as a cardiovascular risk factor: A meta-analysis and review of the literature. *Annals of Internal Medicine, 118,* 956–963.

Everson, S. A., Kauhanen, J., & Kaplan, G. A. (1997). Hostility and increased risk of mortality and acute myocardial infarction: The mediating role of behavioral risk factors. *American Journal of Epidemiology, 146*(2), 142–152.

Folsom, A. R., Daye, S. S., Sellers, T. A., Hong, C. P., Cerhan, J. R., Potter, J. D., & Prineas, R. J. (1993). Body fat distribution and 5-year risk of death in older women. *Journal of the American Medical Association, 269*, 483–487.

Francis, C. D., Go, A. S., & Dauterman, K. W. (1999). Outcome following acute myocardial infarction: Are differences among physician specialties the result of quality care or case mix? *Archives of Internal Medicine, 159*, 1429–1436.

Franklin, S. S., Khan, S. A., & Wong, N. D. (1999). Is pulse pressure useful in predicting risk for coronary heart disease? The Framingham Heart Study. *Circulation, 100*, 354–360.

Gorman, J. M., & Sloan, R. P. (2000). Heart rate variability in depressive and anxiety disorders. *American Heart Journal, 140*(4 Suppl), 77–83.

Grodstein, F., Stampfer, J. I., & Colditz, G. A. (1997). Post-menopausal hormone therapy and mortality. *New England Journal of Medicine, 336*, 1769–1775.

Grundy, S. M. (1999). Primary prevention of coronary heart disease: Integrating risk assessment with intervention. *Circulation, 100*, 988–998.

Grundy, S. M., Balady, G. J., Criqui, M. H., Fletcher, G., Greenland, P., Hiratzka, L. F., Houston-Miller, N., Kris-Etherton, P., Krumholz, H. M., LaRosa, J., Ockene, I. S., Pearson, T. A., Reed, J., Washington, R., & Smith, S. C. (1998). Primary prevention of coronary heart disease: Guidance from Framingham. A statement for healthcare professionals from the American Heart Association's Task Force on Risk Reduction. *Circulation, 97*, 1876–1887.

Grundy, S. M., Benjamin, I. J., Burke, G. L., Chait, A., Eckel, R. H., Howard, B. V., Mitch, W., Smith, S. C., & Sowers, J. R. (1999). Diabetes and cardiovascular disease: A statement for healthcare professionals from the American Heart Association. *Circulation, 100*, 1134–1146.

Guetta, V., & Cannon, R. O. (1996). Cardiovascular effects of estrogen and lipid-lowering therapies in postmenopausal women. *Circulation, 93*, 1928–1937.

Halm, M. A., & Penque, S. (2000). Heart failure in women. *Progressive Cardiovascular Nursing, 15*(4), 121–133.

Heim, L. J., & Brunsell, S. C. (2000). Heart disease in women. *Primary Care, 27*(3), 741–766.

Hochman, J. S., Tamis, J. E., Thompson, T. D., Weaver, W. D., White, H. D., Van De Werf, F., Aylward, P., Topol, E. J., & Califf, R. M. (1999). Sex, clinical presentation, and outcome in patients with acute coronary syndromes. *New England Journal of Medicine, 341*, 226–232.

How well do stents work? (2000). *Heart Watch, 4*(2), 1–2

Hormone replacement and your heart. (2001). *Women's Health Advisor, 5*(9), 1–7.

Hunter, G. C. (2001). Are genes to blame for unstable carotid artery plaque? *Clinician Reviews, 11*(1), 104.

Iribarren, C., Sidney, S., Bild, D. E., Liu, K., Markovitz, J. H., Roseman, J. M., & Matthews, K. (2000). Association of hostility with coronary artery calcification in young adults: The CARDIA study. Coronary Artery Risk Development in Young Adults. *Journal of the American Medical Association, 283*(19), 2546–2551.

Jenkins, J. S., Flaker, G. C., Nolte, B., Price, L. A., Morris, D., Kurz, J., & Petroski, E. (1994). Causes of higher in-hospital mortality in women than in men after acute myocardial infarction. *American Journal of Cardiology, 73*(5), 319–322.

Kannel, W. B. (1999). Historic perspectives on the relative contributions of diastolic and systolic blood pressure elevation to cardiovascular risk profile. *American Heart Journal, 138*(3), 5205–5210.

Knox, S. S., Adelman, A., Ellison, R. C., Arnett, D. K., Siegmund, K., Weidner, G., & Province, M.A. (2000). Hostility, social support and carotid artery atherosclerosis in the National Heart, Lung and Blood Institute Family Heart Study. *American Journal of Cardiology, 86*(10), 1086–1089.

Kubzansky, L. D., Kawachi, I. (2000). Going to the heart of the matter: Do negative emotions cause coronary heart disease? *Journal of Psychosomatic Research, 48*(4-5), 323–337.

Kubzansky, L. D., Kawachi, I., Spiro, A., Weiss, S. T., Vokonas, P. S., & Sparrow, D. (1997). Is worrying bad for your heart? A prospective study of worry and coronary heart disease in the Normative Aging Study. *Circulation, 95*(4), 818–824.

Kudenchuk, P., Maynard, C., Martin, J., Wirkus, M., & Weaver, W. D. (1996). Comparison of presentation, treatment and outcome of acute myocardial infarction in men versus women (The Myocsrdial Infarction Triage and Intervention Registry). *American Journal of Cardiology, 78*, 9–14.

Laurienzo, J. M. (1997). Detection of coronary artery disease in women: The pitfalls of noninvasive tests. *Critical Care Nursing Clinics of North America, 9*(4), 469–474.

Lederbogan, F., Gilles, M., Maras, A., Hamann, B., Colla, M., Hevser, I., & Deuschle, M. (2001). Increased Platelet Aggregability in Major Depression? *Psychiatry Research, 102*(3), 255–261.

Legato, M. J., Padus, E., & Slaughter, E. (1997). Women's perceptions of their general health, with special reference to their risk of coronary artery disease: Results of a national telephone survey. *Journal of Women's Health, 6*, 189–198.

Lenfant, C. (1986). A new challenge for America: The National Cholesterol Education Program. *Circulation, 73*, 855–856.

Lerner, D. J., & Kannel, W. B. (1986). *American Heart Journal, 111*(2), 383–390.

Libby, P. (1995). Molecular bases of the acute coronary syndromes. *Circulation, 91*, 2844–2850.

Lindahl, B., Henrik, T., Siegbahn, A., Venge, P., & Wallentin, L. (2000). Markers of myocardial damage and inflammation in relation to long-term mortality in unstable coronary artery disease. *New England Journal of Medicine, 343*, 1139–1147.

Linden, W., Stossel, C., & Maurice, J. (1996). Psychosocial intervention for patients with coronary artery disease: A meta-analysis. *Archives of Internal Medicine, 156*, 745–752.

Lloyd-Jones, D. M., Evans, J. C., & Larson, M. G. (1999). Differential impact of systolic and diastolic blood pressure level on JNC-VI staging. Joint National Committee on Prevention, Detection, Evaluation, and Treatment of High Blood Pressure. *Hypertension, 34*, 381–385.

Looking beyond LDL cholesterol. (2001). *Heartwatch, 3*(1), 2–4.

Manson, J. E., & Lee, I. M. (1996). Exercise for women: How much pain for optimal gain? *New England Journal of Medicine, 334*, 1325–1327.

Marwick, T. H., Anderson, T., Williams, M. J., Haluski, B., Melia, J. A., Pashkow, F., & Thomas, J. D. (1995). Exercise echocardiography is an accurate and cost-efficient technique for detection of coronary artery disease in women. *Journal of the American College of Cardiology, 26*, 335–341.

Matthews, K. A., Kuller L. H., Sutton-Tyrrell, K., & Chang, Y. F. (2001). Changes in cardiovascular risk factors during the perimenopause and postmenopause and carotid artery atherosclerosis in healthy women. *Stroke, 32*(5), 1104–1111.

McCance, K. L., & Heuther, S. E. (1998). *Pathophysiology: The biologic basis for disease in adults and children* (3rd ed.). New York: Mosby.

McGrath, D. (1998). Coronary artery disease in women. *American Journal for Nurse Practitioners, 2*(6), 7–23.

Mosca, L., Grundy, S. M., Judelson, D., King, K., Limacher, M., Oparil, S., Pasternak, R., Pearson, T. A., Redberg, R. F., Smith, S. C., Winston, M., & Zinberg, S. (1999). AHA/ACC scientific statement: Consensus panel statement: Guide to preventive cardiology for women. *Circulation, 99*, 2480–2484.

Mosca, L., Jones, W. K., King, K. B., Ouyang, P., Redberg, R. F., & Hill, M. N. (2000). Awareness, perception, and knowledge of heart disease risk and prevention among women in the United States. *Archives of Family Medicine, 9*, 506–515.

Mosca, L., Manson, J. E., Sutherland, S. E., Langer, R. D., Manolio, T., & Barrett-Connor, E. (1997). Cardiovascular disease in women: A statement for healthcare professionals from the American Heart Association. *Circulation, 96*, 2468–2482.

NIH News Release (2001). NCEP Issues Major New Cholesterol Guidelines. [Online]. *National Institutes of Health, National Heart, Lung and Blood Institute.* Accessed August 28, 2002. Available: http://nhlbi.nih.gov/new/press/01-05-15.htm.

News. (2002). Cutting Through the HRT Confusion. *American Journal of Nursing, 102*(9), p. 20.

Ornish, D. (1998). *Love and survival.* New York: Harper Perennial.

Packard, C. J., O'Reilly, D. S., & Caslake, M. J. (2000). Lipoprotein-Associated Phospholipase A$_2$ as an independent predictor of coronary heart disease. *New England Journal of Medicine, 243*(16), 1448–1455.

Packer, M., Cohn, J. N., Abraham, W. T., Greenberg, B. H., Leier, C. V., Massie, B. M., & Young, J. B. (1999). Consensus recommendations for the management of chronic heart failure. *American Journal of Cardiology, 83*(2A), 1A–38A.

Pay, S., Ozcan, N., & Tokgozoglu, S. L. (1997). Elevated Lp(a) is the most frequent familial lipoprotein disorder leading to premature myocardial infarction in a country with low cholesterol levels. *International Journal of Cardiology, 60*(3), 301–305.

Penninx, B. W., Beekman, A. T., Honig, A., Deeg, D. J., Schoevers, R. A., van Eijk, J. T., & van Tilburg, W. (2001). Depression and cardiac mortality: Results from a community-based longitudinal study. *Archives of General Psychiatry, 58*(3), 221–227.

Philpott, S., Boynton, P. M., Feder, G., & Hemingway, H. (2001). Gender differences in descriptions of angina symptoms and health problems immediately prior to angiography: The ACRE (Appropriateness of Coronary Revascularisation) study. *Social Science and Medicine, 52*(10), 1565–1575.

Rexrode, K. M., Carey, V. J., Hennekens, C. H., Walters, E. E., Colditz, G. A., Stampfer, M. J., Willett, W. C., & Manson, J. E. (1998). Abdominal adiposity and coronary heart disease in women. *Journal of the American Medical Association, 280*(21), 1843–1849.

Rich-Edwards, J. W., Stampfer, M. J., Manson, J. E., Rosner, B., Hankinson, S. E., Colditz, G. A., Willet, W. C., & Hennekens, C. H. (1997). Birth weight and risk of cardiovascular disease in a cohort of women followed up since 1976. *British Medical Journal, 315*, 396–401.

Ridker, P. M., Manson, J. E., Buring, J. E., Shih, J., Matias, M., & Hennekens, C. H. (1999). Homocysteine and risk of cardiovascular disease among post-menopausal women. *Journal of the American Medical Association, 281*(19), 1817–1821.

Roger, V. L., Farkouh, M. E., Weston, S. A., Reeder, G. S., Jacobsen, S. J., Zinmeister, A. R., Yawn, B. P., Kopecky, S. L., & Gabriel, S. E. (2000). Sex differences in evaluation and outcome of unstable angina. *Journal of the American Medical Association, 283*(5), 646–652.

Rossouw, J. S., Lewis, B., & Rifkind, B. M. (1990). The value of lowering cholesterol after myocardial infarction. *New England Journal of Medicine, 323*, 1112–1119.

Schenck-Gustafsson, K. (1996, August 17). Risk factors for cardiovascular disease in women: assessment and management. *European Heart Journal*, pp. 2–8.

Siegman, A. W., Townsend, S. T., Civelek, A. C., & Blumenthal, R. S. (2000). Antagonistic behavior, dominance, hostility and coronary heart disease. *Psychosomatic Medicine, 62*(2), 248–257.

Sinatra, S. (2000). *Heart sense for women.* Washington, DC: LifeLine Press.

Sixth report of the Joint National Committee on Prevention, Detection, Evaluation, and Treatment of High Blood Pressure. (1997). *Archives of Internal Medicine, 167*, 2413–2446.

Stevenson, C., Pitler, M. H., & Earnst, E. (2000). Garlic for treating hypercholesteremia. A meta-analysis of randomized clinical trials. *Annals of Internal Medicine, 133*(6), 420–429.

Tikkanen, M. J. (1993). Mechanisms of cardiovascular protection by postmenopausal hormone replacement therapy. *Cardiovascular Risk Factors, 3*, 138–143.

Uchino, B. N., Cacioppo, J. T., & Keicolt-Glaser, J. (1996). The relationship between social support and physiological processes: A review with emphasis on underlying mechanisms and implications for health. *Psychological Bulletin, 119*, 488–531.

Vaccarino, V., Parsons, L., Every, N. R., Barron, H. V., & Krumholz, H. M. (1999). Sex-based differences in early mortality after myocardial infarction. *New England Journal of Medicine, 341*, 217–225.

Wenger, N. K. (1996a). Coronary heart disease in women. *Seminars in Reproductive Endocrinology, 14*(1), 4–14.

Wenger, N. K. (1996b). The high risk of CHD for women: Understanding why prevention is crucial. *Medscape Women's Health, 1*(11), 6.

Wexler, L. F. (1999). Studies of acute coronary syndromes in women—lessons for everyone. *New England Journal of Medicine, 341*(1), 275–276.

What is unstable angina? (2000). *Heart Watch, 4*(2), 4.

Whelton, P. K., & Appel, L. J. (1996). Treatment and prevention of hypertension. In J. E. Manson, P. M. Ridker, J. M. Gaziano, & C. H. Hennekens (Eds.), *Prevention of myocardial infarction* (pp. 312–324). New York: Oxford University Press.

Wilson, P. W., D'Agostino, R. B., Levy, D., Belanger, A. M., Silbershatz, H., & Kannel, W. B. (1998). *Circulation, 97* (18), 1834–1847.

Wingate, S. (1997). Cardiovascular anatomy and physiology in the female. *Critical Care Nursing Clinics of North America, 9*(4), 447–453.

Yu, H. H., Pasternak, R. C., & Ginsburg, G. S. (2000). Dyslipidemia in patients with CAD: How to make best use of drug therapy. *Consultant, 2*, 2097–2109.

13

Respiratory Wellness and Illness

Mark Simmons, Vickie Zeiler, and James Heindel

CHAPTER OUTLINE

Objectives

1. *Identify anatomical, physiological, and functional characteristics associated with respiratory wellness.*
2. *Discuss selected environmental pollutants in terms of their potential for compromising pulmonary function and strategies for avoiding them.*
3. *Identify self-care activities that promote respiratory wellness.*
4. *Identify gender differences regarding risks posed by environmental pollutants and susceptibility to respiratory diseases.*

Introduction

Respiratory wellness is a vital component of general good health. The respiratory system provides for both the intake of oxygen into the body and the elimination of carbon dioxide from it, and it plays an indispensable role in the maintenance of acid-base balance. The respiratory tract also constitutes an open passage by which various toxins and contaminants can enter the body. This chapter will address the markers of respiratory wellness and the ways in which respiratory wellness can be promoted. Selected respiratory illnesses will be discussed in terms of gross pathophysiology, signs and symptoms, diagnosis, and treatment.

Markers of Respiratory Wellness

Many assessments can be done to evaluate wellness. The major hallmarks, or markers, of respiratory wellness include vital signs that are within normal limits, normal values on certain blood and pulmonary function tests, normal patterns of sputum production, the absence of chest pain, normal skin and mucous membrane coloration, the absence of headache and altered mental status, the absence of edema, stable weight, and normal exercise tolerance.

Normal Vital Signs

The **vital signs** include the respiratory rate, heart rate, blood pressure, and temperature. Individuals and healthcare providers can monitor these signs in order to determine the status of the vital organs, including the lungs. The vital signs are also checked to identify physiological problems or improvements, to monitor treatment response, and to determine the need for further evaluation and treatment. A single check of the vital signs reveals information only for that moment in time. Multiple checks are customarily done over a period of time to establish a baseline and identify trends. Whereas healthy individuals rarely check their own vital signs, healthcare providers customarily do so during routine office visits. Individuals with abnormal measurements may need to have their vital signs followed more closely and checked on a regular basis. *Heart rate* and *respiratory rate* are more affected by the status of the respiratory system than is blood pressure, and body temperature can be affected if fever is present.

RESPIRATORY RATE

Respiratory rate varies with age, being higher in children (20–30 breaths per minute) and lower in adults (10–16 breaths per minute). When at rest, respiratory rates *greater than 25 for adults* and *50 for children* should be considered abnormal. **Tachypnea,** an increased respiratory rate, may be due to exercise, fever, decreased blood oxygen levels, acidosis, anxiety, or pain. **Respiratory cycles** (the rising of the chest or abdomen with the intake of each breath) should be counted for one full minute. Older adults tend to have an *increased respiratory frequency* of 16–25 breaths per minute. The higher frequency compensates for the decreased **tidal volume** (normal breath size) due to the lung and chest wall changes that occur with age.

HEART RATE

The normal adult heart rate is *60–100 beats per minute* and the rhythm is regular. **Tachycardia,** a heart rate of greater than 100 beats per minute, may be caused by decreased blood oxygen levels, as well as many other things. The amount of oxygen delivered to the tissues of the body is dependent on the heart's ability to pump blood. When oxygen levels are low in arterial blood, the heart beats faster to compensate. Because individuals with pulmonary (lung) disease often have decreased oxygen levels, it is not uncommon for their heart rates to be increased.

TEMPERATURE

Normal body temperature is 98.6°F (37°C), with a range of 97–99.5°F and a daily variation of 1–2°F. Body temperature is usually *lowest in the morning* and *highest in the late afternoon.* Temperature will rise with exercise to between 99° and 100°F. In women, normal temperature increases approximately 1°F during ovulation and during the first four months of pregnancy. Body temperature is maintained by balancing heat production and heat loss. Metabolism produces heat, and the hypothalamus helps regulate heat loss by initiating vasodilation and sweating to dissipate heat. The respiratory system also helps remove heat through ventilation. This warm, moist exhaled air is evident on a cold day, when one can see one's breath.

An elevation of body temperature above normal is called **fever** when caused by disease. A fever increases body metabolism and often results in an increased heart rate and respiratory rate. A fever is not specific for a given disorder and may be caused by both pulmonary and nonpulmonary diseases. Common pulmonary conditions causing fever include lung abscess, bronchitis, tuberculosis, and various forms of pneumonia. The ability to regulate body temperature is somewhat decreased in older adults, and it is not uncommon for older adults to have body temperatures of 96–97°F.

A common site to measure temperature is in the mouth under the tongue. To identify changes in temperature over time, the same device and same site should be used. An oral temperature measurement should not be taken within 15 minutes of ingesting a hot or cold liquid, lest a falsely high or low reading be obtained. It is important to allow ample time for the temperature probe to register a stable reading. Electronic devices require little time to stabilize and are increasingly being chosen over glass mercury thermometers, which require 3–4 minutes to register an accurate reading and may break and pose a risk of mercury poisoning.

Normal Values on Blood and Pulmonary Function Tests

The blood test most often used in the evaluation of respiratory status is arterial blood gas analysis. Pulmonary function tests are noninvasive tests that reflect an individual's ability to move air in and out of the lungs.

NORMAL ARTERIAL BLOOD GAS VALUES

In a healthy person, arterial blood contains an optimal amount of oxygen and carbon dioxide, and it is within an optimal pH range. Arterial blood may be withdrawn for analysis via a procedure known as arterial blood sampling, or taking an **arterial blood gas (ABG),** as it is better known. In this procedure, an artery is punctured with a needle and a small amount of arterial blood is removed. The radial artery in the wrist is a common site for the arterial puncture. ABG reports are used to evaluate the body's acid-base balance and the ability of the lungs to provide oxygen to the blood and to remove carbon dioxide. Three major parameters are measured when arterial blood is analyzed: pH, $PaCO_2$, and PaO_2.

Arterial pH is a reflection of the acid-base status of the body. pH is inversely proportional to the hydrogen ion concentration (H^+) in blood. The normal arterial blood pH value is 7.35 to 7.45. The body is an acid producer and maintains equilibrium by excreting as much acid as it produces. The two main pathways by which acid is removed from the body include the kidneys, which excrete H^+, and the lungs, which give off CO_2. Low pH, or **acidosis,** results in the depression of the central nervous system, starting with lethargy and disorientation. As the acidosis progresses, the patient becomes comatose and dies if not treated properly. Examples of patients at risk for developing acidosis include those with renal disease, which causes the decreased excretion of acid, and those with certain kinds of coronary heart disease or lung disease, both of which cause increased acid production due to the decreased availability of oxygen to the tissues.

$PaCO_2$ is the pressure (P) of carbon dioxide (CO_2) dissolved in arterial (a) blood. It reflects the amount of CO_2 present. Carbon dioxide is a product of cell metabolism throughout the body. CO_2 is transported to the lungs by the venous blood and is excreted on exhalation. Normal values for $PaCO_2$ are 35–45 mm Hg. **Hyperventilation** results in $PaCO_2$ values less than 35 mm Hg and may occur due to anxiety, fear, or **hypoxemia** (decreased blood oxygen levels). **Hypoventilation,** or respiratory failure, results in $PaCO_2$ values greater than 45 mm Hg and can be due to many factors, such as drug overdose, lung disease, or neuromuscular disease, all which result in decreased lung ventilation. Carbon dioxide is an acid; when it builds up in the blood because the lungs are unable to excrete it, pH decreases and the patient develops acidosis. Conditions such as drug overdose and head trauma depress the respiratory drive and are acute situations resulting in a temporary increase in $PaCO_2$. Patients with severe lung disease or **chronic obstructive pulmonary disease (COPD)**—that is, emphysema, bronchitis, and bronchiectasis—may have chronically elevated CO_2 levels. Elderly persons without pulmonary disease tend to maintain normal carbon dioxide levels.

PaO_2 is the measure of the pressure (P) of oxygen (O_2) dissolved in arterial (a) blood. It reflects the amount of oxygen present. The normal PaO_2 is 80–100 mm Hg. PaO_2 is usually not much greater than 100 mm Hg while breathing room air but can increase if a person hyperventilates. PaO_2 can also increase above 100 mm Hg if supplemental oxygen is administered. Low oxygen levels are often seen in patients with lung disease, and, in most cases, PaO_2 levels less than 60 mm Hg should be treated with supplemental oxygen. The lungs provide the only pathway by which oxygen can enter the bloodstream. Oxygen enters the *alveoli* of the lungs during ventilation and then diffuses across the *alveolar-capillary membrane* into the *pulmonary capillaries,* which can be thought of as the bloodstream of the lungs. Any situation that prevents oxygen from entering the alveoli or diffusing into the pulmonary capillaries will result in hypoxemia. If hypoxemia becomes severe, the bodily tissues will suffer due to a lack of oxygen. This is called **hypoxia.** A lack of oxygen at the cellular level causes the cell to begin anaerobic metabolism and the production of *lactic acid.* This also results in acidosis.

Lung diseases such as COPD, atelectasis (collapsed alveoli), asthma, pneumonia, or pulmonary emboli (blood clots in the arteries of the lungs) result in diminished PaO_2 levels, and the entire body will suffer from a lack of oxygen. Due to the lung changes that occur in older adults, which include decreased surface area for gas diffusion and increased thickness of the pulmonary capillary membrane, PaO_2 levels are often somewhat decreased. An estimate of an acceptable PaO_2 level for a given age in years can be calculated by the following formula: $105 - \frac{1}{2}$ the age.

Although some oxygen is dissolved in the blood (PaO_2), most of the oxygen carried in the bloodstream is attached to **hemoglobin,** which is inside the red blood cell. The measurement of the amount of hemoglobin that is carrying oxygen is called the arterial oxygen saturation (SaO_2). This value can be measured during the analysis of an ABG, but it can also be measured noninvasively using a pulse oximeter. A **pulse oximeter** uses a probe, which shines light waves through a vascular bed—most commonly, the tip of a finger or the earlobe. It is calibrated to record arterial saturation or, in this case, pulse oximetry saturation (SpO_2). The normal saturation is 97 to 98 percent. As with PaO_2, if SpO_2 decreases, hypoxia may occur. A saturation of less than 90 percent should be considered low and may require the administration of supplemental oxygen. Not only will readings tend to be a bit lower in older adults (< 97 percent) due to decreased PaO_2 levels, but readings may also be difficult to obtain if poor circulation is present.

NORMAL PULMONARY FUNCTION TESTS

Pulmonary function tests (PFTs) are breathing tests performed to check lung volumes and flow rates. The reasons for obtaining PFTs include screening for the presence of pulmonary disease (especially from smoking), documenting the progression of pulmonary disease (for example, cystic fibrosis), doing a presurgical evaluation for high-risk patients, and evaluating the effectiveness of treatment. Performing PFTs is an easy and inexpensive method of identifying most cases of COPD. The normal values for lung volume vary from one person to another, based on the following: *height* (increased height results in increased volume and flow rates), *sex* (males have larger lung volumes than females of the same size), and *age* (increased age results in changing lung volumes and decreased flow rates). Other considerations include *ethnic background* and *body surface area.* In general, as weight increases, lung volumes decrease. Euro-Americans tend to have somewhat higher lung volumes than individuals belonging to other ethnic groups.

Although many lung volumes and flow rates can be measured, only three will be discussed here. These include peak flow (PF), forced vital capacity (FVC), and forced expiratory volume in one second (FEV_1), the most commonly measured values for identifying airway dysfunction.

Peak Flow   Peak flow (PF) is the maximum flow rate generated during a forced exhalation. It occurs early during expiration and is very effort-dependent. Low values in the face of good effort and normal muscle strength indicate *airway obstruction.* Peak flow is easily measured by using an inexpensive peak flow meter. Asthmatics routinely use peak flows to monitor their lung function and to help guide their treatment management.

Forced Vital Capacity   Forced vital capacity (FVC) is the total amount of air that can be forcibly exhaled following a maximal inspiration. It can be decreased in both *obstructive disorders* (such as emphysema or bronchitis) and *restrictive* disorders (such as pulmonary fibrosis or obesity).

Forced Expiratory Volume in One Second   Forced expiratory volume in one second (FEV_1) is the maximum amount of air that can be exhaled during the first second of the FVC maneuver. In general, a decreased FEV_1 value is a good indicator of airway obstruction, but it can also be reduced in moderate to severe restrictive diseases.

The FEV_1/FVC ratio helps distinguish between patients with restrictive lung disease and those with obstructive lung disease. The normal value for the FEV_1/FVC ratio is greater than or equal to 0.75, or 75 percent. Patients with restrictive lung disease will have normal values, whereas patients with obstructive lung disease will have decreased ratios.

A NORMAL CHEST RADIOGRAPH

Chest X rays, also known as **radiographs,** allow clinicians to visualize structures inside the chest. Normal chest films reveal white bones and black lungs. Increased whitened areas in the lungs, indicating **opacities** (the presence of solid matter) and **infiltrates** (the presence of fluid) are abnormal and may be due to many different conditions. Some of these include lung cancer, atelectasis, pneumonia, tuberculosis, fungal infections, and congestive heart failure.

NORMAL BLOOD COUNTS

A **complete blood cell count (CBCC)** includes an evaluation of the number of *red blood cells (RBCs)*, the amount of hemoglobin (Hb), and the number of *white blood cells (WBCs)*, including their types. RBCs are produced by the bone marrow, have the shape of a biconcave disk, and carry hemoglobin. The hemoglobin molecules on the surface of RBCs are responsible for carrying 98 to 99 percent of the oxygen present in arterial blood. It is the oxygenated hemoglobin that gives arterial blood its red color. Normal hemoglobin concentration is 11–15 g/dL in women and 12–16 g/dL in men. Men have slightly more RBCs than women. A low RBC count is called **anemia.** There are five basic types of WBCs, or *leukocytes,* that work together to fight infection as part of the body's immune system. These WBC types and the reasons for their increased blood levels are listed in Table 13–1. A WBC count is helpful in evaluating the presence of infection, because infections usually result in an increased WBC count. A normal WBC count is 4,500–11,500/mm^3. The CBCC remains relatively stable during the process of aging.

ABSENCE OF COUGH

Coughing is a protective reflex intended to clear the airway. Stimulation of the cough may arise from receptors in the

TABLE 13–1	Types of leukocytes and reasons for elevation in cell counts.

Type of Leukocyte	Reasons for Elevation in Cell Counts
Neutrophil	Bacterial infection, inflammation
Eosinophil	Allergic reaction, parasitic infection
Lymphocyte	Viral infection
Monocyte	Chronic infections, malignancies
Basophil	Myeloproliferative disorders

pharynx, larynx, trachea, or lung. Coughing can be voluntary or involuntary and occurs occasionally in everyone. Although a cough can be a normal occurrence, coughing is also the *primary symptom* in patients with pulmonary disease. If a cough is present, it may be mild and occasional, which is normal, or acute (sudden and severe), as with the common cold. It may also be *chronic* (persistent), lasting for weeks and months. Persistent coughs generate the most concern and may be due to conditions such as postnasal drip, asthma, gastroesophageal reflux, chronic bronchitis (especially from smoking), bronchiectasis, and lung cancer. Severe bouts of coughing can result in complications, including urinary incontinence, dizziness and fainting, **pneumothorax** (collapsed lung), **hemoptysis** (the presence of blood in the sputum), heart dysrhythmias, and rib fractures.

Protective reflexes, such as cough, become less effective with age. Older people may also have swallowing difficulties due to pharyngeal muscle weakness (Pruitt, 2000). Together, these changes may contribute to the increased incidence of **aspiration** (the inhalation of food, liquids, and so on), and the resulting pneumonia, in the elderly.

ABSENCE OF DYSPNEA

The term **dyspnea** refers to the subjective feeling of being short of breath (SOB). Dyspnea may occur in individuals who have respiratory disease and in those who have cardiovascular disease. Dyspnea is very distressing to individuals who have it, as it limits their activities of daily living; it is often the reason they seek medical attention. In that dyspnea is a subjective feeling of SOB, patients' perceptions of dyspnea vary. Patients who suffer from dyspnea are often helped by both relaxation techniques and special breathing techniques. Individuals who experience acute dyspnea should try to document the activity they were engaged in, their body position, and any other significant circumstances during the episodes. This record may be helpful in diagnosing the reasons for the attacks, may assist in selecting proper treatment, and may aid in preventing future attacks. Dyspnea is *not* as-

sociated with normal aging. If dyspnea is present in older individuals, an underlying cause should be investigated.

NORMAL BREATH SOUNDS

The term *breath sounds* refers to the sounds produced during the respiratory cycle. It is necessary to use a stethescope to hear them clearly. Breath sounds can be divided into two general classifications: normal and abnormal. Normal breath sounds include those characterized as tracheal, bronchial, bronchovesicular, and vesicular. Tracheal and bronchial sounds are loud, harsh, and high-pitched and are normally heard over the trachea and large bronchi. Bronchovesicular and vesicular breath sounds are softer and lower-pitched and are normally heard over most of the rest of the lung fields.

Abnormal, or **adventitious,** breath sounds include rhonchi, wheezing, crackles, and stridor. **Rhonchi** are low-pitched, continuous sounds heard mostly during exhalation and are caused by airway obstructions, including secretions, edema, and tumors. **Wheezing** is a type of noisy, high-pitched breathing with a musical sound and is due primarily to narrowing of the bronchi or bronchioles due to spasm (as in asthma), edema (caused by infections), or other causes. Wheezing can also occur due to congestive heart failure, in which extra fluid accumulates in the lungs and compresses the airways. Although primarily an *expiratory* noise, wheezing can be heard during inspiration, especially in patients with severe asthma. A stethoscope is required to hear mild wheezing, whereas severe wheezing can be heard without the aid of a stethoscope. **Crackles** are discontinuous sounds heard most often during *inspiration*. The sound resembles Velcro being pulled apart. Crackles are associated with the sudden opening of airways and are present in patients with atelectasis or pulmonary fibrosis, as well as in patients with congestive heart failure or pneumonia. **Stridor** is heard as a high-pitched sound, usually during inspiration, when there is an upper airway obstruction. *Diminished breath sounds* occur when atelectasis, pneumonia, or other causes of **consolidation** (a lack of air exchange due to the presence of fluid or a mass) occur in the lung. Diminished breath sounds also occur during shallow breathing and in patients with COPD because of the poor distribution of ventilation and smaller tidal volumes associated with their lung disease.

Normal Patterns of Sputum Production

Sputum is a term used to describe secretions and particulate matter that come from the lungs and upper airway, the pharynx, nose, and mouth. The secretions that come only from the lungs are referred to as **phlegm.** The lungs normally produce up to 100 mL of phlegm each day. Tiny, hairlike projections lining the airways, called **cilia,** propel the secretions toward the upper airway, where they are often swallowed. Normally, sputum is clear and watery and is referred to as **mucoid.** When pulmonary infections are present, as in pneumonia, sputum is often thick, has an odor, and becomes colored, often green and yellow. This type of sputum is said to be **purulent.** Smokers with chronic bronchitis often cough up increased amounts of sputum each morning due to increased mucus production and an accumulation of sputum during the sleeping hours. Patients with chronic lung disease, such as bronchiectasis or cystic fibrosis, have *excessive* production of sputum that is often foul-smelling and discolored, due to chronic pulmonary infections.

The presence of a cough that produces *bloody sputum* is called **hemoptysis.** The amount of blood present may be minimal (blood streaking) or massive (frank hemoptysis). Massive hemoptysis is an emergency situation and requires immediate medical intervention. Massive hemoptysis is associated with lung cancer, tuberculosis, bronchiectasis, and trauma. Although blood streaking is not an immediate life-threatening situation, it is not normal and should be investigated. Blood streaking can occur because of severe coughing, pulmonary infections, lung cancer, or pulmonary emboli.

Absence of Chest Pain

There are various types of chest pain and many causes of it—one of which is pulmonary disease. Because the lung **parenchyma**—the small airways and alveoli—has no pain receptors, pulmonary diseases that cause chest pain usually involve the chest wall or the **pleura** (membranous lining) of the thorax. **Pleurisy,** which is an inflammation of the pleura, is a common cause of pulmonary chest pain. Recurring chest pain should not be taken lightly and should be evaluated by a healthcare professional.

Normal Skin and Mucous Membrane Coloration

Mucous membrane and skin *color* is an important indicator of pulmonary status. Regardless of ethnicity, the mucous membranes of a person whose blood is well oxygenated are normally pink, due to the bright red blood flowing through them. The skin of lightly pigmented individuals should look healthy rather than pale or bluish, and darker skin should have no grayish undertones. When oxygen levels decrease in arterial blood, it becomes darker—more like venous blood—and causes the mucous membranes and, in some individuals, the skin, to become pale. When oxygen levels become dangerously low, a bluish-gray hue, known as **cyanosis,** may develop. Cyanosis can also be due to the presence of abnormal types or amounts of hemoglobin or to poor perfusion (blood flow to an area of the body). An example of poor perfusion leading to cyanosis is the bluish hue sometimes seen in chilled fingers and nail beds during the winter. Similarly, children swimming in cold water may have blue lips due to the decreased perfusion to the mucous membranes as the body tries to conserve heat. Cyanosis in patients with pulmonary disease, however, is usually due to decreased oxygen levels. Although the presence of cyanosis is not an absolute indicator that hypoxia is present, it is a strong indicator that a problem exists. A sample of arterial blood can be taken to document the blood oxygen level and to determine whether supplemental oxygen is required.

Absence of Headache and Altered Mental Status

Although headache is a common symptom in many individuals, it can also be an important finding in patients with pulmonary disease. Both hypoxemia and **hypercapnia** (increased blood carbon dioxide levels) will dilate cerebral blood vessels and cause headache, and both are common in patients with chronic obstructive pulmonary disease. Morning headaches may indicate altered blood gases during the night and may require nighttime assessment and treatment. If hypoxemia and hypercapnia become severe, the signs and symptoms can become worse and include tremors, hallucinations, disorientation, stupor, and coma. Although aging can result in neurologic changes, it should be noted that the signs of *dementia* can be mimicked by decreased cerebral perfusion and/or decreased cerebral oxygenation.

Absence of Edema

Abnormal fluid accumulation in the body results in soft-tissue swelling, or edema. Gravity-dependent edema occurs in patients with pulmonary disease when the pulmonary blood vessels become constricted due to hypoxemia or are destroyed due to the disease process. This vasoconstriction or destruction of blood vessels causes an increased resistance to blood flow and makes the *right ventricle of the heart,* which pumps blood to the lungs, work much harder. As the disease progresses, the right ventricle weakens and becomes unable to empty itself sufficiently with each contraction. The residual blood volume causes the pressure in the right heart to increase. This pressure makes it more difficult for blood from the venous system to flow back to the right ventricle. As blood backs up in the venous system, the pressure in the veins builds, and some of the fluid portion of the blood is forced out of them and into the interstitial space, where it causes swelling. This is most noticeable in the **dependent** (lower than the heart) areas of the body, such as the feet, ankles, and legs.

Stable Weight

Although there are many factors that influence body weight, *unintentional* weight loss, or noticeable weight gain, should be brought to the attention of a healthcare provider, particularly if they occur in conjunction with symptoms such as shortness of breath and easy fatigue. Changes in weight can signal the presence of diseases such as emphysema and cancer.

Patients with emphysema often have weight loss, because their dyspnea causes them to expend so much energy simply breathing that they have little left for eating. Their nutritional status suffers, and their body weight decreases. Unexplained weight loss may also be a sign of lung cancer. Conversely, some patients with pulmonary disease, such as chronic bronchitis, may have weight gain due to edema and fluid retention.

Normal Exercise Tolerance

Individuals with healthy respiratory systems are able to tolerate a reasonable amount of exercise, or physical exertion, without becoming markedly fatigued or short of breath. Both easily induced fatigue and exercise intolerance are common among patients with cardiopulmonary disease; low oxygen levels result in limited oxygen availability for cell consumption and energy production. Patients with lung disease often need to take rest periods when performing their normal daily activities. The sensation of dyspnea, even when oxygen levels are acceptable, can also be a limiting factor during exercise; the air hunger some patients experience does not allow them to perform routine activities without rest periods.

The process of aging also has effects on exercise tolerance. Diaphragm strength is reduced, resulting in an earlier onset of fatigue. Calcification of the ribs causes increased stiffness of the bony thorax and makes breathing more of an effort (Pruitt, 2000).

Promoting Respiratory Wellness

One of the best ways to promote wellness is to avoid the risk factors leading to respiratory illness. As the old saying goes, an ounce of prevention is worth a pound of cure. Although both young and old are at increased risk for respiratory disease when placed in unhealthy environments, older adults are at particular risk. Although the aging process itself cannot be stopped, some of the effects of aging may be able to be modified by healthy living.

Avoiding Exposure to Environmental Pollutants

Environmental pollutants include potentially harmful substances in the outdoor and indoor environments. Environmental pollutants contribute significantly to the incidence of a variety of respiratory diseases.

AIR POLLUTION

The term *air pollution* refers to the contamination of the *outdoor* environment as a result of human activity—the growth of industry and the like. Pollutants come in three main forms: particles, vapors, and the products of combustion. **Particles,** which can be either solid or liquid, are produced through processes such as sanding, grinding, demolishing, drilling, and spraying. **Vapors** are produced when liquids evaporate into their gaseous forms. Innumerable chemical and industrial processes result in vaporization and pollution. **Combustion,** or the process of burning, produces smoke, which is probably the most common air pollutant. Furnaces, engines, and outdoor burning all contribute to this problem. Smoke is made up of both particles less than 1 micron and gases. The small particles it contains can penetrate deep into the lungs and can act as catalysts for lung damage. Particles come mainly from the fuel combustion used in industrial processes. Noxious and toxic gases come mainly from fuel combustion in vehicles used for transportation. Other sources of air pollution include ozone, carbon monoxide, carbon dioxide, nitrogen dioxide, sulfur dioxide, hydrocarbons, and chlorofluorocarbons, along with many other particles, fumes, gases, and vapors.

Ozone (O_3) is the main ingredient in smog. It is irritating to the eyes and throat and is responsible for causing coughing, bronchoconstriction, possible alveolar damage, and increased shortness of breath. **Carbon monoxide (CO)** can severely reduce the oxygen-carrying ability of the blood and can decrease exercise tolerance. **Sulfur dioxide (SO_2)** causes bronchoconstriction, especially in asthmatics, and exacerbates lung disease. **Nitrogen dioxide (NO_2)** causes bronchitis and bronchoconstriction and increases susceptibility to respiratory infections.

Particles include pollen, bacteria, fungi, dust, soot, and dirt in the air. Inhaled particles can cause pulmonary irritation and infections, breathing difficulties, a predisposition to cancer, and premature death. In several studies, workers in urban settings and in high-pollution areas were found to have a reduced FEV_1 when compared with workers in rural settings and low-pollution areas (Zordis, 1999).

Air pollution decreases blood oxygen levels and ciliary motion, damages lung cells, and impairs the lung's ability to fight infection—all of which contribute to respiratory illness. Pollution has been shown to cause a number of pulmonary diseases, including lung cancer and patients with bronchitis and emphysema experience the exacerbation of their disease when exposed to pollution.

INDOOR/OCCUPATIONAL POLLUTION

Causes of indoor air pollution, also known as **occupational pollution,** include particles, vapors, gases, smoke, and fumes. Occupational pollution results from the use of cooking oils, gas, kerosene, fireplaces, and stoves for heating. Other contributors include automobile exhaust and smoking, the use of air conditioners, certain building materials and chemical cleaners, and the presence of radon.

Radon is a naturally occurring radioactive gas formed by the decay of uranium in the soil. It is tasteless, odorless, and invisible. Radon seeps through gaps in the foundation or the walls of homes and can become trapped inside. As radon continues to decay, the decay products adhere to dust particles. The inhalation of dust particles laden with radon-decay products can cause lung cell damage leading to lung cancer. The long-term exposure to radon-decay products is thought to be the second leading cause of lung cancer, with smoking as the primary cause. It is estimated that up to 30,000 lung cancer deaths may be caused by radon each year in the United States (Mitchell, 1998).

The exposure to indoor pollution can cause general illness, including cough, shortness of breath, headache, sore throat, nausea, burning eyes, and runny nose. It can contribute to premature death in those previously ill from heart or lung disease, and it is responsible for increasing the incidence of allergic disorders, for stimulating asthma attacks, and for producing constricting airway edema. **Occupational asthma** is now the most common form of occupational lung disease in industrialized countries (Zordis, 1999). More than 250 agents have been shown to cause occupational asthma and to contribute to COPD. Agents that can cause occupational asthma include both naturally occurring and synthetic compounds. Some of the most studied agents include the epoxy resins used in plastics and adhesives and red cedar wood dust. New agents are synthesized each year, and the manner in which they affect the respiratory system is unknown. Thus, it is important to try to remove as many of these agents from the environment as possible.

EXPOSURE TO CIGARETTE SMOKE

Smoking is the number one preventable cause of death in men and women in the United States. Of the more than 140,000 women who die prematurely from tobacco-related illnesses each year, 80 percent began smoking while they were adolescents (*Young Women and Smoking*, 2000). Women are taking up smoking at a younger age than ever before, and young girls and teenage women represent the largest growing group of new smokers—approximately *one teenage girl in every five smokes.* Cigarette smoking during adolescence causes cough, phlegm production, an increased number and severity of respiratory illnesses, and the potential retardation of lung growth, and it has been associated with early signs of **periodontal degeneration** and the presence of lesions (abnormal tissues) in the mouth, which can develop into *oral cancer.* Many adolescent smokers report adverse effects on their *mental health,* such as nervousness and depression. Adolescents who smoke tend to engage in more *risky behaviors,* such as fighting, engaging in high-risk sexual behavior, and using alcohol and other drugs, than do adolescents who do not smoke (*Young Women and Smoking*, 2000) and there is a strong link between illicit drug use and respiratory problems (Wilkins, Krider, & Sheldon, 2000). Smoking negatively affects young women's *appearance* and overall appeal, as it leads to wrinkled skin, stained teeth, and bad breath. Smoking may also be damaging to women's *reproductive health*; it is associated with infertility, complications during pregnancy, and an earlier onset of menopause (*Young*

Women and Smoking, 2000). Expectant mothers who smoke increase their likelihood of experiencing miscarriage and stillbirth and of having a child with birth defects or one that is premature or small for its gestational age. Smoking during pregnancy also increases the risk of having a child with mental retardation by 50 percent; this risk increases to 85 percent when the mother smokes a pack or more each day (*Young Women and Smoking*, 2000). Smoking while pregnant also contributes to a reduction in neonatal pulmonary function at birth (Zordis, 1999). **Sudden infant death syndrome (SIDS)** is more common in children whose mothers smoked while pregnant, as well as in children who were exposed to environmental tobacco smoke (ETS) following birth. Smoking is also responsible for the majority of the clinically significant cases of chronic obstructive pulmonary disease.

Tobacco smoke contains more than 4,000 compounds, including nicotine, carbon monoxide, and 40 known carcinogens (Mitchell, 1998), and women who smoke have a likelihood of developing lung cancer that is at least 10 times greater than that of nonsmoking women (*Young Women and Smoking*, 2000). In 1996, smoking accounted for approximately 80 percent of all lung cancer cases and resulted in more than 60,000 deaths among women. In 1987, lung cancer surpassed breast cancer as the number one cause of cancer deaths among American women (*Young Women and Smoking*, 2000). The rate at which women die of lung cancer has been increasing steadily over time; lung cancer deaths among women increased by 150 percent between 1974 and 1994. During the same time period, men's death rate increased by only 20 percent (*Tobacco Smoke and Women*, 2000). Between 1960 and 1990, women's death rate from lung cancer increased by more than 400 percent.

The increased number of cases of lung cancer in women parallels the increase in smoking by women over the past 60 years. The tobacco industry has used women's desire for equality with men to lure them into the smoking habit. Cigarette ads bearing such slogans as "You've come a long way, baby," are designed to link smoking and liberation. Tobacco marketers have also capitalized on the twin facts that women in our society are judged more than men on the basis of their appearance and that slender women are seen as more attractive than their more robust counterparts. Brand names such as Virginia Slims link smoking with weight control and exploit women's fear of obesity.

Women may be *genetically predisposed* to develop lung cancer as a result of exposure to tobacco carcinogens. Some studies have shown that, when women are compared with men who have smoked the same amount of cigarettes, women have higher rates of lung cancer (*Tobacco Smoke and Women*, 2000). In addition to lung cancer, tobacco use is a major risk factor for cancers of the mouth, esophagus, larynx, bladder, kidney, pancreas, stomach, and cervix. Smoking has a synergistic effect with other risk factors; women who both smoke and suffer exposure to other pollutants greatly increase their risk of malignancy.

Smoking is also a major contributor to *coronary heart disease* and *stroke*. Studies show that smokers are more likely than nonsmokers to have abnormal lipid levels and to develop coronary artery disease; women who smoke are two to six times more likely to suffer a heart attack than are women who do not smoke (Villablanca, McDonald, & Rutledge, 2000). Each year, about 8,000 women die from strokes attributable to smoking (*Young Women and Smoking,* 2000). According to the American Heart Association, heart attacks and strokes have killed more females than males every year since 1984.

Avoiding **secondhand smoke** is also important, particularly for children. Children who are exposed to environmental tobacco smoke (ETS) have an increased likelihood that they will develop childhood respiratory illnesses and exacerbation of asthma. It is estimated that ETS causes between 150,000 and 300,000 respiratory tract infections, such as bronchitis and pneumonia, each year in children younger than 18 months of age. ETS is also estimated to be responsible for up to 1 million cases of asthma exacerbation each year (Mitchell, 1998). Research has shown that FEV_1 values are decreased in children exposed to secondhand smoke in the home (Zordis, 1999).

Secondhand smoke is also dangerous to adults. In adults, secondhand smoke is responsible for an increased incidence of coronary heart disease, stroke, and lung cancer. Women who are regularly exposed to ETS have a 91 percent greater chance of developing coronary heart disease than women who are not exposed, and it is estimated that 53,000 deaths each year are attributed to ETS (*Secondhand Smoke,* 1998). Although the risk for lung cancer, the leading cause of cancer deaths in women, is slight for nonsmokers, it is estimated that *more than 3,000 nonsmoking women die each year from lung cancer caused by ETS.* The risk of lung cancer is also 30 percent greater among women whose husbands smoke (*Secondhand Smoke,* 1998).

Smoking is not simply a bad habit; it is a serious *drug addiction* that requires an accurate diagnosis and appropriate medical treatment. The addicting ingredient in tobacco smoke is nicotine, which, although not thought to be related to the lung diseases associated with smoking, has been found to decrease HDL cholesterol levels. Moffatt, Biggerstaff, and Stamford (2000) found that the administration of nicotine via skin patch to subjects who had quit smoking inhibited the expected normalization of their high density lipoprotein cholesterol (HDL-C) levels. Seconds after the inhalation of cigarette smoke, nicotine is absorbed into the bloodstream and delivered to the nicotine receptors in the brain. The stimulation of the nicotine receptors results in the secretion of dopamine, resulting in a pleasurable sensation, cognitive arousal, and, for smokers, the rapid relief from nicotine deprivation. Additionally, there is an increased release of norepinephrine, beta-endorphin, acetylcholine, serotonin, glutamate, and vasopressors, chemicals that affect the central nervous system in a way that decreases anxiety and enhances

---

Box 13–1 Symptoms of Nicotine Withdrawal

- Anxiety
- Irritability
- Decreased heart rate
- Difficulty in concentration
- Increased appetite, weight gain
- Restlessness
- Craving for cigarettes
- Depression

---

concentration, alertness, and memory. The overall result is a feeling of well-being. An abrupt discontinuance of tobacco products also has a profound effect on the central nervous system. **Nicotine withdrawal** causes an acute reduction in the levels of dopamine and norepinephrine, leading to the symptoms listed in Box 13–1. The resumption of tobacco products quickly reverses all the symptoms of nicotine withdrawal (Linnington, Leonard, & Sachs, 2000).

The 1980 Surgeon General's Report on the Health Consequences of Smoking concluded that women have greater difficulty quitting tobacco use than men. It has been suggested that this is true because many women smoke to reduce emotional stress (Tanoue, 2000). Moreover, fear of the weight gain associated with smoking cessation stops many women from even attempting to quit (Jeffery, Hennrikus, Lando, Murray, & Liu, 2000). Physicians and other healthcare providers can and should play an important role in guiding nicotine-dependent individuals toward successful smoking cessation. They can make referrals to tobacco cessation programs and/or behavior modification programs and can provide appropriate drug therapy. **Nicotine replacement therapy (NRT)** was the first successful pharmacological treatment used in smoking cessation. NRT's effectiveness is dose-dependent and is inversely proportional to an individual's level of nicotine dependency. NRT's effectiveness is dependent on its ability to reduce withdrawal symptoms, particularly in the first two to four weeks after smoking cessation; the higher the dosage, the higher the rate of successful smoking cessation. The problems most frequently related to nicotine treatment are underdosing and an inadequate duration of therapy. Nicotine replacement is available in a number of modalities, which include transdermal patches, gum (polacrilex), nasal spray, and, most recently, a nasal inhaler. Adequate nicotine replacement has been shown to reduce cessation-related weight gain to negligible levels in women (Moffatt et al., 2000).

Buproprion, or **Wellbutrin SR,** an antidepressant, is also used to relieve or suppress the symptoms of nicotine withdrawal. Buproprion affects *dopamine levels,* thus simulating the same feeling of well-being that nicotine produces. The drug can be used alone or in conjunction with nicotine replacement therapy. Buproprion is contraindicated for patients who have a history of seizures, brain surgery, or eating disorders. It is also contraindicated in alcoholics and in people who are taking medications that lower seizure threshold, such as theophylline. The most recent data indicates that women have the most effective treatment results when using simultaneous buproprion and nicotine replacement therapy (Linnington et al., 2000).

Avoiding Obesity

More than 50 percent of the adult population of the United States is considered overweight, with 25 to 35 percent considered obese (Lesperance, 2000). Obesity is one of the major causes of chronic illness and premature death in the United States, and it can contribute to respiratory disease. Some reports suggest that gaining a pound a year accelerates FEV_1 decrease by another 5–8 mL/year (Wilkins et al., 2000). One study showed that, when a group of volunteers lost an average of 31.2 pounds over a 14-week period, they had a 7.2 percent improvement in their FEV_1 (Lesperance, 2000).

Obese individuals are more likely to suffer from **obstructive sleep apnea (OSA),** which has been documented in 50 percent of all obese men. OSA is due to airway occlusion in the area of the pharynx. Many individuals who suffer from sleep apnea are obese; have a short, thick neck; and snore; however, not all snorers have OSA. OSA is estimated to occur in 4 to 9 percent of middle-aged men and 1 to 2 percent of all women (Olson, King, Hensley, & Saunders, 1995). Although it is estimated that 15 percent of women and 25 percent of men snore, the incidence of OSA is not that high (Wilkins et al., 2000). Sleep apnea is common in women with coronary artery disease (CAD) and remains a significant predictor of CAD in women (Mooe, Rabben, Wiklund, Franklin, & Eriksson, 1996). Individuals with OSA tend to have excessive daytime sleepiness, impaired cognitive and psychomotor function, and hypertension, but they breathe normally during daytime waking hours. They may also experience bed-wetting, impotence, morning headaches (possibly due to hypoxemia), memory loss, and personality changes. Common treatments for OSA include weight loss, nasal CPAP (continuous positive airway pressure) during sleeping hours, and upper airway surgery.

Obesity is classified as a *restrictive lung condition,* resulting in decreased lung volumes and increased respiratory rates. The increased bulk of the chest and abdomen decreases lung volumes, increases the work of breathing, decreases the elasticity of the lungs and increases airway resistance, all of which leads to hypoxemia. Persons with morbid obesity may develop obesity-hypoventilation syndrome, referred to as **Pickwickian syndrome.** Over time, these patients develop hypoxemia and a decreased respiratory sensitivity to increased $PaCO_2$ levels. It takes increasingly high $PaCO_2$ levels to trigger spontaneous respiration, and CO_2 levels build up in the blood.

There is also a possible link between childhood obesity and asthma, with very obese children being two to three times more likely to develop asthma. Evidence indicates that weight loss results in a decrease in asthmatic symptoms (Lesperance, 2000).

Getting Vaccinated Against Flu and Pneumonia

Flu and pneumonia vaccines contain noninfectious, inactive viruses or bacteria, so there is no risk of getting the disease from the shot. New guidelines from the Centers for Disease Control and Prevention (CDC) have lowered the recommended flu and pneumonia immunization age from 65 to 50 years for individuals who are in good health (Connelly, 2000). It is advised that immunization begin much earlier in persons who suffer from a chronic illness or have a compromised immune system: the first flu vaccination should be given at six months of age and the first pneumoccocal pneumonia vaccination at two years of age. Currently, the pneumococcal vaccine (Pneumovax) is ineffective for children under two years old, however, testing is being done on a new vaccine that could be effective. This new vaccine will also give protection against the most common bacterial strains that are responsible for meningitis, as well as for sinus and ear infections (Connelly, 2000).

It has been estimated that half the deaths from pneumococcal pneumonia could be prevented by immunization, which protects against the 23 strains of pneumococcal bacteria, which are responsible for 88 percent of all pneumococcal disease (Cassiere & Fein, 1997). Although the pneumococcal pneumonia vaccination provides protection for 10 years or longer, it is suggested that individuals older than 65 and those with chronic illness receive a booster shot (Cassiere & Fein, 1997). Flu immunizations must be received *annually,* because the vaccine is composed of inactivated viruses from flu strains known to be in circulation during that particular year.

Immunization is particularly important for older individuals. Increased age impairs cell-mediated immunity, making older individuals more susceptible to respiratory infections. In general, the pulmonary defense mechanisms are also impaired in this population. The epithelial cells of the airways show degenerative changes, and the activity of the cilia slows down, decreasing the mucociliary clearance of sputum. The phagocytic activity of macrophages is also decreased, and cough becomes less effective due to respiratory muscle weakness. Each of these changes increases the susceptibility of the lungs to infection (Pruitt, 2000). Even though cell-mediated (humoral) immunity, the acute antibody response, is also reduced in older adults, immunizations, which rely on this response, are still strongly recommended. Because children develop more protective antibodies than older adults, vaccination earlier in life means added protection for 10 years or longer.

Respiratory Illnesses

There are many types of respiratory illness, and it is beyond the scope of this chapter to address most of them. Therefore, the following sections address some of the most common preventable or controllable respiratory disorders: the common cold, influenza, pneumonia, asthma, chronic obstructive pulmonary disease, and lung cancer.

The Common Cold

The common cold (**acute coryza**) is a contagious *viral* infection of the upper respiratory tract that causes inflammation of the mucous membranes. The most common cold viruses are classified as rhinoviruses. Cold viruses are easily passed from one individual to another by sneezing, coughing, or direct contact, as well as via inanimate objects that are contaminated with nasal secretions. Washing hands often, maintaining good nutrition, and decreasing stress help prevent a cold (*Taking the Fight out of a Cold*, 1998). The incubation period is usually 1–3 days, but the contagious period begins *prior* to the onset of symptoms and may last for up to 10 days. Children develop immunity with each viral exposure, resulting in a decreased number of colds as they get older. Colds do not result in death but do result in substantial absenteeism from school or work.

SYMPTOMS

The symptoms of colds include sneezing, tearing, **rhinitis** (runny nose), a sore or scratchy throat, nasal congestion, headache, a possible low-grade fever, and malaise (a "washed-out" feeling). The onset of symptoms begins a day or two *after* infection occurs, with most symptoms resolving in about a week. Unless severe cold symptoms persist, diagnostic tests are seldom done. A healthcare provider should be consulted if symptoms seem abnormal or if the sinuses become infected.

TREATMENT

Because the common cold cannot be cured, treatment is aimed at *symptom relief* and includes rest, plenty of fluids (some prefer hot drinks), gargling with warm salt water, decongestants to relieve a stuffy nose, and analgesics (such as acetaminophen) for pain. If a dry cough is present, an over-the-counter medication that contains a *cough suppressant,* such as *dextromethorphan,* may be helpful. If a productive cough is present, a medication containing **guaifenesin,** which will loosen secretions, may be used. It is not a good idea to suppress a productive cough, as retained secretions encourage the growth of bacteria and subsequent infection. Since the common cold is of viral origin, *antibiotic treatment is unnecessary and unhelpful;* antibiotics do not work against viruses. Colds are usually self-limiting, meaning that, given time, the body's immune system will destroy the virus, and the symptoms will subside.

Influenza

Influenza (the flu) is an acute viral infection of the respiratory tract that is highly contagious. It is spread via airborne droplets from the nose and mouth of infected persons. Infections are most prevalent in the winter and spring months. The causative agent is usually a type of myxovirus. The major viral strains identified include Type A and Type B, but new strains emerge at regular intervals and are named according to their geographic region of origin. The new strains account for the need for yearly vaccinations. Flu viruses are the only organisms that still cause acute nationwide epidemics. The incubation period is usually one to three days following infection; after that, the symptoms manifest. The infection is often self-limiting and lasts two to seven days. In this country, more than 110,000 people are hospitalized each year due to the flu, and more than 20,000 die (Palencia, 2000). Because of their greater susceptibility to infection, older persons with influenza are at risk for developing concomitant respiratory tract infections, such as bacterial pneumonia. Such flu-related infections produce significant morbidity and mortality in the older population. In recent years, 80 percent of deaths related to influenza pneumonia have occurred in persons over 65 years old.

SYMPTOMS

The symptoms of the flu include fever lasting two to three days, chills, headache, *myalgia* (muscular pains), fatigue, cough, weakness, sneezing, stuffy nose, sore throat, chest discomfort, and malaise. Influenza is distinguished from the common cold by the presence of *fever* and the *greater severity of the symptoms*. Diagnostic tests are routinely not performed unless symptoms are severe or continue for a prolonged period of time.

TREATMENT

The best treatment for the flu is *prevention* through use of the influenza vaccine. Although not 100 percent effective, the use of the influenza vaccine is associated with a 50 percent reduction in hospitalizations and a 60 to 70 percent reduction in mortality in high-risk patients (Bartlett, Breiman, Mandell, & File, 1998). A list of conditions designating high-risk individuals is located in Box 13–2. Because a new and different flu vaccine must be administered each year in order to provide adequate protection, vaccination should be annual, rather than intermittent (Ahmed, Nicholson, & Nguyn-Van-Tam, 1995). Unfortunately, surveys indicate that only 50 percent of eligible elderly individuals are receiving the flu vaccine. It should be noted that persons who are *allergic to eggs* should not receive the vaccine, as it is made using chicken embryos.

Once a person has become infected with the flu virus, treatment is aimed mostly at ameliorating the symptoms and includes rest, analgesics, and fluids. Recently, new flu medications have become available that can prevent flu symptoms from developing after an exposure and lessen the severity of

- Age over 65 years
- Residence in a nursing home or chronic-care facility
- Asthma
- Diabetes
- Chronic disorders of the lung, heart, liver, kidney, blood, or immune system
- Pregnancy (in second or third trimester)
- Long-term aspirin therapy (in children)

symptoms once they have occurred. Except in certain unusual situations, however, these antiviral treatments should not be promoted as an acceptable alternative to vaccination (Gross, Hermogenes, Sacks, Lau, & Levandowski, 1995). The reason for this is their limited ability to protect against the yearly viral strains: Symmetrel and Flumodine give protection against only Type A viral strains, whereas Tamiflu offers some protection against both Type A and Type B viral strains. However, as there is no guarantee that the flu season will bring only Types A and B viral strains, the medications may provide little, if any, protection. Relenza is recommended only for lessening flu symptoms. Table 13–2 lists antiviral medications that can help prevent and treat influenza.

Pneumonia

The term *pneumonia* refers to an acute inflammation of the lung tissue or lower airways due to infection. Although viruses, fungi, or protozoa can cause pneumonia, the most common cause is *bacterial contamination*. Lower respiratory tract infections are the sixth most common cause of death in the United States—more than 78,000 a year—with 6 million cases of pneumonia reported annually (Rao & San Pedro, 1996). Pneumonia occurring outside the hospital is termed **community-acquired pneumonia (CAP)** and is most often caused by a pneumococcal bacterium called *Streptococcus pneumoniae*. *Streptococcus pneumoniae* is also responsible for middle ear infections (otitis media), sinus infections (sinusitis), some cases of bacteremia (blood infections), and meningitis (infection of the membranes lining the brain). Other common bacteria that cause pneumonia include *Haemophilus influenza, Staphylococcus aureus, Klebsiella pneumoniae,* and *Legionella pneumophila.* The most serious form of pneumonia is **pneumococcal pneumonea,** caused by the pneumococcal bacterium. Each year, more than 45,000 patients die of pneumococcal pneumonia, making it the most deadly of the vaccine-preventable bacterial diseases (Connelly, 2000). Elderly people are three to five times more likely than persons age 18–40 to get pneumococcal bacteremia, which is fatal in up to 60 percent of cases (Cassiere & Fein, 1997).

Pneumonia occurs when the body's pulmonary defense mechanisms are overcome by an organism, and it usually follows the colonization of the upper airway. The risk factors for developing pneumococcal disease are listed in Box 13–3.

TABLE 13–2   Medications used in the treatment of influenza.

	Flu Medications			
	Relenza (zanamivir)	Tamiflu (oseltamivir)	Symmetrel (amantadine)	Flumodine (rimantadine)
Viral effectiveness	Types A, B	Types A, B	Type A only	Type A only
Administration	Inhalation (diskhaler)	Orally	Orally	Orally
Approved for age	≥ 7 years	≥ 13 years	≥ 1 year	≥ 1 year
Dosage and duration of use	Twice a day for 5 days	Twice a day for 5 days	Twice a day for 10 days	Twice a day for 7 days
When to begin	Within 48 hrs of onset	Within 48 hrs of onset	Within 48 hrs of onset	Within 48 hrs of onset
Approved for	Symptoms (All decrease the duration and severity of symptoms.)	Prophylaxis	Prophylaxis	Prophylaxis
Side effects	Bronchospasm: < 5 percent incidence	Rare	Rare	Rare

Box 13–3 Factors That Place Individuals at High Risk for Pneumococcal Disease

- Age 65 years or older
- Residence in a long-term or chronic-care facility
- Alcohol abuse
- Asthma
- Impaired immunity
- Poor nutritional status
- Chronic illness
- Diabetes
- Cancer
- Heart, lung, kidney, or liver disease
- Positive HIV status or AIDS
- Sickle-cell anemia
- Hodgkin's disease

One study suggests that female sex is a risk factor for predicting a complicated course in some cases of CAP (Porath, Schlaeffer, & Lieberman, 1996).

SYMPTOMS

The symptoms of pneumonia include high fever and chills; rapid heart rate; rapid breathing with a feeling of being short of breath; chest pain on inhalation; a productive cough with yellow, green, or brownish sputum; sweating; muscle aches; fatigue; headache; and lack of appetite. A healthcare provider who examines a person with pneumonia will hear crackles over the area of the lung that is infected.

DIAGNOSIS

Chest radiographs (x-rays) will likely be taken if a diagnosis of pneumonia is suspected (Bartlett et al., 1998) and will reveal the presence of an acute infiltrate (whitened area) if pneumonia is present. After treatment is begun, it may take six weeks or longer for the infiltrate to disappear. A sample of the person's sputum may be cultured to determine the nature of any bacteria present, but controversy exists as to the benefit of this procedure, as antibiotics that will kill the organisms that commonly cause pneumonia are routinely prescribed. If, however, the organisms present prove resistant to the antibiotics prescribed, microbial identification may be needed for proper treatment. Because the presence of pneumonia will cause the body to produce extra white blood cells to fight the infection, blood tests that will reveal any increase in the white blood cell count are sometimes ordered as part of the diagnostic workup.

TREATMENT

It is estimated that 75 percent of patients with CAP can be treated effectively on an outpatient basis (Lucas, 1999). Be-

cause treatment is often done without identifying the microbe and without knowing which antibiotics it is sensitive to, a broad-spectrum antibiotic is used. First-line drugs include members of the macrolide class, such as erythromycin, clarithromycin, or azithromycin. Other first-line drugs include doxycycline and drugs belonging to the fluoroquinolone class. If first-line drugs are contraindicated or ineffective, alternate drugs, such as amoxicillin/clavulanate, second- and third-generation cephalosporins, trimethoprim/sulfamethoxazole, and B-lactam/B-lactamase inhibitors can be used (Lucas, 1999). The treatment for pneumonia also includes medications for pain and fever, plenty of fluids, and rest. The best way to treat pneumococcal disease is to prevent it with a vaccine. The pneumococcal vaccine (Pneumovax) protects against 88 percent of the pneumococcal bacteria types that cause pneumonia. One injection can provide protection for up to 10 years. It is suggested, however, that high-risk patients get a booster shot every six years (Connelly, 2000). The vaccine is considered safe but has some local side effects, including **erythema** (redness) at the injection site and soreness, which may last up to 48 hours.

Patients who cannot be treated on an outpatient base due to the severity of their illness are admitted to the hospital. Treatments there include antibiotics, oxygen therapy for hypoxemia, and, in severe cases, mechanical ventilation if respiratory failure develops.

Asthma

Asthma is a lung disease characterized by episodic bouts of airway inflammation and narrowing due to hyper-responsiveness to various stimuli. In the past, asthma was often called "reversible airways disease" because the signs and symptoms would intermittently appear and disappear and because the pathophysiology was not well understood. It is now known, however, that an asthma attack involves a very complex set of events that occur simultaneously: A stimulus causes the mucosal lining of the airways to become infiltrated with inflammatory cells. These cells cause the small blood vessels in the mucosa to leak fluid into the surrounding tissues, causing them to swell and produce excess *mucus*. At the same time, the smooth muscles around the airway go into *spasm*. Together, these events cause the airway to become not only smaller but partially obstructed as well. Taking a breath becomes increasingly difficult, and the person becomes more and more short of breath. Currently, asthma is seen as a *chronic* condition that can be managed with various therapies, but not cured.

It is estimated that asthma affects 5 to 7 percent of the U.S. population, or approximately 14.6 million people (Weil, 1997). The cases of reported asthma more than doubled from 1982 to 1994. Women's risk of developing asthma varies with age: In childhood, girls appear to have a lower risk of developing asthma than boys. Around the age of puberty, however, the incidence of asthma in males and females is about equal, and, after puberty, women are at significantly *higher* risk of developing asthma than men. Currently, about

60 percent of adult asthmatics are women (de Marco, Locatelli, Sunyer, & Burney, 2000). No definite cause for the higher incidence in women has been identified, but the major theories include the hypotheses that (1) women's asthma is related to their smaller airway diameter, (2) women tend to be more hyper-responsive than men to various stimuli, (3) women have a genetic predisposition to asthma, and (4) women's fluctuating hormone levels (estrogen and progesterone) are somehow involved.

Two forms of asthma are often identified, extrinsic and intrinsic. **Extrinsic asthma** is associated with allergic reactions, and specific allergens can usually be identified. Individuals can be allergic to viruses, dust, smoke, various chemicals, drugs, foods, food additives, and food preservatives. Asthma can also be induced by chemical changes in the body related to exercise and emotional arousal. **Intrinsic asthma** is said to occur when no specific causes of the disease can be identified.

SYMPTOMS

The most common symptoms of asthma are difficulty taking in a breath, difficulty exhaling, wheezing, and cough.

DIAGNOSIS

Diagnosing asthma can be a long and involved process. The medical history and physical exam are both important components of the diagnostic workup. Answers to questions about seasonal allergies, exposure to irritants, the timing of attacks, and so on can provide valuable clues to diagnosis. Pulmonary function tests, particularly the FEV_1, are used to determine if airflow obstruction is occurring during exhalation. The peak flow measurement will reveal airway narrowing. In some cases, a **bronchial provocation test** may be needed to make the diagnosis. This test involves delivering an agent that produces bronchospasm (under controlled conditions) and performing PFTs to demonstrate airflow obstruction. The most common drug used for bronchial provocation is methacholine.

TREATMENT

The *prevention of asthma attacks* is the primary goal in the treatment of asthma. It is important to eliminate or avoid irritants and known triggers that aggravate bronchial hyper-responsiveness. If, for example, the asthmatic individual is allergic to cats and cat dander, environments in which cats are present must be avoided. Allergists can perform skin testing to determine the nature of specific allergens. A variety of drugs that can decrease airway irritability are also available. Used regularly, **mast cell stabilizers** (such as Intal and Tilade) can prevent the release of histamine and other cellular substances that are known to cause bronchospasm. **Sympathomimetics,** drugs that relax bronchial smooth muscle, are frequently used in inhaler form for the treatment of asthma. Currently available examples of these drugs include Albuterol, Maxair, and Serevent. **Steroids** by inhaler can also be used, because they provide great anti-inflammatory coverage directly to the air-way. Flovent, Azmacort, and Aerobid are all steroid inhalers in common use. During severe attacks, asthmatics may need aerosolized and intravenous medications to bring their symptoms under control. Occasionally, an asthmatic will need to be hospitalized during the acute phase of a severe attack, and sedation and mechanical ventilation may be required.

Chronic Obstructive Pulmonary Disease

Chronic obstructive pulmonary disease (COPD) is characterized by the presence of airflow obstruction. COPD affects approximately 16 million people in the United States. It is the fourth leading cause of death in the United States, resulting in approximately 105,000 deaths per year (Scanlan, Wilkins, & Stoller, 1999). Chronic bronchitis and emphysema are the two most common forms of COPD. Smoking is responsible for most of the clinically significant cases of both.

The term **bronchitis** refers to inflammation of the bronchial tree. In order to be considered chronic, bronchitis must have been present for three consecutive months in two successive years, as evidenced by a productive cough. The leading cause of chronic bronchitis is *smoking*. Other factors leading to chronic bronchitis include recurrent respiratory infections, airway hyperactivity, and air pollution. In this disease process, ongoing changes in the airways damage the lungs over a period of time. These changes include the enlargement of the bronchial glands, an increase in the number and activity of the goblet cells (cells that engulf bacteria), the infiltration of inflammatory cells into the submucosal lining of the airways, and the loss of cilia. The result of these changes is the excessive production of thick mucus, chronic airway narrowing, and bronchoconstriction. The common signs and symptoms of chronic bronchitis are chronic cough with the production of bloody sputum, recurrent lung infections, and severe dyspnea. Patients with chronic bronchitis are often overweight and appear cyanotic (having a blue discoloration of the skin). The *incidence* of bronchitis is higher in women than in men, and, since the 1970s, the *mortality rate* for women with COPD has been strikingly greater than that of men (National Lung Health Education Program Executive Committee, 1998).

Emphysema is a condition in which an abnormal, permanent enlargement of air spaces in the small airways and alveoli occurs. As in the case with chronic bronchitis, the leading cause of emphysema is smoking; however, some types of emphysema are caused by genetic factors. As lung tissue destruction progresses in emphysema, the lung's ability to recoil to its normal resting state is lost. This loss of elasticity can be likened to that of a rubber band that has been overstretched and can no longer return to its original shape. The end result for the patient is incomplete and inadequate exhalation, due to early airway closure and the trapping of increased amounts of air in the lung. This pathology manifests as increasing shortness of breath and difficulty breathing. If a cough is present, it is often dry and nonproductive, unless a respiratory infection is occurring. Emphysematous patients are often thin, pink, and very short of breath.

DIAGNOSIS

The diagnosis of COPD is accomplished by obtaining a thorough medical history and physical exam of the patient. Persons with COPD complain of shortness of breath, productive cough, and a very low exercise tolerance. They also have a characteristic appearance, in that they have what is known as a barrel chest. A **barrel chest** is wider than normal from front to back, due to permanent hyperinflation of the airways. Chest radiographs are diagnostic in themselves, as they show the hyperinflated lungs and the lowered, flattened diaphragm. Pulmonary function testing is a quick and inexpensive method of determining the presence and degree of airway obstruction in COPD. The easily measured spirometric value FEV_1 will be decreased, and lung volumes, especially the residual volume and functional residual capacity, will be increased. It is of interest that, FEV_1, which normally *decreases* at a rate of approximately 25 mL/year in women and 31 mL/year for men after age 25, does so even more rapidly in smokers. Smokers may have a deterioration rate four times the normal, resulting in a decrease of over 100 mL/year in their FEV_1 (Wilkins et al., 2000). Individuals who stop smoking show a less severe rate of decline in their pulmonary function, often returning to the normal rate of decline.

TREATMENT

The treatment of COPD involves managing the signs and symptoms of the underlying diseases. Unfortunately, most of the underlying tissue damage cannot be reversed; therefore, treatment focuses on making patients as comfortable as possible and providing them with information about how best to cope with the disease. A treatment priority is to help patients with COPD stop smoking. Teaching them how to avoid respiratory irritants and infections is another key to successful treatment. As the disease progresses, patients will need to use inhaled drugs, such as steroids and bronchodilators, and some patients may need to be on supplemental oxygen at home. Fortunately, pulmonary rehabilitation programs are now available to COPD patients. The goal of such programs is to train patients and their families to cope with the disease and the treatment regimen. Some individuals with severe COPD require a period of hospitalization and possibly mechanical ventilation. In some cases, surgery to remove a portion of the diseased lung may be necessary for symptom relief and a better quality of life.

Lung Cancer

In the United States, lung cancer ranks only second to coronary heart disease as a cause of death (American Cancer Society, 2000). There were an estimated 156,000 deaths due to lung cancer in 2000, which accounted for 28 percent of all cancer deaths. During the years 1992–1996, the mortality rates due to lung cancer declined in men, whereas the rates for women *rose significantly* by 0.9 percent per year.

The decline in men's mortality can be attributed to an overall reduction in their smoking habits, but women have not been as successful as men in breaking the smoking habit. Since 1987, more women have died each year from lung cancer than breast cancer, which had been the leading form of cancer in women (Winawer & Shike, 1995). There were an estimated 164,100 new cases of lung cancer diagnosed in 2000, accounting for 28 percent of all cancer diagnoses.

Cancer develops in the body's cells, the basic units of life. Normally, cells grow, divide, and produce more cells to keep the body functioning in a healthy manner. Sometimes, however, the cells continue to divide even when new cells are not needed; such a mass of new cellular growth is called a **tumor.** **Benign** tumors are noncancerous, do not spread to other parts of the body, and are rarely life-threatening. However, **malignant** tumors are cancerous; that is, they are made up of abnormal cells, which divide uncontrollably, sometimes invading other tissues around them. Half of all lung tumors contain a defective tumor suppressor gene, called p53, that permits uninhibited cell growth (American Cancer Society, 2000). Cancer cells can also break away from the tumor site, enter the bloodstream and lymphatic system, and spread to other tissues and organs of the body in a process called **metastasis** (Cancer Institute, 1999). Lung cancer develops when a carcinogen damages a lung cell's DNA. The suspected causes of lung cancer are numerous and include the following:

- *Smoking.* Smoking accounts for approximately 87 percent of all lung cancers (Winawer & Shike, 1995). Cigarette smokers' risk of developing lung cancer is about 10 times that of nonsmokers (Kramer, Gohagan, & Prorok, 1999), and lung cancer mortality rates are 13 times higher in women who smoke than in women who have never smoked. Tobacco contains cancer-causing substances, called **carcinogens,** which damage lung cells. The ways in which carcinogens affect lung cells differ in men and women. Women are more susceptible to these tobacco-related carcinogens and sustain damage to the peripheral, or outer, parts of their lungs. In contrast, men who smoke are less likely to develop cancer, and, when they do, they sustain injury in the larger, more centrally located airways (Stieglitz, 1999). The risk of developing lung cancer is affected by the age at which smoking begins, the length of time a person smokes, the number of cigarettes consumed daily, and how deeply a person inhales when smoking. Individuals who smoke cigars and pipes in addition to cigarettes are at an even greater risk of developing lung cancer.
- *Environmental tobacco smoke.* Environmental tobacco smoke (ETS) exposure, often referred to as involuntary or passive smoking, is responsible for lung cancer in about 3,000 nonsmoking adults each year (Winawer & Shike, 1995).
- *Radon.* Radon is considered to be the cause of 10 percent of all lung cancer deaths and an estimated 30

percent of deaths in those who have never smoked (Kramer et al., 1999). In some parts of the country, excessive radon is found in homes. Radon test kits, which measure levels of radon, are available in many hardware stores. If increased radon levels are found, steps must be taken to reduce the levels. Once radon levels are corrected to acceptable levels, the hazard is gone.

- *Asbestos.* Asbestos is a type of natural fiber used in certain industries. These fibers tend to break off into fine particles, which float in the air and subsequently are easily inhaled. The particles can lodge in the lung and cause damage to cells, thus increasing the risk for lung cancer. Research has shown that workers exposed to asbestos are three to four times more likely to develop lung cancer, although it may have a latent period of over 30 years. Asbestos workers are encouraged to wear protective equipment while working.
- *Lung disease, such as tuberculosis.* Having tuberculosis (TB) increases a person's risk for lung cancer as a result of lung scarring (Cancer Institute, 1999). About 1 in 100 patients with chronic obstructive pulmonary disease develop lung cancer. Also, a person previously diagnosed with lung cancer is more likely to develop a second lung cancer (American Cancer Society, 2000).
- *Genetic predisposition.* There have been observations that lung cancer does not always develop in smokers and is sometimes detected in family clusters. This has led to a search for markers, focusing on genetically determined enzymes of metabolism and DNA repair. An increased incidence of lung cancer has been associated with the activity of cytochrome P-450 enzymes, which are known to activate certain carcinogens (Kramer et al., 1999).

Lung cancer can be grouped into two major types: nonsmall cell and small cell lung cancer. **Nonsmall cell lung cancer** occurs more commonly but typically grows and spreads more slowly. There are three types of nonsmall cell lung cancers, named after the types of cells in which the cancer develops: squamous cell carcinoma, adenocarcinoma, and large cell carcinoma. **Small cell lung cancer,** often referred to as oat cell carcinoma, is less common but grows more quickly and is more likely to spread to other organs (Cancer Institute, 1999).

SYMPTOMS

Lung cancer rarely produces symptoms until the disease is advanced, making early detection difficult. By the time of the diagnosis, the cancer has often metastasized to other parts of the body. Fewer than one in five lung cancers are detected early. The most common signs and symptoms of lung cancer are listed in Box 13–4. These symptoms are not specific to lung cancer and can be caused by a variety of other conditions.

DIAGNOSIS

To determine the cause of symptoms, a provider will evaluate the patient's family, medical and smoking history, and

---

Box 13–4   Signs and Symptoms of Lung Cancer

- Fatigue
- Persistent cough that doesn't go away and worsens over time
- Chronic chest pain
- Shortness of breath, wheezing, or hoarseness

---

any relevant environmental and occupational exposures to potential carcinogens. Along with the history and physical exam, a chest radiograph and other diagnostic tests are often required. If lung cancer is suspected, a **sputum cytology,** a microscopic examination of the sputum produced by a deep cough, is done. To confirm the presence of lung cancer, however, a **biopsy** is necessary. This involves removing a small sample of tissue for a microscopic exam. A biopsy can be performed in a variety of ways:

- *Bronchoscopy.* A bronchoscope is a thin, lighted tube that is inserted through the mouth or nose, passing through the trachea (windpipe), to visualize the breathing passages. Samples of cellular material can be collected through the bronchoscope.
- *Needle aspiration.* A needle is inserted through the chest wall *into* the lung, and a sample of tissue is removed.
- *Thoracentesis.* Fluid from *around* the lung is removed, using a needle inserted through the chest wall.
- *Thoracotomy.* A thoracotomy is a major surgical procedure, which involves surgically opening the chest.

TREATMENT

The treatment of lung cancer is dependent on a number of factors. These include the type of lung cancer present, the size, the location and extent of tumor growth, and the general overall health of the patient. Treatment options include the surgical removal of the tumor, chemotherapy, radiation therapy, and photodynamic therapy (PDT) (Cancer Institute, 1999). **Surgery** is considered the primary treatment when the tumor is confined to one lung. **Chemotherapy,** the use of anticancer drugs to kill cancer cells, and/or **radiation,** the use of high-energy rays that do the same thing, are often used as a follow-up to surgery to eradicate any malignant cells that still may be present. In cases of inoperable cancer (50 percent of all lung cancer), a combination of radiation and chemotherapy is used to control cancer growth or to relieve shortness of breath. Radiation is often the treatment of choice for small cell lung cancer (American Cancer Society, 2000); the simultaneous administration of radiation and chemotherapy has resulted in slightly improved survival rates. **Photodynamic therapy** involves injecting a chemical into the bloodstream, which is absorbed by all cells but remains in cancer cells for a longer time. A laser light is then directed at the site of the cancerous lesion, killing the cancer cells that have absorbed the chemical. In inoperable cancer, photodynamic therapy may be used along with other therapies to reduce bleeding or to relieve breathing difficulties that occur when the tumor mass blocks the airways (Cancer Institute, 1999).

Unlike some other forms of cancer, which are now considered highly curable, lung cancer remains a deadly disease. Although the one-year survival rate has increased from 34 percent in 1975 to 41 percent in 1995 as a result of improvement in surgical techniques, the five-year survival rate for all stages combined is only 14 percent and has not changed over the past three decades (Winawer & Shike, 1995). Patients who have been previously diagnosed with lung cancer are encouraged to have regular checkups, especially if changes in health status have been noticed, to determine if the cancer has returned or if a new cancer has developed. Screening for lung cancer, which generally includes an annual chest X ray, is also advised for high-risk individuals (American Cancer Society, 2000).

The most effective strategy for reducing one's risk for lung cancer is avoiding all forms of tobacco. Research also suggests that consuming several servings of fruits and vegetables provides protection against lung cancer in both smokers and nonsmokers. Most studies attribute this to a strong association with beta-carotene. Retinol, a form of vitamin A, may also have some protective properties.

Respiratory Wellness Self-Assessment

Use the following questions to estimate your level of respiratory wellness. The more questions to which you can answer a definite yes the better.

1. *Are you a nonsmoker?*
2. *Is the space in which you live or work smoke-free?*
3. *Are you careful not to walk or jog alongside heavily trafficked roads or highways?*
4. *Do you know whether you are exposed to environmental pollutants at work? If you are, do you take measures to protect yourself?*
5. *Is your home free of radon?*
6. *Are you free of chronic cough and/or wheezing?*
7. *Are you generally able to walk quickly and climb a flight of stairs without becoming markedly short of breath?*
8. *Are you at a reasonable weight?*

New Directions

As is the case with most health problems, there are no known magic cures on the horizon for respiratory diseases. Ongoing research, however, offers the promise of new treatments. For example, pharmacological research into better treatments for the common cold is focusing on ways of enhancing the im-

mune system to make it better able to ward off colds, and influenza researchers are working on developing a means of producing an influenza vaccine without the use of eggs. This will allow for the vaccination of a greater number of people, because egg allergy will no longer be a barrier.

Current efforts to decrease the morbidity and mortality associated with pneumonia include educating the public about the disease and taking environmental measures to limit its spread. Efforts are also being made to identify the risk factors that are amenable to intervention and to develop more effective antibiotics. The latter is particularly important, considering the recent emergence of resistant bacterial strains. Researchers are also working on new and improved vaccines, particularly oral vaccines that will increase the number of people willing to be vaccinated.

Developing new and better ways of preventing and treating asthma is a priority among researchers who focus on respiratory diseases. More effective ways of identifying the instability and progression of the disease among asthmatics are needed, as well as more effective strategies for identifying and avoiding triggers. New beta-adrenergic and nonbeta adrenergic drugs to prevent and treat asthma attacks are currently under development. Another innovation in drug therapy has to do with decreasing the environmental impact of metered dose inhalers (MDIs). Currently, most MDIs use the ozone-depleting propellant chloroflurocarbon. In the future, however, drug manufacturers will be substituting a less harmful propellant, hydrofluoroalkane.

Convincing a greater percentage of the populace—particularly, young women—to avoid or stop smoking remains a priority goal. The approaches include education, counseling, behavior modification, and pharmacological intervention using both nicotine and nonnicotine drug treatments. New, palliative treatments for lung cancer patients are also being developed. For example, stents are now being used to hold airways open and improve ventilation.

QUESTIONS FOR REFLECTION AND DISCUSSION

1. *What factors may be related to the increasing rates at which girls and women are taking up smoking?*
2. *If you smoke, what are the factors that stop you from quitting? If you do not smoke, what factors might stop a person from quitting?*
3. *To what degree are people responsible for their own respiratory wellness?*

RESOURCES

Books

Barger, W. E. (2000). *Allergies and asthma for dummies.* Hungry Minds, Inc.

Brostoff, J. (2000). *Asthma: The complete guide to integrative therapies*. Inner Traditions International, Limited.

Fisher, E. (1999). *American Lung Association 7 steps to a smoke-free life*. John Wiley & Sons.

Websites

Allergy and Asthma Network
www.aanma.org

American Association of Cardiovascular and Pulmonary Rehabilitation
www.aacvpr.org

American Association for Respiratory Care
www.aarc.org

American Lung Association
www.lungusa.org

REFERENCES

Ahmed, A. E., Nicholson, K. G., & Nguyn-Van-Tam, J. S. (1995). Reduction in mortality associated with influenza vaccine during 1989–90 epidemic. *Lancet, 346*(8975), 591–595.

American Cancer Society. (2000). *Cancer facts & figures 2000.* (Publication No. 5008.00). New York: National Media Office.

Bartlett, J. G., Breiman, R. F., Mandell, L. A., & File, T. M. (1998). Community-acquired pneumonia in adults: Guidelines for management. *Clinical Infectious Diseases, 26,* 811–838.

Cancer Institute. (1999, August 2). *Lung cancer* [On-line]. Available: http://cancernet.nci.nih.gov/wyntk_pubs/lung.htm

Cassiere, H. A., & Fein, A. M. (1997, July). Pneumonia in the elderly: An update. *Emergency Medicine, 29*(7), 41–52.

Connelly, C. (2000). Flu and pneumonia vaccination: your best shot. *Breathe Well, 4*(4), 9–11.

de Marco, R., Locatelli, R., Sunyer, J., & Burney, P. (2000). Differences in incidence of reported asthma related to age in men and women. *American Journal of Medicine, 162*(1), 68–74.

Gross, P. A., Hermogenes, A. W., Sacks, H. S., Lau, J., & Levandowski, R. A. (1995, October). The efficacy of influenza vaccine in elderly persons. A meta-analysis and review of the literature. *Annals of Internal Medicine, 123*(7), 518–527.

Jeffery, R. W., Hennrikus, D. J., Lando, H. A., Murray, D. M., & Liu, J. W. (2000). Reconciling conflicting findings regarding post cessation weight concerns and success in smoking cessation. *Health Psychology, 19*(3), 243–246.

Kramer, B., Gohagan, J., & Prorok, P. (1999). *Cancer screening.* New York: Marcel Dekker.

Lesperance, K. (2000). On the trail of obesity's impact on breathing. *Advance for Respiratory Care Practitioners, 13*(24), 10, 15.

Linnington, G. A., Leonard, C. T., & Sachs, D. P. (2000). Smoking cessation. In J. Rusko (Ed.), *Clinics in chest medicine* (pp. 322–328). Philadelphia: William B. Saunders.

Lucas, B. D. (1999, January). Respiratory infections: Which antibiotics for empiric therapy? *Patient Care for the Nurse Practitioner,* pp. 30–45.

Mitchell, T. (1998). Clearing the air. *Journal for Respiratory Care Practitioners, 3,* 81–83.

Moffatt, R. J., Biggerstaff, K. D., & Stamford, B. A. (2000). Effects of the transdermal nicotine patch on normalization of HDL-C and its subfractions. *Preventive Medicine, 31* (2 Pt. 1), 148–152.

Mooe, T., Rabben, T., Wiklund, U., Franklin, K. A., & Eriksson, P. (1996). Sleep-disordered breathing in women: Occurrence and association with coronary artery disease. *American Journal of Medicine, 101*(3), 251–256.

National Lung Health Education Program Executive Committee. (1998). Strategies in preserving lung health and preventing COPD and associated disease. *Respiratory Care, 43*(3), 185–216.

Olson, L. G., King, M. T., Hensley, M. J., & Saunders, N. A. (1995). A community study of snoring and sleep-disordered breathing prevalence. *American Journal of Respiratory Critical Care Medicine, 152*(2), 711–716.

Palencia, S. (Fall 2000). Treating the flu: Available medications. *Allergy and Asthma Health,* pp. 30–32.

Porath, A., Schlaeffer, F., & Lieberman, D. (1996). Appropriateness of hospitalization of patients with community-acquired pneumonia. *Annals of Emergency Medicine, 27*(2), 176–183.

Pruitt, B. (2000). Special considerations for the geriatric patient: Changes in the cardiopulmonary system. *AARC Times, 24*(10), 17–20.

Rao, V. T. V., & San Pedro, G. S. (1996, October). Nonresolving pneumonia: What to do when pneumonia lingers. *Consultant,* pp. 2191–2199.

Scanlan, C., Wilkins, R., & Stoller, J. (1999). *Fundamentals of respiratory care* (7th ed.). St. Louis: Mosby.

Secondhand smoke. (1998, September). *Women's Health Watch,* p. 6.

Stieglitz, H. (1999, April 21). *Men and women differ in lung cancer lesions* [On-line]. Available: http://unisci.com/stories/19992/04211992.htm

Taking the fight out of a cold. (1998, September). *Health,* p. 36.

Tanoue, L. T. (2000). Cigarette smoking and women's respiratory health. In J. Rusko (Ed.), *Clinics in chest medicine 21*(1), pp. 239–248. Philadelphia: William B. Saunders.

Tobacco smoke and women: A special vulnerability. (2000, May). *Women's Health Watch,* p. 1.

Villablanca, A. C., McDonald, J. M., & Rutledge, J. C. (2000). Smoking and cardiovascular disease. In J. Rusko (Ed.), *Clinics in chest medicine 21*(1), pp. 121–128. Philadelphia: William B. Saunders.

Weil, A. (1997, June). Breathing easier with asthma. *Self Healing,* pp. 1–7.

Wilkins, R. L., Krider, S. J., & Sheldon, R. L. (2000). *Clinical assessment in respiratory care*. St. Louis: Mosby.

Winawer, S. J., & Shike, M. (1995). *Cancer free.* New York: Simon & Schuster.

Young women and smoking [On-line]. (2000, November 11). Available: http://www.inwat.org/young.htm

Zordis, J. D. (1999). The impact of air pollution on COPD. *Journal for Respiratory Care Practitioners, 4,* 43–45, 63.

14

Musculoskeletal Wellness and Illness

Kay L. Huber

Objectives

1. *Identify the markers of musculoskeletal wellness.*
2. *List strategies for promoting musculoskeletal wellness.*
3. *Describe four disorders of the musculoskeletal system that commonly affect women.*
4. *Identify new directions in research for osteoarthritis and osteoporosis.*

Introduction

This chapter addresses musculoskeletal wellness, in terms of its markers, and strategies for promoting it and musculoskeletal illness. Four disorders of the musculoskeletal system of particular concern to women—osteoarthritis, osteoporosis, bunions, and hammer toe—are explored and the related risk factors, pathophysiology, signs and symptoms, diagnostic tests, and treatment options are described. (Rheumatoid arthritis is addressed in Chapter 20.) New directions in research and treatment for the major disorders osteoarthritis and osteoporosis are discussed.

Markers of Musculoskeletal Wellness

The musculoskeletal system, one of the body's largest systems, accounts for over 50 percent of the body's weight. Bones, joints, muscles, and supporting structures provide the stability and mobility necessary for physical activity as all of these components work together to produce movement and to supply structure and support. Muscles pulling on bones produce body movement; the bones serve as levers, and the joints serve as fulcrums for the levers. Because the musculoskeletal, circulatory, and nervous systems are interrelated, any problem that causes disruptions in innervation, circulation, muscle contraction, joint articulation, or support results in musculoskeletal dysfunction. The proper functioning of the musculoskeletal system enables human beings to perform complex and precise movements and to interact with and adapt to the environment. Injuries to this system are common because it serves as the body's first line of defense against external forces. These forces can cause alterations in the structure of bone or soft connective tissue, with functional disability as the result (Lewis, Heitkemper, & Dirksen, 2000). The markers, or indicators, of musculoskeletal wellness are related to muscle strength, joint mobility and function, posture, bone integrity, and feet that are free of soreness and deformity.

Normal Muscle Strength

Skeletal muscle constitutes the largest mass of tissue in the body. Skeletal muscle contractions are responsible for posture and movement. **Isotonic contractions,** such as those that allow an object to be lifted, produce movement, whereas **isometric contractions,** such as pushing against a wall, increase the tension within a muscle but do not produce movement. Most muscle contractions are a combination of both isotonic and isometric. When there is no muscle contraction, **atrophy** (a decrease in size) of the muscle occurs, with resultant loss of function and muscle strength. Healthy muscles are usually *symmetrical bilaterally,* unless the excessive use of a muscle group on one side of the body causes a predictable disproportion. The development of unexplained muscular weakness is cause for concern and investigation.

Normal Joint Mobility and Function

All joints have a normal range of motion, and limitation of joint motion results in some degree of functional loss. Normal joint motion should be symmetrical—that is, the range of motion of a joint on one side of the body should be equal to the range of motion of the same joint on the other side. Joints should move freely throughout their range of motion without pain and without producing the grating sound known as **crepitus.** The presence of *pain and/or swelling* in any joint signifies the presence of a musculoskeletal problem.

Good Posture

The back can be seen as scaffolding on which the body is hung. The spine, or vertebral column, provides strength and mobility and protects the spinal cord. The vertebrae, identified in groups labeled cervical, thoracic, lumbar, and sacral, bend and rotate on discs in the front and joints in the back. The back has natural curves—a gentle concave curve in the lumbar spine and a gentle convex curve in the thoracic spine. The discs provide flexibility and act as shock absorbers. Groups of muscles control movements and support the vertebral column to keep it upright. The *abdominal muscles* are also very important in maintaining good posture and a healthy back.

An easy way to evaluate posture is to stand sideways in front of a full-length mirror wearing tight-fitting clothing, such as a swimsuit. If posture is optimal, it should be possible to visualize a *straight line* running through the front of the earlobe, the front of the shoulder, the center of the hip, just behind the kneecap, and just in front of the ankle bone. The chin should be parallel to the floor. Sitting posture can be evaluated while sitting sideways in an armless chair and visualizing a line running through the same points and out from the center of the hip (Margolis & Kostuik, 1999).

Bone Integrity

Bone is living tissue. It is remodeled constantly by the body, with the rates of **resorption** (loss) and **deposition** (formation of new bone) being equal, so that the total bone mass remains constant. A healthy human skeleton supports good posture and allows strenuous activities, such as running and lifting, to be undertaken without pain or injury. Healthy adult bones do not fracture easily. A pattern of easily sustained fractures suggests the presence of bone disease. This chapter's section on Musculoskeletal Problems and Diseases contains further discussion of bone physiology.

Foot Integrity

Feet may be seen as platforms that provide support for the weight of the body and absorb shock during walking. As such, they undergo a great deal of use, misuse, trauma, and neglect as part of everyday living. The feet have many important functions. They carry the body's weight, hold it erect in an upright and stationary position, coordinate and maintain balance in walking, and conform to the surfaces underfoot. Feet influence physical, psychological, and social well-being. They have a significant effect on the amiability, productivity, and mobility of an individual, as discomfort may cause irritability, fatigue, and loss of mobility (Ebersole & Hess, 1998). Foot problems may increase older adults' risk of falling. The feet can also reflect systemic diseases; sudden or gradual changes in the condition of the skin or nails, and/or recurring infection, may herald the advent of more serious health problems. An important indicator of foot health is *comfort*. Walking reasonable distances in well-fitting, flat or nearly flat shoes should not produce foot pain. Healthy feet are also free of deformities and the painful, built-up calluses known as *corns*. Finally, healthy feet are free of thickened, discolored, or ingrown toenails, as well as itchiness and lesions of any kind.

Promoting Musculoskeletal Wellness

Musculoskeletal wellness is promoted by regular exercise that strengthens muscles and places growth-producing stress on bones. It is also promoted by activities that strengthen the muscles that support the back and by conscious efforts to maintain good posture. Also, musculoskeletal wellness is supported by the regular consumption of a diet that supports bone integrity. Taking measures to protect the feet is also very important.

Maintaining Muscle and Bone Strength Through Exercise

Muscle strength and tone are maintained by the usual activities of daily living and regular exercise. The range of motion of the joints is maintained by regular physical activity in which the joints are fully used. The preservation of bone mass depends on skeletal stress through muscle contraction and weight bearing. The mechanical stress of exercise stimulates bone formation. Unfortunately, women's levels of physical activity are generally lower than are those of similarly aged men and become progressively lower as women age (Gallant, Keita, & Royak-Schaler, 1997). Also, African American women and other ethnic minority populations tend to be less active than Euro-American women. Men are more likely to engage in vigorous exercise and sports; however, both sexes are more likely to continue low- to moderate-intensity physical activities across time. Women's lower level of physical activity puts them at risk for cardiovascular and other chronic diseases. Because regular physical exercise is such a major determinant of health and functioning in women, the importance of its initiation and continuation cannot be understated.

Strengthening and Supporting the Back

Preventive measures that can reduce the risk of damage to the spine and its supporting structures include maintaining correct posture, engaging in regular exercise to strengthen the back and abdominal muscles, and, if needed, using special products that can help reduce back strain.

Maintaining correct posture is a matter of allowing the body to follow the natural S-shaped curves of the spine (Margolis & Kostuik, 1999). A common type of incorrect posture, perpetual slouching with the shoulders rolled forward, causes **kyphosis,** an abnormal accentuation of the usual convex curve of the thoracic spine. Another postural problem, **lordosis** (swayback), in which the abdomen is thrust too far forward and the buttocks too far to the rear, is common in overweight people with weak abdominal muscles. Strengthening the abdominal muscles is especially important for good posture and the prevention of back pain. A protruding abdomen contributes to back pain by pulling the spine out of proper alignment and placing strain on muscles. Mild kyphosis and lordosis can usually be corrected by following an exercise program and, for persons who are overweight, a weight-loss program.

Regular exercise, in addition to helping with weight loss and improving overall health, tones and strengthens the muscles that hold the back in proper alignment. One of the best exercises for improving posture is walking. Walking, running, using a treadmill, and bicycling are types of general conditioning exercises that are beneficial for muscle strength and cardiovascular fitness. Although bicycling provides aerobic exercise, weight-bearing exercises are essential for women who want to prevent osteoporosis.

Various tasks that are performed at work and in the home can place excessive strain on the lower back. Sitting behind a desk or standing all day has as much potential to cause back pain as does lifting heavy objects. Even if sitting posture is correct, it is essential to get up and move around every half-hour or so. Avoiding back strain involves learning to change the way in which many everyday activities are carried out. Box 14–1 contains examples of ways to avoid back strain by maintaining correct posture or improving it.

A variety of exercises can be done to strengthen the back. Exercises should be done at least three times each week for 30 to 60 minutes each time for the best effect (Lueckenotte, 2000). Beneficial weight-bearing exercises that do not stress the joints include walking, low-impact aerobics, and vigorous water exercises. Margolis and Kostuik (2000) point out that women who simply do more gardening and other household chores, as well as spend fewer hours sitting each day, significantly reduce their risk of a hip fracture. Box 14–2 contains examples of muscle-strengthening exercises for the back.

Box 14-1 *Tips for Maintaining and Improving Posture and Avoiding Back Strain*

Sitting Posture

♦ Sit in a straight-backed chair with your hips to the rear of the chair and your shoulders against the chair back, chest lifted, and upper back straight. Place your feet comfortably on the floor, with your knees slightly above your hips (use a small footstool if you need to elevate your feet).

♦ Choose straight-backed chairs with armrests to support the weight of your arms and reduce pressure on your back.

♦ Don't sit for long periods of time; stand while talking on the phone to vary your routine.

♦ Don't cradle the telephone between your neck and shoulder (this can lead to neck and shoulder pain).

♦ If you must sit for prolonged periods, shift your weight occasionally.

♦ Stretch while sitting in a chair by sitting up straight, bending at your waist, and placing your fingers on the floor (repeat five times).

♦ Use a lumbar cushion or portable backrest for extra support and alignment of the spine when sitting or driving.

Standing Posture

♦ Keep your body weight evenly distributed by standing straight and relaxed, maintaining the spine's natural S-curve.

♦ To ease pressure on your back, rest one foot on a raised object, such as a stool, ledge, or chair.

♦ Another way to ease pressure on your back is to stand with one foot in front of the other, with knees slightly bent, while resting your hand or elbow on a ledge or an object at waist level.

♦ Occasionally shift your weight from one leg to the other.

♦ Don't stand in one position for long periods of time.

♦ Try simple stretching exercises when your back feels stiff.

♦ Try to keep one or both knees flexed when sweeping, mopping, vacuuming, or raking.

♦ Stop activities frequently to allow your back to rest.

Lifting

♦ Never bend at the waist to pick up objects, even lightweight ones.

♦ Always bend at the knees when picking up objects.

♦ Carry objects close to your body, and never stoop or twist while carrying a load.

♦ Face the object you intend to lift straight on.

♦ When moving an object, always push it rather than pull it to make better use of your leg and stomach muscles.

♦ Store items at a comfortable height to avoid having to bend over.

♦ Wearing a back support belt may serve as a reminder to bend and lift using proper body mechanics.

Source: Margolis & Kostuik, 1999; Margolis & Kostuik, 2000; Puppione, 1999.

Supporting Bone Strength and Joint Integrity Through Diet

A healthy diet is vital to the development and maintenance of a strong skeletal bone mass. Adequate amounts of calcium, phosphorus, magnesium, and vitamin D are essential for the ongoing synthesis of bone, and protein, vitamin C, and iron are needed for the synthesis of **collagen,** the protein matrix on which bones and teeth are formed. Women attain their peak bone mass by the age of 30–35; however, in the absence of adequate amounts of **calcium,** the bone mass formed is relatively light and insufficiently dense to withstand the demineralization that occurs during and after menopause. Unfortunately, many adolescent women in this culture do not take in sufficient amounts of calcium to build a strong skeleton. An obsession with body image and weight loss gives rise to perpetual dieting, which often means the avoidance of milk, cheese, and other calcium-rich dairy products. Girls who are dieting are also liable to consume large amounts of carbonated diet sodas, which are high in **phosphorus.** The excessive consumption of phosphorus can affect calcium metabolism and bone mass. Additional information on the importance of calcium to bone integrity is provided in the section on Musculoskeletal Problems and Diseases.

Another diet-related problem, **overweight,** is believed to be a leading factor behind the high rates of osteoarthritis in women (Margolis & Flynn, 2000). The joints affected are often weight-bearing joints, and they are stressed and irritated by having to carry excess poundage. Persons with a body mass index (BMI) of 25 or above have an increased risk of osteoarthritis (OA); therefore, keeping BMI below this level can help prevent OA. Body mass index is calculated by dividing body weight in kilograms by squared height in

Box 14–2   Back Exercises

Please note: All exercises should be conducted on a firm surface.

Exercise 1

Lie on back, with knees bent, feet flat on the floor.

Grasp one leg while inhaling.

While exhaling, roll head and shoulders forward, bringing knee to chin—hold 5 seconds.

Inhale; then release and exhale.

Work up to 10 repetitions for each leg.

Exercise 2 (to Stretch Hip, Buttock, and Lower Back Muscles)

Lie on back, with knees bent, feet flat on the floor.

Draw both knees up to chest.

Place both hands around knees and pull them firmly against chest—hold for 30 seconds.

Lower legs and return to starting position.

Repeat 5–10 times.

Exercise 3

Lie flat on back and slowly lift legs until feet are 12 inches from the floor.

Keep legs straight and hold this position for a count of 10.

Lower legs to floor.

Repeat 5 times.

Exercise 4 (to Strengthen Abdominal Muscles)

Lie flat on back, with knees bent, feet flat on the floor, and hands on chest.

Slowly raise head and neck to top of chest.

Reach both hands forward and place on knees—hold for a count of 5 and return to starting position.

Repeat 5–10 times.

Box 14–3   Choosing Footwear

- The shoe must be long and wide enough to prevent crowding the toes and forcing the great toe toward the second toe.
- The width of the shoe at the metatarsal head (the widest area behind the toes) should be sufficient to allow free movement of the foot muscles and to permit the bending of the toes.
- The shank of the shoe should be rigid enough to offer optimum support.
- The height of the heel should be realistic in terms of the purpose for which the shoe is worn.
- The heel should be no more than one inch higher than the forefoot support.

Hints for Buying Comfortable Shoes

- Buy shoes in the afternoon.
- Always try on both shoes before purchasing.
- Don't make impulsive purchases—take the time to find a good fit.
- Allow ¼ to ½ inch between the longest toe and the tip of the shoe.
- Look inside the shoes for cushioning that will increase shock absorption.
- Avoid heels higher than one inch.
- Be certain the shoes are comfortable before purchasing.

Source: Adapted from Lewis, S., Heitkempter, M., & Dirksen, S. (2000). *Medical-surgical nursing* (5th ed.). St. Louis: Mosby; and Ebersole, P. & Hess, P. (1998). *Toward healthy aging* (5th ed.). St. Louis: Mosby.

meters. The following steps can be used to determine personal BMI using pounds and inches:

1. *Multiply your weight in pounds by 704.*
2. *Square your height in inches by multiplying the number by itself.*
3. *Divide the result of step 1 by the result of step 2.*

A person is considered to be overweight when the BMI is between 25 and 29.9 and obese when the BMI is 30 or higher

(Margolis & Flynn, 2000). Persons who have low back pain should be evaluated by a healthcare provider prior to beginning an exercise program. Some forms of exercise may be harmful if an unrecognized musculoskeletal problem exists.

Promoting Foot Health

Many disorders of the feet can be directly attributed to or exacerbated by the type and fit of shoes. Improperly fitted shoes

Box 14–4 Essentials of Good Foot Care

- Wash and inspect your feet daily—use a mirror or magnifying glass, if necessary.
- Dry your feet by blotting, rather than rubbing; pay particular attention to the area between the toes.
- Use emollients, such as cocoa butter, lanolin, or mineral oil, to soften dry skin, but *do not* apply between the toes.
- Cut toenails straight across shortly after bathing or showering; never cut down the corners.
- Wear clean hose or socks daily.
- Avoid shoes that are uncomfortable or ill-fitting.
- Do not open blisters.

- Avoid wearing tight-fitting hose or socks. Be sure support garments have adequate toe room.
- Do not sit with your legs crossed.
- Stop smoking.
- Walk regularly.
- If your feet perspire a lot, dust them with talc or hygienic foot powder.
- Do not go barefoot outdoors.
- Massage your feet daily to improve circulation and promote relaxation.
- If you walk on hard surfaces for long periods of time, wear heel pads or cushions in the bottom of your shoes.

Source: Adapted from Ebersole, P. & Hess, P. (1998). *Toward healthy aging* (5th ed.). St. Louis: Mosby; and Phipps, W., Sands, J., & Marek, J. (1999). *Medical-surgical nursing* (6th ed.). St. Louis: Mosby.

can cause crowding and angulation (unnatural bending) of the toes and can inhibit the normal movement of the foot muscles. It is essential to wear well-constructed and properly fitted shoes in order to have healthy, pain-free feet. Women often select footwear on the basis of fashion rather than on the basis of comfort and support. Only shoes that conform to the feet should be purchased (see Box 14–3). Other essential components of good foot care are highlighted in Box 14–4.

Musculoskeletal Problems and Diseases

The musculoskeletal problems and diseases that affect women's lives most frequently include osteoarthritis, osteoporosis, and common foot problems such as bunions and hammertoe.

Osteoarthritis

Primary osteoarthritis, also known as **degenerative joint disease,** is one of the most prevalent chronic diseases in the older adult population, and the tendency to develop it increases with age. The disease affects men and women equally, but women are more likely to have symptoms. Osteoarthritis is distributed throughout the central and peripheral joints, usually affecting the joints of the hand, wrist, neck, lumbar spine, hip, knee, and ankle. The pattern of joint involvement differs with gender, with women having more joints involved and more frequent complaints of morning stiffness, joint swelling, and nighttime pain. Women tend to have osteoarthritis more often in their hands and knees, whereas men typically develop the disease in their hips (Harris, 1993). Although this disease has little

or no impact on life span, severe involvement of the knees, hips, and spinal column can greatly affect activity levels and quality of life.

Osteoarthritis is generally termed "non-inflammatory arthritis" to distinguish it from rheumatoid arthritis (Phipps, Sands, & Marek, 1999). Although there is no known cause for primary osteoarthritis, the **articular cartilage,** the connective tissue that covers the articulating surfaces of the joints, is affected, whether osteoarthritis is primary or secondary. Degenerative changes in the joint over time cause the joint cartilage to have a rough surface and areas of softening. This process is believed to occur as a result of the digestion of the cartilage by an enzyme, hyaluronidase, normally found in the *synovial fluid,* which is a clear, lubricating fluid secreted by the inner layer of the capsule that surrounds freely movable joints. The layers of cartilage become thinner, and the bony surfaces are drawn closer together. As the cartilage continues to break down, fissures may occur, and fragments of the cartilage become loose. When the cartilage is totally gone from the articular surface, subchondral bone (bone normally covered by cartilage) increases in density and becomes **sclerotic**—that is, **osteophytes** (bone spurs) form at joint margins and at the attachment sites of ligaments and tendons. The osteophytes may break off and appear in the joint cavity as "joint mice."

RISK FACTORS

The risk factors for osteoarthritis can be divided between those that can be modified and those over which individuals have no control (see Table 14–1). There is increasing evidence that osteoarthritis can be inherited through a recessive gene passed down from either parent; however, postmenopausal women taking hormone replacement therapy appear to have a lower risk of developing the disease. The primary risk factor appears to be age because of the gradual,

TABLE 14–1	Risk factors for osteoarthritis.	
Modifiable	**Nonmodifiable**
Obesity	Age
Repetitive joint stressors	Gender
Postmenopausal bone loss	Family history
	Trauma, fractures, infection

Source: Adapted from Arthritis Foundation. (1996, July). *Living Well with Osteoarthritis*. Atlanta, GA: Author.

age-related breakdown of cartilage. Activities and occupations that cause excessive or repetitive stress on knees, hips, and other joints can also cause osteoarthritis and obesity is a predictor for osteoarthritis of the hips and knees. Osteoarthritis caused by repetitive stress and obesity is known as **secondary osteoarthritis.** Regular moderate exercise does not seem to cause osteoarthritis in normal joints.

SYMPTOMS

People rarely have symptoms of primary osteoarthritis before they are in their forties or fifties; however, by age 40, about 90 percent of all people have X-ray evidence of osteoarthritis in weight-bearing joints (Margolis & Flynn, 1999). Systemic symptoms, such as fever and fatigue, are not present in osteoarthritis. Joint involvement is usually asymmetrical (one-sided) but may be symmetrical. **Heberden's nodes** are a common sign of osteoarthritis, especially in women who have primary osteoarthritis. These nodes are bony overgrowths located at the distal interphalangeal (first) joints of the fingers and are often associated with flexion (downward bending) and lateral deviation (sideward bending). **Bouchard's nodes,** seen less often in osteoarthritis, involve the proximal interphalangeal (middle) joints of the fingers. Both types of nodes can cause redness, swelling, tenderness, and aching.

An early symptom related to joint involvement is morning stiffness, usually lasting less than 30 minutes. Joint stiffness may also occur after periods of rest or after being in the same position for an extended period of time. Rest generally relieves the pain caused by motion and weight bearing, but, as the disease progresses, sleep may be disrupted by joint pain. Rising humidity and falling barometric pressure often aggravate the symptoms of osteoarthritis. Audible or palpable crepitus and a limited range of motion are commonly found in affected weight-bearing joints (Kee, Harris, Booth, Rouser, & McCoy, 1998). In many people, the symptoms progress no further, but in others the pain and stiffness gradually worsen until they limit daily activities, such as walking and going up stairs. Gross deformity and partial dislocation of the joint characterize advanced osteoarthritis.

Osteoarthritis of the hip, either unilateral or bilateral, is often extremely disabling. Although men are more often affected than women, osteoarthritis of the hip does occur in many women. The associated pain may be felt in the groin, buttock, or medial side of the thigh or knee, making localization difficult. Pain experienced during standing and walking may become progressively severe, culminating in pain that occurs while sitting or lying down. As osteoarthritis of the hip progresses, lowering the body into chairs and rising from chairs becomes difficult—especially when the chairs are designed so that the hips are lower than the knees while sitting. Loss of motion and gait changes become progressively more significant, and it is more difficult to extend and internally rotate the hip joint.

Persons with osteoarthritis of the knee usually have pain with motion, stiffness after periods of inactivity, and decreased flexion. In the knee, a **varus deformity,** in which part of the limb is turned inward toward the midline of the body, is common. The degeneration of the weight-bearing surfaces, usually seen in older women, is associated with the limitation of motion, crepitus, and a deformity that prevents full extension of the knee or complete movement of the hip.

Osteoarthritis of the spine is the *most common cause of low back pain*. It can also cause stiffness and muscle spasm and can result in an extreme sensitivity of the touch receptors in the skin, weakness in lower extremity muscle groups, decreased or absent reflexes, and pain in the lower leg, as well as other neurological symptoms.

DIAGNOSIS

There are no specific laboratory tests used to diagnose osteoarthritis, but laboratory studies may be ordered to differentiate this disorder from other common diseases that cause swelling and tenderness around joints. The diagnosis of osteoarthritis is usually made on the basis of the person's history and the results of physical assessment and X rays. Some questions that a healthcare provider may ask about symptoms include which joints are involved, when pain is most severe, what is effective for pain relief, whether or not there is any joint inflammation or swelling, and if there is morning stiffness and the length of time it lasts. The physical assessment includes an inspection of all the joints of the hands, arms, legs, feet, and spine to determine how many are affected and whether any joint involvement is symmetrical. It may be useful to obtain synovial fluid from the affected joint when the diagnosis is in doubt. A healthcare provider may also perform an **arthroscopy,** an examination of the interior of a joint by inserting a scope through a small incision, as it allows the direct visualization of the articular surfaces and may detect early disease.

X rays may show joint space narrowing, spur formation, and a partial abnormal separation of the articular surfaces of the joint in the later stages of osteoarthritis. The radiologic findings do not necessarily correlate with the degree of pain

Box 14-5 Recommendations for Joint Protection and Exercise

- Reduce the weight load on joints, such as through a weight management program or aquatic exercise.
- Reduce compressive forces—for example, use a cane, avoid stairs.
- Choose shoes and insoles for their shock reduction benefit.
- Alternate weight-bearing and nonweight-bearing activities.
- Choose exercises to improve and maintain flexibility, strength, endurance, and neuromuscular conditioning.
- Choose nonweight-bearing exercises (such as bicycling or rowing) or partial nonweight-bearing exercises (such as aquatic exercises) when weight-bearing activity must be limited due to pain or joint vulnerability.
- Gradually increase the duration of aerobic exercise.
- Choose a walking speed that does not make joint pain worse.

- Recognize that postexercise joint pain or swelling signals overuse.
- Modify the current exercise program to avoid injury or reinjury.
- Use conditioning exercises as injury prevention and joint protection measures.
- Set realistic exercise goals.
- Learn exercise self-management.
- Take the talk test (if you can talk comfortably while you are exercising, you are not doing too much).
- Exercise at the time of day when you have the least pain and stiffness.
- If pain suddenly gets worse, stop the exercise.
- Avoid being in the same position for a long time.
- Sit in chairs that have a straight back, arms, and a high seat.

Source: Adapted from Minor, M. (1994). Exercise in the management of osteoarthritis of the knee and hip. *Arthritis Care and Research* 7(4), 198–205; & Arthritis Foundation. (1996, July). *Living well with osteoarthritis*. Atlanta: GA. Reprinted with permission of Wiley-Liss., Inc. a subsidiary of John Wiley & Sons, Inc.

or the amount of function, as only 50 to 60 percent of persons with radiographic changes are symptomatic.

TREATMENT OPTIONS

There are currently no specific treatments for osteoarthritis, and there is no evidence that treatment alters the progression of the disease. Therapy is focused on controlling pain, preventing disability, and maintaining or restoring joint function. Controlling pain is important, because, if pain is not effectively managed, the person with osteoarthritis may favor the affected joint, causing surrounding muscles to weaken; immobility, misery, and dependence may result (Kee et al., 1998). The use of Nonsteroidal Anti-inflammatory Drugs (NSAIDs) for pain control is not recommended as first-line treatment. The reasons for this are discussed in the sections on Nondrug Treatments and Drug Therapy.

Nondrug Treatments   The focus and goal of nondrug treatments include maximizing functional capacity and independence, as well as minimizing pain and joint degradation (Ross, 1997). Early treatment can make a significant improvement in quality of life and may alter the course of the disease. An early consultation with a physical therapist may be beneficial in increasing joint movement (Creamer, Flores, & Hochberg, 1998) and may provide a foundation that will encourage lifestyle adaptation. Consultation with an occupational therapist may be helpful in determining the assistive devices that are most effective in maximizing functional ability (Puppione,

1999). A nutritionist is a valuable member of the treatment team for persons whose osteoarthritis is worsened by obesity.

One of the most important nondrug treatments is striking a balance between *rest* and *exercise*. This is crucial for a person with osteoarthritis. Exercise programs should be started with the approval of a healthcare provider and, if possible, under the direction of a physical therapist, who can design and teach exercises to be done at home. Aquatic exercise can increase joint flexibility, strengthen muscles, provide an effective aerobic workout, and increase self-confidence while enabling the person to move about with minimal stress on the joints. Walking while wearing comfortable, supportive exercise shoes helps improve overall body fitness and builds strength while providing potential weight control. Other types of exercise include putting joints through their full range of motion to help maintain healthy cartilage and to prevent **contractures,** or "frozen" joints. Stretching exercises help preserve and increase joint mobility, and isometric, isotonic, and isokinetic exercises increase joint strength and stability (Murphy & Jurisson, 1998). **Isometric exercises** involve increasing muscle tension by applying pressure against a stable resistance, such as a wall or doorframe. **Isotonic exercise,** such as walking, is active exercise during which the muscle contracts and causes movement. In **isokinetic exercise,** such as weight lifting, muscles contract and stretch against resistance. All types of regular exercise have been shown to decrease the long-term disability associated with osteoarthritis. Recommendations for joint protection and exercise are shown in Box 14–5.

Other nondrug approaches to treatment include the use of heat and cold. The appropriate use of *heat,* in the form of a warm bath or shower or warm compresses, may relieve pain and reduce stiffness by relaxing the muscles and stimulating circulation. Other types of heat treatments range from diathermy, the production of heat in the tissues from high-frequency currents, and paraffin dips, usually done by physical therapists, to hot water bottles, electric heating pads, and packs warmed in the microwave. Starting the day with a hot bath or shower may alleviate morning stiffness. Approximately 20–30 minutes of heat is sufficient for relief, and care should be taken against burns.

The application of *cold packs* provides better pain relief than heat for some persons, especially when pain, swelling, and inflammation follow activity or exercise. However, *ice* should never be applied directly to the skin and should be removed before the area becomes numb.

Nutrition provides yet another avenue for nondrug treatment. Diet can be a major component of nondrug therapy for persons who are overweight, as weight loss decreases joint load and therefore joint pain and destruction (Ross, 1997). There are no studies that examine the relationship of diet (other than for weight loss) and osteoarthritis, and the Arthritis Foundation, while acknowledging that some special diets seem to be efficacious, attributes their success to the placebo effect.

Glucosamine and **chondroitin sulfate** are two dietary supplements that have received attention as potential treatments for osteoarthritis and are often taken together. These substances—derived from crustacean shells and animal organs, respectively—are thought to help restore and maintain cartilage (*A "Natural" Approach to Treating Osteoarthritis,* 2000), as well as to relieve pain. Researchers from the Boston University School of Medicine did a systematic analysis of clinical trials on glucosamine and chondroitin sulfate for treating osteoarthritis and concluded that these compounds may have some efficacy against the symptoms of OA (McAlindon, LaValley, Gulin, & Felson, 2000). To date, there is no solid evidence that these two supplements can rebuild cartilage or slow or reverse cartilage loss; however, a major four-year study, started in 1999, is being conducted under the auspices of the National Institutes of Health National Center for Complementary and Alternative Medicine to explore the efficacy of glucosamine and chondroitin in treating osteoarthritis of the knee. Persons with shellfish and/or sulfate allergies and persons with other health problems should consult their healthcare providers prior to taking these supplements. Because dietary supplements are not regulated, consumers need to be mindful that the quality and amount of labeled ingredients may not be accurate. Further information can be obtained from The Arthritis Foundation, the National Institute of Arthritis and Musculoskeletal Diseases of the National Institutes of Health, or the National Center for Complementary and Alternative Medicine of the National Institutes of Health.

Drug Therapy　The drug information in this section is insufficient for making treatment decisions. All drug therapy should be considered in consultation with a healthcare provider.

The first-line drug of choice for treating the pain of osteoarthritis is **acetaminophen** (such as Tylenol). Acetominophen is a relatively safe pain reliever that has no anti-inflammatory effect. Because inflammation plays a minor role in osteoarthritis, treatment with anti-inflammatory medications such as ibuprofen (e.g., Motrin, Advil), naproxen (e.g., Aleve), and ketoprofen (e.g., Orudis KT), which can cause stomach problems, is not usually necessary. Acetaminophen in a daily dose of 2,600–4,000 milligrams is usually as effective in reducing pain as are nonsteroidal anti-inflammatory drugs (NSAIDs). Acetaminophen must, however, be used cautiously by persons who have kidney or liver disease, because serious and permanent liver and kidney damage can result from prolonged use or high doses taken for even short periods of time. All persons should take NSAIDs with caution, because long-term use of these drugs can cause side effects, such as peptic ulcers and stomach irritation and bleeding. NSAIDs interfere with the production of the protective mucus that normally coats the lining of the stomach. Nonsteroidal anti-inflammatory drugs should be taken with food to reduce the risk of adverse effects. All persons taking NSAIDs over a long period of time should have blood tests after the first month and every six months thereafter, to check for bleeding from the stomach and to monitor kidney function (Margolis & Flynn, 1999). The risk of adverse effects from NSAIDs can be minimized by taking those with fewer side effects, such as salsalate, low-dose naproxen, or Arthrotec, which contains a combination of an NSAID and misoprostol, a drug that protects the stomach. Medications that protect the stomach, such as omeprazole (Prilosec), sucralfate (Carafate), or cimetidine (Tagamet) can also be taken concurrently with NSAIDs. Misoprostol (Cytotec) is the only drug currently approved by the Food and Drug Administration for use with NSAIDs to prevent stomach ulcers.

COX-2 inhibitors, among the newest drugs available to treat arthritis, appear to be less likely than NSAIDs to cause gastrointestinal bleeding or peptic ulcers. These drugs selectively target an enzyme that triggers pain and inflammation. The drug specifically recommended for osteoarthritis is rofecoxib (Vioxx), which is usually taken only once a day.

Osteoarthritis of the knee can be treated with a new therapy called **viscosupplementation,** which reduces joint pain by supplementing the natural lubricating and shock-absorbing properties of synovial fluid. Viscosupplementing agents, such as Hyalgan and Synvisc, are derived from hyaluronan, a substance found naturally in synovial fluid. They are introduced directly into the knee joint via a series of injections over a specific period of time. Whether they are effective on other joints or in other forms of arthritis is not yet known. Hyalgan and Synvisc have anti-inflammatory effects, a short-term lubricant effect, and an analgesic effect, and they stimulate the synovial lining cells to produce normal hyaluronan (Leslie, 1999). Both drugs provide pain relief for about six months with few side effects, but there is no information on their long-term effects or evidence that they will alter the progression of osteoarthritis of the knee.

Topical products, products applied to the skin, for osteoarthritis can also provide temporary pain relief. Some of these products, called *counter-irritants,* mask pain by stimulating a warm or cool sensation, which may distract users from the underlying discomfort. The active ingredient in these preparations is usually camphor, menthol, or turpentine oil. Other topical preparations offer limited direct pain relief by reducing the amount of specific neurotransmitters, chemicals that transmit pain impulses to the central nervous system, inside an aching joint (Margolis & Flynn, 1999). Neurotransmitters may encourage inflammation. **Capsaicin** is a compound that reduces the amount of a specific neurotransmitter called substance P. Substance P is thought to be responsible for enhancing cartilage destruction, releasing inflammation-causing enzymes, and carrying pain impulses to the nervous system. One group of researchers (Altman et al., 1994) found 0.025% capsaicin cream to be so effective and safe that they recommended that it be used as first-line therapy for osteoarthritis. Numerous preparations are now available over-the-counter that contain varying amounts of capsaicin. All of the preparations must be applied to the affected joints three or four times a day, and the effects of the preparations disappear if use is discontinued. It is important that persons using topical preparations follow the package directions and stop using the product immediately if skin irritation develops.

Joints can be injected with **corticosteroids** to provide temporary pain relief and increased mobility. Pain relief lasts from several weeks to several months, but an individual joint should not be injected more than three times a year, because the accelerated deterioration of bone and cartilage can occur when frequent injections are administered over an extended period. Steroid injection should not be used on joints that are infected.

Surgical Options   A number of surgical procedures can relieve pain, improve function, or correct deformities when osteoarthritis becomes disabling. Surgery can be performed to preserve or restore articular cartilage or to realign, fuse, or replace joints. These procedures are usually performed when drug therapy and physical therapy have been unsuccessful and should be done before severe deformity, joint instability, contractures, or severe muscle atrophy develop.

Arthroscopy can be performed on the knee, shoulder, wrist, elbow, and hip. It can be used to *inspect the joint* and confirm the diagnosis of arthritis or therapeutically to *repair torn cartilage.* Arthroscopy can also be used to abrade rough cartilage in order to stimulate its growth and to remove loose bone fragments.

Osteotomy, or the surgical incision of bone, can be done in order to realign a joint or bone or to redistribute the load-bearing surface of a joint. In osteoarthritis cases, osteotomy is used to remove areas of bone that cause joint misalignment.

Arthrodesis, or the fusing of two bones to form a single bone, is done to relieve pain and to restore joint stability and alignment. The procedure has limited use because the fusion results in lost motion. Arthrodesis is most commonly performed on the cervical and lumbar spine and the joints of the fingers, wrists, and ankles.

Arthroplasty, or joint replacement, involves removing the entire damaged joint and replacing it with a mechanical one. Most joint replacements involve the hip and the knee; however, joints in the elbows, shoulders, hands, and feet can also be replaced. Joint replacement may be indicated when joint pain is severe enough to cause awakening at night or when it limits walking to about one block. It is also used when there is severe pain and evidence of substantial joint degeneration on an X ray (Margolis & Flynn, 1999). The decision to consider surgery should be made only after more conservative treatments have been unsuccessful.

Alternative Therapies   Alternative therapies for osteoarthritis include acupuncture, aromatherapy, massage therapy, relaxation techniques, imagery, distraction, and music (see Chapter 11). The potential usefulness of these therapies can be determined following an evaluation of the coping strategies currently being used by the person with osteoarthritis. In no case should the person discount the value of other nondrug approaches or the use of medication for pain relief.

PSYCHOSOCIAL CONSIDERATIONS

Learning to cope with osteoarthritis leads to fewer feelings of stress or depression, a greater feeling of control, and a more positive outlook (Arthritis Foundation, 1996). There is, however, little information available about psychosocial factors and their influence on coping with osteoarthritis. Interventions supported by the few studies that have been done include helping the person understand the nature of osteoarthritis, explaining the physiological effects of the disease in understandable terms, and teaching strategies for maintaining function. A recent study by Blixen and Kippes (1999) explored depression, social support, and the quality of life in older adults with osteoarthritis. They found that, although depression was present in almost half the sample, the self-reported quality of life was extremely high in the group of people who had large, informal social support networks made up of family and friends. The researchers concluded that *social support* appeared to play an important role in moderating the effects of pain, functional limitation, and depression on the quality of life.

Osteoporosis

Osteoporosis is a disease characterized by *low bone mass* and the *structural deterioration* of bone tissue. It leads to bone fragility and an increased susceptibility to fractures of the hip, spine, and wrist. This major health problem is defined by The National Osteoporosis Foundation (NOF) as the most common bone disorder in the Western world. It affects more than 28 million Americans, 80 percent of whom are women. The NOF estimates that between 13 percent and 18 percent of postmenopausal Euro-American women in America (4 to 6 million) have osteoporosis, and an additional 30 to 50 percent (13 to 17 million) have low bone mineral density at the hip (National Osteoporosis Foundation, 1999a). The foundation also indicates that approximately 10 percent of African American women over age 50 have osteoporosis, and an additional 30 percent have low bone mineral density. The average age of onset for women is 55 years. The National Osteoporosis Foundation estimates that one in two women and one in eight men over the age of 50 will have an osteoporosis-related fracture in their lifetimes, and the prevalence of this health problem will *increase,* because elderly women are the fastest growing segment of the U.S. population. Attention is also beginning to be focused on the development of osteoporosis in men, as it is believed that, by age 75, nearly one-third of all men have the disease (Beier, Maricic, & Staats, 1998).

Osteoporosis is classified as either a primary age-related disease or as a secondary disease related to another cause or medical condition. Primary osteoporosis can be further subdivided into Type I and Type II. **Type I** is the estrogen deficiency–induced bone loss of early menopause. **Type II** is the more severe bone loss seen in older people. Type II osteoporosis is thought to be caused by an age-related decline in vitamin D production and the development of intestinal resistance to vitamin D. Resistance to vitamin D leads to decreased intestinal calcium absorption (Burki, 1999).

Bone is remodeled constantly by the body, with the rates of resorption and deposition being equal (during youth), so that the total bone mass remains constant. Peak bone mass occurs during adolescence, but later bone loss is inevitable. Rapid bone loss often occurs in women at menopause. By the time a person reaches age 75, the skeletal mass is reduced about 50 percent from age 30 levels. When osteoporosis occurs, bone resorption greatly exceeds bone deposition, and the resultant weakening of the bone occurs most commonly in the spine, hips, and wrists.

The vertebrae, pelvis, flat bones, and ends of the long bones are made up of predominantly **trabecular bone,** which is more metabolically active than **cortical bone,** which is found in the shafts of the long bones. Cortical thinning begins around age 40, increases with aging, and almost ceases in late life. Postmenopausal women lose cortical bone at a rate of 2 to 3 percent per year, returning to normal levels about 10 years after menopause (Phipps et al., 1999). Trabecular bone loss begins even earlier in both sexes, and is lost in greater amounts. The rate of trabecular bone loss is as high as 8 percent annually following menopause. As bone density decreases, the ability of trabecular bone to withstand mechanical stressors also decreases. Women eventually lose about 35 percent of their cortical bone and approximately 50 percent of their trabecular

TABLE 14–2 Risk factors for primary osteoporosis.	
Nonmodifiable	**Potentially Modifiable**
• Aging • Female sex • Euro-American ethnicity • Thin, small frame • Family history of osteoporosis	• Chronic calcium deficiency • Vitamin D deficiency • Sedentary lifestyle • Smoking • Excessive use of alcohol • Diet high in protein and fat • Menopause—surgical or natural

Source: Adapted from *Physician's Guide to Osteoporosis Prevention and Management* (Copyright NOF, 1998). Reprinted with permission from the National Osteoporosis Foundation, Washington, DC 20037.

bone, whereas men lose about 23 percent and 33 percent, respectively (Whitmore, 1998).

The National Osteoporosis Foundation (1998) states that all women should be counseled regarding the risk factors for osteoporosis because there are no warning signs until a fracture occurs. It appears that there is significant risk for developing osteoporosis in people of all ethnic backgrounds, even though the majority of persons currently affected with the disease are Euro-Americans. The risk factors for primary osteoporosis can be divided into the categories of nonmodifiable and potentially modifiable (see Table 14–2).

It has recently been suggested that vitamin k may play a role in bone health (Olson, 2000). Lark (2001) suggests that a diet too high in acid-forming foods (such as red meat and pork) can contribute to osteoporosis because in order to balance the extra acid in the blood, the alkaline mineral calcium is released from bone into the blood. Indeed, a 1999 study (Tucker et al.) indicated that elderly people who consume a diet rich in alkaline-forming fruits and vegetables have higher bone mass than those who do not. Caffeine intake has not been found to be related to bone mass (Chinchilli, 1997).

The risk factors for secondary osteoporosis are numerous and include endocrine disorders, such as diabetes and the chronic, exercise-related suppression of menstruation, as well as prolonged drug therapy with corticosteroids, certain anti-seizure medications, aluminum-containing antacids, and certain diuretics. Disuse of extremities due to paralysis or prolonged bed rest can also cause osteoporosis, as can anorexia nervosa and gastrointestinal diseases that cause diarrhea or decreased absorption of nutrients.

SYMPTOMS

Osteoporosis is sometimes called the "silent thief" because most persons who are affected have no outward signs of the

TABLE 14–3	Risk factors for fracture in persons with osteoporosis.

Nonmodifiable	Modifiable
• Experienced fracture as an adult	• Currently smokes cigarettes
• Has first-degree relative with history of fracture	• Has low body weight
• Is a Euro-American female	• Has an untreated estrogen deficiency
• Is of advanced age	• Has lifelong low calcium intake
• Has dementia	• Uses alcohol excessively
• Is frail and in poor health	• Has recurring falls
• Has decreased visual acuity despite correction	• Has decreased or inadequate physical activity

Source: Adapted from Physician's guide to Osteoporosis prevention and treatment (Copyright NOF, 1998). Reprinted with permission from the National Osteoporosis Foundation, Washington, DC 20037.

Box 14–6 Screening Guidelines for Bone Mineral Density Assessment

- ♦ All postmenopausal women under the age of 65 who have one or more risk factors for osteoporotic fractures in addition to menopause
- ♦ All women age 65 and older, regardless of additional risk factors for fracture
- ♦ All postmenopausal women who present with a fracture
- ♦ Women considering treatment for osteoporosis when BMD would facilitate the decision
- ♦ Women who have been on hormone replacement therapy for a long period of time

Source: Adapted from Physician's guide to Osteoporosis prevention and treatment (Copyright NOF, 1998). Reprinted with permission from the National Osteoporosis Foundation, Washington, DC 20037.

disease. A person with osteoporosis is free of symptoms until fractures occur. The earliest manifestations of the disease may be acute back pain, as a result of a vertebral fracture, or a fracture of the wrist after a fall on an outstretched hand. Fractures of the hip may occur with little or no trauma. Vertebral fractures may result in restricted motion of the spine, thoracic kyphosis (**dowager's hump**), loss of height, and a protruding abdomen. At the time of a fracture, the person may experience paravertebral muscle spasms. The consequences of osteoporotic fractures include chronic pain, loss of physical function, body deformity, muscle weakness, social isolation, and loss of independent living (McClung, 1999).

All women should be evaluated for fracture risk after menopause. The National Osteoporosis Foundation (1998) separates the risk factors for osteoporotic fracture into nonmodifiable and modifiable categories (see Table 14–3). The primary factors associated with fracture include a decrease in bone mass and bone strength, impaired bone quality, and poor bone mineralization accompanied by an injury. Decreased bone mineral density (BMD) is one of the most important factors that contribute to fracture risk in older adults. Bone density in the hip is more strongly related to the subsequent risk of hip fracture than is bone density in the spine, wrist, or heel (Notelovitz, 1997). A risk factor assessment for osteoporosis can be obtained from the National Osteoporosis Foundation (see the Resources section at the end of this chapter).

DIAGNOSIS

The evaluation of a person for the diagnosis of osteoporosis will begin with a thorough history and a physical examination to identify the nutritional, genetic, and lifestyle factors that may affect bone mass and fracture risk. All present and past use of medications will be documented, including over-the-counter preparations and any drugs associated with an increased risk of osteoporosis. During the physical examination, height will be measured and compared with the self-reported maximum height in young adulthood, as loss of height may suggest that vertebral fractures have occurred. There will also be an assessment for chronic low back pain and lower-extremity muscle weakness. Laboratory tests may be used to check for the possible secondary causes of bone loss.

Routine X rays have limited sensitivity for assessing BMD, because 30 to 40 percent of bone mineral must be lost before X rays can detect a change in density. The National Osteoporosis Foundation's (1998) guidelines as to who should be tested for bone mineral density are shown in Box 14–6.

According to the World Health Organization standard, osteoporosis is diagnosed by BMD when bone mass is less than 2.5 standard deviations below the average values measured in young women. The National Osteoporosis Foundation uses 2 standard deviations or more below the peak adult range (Phipps et al., 1999).

All the types of bone density tests available are safe, have acceptable precision and accuracy, and have been demonstrated to predict fracture risk. The gold standard for hip fracture prediction is **dual energy X ray absorptiometry (DEXA)** of the proximal femur (thigh bone). This technique can also measure BMD at other sites, such as the spine and forearm. Less precise screening can be done using sites such as the finger and the heel, but definitive testing using the gold standard should be considered for postmenopausal women. As of July 1, 1998, the Medicare Bone Mass Measurement

TABLE 14–4 Prevention and treatment of osteoporosis.

Nonpharmacologic Therapy	Pharmacologic Therapy
• Adequate dietary intake of calcium and vitamin D • Regular weight-bearing exercise • Avoidance of tobacco smoking • Alcohol use in moderation only	• Estrogen/hormone replacement • Alendronate (Fosamax) • Calcitonin • Raloxifene (Evista)

Source: Adapted from Physician's Guide to Osteoporosis Prevention and Management (Copyright NOF, 1998). Reprinted with permission from the National Osteoporosis Foundation, Washington, DC 20037.

Coverage Standardization Act established the national criteria for bone density test reimbursement in the Medicare program (Centers for Disease Control and Prevention, 1998). There is now standardized coverage for persons at high risk for osteoporosis.

PREVENTION AND TREATMENT OPTIONS

The prevention and treatment options are frequently one and the same. Interventions to maximize and preserve bone mass can be universally recommended for all persons (see Table 14–4).

Nonpharmacologic Treatment and Prevention Options

The nonpharmacologic options include calcium and vitamin D supplementation, exercise, and avoidance of smoking and excess alcohol intake.

Calcium and vitamin D The National Osteoporosis Foundation (1998) recommends that all persons obtain an adequate intake of dietary calcium (at least 1,200 mg/day, including supplements if necessary) and vitamin D (400–800 IU/day for persons at risk of deficiency). Many healthcare providers recommend at least 1,500 mg per day of calcium, especially for postmenopausal women who are not taking estrogen or who are over age 65. The typical American diet commonly provides only 400 to 600 mg/day, so the use of calcium supplements to make up the difference is usually necessary. The current emphasis on avoiding high-fat dairy products to lower blood cholesterol levels contributes to a reduction in dietary calcium. The best sources of calcium are low-fat milk and other dairy products, canned salmon with bones, calcium-fortified orange juice, leafy green vegetables, almonds, breads, cereals, pastas, and other grain products.

There are many nonprescription calcium supplements available, and consumers must make informed choices when purchasing any supplement. Although most brand-name calcium products are easily absorbed, some may not be. If there is no information about absorption on the package, a simple at-home test can be performed: Place the tablet in a small amount of warm water and allow it to remain for 30 minutes, stirring it occasionally. If the tablet has not dissolved within this time, it probably will not dissolve in the stomach (National Osteoporosis Foundation, 1999b). Chewable and liquid calcium supplements dissolve well and are easy preparations to use for people who have difficulty swallowing pills. Calcium *carbonate* contains about 40 percent calcium in each tablet and is best absorbed when taken with food. Calcium *citrate*, which contains about 50 percent calcium in each tablet, can be taken at any time. Consumers should avoid calcium derived from unrefined oyster shell, bone meal, or dolomite, unless the package bears the United States Pharmacopeia symbol. These substances historically have contained higher levels of lead and other toxic metals.

It is advisable to discuss calcium supplementation with either a pharmacist or a healthcare provider because of possible interactions between calcium and prescription or other over-the-counter medications. For example, calcium interferes with iron absorption, so a calcium supplement should not be taken at the same time as the iron supplement (Priestwood & Weksler, 1997).

Vitamin D plays a major role in the absorption of calcium. A daily intake of 400 to 800 IU of vitamin D is recommended for persons at risk of deficiency, such as older adults and persons who are chronically ill, homebound, or institutionalized. Major dietary sources of vitamin D include vitamin D–fortified milk and cereals, egg yolks, saltwater fish, and liver. Most multiple vitamin preparations and many calcium supplements also contain vitamin D. Both vitamin D and calcium are necessary for the optimal treatment of osteoporosis in women who are taking prescription medications for the prevention or treatment of this health problem (Osteoporosis, 2000).

Regular Weight-Bearing Exercise Weight-bearing exercise is an integral part of all osteoporosis prevention and treatment strategies. Weight-bearing and muscle-strengthening exercise can improve agility and flexibility, strength, coordination, and balance, all attributes that can reduce the risk of falls. Additionally, regular weight-bearing exercise, such as walking and stair climbing, may produce a modest increase in bone density (National Osteoporosis Foundation, 1998). More strenuous exercise, such as jogging or dance aerobics, is also effective at preserving bone mass, but it may be too jarring for some persons who already have osteoporosis. Golf and tennis, which twist the back, may add undue stress to already weakened bones. Persons with osteoporosis should avoid rowing machines, because the bending required to operate the machine may cause a low-back sprain or vertebral fracture (Margolis & Kostuik, 1999). Exercise is most beneficial when it is performed three or four times a week for at least 20 minutes.

Avoidance of Tobacco Use and Excess Alcohol Intake Smoking increases the metabolism of estrogens in the liver and lowers active hormone levels (Prestwood & Weksler, 1997). This is undesirable because estrogen contributes to bone strength. Women who smoke tend to begin menopause, and the associated bone loss, at an earlier age than women who do not smoke. Also, postmenopausal women who smoke *do not get the same benefit from hormone replacement therapy* as women who do not smoke. Smoking cessation is highly recommended for all persons who smoke, because the use of tobacco is detrimental to general health as well as to the skeleton. Alcohol abuse is also associated with decreased bone mass and increased fractures.

A substance called **ipriflavone,** a synthetic isoflavone structurally similar to soy isoflavones and sold as a dietary supplement, showed early promise as an alternative therapy for osteoporosis. In small trials conducted in Asia and Europe, it appeared to stimulate bone formation and inhibit bone resorbtion (Margolis & Konstuik, 2000). However, a larger, well-controlled trial involving 474 postmenopausal Euro-American women failed to demonstrate that taking 200 mg. of ipriflavone for three years improved bone mineral density (Alexanderson et al., 2001).

Pharmacologic Prevention and Treatment Options
Taking **antiresorptive drugs** reduces fracture risk in postmenopausal women who are at risk for or who have osteoporosis. Antiresorptive drugs preserve or increase bone density while decreasing the rate of bone resorption. The antiresorptive drugs include estrogen, bisphosphonates, calcitonin, and selective estrogen receptor modulators.

Hormone Replacement Therapy Hormone replacement therapy (HRT) is the most frequently used intervention in preventing and treating osteoporosis because of estrogen's proven ability to prevent and stabilize bone loss and to prevent osteoporotic fractures (Beier et al., 1998). All women should discuss the appropriateness of hormone replacement therapy with their physician at the time of menopause or when ovarian function is lost. The National Osteoporosis Foundation (1998) points out that epidemiological studies of HRT indicate a 50 to 80 percent decrease in vertebral fractures and a 25 percent decrease in nonvertebral fractures after a woman takes HRT for five years. The sooner HRT is started after menopause, the greater the preservation of bone. Several studies suggest that some lessening of bone loss is possible even when HRT is started some years after menopause (Margolis & Kostuik, 1999).

Bisphosphonates Bisphosphonates are antiresorptive agents that bind to the surface of bone and inhibit bone resorption by mechanisms that are not well understood. There are four oral bisphosphonates available in the United States, and **alendronate (Fosamax)** is the one most commonly prescribed for the prevention and treatment of osteoporosis.

Treatment with alendronate reduces the incidence of fracture of the spine, hip, and wrist by 50 percent in persons with osteoporosis. According to the National Osteoporosis Foundation (1998), alendronate is a powerful option for those women who meet BMD criteria for treatment but who are unwilling or unable to take HRT. Alendronate is available in both daily and weekly dosing formulations. The drug must be taken on an empty stomach, first thing in the morning, with a full glass of water, at least 30 minutes before eating or drinking. It cannot be taken with other beverages, medications, or nutritional supplements, and an upright posture must be maintained for 30 minutes to speed absorption. A significant proportion of persons who take this drug experience upper gastrointestinal disturbance, especially chest pain, heartburn, and painful or difficult swallowing.

Calcitonin Calcitonin is another substance that inhibits bone resorption. It is synthesized and secreted by the thyroid gland. Calcitonin is effective in decreasing spinal bone loss during menopause, but it does not decrease cortical bone loss in the extremities (Notelovitz, 1997). This drug has a central analgesic effect, which may be useful in managing the pain of an acute vertebral fracture. Calcitonin was available only in an injectable form for many years, but it is now available as a nasal spray. The recommended dose of nasal spray is 200 IU/day in alternating nostrils. The principal side effects from the nasal spray include rhinitis and irritation of the nasal mucosa.

Raloxifene Raloxifene is classified as a **selective estrogen receptor modulator (SERM).** It confers the beneficial effects of estrogens without stimulating breast and uterine tissues. Because raloxifene blocks estrogen receptors in the uterus and in the breast, it causes neither bleeding nor sore breasts. However, it does not treat vasomotor symptoms and urogenital atrophy, as estrogen does, so it is not ideal for the treatment of early menopausal symptoms. Raloxifene can be administered without concurrent progesterone therapy. It has been shown to prevent bone loss and to reduce the risk of vertebral fracture by 40 to 50 percent. The side effects are generally mild—primarily, hot flashes, leg cramps, and sinus inflammation—with the most serious adverse effect being a greater risk of deep vein thrombosis. Persons with congestive heart failure or who are at risk for blood clots should not take the drug. Therapy should be discontinued at least 72 hours prior to any anticipated period of prolonged immobilization (bed rest or a long airplane flight), which raises the risk of blood clots (Margolis & Kostuik, 1999). The long-term effectiveness and safety of raloxifene remain unknown at this time.

Common Foot Problems

Disorders of the human foot, particularly the female foot, are often caused by poorly fitted shoes. Modern civilization has disregarded the physiology of the foot, and fashion, vanity, and visual appeal, rather than function, dictate women's choices of footwear.

BUNIONS

The term *bunion* refers to a combination of two related pathologies: a deformity of the great toe and first metatarsal head (**hallux valgus**), which causes the great toe to progressively deviate laterally toward the second toe, and the concomitant development of metatarsal **bursitis.** Bursae are disc-shaped, fluid-filled structures that naturally surround some joints and that form around others as a response to ongoing pressure and irritation. Their purpose is to decrease friction and promote ease of motion. Bursae are made of connective tissue and can become inflamed and painful. Women experience hallux valgus deformity 10 to 15 times more frequently than men, most commonly in the sixth decade of life. Factors that contribute to the development of hallux valgus and bunions include familial tendency, narrow shoes that cause crowding and angulation of the toes, and the age-related gradual widening and lengthening of the foot.

Treatment is based on the age of the person, the degree of the deformity, and the severity of the symptoms. Wearing properly fitted shoes that allow room for the toes and that do not exert pressure on the protruding bunion may be all the treatment that is needed. Corticosteroids can be injected directly into the joint to decrease the acute inflammation. Acetaminophen or nonsteroidal anti-inflammatory medications can be taken to relieve pain. Protective padding can be taped under the metatarsal head (ball of the foot) to ease the weight-bearing pressure.

If conservative treatment fails, the surgical removal of the bunion and the realignment of the toe may be necessary to improve function and appearance. Numerous types of surgical procedures can be used to correct this deformity, and they all involve the resection of bone, fixation of the joint, and revision of the soft tissue structure. Following surgery, wearing certain types of shoes may no longer be possible.

HAMMER TOE

A hammer toe is a flexion deformity of the proximal interphalangeal joint. It may involve several toes and often accompanies hallux valgus. Hammer toe deformity is usually acquired by wearing tight shoes or socks that push an overlying toe back into the line of the other toes. The toes are usually pulled upward, forcing the ball of the foot downward. Corns can develop on the tops of the toes, along with calluses under the metatarsal area. Treatment consists of conservative measures, such as using pads to cushion the foot from the shoe, removing corns, performing manipulative or passive stretching exercises, and wearing open-toed sandals or shoes that conform to the shape of the foot. Surgery may be necessary to correct an established deformity.

Musculoskeletal Wellness Self-Assessment

Use your answers to the following statements to assess your musculoskeletal wellness. Answer each question with a yes or no. The more questions to which you can honestly answer yes, the greater your degree of musculoskeletal wellness.

1. *I walk or engage in other weight-bearing exercise at least four days a week.*
2. *I regularly engage in activities or exercises that strengthen my arms and back.*
3. *My spinal column is straight when viewed from the rear, and my upper back is bilaterally symmetrical when viewed from the side.*
4. *I seek to maintain proper posture at all times.*
5. *I almost always wear comfortable, supportive, low or no-heel shoes.*
6. *I make certain my dietary intake of calcium is sufficient.*
7. *I consume carbonated beverages only occasionally.*
8. *My weight is within the normal range for my height and build.*
9. *I have no pain, redness, or swelling in any of my joints.*
10. *The range of motion in the joints in my extremities is symmetrical bilaterally.*
11. *I am aware of no unusual weakness in any muscle or muscle group.*
12. *My bones do not fracture easily, and I do not have dowager's hump.*
13. *Walking is not painful for me.*

New Directions

Researchers are currently investigating new methods that may halt or repair the joint damage that occurs from osteoarthritis. Treatments currently under investigation include a new class of medications called disease-modifying drugs for osteoarthritis, cartilage transplants, and genetic therapy.

Some non-FDA-approved drugs currently exist that are used for the prevention and treatment of osteoporosis. These nonapproved agents include sodium fluoride, calcitriol, and bisphosphonates other than alendronate and risedronate. The National Osteoporosis Foundation (1998) does not advocate the use of nonapproved drugs at this time. However, there are two other bisphosphonates that are currently being prescribed (etidronate disodium, pamidronate disodium) to treat postmenopausal osteoporosis (Kleerekoper, 1999).

Parathyroid hormone may be the first true **anabolic** (tissue-building) substance to be used to treat osteoporosis. This substance, when given by daily injection together with oral estrogen, may increase bone formation. Because the drug cannot be given orally, studies will need to demonstrate that it provides substantial improvement over oral preparations.

Other new agents that may prove effective in the prevention and treatment of osteoporosis include a new formulation of alendronate, new and improved selective estrogen response modifiers, a new bisphosphonate that would require one injection every three months, and a nasal spray containing parathyroid hormone. Researchers are also working on the development of a safe and effective sodium fluoride regimen (Kleerekoper, 1999).

QUESTIONS FOR REFLECTION AND DISCUSSION

1. *What elements would you include in a musculoskeletal wellness program for adolescent girls?*
2. *What elements would you include in a musculoskeletal wellness program for middle-aged women?*
3. *Why are prevention and treatment regimens for osteoporosis often identical?*
4. *Why are women especially susceptible to the musculoskeletal disorders covered in this chapter?*

RESOURCES

Books

Good Living with Osteoarthritis (2000), a publication of the Arthritis Foundation. Longstreet Press.

The Osteoporosis Book: A Guide for Patients and Their Families (2001), by Nancy E. Lane, MD. Oxford University Press.

Strong Women, Strong Bones (2000) by Miriam Nelson. Putnam Publishing Group.

Organizations

American Academy of Orthopaedic Surgeons
American Association of Orthopaedic Surgeons
6300 N. River Rd.
Rosemont, IL 60018-4262
Web: www.aaos.org

Arthritis Foundation
1330 Peachtree St.
Atlanta, GA 30309
Phone: 1-800-283-7800
Web: www.arthritis.org

American Orthopaedic Foot and Ankle Society
1216 Pine St., Suite 201
Seattle, WA 98101
Web: www.aofas.org

Creighton University Osteoporosis Research Center
2500 California Plaza
Omaha, NE 68178
Web: www.osteoporosis.creighton.edu

National Arthritis and Musculoskeletal and Skin Diseases Information Clearinghouse
NAMSIC AMS Circle
National Institutes of Health
9000 Rockville Pike, Bldg. 31, Room 4C32
Bethesda, MD 20892-3675
Web: www.nih.gov/niams

National Institutes of Health
Osteoporosis and Related Bone Diseases—National Resource Center
1232 22nd St., NW
Washington, DC 20037-1292
Phone: 1-800-624-BONE
Web: www.osteo.org/index.html

National Osteoporosis Foundation
1232 22nd St., NW
Washington, DC 20037-1292
Web: www.nof.org

Townsend Design
4615 Shepard St.
Bakersfield, CA 93313
Phone: 1-800-432-3466
Web: www.townsenddesign.com

U.S. Food and Drug Administration
Center for Food Safety and Applied Nutrition
200 C St., SW
Washington, DC 20204
Web: http://vm.cfsan.fda.gov/list.html

Websites

American Association of Othopaedic Foot and Ankle Surgeons
www.footdocs.org

Arthritis Connection
www.arthritisconnection.com

Fitness Link
www.fitnesslink.com

International Osteoporosis Foundation
www.effo.org

REFERENCES

Alexanderson, P., Toussaint, A., Christiansen, C., Devogelaer, J.P., Roux, C., Fechtenbaum, J., Gennari, C., Reginster, J. Y., (2001). Ipriflavone in the treatment of postmenopausal osteoporosis. *Journal of the American Medical Association, 285*(11), 1482–1488.

Altman, R., Aven, A., Holmburg, C., Pfeifer, L., Sack, M., & Young, G. (1994). Capsaicin cream 0.025% as monotherapy for osteoarthritis: A double-blind study. *Seminars in Arthritis and Rheumatism, 23*(6), 25–33.

Arthritis Foundation. (1996). *Living well with osteoarthritis.* Atlanta: Author.

Beier, M., Maricic, M., & Staats, D. (1998). Management of osteoporosis and risk assessment for falls in long-term care. *Annals of Long-Term Care, 6*(Suppl. D), 1–16.

Blixen, C. E., & Kippes, C. (1999). Depression, social support, and quality of life in older adults with osteoarthritis. *Image Journal of Nursing Scholarship, 31*(3), 221–226.

Burki, R. (1999). Trends in osteoporosis management. *The Clinical Advisor, 2*(2), 22–29.

Centers for Disease Control and Prevention. (1998). Osteoporosis among estrogen-deficient women—United States, 1988–1994. *Mortality and Morbidity Weekly Report, 47*(48), 478.

Creamer, P., Flores, R., & Hochberg, M. (1998). Management of osteoarthritis in older adults. *Clinics in Geriatric Medicine, 14,* 435–454.

D'Epiro, N. (1998). HRT: New data, continuing controversies. *Patient Care Nurse Practitioner, 1*(10), 18–20, 25–34.

Ebersole, P., & Hess, P. (1998). *Toward healthy aging* (5th ed.). St. Louis: Mosby.

Gallant, S., Keita, G., & Royak-Schaler, R. (1997). *Health care for women*. Washington, DC: American Psychological Association.

Harris, C. (1993). Osteoarthritis: How to diagnose and treat the painful joint. *Geriatrics, 48*(8), 39–46.

Kee, C., Harris, S., Booth, L., Rouser, G., & McCoy, S. (1998). Perspectives on the nursing management of osteoarthritis. *Geriatric Nursing, 19*(1), 19–26.

Kleerekoper, M. (1999). Osteoporosis: Protecting bone mass with fundamentals and drug therapy. *Geriatrics, 54*(7), 38–43.

Lark, S. (2001, May). Bountiful bone, part 1. *The Lark Letter, 2–3.*

Leslie, M. (1999). Hyaluronic acid treatment for osteoarthritis of the knee. *The Nurse Practitioner, 24*(7), 38–48.

Lewis, S., Heitkemper, M., & Dirksen, S. (2000). *Medical-surgical nursing* (5th ed.). St. Louis: Mosby.

Lloyd, T., Rollings, N., Eggli, D., Kieselhorst, K., & Chinchilli, V. (1997). Dietary caffeine intake and bone status of post-menopausal women. *American Journal of Clinical Nutrition, 65,* 1826–1830.

Lueckenotte, A. (2000). *Gerontologic nursing* (2nd ed.). St. Louis: Mosby.

Margolis, S., & Flynn, J. (1999). *Arthritis*. Baltimore: The Johns Hopkins Medical Institutions.

Margolis, S., & Flynn, J. (2000). *Arthritis*. Baltimore: The Johns Hopkins Medical Institutions.

Margolis, S., & Kostuik, J. (1999). *Low back pain and osteoporosis*. Baltimore: The Johns Hopkins Medical Institutions.

Margolis, S., & Kostuik, J. (2000). *Low back pain and osteoporosis*. Baltimore: The Johns Hopkins Medical Institutions.

McAlindon, T., LaValley, M., Gulin, J., & Felson, D. (2000). Glucosamine and chondroitin sulfate for treatment of osteoarthritis: A systematic quality assessment and meta-analysis. *Journal of the American Medical Association, 283,* 1469–1475.

McClung, B. (1999). Using osteoporosis management to reduce fractures in elderly women. *The Nurse Practitioner, 24*(3), 26–47.

Murphy, S., & Jurisson, M. (1998). Putting exercise to work for your patients with osteoarthritis: Reduced pain and improved mobility are among benefits. *Journal of Musculoskeletal Medicine, 15*(6), 26–34.

National Osteoporosis Foundation. (1998). *Physician's guide to osteoporosis prevention and treatment*. Washington, DC: Author.

National Osteoporosis Foundation. (1999a). *Osteoporosis Report*. Washington, DC: Author.

National Osteoporosis Foundation. (1999b). *Osteoporosis Report*. Washington, DC: Author.

Notelovitz, M. (1997). Osteoporosis: Alternatives for keeping bones strong. *Contemporary Nurse Practitioner, 2*(1), 7–19.

A "natural" approach to treating osteoarthritis. (2000, May). *Healthnews, 6,* 1–2.

Olson, R. E. (2000). Osteoporosis and vitamin k intake. *American Journal of Clinical Nutrition, 71*(5), 1031–1032.

Osteoporosis. (2000). *Prescriber's Letter, 17*(8), 32–36. Author.

Patient Health Network. (1984). *Your neglected back*. Brooklyn, NY: Author.

Phipps, W., Sands, J., & Marek, J. (1999). *Medical-surgical nursing, concepts and clinical practice* (6th ed.). St. Louis: Mosby.

Prestwood, K., & Weksler, M. (1997). Osteoporosis: Up-to-date strategies for prevention and treatment. *Geriatrics, 52,* 92–94, 97–98.

Puppione, A. (1999). Management strategies for older adults with osteoarthritis: How to promote and maintain function. *Journal of the American Academy of Nurse Practitioners, 11,* 167–171.

Ross, C. (1997). A comparison of osteoarthritis and rheumatoid arthritis: Diagnosis and treatment. *The Nurse Practitioner, 22*(9), 20–39.

Tucker, K. L., Hannan, M. T., Chen, H., Cupples, L. A., Wilson, P. W., Kiel, D. P. (1999). Potassium, magnesium, and fruit and vegetable intakes are associated with greater bone mineral density in elderly men and women. *American Journal of Clinical Nutrition, 6a*(4), 727–736.

Whitmore, S. (1998, October 3). Rebuilding bone . . . renewing lives. *Advance for Nurse Practitioners,* 30–35.

15

Gastrointestinal Wellness and Illness

Kathleen M. Blade

Objectives

1. *List at least five lifestyle choices that promote gastrointestinal wellness.*
2. *Identify the indicators that the gastrointestinal system is functioning normally.*
3. *Compare the manifestations of heartburn and peptic ulcer disease.*
4. *Discuss the symptoms of and self-care related to irritable bowel syndrome.*
5. *Discuss the factors related to the development of gallstones.*

Introduction

Problems with the gastrointestinal (GI) system are common. Most people have experienced some form of stomach upset, such as nausea, vomiting, or diarrhea. It is estimated that over 95 million Americans per year have some kind of digestive problem, with care costs exceeding $40 billion (Common GI Problems—United States, 2000). Proper functioning of the GI system is essential to health because the GI system is responsible for providing nutrients to the body and eliminating wastes. Gastrointestinal wellness and four conditions that commonly concern women, gastroesophageal reflux disease, peptic ulcer disease, irritable bowel syndrome, and gallbladder disease, are discussed in this chapter.

Markers of Gastrointestinal Wellness

The gastrointestinal tract (see Figure 15–1) is a hollow tube that extends from the mouth to the anus. It provides the body with nutrients and fluid and eliminates waste products. The upper portion of the GI tract is composed of the mouth, esophagus, and stomach. The structures of the lower GI tract are the intestines, rectum, and anus. The accessory organs of the GI system are the gallbladder, pancreas, and liver.

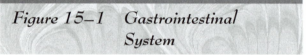

Figure 15–1 Gastrointestinal System

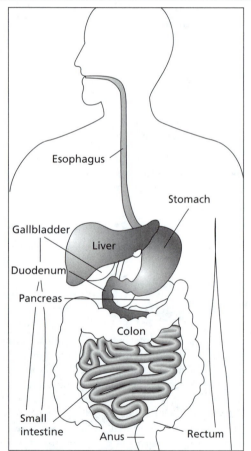

Used with permission by the National Digestive Diseases Information Clearinghouse.

Normal Digestion

Digestion is the process by which the nutrients in food are made available to the body. Digestion begins in the mouth, where saliva is secreted to soften food as it is chewed. The normal mouth is pink, moist, and free of sores. Teeth should be free of cavities. Gums should be light pink and should not bleed when the teeth are brushed. Gums that are reddish and bleed easily signal the presence of **gingivitis,** an inflammatory condition that can cause tooth loss and even contribute to coronary heart disease (see Chapter 12).

When chewing has been completed, food is pushed to the back of the throat and down the esophagus to the stomach. This passage, swallowing, should proceed easily, without discomfort, pain, or any sensation of blockage or choking.

The stomach is a temporary reservoir for food. It secretes acid and enzymes that further help break down food for digestion. The stomach lining is protected from the acid by a thick layer of mucus. Food is mixed and churned in the stomach, breaking into smaller particles, called **chyme,** which is propelled into the small intestine. There should be no sensations of **gastritis,** commonly called heartburn, before, after, or between meals.

The small intestine has three main functions: the movement, digestion, and absorption of nutrients. Muscular contractions, called **peristalsis,** mix and transport the chyme. It takes an average of 3 to 10 hours for the chyme to pass through the small intestine and for the nutrients to be absorbed. The liquid chyme residue that is left is next passed to the large intestine.

Normal Elimination

The main function of the large intestine is elimination. The large intestine absorbs water from the nutrient-depleted chyme residue, thereby creating the firm food waste known as **feces,** and stores it to be eliminated in what is commonly known as a bowel movement, or **defecation.** Transit time through the large intestine is slow—approximately 12 hours. Fecal contents are propelled toward the rectum a few times each day. Bowel movements are initiated when food enters the upper small intestine, especially after the first meal of the day. It is normal to notice occasional "rumbling" sounds related to intestinal motility and occasionally to pass air, or gas, via the rectum.

Elimination patterns vary among healthy people. Alterations in a person's normal elimination patterns usually are related to gastrointestinal illness or a change in dietary or activity patterns. An example of an alteration in elimination is **constipation,** a decrease in the frequency of bowel movements. Constipation is accompanied by the prolonged passage of small, hard stools (feces). Stools should be brown and soft enough to be passed easily and without discomfort. **Diarrhea** is an increase in the number of stools and the passage of mushy or semi-liquid, unformed feces (Potter & Perry, 1997).

The gallbladder, liver, and pancreas also contribute to digestion. The major function of the gallbladder is to store and concentrate **bile.** Bile is formed in the liver and contains bile salts, which facilitate *fat digestion* in the small intestine. When fat enters the duodenum, a chemical called cholecystokinin is released, causing the gallbladder to contract and squirt bile into the duodenum. At the same time, the pancreas is secreting its fat digestion enzyme, called lipase. Normal digestive and eliminative processes do not cause pain or bloating.

Promoting Gastrointestinal Wellness

A variety of strategies can be used to promote gastrointestinal wellness. They include avoiding substances that are irritating to the stomach, fostering optimal elimination, and undergoing age-appropriate screening tests.

Avoiding Stomach Irritants

Certain habits have a known effect on the integrity of the GI system. For example, smoking, drinking alcohol, and experiencing stress have negative effects, whereas eating a high-fiber diet has positive ones. The hazards of smoking are well known, yet millions continue to do so. Nicotine irritates the gastrointestinal mucous lining and is linked to oral and esophageal cancers. There is also a strong association between smoking and the occurrence of **peptic ulcer,** as well as ulcer complications and recurrence. An ulcer is an open sore. A *peptic* ulcer is a sore in the lining of either the stomach or the duodenum, which is the part of the small intestine into which the stomach empties. Current smokers are twice as likely to develop ulcers as are nonsmokers (Black & Jacobs, 1997; Phipps, Sands, & Marek, 1999).

The ingestion of alcohol causes irritation of the inner surface of the stomach and can lead to inflammation (gastritis). Wine and beer stimulate acid secretion, and heavy beer drinkers are more prone to colorectal cancer. Alcohol ingestion also causes changes in the intestinal mucosa, which can lead to the malabsorption of many nutrients. Persons with these changes are two to four times more likely to undergo changes in the esophageal mucosa as well, and develop esophageal cancer (Lutz & Przytulski, 1997; Mahan & Stump, 1996).

Many women are concerned about their caffeine intake, yet there is no substantial link between caffeine use and gastrointestinal illness. However, both coffee and tea are recognized as gastric acid stimulants. Therefore, caffeine should be consumed in moderation. Thus far, the consumption of as many as three 8 ounce cups of caffeinated beverages per day has been shown not to be related to any known health risk (*Caffeine—United States,* 2000).

Whether or not spices used in cooking irritate the GI tract still is unclear. Relative tolerance of spicy foods appears to be highly variable; some individuals develop indigestion after consuming spices, whereas others do not (Phipps et al., 1999). However, it has been shown that red or black pepper ingested into an empty stomach can cause increased secretion of gastric acid, as well as superficial damage to the mucosal lining of the GI system (Mahan & Stump, 1996).

Some food substances, such as fatty, pickled and smoked foods are associated with **cancer** when eaten frequently, so moderating intake of such foods is advisable. Cooking methods can also influence the development of cancer.

Diets high in fat seem to be related to colon cancer because certain end products of fat metabolism are thought to be carcinogenic (Black & Jacobs, 1997; Mahan & Stump, 1996). The frequent consumption of fat subjects the intestinal walls to prolonged exposure to those end products because the transit time of fatty foods through the intestines is slow. It is currently recommended that calories from fat be limited to 30% of the daily total (Lutz & Przytulski, 1997).

Pickled and smoked foods have been linked to esophageal and stomach cancers because they contain significant amounts of carcinogenic substances known as **nitrates and nitrites.** The process of smoking foods such as meats and fish is thought to cause the formation of carcinogenic **tars,** similar to those found in tobacco. Recent data shows that methods of meat cooking that require high temperatures, such as searing and broiling, cause carcinogens known as **nitrosamines** to form on the surface of foods (Lutz & Przytulski, 1997).

Promoting Optimal Elimination

Effective bowel elimination is essential if the body is to rid itself of food wastes. Many factors, such as fiber and water intake, exercise level, and emotional states can influence elimination patterns.

The food choices a person makes have a direct influence on elimination. A diet rich in fiber stimulates intestinal motility, or peristalsis (see Table 15–1). When peristalsis is stimulated, foods pass through the large intestine at a normal rate, and soft stools are produced. On the other hand, the slow passage of fecal material causes hard stools, because it is in the large intestine that the water content of stool is absorbed through the intestinal wall. The consumption of gas-producing foods, such as onions, cauliflower, and beans, also can support the

---

TABLE 15–1   High fiber foods.

- Raw fruits and vegetables (apples, lettuce, celery)
- Greens (spinach, cabbage)
- Whole grains (bran cereal, whole wheat, waffles, oatmeal)
- Legumes (beans and lentils)
- Popcorn and nuts
- Cooked fruits and vegetables (brussel sprouts, corn, broccoli)

peristaltic process and a normal elimination pattern (Lutz & Przytulski, 1997; Potter & Perry, 1997).

Fluid intake also influences bowel elimination. A decreased intake of fluids slows the passage of food through the intestines, which leads to increased water absorption by the large intestine and the subsequent hardening of feces. To keep feces soft, it is recommended that adults drink six to eight glasses of fluid daily (Potter & Perry, 1997).

Physical activity promotes peristalsis, whereas a sedentary lifestyle depresses it. Even physical activities such as raking leaves, dancing, and gardening will suffice to influence regular bowel elimination (Cadoff, 1999).

Negative emotional states, such as anxiety and depression, can impair proper elimination. When a person becomes anxious, the GI system is stimulated, resulting in increased peristalsis and diarrhea. When a person becomes depressed, the reverse happens, and constipation can result (Potter & Perry, 1997). Decreasing stress through the use of stress-reduction techniques (see Chapter 7) can help promote proper elimination.

Undergoing Screening Tests

Screening tests for **colorectal cancer** are done as part of a routine physical exam. Colorectal cancer is the 2nd leading cause of cancer-related death in the population, and a significant killer of women. Women who have a history of breast, ovarian or uterine cancer are at increased risk for developing colorectal cancer, as are women who have a 1st degree relative who has had it. (What You Need to Know About Colorectal Cancer, 1999).

The screening tests for colorectal cancer include the **fecal occult blood test (FOBT),** the **proctosigmoidoscopy** and the **colonoscopy.** The FOBT is useful in determining any bleeding in the GI tract. A smear of stool is placed on filter paper and exposed to a blood-sensitive solution. When stool is positive for blood, the paper turns blue. A proctosigmoidoscopy is a visual examination of the rectum and sigmoid colon using a lighted flexible tube called a scope. A colonoscopy is a similar examination of the entire large intestine. An annual FOBT and a proctosigmoidoscopy or colonoscopy every three to five years are recommended for all women over the age of 50. Unfortunately, women of higher socioeconomic status are more likely to have these tests than are women of lower socioeconomic status (Allen & Phillips, 1997).

Gastrointestinal Illnesses and Problems

Gastrointestinal illnesses and problems are common in our society. Over-the-counter and prescription drugs used to treat constipation, diarrhea, gastroesophageal reflux disease, and irritable bowel syndrome are advertised heavily on television and in the print media. Gallbladder disease is also a significant cause of illness.

TABLE 15–2   Common medications used to manage constipation.

Bulk Formers
- Methalcellulose (Citrucil)
- Psyllium (Metamucil)

Emollients
- Ducosate Sodium (Colace)

Lubricants
- Mineral Oil

Saline Laxatives
- Magnesium Hydroxide (Milk of Magnesia)
- Magnesium Citrate (Citromag)
     (Citrate of Magnesium)
- Magnesium Sulfate (Epsom Salts)

Combinations
- Magnesium Hydroxide/Mineral Oil (Haley's MO)

Stimulants
- Senna (EXLAX)
     (Senokot)
- Castor Oil

Constipation

Constipation can result from lack of fiber in the diet, lack of exercise, or insufficient water intake. Constipation occurs when feces remain in the large intestine for long periods of time and water continually is absorbed, making the stool hard and difficult to pass.

Occasional constipation is common and not detrimental to health. It can be managed easily by using over-the-counter medications called **laxatives.** However, an overuse of laxatives can lead to dependency; the decreased absorption of the fat-soluble vitamins, A, D, E, and K; and chronic constipation (Phipps et al., 1999).

Different laxatives exert their effects in different ways. *Bulk formers* act by mixing with intestinal fluids, swelling, and stimulating the movement of the large intestine. *Emollients* incorporate liquid and fat into the stool, thereby softening it and allowing for easier passage. *Oils* lubricate the intestine to facilitate stool passage. *Saline* laxatives lead to fluid retention, which distends the large intestine and increases movement, while *stimulants* irritate the intestine to promote movement (Deglin & Vallerand, 1999). Table 15–2 lists examples of medications commonly used to manage occasional constipation.

Diarrhea

One of the most classic symptoms of GI illness, diarrhea, usually represents an increase in the number of stools and/or a change in stool consistency. Diarrhea can be acute, lasting for less than 3 days, or chronic, related to changes within the GI system (Phipps et al., 1999). **Acute diarrhea** is the more common form and usually is the result of infectious agents, such as viruses or bacteria, that enter the body because of the improper handling and storage of food, contaminated water, or poor hygiene after using the toilet.

When infectious agents enter the GI tract, large amounts of water and electrolytes are secreted by the intestinal lining. The movement of the intestines increases, thereby decreasing the time fecal material is in the GI tract. This process leads to large volumes of watery stool being passed. Diarrhea may be accompanied by abdominal cramping and distention and loud bowel sounds. Depending on its severity, diarrhea can lead to electrolyte disturbances and dehydration.

The treatment of diarrhea includes fluid replacement, temporary changes in diet, and the use of antidiarrheal medications. Oral replacement solutions, such as Resol and Rehydralate, are recommended to replenish electrolytes and glucose. Fruit juices and carbonated drinks should be avoided because they stimulate the intestinal tract (Phipps et al., 1999). Dietary intake should consist of small volumes of clear liquids for the first 24 hours. Chicken broth made from bouillon cubes or granules is an excellent source of replacement for the lost sodium. Ingesting water should be avoided because it lacks the needed electrolytes. After 24 hours, the diet can be advanced to foods such as toast with jelly or saltine crackers. If these foods are tolerated, bland foods, such as nonfatty soups, yogurt, cottage cheese, mashed potatoes, or cooked vegetables, can be added (Ignatavicius, Workman, & Mishler, 1999).

The use of antidiarrheal medications for bacterial or viral diarrhea is controversial. Some believe that the infecting organisms need to be eliminated from the body to prevent worsening of the invasion (Phipps et al., 1999). However, in some cases, certain medications may be helpful. Loperamide (Imodium), a systemic acting antidiarrheal, which decreases central nervous system stimulation of the intestines has proven to be more effective than local acting medications, such as Kaopectate, which absorb irritants and soothe the intestinal walls directly (Deglin & Vallerand, 1999). Table 15–3 lists commonly used over-the-counter antidiarrheal medications.

Measures can be taken to help prevent diarrhea. Extreme cleanliness in all aspects of food preparation is crucial, including making sure that utensils and surfaces are washed well before and after all food preparation. Food should be defrosted in the refrigerator, rather than on counters. Leftovers should be returned to the refrigerator while still warm to prevent organism growth. Eating raw meats and seafood should be avoided. Ground beef always should be cooked well. When traveling, caution should be used in drinking local water and eating raw fruits and vegetables.

Gastroesophageal Reflux Disease

Gastroesophageal reflux disease (GERD), also known as heartburn, is caused by the backward flow of acid from the

TABLE 15–3 Medications used to manage diarrhea.

Systemic Acting
- Loperamide (Imodium)
    (Pepto Diarrhea Control)
    (Maalox Anti-diarrheal Caplets)
- Tincture of Opium (Paragoric)

Local Acting
- Kaolin and Pectin (Kaopectate)
    (Donnagel-MB)
    (Parapectolin)
- Bismuth Subsalcylate (Pepto-Bismol)
    (Bismed)

stomach into the esophagus. It can occur at any age, but it is more common in people over 50 (Ignatavicius et al., 1999). The actual incidence of heartburn is unknown because many people accept it as a normal response to overindulgence, and it is easily treated with over-the-counter drugs. There also are no associated gender patterns; equal numbers of women and men suffer from heartburn.

Normally, the reflux of acid from the stomach into the esophagus is prevented by a structure known as the **lower esophageal sphincter (LES).** The LES is located at the juncture of the esophagus and the stomach. Reflux occurs when either the stomach volume or pressure in the abdomen is increased or when the sphincter is relaxed. With repeated exposure to acid, the normal lining of the esophagus breaks down and becomes inflamed. The degree of inflammation depends on the extent and duration of the exposure to acid. If the inflammation is of a long duration, the surface of the esophagus becomes eroded, leading to serious complications, such as bleeding, difficulty swallowing, and shortness of breath (Phipps et al., 1999).

SYMPTOMS

The symptoms of GERD are generally described as a feeling of burning pain and warmth behind the breastbone, which extends upward toward the neck. The pain occurs in waves and typically begins 20 minutes to 2 hours after eating. It usually is worsened by activities that increase abdominal pressure, such as bending over, straining, or lying down. At times, it is accompanied by a bitter or sour taste in the mouth. Discomfort can be relieved by standing or drinking fluids.

DIAGNOSIS

The diagnosis of GERD is made on the basis of classic symptoms and the results of tests such as a barium swallow, 24-hour pH monitoring, esophageal manometry, and upper endoscopy. During a **barium swallow,** or upper GI examination, the person being tested is given a thick, white, milkshake-like liquid, called barium, to drink. This liquid is radio-opaque

TABLE 15–4 Recommended dietary modifications for GERD.

- Avoid extremely hot, cold, or spicy foods; plus fats, alcohol, coffee, chocolate, citrus juices, and tomato products.
- Eat 4–6 small meals per day rather than 3 large ones.
- Avoid carbonated beverages.
- Reduce weight if overweight.
- Drink enough fluids at meals to help with food passage.
- Eat slowly and chew thoroughly.
- Do not eat or drink before going to bed.

TABLE 15–5 Common NSAIDS.

Generic Name	Trade Name
Over the Counter Drugs	
Ibuprofen	Motrin; Advil; Nuprin; Trendar
Naproxen Sodium	Aleve
Ketoprofen	Orudis
Prescription Drugs	
Diclofenac	Voltaren
Indomethicin	Indocin
Naproxen	Naprosyn
Piroxicam	Feldene
Sulindac	Clinoril

TABLE 15–6 Medications used to treat heartburn and GERD.

Antacids	Action	Side Effects
Magnesium based (Milk of Magnesia)	Neutralize acid secretions	Diarrhea
Aluminum based (Amphogel)		Constipation
Magnesium + Aluminum based (Malox, Mylanta, Riopan)		
Calcium Carbonate (Tums, Rolaids)		Constipation
Histamine Receptor Antagonists		
Cimetidine (Tagamet)	Inhibit acid secretion	Headache, diarrhea
Ranitidine (Zantac) Famotidine (Pepcid)		

and coats the surfaces with which it comes into contact. X rays then are taken to visualize the esophagus and stomach. The **24-hour pH monitoring test** is the most accurate tool for diagnosis. In this test, probes that analyze the acidity of gastric secretions are placed above the lower esophageal sphincter. Serial measurements can be made by leaving the electrode in place for a 24-hour period. **Esophageal manometry** involves the insertion of a small, flexible tube through the nose and into the esophagus in order to measure pressures in, and evaluate the function of, the esophagus. It can also measure the degree of acid refluxed into the esophagus. **Upper endoscopy** involves the insertion of a small, lighted tube into the esophagus through the mouth in order to detect any abnormalities. Medicines to numb the throat and relax the person being tested are given prior to the examination (Phipps et al., 1999).

TREATMENT

In mild cases of GERD, dietary modifications, as noted in Table 15–4, may be the only treatment necessary because some foods and beverages may contribute to the formation of acid or increased abdominal pressure.

Certain lifestyle changes are also encouraged to control GERD. One of the most important things persons suffering from GERD can do is to stop smoking. Tobacco both stimulates acid production and relaxes the sphincter between the esophagus and stomach, thus making it more likely that acid reflux will occur (Ignativicus et al., 1999). It is important to avoid wearing constrictive clothing, lifting heavy objects, straining, and working in a bent-over position because these activities will increase abdominal pressure. Also, people with GERD should *refrain from taking aspirin and nonsteroidal anti-inflammatory drugs (NSAIDs)* (see Table 15–5), as they can be irritating to the gastrointestinal mucosa, especially if taken on an empty stomach. Acetaminophen (such as Tylenol) can be taken, for it does not irritate the GI mucosa.

Drug therapy for GERD is usually self-initiated and consists of **antacids,** such as Tums or Maalox—or **histamine receptor antagonists (H_2 blockers),** such as Pepcid, Taga-

met, or Zantac. Antacids neutralize the acid in the stomach and provide prompt relief; however, their action is short and they provide only minimal nighttime protection. Either aluminum- or magnesium-containing antacids can be used, but aluminum-containing products can cause constipation, and magnesium-containing products can cause diarrhea. The use of combination products, which contain both magnesium and aluminum, seems to minimize these side effects. H_2 blockers, now available over-the-counter in lower dosages than prescription preparations, decrease the symptoms of acid reflux by inhibiting gastric acid secretion (Deglin & Vallerand, 1999) (see Table 15–6).

Peptic Ulcer Disease

Peptic ulcer disease occurs in approximately 10 percent of the population (Black & Jacobs, 1997). Currently, both forms of peptic ulcers, (stomach and duodenal) are equally common, and the incidence of both types continues to increase with age (Phipps et al., 1999).

It is thought that most ulcers are caused by infection with the bacterium *Helicobacter pylori (H. pylori)*. *H. pylori* is one of the most common bacteria; it resides naturally within the stomachs of approximately 30 to 50 percent of all people worldwide (Christensen, 1999). It is found in 90 percent of the people who develop duodenal ulcers and 70 percent of the people with gastric ulcers (Fedotin, 1993). However, not everyone who has *H. pylori* develops a peptic ulcer, so it is clear that other factors affect ulcer development. For example, the relationship between the use of NSAIDs and the development of gastric ulcers increasingly is being recognized. These substances may damage the protective mucous lining of the stomach by stimulating acid secretion while suppressing mucus secretion (Black & Jacobs, 1997).

Another factor that seems to play a role in the development of peptic ulcers is stress. Emotional stress has been shown to increase gastric secretion and motility, causing food to leave the stomach more quickly, thus leaving the mucosa in contact with acid undiluted by food (Ignatavicius et al., 1999).

Cigarette smoking and alcohol also are thought to contribute to the development of peptic ulcers. A strong association exists between smoking and ulcer incidence. Although the pathology has not been well identified, it is thought that smoking increases the risk of infection by *H. pylori* (Soll, 1998). Alcohol stimulates gastric acid production, irritates the GI mucosa, and can cause constipation and diarrhea (Phipps et al., 1999).

SYMPTOMS

The most common symptom of ulcer disease is an aching, burning, gnawing pain in the abdomen, usually between the navel and breastbone. It ordinarily occurs on an empty stomach and awakens people at night. When the ulcer is in the duodenum, the ingestion of food or an antacid will relieve the pain. However, with a gastric ulcer, the ingestion of food may cause the pain. Rarely, nausea, vomiting, and loss of appetite are also present.

DIAGNOSIS

The most common diagnostic tests used to confirm the presence of an ulcer are the **upper GI series (UGI)** and an endoscopic exam, **esophagogastroduodenoscopy (EGD).** The UGI is an X-ray test in which the person is given a thick, white liquid (barium) to drink while X rays are taken to visualize the gastrointestinal tract. An upper GI series takes approximately one to two hours. It is not uncomfortable, but the barium may cause constipation and white-colored stools for a few days after the procedure. An EGD involves the insertion of a small, flexible, lighted tube into the esophagus, stomach, and duodenum via the mouth. Then the gastrointestinal lining is examined carefully. During the test, samples of tissue are taken and tested for possible malignancy.

Patients with ulcer disease are tested for the presence of *H. pylori*. There are several tests currently available. Blood tests for specific antibodies reveal previous exposure to the bacteria. A **urea breath test** is used for mass screening. This test involves the use of a capsule that dissolves in the presence of *H. pylori*. The capsule contains carbon dioxide gas (CO_2). The person being tested swallows the capsule, and, if it dissolves, the amount of CO_2 released can be measured via spectrometry (Phipps et al., 1999).

TREATMENT

The treatment of most ulcers involves the use of medications. The main objective of treatment is to protect the stomach from acid long enough for it to heal. Although recent research has identified the role of *H. pylori* in the causation of ulcers, increased acid secretion continues to be a major factor. Therefore, medications that decrease acid secretion are used in conjunction with antibiotics (to kill H. pylori) as first-line therapy.

The types of medications most often prescribed to reduce the amount of acid in the stomach are antacids, H_2 antagonists, and proton pump inhibitors (Ignatavicius et al., 1999). **Proton pump inhibitor drugs,** such as omeprazale (Prilosec), have been found to be more effective than H_2-antagonists in impeding acid secretion and healing duodenal ulcers. **Cytoprotective,** or **mucosal protective, agents** are used to support the mucosal barrier of the stomach. These drugs include sulcrafate (Carafate) and misoprostol (Cytotec). Sulcrafate provides a sealant protection against acid irritation at the ulcer site. It neither inhibits acid secretion nor neutralizes it. Misoprotol both suppresses the secretion of gastric acid and stimulates the production of cytoprotective mucus (Deglin & Vallerand, 1999).

There is no single medication that can eradicate *H. pylori;* therefore, a combination of drugs is used. Protocols continue to change as new research findings accumulate. At present, the combination of an antibiotic, such as clarithromycin (Biaxin), and the antifungal drug metronidazole (Flagyl) is being recommended.

Lifestyle changes also are indicated in the management of peptic ulcer disease. In addition to drug therapy, it is necessary to eliminate smoking. Alcohol also should be avoided. Controversy still exists regarding the role of diet in ulcer disease. There is little evidence that restricting the diet promotes healing; food, after all, acts as an antacid by neutralizing acid. However, it is advisable to avoid foods that cause discomfort. Some likely candidates are coffee, colas, and teas, which promote acid secretion (Lutz & Przytulski, 1997; Mahan & Stump, 1996).

Irritable Bowel Syndrome

Irritable bowel syndrome (IBS), sometimes known as **spastic colon,** is a chronic disorder of the colon that causes abdominal pain and altered bowel habits that occur in the absence of any identifiable organic disease. IBS is the most common gastrointestinal disorder. It usually begins in early adult life and affects women twice as often as men (*NIH [Irritable Bowel Syndrome]*, 2000).

IBS is called a **functional disorder** because there is no sign of disease when the colon is examined. The diagnosis is made when other conditions have been excluded. However, studies strongly suggest that IBS is a disorder of abnormal muscle movement of the lower intestine (Ignatavicius et al., 1999). The alterations in muscle movement can result in diarrhea, constipation, or alternating diarrhea and constipation.

IBS causes discomfort and distress, but it does not lead to permanent harm, intestinal bleeding, or cancer. The cause of the problem is specific to the person, and most can identify factors that help contribute to an attack, such as a certain food, stress, or anxiety. Chocolate, caffeine, milk products, or large amounts of alcohol are frequent offenders. Researchers have found that women appear to have an increase in symptoms during their menstrual periods, which suggests a link to reproductive hormones (*NIH [Irritable Bowel Syndrome]*, 2000).

SYMPTOMS

The most common symptom of IBS is pain in the lower left abdomen, which increases after a meal and is relieved by a bowel movement. Diarrhea tends to be the major problem, but not usually at night. If stools are constipated, they are small and hard (pelletlike) and usually followed by softer movements. Other manifestations include belching, gas, decreased appetite, and bloating. Associated behavioral changes, such as anxiety, nervousness, or depression, also may be present.

DIAGNOSIS

Techniques for the diagnosis of IBS include a complete medical history with a careful description of symptoms, and a physical examination. Routine laboratory work is done to evaluate the general condition of the person, including a stool examination for blood. At times, the healthcare provider may order a **barium enema,** or **lower GI series,** because colon spasm can be detected during the procedure. A barium enema consists of introducing barium into the rectum through a small tube. During the procedure, which lasts about 45 to 60 minutes, the person having the procedure is asked to assume several different positions to help with the visualization of the colon. After the procedure, a laxative is given to prevent the constipating effect of the barium.

TABLE 15–7 Recommended dietary modifications for IBS.

- Avoid alcohol and excess caffeine.
- Eat regular meals.
- Drink 8–10 cups of liquid daily.
- Chew food slowly.
- Eat smaller meals more frequently.
- Check with your health care provider about following a high fiber diet to decrease episodes of constipation or loose stools.

TREATMENT

There is no standard treatment for IBS, but lifestyle modifications and medications can control the symptoms. The medications most commonly prescribed are a combination of antidiarrheals, bulk-forming agents, and antispasmodics. Antidiarrheals, such as loperamide (Imodium) and attapulgite (Kaopectate), help decrease cramping and the frequency of stools. The bulk-forming agents, such as psyllium hydrophilic mucilloid (Metamucil), help prevent dry, hard, or liquid stools. Antispasmodics, such as the drugs decyclomine (Bentyl) and hyoscamine (Cytospay), help relieve cramping and intestinal spasm (Deglin & Vallerand, 1999). When the symptoms of IBS are accompanied by anxiety or depression, tranquilizers and antidepressants may be prescribed. A proper diet also can help lessen the symptoms of IBS. People who suffer from IBS often are counseled to keep a food-symptom diary to identify foods that trigger discomfort. A consultation with a dietitian can help with meal planning. Further dietary guidelines can be found in Table 15–7. Relaxation techniques and personal counseling can assist with stress management. (The use relaxation techniques is discussed in Chapter 7.)

Gallbladder Disease

Disorders of the biliary tract (the gallbladder and associated ducts) are common health problems in the United States, with the two most prevalent conditions being **cholecystitis,** or inflammation of the gallbladder, and **cholelithiasis,** or gallstones. The incidence of gallbladder problems is higher in women, especially among those of European American decent. Predisposing factors include a family history of gallbladder disease, a sedentary lifestyle, and obesity. By age 60, almost one-third of obese women have had gallbladder disease (Allen & Phillips, 1997).

Cholecystitis is usually caused by a blockage in the duct leading from the gallbladder to the intestine. The most common cause of such a blockage is the presence of a gallstone. Table 15–8 lists other causes of cholecystitis.

TABLE 15–8 Potential causes of cholecystitis.

- Trauma
- Inadequate blood supply
- Prolonged immobility
- Swelling
- Prolonged dehydration
- Excessive opiate use
- Bacterial invasion

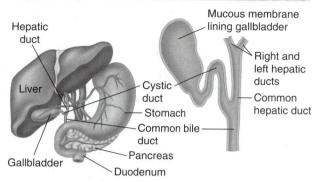

Figure 15–2 Biliary Ducts

Source: HUMAN DISEASES: A SYSTEMIC APPROACH 5e by Mulvihill/Zelman/Holdaway/Tompary/T, © 2000. Reprinted with permission of Pearson Education, Inc., Upper Saddle River, NJ.

When the gallbladder cannot empty its contents into the small intestine, it becomes inflamed by the irritating liquid, (bile), it stores. The inflammation leads to the swelling of involved tissues, distention of the gallbladder, and impairment of circulation.

SYMPTOMS

The symptoms of cholecystitis vary in intensity and frequency. The most common symptom is episodic or vague upper right abdominal pain. The pain usually follows the ingestion of a high-fat meal, as fat stimulates gallbladder activity. Other symptoms, such as nausea, vomiting, belching, and gas, may be present.

Cholelithiasis is the formation of one or more stones within the gallbladder. Women have a higher incidence of cholelithiasis, as do Euro-Americans and Native Americans. Pregnancy, the use of birth control pills, and hormone replacement therapy all can accelerate gallstone formation in susceptible individuals. The higher estrogen levels associated with these factors cause the bile to contain more cholesterol, which is a major component of many gallstones (Ignatavicius et al., 1999; *NIH [Gallstones],* 2000). The mechanism by which gallstones are formed is not clearly understood. Bile, which is made in the liver, is composed of water, cholesterol fats, and bilirubin. Bilirubin is produced when red blood cells die and the hemoglobin (oxygen-carrying component) is broken down. When the balance of bile contents is disturbed, the cholesterol component can harden into stones. Gallstones can stay dormant inside the gallbladder or move to other areas within the connecting ducts. If a stone becomes lodged anywhere within this ductal system (see Figure 15–2), the flow of bile is blocked. If the ducts remain blocked for any length of time, the stasis of bile leads to cholecystitis and/or damage to the liver and pancreas.

The severity of the symptoms of cholelithiasis depends on such factors as whether or not the stone moves, the size of the blockage, and the amount of inflammation (Phipps et al., 1999). Most commonly, the symptoms occur suddenly and are referred to as a "gallstone attack" (*NIH [Gallstones],* 2000). The pain of cholelithiasis is steady, severe, and located in the upper right abdomen. It frequently radiates to the right shoulder or back and is often triggered by the ingestion of a meal containing a large amount of fat. Persons who experience gallstone attacks often are awakened at night by pain that lasts from one to three hours. Other symptoms include nausea, vomiting, and gas. If there is accompanying cholecystitis, the symptoms may include chills and fever.

DIAGNOSIS

The diagnosis of cholelcystitis and cholelithiasis is fairly straightforward when the classic symptoms are present. To verify the presence of stones, an ultrasound examination is performed. An **ultrasound machine** uses sound waves to visualize organs. The sound waves are directed into the body and are reflected in different ways, depending on the tissue structures. If stones are present, their location will be shown on the screen. Another test that may be performed is the **endoscopic retrograde cholangiopancreatography (ERCP).** In this examination, a long, flexible tube with a light on the end is passed through the mouth and guided into the ducts of the biliary system. Dye is injected into the tube to aid in visualizing the area on the X rays (*NIH [Gallstones],* 2000).

TREATMENT

The treatment of cholecystitis depends on the cause. For example, if the inflammation is due to the presence of bacteria, an antibiotic may be prescribed and a low-fat diet recommended in order to avoid stimulation of the gallbladder. If cholecystitis is due to the presence of gallstones, the most common treatment is **cholecystectomy,** surgical removal of the gallbladder. The standard surgical procedure is called **laparoscopic cholecystectomy** (Ignatavicius et al., 1999). In this operation, the surgeon makes four or five tiny incisions in the abdomen and inserts various instruments and a miniature video camera. The camera sends a picture of the inside of the body to a monitor. While watching the monitor, the surgeon dissects the gallbladder with a laser and removes it through one of the incisions. Under certain circumstances, however, the laparoscopic procedure is contraindicated, and the patient must undergo the older cholecystectomy procedure, which involves a large incision that severs abdominal muscles. Patients who have the laparoscopic procedure enjoy a shorter healing period and have less scarring and pain (Gauwitz, 1992).

The *non-surgical* management of cholelithiasis is used when someone is a poor surgical risk or refuses surgery. The two most common types of treatments are **oral dissolution therapy** and **extra corporeal shockwave lithotripsy (ESWL).** Drugs for oral dissolution are made from bile acid and work best on small cholesterol stones. However, months of treatment are usually necessary in order to dissolve stones fully, and recurrence within five years is common (Deglin & Vallerand, 1999). ESWL is a process wherein sound waves are used to break up gallstones into tiny pieces, which can be passed through the bile ducts and excreted via the intestines. The recurrence of stones is a problem and the treatment is five times more expensive than surgery (Phipps et al., 1999).

Gastrointestinal Wellness Self-Assessment

Use the following statements to assess your gastrointestinal health. The more statements that apply to you, the higher your level of gastrointestinal wellness is likely to be.

1. *I limit my consumption of alcoholic beverages.*
2. *I seek medical help for frequent episodes of heartburn.*
3. *I limit the amount of fat in my diet.*
4. *I refrain from smoking cigarettes.*
5. *I limit my caffeine intake.*
6. *I do not suffer abdominal pain after eating fatty meals.*
7. *I do not suffer from constipation, diarrhea, or abdominal cramps frequently.*
8. *I undergo appropriate screening tests for colorectal cancer.*
9. *I do not include pickled and smoked foods in my diet on a regular basis.*
10. *I do not frequently barbecue my food.*

New Directions

Research that focuses on the causes and optimal treatment of gastrointestinal disease is ongoing. A number of studies on GERD are underway. One is intended to provide information about the relationship between hiatal hernia and esophageal reflux. A hiatal hernia is a defect in the diaphragm that allows a portion of the stomach to protrude upward through it. The normal opening in the diaphragm allows only the esophagus to pass through it. Existing studies suggest, but do not confirm, that the presence of a hiatal hernia contributes to the reflux of stomach acid into the duodenum (*GERD—United States*, 2000). Current research is also being conducted on the nonesophageal symptoms of reflux, such as laryngitis, chronic cough, and cancer of the larynx (*GERD—United States,* 2000). In June and August 1999, the U.S. Food and Drug Administration (FDA) approved two new proton pump inhibitor drugs, Protonix (pantotrazole) and Aciphex (rabeprazole sodium). They can be prescribed for the healing of GERD, the maintenance of healed erosive GERD, and the healing of duodenal ulcers (*Ulcers— United States*, 2000).

Other promising new research is being conducted in the area of *H. pylori* eradication. Researchers from around the world are evaluating the effectiveness of triple therapy treatment. Although the specific drugs and length of treatment may vary, the triple therapy regime generally involves pairing an anti-infective drug with one or more gastroprotective agents. Results have been promising, with 75 to 85 percent eradication rates (*Duodenal Ulcers—United States*, 2000; *Ulcers—United States*, 2000). Another area being evaluated is the association between the decreased incidence of *H. pylori* and the increased occurrence of GERD and its complications. Some researchers have questioned the wisdom of eradicating *H. pylori*. Martin Blaser of Vanderbilt University notes that, as *H. pylori* has been disappearing, the occurrence of GERD, **Barrett's esophagitis** (an ulcerlike disease of the esophagus), and cancers of the lower esophagus and upper stomach have been increasing (Christensen, 1999). While some researchers agree with Blaser, others argue that the rise of esophageal cancer may be associated with diet, body weight, or environmental exposure. More research is needed in this area. Research projects evaluating the effectiveness of preventive measures, such as avoiding heavy smoking, not overusing alcohol and coffee, and discontinuing the use of aspirin and related drugs, are also being conducted. The effects of stress and the practice of taking meals in a hurried manner also are being investigated (*Duodenal Ulcers—United States*, 2000).

Researchers at the Mayo Clinic have found that a new drug, **alosetran,** significantly improves both pain and bowel function in women with IBS (Camilleri et al., 1999). Research is also being done on the effectiveness of certain drugs and *herbal medicines* in the treatment of IBS. At the University of Western Sydney, researchers found that the use of certain Chinese herbal medicines significantly improved the bowel symptoms associated with IBS (Bensoussan et al., 1998). The usefulness of *hypnotherapy* in IBS also is being investigated. Previous research from the United Kingdom concerning the use of hypnotherapy in IBS has been replicated at the University of Albany in New York with promising results. All subjects treated with hypnosis reported improvement in the symptoms of abdominal pain, constipation, and flatulence (Galovski & Blanchard, 1999).

New research is being conducted on the treatment of gallstones. Researchers in both Japan and Finland have found that combining a cholesterol-lowering agent with a stone-dissolution drug is more effective in dissolving stones than is the use of a dissolution agent by itself (Miettinen & Vuoristo, 1998; Tazuma et al., 1999).

QUESTIONS FOR REFLECTION AND DISCUSSION

1. *What would you tell a friend who has confided to you that she takes antacids to relieve stomach pain that awakens her at night?*
2. *You've been asked to speak to a group about preventing peptic ulcer disease. What lifestyle modifications will you discuss?*
3. *Which categories of foods would you include in a menu plan for a person with irritable bowel syndrome?*
4. *What are the relative merits of lifestyle changes versus taking medication for people with GERD?*

RESOURCES

Books

Berkson, D. Lindsey (2000). *Healthy digestion the natural way: Preventing and healing heartburn, constipation, gas, diarrhea, inflammatory bowel and gallbladder diseases.* John Wiley & Sons.

Nichols, T. W., & Faass, N. (1999). *Optimal digestion—new strategies for achieving digestive health.* New York: HarperCollins.

Organizations

Digestive Disease National Coalition
507 Capitol Court NE., Suite 200
Washington, DC 20002
Phone: 202-544-7497
Web: *http://www.ddnc.org*

National Digestive Diseases Information Clearing House
2 Information Way
Bethesda, MD 20892
Phone: 301-654-3810
Web: *http://www.niddk.nih.gov/health/digest/nddic.htm*

Pediatric/Adolescent Gastroesophageal Reflux Assoc., Inc.
P.O. Box 1153
Germantown, MD 20875-1153
Phone: 301-601-9541

Websites

Med Help International—*http://medhlp.netusa.net* A non-profit site that provides articles, support groups and resources on a wide variety of health concerns. The site is run by two lay persons and supported by a large medical advisory board and a board of directors comprised mainly of medical professionals.

REFERENCES

Allen, K. M., & Phillips, J. M. (1997). *Women's health across the lifespan: A comprehensive perspective.* Philadelphia: J. B. Lippincott.

Bensoussan, A., Talley, N. J., Hing, M., Menzies, R., Guo, A., & Ngu, M. (1998). Treatment of irritable bowel syndrome with Chinese herbal medicine: A randomized control trial. *Journal of the American Medical Association, 280*(18), 1585–1589.

Black, J. M., & Jacobs, E. M. (1997). *Medical-surgical nursing: Clinical management for continuity of care* (5th ed.). Philadelphia: W. B. Saunders.

Cadoff, J. (1999, September/October). Just move it. *Remedy,* pp. 39–42.

Caffeine—United States [On-line]. (2000). Available: http://www.healthcentral.com/mhc/top/002445.cfm

Camilleri, M., Mayer, E. A., Drossman, D. A., Heath, A., Dukes, G. E., McSorley, D., Kong, S., Mangel, A., & Northcutt, A. R. (1999). Improvement in pain and bowel function in female irritable bowel patients with alostron. *Alimentary Pharmacology and Therapeutics, 13*(9), 1149–1159.

Christensen, D. (1999, October). Is your stomach bugging you? *Science News,* pp. 234–237.

Common GI problems—United States [On-line]. (2000). Available: http://www.acg.gi.org/patientinfo/cgp/cgvoll.htm/#gerd

Deglin, J. H., & Vallerand, A. H. (1999). *Davis's drug guide for nurses* (6th ed.). Philadelphia: F. A. Davis.

Duodenal ulcers—United States [On-line]. (2000). Available: http://www.lifestages.com/health/duodenal.html

Fedotin, M. (1993). *Helicobacter pylori* and peptic ulcer disease: Re-examining the therapeutic approach. *Postgraduate Medicine, 94*(8), 38–45, 139–140.

Galovski, T. E., & Blanchard, E. B. (1999). The treatment of irritable bowel syndrome with hypnotherapy. *Applied Psychophysiology and Biofeedback, 23*(4), 219–232.

Gauwitz, D. F. (1992). Endoscopic cholecystectomy: The patient friendly alternative. *Nursing, 92, 20*(12), 58–59.

GERD—United States [On-line]. (2000). Available: http://www.drkoop.com/conditions/GERD

Ignatavicius, D. D., Workman, M. L., & Mishler, M. A. (1999). *Medical-surgical nursing across the health care continuum* (3rd ed.). Philadelphia: W. B. Saunders.

Lutz, C. A., & Przytulski, K. R. (1997). *Nutrition and diet therapy* (2nd ed.). Philadelphia: F. A. Davis.

Mahan, L. K., & Stump, S. E. (1996). *Krauese's food, nutrition & diet therapy* (9th ed.). Philadelphia: W. B. Saunders.

Miettinen, T. E., & Vuoristo, M. (1998). The sedimentable sterols in gallstone patients before and during ursodeoxycholic acid and simvastatin treatments. *Scandinavian Journal of Gastroenterology, 33*(12), 1297–1302.

NIH (gallstones) [On-line]. (2000). Available: http://www.nih.gov/health/

NIH (irritable bowel syndrome) [On-line]. (2000). Available: http://www.nih.gov/health/

Phipps, W. J., Sands, J. K., & Marek, J. F. (1999). *Medical-surgical nursing: Concepts and clinical practice* (6th ed.). St. Louis: Mosby.

Potter, P. A., & Perry, A. G. (1997). *Fundamentals of nursing: Concepts, process and practice* (4th ed.). St. Louis: Mosby.

Soll, A. H. (1998). Peptic ulcer and its complications. In Sleisinger, M. & Fortrans, J. (Eds.), *Gastrointestinal and liver disease* (6th ed., pp. 428–437). Philadelphia: W. B. Saunders.

Tazuma, S., Kajiyama, G., Mizuno, T., Yamashito, G., Miura, H., Kajihara, T., Hattori, Y., Miyake, H., Nishioka, T., Hyogo, H., Sunami, Y., Yasumiba, S., Ochi, H., Matsumoto, T., Abe, A., Adachi, K., Omati, F., Veno, S., Sugata, F., Ohguri, S., Shibata, H., & Kikubee, S. (1999). A combination therapy with simvastatin and ursodeoxycholic acid is more effective for cholesterol gallstone dissolution than is ursodeoxycholic acid monotherapy. *Journal of Clinical Gastroenterology, 26*(4), 287–291.

Ulcers—United States [On-line]. (2000). Available: http://www.wellweb.com/INDEX/QDUODEN.HTM

What You Need To Know About Colorectal Cancer [On-line]. (1999). National Cancer Institute Cancernet. Retrieved December 10, 2001. Available: http://www.cancernet.nci.nih.gov/wyntk_pub./colon.htm#5

16

Urinary Tract Wellness and Illness

Jeanie Krause Bachand

Objectives

1. *Identify the normal and abnormal characteristics of urine.*
2. *Describe practices that enhance urinary tract wellness.*
3. *Compare and contrast the symptoms of kidney infection and urinary tract infection.*
4. *Discuss the prevention and treatment of urinary incontinence.*

Introduction

This chapter addresses the urinary tract and the structures and processes associated with it. The markers, or indicators, of urinary wellness (normal voiding patterns and urine that is normal in color and consistency) are described and strategies for promoting urinary wellness (drinking enough water, avoiding substances that are toxic to the kidneys, and practicing good personal hygiene) are outlined. Illnesses and problems that commonly affect the urinary tract (infections, interstitial cystitis, and incontinence) are discussed in terms of incidence, pathophysiology, diagnosis, and treatment.

Markers of Urinary Tract Wellness

The basic functions of the urinary tract are to regulate the composition and volume of body fluids and to eliminate waste materials, such as urea, creatinine, uric acid, sulfate,

Figure 16–1 The Urinary Tract

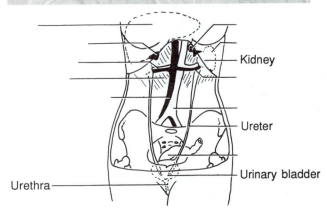

Source: Chapter title and author in Burrell/Gerlach/Pless, *Adult nursing: Acute and community care* (2nd ed., © 1997, p. 1199, F. 47–1). Reprinted by permission of Pearson Education, Inc., Upper Saddle River, NJ.

and phosphate. The urinary tract consists of two kidneys, two ureters, the bladder, and the urethra (see Figure 16–1). The kidneys remove the wastes and some of the water from the blood to make urine. Two tubes, the ureters, transport the urine to the bladder, where it is stored. The urine remains there until the bladder is full and the urge to urinate develops. The urine then flows through the urethra, another tube, and leaves the body.

A variety of factors affect the volume and quality of urine excreted and an individual's ability to urinate. These include fluid intake volume and the individual's ability to release urine, hold urine, and be comfortable while urinating. Other factors that affect urination include the structural integrity of the kidneys and urinary tract and the presence of diseases, such as infection or kidney stones. Knowing what is considered normal regarding urinary elimination allows individuals to be aware of changes that may indicate that an abnormal condition is developing.

Normal Color, Smell, and Amount of Urine

Normal urine can be pale, straw-colored, or amber, depending on the amount of fluid ingested and the pigments present in the urine. The urine is usually darker in the morning and becomes lighter as the individual drinks more fluids. Pink, red, or red-brown urine indicates bleeding from one of the structures in the urinary tract. A yellow-brown or green-brown color is usually a sign that bile pigments are present in the urine. Foods high in riboflavin, such as beets, rhubarb, and blackberries can also cause orange or red urine (Parker & Berding, 1997). Numerous

Box 16–1 Medications That Change the Color of Urine

- ◆ Dark Yellow to Orange Urine

  Azulfidine

  Pyridium

  Vitamin B-2

- ◆ Pink to Reddish Urine

  Cascara

  Ex-lax

  Dilatin

  Thorazine

- ◆ Green to Blue Urine

  Dyrenium

  Methylene blue

  Mitoxantrone

- ◆ Rust to Brown Urine

  Doxorubicin

  Flagyl

  Levodopa

  Furadantin

medications can also affect the color of urine (see Box 16–1). Fresh urine has a characteristically aromatic smell. Urine that is left standing has an ammonia smell, which is common in individuals who have **urinary incontinence,** the inability to hold urine. Urine that contains microorganisms because of an infection may have an offensive smell. Urine with a sweet, fruity smell is associated with diabetes mellitus, dehydration, and starvation.

The amount of urine produced depends on an individual's fluid intake. Generally, a normal adult produces 1,500 ml of urine in a 24-hour period. The production of large amounts of urine is seen in individuals with diabetes mellitus, a disorder of glucose metabolism, or diabetes insipidus, a neurological disorder. The urinary bladder of a normal adult has the capacity to hold 350–600 ml of urine; however, the desire to urinate is usually sensed when the urinary bladder contains 150–250 ml of urine. Normal adults, therefore, urinate an average of five or more times per day. Urinating at frequent intervals in small amounts may indicate that a urinary tract infection is present.

Normal Voiding Patterns

Normal daily urination (also called voiding or micturition) patterns, including the volume produced with each urination and the frequency of urination, are markers of urinary tract wellness. Most individuals with a normal fluid intake void five or six times a day. The usual times for voiding are on awakening, before meals, and at bedtime. An increase in the frequency of urination can be caused by inflammation, infection, pregnancy, or a decreased bladder capacity due aging, neurological disorders, or obstruction.

Most healthy individuals sleep through the majority of their nights without having to get up to void. **Nocturia,** excessive or frequent urination at night, can be caused by a variety of factors. The most common causes in women include taking fluids before going to bed (particularly coffee and alcohol) and being pregnant. The need to urinate during the night may also arise as a result of the normal aging process.

Healthy individuals can usually control the urge to void, do not "leak" urine when they cough or sneeze, and empty their bladders completely when they void. **Urgency,** or feeling the need to void immediately, is normal if caused by a full urinary bladder but is pathological if caused by irritation and inflammation from an infection or by a weak urethral sphincter (muscle). Urination is normally a painless and comfortable process. Painful or difficult urination, known as **dysuria,** is most commonly caused by a urinary tract infection.

Older women often have a problem with loss of urinary bladder muscle (detrusor muscle) tone. Loss of detrusor tone can lead to the incomplete emptying of the urinary bladder and the growth of bacteria in the retained, stagnant urine. Poor detrusor muscle tone may also cause a **cystocele** (an outpouching of the urinary bladder through a weakness in the vaginal wall) to develop. Cystoceles cause a bulge in the anterior vaginal wall and are readily detected during pelvic examination (see Figure 16–2).

Older women often experience some loss of urinary bladder tone; 37 percent of women age 60 and over have some degree of urinary incontinence (Newman, 2001). There are several types of urinary incontinence, some of which are particularly common in women. **Stress incontinence** occurs with straining—for example, during coughing or sneezing. In women, stress incontinence is usually related to pelvic muscle relaxation as a consequence of childbirth. **Urge incontinence,** the inability to hold urine when a strong urge to void is experienced, is common in women with multiple sclerosis and dementia. When **total incontinence** is present, urine is leaked continuously. This type of incontinence is related to damage to the urethral sphincter or to the presence of a fistula, or opening, between the vagina and the urinary bladder.

Urinary retention, the inability to empty the bladder or to empty it completely, is most often caused by an obstruction in the urinary tract or by a neurological disorder. **Acute** (sudden) **retention** causes urgency and discomfort and needs to be relieved before serious complications occur.

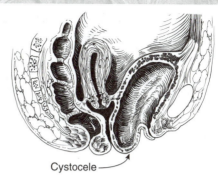

Figure 16–2   Cystocele

Cystocele —

Source: *Adult Nursing: Acute and Community Care* by Burrell/Gerlach/Pless. Copyright 1997. Reprinted by permission of Pearson Education, Inc., Upper Saddle River.

Chronic (long-standing) **retention** develops over a period of time and may be accepted as normal. The individual continues to urinate but does not empty the bladder completely. This puts her at risk for developing a urinary tract infection.

Promoting Urinary Tract Wellness

Many factors, including fluid intake, environmental toxins and medications, and personal hygiene practices, can affect the health of the urinary system. Each of these is briefly addressed in this section.

Drinking Enough Water

The kidneys are responsible for maintaining a balance between the retention and excretion of fluids. An increase in fluid intake causes an increase in the amount of urine that is produced by the kidneys. In healthy individuals, the amount of water ingested is approximately equal to the volume of urine that is excreted. Taking in a sufficient amount of fluid prevents the urine from becoming too concentrated and helps flush mucus and other debris from the urinary bladder. Keeping the urine relatively dilute and flushing the bladder frequently are helpful in preventing urinary tract infections and kidney stones. Toward those ends, women should drink a minimum of eight glasses of water or other liquids per day.

Water has been shown to lower the risk of bladder cancer, if taken in sufficient amounts. In one study, the men who drank at least six glasses of water per day had a 50 percent lower risk of bladder cancer then the men who drank less than one glass (Michaud et al., 1999). A similar study done on women (Koivusalo et al., 1998) did not include enough cases of bladder cancer to yield statistically significant results.

Avoiding Substances Toxic to the Kidneys

A variety of agents have been identified that are potentially toxic to the **nephrons,** the functional units of the kidneys. Exposure to cigarette smoke has been associated with an increased risk for bladder cancer. Michaud et al. (1999) found that the risk of bladder cancer was almost four times higher among men who were heavy smokers. Certain dyes, rubber, paint, cleaning solvents, pesticides, and organic chemicals are also capable of causing kidney damage (Berding, 1997). See Box 16–2 for a list of nephrotoxic substances.

Both over-the-counter and prescription **drugs** can also be nephrotoxic. Drugs can injure the kidneys through a variety of mechanisms. Some are directly toxic. Others cause a hypersensitivity reaction or constrict the blood vessels that feed the kidney. Still others precipitate (form solids) and cause kidney stones that can impair renal function to form. See Table 16–1 for a list of nephrotoxic medications.

Practicing Good Personal Hygiene

A woman has a one in two chance of acquiring a urinary tract infection (UTI) in her lifetime. UTIs are more common in women because the female urethra is shorter and closer to the anus than is that of the male (Berding, 1997). Washing the hands frequently and observing certain rules of good personal hygiene are the best ways to lessen the chance that bacteria will be introduced into the bladder through the urethra. The following are some good hygiene practices (Parker, 1997; Potter & Perry, 1997):

- Clean the genitals from front to back after urinating or having a bowel movement. This will reduce the chance that bacteria will be spread from the anus to the urethra.
- To avoid irritation, use nonperfumed soap and water to cleanse the genital area and avoid colored toilet paper, bubble bath, douches, feminine hygiene deodorants, and deodorant tampons and napkins.
- Change menstrual pads at least twice a day.
- Avoid sugar, chocolate, alcohol, and caffeine, as they can depress the immune system.
- To encourage good drainage and air circulation in the genital area, wear underwear made from cotton rather than synthetic material.
- Avoid using strong detergents and bleaches when washing underwear.
- Avoid bodysuits, panty hose, and other clothing that is tight in the crotch area.
- Urinate when the urge is felt, because holding urine increases the chance of developing an infection.
- Urinate before and after sexual intercourse.
- Drink at least eight glasses of fluid a day to prevent urine from becoming too concentrated and to flush out the bladder.
- Acidify the urine by including meats, eggs, whole grain breads, cranberry juice, prunes, and plums in the diet. This may reduce the number of bacteria in the urine.
- If prone to infections, avoid activities that tend to irritate the genital area, such as bicycling, horseback riding, motorcycling, and driving for long periods of time.

TABLE 16–1 Nephrotoxic medications.

Antibiotic/Antifungal Agents	Antineoplastic Agents	Miscellaneous
Amphotericin B	Altretamine	Acetaminophen
Amikacin	Carboplatin	Cyclosporine
Gentamicin	Cisplatin	Ibuprofen
Kanamycin	Doxorubicin	Indomethacin
Netilmicin	Hydroxyurea	Radiographic dyes
Streptomycin	Ifosfamide	Toradol
Tobramycin	Mitomycin	
Zithromax	Mitoxantrone	
	Plicamycin	

Source: *Adult Nursing: Acute and Community Care* by Burrell/Gerlach/Pless. Copyright 1997. Reprinted by permission of Pearson Education, Inc., Upper Saddle River, NJ.

Urinary Tract Illnesses and Problems

Women are at higher risk than men for developing some disorders of the urinary tract. This section will address lower urinary tract infection, interstitial cystitis, kidney infection, and urinary incontinence.

Lower Urinary Tract Infection

The terms **urinary tract infection (UTI)** and **cystitis** both refer to the inflammation and infection of the urinary bladder. UTIs are caused when microorganisms, such as bacteria, enter the urinary bladder, usually by ascending the urethra. UTI is responsible for more than 5 million physician visits per year (Parker & Berding, 1997) and is the most common **nosocomial** (hospital-acquired) infection in the United States. Diabetic women, pregnant women, elderly women, and women who are sexually active are especially vulnerable to UTI.

The microorganism that most often causes UTIs in women is *Escherichia coli (E. coli)*. Normally present in feces, *E. coli* is easily transmitted from the anus to the vaginal and urethral openings. The short length of the female urethra makes it easy for *E. coli* bacteria to ascend the urethra and invade the urinary bladder. A related factor that may also play a part in women's susceptibility to UTI is the presence of a compound called **glycosphingolipid** in at least some women's urinary tracts. This compound, discovered in 1998, seems to have the property of binding strongly with *E. coli*. Scientists are presently working to develop a substance that will inhibit *E. coli* from binding with glycosphingolipid.

Up to 10 percent of women who experience UTIs have three to five infections a year. These recurring infections are difficult to treat, and, until recently, it was not known why they occur. Recently, it has been discovered that, in some women, *E. coli* evades antibiotics by penetrating the immune cells that line the bladder (Baorto et al., 1997). It is anticipated that many cases of recurrent UTI can be halted by the use of antibiotics that more thoroughly penetrate these cells.

Innate mechanisms exist to protect the urinary tract from bacterial invasion. For example, the chemical nature of urine is such that the bacteria that are normally found in the urethra do not usually grow well in it, and bacterial growth is most inhibited when the pH of the urine is low. In addition, the flow of urine flushes bacteria from the urinary bladder. These defense mechanisms serve as natural protective measures against urinary tract infections (Berding, 1997).

Cystitis is a very common infection, occurring in 2 out of 100 people. Among the elderly, the incidence is 30 out of 100 people (Parker & Berding, 1997). UTIs are more common in **women** than men; on average, 10 to 20 percent of younger women and over 30 percent of elderly women experience a UTI at least once (Stein, 1994).

A number of risk factors increase a woman's chances of developing a UTI. Having an instrument inserted into the urinary tract (as during catheterization), pregnancy, and diabetes, all increase the risk. Having an obstruction of the bladder or urethra is also a risk factor, as it can cause the incomplete emptying of the urinary bladder, with subsequent retention and stagnation. Sexual intercourse increases a women's risk for developing a UTI, because bacteria can be introduced into the urethra. Postmenopausal status also increases the risk, because the drop in estrogen levels lower the acidity of the vaginal canal, making it easier for bacteria to adhere to the vaginal wall, and migrate into the urethra (Bladder Trouble?, 2001).

SYMPTOMS

The symptoms most commonly experienced by women with a UTI are **dysuria** (painful urination), **frequency** (urinating frequently in small amounts), urgency, and nocturia. Irritation and inflammation of the urethra and urinary bladder may also cause pain, and a feeling of pressure, in the lower abdomen. The color of the urine may be abnormal, and it may appear cloudy and have a strong, foul odor. If there is severe irritation and inflammation of the bladder lining, the urine may be blood-tinged or may be grossly bloody (hematuria). Although many women do not experience a fever, many do complain of fatigue, nausea, vomiting, or painful sexual intercourse. Table 16–2 summarizes the common signs and symptoms of lower urinary tract infection. In elderly women, the initial symptoms may be mental changes and confusion. This is because age-related physiological changes in the urinary tract may mask the usual signs and symptoms of a UTI. In that event, the infectious process will go unnoticed until it becomes systemic and produces a change in the level of consciousness, disorientation, and confusion.

TABLE 16–2 Symptoms of lower urinary tract infection.

Pressure in the lower pelvis	Cloudy urine
Painful sexual intercourse	Bloody urine
Painful urination	Foul or strong urine odor
Frequency	Fever
Frequent voiding at night	Vomiting
Urgency	Mental changes or confusion
Fatigue	(elderly women)
Chills	

DIAGNOSIS

The diagnosis of a urinary tract infection depends on the persistence of the signs and symptoms and the isolation of the offending bacteria from the urine. Any woman with the signs and symptoms of a UTI should contact her doctor immediately for a medical evaluation. The laboratory tests that are most often done include a **urinalysis** and a **urine culture**. The urinalysis may reveal a higher than normal number of white blood cells in the urine, which is indicative of a possible infection. Normally, urine contains less then 10,000 organisms per milliliter of urine; the diagnosis of UTI is usually made when there are 100,000 or more (Stein, 1994). The urine may also contain red blood cells, which, if present in sufficient amounts, causes the urine to appear cloudy or pink.

A urine culture is done to identify the specific bacterium that is causing the infection. A **clean catch** (collected after the urinary opening has been cleansed) or **catheterized** (collected via a sterile tube inserted into the bladder) urine specimen is necessary, so that the urine will not be contaminated by organisms commonly found on the skin near the vaginal opening. The identification of the offending organisms is useful in ensuring that the appropriate antibiotic therapy is used to eradicate the infection.

TREATMENT

The goals of treatment are to eradicate the invading bacteria and to prevent a reccurrence of the infection. Antibiotics are used to rid the urinary bladder of bacteria. Forty-eight hours of treatment with antibiotics usually reduces significantly the number of bacteria present in the urinary bladder. The antibiotics most commonly used to treat UTIs include cephalosporins and sulfa drugs (see Table 16–3). Antibiotics are usually prescribed for three to seven days. *It is important to complete the entire course of medication, even if the symptoms have disappeared.* Interrupting drug therapy prematurely may allow the regrowth of bacterial strains resistant to the antibiotic. A new, single-dose antibiotic (Monurol) that remains concentrated in the urinary bladder for more then three days is now available (Bladder Trouble?, 2001). The drug Pyridium or (Uristat) may be used to calm urgency and burning until the antibiotics take effect.

Recurrent UTIs must be treated thoroughly to prevent the development of a **kidney infection.** Antibiotic therapy may be needed for as long as six months to two years, and stronger antibiotics than those used for single episodes may be necessary. After the acute symptoms of a recurrent infection have subsided, the healthcare provider may use preventive low-dose therapy for an extended period of time.

The practice of increasing fluid intake (forcing fluids) to flush the bacteria from the urinary bladder when an infection is present is controversial. Forcing fluids may actually hinder treatment by lowering the concentration of the antibiotic in the urinary tract. Women should discuss the advisability of forcing fluids with their healthcare providers.

TABLE 16–3 Medications used to treat UTI.	
Anti-infective/Sulfa Medications	**Cephalosporins**
Amoxicillin	Duricef
Ampicillin	Ancef
Ampicillin/sulbactam (Unasyn)	Keflex
Furadantin	Mandol
Sulfamethethoxazole (Grantanol, Urobak)	Cefotan
	Zinacef
Trimethoprim (Proloprim, Trimpex)	Maxipime
Trimethorprim/sulfmethoxazole (Bactrim, Septra, TMP/SMX)	Claforan
	Rocephin
	Fortaz

Avorn (1994) reported that drinking cranberry juice decreases the risk of recurrent UTIs in elderly women. The researchers found that women who drank 10 ounces of cranberry juice a day for six months were 58 percent less likely to have recurrent infections than were those who drank a placebo. A more recent study (Kontiokari et al., 2001) also supports cranberry juice as an agent that is effective in preventing UTI. Cranberries, and to a lesser extent blueberries, contain a substance that prevents *E. coli* bacteria from adhering to the cells that line the urinary bladder, thus enabling the bacteria to be flushed out in the urine. Ingesting cranberry juice or dry cranberry juice extract (300 to 500 milligrams in one to two capsules a day) is an alternative therapy for women who suffer from recurrent infections and are on almost continuous antibiotic therapy. Cranberry juice *without sugar* should be used, as sugar is a good growth medium for bacteria. Although cranberry is usually a safe therapy, it should be used cautiously by women who are taking antidepressants or pain medication, as the cranberry may cause the medications to be excreted more rapidly (How to Eradicate Bladder Infections (2000)).

The thinning of the urinary bladder lining that gradually develops after menopause decreases the bladder's ability to resist bacterial infections. A topical estrogen cream can enhance the health of urinary tissue and prevent recurrent urinary tract infections (Northrup, 2001).

Natural products, such as herbs, have been used to treat UTIs in Europe for decades. *Echinacea* (*E. purpurea radix*) has been shown to have antibacterial and immune-modulating properties. It is said to promote the destruction of bacteria and to inhibit the action of a substance secreted by the bacteria that helps them gain access to healthy cells. Echinacea is available as an extract (1–2 milliliters three times a day) or in capsule form (300 milligrams three times a day). *Nettle* is another herb that has been used to treat urinary tract infections. It should be avoided during pregnancy and in women with cardiac or renal disease. Nettle is available as a dried extract (770 milligrams twice a day) and as a liquid extract (3–4 milliliters three times a day) (Bladder Trouble?, 2001). *Uva ursi* is another herb used to treat urinary tract infections. The active ingredient in uva ursi is arbutin, which is converted into the antiseptic **hydroquinone,** which has antibacterial effects when it reaches the urinary bladder. Uva ursi should not be used during pregnancy or when concurrent kidney or gastrointestinal disorders are present. Generally, a tea is made from the dried leaves and a cup consumed up to four times daily. Uva ursi should be used for only one week at a time and no more then five times a year (Bladder Trouble?, 2001). Before using herbal therapies, women should discuss the matter with their healthcare providers, as there may be a potential interaction between the herb and the antibiotic therapy.

Interstitial Cystitis

Interstitial cystitis is a chronic, inflammatory bladder condition that primarily affects middle-aged women. It is a non-bacterial form of cystitis that causes a decrease in bladder capacity and a thickening of the bladder lining. The cause, or **etiology,** of interstitial cystitis is unknown. Various factors have been implicated, including a neurogenic inflammatory response, allergies, autoimmune disease, defects in or damage to the urinary bladder, and an obstruction of the blood vessels and lymph system of the bladder (Berding, 1997).

There are approximately 700,000 cases of interstitial cystitis in the United States, with 90 percent of the affected individuals being women. Interstitial cystitis is three times more prevalent in the United States than in Europe (Ratner, 2001). The National Institutes of Health have allocated $7.5 million for research on this condition.

SYMPTOMS

The symptoms of interstitial cystitis include complaints of frequency, urgency, nocturia, and pain; the urine, however, is clear of infection. Additional complaints include severe pain with sexual intercourse, lower back and thigh pain, sleep deprivation, and depression. The symptoms may disrupt women's personal and professional lives. Some women are unable to work full-time, and others are so disabled by this condition that they are unable to work at all.

DIAGNOSIS

A woman complaining of symptoms suggestive of interstitial cystitis will be given a physical examination, and her lower abdomen will likely be found to be tender. Her urine will be examined microscopically for the presence of red blood cells, which may be found if the bladder is overdistended. **Cystoscopy** (using an instrument to examine the inside of the urinary bladder) will also be done. The diagnosis of interstitial cystitis is confirmed if hemorrhages known as **Hunner's ulcers** are present (Ratner, 2001).

TREATMENT

Treatment is aimed at relieving the symptoms. It requires active participation by the woman and may be prolonged. Nonsteroidal anti-inflammatory drugs, such as ibuprofen, may be used to decrease inflammation and provide pain relief. Anticholinergic drugs, (such as Atropine, Robinul, and Probanthel) may help reduce bladder spasms. **Pentosan polysulfate sodium** is currently the only drug specifically approved for the treatment of interstitial cystitis. It is thought to promote the restoration of the bladder lining and has been demonstrated to be effective (Bladder Trouble?, 2001). The amino acid L-arginine is thought by some to have antibacterial, smooth muscle relaxant and immune-modulating effects on the lining of the bladder, and, in one clinical trial (Smith, Wheeler, Foster, & Weiss, 1996), it was found to decrease pain on urination, lower abdominal pain, urinary frequency, and nocturia. Unfortunately, a subsequent study done in Sweden (Ehren, Lundgerg, Adolfsson, & Wiklund, 1998) did not support the original findings. The use of L-arginine in interstitial cystitis remains controversial and is not considered accepted therapy at the present time. More studies on herbs are necessary to further evaluate their effectiveness.

Methodologies other than oral drug therapy are also used to treat interstitial cystitis. The liquid **dimethyl sulfoxide (DMSO)** can be instilled directly into the bladder in an attempt to enlarge its capacity. DSMO has analgesic, anti-inflammatory, and smooth muscle relaxant effects. It must be instilled regularly, however, usually on a weekly basis, to be effective (Berding, 1997). **Transcutaneous electrical nerve stimulation (TENS)** during which mild electrical current is applied to the skin has been used to treat the pain associated with interstitial cystitis. Battery powered implants that stimulate the sacral nerve have been evaluated in clinical trials (Maher, Carey, Dwyer, & Schluter, 2001) and have been found to increase urine volume, decrease in urinary frequency, and decrease in bladder pain. Further studies are being carried out on this promising experimental therapy. Laser surgery has been used to treat Hunner's ulcers. Although it is not considered a cure, it can alleviate symptoms for a long period of time (Ratner, 2001). Stress reduction, exercise, and bladder retraining are adjunct therapies that may provide symptom management for some women. Avoiding caffeine, artificial sweeteners, alcohol, and tobacco can also reduce symptoms, as can a diet low in acidic foods and the amino acids tyramine, tyrosine, and trytophan. Some women find that restricting their intake of salt and sugar and avoiding foods that contain yeast is beneficial (Ratner, 2001). Box 16–3 lists the foods and beverages that seem to exacerbate interstitial cystitis in some women.

Kidney Infection

A kidney infection, or **acute pyelonephritis,** is caused by bacteria that invade the kidney tissue and the renal pelvis. The infection usually begins in the lower urinary tract and

Figure 16–3   Pathological Changes in the Kidney from Acute Pyelonephritis

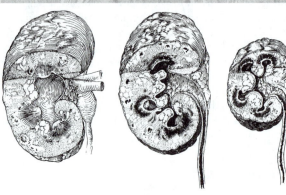

| Severely enlarged kidney | Moderately enlarged kidney | Normal kidney |

Source: Chapter title and author in Burrell/Gerlach/Pless, *Adult nursing: Acute and community care* (2nd ed., © 1997, p. 1279, F. 48-7). Reprinted by permission of Pearson Education, Inc., Upper Saddle River, NJ.

ascends from the bladder to a ureter, and then to the kidney itself. When bacteria reaches the kidney, the infection becomes more severe and more difficult to cure with antibiotics. Because women are more susceptible than men to UTIs, their risk for developing kidney infections is also greater.

Acute pyelonephritis affects approximately 3 to 7 people out of 10,000 at some point in their lives and physicians treat about 375,000 cases of kidney infection annually in the United States (Parker, 1997). Women are markedly susceptible to acute pyelonephritis due to urethral trauma sustained during intercourse and the short length of their urethra. Other factors that increase the risk of kidney infection include a history of cystitis, kidney stones, injury to the kidney, or problems that interfere with the flow of urine.

In healthy individuals, the urinary bladder, kidneys, and urine are **sterile.** Urine stored in the bladder is known to be a good environment for the growth of the bacteria that cause UTIs. Kidney infections caused by bacteria ascending from the urinary bladder are usually caused by the **reflux** (backward flow) of infected urine from the bladder to the ureters and kidneys (Parker, 1997). The infected kidney tissues swell, and the flow of urine from one or both of the kidneys becomes increasingly obstructed. The infected kidney becomes enlarged (see Figure 16–3), and localized destruction of renal structures occurs. The acute inflammation usually subsides after 1 to 3 weeks. After 6 to 10 weeks a scar develops and the kidneys become sterile again.

SYMPTOMS

The major symptoms of kidney infection are high fever, 102°F or higher, that persists for more than two days; flank or back pain, which may radiate to the front; painful or difficult urination; and frequency. Other symptoms that may be present include chills; moist skin (diaphoresis); flushed, warm skin; nausea and vomiting; fatigue; and malaise. The urine may be cloudy or have an abnormal color, with a foul or strong odor. **Hematuria** (red blood cells in the urine) may be present. In the elderly population, acute pyelonephritis may cause acute confusion with urinary incontinence or the deterioration of physical, mental, and behavioral abilities (Matsumoto & Kumazawa, 1999).

DIAGNOSIS

A physical examination may reveal tenderness on palpation over the affected kidney. When the urine is analysed (urinalysis) blood, pus, and white blood cells are usually found to be present in the urine. A urine culture on a clean catch or catheterized specimen will identify the offending bacteria. Blood work usually shows an elevated white blood count, and a blood culture often reveals infection with **gram-negative bacteria,** such as *Escherichia coli.* Uncomplicated acute pyelonephritis does not affect kidney function; therefore, the **blood urea nitrogen level (BUN)** is normal. A severe infection will result in an elevated BUN and **proteinuria** (protein in the urine) and may cause kidney damage. An intravenous pyelogram **(IVP)** (an X ray of the kidneys using a radiographic dye) or a CT scan of the abdomen will reveal enlarged kidney.

TREATMENT

The treatment goals for acute pyelonephritis include eradication of the infection and the reduction of the symptoms. The initial symptoms may persist for more than 48 hours after treatment has been started. Due to the risk for permanent kidney damage and a high mortality in the elderly from acute pyelonephritis, prompt treatment is recommended. The individual is usually given broad-spectrum antibiotics IV (intravenously) until the causative bacterium is identified. After 3 to 5 days of IV antibiotic therapy, oral medication can usually be started. Antibiotic therapy is continued for 10 to 14 days, and it is imperative that the entire course of therapy be finished. Antipyretics, such as Tylenol and Motrin, are given to control the fever. An increased fluid intake of 2,000 to 4,000 cc (8 to 10 eight ounce glasses) per day will cause frequent urination and will flush bacteria from the bladder (Parker, 1997). Most cases of acute pyelonephritis resolve without complication when treated effectively, but the therapy may need to be aggressive and/or prolonged.

Urinary Incontinence

Urinary incontinence, is defined as a condition in which involuntary loss of urine is objectively demonstrable, resulting in a social or hygiene problem (Hagglund, Olsson, & Leppert, 1999). Urinary incontinence can result from a number of factors that affect the urinary tract itself, as well as from extraneous factors, such as infection, the effects of menopausal estrogen loss, dementia, impaired mobility, fecal impaction (a buildup of fecal material in the rectum), and side effects of medications. Fortunately, many intrinsic and extrinsic causative factors can be reversed.

Approximately 11 to 17 million adults in the United States have urinary incontinence, and about 85 percent of them are women (Swithinbank & Abrams, 1999). The prevalence of urinary incontinence in women ages 42 to 50 is approximately 30 percent. Prevalence increases as women age, and it has been estimated that 45 percent of noninstitutionalized women over 65 years of age suffer from incontinence (Johnson, 2000). Urinary incontinence is a major cause of disability and dependence in the United States. Cummings and Houston (1994) report that incontinence is the most common reason for institutionalizing elderly individuals, and many of the 1.5 million nursing home residents have one or more episodes of urinary incontinence per day.

Americans spend more than $15 million annually to manage urinary incontinence, and approximately 40 percent of the sanitary pads purchased in this country are used by incontinent, rather than menstruating, women (Johnson, 2000). Urinary incontinence is embarrassing for women; their clothing may become wet with urine, resulting in an offensive odor. Incontinence can impair body image and cause a loss of self-esteem and dignity (Swithinbank & Abrams, 1999), and incontinent women may feel that they have no control over their bodies. Many experience feelings of frustration and despair, and some even avoid social situations and become recluses.

The urinary bladder is a muscular sac, which sits in the pelvis and stores urine received from the kidneys via the ureters. When the bladder is full of urine, it should remain relaxed until the individual wishes to void. At that time, it should contract in order to squeeze the urine into the urethra. Sphincter muscles, which prevent the leakage of urine from the bladder, encircle the urethra. When the bladder becomes full, the individual experiences the desire to void. When she is ready to do so, nerve signals cause the bladder to contract and the urethral sphincter to relax. Normally, squeezing urine out of the bladder into the urethra is under **voluntary** control. However, incontinence can develop if the bladder muscle becomes overactive, particularly if the urethral spincter muscles have become weak. Urinary control problems can also occur when the bladder muscle becomes too weak to contract properly, or when signals from the nervous system to the urinary structures are interrupted. The three types of incontinence that most frequently afflict women are stress incontinence, urge incontinence, and overflow incontinence.

Stress incontinence is the involuntary loss of urine due to a sudden increase in intra-abdominal pressure, usually related to coughing or lifting (Parker & Berding, 1997). It is the most common type of incontinence in women age 45 to 54 years (Newman, 2001). Common causes of stress incontinence include pelvic muscle relaxation due to pregnancy and childbirth and weakening of the spincter muscles after menopause due to the loss of estrogen. The relaxation of the pelvic muscles results in hypermobility or displacement of the urethra and bladder neck, causing them to drop and open during exertion (Butler, Maby, Montella, & Young, 1999).

Urge incontinence is the involuntary loss of urine associated with a sudden, strong desire to void (Parker & Berding, 1997). Involuntary detrusor (bladder) muscle contraction, known as **detrusor overactivity,** is commonly associated with urge incontinence. Detrusor overactivity is frequently seen in women with neurological conditions, such as those who have had a stroke, and those who suffer from multiple sclerosis or dementia (Newman, 2001). When no neurological impairment is present, patients with urge incontinence are said to have **detrusor instability,** also known as an unstable bladder and overactive bladder. The causes of detrusor instability include bladder **calculi** (stones), **diverticuli**

(pouches in the bladder wall), foreign bodies, and tumors (Cummings & Houston, 1994). Smoking and obesity can also contribute to UI. Nicotine enhances bladder contractility, and obesity results in higher intra-abdominal pressures and greater pressure on the bladder (Newman, 2001).

Yet another form of incontinence, **overflow incontinence,** is characterized by intermittent loss of urine associated with overdistention of the bladder (Parker & Berding, 1997). A number of factors can cause a bladder to fail to contract sufficiently to expel urine and become overdistended. These include an underactive detrusor muscle and an obstruction in the urethra or bladder. Anything that impairs the signals sent to the bladder by the nervous system, such as spinal cord injury, pelvic surgery, and diabetes, can also impair the bladder's ability to contract. The bladder may also become underactive as a result of medication and fecal impaction. When the bladder is already overdistended, and additional urine enters from the kidneys, the individual experiences a strong desire to void; if she cannot do so quickly, involuntary leakage of urine results.

Symptoms

Different symptoms are associated with the three types of incontinence. It is vital to determine the type and cause of the incontinence before treatment is initiated.

In stress incontinence, urine leakage occurs with coughing, sneezing, laughing, physical activities, lifting of heavy objects, and other straining. This leakage is the result of the combination of weak pelvic muscles and an increase in abdominal pressure.

The individual with urge incontinence experiences strong, sudden urges to urinate (urgency), even if the bladder contains little urine. There is involuntary loss of urine immediately following this abrupt and strong desire to go to the bathroom.

Women who suffer from overflow incontinence experience an intermittent loss of urine that manifests as frequent or constant dribbling. The bladder becomes overdistended with urine, and, when more urine enters from the kidneys, an abrupt desire to void is experienced. If the woman does not urinate, dribbling occurs.

Diagnosis

It is important to establish which type of incontinence a woman has, so that effective treatment can be provided. An evaluation to determine the type and cause of incontinence will include a history and physical exam, plus a urinalysis, and perhaps more specialized testing as well. The woman will be asked about her medical, neurological, and genitourinary history, as well as what prescription and nonprescription medications and dietary supplements she takes. She will also be asked to describe her symptoms and any related factors. The individual will be specifically questioned about the following (Newman, 2001):

1. *The duration and characteristics of the leakage*
2. *The frequency, timing, and amount of urination (continent and incontinent)*
3. *Any associated symptoms and precipitating factors*
4. *Any other lower urinary symptoms (pain while urinating, bloody urine)*
5. *Daily fluid intake*
6. *Changes in bowel and/or sexual function*
7. *Any previous treatment for incontinence and its effects*
8. *The use of pads, briefs, and other protective supplies*
9. *The use of any food supplements or drugs that affect urinary patterns, such as diuretics, tricyclic antidepressants, and caffeine*

The physical examination of incontinent individuals will include the following components (Newman, 2001):

1. *An abdominal examination to detect masses and bladder fullness or tenderness*
2. *A pelvic examination to assess for skin excoriation, genital atrophy, pelvic masses, or abnormal bulging of the urethral or bladder wall into the vagina, and to evaluate muscle tone*
3. *A general examination intended to detect related or additional health problems, and neurological assess mobility, cognition, and manual dexterity*

After the history and physical exam are completed, several tests may be performed to clarify symptoms, identify specific abnormalities, and determine initial treatment. An estimation of the **post-void residual (PVR)** is recommended for all individuals with incontinence. The PVR is the amount of urine left in the bladder after voiding. The general consensus is that a PVR of less than 50 mL (milliliters) of urine reflects adequate emptying of the bladder and more than 200 mL of urine reflects inadequate emptying.

If stress incontinence is suspected, the individual will be asked to cough vigorously while the physician observes for loss of urine. This test can be done in a standing or **lithotomy** (feet in stirrups) position. If urine leaks immediately when the woman begins coughing, stress incontinence is suspected. When the leakage is delayed or continues after coughing, detrusor overactivity is usually the cause. If the test is initially performed in the lithotomy position and there is no leakage, it will be repeated in the standing position.

A urinalysis is done to assess for associated conditions, such as **hematuria** which suggests infection, cancer, or stones; **pyuria** (pus in urine); **glycosuria** (sugar in urine); and **proteinuria** (protein in urine). The urine may also be examined under a microscope; if white blood cells and/or bacteria are seen, a **urine culture** (allowing a sample of bacteria from the urine to reproduce in a laboratory in order to identify them) is warranted.

If further evaluation is necessary to determine the type and cause of incontinence, a number of urodynamic and endoscopic tests can be performed to determine the anatomical and functional status of the bladder and urethra. **Urodynamic** tests measure such variables as the pressure in the abdomen, the volume of urine in the bladder, the force with which the bladder contracts, and so on. Endoscopic procedures involve threading a hollow, lighted catheter into the urethra, bladder, ureters, and interior of the kidney in order to visualize them directly. Which tests are performed depends on the type of incontinence that is suspected.

Urodynamic and Endoscopic Tests The urodynamic tests used to distinguish among the various types of incontinence include the stress cystourethrogram, cystometrogram, dynamic profilometry, uroflowometry, and videourodynamics. The endoscopic test is known as cystourethroscopy.

A **stress cystourethrogram** is done to measure simultaneously detrusor function and intra-abdominal pressure. This test can assess bladder sensation, capacity, and compliance and can differentiate an involuntary detrusor contraction from increased abdominal pressure.

A **cystometrogram (CMG),** a test of detrusor function, is done by using a catheter to fill the bladder with fluid to capacity, or until involuntary detrusor contraction occurs. If the individual is able to urinate, a voiding CMG may be performed to measure detrusor contractility and detect urethral obstruction.

Dynamic profilometry, also known as **leak point pressure determination,** measures the pressures in the urethra under various conditions, such as being at rest or during coughing or straining. These measures can be used to determine the effect of exertion on the individual's ability to control the flow of urine.

Uroflowometry measures the rate at which the urine flows from the bladder. While it has not been proven to differentiate among the specific types of incontinence in women, and it cannot distinguish between urethral obstruction and detrusor weakness, it can provide useful information in cases in which the individual has difficulty emptying her bladder (Berding, 1997).

Videourodynamics combines various urodynamic tests with simultaneous X-ray visualization. It can be used to differentiate between detrusor overactivity and underactivity, and it can reveal abnormalities and obstructions in the urethra and bladder.

Cystourethroscopy, or direct visualization of the urethra and bladder, is helpful in identifying bladder lesions, foreign bodies, diverticula (pouches in the bladder wall), and strictures (abnormal narrowing).

PREVENTION AND TREATMENT

How urinary incontinence is treated depends on the type of bladder control problem that the individual experiences. Some types of treatment are relatively simple and others are more complex. The treatment options available to a particular woman must be discussed with her and the risks, benefits, and potential outcomes explained. In most cases, the least invasive procedure with the fewest risks is the first choice for treatment. Generally, surgical intervention is used only when other treatment methods have failed.

Stress Incontinence The prevention and conservative (nonsurgical) treatment of stress incontinence includes the following: (1) using pelvic muscle exercises and/or electrical stimulation to strengthen perineal muscles, (2) using various devices to hold the bladder in its proper position or mechanically prevent urine from leaking from it, (3) taking medications that cause the bladder neck to contract and stop the flow of urine, (4) embarking on a program of bladder retraining, and (5) educating the woman about the implications and importance of fluid intake.

Pelvic muscle exercises, called **Kegel exercises,** strengthen the sphincter muscles that surround the urethra. They also increase muscle support to the pelvic structures, thereby enhancing the closing of the urethra. Kegels involve two types of muscle contractions—short and long. Short contractions last 2 seconds and long contractions can last up to 10 seconds, with practice. The steps in performing Kegel exercises are listed in Box 16–5. It is recommended that women begin doing Kegels before menopause and do them on a consistent basis. They should also do Kegels during pregnancy and after childbirth to prevent damage to the pelvic muscles (Johnson, 2000). Kegels are generally most helpful to women with stress incontinence, but they can be useful in cases of urge incontinence (Newman, 2001). A form of biofeedback (see Chapter 11) known as **surface electromyography (sEMG)** has proven

---

Box 16–5 Steps in Performing Kegel Exercises

Step 1

Identify the correct muscles by stopping the flow of urine during voiding and then restarting it.

Step 2

Assume a comfortable position; standing, sitting, or lying down are all acceptable. Squeeze the vaginal muscles (as if you were stopping the flow of urine) and hold them tightly for several seconds. Repeat this 10 times.

Step 3

Squeeze the muscles around the anus (as if holding back gas) and hold them tightly for several seconds. Repeat this 10 times.

Step 4

Repeat these cycles 3 or 4 times a day. The number and duration can be increased as you tolerate the exercises.

to help women learn to strengthen the muscles that control urination. Electrodes are attached to the skin overlying the target muscles, and a visual or an auditory signal alerts the patient when she is targeting the correct muscle group (Woolner, 2001).

Cone-shaped **vaginal weights** can also be used to strengthen the peri-urethral muscles. Contracting the pelvic muscles in order to hold the weight in the vagina for up to 15 minutes strengthens them. Initially, the woman inserts the lightest cone into her vagina and contracts her pelvic floor muscles to keep it in place. If she can hold the weight in place for 60 seconds, she moves to the next heaviest weight. When she finds a weight that she cannot hold for 60 seconds, she will use that one during her exercise periods. This exercise should be done in the sitting position initially; however, once the weight can be retained in this position, the woman can begin to walk, climb stairs, run in place, and cough while holding the weight in place. As a woman's symptoms improve, she can decrease the frequency of her exercise sessions to alternate days or to whenever she feels a need. Vaginal cones are used primarily in premenopausal women and should be used with caution in postmenopausal women who have **vaginal atrophy** (thinning of vaginal tissues due to a lack of estrogen) (Johnson, 2000).

Electrical stimulation involves placing in the vagina a small electrode connected to a generator. The generator produces a small current, which stimulates weakened pelvic muscles to contract (Newman, 2001).

Pessaries are devices designed to hold the bladder in place and to prevent urine leakage when abdominal pressure rises. When inserted high in the vagina, they lift the bladder into a more normal position. Pessaries are made in a variety of shapes and sizes (see Chapter 17) and are composed of flexible or rigid silicone, latex, or acrylic material. Some types can be inserted by the woman herself, but others must be inserted by a health professional (Johnson, 2000). A similar device, **Introl,** is a soft silicone ring which women can insert into their vaginas and removed daily for cleaning. *Introl* has two prongs, which support the junction between the urethra and the bladder neck. Its manufacturer claims a high success rate at controlling incontinence caused by mild structural abnormalities.

Collagen, a bulking agent, can be injected into the tissues surrounding the urethra to help support it. Collagen remains in the tissues for a period of time between six months and two years, and it can be reinjected as necessary. Tschopp, Wesley-James, Spekkens, and Lohfeld (1999) studied the efficacy of collagen injection as a treatment for incontinence, and reported a mean success rate of 56 percent.

A similar approach involves placing a **temporary adhesive patch** over the urethral opening. Patches do not totally eliminate leakage, but they decrease the amount of urine that is leaked from the bladder. They must be replaced after each voiding.

Yet another mechanical option is the **Reliance balloon-tipped catheter.** Women insert this catheter into the urethra and inflate the balloon. The balloon blocks the flow of urine, much like a cork. When the woman wishes to void, she pulls a string to deflate the balloon and remove the catheter (*Controlling Urinary Incontinence,* 2000).

The medications that are used to treat stress incontinence belong to the category of drugs known as **alpha-adrenergic agonists.** They are effective because they stimulate the numerous alpha-adrenergic receptors present in the urethra, bladder neck, and bladder base. Alpha-adrenergic stimulation strengthens muscle contractions in these structures and enhances their ability to hold urine in the bladder. Phenylpropanolamine (Triaminic) and pseudoephedrine (Sudafed) are the two alpha-adrenergic agonists currently prescribed for women with stress incontinence.

Estrogen replacement therapy can be used to help maintain vaginal and bladder muscle control in postmenopausal women. The exact mechanism of action is unknown, but it is believed that estrogen increases bladder outlet resistance, thereby decreasing stress incontinence. Estrogen therapy by mouth or in the form of a vaginal cream may benefit some women with stress incontinence (Parker & Berding, 1997).

Bladder retraining involves placing the incontinent woman on a voiding schedule. She is taught to resist the feeling of urgency, to consciously postpone voiding, and to urinate on schedule, rather than when she has the urge to void. The time between scheduled voidings is gradually increased, until a reasonable frequency pattern has been achieved. Distraction and/or relaxation procedures are often used to help women resist the urge to void (Newman, 2001). Eventually, the bladder begins to respond to the schedule and contracts at the appointed times, rather than haphazardly. Fantl et al. (1991) studied the efficacy of bladder retraining in a population of elderly women with incontinence and found that the number of incontinent episodes was reduced in most subjects and that 75 percent of the women improved by more than 50 percent. The steps of a bladder-retraining program are outlined in Box 16–6.

Women who are incontinent must be educated about the importance of taking in an optimal amount of **fluid** in the course of a day. Many incontinent women mistakenly believe that limiting fluid intake will help them remain dryer, but this is a misconception. *Concentrated* urine is more irritating to the bladder than more dilute urine, and restricting fluids to the point below 1,500 mL/day will only aggravate incontinence. Many authorities recommend that incontinent women take in 2,400 mL/day (Newman, 2001).

If conservative treatment of stress incontinence fails, **surgical repair** may be necessary. The most common procedure for stress incontinence is bladder neck suspension, which restores a sagging bladder to its proper position. In some cases, a sling is placed under the urethra and bladder to provide extra support. Surgery for stress incontinence

Box 16–6   Steps in Bladder Retraining

Step 1

Perform Kegel exercises as described in Box 16–5.

Step 2

Develop a toileting schedule. Begin with on arising, every two hours during the day and evening, before going to bed, and every four hours during the night.

Step 3

Make an effort to void at the specific times, even if you don't have the urge. Try running the water or drinking cold water.

Step 4

Relax and try to empty your bladder each time you void. Try reading a book or doing deep-breathing exercises.

Step 5

Drink some liquids about 30 minutes before each planned voiding.

Step 6

Avoid tea, coffee, alcohol, and other liquids that contain caffeine.

Step 7

Take diuretics and liquids that increase urination (such as coffee or tea) early in the day.

Step 8

Limit liquids after supper until bedtime.

Step 9

Gradually lengthen or shorten the time periods between voiding, depending on your degree of continence.

Step 10

Have a positive outlook and don't become discouraged. Becoming continent may take several weeks or months.

generally requires two or more days of hospitalization. Surgical intervention for stress incontinence, and other forms of incontinence as well, should be performed only after a thorough medical evaluation and discussion between the woman and her physician. The evaluation and discussion should include confirmation of the type of incontinence, its severity, the nature of the planned procedure and the risks involved, and the potential impact of the procedure on the woman's quality of life.

Urge Incontinence   The prevention and treatment of urge incontinence includes bladder retraining, electrical stimulation, medications to treat detrusor overactivity, and surgery for severe bladder instability or poor compliance. Several lifestyle changes can also be beneficial in the treatment of urge incontinence. Limiting fluid intake and avoiding **caffeine,** a known stimulant for an unstable bladder, can reduce the frequency of incontinent episodes. Acidic and spicy foods, alcohol, and artificial sweeteners may also irritate the bladder (*Controlling Urinary Incontinence*, 2000).

The medications used to treat urge incontinence generally relax the bladder and thereby increase bladder capacity, to some degree (Jay & Staskin, 1998). The **anticholinergic** medications Ditropan, Levbid, and Detrol are commonly used for this purpose. Women should think carefully about taking them, however, because bladder contractions are usually not completely abolished, and improvement is modest. Studies indicate that the use of these medications typically results in only about a 20 percent reduction in the total number of voidings over 24 hours. These medications are costly, and most have annoying side effects (*Controlling Urinary Incontinence*, 2000).

Overflow Incontinence   Overflow incontinence in women is most commonly caused by obstruction of the urethra or another reversible condition. Treatment generally involves identifying and treating the underlying cause. If the underlying cause is a displaced bladder or an obstruction, surgery is recommended. When overflow incontinence results from an underactive detrusor, bladder retraining, timed voiding, and insertion of a pessary comprise the treatment choices. There are no medications that increase the strength of the bladder muscles.

Timed voiding, also known as habit training, means urinating at scheduled times on a routine basis. An effort is made to identify the individual's normal voiding schedule and plan the voiding routine based on it. Timed voiding has been shown to be effective in dependent and cognitively impaired women, because women who need assistance to get to the bathroom, or who forget to go, often have overdistended bladders, and leakage occurs as urine continues to enter the bladder from the kidneys. Having such women empty their bladders at scheduled times prevents overdistention and encourages continence. To achieve success with timed voiding, dependent or cognitively impaired women must have a caregiver who will assist with maintaining the voiding schedule (Newman, 2001).

PROTECTIVE PRODUCTS

Long-term use of protective products for all types of incontinence should be considered only after the individual's incontinence has been evaluated by a healthcare professional.

Protective pads and special panties should be offered as a choice only after other treatment options have failed. Dependence on pads and panties may be a detriment to continence because it gives the individual a sense of security. Accepting incontinence decreases the individual's motivation to seek evaluation and treatment (Starer & Libow, 1985). When used improperly, pads can contribute to skin breakdown and urinary tract infection. Pads must be changed frequently; meticulous hygiene must be maintained. The quality and cost of protective products vary greatly, and there is a lack of research comparing the quality and effectiveness of various products. Finally, the cost of pads and panties can be a burden for women on a fixed income (Hu, Kaltreider, & Igou, 1989).

 ## Urinary Tract Wellness Self-Assessment

Considering your answers to the following questions in light of the information provided in this chapter will help you evaluate the functioning of your urinary tract.

Urinary Wellness

1. Is your urine clear and yellow, with an aromatic odor?
2. Do you urinate more than five times during the day?
3. Do you frequently have to get up more then twice at night to urinate?
4. Do you drink at least six to eight eight ounce glasses of water per day?
5. Do you practice good perineal hygiene?

Lower Urinary Tract and Kidney Infections

1. Do you experience pain or burning on urination?
2. Do you void frequently in small amounts?
3. Is your urine cloudy or blood-tinged?
4. Do you have pain in your flank area that radiates to your abdomen or pelvis?
5. Do you also have a fever, nausea, vomiting, loss of appetite, or malaise?

Urinary Incontinence

1. Do you have any problem holding your urine or emptying your bladder?
2. Do you wear protective products?
3. Does your bladder control problem interfere with daily activities?
4. Do you often have a strong, sudden urge to urinate?
5. Do you void more than eight times in 24 hours?
6. Do you urinate so frequently that it interferes with normal life?
7. Do you have a warning before you experience leakage?
8. Do you leak with strenuous activity, such as coughing or sneezing?

New Directions

Tension-free vaginal taping, in which a section of polypropylene tape is placed around the mid-urethra via a small vaginal incision, is a promising procedure for women with stress incontinence. The procedure is done under local anesthesia, and the majority of women are discharged within 24 hours. A study conducted on women who had this procedure in Norway (Schiotz, 1999) showed that 85 percent of the subjects were cured of their stress incontinence, and 10 percent continued to have slight incontinence.

Davila et al. (1999) evaluated the safety and efficacy of a bladder-neck support device for women with stress incontinence due to urethral hypermobility. With the device in place, urodynamic testing indicated normal urethral function and no evidence of obstruction. The subjects reported that the device is comfortable, easy to use, and convenient. The findings included a statistically significant reduction of incontinence on pad testing, mean 46.6–16.6 g and, in a bladder diary, mean 28.6–7.8 losses per week.

Schurch, Suter, and Dubs (1999) assessed the efficacy and safety of an intraurethral sphincter device as a treatment option for overflow. The prosthesis consists of a valve and pump inside a short, self-retaining silicone device, which is activated by a magnetic remote control device. Unfortunately, the results of this study were disappointing; eight of the 18 subjects experienced worsened incontinence, and technical problems with the device or the remote control unit were common. Six of the women showed some widening of the urethra, indicating that it is not suitable for long-term use. Attempts to refine mechanical devices such as the intraurethral spincter are continuing.

Although some of the newer research shows promise, science still has a long way to go in the treatment of urinary incontinence in women. Prevention, an awareness of the signs and symptoms of a bladder control problem, and early medical evaluation and intervention are the best strategies at the present time. The continued investigation of pharmacological alternatives, prosthetic devices, and surgical procedures will hopefully provide women with more options.

QUESTIONS FOR REFLECTION AND DISCUSSION

1. What are the four structures that constitute the urinary tract?
2. What is the bacterium that most commonly causes urinary tract infections in women?
3. Why are women at higher risk to develop urinary tract infections than men?
4. How does interstitial cystitis differ from urinary tract infection?

5. *How are most kidney infections in healthy women acquired?*
6. *Why is it important to complete the course of antibiotic therapy for the treatment of a urinary tract or kidney infection?*
7. *How do the three most common types of incontinence in women differ?*
8. *Why are women sometimes reluctant to seek treatment for urinary incontinence?*
9. *What is the most common cause of stress incontinence?*
10. *What is the physiological mechanism whereby overflow incontinence occurs?*

RESOURCES

Organizations

Agency for Health Care Policy and Research (AHCPR)
P.O. Box 8547
Silver Spring, MD 20907-8547
Phone: 1-800-358-9296 or 410-381-3150

American Foundation for Urologic Disease
The Bladder Health Council
300 West Pratt St., Suite 401
Baltimore, MD 21201
Phone: 1-800-242-2383

American UroGynecologic Society
401 North Michigan Ave.
Chicago, IL 60611-4267
Phone: 1-800-644-6610

National Association for Continence
P.O. Box 8306
Spartanburg, SC 29305
Phone: 1-800-252-3337 or 864-579-7900

National Kidney Foundation, Inc.
2 Park Ave.
New York, NY 10016
Phone: 212-889-2210

National Kidney and Urologic Diseases
Information Clearinghouse
3 Information Way
Bethesda, MD 20892-3580
Phone: 301-654-4415

Simon Foundation for Continence
P.O. Box 835
Wilmette, IL 60091
Phone: 1-800-237-4666 or 847-864-3913

REFERENCES

Avorn, J. (1994). Reduction of bacteria and pyuria after ingestion of cranberry juice. *Journal of the American Medical Association, 271*(10), 751.

Baorto, D. M., Gao, Z., Malaviiya, R., Dustin, M. L., Vander-Merue, A., Lubin, P. M., & Abraham, S. N. (1997). How E. coli evades antibiotics by penetrating immune cells. *Nature, 389*(6652), 636–639.

Berding, C. (1997). Disorders of the ureters, bladder and urethra. In L. O. Burrell, M. J. Gerlach, & B. S. Pless (Eds.), *Adult nursing: Acute and community care.* Stanford, CT: Appleton & Lange, pp. 1291–1313.

Bladder Trouble? (2001). *Women's Health Advisor, 5*(5), 6–7.

Butler, R. N., Maby, J. I., Montella, J. M., & Young, G. P. (1999). Urinary incontinence: Keys to diagnosis of the older woman. *Geriatrics, 54*(10), 22–26, 29–30.

Cummings, J. M., & Houston, K. (1994). The treatment of urinary incontinence. *Hospital Practice, 29*(2), 97.

Davila, G. W., Neal, D., Horbach, N., Peacher, J., Doughtie, J. D., & Karram, M. (1999). A bladder-neck support prosthesis for women with stress and mixed incontinence. *Obstetrics and Gynecology, 93*(6), 938–942.

Ehren, I., Lundgerg, J. O., Adolfsson, J., & Wiklund, N. P. (1998). Effect of L-arginine treatment on symptoms and bladder nitric oxide levels in patients with interstitial cystitis. *Urology, 52*(6), 1026–1029.

Fantl, J. A., Wyman, J. F., McClish, D. K., Harkins, S. W., Elswick, R. K., Taylor, J. R., & Hadley, S. C. (1991). Efficacy of bladder training in older women with urinary incontinence. *Journal of the American Medical Association, 265*(5), 609–613.

Hagglund, D., Olsson, H., & Leppert, J. (1999). Urinary incontinence: An unexpected large problem among young females. Results from a population-based study. *Family Practice, 16*(5), 506–509.

How to eradicate bladder infections (2000, May). *The Lark Letter,* 1–2.

Hu, T. W., Kaltreider, D. L., & Igou, J. (1989). Incontinence products: Which is best? *Geriatric Nursing, 10*(4), 184–186.

Jay, J. & Staskin, D. (1998). Urinary incontinence in women. *Advanced nursing practice, 6*(10), 32–37.

Johnson, S. T. (2000). From incontinence to confidence. *American Journal of Nursing, 100*(2), 69–76.

Koivusalo, M., Hakulinen, T., Vartiainen, T., Pukkala, E., Jaakkola, J. J., & Tuomisto, J. (1988). Drinking water mutagenicity and urinary tract cancers: A population-based, case-controlled study in Finland. *American Journal of Epidemiology, 147*(7), 704–712.

Kontiokari, T., Sundquist, K., Nuutinen, M., Pokka, T., Koskela, M., & Uhari, M. (2001). Randomized trial of cranberry-lingonberry juice and *Lactobacillus* drink for the prevention of U.T.I. in women.

Maher, C. F., Carey, M. P., Dwyer, P. L., & Schluter, P. L. (2001). Percutaneous sacral nerve root neuromodulation for intractible cystitis. *Journal of Urology, 165*(3), 884–886.

Matsumoto, T., & Kumazawa, J. (1999). Urinary infections in geriatric patients. *International Journal of Antimicrobial Agents, 11*(3–4), 269–273.

Michaud, D. S., Spiegelman, D., Clinton, S. K., Rimm, E. B., Curhan, G. C., Willett, W. C., & Giovannucci, E. L. (1999). Fluid intake and the risk of bladder cancer in men. *New England Journal of Medicine, 340*(18), 1390–1397.

Newman, D. K. (2001). [On-line]. Urinary incontinence and overactive bladder: A focus on behavioral interventions. *Medscape Nursing, 1*(1). Available: http://womenshealth.medscape.com/Me...15.03newm/pnt-mns0515.03.newm.html.

Northrup, C. (2001). *The wisdom of menopause*. New York: Bantam Books.

Parker, K. P. (1997). Disorders of the kidneys. In L. O. Burrell, M. J. Gerlach, & B. S. Pless (Eds.), *Adult nursing: Acute and community care* (2nd ed., pp. 1239–1290). Stanford, CT: Appleton & Lange.

Parker, K. P., & Berding, C. (1997). Nursing assessment and common urinary interventions. In L. O. Burrell, M. J. Gerlach, & B. S. Pless (Eds.), *Adult nursing: Acute and community care* (2nd ed., pp. 1198–1238). Stanford, CT: Appleton & Lange.

Ratner, V. (2001). Interstitial cystitis: A chronic, inflammatory bladder condition. *World Journal of Urology, 19*(3), 157–159.

Schiotz, H. A. (1999). Tension free vaginal tape—A new surgical method for stress incontinence in women. *Tidsskr Nor Laegeforen, 119*(16), 2338–2341.

Schurch, B., Suter, S., & Dubs, M. (1999). Intraurethral sphincter to treat hyporefexic bladders in women: Does it work? *British Journal of Urology International, 84*(7), 789–794.

Smith, S. D., Wheeler, M. R., Foster, H. E., & Weiss, R. M. (1996). Urinary nitric oxide synthase activity and cyclic GMP levels are decreased with interstitial cystitis and increased with urinary tract infections. *Journal of Urology, 155*(4), 1432–1435.

Starer, P., & Libow, L. S. (1985). Obscuring urinary incontinence: Diapering the elderly. *Journal of the American Geriatrics Society, 33*(12), 842–846.

Stein, J. H. (Ed.). (1994). *Internal medicine* (4th ed.). St. Louis: Mosby.

Swithinbank, L. V., & Abrams, P. (1999). The impact of urinary incontinence on the quality of life in women. *World Journal of Urology, 17*(4), 225–229.

Tschopp, P. J., Wesley-James, T., Spekkens, A., & Lohfeld, L. (1999). Collagen injections for urinary stress incontinence in a small urban urology practice: Time to failure analysis of 99 cases. *Journal of Urology, 162*(3 Pt. 1), 779–783.

Woolner, B. (2001, February 12). Using sEMG biofeedback to treat patients with urinary incontinence. *Advance for Nurses,* pp. 16–18.

17

Gynecological Wellness and Illness

Christine Gold, Teresa Nardontonia, and Marian C. Condon

CHAPTER OUTLINE

Objectives

1. *Differentiate normal from abnormal phenomena associated with the female reproductive anatomy and reproductive cycle.*
2. *Identify safe and unsafe practices regarding the prevention of unwanted pregnancy and sexually transmitted diseases.*
3. *Discuss the implications of selected contraceptive modalities for women's overall health.*
4. *Identify the signs and symptoms of breast, cervical, uterine, and ovarian cancer.*
5. *Discuss the theory of PMS as a culture-bound phenomenon.*
6. *Discuss the symptoms, diagnosis, and treatment of selected benign gynecological conditions.*

Introduction

This chapter addresses the identification and promotion of gynecological wellness and the identification and prevention of gynecological illness, disease, and unwanted pregnancy. Strategies for supporting the health of the female reproductive system are presented, and common gynecological problems and illnesses are addressed in terms of symptoms, diagnostic procedures, and treatment. Infertility is an extremely complex problem and will not be addressed in this chapter. Books and websites that address the problem of infertility are listed in the Resources section at the end of the chapter. Sexually transmitted diseases are discussed in Chapter 22.

Markers of Gynecological Wellness

Women who are free of illness or pathology in the organs and processes associated with reproduction have normal breast tissue, normal menstrual cycles, and a normal vaginal discharge.

Normal Breast Anatomy

Breasts are made up of fat, lobules (milk-producing glands), fibrous tissue, and ducts, and they rest on underlying muscle and bone (see Figure 17–1). They are not necessarily symmetrical bilaterally, and it is not unusual for one to be slightly larger than the other. Contrary to popular belief, it is normal for the breasts to feel somewhat lumpy and uneven in texture, and

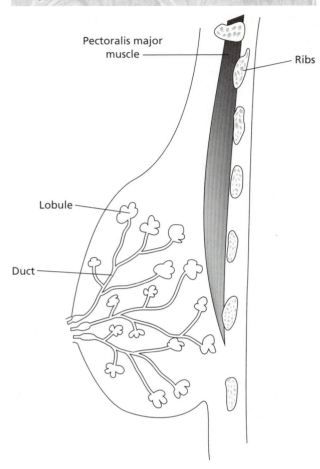

Figure 17–1 Side View of the Breast

Pectoralis major muscle

Ribs

Lobule

Duct

more so at some times than others. For example, in the two weeks before and during the **menses** (menstrual periods), fluid may collect in the breasts, producing extra lumps. The breasts may also be somewhat tender at this time, although breast tenderness that continues throughout the menstrual cycle is not normal and should be brought to the attention of a healthcare provider. Age, pregnancy, birth control pills, hormone replacement therapy, and diet can also cause changes in the way the breasts feel. Younger women's breasts are generally more dense and contain more fatty tissue, than the breasts of older women. Pregnancy causes the breasts to enlarge (see Chapter 23), and birth control pills and hormone replacement therapy can cause breast swelling and tenderness.

A Normal Menstrual Cycle

The term *menstrual cycle* refers to the recurrent changes occurring in the uterus, ovaries, cervix, and vagina associated with menstruation and the period of time in between menses. A marker for wellness in a sexually mature woman is cyclical menstrual bleeding, which starts with **menarche** (first menstruation) and ends with menopause, (the permanent cessation of menstruation). In the United States, the average age of onset is 12.5 years, with a range from 9 to 17 years. Initially, the cycles are **anovulatory** (without ovulation) and vary in length from 10 to 60 days or more. During the adolescent years, a regular pattern of menstruation is established, with 30- and 35-day intervals. In adulthood, an average cycle lasts 28 days, with intervals of 21 to 35 days considered normal, and the menstrual cycle has developed characteristics, patterns, and intervals specific to each woman (Robinson & Huether, 1998).

The menstrual cycle is divided into three specific phases: **menstruation** (bleeding); the **follicular/proliferative phase,** during which the **endometrium** (uterine lining) builds up; and the **luteal/secretory phase,** during which the hormone progesterone stabilizes the endometrium in readiness to receive a fertilized egg (see Figure 17–2). In order for women to have regular and predictable menstrual cycles, the sequential secretion of specific hormones must occur. **Gonadotropin-releasing hormone (GnRH),** secreted by the hypothalamus gland in the brain, stimulates the anterior pituitary gland, also located in the brain, to secrete **follicle-stimulating hormone (FSH)** and **lutenizing hormone (LH).** These hormones then stimulate special cells of the ovary to secrete estrogen and progesterone.

At birth, the **ovaries,** or the female gonads, each contain approximately 1 million ova (eggs) within the immature ovarian follicles. At puberty, the number of ova-containing follicles ranges between 200,000 and 400,000 (Robinson & Huether, 1998). FSH acts directly on specific types of follicular cells and causes them to grow. As each follicle grows, it secretes estrogen, which stimulates the endometrium to grow. The increase in FSH, the growth of the ovarian follicle, the rise in estrogen level, and the growth of the endometrium constitute the follicular/proliferative phase of the menstrual cycle.

A midcycle surge of LH causes ovulation to occur in response to the increase in estrogen level. Ovulation marks the beginning of the luteal/secretory phase of the menstrual cycle. When ovulation occurs, there is a drop in the estrogen level. The ovarian follicle transforms into what is known as the **corpus luteum** and secretes high levels of progesterone. Progesterone causes the endometrium to become thick and rich with engorged blood vessels, and a glycogen-containing fluid is produced. These changes make the endometrium ripe for the implantation of a fertilized egg. Ovulation and the changes within the endometrium are known as the luteal/secretory phase of the menstrual cycle (Robinson & Huether, 1998).

If conception and the implantation of an egg does not occur, the corpus luteum on the ovary deteriorates, and there is a decline in progesterone and estrogen levels. This interferes with the blood supply to the endometrium, causing the thickened tissue to begin to shrivel and slough off.

Figure 17–2   The Menstrual Cycle

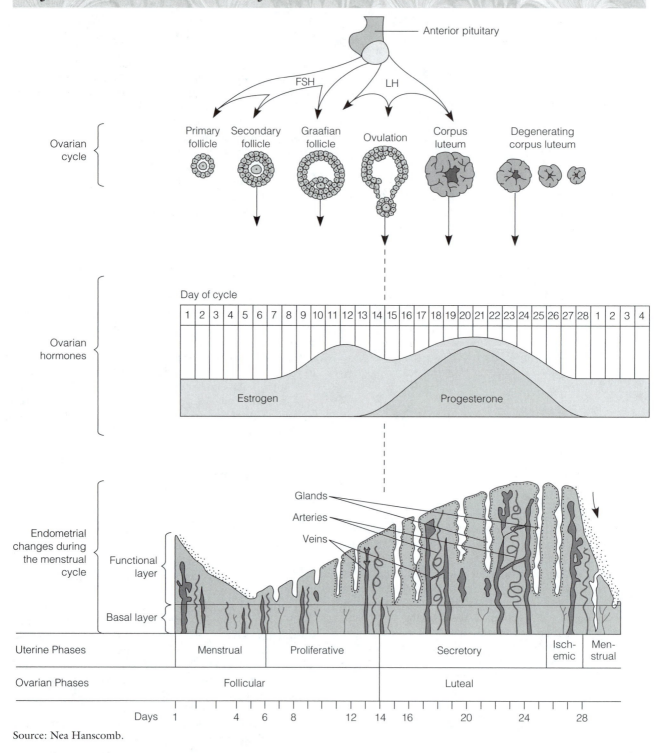

Source: Nea Hanscomb.

Menstruation occurs, marking the beginning of the next menstrual cycle (Robinson & Huether, 1998).

NORMAL CYCLICAL BLEEDING

Menstrual bleeding begins about 14 days after ovulation. The duration of bleeding is different for each woman, but it should be similar from cycle to cycle. An average range is 2 to 8 days (Murphy, 1990). Factors such as stress, illness, nutrition, and medication can influence the length of the menstrual cycle. Menstrual blood is composed of the shed endometrial tissue and blood, mucus, and vaginal/cervical cells. The average blood loss during a cycle ranges from 30 to 100 cc. The flow is heaviest during the first 3 days and will taper to spotting or staining before it ends. The color of the menstrual flow gradually changes from bright red to dark brown. A musty odor is characteristic (Robinson & Huether, 1998). Clots may be present but are not usual. Once the menstrual pattern has been established, unusual or irregular vaginal bleeding should prompt a phone call or visit to a healthcare provider.

Women who think they may have a minor menstrual problem should keep a calendar of their menstrual cycles with notations regarding their characteristics: timing, amount, color, character, onset, and duration. The calendar will assist the provider in assessing the problem.

ABSENCE OF ABNORMAL PAIN

Many women experience some discomfort with their menstrual periods. Menstrual cramping can be mild to severe. Another type of pain, called **mittelschmerz**, or intermenstrual pain, may occur at midcycle and last from a few hours to a day or so. Mittelschmerz generally consists of crampy pain, or sudden sharp pain, in the right or left side of the lower abdomen, depending on which ovary is ovulating during that cycle. It may also radiate into the groin area. The cause is unclear, but some theorize that it is caused by rhythmic contractions of the fallopian tube or increased peritoneal fluid (Murphy, 1990). The **peritoneum** is a serous membrane that protects the abdominal and pelvic organs and lines the abdominal cavity.

Normal Vaginal Discharge

Another marker of wellness in a mature woman is a normal vaginal discharge. Normal vaginal discharge has an off-white color and is initially without odor. Odor develops only after bacteria or other foreign organisms, such as trichomonas or *E. coli,* have had time to interact with it.

Vaginal discharge begins as cervical mucus, which undergoes cyclic changes in response to the hormones of menstruation. Cervical secretions produced after menstruation, are sticky and thick. As ovulation approaches, the amount of secretions increases and the character of the secretions changes. The mucus becomes more watery, clear, thin, and stretchy—

resembling raw egg whites. The purpose of this type of mucus is thought to be to enhance sperm motility. Its presence is an indication that ovulation is occurring. It is important that women who use fertility awareness (discussed in the section on avoiding unplanned pregnancy) for pregnancy prevention be able to recognize this type of mucus. If pregnancy is not desired, it is wise to use a method of protection when this mucus is present. Days after ovulation, the mucus again becomes sticky and thick until menstruation.

Vaginal discharge should not be bothersome, except for the fact that it is present. Should the discharge be malodorous or discolored; cause irritation, itching, or burning to the vulvar area, or cause pain with intercourse, a call to a nurse practitioner or physician may be warranted to rule out an infection.

Promoting Gynecological Wellness

Two important aspects of wellness for women are reducing one's risk factors for cancer and taking steps to detect cancer, should it develop. The value of early detection is suggested by the declining *mortality rates* for breast and cervical cancer, even though the *incidence* of both is rising. According to Blackman, Bennett, and Miller (1999), in the United States the incidence of breast cancer increased 25.3 percent from 1973 through 1996 (whites: 26.2 percent; blacks: 36.7 percent), with most of the increase occurring from 1973 to 1991. The age-adjusted mortality rate during that period of time, however, declined from 26.9 to 24.3 per 100,000 women. The same pattern of increased incidence but decreased mortality was seen in cervical cancer. The decrease in breast and cervical cancer mortality can be partially attributed to early disease detection and treatment due to greater use of screening. Much of the reduction in cervical cancer mortality has been associated with the increased use of Pap tests. An estimated 37 to 60 percent reduction in cervical cancer mortality could be achieved with regular screening for all women. Another important aspect of wellness promotion is the prevention of sexually transmitted diseases (see Chapter 22) and undesired pregnancy.

Performing Breast Self-Examination

Learning how breasts feel and what is normal for each woman can be achieved by performing **breast self-examination (BSE)**. The ability to notice changes within the breast is very important in the early detection of breast disease. If breast implants are present, BSE still needs to be performed, especially over the areas of chest wall surrounding the breast.

When breast cancer is detected in its early stages, the rate of cure is increased. Performing BSE, seeing a healthcare provider for a breast examination regularly, and following the recommendations for mammography screening are important steps women can take to protect themselves against breast cancer. About 90 percent of all breast lumps are found through BSE.

BSE takes only about 10 minutes, once a month. The best time to perform BSE is *two or three days after the menstrual period*, when the breasts are least lumpy and tender. Women whose periods are irregular, or who are menopausal, should pick a day of the month that is easy for them to remember, such as the first day of each month, and do BSE on that day each month.

The technique for BSE is as follows:

1. *Begin by* inspecting your breasts. *The exam should always be done in good light. Stand or sit in front of a mirror. Place your arms at your sides. Observe the natural contours of the breasts, and look for dimpling, puckering, or redness of the breast skin, discharge from the nipple, and changes in breast size and shape. This inspection should then be repeated, with the hands pressed tightly on the hips and then with the arms raised high above the head.*

2. *The next step is* palpating the lymph nodes *that drain the breast. In a sitting or standing position, begin by observing and then palpating the* **axillae** *(underarm areas). The axillary examination provides an assessment of the breast tissue in the tail of Spence, the portion of breast tissue that extends into the armpit. It also provides for an examination of the axillary lymph nodes. Remember to examine yourself on both sides.*

3. *To examine the breasts themselves, lie flat on your back. Place a folded towel or pillow under the left shoulder and your left arm above your head. Use your right hand to examine the left breast, and vice versa. Hold the first three fingers of the hand together, use the balls of the fingers, and press firmly and carefully. Picture the breast as a face on a clock, with 12:00 being at the very top of the breast. Begin the examination by placing the fingers on the uppermost part of the breast at the 12:00 position. Use small, circular motions at 12:00 and then repeat the circular motion at 1:00, 2:00, and so on until you reach the 12:00 position again. Use the same technique, in smaller and smaller circles, until you reach the nipple and have examined the entire breast.*

4. *An* examination of the areola (the darker area surrounding the nipple) and the nipple *should include an inspection of the size and color of the areola and characteristics of the nipple.* **Nipple inversion** *(retraction of the nipple into the breast tissue) may be normal, however, nipple inversion is considered a normal variation only before puberty. The inverted nipple should not be fixed; it should be capable of becoming erect and protruding from the breast tissue.*

5. *Lower the left arm and remove the towel or pillow from behind the left shoulder. Repeat the same examination technique for the right breast, beginning with the placement of the towel or pillow under the right shoulder. Examine the right breast with the left hand.*

The examination technique can also be performed while taking a shower or bath. It may be easier to examine the breasts when they are smooth and wet with soap and water.

Having Mammograms

Mammography is a low-dose X ray study of the breast that can detect changes in the breast tissue. It is the best method of screening for the presence of a small lump or tiny group of microcalcifications—which may be the only sign of breast cancer. Studies show that the early detection of breast cancer through regular screening increases the chance of cure—often through a form of treatment that allows for the preservation of the breast.

Women who are preparing for a mammogram should dress comfortably, preferably in a two-piece outfit, as the test will require being undressed from the waist up. Deodorants and powders should not be used prior to the test, as they may interfere with the reading of the mammogram.

Mammography takes only a few minutes and involves two views of the breast, one from above and one from the side. Two smooth, flat plastic plates are placed on either sides of the breast and pressed together to flatten out the breast tissue, so that the most tissue can be examined with the least radiation. An X ray is then taken and processed. The radiologists will review and read the X ray and prepare a written report on the findings. Mammography may be mildly uncomfortable for women with tender breasts, but it is seldom painful.

The American Cancer Society recommends an annual screening mammogram, plus a **clinical breast exam (CBE)** done by a healthcare provider, for women age 40 years and older. The American Medical Association recommends an annual or biennial screening mammogram and an annual CBE for women age 40–49 years and an annual mammogram with CBE for women aged 50 years and older (Blackman et al., 1999). However, some (Lark, 2002) argue that mammography is overused in young women, and that overuse leads to too many false positive results and excessive exposure to ionizing radiation, without clear benefits.

Having Gynecological Checkups

Having routine, screening gynecological and breast examinations at regular intervals is important for women because some potentially serious problems, such as breast and cervical cancer, produce no symptoms in their early, treatable stages. Routine visits also provide nurse practitioners and physicians with an opportunity to offer counseling about general health maintenance and prevention of illness (Papera, 1990).

Gynecological examinations should be scheduled for a time when menstruation is *not* likely to occur because bleeding would interfere with the collection of the Pap smear and necessitate a return visit. Women should refrain from using intravaginal medications for at least *one week* prior to the examination, and should not have sexual intercourse, douche, or use tampons within *24 hours* of the exam (Heggins & Smith, 1997). Such activities might alter cervical and vaginal cells, and invalidate the results of the Pap test.

It is helpful to write down in advance any information the health care provider is certain to request, such as family and personal medical history—including past illnesses and surgeries, and the characteristics of the menstrual cycle. The provider will also request the date of the last menstrual period and the names of any medications currently being taken.

A gynecological visit usually begins with questions about general lifestyle; the reason for the visit; and past patterns of menstruation, sexual activity, contraception, and childbirth. Women are routinely asked about dietary habits, substance use (smoking, alcohol, caffeine, drugs) and exercise and activity level (Lichtman, 1990).

The physical examination detects abnormalities suggested by the history or symptoms the woman may be experiencing. The bladder and bowel should be emptied, if necessary, prior to the examination. It will be necessary to undress completely and put on a gown or paper drapes; this allows for optimal assessment of the body. Many of the major organs of the body will be assessed—such as the heart and lungs—as well as the organs of the reproductive system. This more comprehensive examination is intended to provide baseline information and important clinical data related to general health and well-being, as many women use their gynecological provider as their primary care provider (see Chapter 9).

A **breast examination** is a vital part of the physical and gynecological examination. The healthcare provider will observe and palpate the breasts themselves, as well as the surrounding lymph nodes. The armpits will be examined as well, because breast tissue is found there.

The **pelvic examination** (internal exam) is used to detect female genital tract problems, such as cancers of the cervix, uterus, and ovaries. It also assists in the evaluation of other conditions, such as vaginal and pelvic infections, abnormal uterine bleeding, pelvic pain, and endometriosis. A Pap smear will also be done to test for premalignant lesions of the cervix and cervical cancer.

The pelvic examination is performed with the woman lying on her back with her feet in the stirrups. The exam includes inspection and palpation of the external female genitalia (pubic region, clitoris, labia, rectum, and so on) and surrounding lymph nodes. After a thorough inspection and palpation of the external genitalia, the vagina and cervix should be assessed. A warmed **speculum** (an instrument used to separate the vaginal walls) will be used to inspect the vagina and cervix. The speculum is inserted carefully into the vagina and opened slowly and just enough to allow an inspection of the vaginal walls and location of the cervix. Discharge that obscures the vaginal walls or cervix will be removed with a cotton-tipped applicator, and cultures will be obtained if an infection is suspected. A **Pap smear** (a sample

of cervical and vaginal cells) will likely be taken at this point, after which the speculum will be withdrawn.

A **bimanual examination** is then performed to assess the internal organs of the pelvis. Water-soluble lubricant is placed on the index and middle fingers of the examiner's gloved hand, and two fingers are inserted into the vagina. The cervix, uterus, ovaries, and adnexal (adjacent) regions are assessed for normality or abnormalities. Vaginal tone is noted and the presence of a cystocele (a bulge caused by a weakness in the wall between the bladder and vagina) or rectocele (a bulge caused by a weakness in the wall between the rectum and the vagina) will be detected at this time.

A **rectovaginal examination** in which the uterus is palpated via the rectum, is performed next to assess the uterus and the tissue that separates the vagina and the rectum. In obese women, or women whose uterus is **retroverted** (tipped backward), the rectovaginal examination allows more complete palpation of the uterus and surrounding structures. Any stool present in the rectum is tested for *occult* (hidden) *blood*, which can signal the presence of bowel disease. The American Cancer Society advises annual rectal examinations from age 40 onward and an annual examination of stool for occult blood after age 50 (Papera, 1990).

The National Cancer Institute, the American Cancer Society, the American College of Obstetricians and Gynecologists, and the American Medical Association endorse annual Pap smears for women who are sexually active or have reached 18 years of age (Blackman et al., 1999).

Avoiding Unplanned Pregnancy and Sexually Transmitted Diseases

Controlling fertility (if desired) and preventing disease are absolutely essential to women's welfare. Currently, over the course of their reproductive lives, U.S. women have an average of 3.2 pregnancies. Statistically, two of these result in live births, 0.7 in induced abortions, and 0.5 in miscarriages and stillbirths. According to recent estimates, however, only 1.8 of these pregnancies are desired by the woman (Centers for Disease Control and Prevention, 2000). Teen pregnancy and teen births are generally considered undesirable, from both a health and a social welfare standpoint. In 1997, the birth rate for teenagers was 52.3 births per 1,000 women age 15–19 years (Ventura, Martin, Curtin, & Mathews, 1999).

There is a great need around the world for reliable contraception. Some individuals and couples do not desire children, and individuals and families who do wish to rear children are often limited in the number of children they can care for. Many people desire no more children once they have completed their families or have reached a certain age. Healthy women are fertile until about age 50 to 51, and healthy men are fertile essentially throughout their lifetimes, although men's fertility does decline with age (Ford et al., 2000). Most people, however, have given birth to or have sired all the children they desire before the end of their reproductive years (Stewart & Carignan, 1998). No matter what contraceptive method is ultimately chosen, it is important that women make an informed decision. Gynecologists, nurse practitioners, and other providers who offer healthcare to women can be invaluable sources of information.

The Department of Health and Human Services estimates that 12 million new cases of sexually transmitted diseases (STDs) appear each year (see Chapter 20). According to the American Academy of Family Physicians, the American College of Obstetricians and Gynecologists, and the U.S. Preventive Services Task Force, counseling regarding the prevention of unintended pregnancy and sexually transmitted diseases is important for all sexually active women and men (Clinical Guidelines, 1995).

Some of the methods of contraception described in this section prevent the transmission of STDs, but some do not. It is important for all sexually active women to understand the purpose and limitations of contraceptive drugs and devices.

ABSTINENCE

The only absolutely certain method of preventing both pregnancy and the transmission of sexually transmitted diseases is to refrain from having any form of sexual contact with another person. Historically, sexual abstinence has probably been the single most important factor in curtailing human fertility (Kowal, 1998). The term *abstinence* has several definitions; it can refer to refraining from all sexual behaviors, including masturbation, or to refraining from only sexual behavior involving genital contact and/or penetration.

It is important to know one's own thoughts and feelings regarding sexual activity and sexual expression. Women of all ages must make decisions pertaining to these matters for themselves and not allow others to make those decisions for them.

It is important for women to decide in advance what sexual activities they are willing to participate in and to convey this decision to their partners. Women who choose abstinence are wise to avoid places or situations that might compromise their decision; however, they should still learn about contraception and safer sex, in case they change their minds (Kowal, 1998).

FERTILITY AWARENESS METHOD

Fertility awareness-based methods of family planning involve identifying the days during each menstrual cycle when intercourse is most likely to result in conception and taking steps to avoid it. During the fertile period, couples can abstain from sex, use a barrier method, or practice withdrawal. The success of the fertility awareness method hinges on the female partner's ability to accurately identify the potentially fertile days of her cycle. There are two variants on the fertility awareness method: if the couple uses barriers or withdrawal during the fertile time, they are using **fertility**

awareness–combined methods (FACM), and, if they abstain, they are using **natural family planning (NFP)** (Jennings, Lamprecht, & Kowal, 1998).

To identify the start of her fertile period, a woman can observe the consistency of her cervical secretions, monitor changes in the position and feel of her cervix, or use a calendar calculation. To mark the end of the fertile period, a woman can use the same indicators, as well as monitor changes in her basal body temperature (BBT), or temperature at rest (Jennings et al., 1998).

The practice of monitoring cervical secretions in order to track the fertile period is grounded in reproductive physiology, as are the other fertility awareness techniques. As the ovarian follicle grows during the menstrual cycle and releases more estrogen, cervical secretions appear that are initially sticky, thick, and cloudy. As estrogen peaks at midcycle, the secretions become clear, stretchy, and slippery. These cervical secretions facilitate sperm transport and indicate that the woman is fertile (Jennings et al., 1998). The last day on which this type of secretion is observed is known as the *peak day*. If pregnancy is not desired, the appearance of sticky mucus heralds the time frame during which to use abstinence or another method of contraception.

After ovulation, progesterone counteracts the effects of estrogen and causes the cervical secretions to dry up and form a mucous plug, which prevents sperm from traveling through the cervix (Jennings et al., 1998). Knowing one's basal body temperature is useful in determining the end of the fertile period because progesterone causes the BBT to rise around the time of ovulation.

Women may also keep track of their fertile periods by noting the position and consistency of the cervix. As ovulation approaches, the opening to the cervix becomes softer and wider, and the cervix pulls up higher in the vaginal vault. After ovulation, the cervix returns to a lower position, and its opening closes and feels more firm (Jennings et al., 1998). The rise and fall of estrogen and progesterone cause these changes to occur.

A woman's cycle can vary according to her nutritional status, weight, psychological or physical condition, and age (Fonte, 1997). These factors can influence how the observations made during each cycle are interpreted. Women wishing to use the fertility awareness method should consult a healthcare provider for more detailed and personalized information.

The fertility awareness method is free of medical side effects because it does not require any chemicals or devices. It is also reversible, easily learned, inexpensive, and approved by all major religions (Fonte, 1997). The successful use of fertility awareness–based methods depends on the accuracy of the method in identifying the actual fertile days, the couple's ability to correctly identify the fertile time, and their ability to follow the rules of the method they are using (Jennings et al., 1998). Among *typical* users of these methods, about 25 percent experience an unintended pregnancy during the first year of use. Among *perfect* users, the first-year probabilities of pregnancy are substantially lower, ranging from 1 to 9 percent (Jennings et al., 1998).

STERILIZATION VIA TUBAL LIGATION

Since 1970, approximately 1 million sterilizations have been performed annually in the United States. Nearly 15 million women rely on sterilization as their contraceptive method; 10.7 million rely on female sterilization, and 4.2 million on vasectomy (Stewart & Carignan, 1998). In the United States, sterilization is now the contraceptive method of choice for 27.5 percent of all women age 15 to 44 (Christman & Uechi, 2000).

For women, sterilization involves mechanically blocking the **fallopian tubes** (the structures through which the eggs must pass in order to reach the uterus) to prevent the egg and sperm from uniting and thus preventing conception. Sterilization procedures can be done via a surgical incision in the abdomen (**laparotomy**) or via **laparoscopy,** which involves inserting small, lighted instruments into the abdominal cavity through several small openings about the size of a dime. Sterilization via laparoscopy generally does not require an overnight stay in the hospital. Sterilization can be performed immediately after childbirth without increasing the health risks to the woman. Sterilization is generally considered to be a safe operative procedure for women.

The failure rates associated with sterilization are lower than those associated with most temporary contraceptive methods during the first year of use. The Collaborative Review of Sterilization (CREST) study found the first-year probability of pregnancy to be 5.5 for every 1,000 procedures and the 10-year cumulative probability to be 18.5 pregnancies for every 1,000 procedures (Stewart & Carignan, 1998).

Sterilization is ideal for women who are certain they want no more children and need a reliable contraceptive method. It is permanent, private, highly effective, and cost-effective, and it has no side effects. There is nothing to buy or remember, and partner compliance is not required. Moreover, there is no interruption in lovemaking (Stewart & Carignan, 1998). Sterilization, however, is not recommended for anyone who is not absolutely certain she wants no more children. Reversing sterilization procedures is difficult and expensive, and, of course, requires surgery and anesthesia.

Sterilization also has other drawbacks. It is expensive at the time of the procedure, and, if sterilization fails, there is a high probability that an **ectopic pregnancy** will occur. In an ectopic pregnancy, the embryo begins to grow in the fallopian tube, which will eventually rupture if surgical intervention is not obtained. Morbidity and mortality related to ectopic pregnancy are high. Another drawback to sterilization is that it confers no protection against STDs, including HIV (Stewart & Carignan, 1998).

Complications during or shortly after the actual procedure occur in less than 1 percent of all sterilization cases (Christman & Uechi, 2000). Death as a result of female sterilization is extremely rare: A large U.S. study found 13 deaths among more than 900,000 procedures (Christman & Uechi, 2000). Most of the complications can be prevented by careful screening, good preoperative education, close monitoring of vital signs, and careful surgical and anesthesia techniques (Stewart & Carignan, 1998). Long-term morbidity associated with the procedure includes chronic pelvic pain and abnormal menstrual bleeding.

The recent trend toward cost-cutting mergers among hospitals and other healthcare agencies has resulted in a reduction in women's access to some medical services, such as sterilization procedures, contraception, abortion, infertility treatment, and emergency contraception—even for rape victims. Some religious doctrines forbid such services, and, when religiously affiliated hospitals merge with secular organizations to form new agencies, they often insist that the new agency refrain from providing services to which they object. This phenomenon has been most frequently documented in relation to Catholic institutions (Gallagher, 1997) but may occur in others as well. In such scenarios, women are often denied optimum healthcare. For example, if a woman who wants no more children is denied a sterilization procedure after a cesarean delivery, she is forced to undergo a second operation at a different institution, with the attendant inconvenience, additional expense, and anesthesia risk. Because of the trend toward consolidation, neighborhood hospitals are disappearing, and a woman may not have geographical access to an institution that provides the procedure she desires.

THE PILL

The many different contraceptive formulations available in pill form fall into two major categories: combination oral contraceptives and progesterone-only contraceptives.

Combination Oral Contraceptives (OCs) Combination oral contraceptives are pills that contain both estrogen and progestin. They prevent pregnancy by suppressing ovulation through the combined action of estrogen and progestin. Estrogen inhibits ovulation in part by suppressing FSH and LH and alters the makeup of the endometrial lining within the uterus. Progestin inhibits ovulation by suppressing LH and causes the cervical mucus to become thick, thereby hindering sperm motility. It also hinders implantation by producing an endometrium that is unreceptive to ovum implantation (Sherif, 1999).

Currently in the United States, only two estrogenic compounds are used in OCs—ethinyl estradiol (EE) and mestranol. There are several progestins found in OCs—norethindrone, norethindrone acetate, ethynodiol diacetate, norgestrel, levonorgestrel, norethynodrel, desogestrel, norgestimate, and gestodene (Hatcher & Guillebaud, 1998). The estrogens and progestins in birth control pills are *non-bioidentical*—they are not molecularly the same as the estrogen and progesterone produced in women's bodies. Controversies related to the use of non-bioidentical hormones are discussed in Chapter 24.

The effectiveness of OCs among *perfect* users is such that only about 1 in 1,000 women (0.1 percent) is expected to become pregnant within the first year. Among *typical* pill users, about 1 in 20 women (5 percent) will become pregnant during the first year (Hatcher & Guillebaud, 1998). OCs are taken every day at about the same time. Missing a pill or taking it late lessens the effectiveness of the pill and therefore increases the risk of a pregnancy.

The pill is effective, is generally considered to be safe, and can be used for years. Its effects are reversible, and it can normalize problematic menstrual periods. Birth control pills are also used to control acne and the excessive growth of facial hair. They can also ease dysmenorrhea and mittelschmerz (Hatcher & Guillebaud, 1998; Sherif, 1999). There are many noncontraceptive benefits of the pill as well: It has protective effects against endometrial cancer (50 percent reduction), ovarian cancer (40 percent reduction), benign breast disease (50 percent reduction), ovarian cysts, ectopic pregnancy, pelvic inflammatory disease, and anemia (Hatcher & Guillebaud, 1998; Gallagher & Fuller, 1997; Sherif, 1999).

There are also some disadvantages to OC use. Pills offer no protection against STDs. Moreover, they are expensive and must be taken daily. Pills can also cause unwanted menstrual cycle changes, nausea or vomiting, headaches, breast tenderness, and weight gain. They can cause or worsen depression and sometimes decrease libido. The pill increases the incidence of **cervical ectopia,** a condition in which the cells that normally line the cervical canal are present on the surface of the cervix near the opening of the canal. When ectopia are present, the cervix is more vulnerable to infections. The pill can also increase the risk of cardiovascular diseases, such as hypertension, deep vein thrombosis, stroke, and heart attack, and can accelerate gallbladder disease. Smoking also increases the risk of myocardial infarction, thrombotic stroke, and hemorrhagic stroke. *Women who smoke should probably stop taking the pill at age 35 and should definitely stop by age 40* (Hatcher & Guillebaud, 1998). There is some evidence that the pill increases blood sugar levels in some individuals. The pill also decreases blood levels of some important vitamins, such as B-2, B-6, B-12, and C. It also lowers levels of folic acid, magnesium, and zinc (Pelton, Lavalle, Hawkins, & Krinsky, 2001). Women who use OCs must take care to consume extra amounts of the foods that contain these nutrients.

Because oral contraceptives (OCs) contain estrogen, there has been some concern that taking birth control pills might increase a woman's risk of developing breast cancer. Indeed, women who took oral contraceptives prior to 1975 (when OCs contained up to 150 micrograms of the synthetic estrogen *mestranol*) are known to be at a substantially higher risk than women who have never taken OCs, particularly if they have a family history of breast cancer (*Contraceptive Update: Oral Contraceptives and Breast Cancer Risks,* 2001). The birth control pills most commonly prescribed in the United States today, however, contain much smaller amounts of a different estrogen—50 micrograms or less of *ethinyl estradiol*. The authors of a recent comprehensive analysis of the literature on the relationship between OCs and breast cancer risk concluded that taking OCs increases breast cancer risk only slightly and that, when breast cancer does develop in a woman on OCs, it usually does so while she is still taking them, or within 10 years after she stops (*The Collaborative Group on Hormone Factors in Breast Cancer,* 1997). Because the development of cancer is generally a slow process, and it is more typical for cancer risk to peak decades after exposure to a carcinogen, the authors theorized that the estrogen in OCs may escalate the growth of existing cancers rather than initiating new ones.

The slightly higher breast cancer risk that taking OCs confers must be weighed against the facts that women in their childbearing years are at low risk for breast cancer to start with, that OCs offer some protection against ovarian cancer, and that unwanted pregnancy may undermine a woman's physical and emotional health. Whether to take birth control pills is a decision that each woman must make for herself, in consultation with her healthcare provider.

Before she can start taking birth control pills, a woman must have a thorough medical examination. There are several absolute contraindications for the use of OCs: pregnancy, a past or current problem with blood clots, stroke or coronary artery disease, breast cancer or other estrogen-dependent cancer, benign or malignant liver tumor, and undiagnosed abnormal vaginal bleeding (Sherif, 1999). Women who are taking drugs that stimulate the metabolic capacity of the liver, such as rifampin, penicillin, tetracycline, phenobarbital, phenytoin, primidone, or carbamazepin, are not good candidates for oral contraception because these drugs can adversely affect the efficacy of OCs. *Women who take birth control pills and need a short course of an antibiotic or another medication that can interfere with the effectiveness of the pill must use an additional method of protection.* Birth control pills may potentiate the action of some anti-anxiety medications and antidepressants, as well as the asthma medication theophylline (Sherif, 1999). Again, informing one's healthcare provider about current use of medications is important.

It is important to know the warning signs that a pill-related complication may be occurring: severe abdominal pain, chest pain, shortness of breath, a sharp pain felt on breathing in, headache, dizziness, weakness or numbness, problems with vision, and severe leg pain (Hatcher & Guillebaud, 1998). Should any of these symptoms occur, a healthcare provider must be notified immediately.

Progesterone-Only Pills The **minipill** contains a small dose of progestin and no estrogen. It must be taken daily, with no interruptions in dosage (Speroff & Darney, 1996). The contraceptive effect of this type of pill is related to its effects on the endometrial and cervical mucus. The minipill causes the endometrial lining to become thin and hostile to implantation and the cervical mucus to become thick and impermeable. Approximately 40 percent of women who take this type of pill ovulate normally (Speroff & Darney, 1996).

The minipill contains a low dose of hormones and therefore must be taken every day at the same time of day. When a dose is more than 3 hours late, the woman must use a back-up method of birth control for 48 hours after the time of the last dose (Speroff & Darney, 1996). The minipill causes no significant metabolic effect on lipid levels, carbohydrate metabolism, or coagulation factors and therefore does not raise the risk of cardiovascular disease. There is an immediate return to fertility on discontinuation (Speroff & Darney, 1996).

Failure rates have been demonstrated to range from 1.1 to 9.6 per 100 women in the first year of use. The failure rate is higher in younger women (3.1), compared with women over age 40 (0.3). In motivated women, the failure rate is comparable to that of combination oral contraceptives (less than 1 out of 100 women) (Speroff & Darney, 1996).

The minipill should be started initially on the first day of menses. A back-up method of birth control must be used for the first seven days because some women ovulate as early as seven to nine days after the onset of menses. If a pill is missed or GI illness alters absorption, the pill should be resumed as soon as possible, and a back-up method should be used immediately and until the pills have been resumed for at least two days. If two or more pills are missed in a row and there is no menstrual bleeding in four to six weeks, a pregnancy test should be taken (Speroff & Darney, 1996).

The minipill is a good choice for women who are breast-feeding. Lactating women produce high levels of prolactin, which suppresses ovulation, and, in combination with the minipill, a level of effectiveness nearing 100% is achieved (Hatcher, 1998). Also, there is no evidence for any adverse effect on breast-feeding (Speroff & Darney, 1996). The minipill is also a good choice for women over 40, who tend to be less fertile than younger women, and in situations in which estrogen is contraindicated.

Women using medications that increase liver metabolism (such as phenobarbital, Dilantin, and Tegretol) should avoid this method of contraception because of the relatively low doses of progestin administered (Speroff & Darney, 1996). The increased liver metabolism may clear the drug from the body before it can exert its full effect on fertility.

Emergency Contraception (EC) There are approximately 3.2 million unplanned pregnancies in the United States each year. It is estimated that half of the couples who experience unplanned pregnancy did not use any contraception and that half experienced contraceptive failure (Chez & Chapin, 1997). Emergency contraception could potentially prevent up to 1.7 million unintended pregnancies per year (Van Look & Stewart, 1998).

The two methods of EC now available in the United States are oral contraceptive pills and copper-T intrauterine devices (see Figure 17–7). There are two types of emergency contraceptive pills (ECP): the Yuzpe regimen (combinations of estrogen and progestin) and oral contraceptives.

The Yuzpe regimen, a combination of estrogen and progestin, was introduced in the early 1970s (Van Look & Stewart, 1998). Today, *Preven*, a specially packaged and labeled form of EC, is available with a prescription from a healthcare provider. When given before ovulation, this estrogen-progestin combination disrupts normal follicular development and maturation, resulting in anovulation or delayed ovulation with deficient luteal function. Treatment that is administered after ovulation has occurred and fertilization may have taken place has no effect on ovarian hormone secretion and only a limited effect on the endometrium (Van Look & Stewart, 1998). Therefore, emergency contraception has no effect if pregnancy has already occurred. Another type of emergency contraceptive pill that contains only progestin is available.

Oral contraceptives for EC can be offered to any woman of reproductive age who has had unprotected sexual intercourse and appears for treatment within 72 hours of that unprotected intercourse. What phase of her menstrual cycle she is in is not a consideration in deciding whether EC should be prescribed. A confirmed pregnancy is the only specific contraindication to the method because treatment would be of no value (Chez & Chapin, 1997). There are no data that suggest that the contraindications that apply to birth control pills apply to EC, which is taken for a very brief period of time. No major cardiovascular or neurological side effects of ECs have been reported to date (Chez & Chapin, 1997). Minor side effects, such as nausea, vomiting, and breast tenderness, have been noted. No evidence suggests an increase in ectopic pregnancy associated with EC use (Davies, 1997).

After EC treatment, pregnancy rates are typically in the range of 0.5 to 2.5 percent (Van Look & Stewart, 1998). According to the American College of Obstetricians and Gynecologists (ACOG), the efficacy of ECPs is not affected by whether the first dose is taken 24, 48, or 72 hours after exposure (Chez & Chapin, 1997). On average, menstruation can be expected to begin within seven to nine days after treatment and typically is of normal duration. Approximately 98 percent of women who take EC have menses within 21 days of treatment (Chez & Chapin, 1997). *EC is not intended to be a method of family planning.* It is neither as effective as nor as free of side effects as other methods on the market, and it will not prevent or treat sexually transmitted diseases (Chez & Chapin, 1997).

The second type of emergency contraceptive is the copper T-intrauterine device (IUD). This device prevents the implantation of the fertilized egg and can be inserted up to five days after unprotected intercourse, or five days after the expected date of ovulation, which ever is later, to prevent pregnancy. The insertion of the copper T-intrauterine device is much more effective than the use of emergency contraceptive pills; it reduces the risk of pregnancy following unprotected intercourse by more than 99 percent. The copper T-intrauterine device can be left in place to provide continuous contraception for up to 10 years. However, it is not suitable for women who are not candidates for intrauterine contraception (Speroff & Darney, 1996).

BARRIER METHODS

Barrier methods, which include condoms (male or female), diaphragms, cervical caps, and contraceptive sponges provide about a 50 percent reduction in the incidence of STDs and pelvic inflammatory disease (PID). Although most barrier methods block infections, such as chlamydia, gonorrhea, herpes, cytomegalovirus, and human papillomavirus, only condoms have been proven to prevent *HIV infection* (Speroff & Darney, 1996). Vaginal barrier methods have many advantages that make them reasonable for short- and long-term contraception. They do not cause systemic side effects and do not alter a woman's hormonal pattern (Stewart, F., 1998).

Male Condoms   The male condom remains the most widely available and popular contraceptive method in the United States. More than 9 million reproductive-age women in the United States report using male condoms for contraception or protection from sexually transmitted disease (Warner & Hatcher, 1998). The male condom acts as a physical barrier when placed over the glans and shaft of the penis. It prevents pregnancy by blocking the passage of sperm and is effective only when used from "start to finish" during every act of intercourse (Warner & Hatcher, 1998). *Pre-ejaculatory fluid contains sperm;* therefore, the condom must be applied before the penis comes close to the vagina and before penetration.

Some condoms are lubricated with a small amount of nonoxynol-9, a spermicide. There is no evidence, however, that these condoms are more effective than those without spermicide (Warner & Hatcher, 1998). The concurrent use of a separate vaginal spermicide is recommended as a backup, in case the condom breaks or falls off. The estimated failure rate of the male condom among couples using condoms consistently and correctly is about 3 percent during the first year of use (Warner & Hatcher, 1998).

A few of the advantages of condoms include protection against pregnancy and STDs, accessibility, low cost, and the prevention of sperm allergy. There are also disadvantages, such as reduced sensitivity for males, decreased spontaneity, potential interference with erection, and latex allergy. Some feel that condoms make intercourse unnatural and imply a lack of trust between partners (Warner & Hatcher, 1998).

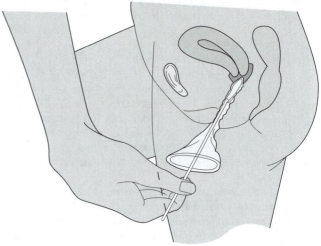

Figure 17–3   Reality Female Condom

Source: Precision Graphics.

Female Condoms   The female condom provides a physical barrier that lines the vagina entirely and partially shields the external genitalia. The Reality Female Condom (see Figure 17–3) is a soft, loose-fitting polyurethane sheath, 7.8 cm in diameter and 17 cm long. One ring lies inside the condom, at the closed end of the sheath, and serves as an insertion mechanism and internal anchor. The other ring forms the external, open edge of the device and remains outside the vagina after insertion (Stewart, F., 1998).

The sheath is lubricated with a substance that has no spermicidal activity. It can be inserted up to eight hours before intercourse; however, each condom is intended for one-time use only. The sheath is made of a material that is thinner, yet stronger, than latex and less likely to tear or break. With the typical use of the female condom, a failure rate of 21 percent has been noted (Stewart, 1998). *Female and male condoms should not be used together;* they can adhere to each other, causing slippage or the displacement of one or both devices (Stewart, 1998).

Diaphragms   A diaphragm (see Figure 17–4) is a dome-shaped, soft, rubber or latex cup with a flexible rim. It is inserted into the vagina before intercourse. The anterior rim fits snugly behind the pubic bone, and the posterior rim rests along the rear wall of the vagina. When properly in place, the diaphragm covers the cervix and acts as a barrier that prevents sperm from entering it. Prior to insertion, a spermicidal cream or jelly is placed inside the dome of the diaphragm and around the rim, in case any sperm make their way to the cervix.

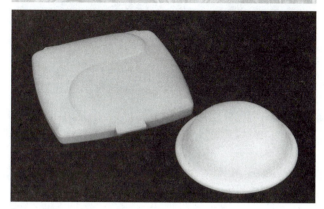

Figure 17–4   Types of Diaphragms

Source: Planned Parenthood.

Diaphragms are available in different sizes and in several styles. They must be fitted for size by a healthcare provider and require a prescription for purchase. Once in position, the diaphragm provides contraceptive protection for 6 hours. If a longer time between insertion and intercourse has elapsed, additional spermicide should be inserted into the vagina with a special applicator (leaving the diaphragm in place). *After intercourse has occurred, the diaphragm must be left in place for at least 6 hours.* If intercourse is repeated during this 6-hour time frame, the diaphragm is left in place, and an additional application of spermicide is instilled into the vagina for additional protection. Wearing a diaphragm for longer than 24 hours is not recommended because of the possible risk of toxic shock syndrome (Stewart, 1998).

Each time the diaphragm is used, it should be checked for holes or tears prior to insertion, and it should be replaced every two years. The fit of the diaphragm should be checked annually by a healthcare provider, after a pregnancy, and after a gain or loss of more than 10 pounds. Failure rates vary from as low as 2 percent per year to 23 percent, with a typical failure rate of 18 percent after one year of use (Speroff & Darney, 1996).

Cervical Caps   The cervical cap is a smaller version of the diaphragm. It is made of slightly thicker rubber and fits snugly around the base of the cervix. As is the case with diaphragms, cervical caps must be fitted by a healthcare provider. The dome of the cap is one-third filled with spermicide prior to insertion (Stewart, 1998).

Although not frequently chosen as a method of contraception, the cap provides continuous protection for 48 hours, no matter how many times intercourse occurs (Stewart, 1998). Additional spermicide is not necessary for re-

peated intercourse. Because of the possible risk of toxic shock syndrome, caps, like diaphragms, should not be worn longer than 48 hours. Some women experience odor problems with prolonged cap use. The cervical cap is as effective as the diaphragm (20 percent failure rate) in women who have not had children. In women who have given birth, however, the failure rate is 40 percent (Stewart, 1998). As with a diaphragm, the cap should be checked for cracks or tears prior to each use. If there are signs of deterioration, it should be replaced. The fit should be checked annually and after pregnancy. It is important to have a Pap smear within a few months of starting the use of the cap, as certain types of infection and inflammations are more likely among users of this device.

Contraceptive Sponges   The Today Sponge is a small, pillow-shaped, polyurethane sponge containing 1 gm of nonoxynol-9 spermicide. It provides a barrier to conception when inserted deep into the vagina. The concave, dimpled side is designed to fit over the cervix and to decrease the chance of dislodgement during intercourse (Stewart, 1998). The sponge is a one-size-fits-all, over-the-counter product that does not require a prescription. Sponges should be moistened with tap water prior to use.

Sponges protect for up to 24 hours, no matter how many times intercourse occurs, and must be left in place for at least 6 hours after the last act of intercourse. Like the diaphragm and cervical cap, the sponge is not to be worn longer than 24 hours because of the possibility of toxic shock syndrome (Stewart, 1998). The failure rate is 40 percent for women who have borne children and 20 percent for those who have not. Sponges are among the less popular method of birth control.

There is controversy regarding the overall effect of contraceptive sponge use on women's health. The National Women's Health Network recently petitioned the FDA not to allow the contraceptive sponge to be sold because it is a high-dose delivery system for nonoxynol-9—a spermicide that has been found in some studies to be irritating to vaginal and cervical tissues, particularly when in contact with them for a lengthy period of time. The network's concern is that such tissue damage may increase the likelihood that the organisms that cause toxic shock and acquired immunodeficiency syndrome (AIDS) will enter the body (Braiman & Lione, 2000). Gollub (2000), however, argues that the studies that showed nonoxynol-9 to increase infection rates suffered from a number of design flaws and maintains that the availability of the sponge increases women's autonomy and decreases their risk of infection and unwanted pregnancy. More research is needed to resolve this issue.

When using any vaginal barrier device that will be left in place for awhile (diaphragm, cervical cap, sponge), it is important to recognize the warning signs of a serious bacterial infection known as **toxic shock syndrome:** sudden high fever, vomiting, diarrhea, dizziness, faintness, weakness, sore throat, aching muscles and joints, and rash (like a sunburn). Should any of these symptoms occur, a healthcare provider must be notified immediately.

OTHER CHEMICAL OR MECHANICAL METHODS OF CONTRACEPTION

In addition to the drugs and devices already discussed, women can choose from among spermicidal products that can be purchased over-the-counter and products that must be obtained from a healthcare provider, such as devices that are inserted into the uterus, and long-acting drug-delivery systems.

Vaginal Spermicides Spermicidal products are easy to use, free of systemic side effects, and available without a prescription. They can be used alone, with a vaginal barrier method, or as an adjunct to any other contraceptive method for added protection against both pregnancy and some sexually transmitted diseases (Cates & Raymond, 1998).

Nonoxynol-9, the active chemical agent in spermicide products available in the United States, is a surfactant that destroys the sperm cell membrane. In the laboratory, nonoxynol-9 is lethal to organisms that cause gonorrhea, genital herpes, trichomoniasis, syphilis, and AIDS. Microbicide activity in the test tube, however, does not guarantee that spermicides provide reliable protection during actual human use (Cates & Raymond, 1998). In 1998, there were more than 20 chemical barrier methods in various stages of development and evaluation (Cates & Raymond, 1998).

Spermicides come in the form of gels, creams, suppositories, and film, or are instilled in spermicidal condoms. Pregnancy rates among typical users vary widely, from less than 5 percent to more than 50 percent in the first year of use (Cates & Raymond, 1998). The effectiveness of a spermicide, like that of a barrier, depends on the consistent and correct use. For a spermicide to be effective, it must be placed high enough in the vagina to make contact with the cervix. This must be done no more than one hour prior to intercourse. Using a physical and a chemical barrier method *together* increases contraceptive efficacy. It is important to follow the directions on the label when using a spermicide. Spermicides may cause temporary skin irritation of the vulva, vagina, or penis because of an allergy or a sensitivity to the spermicidal agent. An increased incidence of yeast vaginitis and bacterial vaginosis has been noted among spermicide users (Cates & Raymond, 1998).

Intrauterine Devices (IUDs) In 1970, approximately 10 percent of American women using artificial contraception used an IUD. By 1998, however, this number had dropped to 2 percent. According to Haas (1998), this decrease was linked to the misconceptions regarding the IUD that were held by both healthcare providers and women. Widely publicized

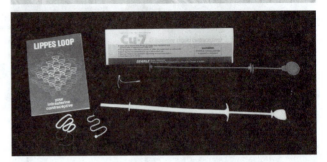

Figure 17–5 Three Currently Used IUDs

Source: Planned Parenthood.

problems with one type of IUD, the Dalkon Shield, cast a shadow over all IUDs. Currently, three FDA-approved IUDs are marketed in the United States: the ParaGard T 380A (Copper-T 380A), available since 1988, Progestasert (a progesterone-releasing device), available since 1976 (Haas, 1998), and the *Levonorgestral IUD* (see Figure 17–5).

The ParaGard T 380A is a T-shaped device made of polyethylene and wrapped with copper wire. It prevents pregnancy due to the directly toxic effect that copper has on sperm, and because its presence makes cervical mucus thicker, thereby retarding the mobility of sperm. This mucosal modification is also thought to cause high concentrations of white blood cells in the uterus and fallopian tubes (Haas, 1998) which may also be inhospitable to sperm. The failure rate during the first year of use is only 0.8 percent (Haas, 1998). The device can be used continuously for 10 years.

The Progestasert (see Progesterone T in Figure 17–7), is impregnated with progesterone, which is released daily. It also modifies the cervical mucus. Additionally, the systemic effect of progesterone blocks ovulation. Progestasert has a failure rate of 2 percent during the 12-month postinsertion period and must be replaced yearly (Haas, 1998). A similar device, the *Levonorgestrel* IUD, contains a form of progesterone known as levonorgestrel. This device strongly suppresses endometrial growth and therefore decreases menstrual blood loss and dysmenorrhea. It also protects against ectopic pregnancy and pelvic inflammatory disease (PID). The failure rate is low at approximately 0.2 percent (Luukkain & Toivonen, 1995).

The most common adverse effect associated with IUDs in general is pelvic inflammatory disease due to infection. Women who have multiple sexual partners are at higher risk for PID and may not be good candidates for an IUD. Another concern with the IUD is expulsion. In one study, the women using the ParaGard T 380A had an expulsion rate of

3.3 to 7.1 percent in the first year; the Progestasert rates were lower, at 1.2 to 4.2 percent (Haas, 1998). Expulsion commonly occurs during the first postinsertion menses or during the first three months of use. Periodically checking for placement, especially after the menses, can help ensure that the IUD is still properly placed. Uterine perforation is a potential risk associated with IUD insertion. The healthcare provider's skill and degree of experience are directly correlated with the rate of perforation associated with insertion (Haas, 1998). IUDs can also cause dysmenorrhea and other menstrual problems. On average, about 10 to 15 percent of copper IUD users have their IUDs removed because of abnormal bleeding or spotting (Stewart, G. K., 1998).

IUDs offer no protection from sexually transmitted disease. The preferred candidate for an IUD is a woman who has already had children, does not have a history of PID, has normal genitalia, is in a monogamous sexual relationship, and desires a long-term method of birth control. IUDs are also appropriate for women who smoke or have other contraindications to hormonal contraceptives, as long as they are at low risk for acquiring an STD. The contraindications for IUD use include menorrhagia (excessive menstrual bleeding), suspected uterine malignancy, severe anemia, undiagnosed vaginal bleeding, severe dysmenorrhea, suspected pregnancy, and valvular heart disease, among others.

It is important for women who choose to wear an IUD to learn, and to pay attention to, the signs that warn that an IUD-related problem may be developing. These signs include a late period, abnormal spotting or bleeding, abdominal pain, pain with intercourse, abnormal discharge, fever, chills, or a string that has suddenly become longer or shorter, or is missing. A healthcare provider should be notified immediately, should any of these occur. It is also important for women who are wearing an IUD to notify their healthcare providers if they know they have been exposed to an STD (Stewart, G. K., 1998). Proper screening and education regarding this method of birth control are imperative if a women is to succeed in using an IUD as her long-term method of contraception (Haas, 1998).

Injectable Depo-Provera *Depo-Provera*, a long-acting progestin (Depo-medroxyprogesterone) administered by injection, was approved for contraception in the United States in 1992, although it has been available in some countries since the mid 1960s (Speroff & Darney, 1996). Much of the information regarding its safety, efficacy, and acceptability comes from Thailand and Mexico, where it has been studied for decades (Speroff & Darney 1996).

A fairly large dose, 150 mg, of Depo-medroxyprogesterone acetate is administered via intramuscular injection every 12 weeks. Depo-Provera's mode of action is different from that of the low-dose, progestin-only preparations because, in addition to thickening the cervical mucus and altering the endometrium, it provides levels of circulating progestin that are high enough to effectively block the LH surge; therefore, ovulation does not occur (Speroff & Darney, 1996).

The injection must be given within the first five days of the menstrual cycle; otherwise, the use of a back-up method is necessary for two weeks (Speroff &Darney, 1996). The efficacy of this method is equal to that of sterilization and better than that of all the other temporary methods. Its efficacy is not influenced by weight or by the use of medications that stimulate liver enzymes (Speroff & Darney, 1996).

Some of the advantages of Depo-Provera are that it is very effective, easy to use, and safe, in that it produces no serious health effects. It is free from estrogen-related problems, and it enhances lactation in new mothers. It also has additional benefits attractive to some women: It produces scanty menses and decreases both menstrual cramps and the pain associated with endometriosis (Speroff & Darney, 1996).

The major problems with this method of birth control are irregular menstrual bleeding, breast tenderness, weight gain, depression, and the inability to discontinue the treatment should problems develop. The most common problem is irregular menstrual bleeding. The incidence of this is 70 percent in the first year of treatment and 10 percent thereafter. If necessary, the bleeding can be treated with the addition of estrogen, given daily for seven days. Nevertheless, up to 25 percent of women who begin contraception with Depo-Provera go off it within the first year. The impact of this medication on lipoprotein profile is uncertain. There are no clinically significant changes in carbohydrate metabolism or in coagulation factors (Speroff & Darney, 1996).

The delay in becoming pregnant after ceasing the use of Depo-Provera is a problem unique to injectable contraception. About half of the women who discontinue Depo-Provera can expect normal menses to return in 6 months after the last injection, but 25 percent will wait a year before the resumption of a normal pattern. On average, 90 percent of Depo-Provera users who desire to become pregnant will do so within 18 months of their last injection (Speroff & Darney, 1996).

Implant Contraception *Norplant* is a progestin-only implant system that consists of six silastic (a flexible plastic) tubes about the size of toothpicks. The tubes, which are surgically implanted under the skin, contain progesterone, which is gradually released into the user's system (Speroff & Darney, 1996). Norplant was first introduced into clinical trials in Chile in 1972 and was approved for marketing in the United States in 1999. The implants must be inserted and removed by trained personnel; women cannot initiate or discontinue this method without the assistance of a healthcare provider. The implants may be left in place for up to five years, and then they need to be removed and replaced. If the capsules are not replaced, an alternative method of birth control must be used.

Norplant is a highly effective birth control method. It is as effective as sterilization and IUDs and more effective than oral and barrier contraceptives. The failure rate is estimated to be less than 0.2 pregnancies per 100 women-years of use. (Ten women, each using a method for 10 years, would equal 100 woman-years of use). Within 24 hours after insertion of the capsules, the plasma concentration of the progestin is high enough to prevent conception (Speroff & Darney, 1996).

Norplant is a safe, highly effective, continuous method of contraception. Because the serum levels of progestin remain low and there is no estrogen administered with this form of birth control, this method does not cause any serious health effects. There are no long-term effects on future fertility, the return of fertility after Norplant removal is prompt, and pregnancy outcomes are within normal limits (Speroff & Darney, 1996).

Norplant does, however, cause the same side effects as other progestin-based systems. In addition, hyperpigmentation over the implant sites can occur (Speroff & Darney, 1996). Although most of these side effects are considered minor by providers, they are upsetting to many women.

Gynecological Illnesses and Problems

If the reproductive system is to function normally, there must be an exquisite integration of function among the hypothalamus, pituitary, ovary (including the follicle), ovum, and corpus luteum, as well as the uterus, endometrium, cervix, and vagina (Shulman, 1990). Most women experience some malfunctioning of this system at various points in their lives. Problems related to the internal reproductive organs that are commonly experienced by women include abnormal bleeding patterns, menstrual difficulties, endometriosis, pelvic relaxation, infections, and benign and malignant growths in the uterus and ovaries. Problems with women's external genitalia, known collectively as the **vulva,** also occur. A commonly used medical term for the vulva, is *pudendum*, which is derived from the Latin *pudendus*, meaning something of which one should be ashamed (Fogel & Woods, 1995) (see Chapter 1 for a discussion of ways in which societal views of women influence women's health and healthcare).

In this section, the following problems will be addressed: dysfunctional uterine bleeding, amenorrhea, premenstrual syndrome, dysmenorrhea, endometriosis, pelvic floor relaxation, yeast vaginitis, bacterial vaginosis, pelvic inflammatory disease, cervical polyps, cervical cancer and uterine fibroids, uterine cancer, benign ovarian cysts and tumors, ovarian cancer, Bartholin's duct cysts, lichens sclerosus, vulvar intraepithelial neoplasia, and benign and malignant conditions of the breast (mastalgia, benign breast tumors, and breast cancer).

Dysfunctional Uterine Bleeding

Uterine bleeding beyond what is considered normal can be caused by relatively benign physiological aberrations or by more serious pathologies. Differentiating between the two requires a thorough physical examination and testing of various kinds. Vaginal bleeding that is menstrual may be considered abnormal because it is excessive or insufficient or because it occurs too soon, too late, or too often in the cycle. Often, a cause can be found for such abnormal patterns. If no cause can be found, the problem is referred to as **dysfunctional uterine bleeding (DUB)** (Shulman, 1990).

Most DUB is associated with an alteration in the hypothalamic-pituitary-ovarian axis, resulting in a failure to ovulate (**anovulation**). When ovulation does not occur, estrogen continues to build up the endometrial lining. When the lining eventually outgrows its blood supply and loses nutrients, it is shed and bleeding occurs. This can result in short cycles, long cycles, heavy flow, or intermenstrual bleeding (Mehring, 1997). Anovulatory DUB is most common at either end of the reproductive years, with adolescents accounting for about 20 percent and perimenopausal women accounting for approximately 50 percent of cases (Mehring, 1997). There are many other possible causes of DUB, including reactions to drugs, hormonal imbalances, malignant and nonmalignant tumors, and infections. DUB can also be caused by **systemic diseases,** such as hypothyroidism, cirrhosis of the liver, and disease states in which blood does not clot normally (Brenner, 1996).

SYMPTOMS

Abnormal uterine bleeding is said to be present when the interval between the start of successive menses is ≤ 21 days, the duration of menstrual flow is > 7 days, or the menstrual blood loss is > 80 cc. A deviation from a previously established menstrual pattern, a sudden increase of two or more sanitary pads per day, menses lasting ≥ 3 days longer than usual, intermenstrual bleeding, or an interval between menses ≥ 4 days less than usual, should be considered abnormal for that woman (Brenner, 1996).

DIAGNOSIS

It is important for women who think they may be experiencing a menstrual abnormality to keep a record of the onset, duration, amount, color, and character of their bleeding. They should also record any accompanying odor, pain, fever, nausea, vomiting, diarrhea, constipation, or painful bowel movements, as well as problems with urination or sexual activity (Shulman, 1990). Potential precipitating events, such as trauma, must be confided.

The history and physical examination together will narrow the possible diagnosis, but additional tests may be necessary in order to reach a final diagnosis. A urine pregnancy test can rule out the complications of pregnancy as the source of irregular bleeding. Other laboratory tests to rule out infection, anemia, or problems with blood clotting may also be done. Tests to determine blood levels of various hormones may be needed. In some cases, procedures such as endometrial biopsy or pelvic ultrasound may be necessary. Sometimes, surgical procedures, such as dilatation and curettage, hysteroscopy, laparoscopy, or laparotomy may be needed (Shulman, 1990).

An **endometrial biopsy** involves inserting a thin, hollow, flexible tube through the cervix into the uterine cavity to obtain a sample of the uterine tissue. **Dilation and curettage (D&C)** involves scraping away tissue from the lining under light general anesthesia. During a **hysteroscopy,** a lighted tube with a lens is inserted into the uterus, enabling the surgeon to see the lining of the uterus. A **laparotomy** is performed by creating a surgical opening of the abdomen; a laparoscopy uses a type of endoscope, called a laparascope, to explore the abdomen. If the irregular vaginal bleeding is chronic, recording basal body temperatures, bleeding patterns, and cervical mucus charts for one to three months can determine if normal hypothalamic-pituitary-ovarian functions are present and perhaps obviate the need for a lengthy and costly diagnostic workup (Shulman, 1990).

TREATMENT

Abnormal bleeding due to infection, anemia, or clotting disorders is treated by eradicating the underlying cause. DUB due to hormonal disturbances is generally treated with an appropriate hormonal regimen, although surgical intervention is indicated in some cases. The objectives in treating DUB are to control the bleeding, prevent recurrence, preserve fertility, correct associated disorders, and induce ovulation in women who desire to conceive. The age of the woman, severity of bleeding, number of children, desire for future fertility, and presence of associated pelvic pathology are factors that influence the selection of therapy (Chuong & Brenner, 1996). Medical, as opposed to surgical, treatment is preferred, especially if more children are desired and there are no associated pelvic lesions.

When bleeding is caused by hormonal imbalance in a woman who is **ovulating,** high-dose estrogen, either oral or intravenous, is the treatment of choice because it promotes rapid endometrial regrowth. Once the bleeding is controlled, oral estrogen is continued for 21 to 25 days, and oral progesterone is given along with the estrogen for the last 7 to 10 days. Then both hormones are discontinued, and a withdrawal bleed occurs that is heavy but rarely prolonged (Chuong & Brenner, 1996). Another option is the use of high-dose estrogen-progestin therapy, achieved by using combined oral contraceptives. Once the bleeding stops, the treatment is continued for at least one more

week and then a standard-dose oral contraceptive regimen can be used for two or three more cycles.

If the DUB is **anovulatory** (associated with failure to ovulate), synthetic progestins (such as Provera, Aygestin, Norlutate, and Norlutin) may be given for 10 days out of each month in order to prevent recurrent episodes. The prolonged use of high-dose progestins can cause fatigue, mood changes, weight gain, and changes in the lipid profile (Chuong & Brenner, 1996). Natural pro-gesterone is made from plant steroids and is an exact chemical duplicate of the progesterone produced by the body; therefore, it is better tolerated. It is also **micronized** (finely ground) to enhance absorption. However, some disadvantages of the natural hormone include a short half-life (three to six hours), which requires that it be taken two or three times a day, and limited availability. Also, as natural progesterone for the treatment of anovulatory bleeding has yet to be approved by the FDA, most insurance companies will not pay for it. Natural hormones are available through compounding pharmacies, which are becoming more numerous. **Compounding pharmacies** are pharmacies that supply custom pharmaceutical products. Perimenopausal women with anovulatory bleeding can be treated with cyclic hormone replacement therapy, and those who do not smoke and have no evidence of vascular disease can be treated with low-dose oral contraceptives (Chuong & Brenner, 1996).

Nonsteroidal anti-inflammatory drugs, such as mefenamic, ibuprofen, and naproxen, have also been shown to be effective in the control of *ovulatory* DUB (Chuong & Brenner, 1996). They can be used alone or in combination with oral contraceptives or progestins to achieve a greater reduction in menstrual blood loss. Androgenic steroids (such as Danazol) and gonadotropin-releasing hormone (such as Lupron and Zoladex) can also be used to reduce menstrual blood loss, but the expense and side effects associated with these drugs limit their use.

Surgical treatment for DUB includes D&C, endometrial ablation, and hysterectomy. D&C is the fastest method of stopping bleeding. It can be both therapeutic and diagnostic, but it does not usually prevent the recurrence of excessive uterine bleeding, unless it is followed by additional hormonal management (Chuong & Brenner, 1996). Hysteroscopic examination allows for the direct visualization of the endometrial cavity and the identification of polyps and submucous fibroids, as well as the directed biopsies of the most suspicious areas. In a newer treatment for DUB, **endometrial ablation,** the endometrium is destroyed by a laser or another source of heat. The procedure is done vaginally, and only a short hospital stay is required. Ablation procedures cause a deep thermal injury, which minimizes the regeneration of the endometrium and usually renders the woman sterile (Mehring, 1997). Ablation is highly effective; up to 90 percent of women who undergo ablation become amenorrheic or at least have an acceptable reduction of menstrual blood loss (Chuong & Brenner, 1996). The long-term effects of endometrial ablation are not yet known, but its use is becoming more frequent, and ablation is now considered a cost-effective alternative to hysterectomy when all other treatment modalities have failed (Chuong & Brenner, 1996). A hysterectomy is done only when all other methods of treatment have failed, or when other pelvic disorders also exist.

Amenorrhea

Amenorrhea means a lack of menstruation and is divided into two categories: primary amenorrhea and secondary amenorrhea. **Primary amenorrhea** is the failure to have menstruated by the age of 14 years (without the development of secondary sex characteristics) or by the age of 16 years (regardless of the presence of secondary sex characteristics) (Robinson & McCance, 1998).

The causes of primary amenorrhea include abnormalities such as congenital defects of the gonadotropin production, genetic disorders, congenital central nervous system (CNS) defects, congenital anatomic malformation of the reproductive system, and acquired CNS lesions (Robinson & McCance, 1998). In some congenital syndromes, the hypothalamic-pituitary-ovarian axis is dysfunctional. The hypothalamus is unable to synthesize GnRH, so the pituitary fails to secrete FSH and LH; then the ovaries do not receive the hormonal signals necessary to initiate the ovarian and endometrial changes of the menstrual cycle, and ovulation and menstruation do not occur (Robinson & McCance, 1998). Anatomic defects of the genitalia, such as a congenital absence of the vagina and uterus and congenital uterine hypoplasia (an abnormally small uterus), are also associated with primary amenorrhea. Females without a uterus or vagina usually have normal ovarian functions; therefore, skeletal growth and secondary sex characteristics develop but menstruation does not occur (Robinson & McCance, 1998). A number of genetic disorders are also associated with primary amenorrhea (Robinson & McCance, 1998).

The term **secondary amenorrhea** refers to the absence of menstruation for three or more cycles, or six months, in women who have previously menstruated. (This is normal during early adolescence, pregnancy, lactation, and perimenopause.) This form of amenorrhea can be caused by elevated or decreased levels of ovarian hormones, by an overproduction of the hormone prolactin, or by structural defects. Such abnormalities may act singly or in combination to cause amenorrhea.

SYMPTOMS

The major clinical manifestation of both primary and secondary amenorrhea is the absence of menses. The cause of the amenorrhea determines whether secondary sex characteristics and height are affected (Robinson & McCance, 1998).

DIAGNOSIS

The diagnosis of primary amenorrhea is based on the medical history and physical examination. The physical exam may reveal abnormal physical immaturity or a structural or physiological alteration. Laboratory tests are done to reveal abnormal levels of hormones, such as gonadotropin and the ovarian hormones. Diagnostic imaging is used to detect internal structural abnormalities (Robinson & McCance, 1998).

The diagnosis of secondary amenorrhea involves identifying the underlying hormonal or anatomic alterations. A complete history and physical examination are, of course, important elements of the diagnostic process. Pregnancy will be ruled out and blood levels of hormones, such as the ovarian hormones, thyroid-stimulating hormone, gonadotropin, and prolactin, will be determined. Additional tests may include X-rays and computerized axial tomography (CAT) scans.

TREATMENT

The treatment of primary dysmenorrhea involves the correction of any underlying disorders and hormone replacement therapy to induce the development of secondary sex characteristics. Surgery may be needed to correct any structural abnormalities of the genitalia (Robinson & McCance, 1998). Depending on the cause, the treatment of secondary dysmenorrhea includes hormone replacement therapy or corrective surgery (Robinson & McCance, 1998).

Premenstrual Syndrome

The term **premenstrual syndrome (PMS)** refers to a constellation of distressing physical, psychological, and/or behavioral changes that recur cyclically during the second half (luteal phase) of the menstrual cycle. These changes are often mild but in some cases are severe enough to cause a deterioration in interpersonal relationships and to interfere with normal activities (Ugarriza, Klinger, & O'Brien, 1998). PMS is estimated to occur in 30 to 40 percent of women of childbearing age; severe symptomatology, however, is limited to less than 10 percent of women in that age range (Ugarriza et al., 1998). The exact cause of PMS is not known, but it seems to involve a combination of physical, psychological, and perhaps social factors.

The hormonal factors implicated in PMS are changes in estrogen, progesterone, and prolactin levels. Higher progesterone levels cause excess aldosterone to be produced by the adrenal cortex. This, in turn, induces the sodium and water retention responsible for the edema (bloating) common in PMS. Progesterone disturbances are also associated with decreased libido and altered mood (Ugarriza et al., 1998). Excessive levels of prolactin can cause breast tenderness and swelling. Altered glucose tolerance, leading to changes in blood sugar levels, may cause the symptoms of PMS that seem to be hypoglycemic—for example, irritability and difficulty concentrating. There is also a possible link between thyroid dysfunction and PMS, as both are characterized by fluctuations in temperature and blood viscosity, as well as weight gain, lethargy, irritability, moodiness, and anxiety (Ugarriza et al., 1998).

Blood levels of vitamins, minerals, and neurotransmitters may also play a role in PMS. Deficiencies in vitamin B-6 and magnesium may contribute to the emotional symptoms associated with PMS. Vitamin B-6 deficiency is specifically associated with the decreased serotonin levels that are noted in depressive syndromes (Ugarriza et al., 1998). Serotonin is a neurotransmitter that influences mood. Ovarian hormones influence calcium and vitamin D metabolism, and low blood levels of calcium and vitamin D have also been implicated in PMS.

Excessive amounts of refined sugars, fat, caffeine, and alcohol in the diet are also thought to cause PMS symptoms or at least to make them worse. Oral contraceptives and tobacco use have also been related to the occurrence of PMS (Ugarriza et al., 1998).

Although there is no known psychological cause of PMS (Ugarriza et al., 1998), the psychological and behavioral changes PMS is said to foster have warranted the inclusion of a severe form of PMS (**premenstrual dysphoric disorder**) as a diagnosis in the *Diagnostic and Statistical Manual of Mental Disorders,* published by the American Psychiatric Association. The inclusion of even severe PMS in a compendium of mental and emotional diseases is controversial. Chrisler (1991) argues that PMS does not meet the criteria of a discrete disease because there is little agreement in the literature on how many symptoms must be experienced, how often, and to what degree of severity in order to warrant the diagnosis. Chrisler also points out that the symptoms of PMS are experienced, to some degree, by the majority of adolescent and adult women and can occur throughout all phases of the menstrual cycle. Chrisler's argument is strengthened by the fact that the presence and severity of PMS symptoms in a given woman may be inconsistent from month to month (Robinson & McCance, 1998). Moreover, many women have reported feeling energized and happy, as well as especially clear mentally, when they are premenstrual (Nicholson, 1995). Chrisler and others (Faludi, 1991) believes PMS to be a **culture-bound syndrome** (see Chapter 1). To say that a physical problem is culture-bound is to suggest that it is related in some way to societal beliefs about and attitudes toward the group that experiences the problem. The belief that women are nervous, irritable, and generally driven mad by their hormones in the days preceding menstruation is rampant in American culture, as exemplified by T-shirts that proclaim, "It's not PMS—I'm psychotic." Such beliefs may influence both women's experiences of their monthly cycles and medical authorities' interpretation of those experiences. The proposition that PMS symptomatology may be influenced by culture is supported by the fact that the menstrual phase in which peak PMS symptom severity occurs differs according to the population studied (Robinson & McCance, 1998).

SYMPTOMS

In American women, the symptoms associated with PMS typically begin 2 to 12 days before the onset of menses and usually disappear within the first 24 hours after it. There are more than 200 physical, emotional, and behavioral symptoms attributed to PMS, but, in making the diagnosis of PMS, the pattern of symptom frequency and severity is more important than the specific complaints (Robinson & McCance, 1998). The common signs and symptoms of PMS include affective (mood), behavioral, cognitive, and physical phenomena. Sadness, anxiety, anger, agitation, decreased motivation, poor impulse control, decreased concentration, sensitivity to rejection, clumsiness, dizziness, bloating, weight gain, insomnia, anorexia, fatigue, libido change, acne, greasy or dry hair, headache, breast tenderness, and joint and muscle pain have all been reported. More serious manifestations, such as paranoia, social isolation, and suicidal thoughts, have also been documented, although they are not common (Ugarriza et al., 1998).

DIAGNOSIS

Many of the symptoms of PMS can be caused by other health problems, such as diabetes, hypoglycemia, thyroid dysfunction, and excessive levels of the hormone *prolactin* in the blood (Moline & Zendel, 2000). Therefore laboratory studies need to be undertaken to assess for these conditions. Many women find that the PMS symptoms disappear after being treated for these medical conditions (Ugarriza et al., 1998).

Currently, in order to warrant a diagnosis of PMS, consistent signs and symptoms that occur in the luteal phase of the cycle and disappear by the end of the first day of menses must be present. They must also be of sufficient severity to disrupt the woman's daily life (Ugarriza et al., 1998). Women can assist healthcare providers in identifying the nature of their problems by recording their symptoms, and their severity, on a daily basis for three months. This will help differentiate between an exacerbation of chronic symptoms, such as that seen in depression, and symptoms appearing solely during the premenstrual interval (Moline & Zendel, 2000).

TREATMENT

Because the causes of PMS are complex, and because the occurrence and severity of PMS are mediated by lifestyle, social, and psychological factors, the current method of treating PMS is *managing its symptoms,* rather than trying to eradicate a root cause (Robinson & McCance, 1998). Therapy generally involves treating the symptoms causing the most distress (Moline & Zendell, 2000). The interventions are individualized to meet each woman's specific issues and needs. A regular program of aerobic exercises, such as walking, aerobics, jogging, bicycling, or swimming, three or four times a week for 45 to 60 minutes is recommended. Dietary modifications, such as reducing intake of salt, refined sugar, red meat, caffeine, chocolate, and fat, may be helpful. Consuming a well-balanced diet high in whole grains, fruits, and vegetables and increasing protein to at least 45 grams per day can stabilize blood sugar levels and minimize cravings and fatigue. Eating small, frequent meals, rather than fewer large ones, and drinking at least eight glasses of water a day are also beneficial (Ugarriza et al., 1998). Although there have been anecdotal reports that supplements such as vitamin E, vitamin B-6, and magnesium can alleviate PMS, controlled studies of the effectiveness of those substances are either lacking or inconclusive (Bendich, 2000). In one large, well-controlled study, however, supplementing the diet with calcium was found to be effective in modulating or abolishing the symptoms of PMS (Thys-Jacobs, 2000).

Herbal medications have long been used in traditional healing to manage PMS and menopausal symptoms. Recently, scientific studies have supported the efficacy of some phytomedicines in treating problems related to women's reproductive system (see Chapter 11). The herb dong quai may have some efficacy for PMS (Hardy, 2000), but studies done on the effectiveness of evening primrose oil have produced conflicting results (Bendich, 2000). Safety data, especially during pregnancy and lactation, are still largely lacking for many herbal medications, and the recommendations for usage and dosage vary (Hardy, 2000).

Psychotherapy may also be helpful in dealing with PMS. Individual, marriage, or family counseling may be indicated, as may counseling regarding anger management and conflict resolution. Stress-reduction techniques, such as biofeedback, relaxation, and imagery, are also recommended (Robinson & McCance, 1998). Medications may be added to the treatment plan if needed. The medications frequently prescribed include antidepressants, antiprostaglandins, and benzodiazepines. In severe cases, menses can be stopped entirely with oral contraceptives, Depo-Provera, or GnRH agonists, in order to eliminate cyclic fluxuations in estrogen and progesterone (Robinson & McCance, 1998).

Dysmenorrhea

The term **dysmenorrhea** refers to difficult and painful menstruation. There are two categories of dysmenorrhea: primary and secondary. **Primary dysmenorrhea** is menstrual pain that is not caused by a structural abnormality or disease process. Primary dysmenorrhea affects 50 to 75 percent of women age 15 to 25—sometimes so severely that they miss work or school (Robinson & McCance, 1998). Primary dysmenorrhea is believed to be related to higher than normal levels of prostaglandins (PG) because symptoms are more intense during the first 2 days of menstruation, when blood levels of prostaglandin are highest (Morrison, Daniels, & Kotey et al., 1999). **Secondary dysmenorrhea** is menstrual pain associated with a known anatomic factor, or pelvic pathology.

SYMPTOMS AND DIAGNOSIS

The main symptom of primary dysmenorrhea is pelvic pain with the onset of menses, although the associated symptoms of backache, nausea, vomiting, diarrhea, and headaches may also occur. No special procedures or tests are usually needed to diagnose primary dysmenorrhea, although pelvic pathology, such as uterine fibroids, pelvic inflammatory disease, endometrial polyps, endometriosis, and endometrial cancer, must be excluded as the cause. The pain of secondary dysmenorrhea can be differentiated from primary dysmenorrhea in that it frequently occurs several days before the onset of menses or during ovulation or intercourse. It can be present at any point in the menstrual cycle (Sullivan, 1990).

TREATMENT

The treatment of primary dysmenorrhea consists of heat, message, relaxation techniques, regular exercise, and medications, such as prostaglandin inhibitors, anti-inflammatory analgesics, and hormones (oral contraceptives). The herb Dong quai has been well established as a useful agent for dysmenorrhea (Limon, 2000). The treatment of secondary dysmenorrhea is essentially the same as for primary dysmenorrhea and may also include the need for additional medications or surgical intervention—depending on the pelvic pathology involved.

Endometriosis

Endometriosis is the presence of endometrial tissue in parts of the body other than the uterine cavity. According to the Endometriosis Association (2000), endometriosis is a painful, chronic disease that affects 5.5 million women and girls in the United States and Canada and millions more worldwide. In endometriosis, aberrantly located endometrial tissue is most commonly present in the peritoneal cavity, or on the surfaces of pelvic structures, such as the ovaries, fallopian tubes, or uterus, or on the bowel (Corwin, 1997).

The cause of endometriosis is unknown, although there are a number of theories about its origin. The first is the **retrograde menstruation theory,** which suggests that, during menstruation, some of the menstrual tissue backs up through the fallopian tubes, implants in the peritoneal cavity, and grows. Retrograde menstruation has been documented to occur in approximately 90 percent of all menstruating women (Corwin, 1997). Another theory holds that endometrial tissue is distributed from the uterus to other parts of the body via the lymphatic system or bloodstream. A third theory is that an immune system or hormonal problem allows endometrial tissue to grow outside the uterus (Endometriosis Association, 2000).

A genetic predisposition has been documented (Robinson & McCance, 1998); studies show there is a sevenfold increase in the risk of endometriosis in sisters and mothers of women with endometriosis. The risk is significantly greater in women of Asian descent (Corwin, 1997).

Endometriosis is uncommon in women who have borne more than one child, with an occurrence rate of only 3.7 percent in that population. It is much more common in infertile women, among which a 30 to 40 percent incidence has been reported (Corwin, 1997). The average age range of women with endometriosis is 20 to 45 years, with the highest incidence found in women between 40 and 44 (Corwin, 1997).

The endometrial tissue located outside the uterus responds to hormonal stimulation, just as the tissue within the uterus does. It proliferates (thickens) and secretes various substances. It also decays when hormonal levels fall, but, because there is no outlet by which this tissue can leave the body, it accumulates locally (Corwin, 1997). The cycles of accumulation, growth, and eventual necrosis lead to inflammation of the peritoneal cavity and ultimately cause the symptoms and pathology associated with the disease (Corwin, 1997).

SYMPTOMS

Women with endometriosis often report a short cycle of less than 28 days, heavy flow lasting 5 or more days, menses that last 7 days or more, and significant cramping (Corwin, 1997). In 1998, the Endometriosis Association conducted a survey of 4,000 women in the United States and Canada who had endometriosis (Endometriosis Association, 2000). The most commonly reported symptoms were worsening menstrual cramps (95 percent), fatigue (87 percent), painful bowel movements and diarrhea (85 percent), abdominal bloating (84 percent), heavy bleeding (65 percent), pain with intercourse (64 percent), stomach upset and nausea (64 percent), and infertility (43 percent). The severity of the symptoms may not reflect the extent of the disease—microscopic lesions may be disabling for one woman, whereas much larger lesions may cause minimal discomfort to another.

A relatively common complication of moderate to severe endometriosis is infertility. Repeated inflammation in the genital tract can lead to scarring and the development of **adhesions,** scar tissue that binds other tissues together, which destroy sperm or block their passage through the fallopian tube. Approximately 50 percent of women with unexplained infertility are found to have endometriosis on visual inspection of the peritoneal cavity (Corwin, 1997).

DIAGNOSIS

A careful history and a complete physical examination are important steps in the diagnosis of endometriosis. Whereas a tentative diagnosis can be made on the basis of these initial steps, a definitive diagnosis requires surgical visualization of the pelvic cavity, via either laparoscopy or laparotomy. A tissue biopsy and pathologic confirmation of suspected lesions are required for confirmation of the disease. During surgery, staging (assigning a "stage" of severity) of the disease is done

based on the size and location of endometrial lesions and the presence and extent of adhesions (Corwin, 1997).

TREATMENT

The treatment goals include relieving or reducing pain, shrinking or slowing endometrial growths, preserving or restoring fertility, and preventing or delaying recurrence of the disease (Endometriosis Association, 2000). Over-the-counter pain medications, such as acetaminophen and ibuprofen, may relieve or reduce pain. In some cases, prescription drugs are required.

More aggressive medical management can also be pursued. The suppression of endogenous estrogen levels with GnRH agonists (such as Lupron, Synarel) can reduce extra- and intrauterine endometrial growth (Corwin, 1997). Treatment usually lasts for six months, and the most common adverse effects mimic many of the symptoms of menopause (hot flushes, vaginal dryness, headache, decreased libido). GnRH agonists, however, do appear to be an effective treatment (Prentice, Deary, Goldbeck-Wood, Farquhar, & Smith, 1999). Androgen derivatives, such as Danazol, can also be used to reduce the size of existing endometrial lesions and to prevent further production of new implants (Corwin, 1997). Danazol is usually administered for six to nine months. Its adverse effects are those of the GnRH agonists plus weight gain, acne, oily skin and hair, and hirsutism (excessive body hair). Although Danazol is effective in treating the symptoms and signs of endometriosis, its use is often limited by the androgenic (testosterone-like) side effects (Selak, Farquhar, Prentice, & Singla, 1999). Neither GnRH agonists nor Danazol render women infertile; a method of birth control must be used when taking these types of drugs, for they have a **teratogenic** (deformity-producing) effect on the fetus. Two other medications, medroxyprogesterone acetate (Depo-Provera) injections and oral contraceptives, can be used to control the symptoms of endometriosis in women unwilling or unable to tolerate the side effects of the GnRH agonists and Danazol. Both cause cessation of menses and alleviate symptoms, but neither has been shown to have a lasting impact on the disease (Corwin, 1997).

More radical treatment is available for women who are severely affected by endometriosis or who do not wish to preserve their fertility. A total **hysterectomy** (surgical removal of the uterus), with the removal of any visible adhesions, is considered the definitive treatment for endometriosis (Corwin, 1997). Treatment with GnRH agonist or Danazol is recommended after surgery if there is concern that some lesions may remain.

Pelvic Floor Relaxation

Pelvic floor relaxation occurs when the supporting muscles, ligaments, and connective tissues can no longer hold the pelvic organs in their correct anatomic location. A downward or forward dislocation of the uterus, bladder, and other pelvic structures results (Berek, Adashi, & Hillard,

Figure 17–6   Cystocele and Rectocele

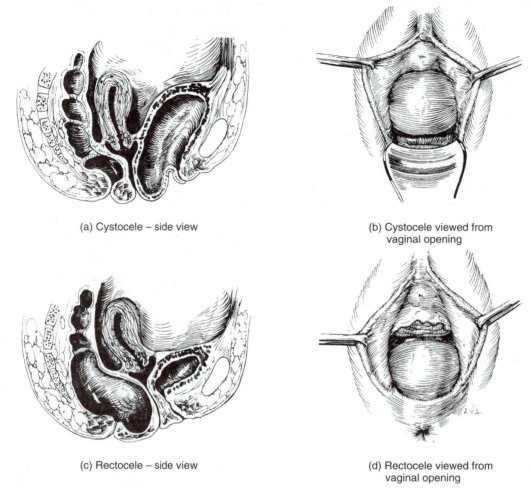

(a) Cystocele – side view

(b) Cystocele viewed from vaginal opening

(c) Rectocele – side view

(d) Rectocele viewed from vaginal opening

Source: DeCherney & Pernoll: *Current Obstetric & Gynecologic Diagnosis & Treatment*, Norwalk, CT, Appleton & Lange, 1994. Reprinted with permission of the McGraw-Hill Companies.

1996; Ryan, Berkowitz, Barbieri, & Dunaif, 1999). Such dislocation is referred to as **prolapse,** and varying degrees of prolapse can occur. In the most severe instances, the uterus can protrude from the vagina, or the bladder or intestine can exert sufficient pressure on the vaginal wall to produce a noticeable bulge. A bulge caused by a descended bladder is called a **cystocele,** and a bulge caused by weakness in the wall between the rectum and the vagina is called a **rectocele** (see Figure 17–6).

Many things can cause the supporting muscles to become weak and fail. The nerves that enervate the muscles and cause them to contract become less efficient with normal aging. Chronic or acute strain on these nerves, such as occurs with constipation or prolonged coughing (such as in

"smoker's cough"), can also lead to nerve degeneration and muscle atrophy. Vaginal birth can also contribute to pelvic relaxation; it can tear the connective tissue that lends additional support to the pelvic floor and surrounding organs. Finally, estrogen deficiency after menopause leaves the tissues of the pelvic floor less elastic and more prone to tearing and trauma. Thousands of surgeries are done each year to correct the problems associated with pelvic floor relaxation (Berek et al., 1996). Despite the prevalence of this condition, beneficial treatments for this disorder evolved slowly during the twentieth century. A greater understanding of the multiple roles of pelvic floor nerves, muscles, and connective tissues is unfolding, and more effective therapies may be forthcoming.

SYMPTOMS

Pelvic floor relaxation may cause no symptoms at all. A bulge at the vagina caused by the downward descent of the uterus or another organ may be the only noticeable sign. When symptoms do occur, they often include stress urinary incontinence (see Chapter 16), back pain, a pulling sensation in the pelvis, or vaginal pressure. Pain, pulling, and pressure sensations are usually worse at the end of the day and can be improved by lying down (Ryan et al., 1999). Severe prolapse can interfere with sexual intercourse by mechanically blocking the vagina. Moreover, as the mucosa of the prolapsed organ is exposed to the air, ulceration of the tissue can form. Pelvic relaxation can also cause urinary retention. If the urethra (the tube by which urine leaves the bladder) becomes kinked, it obstructs the release of urine. Pelvic relaxation can also interfere with defecation. If the rectum is involved, stool can become trapped in the prolapsed area. Women with untreated prolapses of the bladder or rectum must often push up on the bladder or down on the rectum with a finger in order to facilitate emptying.

DIAGNOSIS

Pelvic floor relaxation is diagnosed during physical examination. The examining clinician visualizes the vaginal orifice and asks the patient to bear down. This causes the prolapsed bladder, rectum, or cervix to visibly bulge at the **introitus,** or vaginal opening. A bimanual pelvic (internal) examination is carried out, during which the examiner inserts two fingers into the vagina and the patient is again asked to bear down. The affected organs are felt pressing against the examining fingers. The exam may also be carried out with the patient semiseated or even standing to gain the maximum impact of gravity (Berek et al., 1996). The severity of the prolapse can be mild, with a slight downward movement of the organs during examination, or severe, with the entire uterus protruding out of the vagina.

TREATMENT

The treatment of pelvic floor relaxation is needed only if symptoms are present (Berek et al., 1996). Treatment includes muscle-strengthening exercises, the use of a pessary, and surgery.

Muscle Strengthening   The first line of therapy for a mild prolapse is strengthening of the pelvic floor muscles, especially if stress urinary incontinence is a symptom. Chapter 16 contains a full discussion of Kegel exercises.

Pessaries   Pessaries are diaphragm-like devices that the patient wears inside her vagina (Ryan et al., 1999). They work by mechanically holding the prolapsed organs in place. They are a good choice for elderly or frail patients who cannot withstand surgery. Pessaries come in a variety of shapes and sizes (see Figure 17–7). Because they exert pressure on the vaginal walls, pessaries should always be used in conjunction with estrogen therapy, either oral or locally to the vagina, in postmenopausal women. Postmenopausal women not on estrogen tend to have delicate vaginal tissues prone to ulceration. Pessaries should be removed and cleaned daily with soap and water. However, this requires a lot of manual dexterity, which many elderly patients do not have. Under a clinician's supervision, pessaries can be left in place for several weeks and cleaned in an office setting, as long as an inspection of the vaginal mucosa reveals no sign of erosion or ulceration.

Surgery   The definitive treatment for prolapse of any type is surgery (Ryan et al., 1999). A number of surgical approaches can be used. The type of approach depends on the surgeon's preference and skill, as well as the condition of the patient. The goal of surgery is to relieve the patient of symptoms and to bring the prolapsed organs into a more functional anatomic position. There may be more than one defect in the pelvic floor that needs repair, and many surgical procedures can be done simultaneously. Cystoceles can be repaired through a vaginal or an abdominal incision. Recovery from the latter is longer, however, and there is an associated increase in morbidity, but there is greater long-term success. Laparoscopic approaches using tiny incisions in the umbilical and suprapubic area are currently being investigated. Rectoceles are repaired through an incision in the vaginal mucosa. Muscles and connective tissues are reconstructed in order to provide more support. Vaginal hysterectomy is the treatment of choice for uterine prolapse.

Yeast Vaginitis

Yeast vaginitis (vaginal candidiasis) is one of the most common causes of infection in the female genital tract (Nyirjesy, Seeney, Grody, Jordan, & Buckley, 1995). Yeast infections account for 20 to 25 percent of all cases of vaginitis (Cullins, Dominguez, Guberski, Secor, & Wysocki, 1999). Approximately 75 percent of women will experience such an infection at least once in their lifetime.

Most yeast infections resolve after a single treatment course with common over-the-counter vaginal antifungal preparations. For reasons not yet clear, about 5 percent of women experience unrelenting infections without having other predisposing health factors, such as diabetes or HIV infection (Nyirjesy et al., 1995).

Eighty-five to 90 percent of all vaginal yeast infections are caused by *Candida albicans,* a species of fungus (Nyirjesy et al., 1995). Five to 10 percent of vaginal candidiasis is caused by nonalbicans strains of yeast fungi. Yeast may be part of the woman's normal vaginal milieu, or it may be introduced when there is an imbalance of the bacterial environment of the vagina; for instance, antibiotics destroy the healthy, normal bacteria of the vagina. There are likely other mechanisms of infection involved, which are unknown. The occurrence of

Figure 17–7   Pessaries

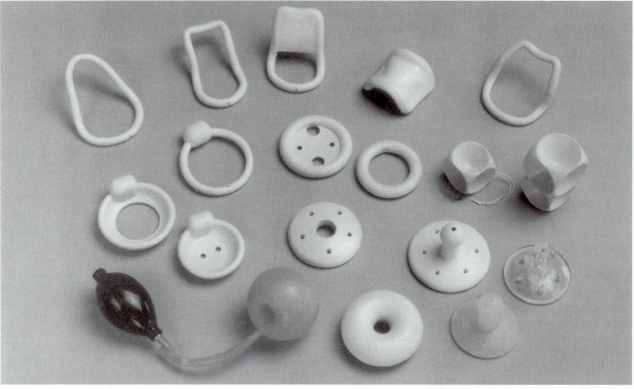

Source: Women's Health: A Primary Clinical Guide, 2e by Youngkin, © 1998. Reprinted with permission of Pearson Education, Inc., Upper Saddle River, NJ.

resistant strains is increasing, perhaps due to the misuse of current therapies (Sinofsky, 1999). Among the risk factors for vaginal candidiasis are recent antibiotic therapy, pregnancy, stress, diabetes, corticosteroid use, obesity, and any disease that compromises the immune system, such as HIV infection (Cullins et al., 1999). Yeast infections are probably not sexually transmitted. Although yeast has been cultured from the penis of male sexual partners (Cullins et al., 1999), treating both women and their partners has not been shown to reduce the rates of recurring infections in women. Many women can be *carriers* of yeast fungus yet have no symptoms, but the nature of this carrier state has yet to be fully elucidated.

SYMPTOMS

The classic symptoms are vaginal itching and a white, cottage cheese–like discharge (Cullins et al., 1999). Other symptoms can be redness and inflammation of the vulva, painful intercourse, and burning of the vulva on contact with semen, urine, or other substances (even water). Sometimes the only symptom a woman has is painful intercourse.

DIAGNOSIS

Yeast infections are diagnosed on the basis of the woman's signs and symptoms, as well as on a microscopic examination of vaginal cells and secretions (Cullins et al., 1999). The clinician looks for spores and hyphae—microscopic yeast forms. However, these yeast forms are not always evident, due to a low number of yeast organisms, a pathogen that is a nonalbicans species, or other factors. If a clinician suspects a resistant strain of yeast, or is unclear of the reason for the woman's symptoms, a culture can be sent to a laboratory to help confirm the diagnosis and guide treatment (Nyirjesy et al., 1995).

TREATMENT

There is a multitude of treatments available for vaginal candidiasis. Over-the-counter products contain a class of drugs called the **azoles.** These include butaconazole, clotrimazole, miconazole, and tioconazole (Cullins et al., 1999). Most of these products are available in suppository, tablet, and cream form and must be used for one, three, or seven days. If used as directed, these treatments are highly effective against the *Candida albicans* strains of yeast. A prescription drug containing terconazole is also used and will destroy some, but not all nonalbicans strains. Recurrent infections are often treated with prolonged courses of suppressive therapy, such as using an azole cream twice weekly for six months after the initial course.

One of the main side effects of the vaginal preparations used to treat yeast infections is vaginal irritation, caused by a local allergic response to the cream (Sinofsky, 1999). When women experience the itching and irritation associated with this side effect, they often assume that their yeast infection hasn't cleared and continue the treatment, which only leads to more irritation. Women who have used an entire course of antiyeast medication and continue to have symptoms beyond two days posttreatment need to be evaluated by their healthcare providers. They may have a resistant strain of yeast, a different infection (such as a sexually transmitted infection), a reaction to the medication used, or a health problem, such as diabetes or immune compromise, that is predisposing them to recurrent yeast infections.

Fluconazole is an oral remedy that is available only by prescription. It is highly effective against the albicans strains of yeast only. A single dose of 150 mg will cure most isolated infections, but dosage over a long period of time may be needed to treat recurrent infections (Nyirjesy et al., 1995). Most people tolerate this medication well; however, potentially serious drug interactions that can cause liver toxicity, among other problems, may occur, so it is imperative that women tell their healthcare providers about any other medications they are taking. Fluconazole should not be taken during pregnancy, as its effect on the fetus has not been determined (Cullins et al., 1999).

Boric acid is the treatment of choice for nonalbicans strains of yeast (Nyirjesy et al., 1995) and has been shown to be as effective as oral prescription anti fungal agents (Guaschino, et al., 2001). A 600 mg boric acid capsule placed in the vagina twice daily for two weeks cures about 85 percent of these infections. Unfortunately, there is a high rate of recurrence among these resistant strains, and a course of suppressive therapy over about six months is often necessary. The most common side effect of boric acid therapy is vaginal irritation. Coating the vulva with A and D ointment frequently can ease this side effect. Most pharmacies, with the exception of compounding pharmacies, do not dispense boric acid capsules. Clinicians prescribe empty gelatin capsules, and the patient must fill them with boric acid acquired in any grocery or hardware store.

The availability of over-the-counter preparations for the self-treatment of yeast infections has been a mixed blessing for women. On the one hand, women have quick access to a remedy that offers relief of their symptoms, especially when a healthcare provider is not immediately available. On the other, women may not always diagnose themselves accurately. In one study of the accuracy of women's self-diagnosis, it was found that 58 percent of the self-diagnoses investigated were found to be incorrect (Sinofsky, 1999). Inaccurate self-diagnosis is costly in terms of dollars and can dangerously delay the diagnosis of other diseases, such as chlamydia or gonorrhea (see Chapter 22). Self-treatment before professional evaluation can also make it more difficult for the clinician to make an accurate diagnosis of the problem. Women who are not sure whether their symptoms stem from a yeast infection should apply A and D ointment to the vulva several times a day to soothe the itching until they can see their healthcare providers. Another pitfall of self-treatment is the tendency women have to use the product only until their symptoms are gone, so as to leave several doses in the tube for "the next time." This common practice leads to an incomplete eradication of the yeast and the potential regrowth of a *more resistant strain*.

PREVENTION

Much has been written about the role of predisposing factors in the occurrence of yeast infections and the strategies for preventing recurrent infection. Although there has been little actual research on these subjects, advice from experienced clinicians can be found in the literature (Northrup, 1994). Many women get yeast infections when stressed, possibly because stress can affect the immune system negatively (see Chapter 27). Exercise, proper sleep, and the resolution of stressful situations often helps reduce the frequency of recurrence. Eliminating concentrated sweets and alcohol from the diet may also help prevent infection.

Wearing sweaty or tight clothing can trigger a yeast infection, as can using harsh chemicals, such as perfumed soaps, and harsh materials, such as scratchy toilet paper, on the vulva. Chafing and irritation make the vulva more prone to infection. Routine douching interrupts the normal cleansing mechanism of the vagina and promotes the growth of pathogens. Minimizing the use of antibiotics is crucial. Antibiotics kill off the normal flora of the vagina, which keep pathogens in check. Antibiotics are frequently prescribed for colds and other viral infections for which they are completely ineffective. If antibiotics must be taken, using a course of antiyeast therapy toward the middle of the antibiotic course may help ward off infection. Unfortunately, many women follow all of these guidelines and still suffer from recurrent yeast infections. Unknown factors that promote this troublesome infection remain.

Bacterial Vaginosis

Bacterial vaginosis (BV) is a disruption of the normal ecological makeup of the vagina (Cullins et al., 1999). There is a decrease in the number of healthy, protective bacteria (*lactobacilli*) present and an abundance of several anaerobic bacterial species that are normally found in the gastrointestinal system. It is believed that these bacteria somehow ascend into the normally sterile cervix, uterus, and upper genital tract. The mechanism of this ascent is still under investigation. The reason this disruption occurs is unknown, although it has been studied for decades. BV was initially classified as a sexually transmitted disease because it occurs more frequently among sexually active women, and the organisms that cause the infection can be isolated from the male urethra of infected partners. However, as studies have progressed, it has been demonstrated that not all male partners harbor the bacteria and that the treatment of male partners does not reduce the rate of recurrent infection (Hillier & Holmes, 1995) and 10 to 31 percent of adolescent virgins also acquire the infection.

Bacterial vaginosis is responsible for 40 to 50 percent of vaginal infections in women (Cullins et al., 1999). BV is the most common cause of vaginal symptoms among childbearing women (Hillier & Holmes, 1995), and pelvic inflammatory disease has also been linked to BV. Recently, BV has been implicated in adverse gynecological and obstetrical events (Hillier & Holmes, 1995). Preterm labor, inflammation and infection of the amniotic fluid during pregnancy, and postpartum (after childbirth) uterine infections have all been linked to BV in some women.

SYMPTOMS

A **malodorous** (foul smelling) vaginal discharge is the most common symptom in women with BV (Hillier & Holmes, 1995). The discharge is often described as white or watery, with a "fishy" smell. Symptoms are usually more prevalent after intercourse without a condom and around menses. Vaginal irritation, if present, is mild and occurs in only 15 percent of cases (Cullins et al., 1999). Approximately 47 percent of women have no symptoms (Hillier & Holmes, 1995).

DIAGNOSIS

The diagnosis of BV is made on the basis of symptoms, a physical examination of the vulva and vagina, and a microscopic evaluation of the discharge. Symptoms alone are not enough to make a reliable diagnosis (Hillier & Holmes, 1995). At least *three* of the following signs must also be present in order for the diagnosis of BV to be made: (1) a white, homogenous vaginal discharge; (2) the release of a fishy odor when potassium hydroxide is added to the vaginal secretions; (3) an elevation in vaginal pH; and (4) microscopic evidence that "clue cells" (abnormal cells present in BV) are present. An evaluation for these diagnostic criteria can be done in the clinician's office; vaginal cultures are rarely of benefit.

TREATMENT

Metronidazole and clindamycin are the two antibiotics currently most effective against the multiple bacteria that cause BV (Sweet & Gibbs, 1995). Both come as oral capsules or tablets and intravaginal creams. The most common side effects of oral metronidazole are headache, nausea and vomiting, and a metallic taste in the mouth. A newer formulation of this drug (*Flagyl ER*) and the vaginal preparation cause fewer problems. Patients must abstain from alcohol during and for 48 hours after oral metronidazole therapy, as severe gastrointestinal problems result from concomitant use. The most common side effect of oral clindamycin is diarrhea (Sweet & Gibbs, 1995). A more serious form of diarrhea occurs less commonly and is associated with frequent, bloody stools.

Because of the recently discovered adverse gynecological and obstetrical outcomes of untreated BV, some clinicians recommend treatment of asymptomatic women (Cullins et al., 1999). Many clinicians are screening pregnant women at least once early in their second trimester, especially if they have a history of adverse pregnancy outcome (Center for Disease Control and Prevention, 2000). Whether all asymptomatic women should be treated is currently being studied (Hillier & Holmes, 1995).

Relapse is quite common in BV, but the reasons for this are unknown. Studies have shown that 80 percent of women treated for BV will have a recurrent infection within nine months (Hillier & Holmes, 1995). Long-term cures have been achieved, however, by an initial course of oral metronidazole followed by metronidazole vaginal cream two times weekly for several months. Because sexual activity has been linked to the infection, either abstaining from intercourse or condom use has been suggested as a means of preventing recurrence (Hillier & Holmes, 1995). Attempts to ward off BV by recolonizing the vagina with lactobacilli have not proven successful (Hillier & Holmes, 1995). The lactobacillus strains found in over-the-counter powders, tablets, and foods (even yogurt with live active cultures) do not readily adhere to the vaginal epithelium and fail to colonize the vagina. There is currently an attempt to produce strains of lactobacillus that will effectively colonize the vagina. Until this is available, the use of such **probiotics** (substances that encourage the growth of friendly bacteria) is probably a waste of money. The prevention strategies for BV are the same as for yeast vaginitis.

Toxic Shock Syndrome

Toxic shock syndrome (TSS) is relatively uncommon. TSS has been linked to tampon use, particularly one brand that was removed from the shelves in the 1980s. TSS is caused by a growth of **Staphylococcus aureus** and the toxins released by this bacterium (Berek et al., 1996). The symptoms of TSS are fever; a generalized, red rash with inflammation of the vaginal mucosa; peeling skin on the palms and soles; extremely low blood pressure; and pathology involving at least three organ systems. Hospitalization and treatment with intravenous antibiotics are usually required.

Pelvic Inflammatory Disease

Pelvic inflammatory disease (PID) is an infection of the upper genital tract (uterus, fallopian tubes, ovaries, and peritoneal cavity). It is estimated that 1 million women are treated for pelvic inflammatory disease each year in the United States (Sweet & Gibbs, 1995). The incidence has been increasing slightly over the past decade, probably due to liberalized sexual behavior and a shift away from contraceptive methods that protect from sexually transmitted diseases. PID is the most important infection among reproductive-age women, as it can result in infertility (20 percent), chronic pelvic pain and scarring, which often require surgical intervention (15 to 20 percent) and ectopic pregnancies (a six- to 10-fold increase). **Hepatitis** (liver infection) occurs in 1 to 10 percent of patients. The direct and indirect costs of treating this problem were estimated to be $4.2 billion per year in 1990 and are expected to approach $10 billion in the near future.

Two types of bacteria, *N. gonorrhoeae* or *C. trachomatis,* have been isolated in the cervix of 65 percent of patients with PID (Sweet & Gibbs, 1995). The inflammation and tissue damage caused by the presence of either organism is felt to enable the entrance of a multitude of other bacteria into the pelvis. The role of bacterial vaginosis in PID is still unclear and is currently under investigation. Viruses such as herpes simplex and cytomegalovirus may play an important role in PID as well, but that mechanism has not been extensively studied.

The colonies of microorganisms that inhabit the upper genital tract in PID can cause progressively worsening degrees of permanent pelvic scarring, fallopian tube occlusion, and even liver involvement. If treatment is delayed longer than three days, the likelihood of severe damage to the reproductive organs is high (Sweet & Gibbs, 1995).

There are multiple risk factors for developing PID. Age is an important one. About 70 percent of women with PID are under age 25 (Sweet & Gibbs, 1995), and 33 percent have their first infection before age 19. Low income, unemployment, and low educational level have also been identified as risks. There are also higher rates of PID in the never married but sexually active population; sexual behavior is strongly associated with risk. Higher rates are found in women who have more than one male sexual partner in 30 days, have acquired a new sexual partner within the previous 30 days, have intercourse frequently, or were young when they first had intercourse. Intercourse during the menstrual cycle and frequent douching have also been associated with PID. The presence of an IUD in a woman who is not in a mutually monogamous sexual relationship renders her prone to PID. Conversely, the correct use of barrier contraceptives, such as condoms and diaphragms, and the use of oral contraceptives reduce the risk. Oral contraceptives make the cervical mucus thicker and act as a barrier to the ascent of microorganisms.

SYMPTOMS

The symptoms of PID can range from mild pelvic cramping to severe abdominal pain, fever, unusual vaginal discharge, painful intercourse, and abnormal vaginal bleeding (CDC, 2000). Many women are **asymptomatic** (experience no symptoms), which is why some women found to have scarring and tubal occlusion during surgery have no known history of pelvic infection.

DIAGNOSIS

Because the symptoms of PID can mimic so many other gynecological and gastrointestinal disorders, such as ovarian cysts, ectopic pregnancy, appendicitis, and even constipation, the diagnosis is very difficult and many times delayed (CDC, 2000). The Centers for Disease Control and Prevention (CDC) has developed a list of criteria that must be met before a diagnosis of PID can be considered. The minimum criterion is tenderness of the lower abdomen in the area of the ovaries and of the cervix on upon palpation. The CDC recommends that all young, sexually active women, and others at risk for PID, be treated for PID if this minimum criterion is met. Often, further diagnostic criteria lend support to the diagnosis. These include a fever of 101° F or higher, the presence of an abnormal cervical or vaginal discharge, elevations in erythrocyte sedimentation rate (ESR) and C-reactive protein (two blood tests that can reveal the presence of inflammation in the body), and positive cervical cultures of *N. gonorrhoeae* or *C. trachomatis*. In a few cases, specific findings from endometrial biopsy, pelvic ultrasound, or laparascopic surgery are needed for a definitive diagnosis.

TREATMENT

The CDC (1998) recommends several regimens of antibiotics for both outpatient and in-hospital treatment of PID. For patients who are likely to take their medicines and who have mild cases with no vomiting, outpatient therapy is suitable. However, if there are severe symptoms, or if the patient is unlikely to comply with treatment, hospitalization with intravenous antibiotics and close observation is recommended. Close observation decreases the likelihood that other serious diseases, such as appendicitis, will be missed. Because PID involves multiple bacterial organisms, a combination of antibiotics is needed to eradicate the infection. The most common outpatient therapies consist of a single intramuscular injection of ceftriaxone plus oral doxycycline for 14 days or oflaxacin plus metronidazole orally for 14 days.

PREVENTION

The best strategy for preventing PID is to obviate as many risk factors as possible. Limiting the number of sex partners, avoiding vaginal douching, using barrier contraceptives along with oral contraceptives, and avoiding intercourse during menses is prudent. Women who are not involved in a mutually monogamous relationship should not use the IUD as a method of birth control.

Cervical Polyps

The cervix can develop benign growths, such as polyps, that are quite common. Polyps are soft, moist, red masses that are a few millimeters to several centimeters in diameter (Ryan et al., 1999). They are diagnosed when the cervix is visualized through a speculum. Most of the time, cervical polyps are asymptomatic; however, they can cause spotting between periods and after intercourse, as well as a profuse vaginal discharge. The polyp is usually painlessly removed at its base, with a small forceps, in a healthcare provider's office.

Cervical Cancer

Both the incidence of and death rate from cervical cancer have dramatically decreased in the United States over the past 40 years (Kurman, Henson, Herbst, Noller, & Schiffman, 1994). This can be largely attributed to the identification of precancerous disease via Pap smear screening. Therefore, women who do not undergo routine Pap smear testing are among those at high risk for cervical cancer. However, Pap smears are not perfect, and a few women develop cancer despite compliance to the recommended screening protocols. It has been estimated that annually in the United States, nearly 13,000 women are diagnosed with cervical cancer and almost 5000 die from it (*Patient Collected,* 2000). Worldwide, 360,000 women develop cervical cancer, and 190,000 die from it each year. The incidence of cervical cancer in the United States is two times higher for African American, Hispanic, and Native American women than for Euro-American women (Ryan et al., 1999).

There is overwhelming evidence that infection with the sexually transmitted **human papillomavirus (HPV)** is the cause of the vast majority of cervical cancer (Ryan et al., 1999). More than 80 strains of HPV have been identified; however, some strains are associated with cancer risk and others are not (for a full discussion of HPV, see Chapter 22). Although it is estimated that at least 60 percent of sexually active women under age 35 have been exposed to HPV (Campion, Ferris, di Paola, Reid, & Miller, 1991), only 10 to 50 percent of women who harbor the virus have HPV changes on their cervix. The exact mechanism by which the virus affects the cervix is not known, but smoking, low levels of folate in the diet, and a history of sexually transmitted diseases, especially HIV, are risk factors for the virus's becoming active (Ryan et al., 1999).

Precancerous changes in cervical tissue are classified according to the degree of dysplasia (see Figure 17–8). The

Figure 17–8 The Cervix and Changes in Cervical Tissue

Pap smear

NORMAL
Large, surface-type squamous cells with small pyknotic nuclei

LOW-GRADE DYSPLASIA

HIGH-GRADE DYSPLASIA: CARCINOMA IN SITU

INVASIVE CARCINOMA

Source: Youngkin & Davis. (1998). *Women's health care: A primary care clinical guide* (2nd ed., p. 94). Orginal source: Chandrasoma, P., & Taylor, C. R. *Concise pathology.* Copyright 1991 The McGraw-Hill Companies, Inc.

continuum of abnormality ranges from low-grade squamous intraepithelial neoplastic lesion (LGSIL) to high-grade squamous epithelial neoplastic lesion (HGSIL) to invasive cancer. It is estimated that 2.5 million women have LGSIL reported on their Pap smears in the United States each year (Kurman et al., 1994). This is about 5 percent of all Pap smears collected. Approximately one-third of all LGSIL cases progress to HGSIL, one-third regress to normal spontaneously, and another one-third remain unchanged for years (Campion et al., 1991). It can take as few as nine months for the transformation from LGSIL to HGSIL to occur. If HGSIL is present, the rate of spontaneous regression is low (about 11 percent). The change from HGSIL to cancer takes from 12 months to as long as 20 years. It is not known why most cervical dysplasia does not progress to cancer, even if not treated. There are most likely other cofactors present that facilitate the expression of the virus.

Once the cervical changes associated with HPV resolve (either with treatment or spontaneously), the virus remains, and the woman can transmit it to future sexual partners. Research is ongoing concerning the nature of "latent" HPV infection and whether the body's immune system is able to rid itself of the virus over time and impart immunity to the invading strain. If allowed to progress, cervical cancer gives rise to a progressively larger tumor, which invades the surrounding organs, such as the uterus and vagina, and eventually the pelvis and lymph nodes.

SYMPTOMS

There are no symptoms of cervical cancer. Even early invasive cancer is usually asymptomatic (Ryan et al., 1999). Irregular vaginal bleeding after intercourse or between menses, or a pink, odorous vaginal discharge, can be present. As the disease progresses, pain that is felt down the buttock, thigh, and knee develops.

DIAGNOSIS

The Pap test remains the best screening tool for cervical cancer and its precursors. During an examination of the cervix, a spatula is used to take a scraping of cells from the outer part of the cervix. A brush is then used to collect cells from the inside canal. The cells are placed on a slide, preserved by the clinician, then sent to a laboratory for interpretation by a cytopathologist.

A recent study revealed that Pap smears are 77.7 percent effective in detecting cervical disease (*Patient Collected,* 2000). In 1995 and 1996, the FDA approved new technologies, AutoPap-300 and Thin Prep, to lower the number of cervical cancers missed by the Pap test (Ryan et al., 1999). AutoPap-300 is a second screening by computer of Pap smears taken in the conventional manner. Currently, this technology is used only if the smear has been initially evaluated as normal. The slide is then sent to a lab, where a second reading is done. Patients or clinicians must make special arrangements for this second screening to be done; however, many insurance companies do not cover this cost. Thin Prep is an improved method of cervical cancer screening. With Thin Prep, the cells collected from the cervix are placed in a vial of liquid instead of directly on a slide. The vial is then sent to a laboratory, where a slide of cervical cells that enables a slightly more accurate reading is created. There is currently no computerized method of reading Pap smears collected with the Thin Prep system. The specimens are still manually screened by cytopathologists specially trained in their interpretation.

If a Pap smear report is abnormal, the next step in the diagnostic workup is **colposcopy** (Ryan et al., 1999) to take a more detailed look at the cervix and to ensure that cancer is not present. This procedure involves washing the cervix with vinegar and examining it with a magnifying instrument called a colposcope. The vinegar causes abnormal areas of the cervix to become more obvious. The clinician then takes tissue biopsies from the abnormal-looking areas and sends them to a laboratory for a definitive diagnosis.

TREATMENT

The treatment of LGSIL is not always necessary (Campion et al., 1991). If a woman is young, is a nonsmoker, and is able to have more frequent Pap smear surveillance, she is a good candidate for management by observation only. After three consecutive normal Pap smears, taken at four- to six-month intervals, have been obtained, she can return to an annual screening schedule. If, however, there are several risk factors present, if the Pap smear progresses to HGSIL, or if the Pap smear doesn't regress after one or two years, colposcopy should be repeated and treatment provided.

If certain criteria are met, cryotherapy is the simplest and safest treatment for LGSIL and HGSIL (Ryan et al., 1999). **Cryotherapy** is usually done in an office setting and involves freezing abnormal tissue in order to destroy it. Freezing gas is applied to the cervix, which regrows normal tissue as it heals. Cramping is the main discomfort women experience during the procedure, which is done in the office. A copious, malodorous, watery discharge is present for two to three weeks after the procedure. Cryotherapy provides a cure rate of about 85 percent.

When LGSIL or HGSIL extends into the cervical canal, other treatments that remove a core of tissue from the cervix are indicated. **Loop excision (LEEP)** is done under a local anesthetic in an office or outpatient setting. In LEEP, an electrified loop is used to burn a core of tissue from the cervix. When more advanced neoplasia (presence of abnormal cells) is present, **laser conization** is performed. A laser is used to cut away a larger amount of cervical tissue than is possible with LEEP.

If invasive cancer is present, a hysterectomy with the removal of all reproductive organs and affected lymph nodes is usually needed (Ryan et al., 1999). Depending on the extent of invasion, chemotherapy and radiation may also be used.

PREVENTION

The prevention of cervical cancer is aimed at reducing sexual behaviors that increase exposure to HPV and at increasing immune functioning. Delaying sexual activity until marriage, having only one lifetime sexual partner, and choosing a partner that has had no other sexual partners greatly reduces the risk for cervical cancer and its precursors. The sexual behavioral patterns common in our culture, however, mean that most women are at significant risk. Stopping smoking and taking a vitamin supplement that contains folate (especially if on oral contraceptives) may reduce the risk by boosting immune resistance to the HPV virus. Limiting the number of future sexual partners reduces risk by limiting potential exposure to the virus. Annual Pap screening with the appropriate follow-up for abnormal findings is the best way to catch the disease well before it turns into cancer. A vaccine against HPV is currently being developed (Human Papilloma Vaccines, 2000). When one will be available is unknown.

Uterine Fibroids

Fibroid tumors, also known as **myomas** and **leiomyomas** are the most common benign neoplasms (abnormal growths) that occur in women of reproductive age (Ryan et al., 1999). They are detected during a vaginal examination in 20 to 25 percent of this group of women. However, it has been estimated that **subclinical** (asymptomatic and undetected on examination) fibroids are present in approximately 80 percent of women. Women of color and those who are overweight have a greater incidence (Ryan et al., 1999). Reduced rates of fibroids are seen in women who have given birth, who smoke, and who take birth control pills.

Fibroids are solid tumors that originate from the smooth muscle of the uterus (Ryan et al., 1999). Their cause is unknown, but it is believed they grow under the influence of estrogen. They can be located inside the uterine cavity (submucosal), in the muscle wall itself (intramural), toward the outside wall (subserosal), or on a narrow stalk from the outside of the uterus (pedunculated). They range in size from a few millimeters in diameter to several centimeters. Giant fibroid tumors that take up the entire pelvic cavity can develop. Growth can occur slowly or rapidly at any time during the reproductive life span. Although many fibroids are not problematic, large ones can obstruct the ureters. Pedunculated fibroids can twist at their stalk and cause pain, resulting from a lack of blood supply to the tissue. If located in the uterine cavity, fibroids can interfere with conception (Berek et al., 1996). Fibroids typically grow during pregnancy and can become so large as to complicate the outcome. However, most women who have fibroids accomplish a healthy pregnancy and delivery, and their tumors generally shrink to their prepregnancy size after delivery. Fibroid-related complications are rare overall, and fibroids generally shrink or disappear after menopause.

SYMPTOMS

Approximately 20 to 25 percent of women with fibroids have symptoms (Ryan et al., 1999). The most common symptom of a submucosal fibroid is heavy, prolonged, or frequent vaginal bleeding. Bleeding can be so heavy as to prohibit activities away from home—forcing women to plan their lives around their periods. Severe anemia can also result. Fibroids can put pressure on the bladder or colon and cause problems with frequent urination, pelvic pressure, or constipation.

DIAGNOSIS

The diagnosis can often be made during a pelvic examination (Ryan et al., 1999). The clinician can feel the enlarged, irregular contour of larger fibroids. Pelvic ultrasound may be required to detect small fibroids or those in the submucosal location.

TREATMENT

There are various surgical and medical treatment options for women experiencing symptoms related to their fibroids (asymptomatic women do not need their fibroids treated). A hysterectomy is considered definitive surgery (Ryan et al., 1999). If bleeding is the main symptom, and surgery is not desired, oral contraceptives or Depo-Provera sometimes offers long-term control of heavy, irregular bleeding (Ryan et al., 1999). This can avoid invasive surgery and the often emotional difficulties women have in undergoing a hysterectomy. Other nonsurgical approaches—such as natural micronized progesterone or herbs—have been used by providers who favor alternative solutions (DeMarco, 1995). No clinical trials of their effectiveness have been conducted thus far.

If the fibroid tumor or tumors are causing problems other than or in addition to bleeding, and the woman wants to continue bearing children, then a **myomectomy,** the surgical removal of the fibroid, can be done. When surgery, whether hysterectomy or myomectomy, has been decided on, GnRH agonists, which induce a reversible menopausal state, are often given temporarily to make bleeding stop and to cause the fibroids to shrink for easier removal. A rapid regrowth of the fibroids ensues if GnRH therapy is discontinued before surgery.

There is controversy as to whether myomectomy is a worthwhile treatment for problematic fibroids in women who do not desire more children. Many, if not most, gynecologists recommend hysterectomy over myomectomy. They maintain that the myomectomy procedure incurs more blood loss, pain, and postoperative complications than hysterectomy and that fibroids return after the procedure in 25 to 51 percent of cases (Vedantham et al., 1999). This perception is not, however, universally supported. Hufnagel (1989) argues that, whereas some fibroid tumors are indeed very difficult to remove, many are not and that many women lose their uterus unnecessarily. She argues further that new fibroids develop in only 30 percent of cases on average and are not always bothersome. **Uterine artery ablation,** a nonsurgical procedure that is now being used to destroy fibroid tumors by depriving them of their blood supply, may render this debate irrelevant. Uterine artery ablation is performed by radiologists (physicians trained in the use of radiation in diagnosis and treatment) who use imaging techniques to facilitate the procedure. The artery that feeds the fibroid is entered with a catheter, and various gelatinous substances are introduced into the artery to occlude blood flow. Ablation procedures are done under heavy sedation and take about 75 minutes. Eighty-five to 95 percent of women have reduced symptoms, and a 39 to 69 percent reduction in fibroid size is seen. However, the long-term results of this procedure are still being studied (Vedantham et al., 1999).

On average, well over a half-million hysterectomies are performed annually in the United States. Statistics indicate that one out of every three women age 60 and one out of every two women age 65 has had a hysterectomy (*Hysterectomy,* 2000). Although it has declined slightly in recent years, the rate at which hysterectomy is performed in this country is still more than twice that of any European country (*Hysterectomy and Its Alternatives,* 1998). Moreover, although about 74 percent of all hysterectomies are performed on relatively young women between the ages of 30 and 54, only about 20 percent are done to treat either life-threatening illnesses, such as uterine or cervical cancer, or intolerable conditions, such as severe uterine prolapse (*Hysterectomy,* 2000). The rest are related to the presence of fibroid tumors, heavy bleeding, endometriosis, or unexplained pelvic pain (*Hysterectomy Surveillance, 1980–1993*). It has been argued that the number of hysterectomies performed in this country is excessive, that hysterectomy is carried out when less drastic measures would suffice, and that relatively radical versions of the operation are too often performed without regard to the overall implications for women's health and well-being (Hufnagel, 1989). Conversely, it has also been argued that, because of its physiology, the uterus is vulnerable to many problems and that U.S. women are fortunate to have ready access to an operation that relieves them of much pain, inconvenience, and worry (Angier, 1999).

The critics of hysterectomy have cited multiple factors for its ubiquity in this culture, including its lucrative appeal for physicians (Hufnagel, 1989), U.S. women's relatively greater propensity for seeking gynecological care (Angier, 1999), and the persistent societal view of women's reproductive organs as inherently pathological (see Chapter 1). Christianne Northrup, a gynecologist, reports that, in the course of her training, she was taught to view the uterus and the other female reproductive organs primarily as sources of potential trouble that are entirely superfluous once childbearing is no longer desired or an option (Northrup, 1994). Indeed, about 50 percent of women who undergo the removal of a problematic uterus are relieved of perfectly healthy *ovaries* at the same time, as a strategy for preventing ovarian cancer (*Hysterectomy and Its Alternatives,* 1998). This practice is condemned by its many critics as analogous to *castrating men* solely for the purpose of preventing testicular cancer. Another practice recently called into question is the routine removal of the cervix, along with the body of the uterus, in order to prevent cervical cancer. The cervix provides support for the bladder and vagina and contains nerves that contribute to the enjoyment of sexual intercourse (*Hysterectomy,* 2000).

The existing literature suggests that hysterectomy can affect women's cardiovascular, sexual, and mental health. What effect a hysterectomy will have on a given woman is not entirely predictable, however, and the effect of hysterectomy on the quality of women's lives overall is not yet clear.

Hysterectomy—whether **subtotal** (in which the body of the uterus only is removed; the cervix and ovaries remain), **total** (the uterus and cervix are removed) or **pan** (the entire uterus, ovaries, and fallopian tubes are removed)—is known to have an adverse effect on women's cardiovascular health. Even women who are treated postsurgically with estrogen have three times the risk of developing cardiovascular disease as women of similar age who still have their uterus and ovaries (Rako, 1998). The reasons for this are not completely understood but are likely related to hormone levels. The uterus produces a hormone called **prostacyclin,** which inhibits blood clotting and may be a factor in younger women's relative immunity to heart attack (see Chapter 12). Both the uterine endothelium and the ovaries produce a natural form of estrogen that is protective against coronary artery disease (CAD). The artificial hormones typically given to women whose uterus and ovaries have been removed seem not to confer the same protection (see Chapter 24) and may even increase the risk for CAD (*Hormone Therapy and Women's Hearts,* 2000). The ovaries also produce over 50 percent of the testosterone in women's bodies, and testosterone may also have important physiological implications for the female cardiovascular system. Testosterone in men has been demonstrated to have beneficial effects on fibrinolysis, blood vessel endothelium, insulin metabolism, and coronary artery circulation (Rako, 1998). Women whose ovaries are not removed are not necessarily spared ovarian dysfunction; the ovaries sometimes lose much of their blood supply due to the surgical disruption of the blood vessels (Rako, 1998). More research on the effects of the various hormones produced in women's reproductive organs is needed.

Hufnagel (1989) has suggested that, because the precise stimuli that produce sexual pleasure and orgasm vary from woman to woman, hysterectomy interferes with sexual gratification in some women. For example, women whose orgasms are enhanced by pressure on the cervix may find that their orgasms are not as intense after surgery. Nevertheless, based on their review of the literature on the subject Farrel and Kieser (2000) concluded that hysterectomy is more likely to have a *positive* impact on women's sexual functioning. They caution, however, that many studies lacked methodological soundness in that they did not control for confounding variables. Helstrom (1994) questioned women about the quality of their sex lives before and after ovary-sparing hysterectomy and found that the most important predictor of the nature of postoperative sexual functioning was preoperative activity and enjoyment. Other determining factors were partner sexual functioning, socioeconomic support from the partner, adaptation to the consequences of hysterectomy (such as sterility), mental status, physical ability, and hormonal status.

Other hysterectomy-related outcomes have also been investigated. In their study of 285 Mexican women who had had total hysterectomies and a similar number who had not, Carranza-Lira, Murillo-Uribe, Martinez-Trejo, and Santos-Gonzales (1997) found that hysterectomy conferred no deleterious effects on lipid levels or bone density but was associated with a frequent incidence of depression. None of the women in the study were on hormone replacement therapy. Farrel and Kieser (2000), however, concluded that hysterectomy tended to *improve* overall well-being, including mood.

Uterine Polyps

Uterine polyps are benign overgrowths of tissue found in the uterine lining. They are present in about 10 to 24 percent of women being evaluated for abnormal bleeding (Ryan et al., 1999). They cannot be detected on physical examination. A surgical procedure called **hysteroscopy** can be done to diagnose and treat polyps. The cervix is dilated, and a lighted tube with a lens is inserted into the uterus, enabling the surgeon to see the lining of the uterus. The polyp can be removed at that time. The procedure is usually accompanied by dilatation and curettage (D&C). Although polyps rarely contain cancer, the tissue is sent for pathological examination. More recently, a type of pelvic ultrasound, called **sonohysteroscopy,** has become available for a nonsurgical diagnosis. A catheter is passed through the cervix into the uterus, and fluid is instilled into the uterine cavity. The fluid in the uterus enables the polyp to be seen clearly on ultrasound.

Uterine Cancer

Uterine cancer is the most common gynecological cancer (Ryan et al., 1999). It is twice as common as ovarian cancer and occurs three times more often than invasive cervical cancer. (Breast cancer is not included in the gynecological cancer category.) Uterine cancer mostly affects women in their perimenopausal and postmenopausal years. The risk factors include obesity, a diet high in fat, a history of infertility, early menarche, a late onset of menopause, the absence of childbearing, hypertension, and diabetes. Women who take estrogen without also taking progesterone after menopause have a slightly increased risk. The antibreast cancer medication tamoxifen has been associated with a slightly increased risk of uterine cancer as well. There is a rare form of uterine cancer that is hereditary and not associated with the above risk factors. Those who have taken oral contraceptives are at reduced risk.

Uterine cancer usually begins as a precancerous condition of the **endometrium** (lining of the uterus) called hyperplasia (Ryan et al., 1999). (For a full discussion of endometrial hyperplasia, see the section on dysfunctional uterine bleeding). If left untreated over time, hyperplasia can convert to uterine cancer. The cancer grows from the uterine lining and continues to extend through the uterine wall and finally to the surrounding organs and lymph nodes.

SYMPTOMS

Over 80 percent of women with uterine cancer have abnormal vaginal bleeding (Ryan et al., 1999). Any bleeding, even spotting, in a postmenopausal woman needs prompt medical attention.

DIAGNOSIS

The diagnosis of uterine cancer is made after an analysis of tissue obtained from the endometrium, either via an endometrial biopsy (see section on dysfunctional uterine bleeding) or D & C (see section on uterine polyps). Pelvic ultrasound can provide more information about the status of the uterine lining.

TREATMENT

Radical hysterectomy, with the removal of involved pelvic lymph nodes, is necessary (Ryan et al., 1999). In radical hysterectomy, the uterus, fallopian tubes, and ovaries are removed. If lymph node involvement is present and/or the cancer is advanced, radiation may be given. Because abnormal bleeding is present in the early stage of cancer and prompts the woman and clinician to initiate testing, a diagnosis is generally made at a stage that has a good prognosis for cure. Overall, 72 percent of women with early stage cancer survive five or more years after diagnosis. If the cancer does recur, it usually does so within three years of diagnosis and is usually located in the vagina. Distant metastasis to such organs as the lungs, liver, and abdomen signals a grim prognosis.

PREVENTION

Maintaining a lifestyle that includes exercise, low-fat eating, and the maintenance of an ideal body weight discourages the hyperestrogenic states that increase the risk that endometrial hyperplasia will develop. Oral contraceptives or progesterone given for 10 to 14 days a month to facilitate the regular shedding of the uterine lining is also protective.

Benign Ovarian Cysts and Tumors

An ovarian **cyst** is a fluid-filled sac that forms on the ovary. A **tumor** is a solid mass. There are two kinds of ovarian cysts: follicular cysts and luteal cysts. A **follicular cyst** forms when the follicle doesn't release the egg in the right way and continues to grow, forming a cyst (Northrup, 1994). A **luteal cyst** results when bleeding from the ovulation site enters the capsule of the ovary, and sometimes the pelvis itself. Ovarian cysts are the most common benign condition of the ovary (Berek et al., 1996).

Dermoid cysts are really ovarian *tumors* that contain a variety of elements; fat, hair, and even teeth can be found in them. They occur when cells of the ovary that are not associated with ovulation begin reproducing. One-third of women under the age of 30 who undergo surgery for a pelvic mass are found to have a dermoid cyst (Berek et al., 1996). Approximately 2 percent of all dermoid cysts undergo malignant transformation; this is more likely to occur in women over 40 (Northrup, 1994).

SYMPTOMS

Many small ovarian cysts and tumors produce no symptoms. If they become large enough, however, they can cause pelvic pain or discomfort due to pressure on nerves and other organs. Cysts can also rupture, causing the sudden onset of severe, sharp pain. Approximately 15 percent of dermoid cysts cause **torsion,** which means that the fallopian tube twists on itself, compressing the blood vessels that feed it and the ovary (Berek et al., 1996). This causes severe pain and threatens the life of the ovary.

DIAGNOSIS

The presence of cysts and tumors is established through a pelvic or ultrasound examination.

TREATMENT

Usually, cysts resolve on their own after four to eight weeks and need no intervention (Berek et al., 1996). Those that persist may require surgical removal. Oral contraceptives can help prevent the formation of cysts, but the dose of hormone in today's low-dose formulations is not high enough to make existing cysts regress (Northrup, 1994). The surgical removal of dermoid cysts is strongly recommended; the ovary can usually be spared.

Ovarian Cancer

Approximately 25,000 cases of ovarian cancer are diagnosed each year in the United States, and 14,000 women die of the disease (DePriest & Nagell, 1997). Ovarian cancer is the fourth leading cause of cancer death among women in the United States. The strongest risk factor for ovarian cancer is maternal and paternal family history (Ryan et al., 1999). If a woman has two first-degree relatives (such as a sister and mother) with the disease, she has a 50 percent chance of developing it herself. Inheriting the BRCA1 or BRCA2 gene, discovered in 1990 and associated with breast cancer, also confers an increased risk of ovarian cancer. Having been exposed to asbestos and talc, pelvic irradiation, and mumps has also been linked to increased risk. Whether taking infertility drugs heightens risk is controversial and still under investigation. *Reduced* rates of ovarian cancer are found among women who have had one or more term pregnancies, have breast-fed, have used oral contraceptives, and have undergone tubal sterilization or removal of the uterus.

The exact mechanism responsible for the development of ovarian cancer is not known. The presence of either of the BRCA genes plays a major role. There are many types of ovarian cancer, and they are classified according to the type of tissue within the ovary that is affected (Ryan et al., 1999). Unlike uterine, cervical, and even breast cancer, ovarian cancer produces no readily detectable precancerous changes in the ovary. Therefore, by the time ovarian cancer is diagnosed, it has usually progressed to an advanced stage with a poor prognosis.

SYMPTOMS

The symptoms of early stage ovarian cancer are subtle and vague, and they mimic several other medical conditions. For example, abdominal swelling, fatigue, and abdominal pain, all symptoms of ovarian cancer (Ryan et al., 1999), can be caused by problems in other organs, too. The establishment of the true diagnosis may be delayed while clinicians search for thyroid or gastrointestinal abnormalities. As the tumor grows and applies pressure on surrounding pelvic organs, there can be constipation and urinary frequency. A sudden onset of pelvic pain can occur if the tumor ruptures or undergoes torsion. Nausea, indigestion, weight loss, anorexia, irregular vaginal bleeding, and shortness of breath can also be symptoms.

DIAGNOSIS

Ovarian cancer is often discovered during a routine pelvic examination; the clinician feels an enlargement in the area of the ovary. This mass must then be differentiated from other structures in the pelvis, such as stool-filled bowel, other ovarian or tubal masses, and uterine fibroids. Ultrasound is done to further assess the mass (Ryan et al., 1999). If it has benign characteristics on an ultrasound, the mass is monitored after a few menstrual cycles. An MRI of the pelvis may be of benefit if the mass looks suspicious. A blood test for the ovarian cancer tumor marker, CA-125, can also be done. Unfortunately, obtaining a CA-125 level is *not* a suitable way of carrying out mass screening for ovarian cancer. CA-125 is useful only if the person has a high risk for cancer or if the tumor has suspicious characteristics on imaging, because benign conditions, such as endometriosis, can cause a false positive result. Also, certain types of ovarian cancer do not give elevations of CA-125, and a false negative result occurs. Moreover, CA-125 is elevated in only about 50 percent of cases of early stage ovarian cancer. If ultrasound and blood tests are inconclusive, surgery in the form of laparoscopy is done to remove the mass and to obtain tissue for laboratory analysis.

There are no good screening tests for the detection of early ovarian cancer. Even pelvic ultrasound has limited value, as there is a high rate of false positive scans. The result of this is that many women undergo surgery for ovarian conditions that turn out to be benign (DePreist & Nagell, 1997). However, when used together for high-risk women, the combination of CA-125 screening and pelvic ultrasound annually can increase the odds of detecting ovarian cancer at an earlier, more curable stage. Currently, most insurance companies do not cover the cost of such screening. Therefore, women from high-risk families are encouraged to enroll in ongoing clinical trials in which free screening is offered. Researchers at the University of Texas have developed a **tumor index** (set of criteria) to assist clinicians in determining if an ovarian mass is cancerous or not (*Tumor Index,* 1999). Clinical trials are being conducted to determine its efficacy. If it proves effective, the index may spare women unnecessary surgery and also enhance the utility of pelvic ultrasound.

TREATMENT

A radical hysterectomy (removal of the uterus, cervix, ovaries, fallopian tubes, part of the vagina, and affected lymph nodes), chemotherapy, and radiation are usually necessary to treat ovarian cancer.

PREVENTION

Conditions that suppress ovulation have been shown to reduce ovarian cancer risk. As women do not ovulate while pregnant or nursing, bearing children and then breastfeeding full-time for several months decrease risk. Suppressing ovulation by using oral contraceptives or Depo-Provera also significantly reduces risk. Because talc (powdered rock) is a possible carcinogen, women should not dust their upper thighs and perineum with talc-based powder; cornstarch-based powders are considered to be safe (Whysner & Mohan, 2000).

Bartholin's Duct Cysts

The **Bartholin's ducts** are two small channels by which the mucus produced by **Bartholin's glands,** which are located near the bottom of the vaginal opening, reaches the external surface of the vulva. The mucus-filled cysts that form when Bartholin's ducts are blocked account for the majority of the symptomatic cysts of the vulva (Wilkinson & Stone, 1995). Cysts can vary in size from one to several centimeters. Bartholin's gland can become infected. When this occurs, *N. gonorrhoeae* is often the pathogen.

SYMPTOMS

Small, uninfected Bartholin's cysts may produce no symptoms or merely a mild sensation of pressure at the vaginal opening. Infected cysts, on the other hand, are quite painful and can cause fever and sometimes systemic infection.

DIAGNOSIS

The diagnosis of a Bartholin's duct cyst is made through the visualization of the bulging cyst at the vaginal orifice where the Bartholin's gland is located.

TREATMENT

Treating asymptomatic, uninfected cysts is not necessary (Wilkinson & Stone, 1995). Symptomatic cysts are **incised** (surgically opened) and drained in the clinician's office. Antibiotics are prescribed if infection is present. If the cyst is large enough, a catheter is inserted into it to allow optimal drainage. A minor surgical procedure called **marsupialization** is done if the cyst is recurrent and not infected; the cyst is incised and drained, and sutures are placed to form an opening which allows the gland to drain properly (Lichtman & Papera, 1990). Marsupialization is usually done as outpatient surgery with light general anesthesia or heavy sedation.

Lichens Sclerosus

In lichens sclerosus, the vulvar skin becomes white, pale, or thickened, with a parchmentlike appearance. The **labia minora** (the small lips of the vulva) eventually become fused with the **labia majora** (the large, hair-bearing lips of the vulva), and the **clitoris** (the structure primarily responsible for orgasm) becomes fused to the tissue covering it, the clitoral hood. As the disease progresses, it can cause a narrowing of the **introitus** (the vaginal opening). The incidence of lichens sclerosus is unknown, but it is the most common vulvar disease seen in vulvar dermatology clinics (Wilkinson & Stone, 1995). It is more common in postmenopausal women but can occur at any age, beginning at infancy (Elchalal et al., 1995). Some estimate that 4 to 6 percent of patients with lichens sclerosus develop vulvar cancer (Elchalal et al., 1995). Whether the condition itself increases the risk of cancer or if the two conditions occur independently of each other is debatable. The cause of lichens sclerosus is unknown.

SYMPTOMS

Severe itching is the major symptom of lichens sclerosus (Wilkinson & Stone, 1995). If the disease is allowed to progress, intercourse may become painful or impossible, and bleeding may occur with bowel movements as splitting of the perineal skin occurs.

DIAGNOSIS

The diagnosis can be made by clinical examination alone. If there is a question of the cause of the symptoms, a vulvar biopsy can confirm the diagnosis (Wilkinson & Stone, 1995).

TREATMENT

There is no cure for lichens sclerosus. It can be well managed, however, and the progression of the disease can be stopped before major scarring of the vulva occurs. A potent topical steroid cream or ointment is applied. In the rare instances in which steroids applied topically do not work, liquid steroid preparations are injected into the skin of the vulva. Because lichens sclerosus is a *chronic* condition, lifelong treatment is generally necessary. As in the case of yeast vaginitis, the use of perfumed soaps and laundry detergents is to be avoided, as is the wearing of sweaty, wet, or tight-fitting clothing.

Vulvar Intraepithelial Neoplasia

The term vulvar intraepithelial neoplasia *(VIN)* refers to the growth of abnormal tissue within the skin of the vulva. One form of VIN is associated with certain strains of the sexually transmitted human papillomavirus (HPV) (see Chapter 22 for a discussion of HPV). The cause of VIN *not* related to HPV is less well understood. VIN is considered a premalignant condition in that it often evolves into invasive cancer if left untreated. Fortunately, the occurrence of actual invasive cancer of the vulva is low. It occurs most commonly in elderly women. The incidence of pre-invasive malignant lesions, however, is rising in younger women (Wilkinson & Stone, 1995). This is most likely due to the epidemic of HPV in the United States among the younger population. VIN is classified according to the degree of dysplasia present. VIN 1 and 2 are considered premalignant stages of the disease, whereas VIN 3 is considered **carcinoma in situ,** cancer that has not yet become invasive.

SYMPTOMS AND DIAGNOSIS

If symptoms of VIN are present, they are most likely to consist of itching and pain during intercourse, which manifest on penetration. (There are many more common reasons for painful intercourse; see Chapter 22.) There may also be red, brown, or white patches present on the vulvar skin. Clinicians can check for the presence of abnormal tissue by applying vinegar to the vulva. Vinegar will make **dysplastic** (abnormal) tissue turn white. Colposcopy can also be done in order to determine the cause of suspicious symptoms.

TREATMENT

Treatment consists of the surgical removal of the involved tissue. If the problem is localized to a few small areas, the diseased tissue can be removed in the office. If larger or multiple areas are involved, the surgery must be done in the operating room. The prognosis is good in VIN, but recurrent disease can be a problem, especially for women who smoke. Therefore, smoking cessation and regular gynecological checkups are crucial for the prevention and early detection of recurrent VIN.

Benign and Malignant Conditions of the Breast

Benign conditions of the breast include mastalgia, nipple discharge, and benign breast tumors. Breast cancer is the major and much feared malignancy.

BENIGN CONDITIONS

Mastalgia Mastalgia, or breast pain, can be either cyclic or continuous. **Cyclic breast pain** afflicts most women at some point during their reproductive lives. It often has its onset at the midpoint of the menstrual cycle and usually ends during the menses (O'Grady, Lindfors, Howell, & Rippon, 1995). Women with **fibrocystic breasts** frequently experience cyclic pain. Fibrocystic breast tissue contains multiple fluid-filled sacs and is part of a woman's normal breast anatomy. Fibrocystic breast tissue does *not* confer an increased risk of cancer. On breast examination, the sacs feel like tiny pebbles or lumpy oatmeal under the skin. One or both breasts may be involved, and any part of the breast, including the areola and even the nipple, can become tender. The pain can be stinging or consist of a dull, aching fullness. The pain is related to hormone level shifts during the menstrual cycle. Women in perimenopause who have more erratic hormonal shifts (see Chapter 22) can experience a worsening of their breast pain or develop it for the first time.

The treatment of cyclic mastalgia requires a combination of approaches. Reducing the amount of caffeine in the diet helps many women. This means avoiding caffeinated soft drinks, chocolate, and drugs containing caffeine (Northrup, 1994). Taking 400 to 600 units of vitamin E daily, or 500 mg of evening primrose oil four times daily, is also an effective strategy. Wearing a supportive bra to prevent undue strain on the ligaments of the breasts is important (O'Grady et al., 1995). If none of these measures works, hormonal manipulation with oral contraceptives, testosterone, or GnRH agonists can be used.

Noncyclic breast pain can result from recent or past trauma, breast cysts, infection, or pain originating from the chest wall muscles, ribs, lungs, and, rarely, the heart. Tumors are infrequently a cause of breast pain; however, a mammogram is warranted to exclude this possibility if the woman is over 30 years of age. A supportive bra and over-the-counter anti-inflammatory agents, such as ibuprofen, can reduce pain and inflammation.

Nipple Discharge Nipple discharge is the third most common breast problem for which women seek breast evaluation (O'Grady et al., 1995). Fluid can be expressed from the nipples of 50 to 60 percent of Euro-American and African American women and 40 percent of Asian American women.

Most experts in the field of breast disease agree that a clear discharge that occurs *only when the breast is squeezed or manipulated* is rarely a sign of disease. However, unless the woman is lactating, nipple discharge that occurs spontaneously needs to be evaluated by a healthcare provider. Bilateral, milky fluid emitted from nonlactating breasts can indicate the presence of a tumor (usually benign) in the pituitary gland of the brain. Discharge that is clear to yellow, green, brown, black, or bloody can be caused by breast cysts or other benign or malignant conditions. Malignancy, however, is found in only 10 to 15 percent of the women experiencing bloody or **serous** (consisting of serum—the yellowish, liquid component of blood) discharge.

Benign Breast Tumors Few health-related occurrences frighten a woman more than finding a mass in her breast. There are a number of types of benign breast masses, including cysts and solid tumors.

Breast cysts occur when tiny sacs, called **alveoli,** in the breast fill up with fluid (see the section on nastalgia) (O'Grady et al., 1995). Breast tissue is influenced by the menstrual hormones estrogen and progesterone. When the levels of these hormones peak at midcycle, fluid and other cellular debris enter the alveoli. During menses, hormone levels fall and the contents of the alveoli drain. If the alveoli are not able to drain properly, they become more and more distended as each menstrual cycle occurs. Several tiny alveoli can enlarge and coalesce into one large cyst. Some breast cysts are too deep or small to be felt and are detectable only by mammography. Others can be readily felt as smooth, spongy, mobile round lumps that are generally tender. A breast mass that has these characteristics can be re-examined after the next menstrual cycle to see if it shrinks or disappears. If the mass persists, ultrasound is the definitive diagnostic tool, along with mammography if the woman is over 30. If the presence of a fluid-filled cyst is confirmed by ultrasound, no intervention is required unless the cyst is painful. Many times, cysts resolve spontaneously after several menstrual cycles. If the cyst is causing discomfort, it can be aspirated using a needle and syringe. Aspirated cysts often come back, and occasionally the surgical excision of the cyst capsule is required. (For information about prevention, see content under mastalgia.)

Fibroadenomas are benign solid tumors frequently found in the breasts of women who are in their teens and twenties (O'Grady et al., 1995). These tumors are smooth, oval, firm, and mobile and rarely become malignant. Removal is not necessary, but they can grow quite large and become disfiguring, especially during pregnancy. Other types of benign lumps that can be found in women's breasts include **hematomas** (collections of semiclotted blood) from a past trauma, fatty tumors, and scar tissue from previous breast surgery.

If a mass is discovered on examination or found with mammography, ultrasound is helpful in determining whether the lump is solid or cystic (fluid-filled). If it is solid or the characteristic is indeterminate, a tissue biopsy is needed to exclude the possibility of cancer (O'Grady et al., 1995). There are several ways to obtain a tissue biopsy. A **fine needle aspiration** is done with a small needle inserted through the skin and into the tumor. Cells and minute bits of tissue are removed. The limitation of this procedure is that many times too few cells are obtained to enable a diagnosis. **Core needle biopsy** uses a larger bore needle, which harvests a core of actual tumor tissue. If the tumor is large and/or fairly superficial (close to the surface of the breast), the needle can be guided into the tumor via ultrasound. If the mass cannot be felt or is small and deep, a **stereotactic core needle biopsy** can be done with imaging equipment. Women who have core needle biopsies with benign results must continue to have follow-up. Only part of the mass has been sampled, and regular examinations are necessary to ensure that the remaining tumor doesn't change. An **excisional biopsy** involves surgical removal of the entire mass. Although this is the most accurate way to biopsy a mass, it leaves a scar and can cause a permanent change in breast contour. In premenopausal women, breast lumps are cancerous in only 1 out of 12 instances. In postmenopausal women, however, 50 percent of lumps found are cancerous (Goldman, 1994).

BREAST CANCER

Although commonly perceived as a result of rapid, disorganized cell growth, clinically significant cancer is actually the end product of a logical, orderly process in which certain cells acquire abilities that render them a danger to the organism in which they arise. Cancer begins when carcinogens enter a cell's nucleus and bind with its DNA. The modified DNA is then replicated and passed to new, "daughter" cells, which divide and multiply more rapidly than other cells of their type. The DNA of these altered cells undergoes still further alteration when it, too, comes into contact with a carcinogen. Eventually, succeeding generations of altered cells develop the ability to invade and change other cells (Marieb, 1989). A proliferating mass of potentially invasive new cells is formed, which, if not detected and eradicated early, can **metastasize** (migrate) to other parts of the body via the blood or lymphatic fluid.

There are few diseases that are more frightening to women than breast cancer. Although breast cancer is a serious and fairly prevalent disease, many women overestimate its incidence and consequences. The oft-cited statistic that "one-in-eight" women will get breast cancer is often interpreted as meaning that one of every eight women has breast cancer right now, or that one in eight women will die of it. What the one-in-eight statistic actually refers to is a woman's lifetime risk *if* she lives to be 85 years old—which only half of all women do (*Breast Cancer,* 1999). Although breast cancer is indeed the *most commonly occurring cancer* among women, it is not the *most lethal;* more women died of lung than breast cancer in 1999. Moreover, cardiovascular disease kills nearly 10 times more North American women than breast cancer (*Breast Cancer,* 1999). Moreover, the threat posed to women by breast cancer is not increasing, as is, for instance, the threat posed by AIDS. The incidence of breast cancer is quite stable (*Breast Cancer,* 1999), and the death rates from breast cancer have been decreasing since 1990 for the Euro-American populations in the United States, United Kingdom, and Canada (*Global Progress,* 1999). However, mortality among African-American women has remained constant, and it is postulated that African-American women do not have the access to healthcare that their white counterparts do (Beaulieu, 2000).

The incidence of breast cancer and the risk of developing it increase incrementally with a woman's age (Ryan et al., 1999). Among women age 30, only about 1 of every 5,900 has the disease; among women age 70, however, 1 in every 330 has it. Seventy-five to 80 percent of breast cancers occur in women over 50 years of age. Women over age 55 tend to develop less aggressive breast cancer tumors than younger patients do. Thus, older women have a more favorable prognosis than younger women, especially if their tumors are found before they reach 2 cm in diameter and before the lymph nodes become involved (Diab, Elledge, & Clark, 2000).

Women with a strong family history of the disease are at relatively greater risk for breast cancer, especially if there is more than one affected relative, if the relative is a mother or sister, or if the relative was premenopausal or had bilateral cancer. A reproductive history that includes early menarche, late menopause, a late first pregnancy, or never having borne children also carries increased risk (Ryan et al., 1999). According to some breast cancer researchers, the risk posed by these four characteristics is related to the fact that a woman's risk of breast cancer is linked to the amount of ovarian hormones (estrogen and progesterone) to which her breasts have been exposed over her lifetime (Spicer & Pike, 1994). According to this theory, the factors that influence the total exposure to these hormones include the amounts of hormone produced by a woman's ovaries and the number of menstrual cycles she experiences—as each menstrual cycle exposes the breasts to a midcycle spike in estrogen and progesterone levels. Both hormones have a stimulating effect on breast tissue and cause breast cells to divide, and it is during cell division that mutant, malignant cells have an opportunity to form. The evidence cited in support of this theory is the lower incidence of breast cancer in rural Africa, where the average woman is either pregnant or nursing throughout most of her adult life, and ovu-

lation, with its hormonal spikes, is a comparatively rare event. One study found that the average woman in a rural North African culture menstruates only about 100 times over her lifetime (Strassman, 1996), in contrast to the average American woman, who menstruates between 350 and 400 times. Additional evidence in support of the hormone level–breast cancer incidence connection is the finding that, because of their largely vegetarian diets, the ovaries of women in rural China and Japan (who have a low incidence of breast cancer) produce only about 75 percent of the estrogen produced by the ovaries of the average American woman (Wang, Key, Pike, Boreham, & Chen, 1991). Rural Asian women's relatively low body weight is also thought to be protective against breast cancer, because fat cells produce small amounts of estrogen.

The widespread use of hormone-modulating chemicals found in insecticides, fungicides, chlorine-based substances, and compounds used in manufacturing has also been suggested as a reason that breast cancer is more common in the modern, developed world than it was in the past or than it is currently in underdeveloped nations (Faloon, 1998). Hormone-modulating substances (see Chapter 5) are substances that mimic and mutate estrogen in the body. Indeed, women with breast cancer have been found to have higher levels of pesticide residue in the fat cells of their breasts than women who do not have breast cancer (Aronsen et al., 2000). The exposure to polycyclic aromatic hydrocarbons (PAH) has also been associated with breast cancer. PAH are found in the exhaust of vehicles and machines that burn gasoline and oil, as well as in cigarette smoke and the brown coating on broiled meat. PAH damages DNA, and, in a recent study, women with breast cancer were found to be four times more likely to have high levels of PAH-induced damage to the DNA in their breasts (Rundle et al., 2000).

Taking hormone replacement therapy for 10 years is also thought to slightly increase the risk of breast cancer (see Chapter 24). Contrary to popular belief, electromagnetic radiation from electric blankets and other household appliances does not appear to increase the risk of breast cancer (Zheng et al., 2000).

Body type and aspects of diet have also been associated with breast cancer incidence: Huang (*Waist Circumference,* 1999) found that postmenopausal women with increased waist circumferences who had never taken hormone replacement therapy have a moderately increased risk. Although there have been conflicting data as to whether dietary fat intake is linked to breast cancer risk among American women (Holmes et al., 1999), recent information suggests that a diet high in saturated fat does not contribute to breast cancer (Velie et al., 2000). The latest data analysis from the Framingham study, a large study conducted over decades in Framingham, Massachusetts, suggests that alcohol intake neither increases nor decreases the risk of breast cancer (*Wellness Facts*, 1999).

Whether a woman has demonstrated a propensity to develop abnormal cells in her breast also affects her risk. A personal history of abnormal cells found upon biopsy confers a higher risk for breast cancer, and a woman who has already had breast cancer is at risk for developing it again (Ryan et al., 1999).

The inheritance of the recently identified BRCA 1 and 2 genes accounts for approximately 10 percent of breast cancer cases. If a woman inherits either of these genes, she has a 55 to 85 percent lifetime risk of developing breast cancer. Carrying the gene does not mean one is definitely going to have the disease. Conversely, the absence of the gene does not guarantee one will not get breast cancer. There may be other genes linked to breast cancer as well. Genetic testing is very costly, and currently insurance does not cover it.

Although many factors that *may* contribute to the development of breast cancer have been identified, the exact mechanisms involved remain unknown. It seems likely, however, that the answer lies in a combination of genetic predisposition and favorable environmental circumstances.

There are two basic types of breast cancer—**ductal** and **lobular.** These designations reflect the part of the breast that is involved. The breasts consist of a branching network of ducts, or pathways via which milk is transported to the nipple, and lobules, which lie at the end of each duct (see Figure 17–1). Most breast cancers originate in the lobules (O'Grady et al., 1995). **Ductal carcinoma in situ (DCIS)** and **lobular carcinoma in situ (LCIS)** are pre-invasive types of cancer (Ryan et al., 1999). If not treated in time, both can progress to invasive cancer, spread to lymph nodes, and cause distant metastasis to other organs.

Cancerous tumors have characteristics that are taken into consideration when prognosis and treatment are determined. The differentiating characteristics identified to date involve cell receptor sites and proteins. Tumors containing **estrogen receptors** (cellular material that prompts growth in response to estrogen) respond to treatment better than those that do not. **Her-2-neu** is a protein associated with a gene for breast cancer. The presence of this protein indicates a less favorable prognosis. Scientists are searching for additional markers.

SYMPTOMS

Early breast cancer has *no* symptoms. If a lump can be felt, the cancer has been present for quite some time. As the tumor grows and invades surrounding tissue, it creates changes in breast appearance and contour. A nipple that has become inverted or retracted, skin that is dimpled, and changes in the contour of the breast are all signs of an advanced tumor. Metastasis creates symptoms that vary according to where the tumor has spread. Metastasis to bone, for example, may cause pain in the back or rib cage.

DIAGNOSIS

It is believed that most forms of cancer are present for a number of years before they are palpable or visible on mammography. Mammography detects most cancers when they are too small to be felt. Cancer often appears as deposits of calcium that are clustered in a characteristic way (most calcium in the breast is benign). The diagnostic tools used for breast cancer are the same as those used for any breast mass.

TREATMENT

Since 1990, the treatment of early breast cancers, such as DCIS and LCIS, has moved away from mutilating radical mastectomy toward lumpectomy (*Breast Conservation,* 1999). **Lumpectomy** conserves the breast and removes only the breast cancer and surrounding tissue. The results are cosmetically less drastic and emotionally less scarring to the individual, and lumpectomy is considered by many to be a safe alternative to mastectomy for small tumors that have not spread widely (Weng, Juillard, Parker, Chang, & Gornbein, 2000). Radiation is used in addition to lumpectomy about 82 percent of the time. For more invasive cancers, mastectomy with concurrent breast reconstruction using either a muscle flap from the abdomen or back, or a saline breast implant, is done. Radiation and/or chemotherapy are also considered. If invasive cancer is present, or if there is doubt about whether the lymph nodes in the axilla (armpit area) have been invaded, **axillary node dissection** is done. This procedure involves removing all or several of the lymph nodes from the underarm on the affected side. Unfortunately, axillary node dissection often results in permanent post-treatment swelling in the affected arm. However, a new, less extensive procedure called **sentinel node biopsy** is being increasingly used to determine whether breast cancer has invaded the lymph nodes. One node is biopsied; if it contains no cancer cells, no further surgery is needed (Ryan et al., 1999). This obviates the need for extensive axillary node dissection in women whose cancer has not spread.

New medical therapies are being used effectively to reduce the recurrence rate of breast cancer. The drug Tamoxifen behaves as an anti-estrogen in breast tissue and is taken for five years after the treatment of estrogen receptor–positive cancer (Ryan et al., 1999). Tamoxifen can cause a slightly increased risk of endometrial cancer, however, and can promote the formation of blood clots. An annoying side effect is hot flashes similar to those experienced by women undergoing menopause. **Herceptin** is a new drug that acts as an antibody against the Her-2 gene. It is used to fight advanced cancer that contains the Her-2 gene and cancer that has spread to other organs. Data continue to be collected on its efficacy, and the therapy seems promising for some women.

Some authorities advocate the use of various nutritional supplements and selected hormones as adjuncts to conventional cancer treatments. Green tea extract, selenium, conjugated linoleic acid, whey protein concentrate, ground flaxseed, garlic, vitamin E, curcumin, concentrates of cruciferous vegetables, soy extracts (not for patients undergoing radiation), and melatonin have all been found to support healthy cells and/or deter the growth of malignant cells (*Protocols: Breast Cancer,* 1999). The research in support of such adjuncts has been conducted on cell cultures, animals, and some women with breast cancer. However, the large, controlled studies needed to establish the efficacy of such adjunctive treatments have not been done to date.

PREVENTION

Adopting a healthy lifestyle that includes exercising; eating a diet rich in vegetables, fruits, and whole grains; and maintaining an ideal body weight are steps all women can take to reduce their risk of breast cancer. The antioxidants present in whole foods are believed to exert a protective effect against breast and other cancers (see Chapter 3). The phytoestrogens present in whole grains have hormonal effects that may protect against hormonally depen-dent cancers, such as breast cancer (Slavin, 2000). A new analysis of the data from the Nurses' Health Study (*Daily Exercise,* 1999) suggests that middle-aged women who exercise daily have a 20 percent lower incidence of breast cancer than women who do not. Monthly breast self-examinations and routine mammography after age 40 should also be part of every woman's health maintenance plan. Some experts recommend that women who are at high risk have twice-yearly breast examinations and start mammography earlier than age 40. The use of tamoxifen has been shown to reduce a woman's risk of developing breast cancer by 50 percent. Another drug that is a cousin to tamoxifen, raloxifene, is being studied to see if it, too, reduces breast cancer risk (Minton, 1999). Raloxifene has an advantage over tamoxifen in that it is not associated with an increased risk of uterine cancer. Raloxifene is currently approved by the FDA for the prevention of osteoporosis in postmenopausal women.

The most radical approach to prevention, **prophylactic bilateral mastectomy** (removal of both breasts to prevent cancer from developing in them), has been shown to reduce the risk of breast cancer by 90 percent in women with a strong family history or who carry the BRCA genes (*Bilateral Mastectomy,* 2000). In a study of 572 women who had undergone this procedure, Frost et al. (2000) found that most of the women (70 percent) were satisfied with the procedure. The majority reported that the procedure either had no effect on or had improved their emotional stability, stress level, self-esteem, sexual relationship,

and sense of femininity. The most striking was that 74 percent reported a lessened degree of concern about the possibility of developing breast cancer. Whether such a drastic protective strategy should be implemented is a decision only women themselves, in consultation with their healthcare providers, can make.

The Challenge of Cancer

A diagnosis of cancer presents a woman with challenges in the physical, emotional, and spiritual domains. In addition to the possibility of death, women who have gynecological or breast cancer may face mutilating surgery, such as vulvectomy and mastectomy, or surgery that will end fertility. They may also face chemotherapy or radiation therapy, which can have unpleasant side effects. As daunting as these potential problems seem, they are by no means insurmountable. Women who have cancer have been shown to benefit from educational and psychotherapeutic interventions, and many cancer survivors report that the experience of having cancer caused them to become aware of their inner strength, to find new meaning in their lives, or to undergo some other positive change (Pelusi, 1997).

Threats to Body Image and Sense of Femininity

Surgical procedures, such as mastectomy and vulvectomy, can undermine a woman's body image and sense of femininity and cause her to worry that her sexual partner may no longer find her attractive (Kraus, 1999). Breast conservation surgery (lumpectomy) plus radiation therapy is an alternative to mastectomy under certain circumstances. Women who choose lumpectomy and radiation, as opposed to mastectomy, tend to be younger, more concerned about body image, and more certain that they would have difficulty adjusting to the loss of a breast. Women who choose more radical surgery tend to be older and more fearful that cancer cells may be left behind (Rowland, Dioso, Holland, Chaglassian, & Kinne, 1995). Whether the quality of life in women who have breast-conserving surgery is higher overall than that of women who have more radical surgery is as yet unclear. A 1997 review of the literature suggested that only scores on body image tend to be more positive in women who have breast-conserving versus radical procedures (Irwig & Bennets, 1997). Pusic et al. (1999) found that age influenced women's degree of satisfaction with breast-conserving and radical procedures: In patients under 55 years of age, quality of life scores were lowest among the women who had had more radical procedures. Among the women older than 55, quality of life was lowest for the lumpectomy patients.

Many women who must undergo more radical surgical procedures elect to have their breast or vulva surgically reconstructed. Such procedures can be done concurrently with the cancer surgery, or at a later date, depending on the nature of the surgery and the woman's preference. In a study done in Sweden on 20 patients who had had a mastectomy with immediate breast reconstruction, 19 of the subjects reported being satisfied with the results of the procedure, and 8 said their result had exceeded their expectations (Rosenqvist, Sandelin, & Wickman, 1996).

Adverse Effects of Chemotherapy and Radiation

The chemotherapy and radiation that can save women's lives often cause nausea, hair loss, fatigue, and a reduced resistance to infection, among other problems (Youngkin & Davis, 1998). Strategies are available, however, for minimizing and coping with the problems related to chemotherapy. Medications can be prescribed that lessen or prevent nausea and vomiting. A special cap can be worn during treatments to reduce hair loss. The cap decreases blood flow to the scalp, so that a lesser amount of the drugs used in chemotherapy reaches hair follicles. Cosmetologists who specialize in helping chemotherapy patients are available to help women use wigs and makeup techniques to restore their normal appearance. Patients with decreased energy can maximize their productivity by allowing for rest periods during the day. Community support groups for women with breast cancer, such as Reach to Recovery, can offer other tips, as well as emotional support, to patients and their families.

Emotional Reactions

Women's emotional reactions to the detection, diagnosis, and treatment of cancer commonly include anxiety, denial, anger, and depression (Oktay, 1998). Friends and relatives may be uncomfortable around the cancer patient and avoid her because of their own fears and because they do not know what to say (Pelusi, 1997). Educational, psychotherapeutic, spiritual, and peer group support have all been reported to improve the quality of life of women with cancer, and some combinations of these interventions have been found to extend their lives.

In their study of more than 300 women with breast cancer, Helgeson, Cohen, Schulz, and Yasko (1999) found that educational programs were consistently beneficial to subjects who participated in them. Stewart et al. (2000) found that most of the 105 women with ovarian cancer in their study wanted detailed information about the disease itself, about its treatment, and about self-care strategies.

In addition to finding that educational programs are of benefit to women with breast cancer, Helgeson et al. (1999) found participation in peer discussion groups generally unhelpful, and even detrimental in some cases. In a later study (Helgeson, Cohen, Schultz, & Yasko, 2000), the same investigators found social support to be the key variable in determining whether the overall well-being of the women in their study was enhanced by participation in a peer discussion group. The women who lacked support from their physicians and/or partners were helped by such participation, but, for women who reported high levels of family, friend, or caregiver support, such participation was detrimental.

There is evidence that groups in which psychotherapy is provided benefit women with breast cancer. Spiegel, Bloom, Kraemer, and Gottheil (1989) provided weekly supportive group therapy for 50 women with metastatic breast cancer and compared their outcomes to those of similar women in a control group. The women who received psychotherapy not only reported a better quality of life but also lived almost twice as long as the women in the control group. Based on a review of the literature on the efficacy of psychotherapy as an adjunctive treatment for cancer and their own experience with cancer patients, Cunningham and Edmonds (1996) recommend that psychotherapy be offered to all patients—not just those with overt psychopathology and the few who specifically request it.

Broader forms of group counseling have also proven beneficial to women with cancer. Shrock, Raymond, Palmer, and Taylor (1999) studied breast cancer patients who participated in six two-hour health psychology classes that included elements of psychotherapy as well as education and guidance in physical, emotional, and spiritual self-care. The classes included a discussion of the effects of beliefs, feelings, and attitudes on health; instruction regarding the value of nutrition and exercise; instruction and practice in mental imagery and relaxation techniques; discussions related to self-esteem and spirituality; and assistance in setting goals and creating a personal health plan. The participants were also asked to do more of whatever brought joy and meaning into their lives. At the end of the four- to seven-year follow-up period, the women who participated in the classes were found to have better overall well-being and significantly higher survival rates than the women in a control group, who did not. Further evidence that spirituality seems to be an important factor in coping with breast cancer is found in Feher and Maly's (1999) study of 33 elderly women newly diagnosed with the disease. The respondents reported that spiritual or religious faith provided them with emotional support (91 percent), social support (70 percent), and the ability to find meaning in their everyday lives.

Gynecological Wellness Self-Assessment

Use the following statements to help you judge how vigorously you are promoting your gynecological and breast health. They can also serve as a lifelong guide to good gynecological health practices.

1. *I do not douche, unless prescribed by my healthcare provider.*
2. *I exercise daily; eat a low-fat, high-fiber diet; and maintain my ideal body weight.*
3. *I do not smoke.*
4. *If premenopausal, I get at least four menstrual periods a year (if not on oral contraceptives or Depo-Provera).*

If Sexually Active

1. *I use condoms when having heterosexual sex unless I am sure I am in a mutually monogamous relationship. If I have homosexual relations, I use a vaginal dam to prevent trichomonas infections.*
2. *I am using a reliable method of birth control if I am at risk for, and do not desire, pregnancy.*
3. *I get a physical examination and Pap smear yearly.*

If Age 18 and Over

1. *I get a physical examination and a Pap smear yearly.*
2. *I examine my breasts monthly.*
3. *I know my family history (if possible) pertinent to breast, ovarian, and uterine cancers.*

If Age 40 and Over

1. *I have mammograms at intervals determined in consultation with my physician.*
2. *I do not experience periods that are closer than 21 days apart (from first day of flow to first day of the next period).*
3. *I do not bleed more than seven or eight days with periods or experience excessively heavy bleeding.*
4. *I do not bleed between periods.*

New Directions

There are many promising research projects underway regarding women's gynecological health. One question investigators are currently attempting to answer is whether bacterial vaginosis plays a role in adverse pregnancy outcomes and in PID. They are also attempting to discover whether a protein called gelsolin plays a role in the regulation of cancerous tumor growth (*Discovery of How Protein Changes Shape Could Lead to New Cancer-Fighting Drugs,* 2000). If it does, it may prove to be a key factor in the mechanism by which breast cancer develops. Another area of inquiry is the effectiveness of tests women can perform at home to detect the presence of high-risk HPV strains (*Patient-Collected,* 2000). Finally, new monoclonal antibody treatments are being developed that may attack cancer cells while sparing the healthy cells and organs of the body (*Monoclonal Antibodies,* 2000).

There are many research projects underway regarding women's gynecological health. The topics currently being investigated include the following:

- The role of bacterial vaginosis in adverse pregnancy outcomes and in PID
- The effectiveness of tests women can perform at home to detect the presence of high-risk HPV strains (*Patient-Collected,* 2000)
- New monoclonal antibody treatments for breast cancer that fight the actual cancerous process itself and spare the healthy cells and organs of the body (*Monoclonal Antibodies,* 2000)

QUESTIONS FOR REFLECTION AND DISCUSSION

1. *What factors most commonly lead to unplanned pregnancy?*
2. *If you had a strong family history of breast or ovarian cancer, would you want to have genetic testing done for BRCA 1 and 2? Why or why not?*
3. *If you were to find that you are a carrier of the BRCA 1 or 2 gene, and were finished with childbearing, would you have your ovaries surgically removed? What factors would influence your decision?*
4. *If you knew yourself to be at high risk for breast cancer, would you have both your breasts removed as a precaution? What factors would influence your decision?*
5. *Under what conditions would you consider having a hysterectomy? What factors would influence your thinking about this?*
6. *Explore your attitudes toward and feelings about each of your reproductive organs. Note any connections you notice between the way you view an organ and its health status.*

RESOURCES

Books

Angier, N. (1999). *Woman: An intimate geography.* New York: Anchor Books.
Boston Women's Health Book Collective. (1998). *Our Bodies, Ourselves.* New York: Touchstone.
Northrup, C. (1996). *Women's bodies, women's wisdom.* New York: Bantam Books.

Websites

Gynecological Health (General Information)

American College of Obstetricians and Gynecologists, www.acog.com. Provides education related to the promotion of health throughout women's lives.
Hardin Internet Library, www.lib.uiowa.edu/hardin/md/obgyn.html. Provides an exhaustive list of links to women's health sites.
New York Times Women's Health Site, www.nytimes.com/specials/women/whome/resources.html. Provides general gynecological information.

Cancer

Association of Cancer On-Line Resources, http://acor.org. Offers a list of on-line resources related to breast and gynecological cancers, as well as other forms of cancer.

Cancerfacts, http://cancerfacts.com. Offers a wide range of information about all aspects of cancer. The site's advisory board is made up of prominent cancer experts and representatives from the National Consumer Advisory Council. Offers the service Breast Cancer Profiler, which provides information about treatment options, drug side effects, and so on, specifically tailored to the circumstances of individuals who submit information.

Dr. Susan Love's Breast Cancer Site, www.susanlovemd.com. Comprehensive information for women recently diagnosed with breast cancer and women who are survivors of breast cancer.

National Cancer Institute Cancer Net, http://cancernet.nci.nih.gov/. Offers information on treatment, prevention, and diagnosis and lists clinical trials in which women can enroll.

National Coalition for Cancer Survivorship, www.cansearch.org. Offers information related to coping with the diagnosis of cancer.

Susan G. Komen Breast Cancer Foundation, www.komen.org. Supports research on breast cancer prevention.

Organizations

The American Cancer Society—Local chapters

Hysterectomy Educational Resources and Services (HERS)
8585 N. 76th St.
Bala-Cynwyd, PA 19004
Phone: 610-667-7757

National Women's Health Network
Web: www.womenshealthnetwork.org
514 10th St. NW, Suite 400
Washington, DC 20004
Phone: 202-347-1140

Y-ME National Breast Cancer Organization (24-hour hot line)
Phone: 1-800-221-2141

References

Angier, N. (1999). *Woman: An intimate geography.* New York: Anchor.

Aronsen, K. J., Miller, A. B., Woolcott, C. G., Sterns, E. E., McCready, O. R., Lickley, L. A., Fish, E. B., Hiraki, G. Y., Holloway, C., Ross, T., Hanna, W. M., SenGupta, S. K., & Weber, J. P. (2000). Breast adipose tissue concentrations of polychlorinated biphenyls and organochlorines and breast cancer risk. *Cancer Epidemiology Biomarkers Preview 2000, 9*(1), 55–63.

Beaulieu, M. (2000). *Racial gap in breast cancer mortality widening.* [On-line]. Available: *http://womenshealth. medscape.com/reuters/prof/1999/11/11.24/ep11249c.html* (1/16/00).

Bendich, A. (2000). The potential for dietary supplements to reduce premenstrual syndrome (PMS) symptoms. *Journal of the American College of Nutrition, 19*(1), 3–12.

Berek, J. S., Adashi, E. Y., & Hillard, P. A. (1996). *Novak's gynecology* (12th ed.). Baltimore: Williams and Wilkins.

Bilateral mastectomy protects BRCA gene mutation carriers from breast cancer. (2000). [On-line]. Available: *http://womenshealth.medscape.com/reuters/prof/2000/04/04.04/c104040c.html* (4/10/2000).

Blackman, D. K., Bennett, E. M., & Miller, D. S. (1999). Trends in self-reported use of mammograms (1989–1997) and papanicolaou tests. (1991–1997). Behavior risk factor surveillance system. [On-line]. Available: *http://www.cdc.gov/epo/mmwr/preview/mmwrhtml/ss4806al.html* [10/8/99].

Braiman, J., & Lione, A. (2000, July/August). The Today contraceptive sponge is inherently dangerous. *The Network News,* p. 1, 7.

Breast cancer: what 1-in-8 means, (1999). *University of California at Berkeley Wellness Letter, 15*(11), 2.

Breast conserving surgery for early-stage cancer increases 65%. (1999). [On-line]. Available: *http://womenshealth.medscape.com/MedscapeWire/1999/08.99/medwire0813.breast.html* (8/13/99).

Brenner, P. F. (1996). Differential diagnosis of abnormal uterine bleeding. *American Journal of Obstetrics and Gynecology, 175* (3, Pt. 2), 766–769.

Campion, M., Ferris, D., di Paola, F., Reid, R., & Miller, M. (1991). *Modern colposcopy: a practical approach.* Augusta, Georgia: Educational Systems, Inc.

Carranza-Lira, S., Murillo-Uribe, A., Martinez-Trejo, N., & Santos-Gonzales, J. (1997). Changes in symptomatology, hormones, lipids and bone density after hysterectomy. *International Journal of Fertility and Women's Medicine, 42*(1), 43–47.

Cates, W. Jr., & Raymond, E. G. (1998). Vaginal spermicides. In Hatcher, R., Trussell, J., Stewart, F., Cates, W. Jr., Stewart, G., Guest, F. & Kowal, D. (Eds.), *Contraceptive Technology* (17th rev. ed.). (pp. 357–369). New York: Ardent Media, Inc.

Centers for disease control and prevention. (2000). *Highlights of Trends in Pregnancy and Pregnancy Rates, 47*(29), 12.

Chez, R. A., & Chapin, J. (1997). Emergency contraception. The pill's little known secret goes public. *Lifelines, 1*(5), 28–31.

Chrisler, J. (1991). PMS as a culture bound syndrome. In Crisler, J., Golden, C. & Rozee, P. (Eds.), *Lectures on the Psychology of Women* (pp. 107–121). New York: McGraw-Hill.

Christman, G. M., & Uechi, H. (2000). Female sterilization. *The Female Patient, 25*(5), 29–36.

Chuong, C. J., & Brenner, P. F. (1996). Management of abnormal uterine bleeding. *American Journal of Obstetrics and Gynecology, 175*(3, Pt. 2), 787–792.

Clinical Guidelines. (1994). Cancer detection by physical examination. *Nurse Practitioner, 19*(10), 20–24.

Clinical Guidelines. (1995). Unintended pregnancy. *Nurse Practitioner, 20*(11), 76–79.

The Collaborative Group on Hormone Factors in Breast Cancer (1997). Breast cancer and hormone replacement therapy: Collaborative re-analysis of data from 51 epidemiological studies of 52,705 women with breast cancer and 108,411 women without breast cancer. *Lancet, 350,* 1047–1059.

Contraceptive Update: Oral Contraceptives and Breast Cancer Risks. (2001). [On-line]. *Network, 20*(4). Quarterly Health Bulletin of Family Health International. Available: http://reproline.jhu.edu/english/6read/6issues/6network/v20-4/nt2048.html

Corwin, E. J. (1997). Endometriosis: Pathophysiology, diagnosis, and treatment. *The Nurse Practitioner, 22*(10), 35–51, 55.

Cullins, V. A., Dominiguez, L., Guberski, T., Secor, M. R., & Wysocki, S. J. (1999). Treating vaginitis. *The Nurse Practitioner, 24*(10), 46–60.

Cunningham, A. L., & Edmonds, P. (1996). Group psychological therapy for cancer patients: a point of view, and discussion of the hierarchy of options. *International Journal of Psychiatry and Medicine, 26*(1), 51–82.

Daily exercise cuts breast cancer risk by up to 20% in middle-aged women. (1999). [On-line]. Available: *http://womenshealth.medscape.com/reuters/prof/1999/10/10.27/ep10279i.html* (11/01/99).

Davies, J. E. (1997). A second chance at preventing pregnancy. Using oral contraceptives for emergency contraception. *ADVANCE for Nurse Practitioners, 5*(11), 43–47.

DeMarco, A. (1995). Hysterectomy alternatives for fibroids and heavy bleeding. *Natural Solutions, 3*(1), 1.

DePriest, P., & Nagell, J. (1997). Current status of ovarian cancer screening. *Contemporary OB/GYN,* September, 151–156.

Diab, S., Elledge, R., & Clark, G. (2000). Tumor characteristics and clinical outcome of elderly women with breast cancer. *Journal of the National Cancer Institute, 92*(7), 550–556.

Discovery of how protein changes shape could lead to new cancer-fighting drugs. (2000). [On-line]. Available: *http://womenshealth.medscape.com/MedscapeWire/2000/0200/medwire.0202.discovery.html* (02/06/2000).

Elchalal, U., Gilead, L., Vardy, D., Ben-Shachar, I., Anteby, S., & Schenker, J. (1995). Treatment of vulvar lichen sclerosus in the elderly: an update. *Obstetrical and gynecological survey, 50*(2), 155–162.

Endometriosis Association. (2000). What is endometriosis? [On-line]. Available: *http://www.EndometriosisAssn.org/endo.html*

Endometriosis Association. (2000). Common symptoms of endometriosis. [On-line]. Available: *http://www.medscape.com/medscape/features/question/1999/08.99/q655.html*

Faludi, S. (1991). Backlash: The undeclared war against American women. New York: Crown.

Farrel, S. A., & Kieser, K. (2000). Sexuality after hysterectomy. *Obstetrics and Gynecology, 95*(6 part 2), 1045–1051.

Feher, S., & Maly, R. C. (1999). Coping with breast cancer in later life: the role of religious faith. *Psychooncology, 8*(5), 408–416.

Fogel, C. I., & Woods, N. F. (1995). *Women's healthcare: A comprehensive handbook.* Philadelphia: Williams & Wilkens.

Fonte, D. R. (1997). The basics of natural family planning. *ADVANCE for Nurse Practitioners, 5*(3), 37–42.

Ford, W. C., North, K., Taylor, H., Farrow, A., Hull, M. G., & Golding, J. (2000). Increasing paternal age is associated with delayed conception in a large population of fertile couples: evidence for declining fecundity in older men. *Human Reproduction, 15*(8), 1703–1708.

Frost, M. H., Schaid, D. J., Sellers, T. A., Slezak, J. M., Arnold, P. G., Woods, J. E., Petty, P. M., Johnson, J. L., Sitta, D. L., McDonnell, S. K., Rummans, T. A., Jenkins, R. B., Sloan, J. A., & Hartman, L. C. (2000). Long-term satisfaction and psychological and social function following bilateral prophylactic mastectomy. *Journal of the American Medical Association, 284*(3), 319–324.

Gallagher, J. (1997). Religious freedom, reproductive health care, and hospital mergers. *Journal of the American Medical Women's Association, 52*(2), 65–68.

Gallagher, R., & Fuller, C. A. (1997). A new generation of oral contraceptives. *ADVANCE for Nurse Practitioners, 5*(11), 39–40, 80.

Global progress: breast cancer mortality rates. [On-line]. (1999). Available: *http://womenshealth.medscape.com/MedscapeWire/1999/05.99/medwire.0511.globalprog.html* (5/21/99).

Goldman, S. (1994). Evaluating breast masses. *Contemporary OB/GYN-NP,* June/July, 8–17.

Gollub, E. (2000, July/August). The Today spermicidal sponge should be available to U.S. women. *The Network News,* p. 1, 7.

Guaschino, S., De Seta, F., Sartore, A., Ricci, G., DeSanto, D., Piccoli, M., & Alberico, S. (2001). Efficacy with maintenance therapy with topical boric acid in comparison with oral intraconazole in the treatment of recurrent vulvo vaginal candidiasis. *American Journal of Obstetrics and Gynecology, 184*(4), 598–602.

Haas, S. L. (1998). The intrauterine device: Dispelling the myths. *The Nurse Practitioner, 23*(11), 58, 63–69, 73.

Hardy, M. L. (2000). Women's health series: Herbs of special interest to women. *Journal of the American Pharmaceutical Association, 40*(20), 234–242.

Hatcher, R. A. (1998). Depo-Provera, Norplant, and progestin-only pills. In Hatcher, R., Trussell, J., Stewart, F., Cates, W. Jr., Stewart, G., Guest, F., & Kowal, D. (Eds.), *Contraceptive Technology* (17th rev. ed.) (pp. 467–509). New York: Ardent Media, Inc.

Hatcher, R. A., & Guillebaud, J. (1998). The pill: Combined oral contraceptives. In Hatcher, R., Trussell, J., Stewart, F., Cates, W. Jr., Stewart, G., Guest, F., & Kowal, D. (Eds.), *Contraceptive Technology* (17th rev. ed.) (pp. 405–466). New York: Ardent Media, Inc.

Helgeson, V. S., Cohen, S., Schulz, R., & Yasko (1999). Education and peer discussion group interventions and adjustment to breast cancer. *Archives of General Psychiatry, 56*(4), 340–347.

Helgeson, V. S., Cohen, S., Schulz, R., & Yasko (2000). Group support interventions for women with breast cancer: who benefits from what? *Health Psychology, 19*(2), 107–114.

Helstrom, L. (1994). Sexuality after hysterectomy: A model based on quantitative and qualitative analysis of 104 women before and after subtotal hysterectomy. *Journal of Psychosomatic Obstetrics and Gynecology, 15*(4), 219–229.

Higgins, P. G., & Smith, P. E. (1997). Assessing cervical cancer risk. *Lifelines, 1*(6), 43–47.

Hillier, S., & Holmes, K. K. (1995). *Sexually transmitted diseases* (2nd ed.). McGraw-Hill, Inc.

Holmes, M., Hunter, D., Colditz, G., Stampfer, M., Hankinson, S., Speizer, F., Rosner, B., & Willett, W. (1999). Association of dietary intake of fat and fatty acids with risk of breast cancer. *The Journal of the American Medical Association* (281), 914–920.

Hormone therapy and women's hearts. (2000, July). *University of California, Berkeley, Wellness Letter, 16*(10), 4–5.

Hufnagel, V. (1989). *No more hysterectomies.* USA: Plume.

Human papillomavirus vaccines. (2000). [On-line]. Available: http://www.medscape.com/medscape/WomensH...rnal/ 2000/ca-who0118.01/ca-who0118.01.html (1/16/00).

Hysterectomy. (2000, April). *Women's Health Advisor, 4*(4), 1, 6–7.

Hysterectomy and its alternatives. (1998). Health Pages. [On-line]. Available: *http://www.thehealthpages.com/articles/ar-hyst.html*

Hysterectomy surveillance–United States. (1980–1993). [On-line]. Available: *http://www.cdc.gov/epo/mmwr/preview/ mmwrhtml/00048898.html*

Irwig, L., & Bennets, A. (1997). Quality of life after breast conservation or mastectomy: a systematic review. *Australian New Zealand Journal of Surgery, 67*(11), 750–754.

Jennings, V. H., Lamprecht, V. M., & Kowal, D. (1998). Fertility awareness methods. In Hatcher, R., Trussell, J., Stewart, F., Cates, W. Jr., Stewart, G., Guest, F. & Kowal, D. (Eds.), *Contraceptive Technology* (17th rev. ed.) (pp. 309–323). New York: Ardent Media, Inc.

Kowal, D. (1998). Abstinence and the range of sexual expression. In Hatcher, R., Trussell, J., Stewart, F., Cates, W. Jr., Stewart, G., Guest, F. & Kowal, D., (Eds.), *Contraceptive Technology* (17th rev. ed.) (pp. 297–302). New York: Ardent Media, Inc.

Kraus, P. L. (1999). Body image, decision-making, and breast cancer treatment. *Cancer Nursing, 22*(6), 421–427.

Kurman, R., Henson, D., Herbst, A., Noller, K., & Schiffman, M. (1994). Interim guidelines for management of abnormal cervical cytology. *JAMA, 271*(23), 1866–1869.

Lark, S. (2002). *Mammography—Is the gold standard fool's gold?* The Lark Letter, August 2002, 7.

Lichtman, R. (1990). The well-women gynecologic interview. In Lichtman, R. & Papera, S. (Eds.), *Gynecology Well-Women Care* (pp. 19–28). Norwalk: Appleton & Lange.

Lichtman, R., & Papera, S. (1990). *Gynecology well woman care.* Norwalk, Connecticut: Appleton & Lange.

Limon, L. (2000). Use of alternative medicine in women's health. *AphA 2000—American Pharmaceutical Association Annual Meeting.* [On-line]. Available: *http://www.medscape.com/ medcape/CNO/2000/APHA/APHA-13.html*

Luukkain, T., & Toivonen, J. (1995). Levonorgestrel-releasing IUD as a method of contraception with therapeutic properties. *Contraception, 52*(5), 269–276.

Marieb, E. (1989). Human anatomy and physiology. Redwood City, CA: The Benjamin/Cummings Publishing Company.

Mehring, P. (1997). Dysfunctional uterine bleeding. Evaluating this common complaint. *ADVANCE for Nurse Practitioners, 5*(11), 27–32.

Minton, S. (1999). *New hormonal therapies for breast cancer.* [On-line]. Available: *http://womenshealth.medscape.com/ moffitt/C...n03/cc0603.03.mint/pnt-cc0603.03.mint.html* (8/2/98).

Moline, M. L., & Zendel, S. M. (2000). Evaluating and managing premenstrual syndrome. *Medscape Women's Health, 5*(2). [On-line]. Available: *http://www.medscape.*

com/medscape/Womens...v05.n02/wh3025.moli/wh3025. moli-01.html

Monoclonal antibodies may offer a magic bullet for treating cancer. (2000). Available: *http://womenshealth.medscape.com/ MedscapeWire/2000/0100/medwire.0118.monoclonal.html* (1/18/00).

Morrison, B., Daniels, S., & Kotey, P., et al (1999). Rofecoxib, a specific Cyclooxygenase-2 inhibitor, in primary dysmenorrhea: A randomized controlled trial. *Obstetrics and Gynecology, 94*(4), 504–508.

Murphy, P. A. (1990). Anatomy and physiology of the female reproductive system. In Lichtman, R. & Papera, S. (Eds.), *Gynecology Well-Women Care* (pp. 3–18). Norwalk: Appleton & Lange.

Nicholson, P. (1995). The menstrual cycle, science and femininity. *Social Sciences and Medicine, 41,* 779–784.

Northrup, C. (1994). *Women's bodies, women's wisdom.* New York: Bantam Books.

Nyirjesy, P., Seeney, S. M., Grody, M. H., Jordan, C. A., & Buckley, H. R. (1995). Chronic focal vaginitis: the value of cultures. *American Journal of Obstetrics and Gynecology, 173*(3), 820–823.

O'Grady, L., Lindfors, K., Howell, L., & Rippon, M. (1995). *A practical approach to breast disease.* New York: Little Brown and Company.

Oktay, J. S. (1998). Psychosocial aspects of breast cancer. *Lippencotts Primary Care Practitioner, 2*(2), 149–159.

Papera, S. (1990). The physical and pelvic examination. In Lichtman, R. & Papera, S. (Eds.), *Gynecology Well-Women Care* (pp. 29–40). Norwalk: Appleton & Lange.

Patient-collected tissue samples may offer effective option to pap smear. (2000). [On-line]. Available: *http://womenshealth.medscape.com/MedscapeWire/2000/ 0100/medwire/0104.patient.html* (1/7/00).

Pelton, R., & Lavelle, J. B. (2000). Heart to heart: A cardiovascular health primer, Pharma, 4(2), 1, 28.

Pelton, R., Lavelle, J., Hawkins, E., & Krinsky, F. (2001). *Drug-induced nutrient depletion.* Andover, MA: Fitzgerald Health Education Association.

Pelusi, J. (1997). The lived experience of surviving breast cancer. *Oncology Nursing Forum, 24*(8), 1343–1353.

Prentice, A., Deary, A. J., Goldbeck-Wood, S., Farquhar, C., & Smith, S. K. (1999). Gonadotropin-releasing hormone analogues for pain associated with endometriosis. The Cochrane Library, (3). [On-line]. Available: *http://www.medscape.com/cochrane/abstracts/ ab000345.html*

Protocols: breast cancer. (January, 1999). *Life Extension,* 33–37.

Pusic, A., Thompson, T. A., Kerrigan, C. L., Sargeant, R., Slezak, S., Chang, B. W., Kelzlsouer, K. J., & Manson, P. N. (1999). Surgical options for the early-stage breast cancer: factors associated with patient choice and postoperative quality of life. *Plastic Reconstructive Surgery, 104*(5), 1325–1333.

Rako, S. (1998). Testerone deficiency: A key factor in the increased C. V. risk to women following hysterectomy or with natural aging? *Journal of Women's Health, 7*(7), 825–829.

Robinson, K. M., & Huether, S. E. (1998). Structure and function of the reproductive system. In McCance, K. L. & Huether, S. E. (Eds.), *Pathophysiology. The Basis for Disease in*

Adults and Children (3rd ed.) (pp. 707–742). Philadelphia: Mosby.

Robinson, K. M., & McCance, K. L. (1998). Alterations of the reproductive system. In McCance, K. L. & Huether, S. E., (Eds.), *Pathophysiology. The Basis for Disease in Adults and Children* (3rd ed.) (pp. 743–811). Philadelphia: Mosby.

Rosenqvist, S., Sandelin, K., & Wickman, M. (1996). Patients' psychological and cosmetic experience after immediate breast reconstruction. *European Journal of Surgical Oncology, 22*(3), 262–266.

Rowland, J. H., Dioso, J., Holland, J. C., Chaglassian, T., & Kinne, D. (1995). Breast reconstruction after mastectomy: Who seeks it, who refuses? *Plastic and Reconstructive Surgery, 95,* 812–822.

Rundle, A., Tang, D., Hibshoosh, H., Estabrook, A., Schnable, F., Cao, W., Grumet, S., & Perera, F. P. (2000). The relationship between genetic damage from polycyclic aromatic hydrocarbons in breast tissue and breast cancer. *Carcinogenesis, 21*(7), 1281–1289.

Ryan, K. J., Berkowitz, R. S., Barbieri, R. L., & Dunaif, A. (1999). *Kistner's gynecology and women's health* (7th ed.). Baltimore: Mosby.

Selak, V., Farquhar, C., Prentice, A., & Singla, A. (1999). Danazol for pelvic pain associated with endometriosis. *The Cochran Library,* (3). [On-line]. Available: *http://www.medscape.com/cochrane/abstracts/ab000068.html*

Sherif, K. (1999). Benefits and risks of oral contraceptives. *American Journal Obstetrics and Gynecology, 180* (6, Pt. 2), S343–S348.

Shrock, D., Palmer, R. F., & Taylor, B. (1999). Effects of a psychosocial intervention on survival among patients with stage 1 breast cancer and prostate cancer: A matched, case-controlled study. *Alternative Therapies in Health and Medicine, 5*(3), 49–55.

Shulman, J. F. (1990). Bleeding disorders. In Lichtman, R. & Papera, S. (Eds.), *Gynecology Well-Women Care* (pp. 355–366). Norwalk: Appleton & Lange.

Sinofsky, F. E. (1999). Vulvovaginal candidiasis: topical versus oral therapy. *The Female Patient, 24.*

Slavin, J. L. (2000). Mechanisms for the impact of whole grain foods on cancer risk. *Journal of the American College of Nutrition, 19*(3 Suppl), 300S–307S.

Speroff, L., & Darney, P. (1996). *A Clinical Guide for Contraception* (2nd ed.). Philadelphia: Williams & Wilkins.

Spicer, D. V., & Pike, M. C. (1994). Sex steroids and breast cancer prevention. *Journal of the National Cancer Institute Monograph,* (16), 139–147.

Spiegel, D., Bloom, P., Kraemer, H. C., & Gottheil, E. (1989). Effect of psychosocial treatment on survival of patients with metastatic breast cancer. *Lancet, 2,* 888–891.

Stewart, D. E., Wong, F., Cheung, A. M., Dancey, J., Meana, M., Cameron, J. I., McAndrews, M. P., Bunston, T., Murphy, J., & Rosen, B. (2000). Information needs and decisional preferences among women with ovarian cancer. *Gynecologic Oncology, 77*(3), 357–361.

Stewart, F. (1998). Vaginal barriers. In Hatcher, R., Trussell, J., Stewart, F., Cates, W. Jr., Stewart, G., Guest, F. & Kowal, D. (Eds.), *Contraceptive Technology* (17th rev. ed.) (pp. 371–404). New York: Ardent Media, Inc.

Stewart, G. K. (1998). Intrauterine devices. In Hatcher, R., Trussell, J., Stewart, F., Cates, W. Jr., Stewart, G., Guest, F., & Kowal, D. (Eds.), *Contraceptive Technology* (17th rev. ed.) (pp. 511–543). New York: Ardent Media, Inc.

Stewart, G. K., & Carignan, C. S. (1998). Female and male sterilization. In Hatcher, R., Trussell, J., Stewart, F., Cates, W. Jr., Stewart, G., Guest, F. & Kowal, D. (Eds.), *Contraceptive Technology* (17th rev. ed.) (pp. 545–588). New York: Ardent Media, Inc.

Strassman, B. (1996). The evolution of endometrial cycles and menstruation. *Quarterly Review of Biology, 71,* 181–220.

Sullivan, N. (1990). Dysmenorrhea. In Lichtman, R. & Papera, S. (Eds.), *Gynecology Well-Women Care* (pp. 345–354). Norwalk: Appleton & Lange.

Sweet, R., & Gibbs, R. (1995). *Infectious diseases of the female genital tract* (3rd ed.). Williams and Wilkins: Baltimore.

Thys-Jacobs, S. (2000). Micronutrients and the premenstrual syndrome: the case for calcium. *Journal of the American College of Nutrition, 19*(2), 220–227.

Tumor index to diagnose ovarian cancer developed. (1999). [On-line]. Available: *http://womenshealth.medscape.com/MedscapeWire/1999/12.99/medwire.1230.tumor.html.* (12/30/99).

Ugarriza, D. N., Klinger, S., & O'Brien, S. (1998). Premenstrual syndrome: Diagnosis and intervention. *The Nurse Practitioner, 23*(9), 40–57.

Van Look, P. F. A., & Stewart, F. (1998). Emergency contraception. In Hatcher, R., Trussell, J., Stewart, F., Cates, W. Stewart, G., Guest, F., & Kowal, D. (Eds.), *Contraceptive Technology* (17th rev. ed.) (pp. 277–295). New York: Ardent Media, Inc.

Vedantham, S., Goodwin, S., McLucas, B., Lee, M., Perrella, R., Forno, A., & DeLeon, M. (1999). *Uterine artery embolization for fibroids: considerations in patient selection and clinical follow-up.* [On-line]. Available: *http://www.medscape.com/medscape/WomensH.../v04.n05/wh3226.good/wh3226.good-01.html* (01/16/2000).

Velie, E., Kulldorff, M., Schairer, C., Block, G., Albanes, D., & Schatzkin, A. (2000). Dietary fat, fat subtypes, and breast cancer in menopausal women: a prospective cohort study. *Journal of the National Cancer Institute, 92*(10), 833–839.

Ventura, S. J., Martin, J. A., Curtin, S. C., & Mathews, T. J. (1999). Births: Final data for 1997. *National Vital Statistics Report, 47*(18).

Waist circumference a risk factor for breast cancer. (1999). [On-line]. Available: *http://womenshealth.medscape.com/reuters/prof/1999/12/12.28/ep12289c.html* (1/16/00).

Wang, D. Y., Key, T. J., Pike, M. C., Boreham, J., & Chen, J. (1991). Serum hormone levels in British and rural Chinese females. *Breast Cancer Research and Treatment, May 18th, Suppl 1,* s 41–45.

Warner, D. L., & Hatcher, R. A. (1998). Male condoms. In Hatcher, R., Trussell, J., Stewart, F., Cates, W. Jr., Stewart, G., Guest, F. & Kowal, D. (Eds.), *Contraceptive Technology* (17th rev. ed.) (pp. 325–355). New York: Ardent Media, Inc.

Wellness Facts. (1999). *University of California, Berkeley Wellness Letter, 15*(8), 1.

Weng, E. Y., Juillard, G. J., Parker, R. G., Chang, H. R., & Gornbein, J. A. (2000). Outcomes and factors impacting local recurrence of ductal carcinoma in situ. *Cancer, 88*(7), 1643–1649.

Whysner, J., & Mohan, M. (2000). Perineal application of talc and cornstarch powders: evaluation of ovarian cancer risk. *American Journal of Obstetrics and Gynecology, 182,*(3), 720–724.

Wilkinson, E. J., & Stone, I. K. (1995). *Atlas of vulvar disease.* Baltimore: Williams and Wilkins.

Youngkin, E., & Davis, M. (1998). Women's health: A primary care clinical guide (2nd ed.). Stamford, Connecticut: Appleton & Lange.

Zheng, T., Holford, T. R., Mayne, S. T., Owens, P. H., Zhang, B., Boyle, P., Carter, D., Ward, B., Zhang, Y., & Zahn, S. H. (2000). Exposure to electromagnetic fields from use of electric blankets and other in-home electrical appliances and breast cancer risk. *American Journal of Epidemiology, 15*(11), 1103–1111.

18

Skin Wellness and Illness

Kathryn Van Dyke Hayes

CHAPTER OUTLINE

Objectives

1. *Describe the markers of healthy skin.*
2. *List methods of promoting skin wellness.*
3. *Discuss the effective use of sunscreen products.*
4. *Identify the manifestations of selected skin problems and diseases.*

Introduction

The skin is the largest organ in the body. It is the protective envelope that surrounds the deeper structures of the body and protects them from microorganisms and trauma. The skin also plays a role in regulating the body's temperature through vasoconstriction and sweating, and manufactures the vitamin D necessary for the absorption of calcium and phosphorous. Although as vital to the functioning of the body as any other organ, the skin is often taken for granted and its contribution to our overall health undervalued. In this chapter, the markers of healthy skin will be identified, and strategies for preserving the health of the skin will be outlined. Common skin problems will be described in terms of symptoms and treatment options.

Markers of Skin Wellness: Skin Color and Texture

The general color and pigmentation of the skin should be uniform over the body surface, except for the vascular areas of the cheeks, upper chest, and genitalia, which may look pink or exhibit a reddish-purple tone (Thompson & Wilson, 1996). The skin color normally ranges from whitish pink to olive tones to deep brown, depending on ethnicity (Thompson & Wilson, 1996).

Persons with darker skin may have lighter pigmentation on the palms, soles, nail beds, and lips and darker pigmentation on the knuckles, elbows, and knees (Thompson & Wilson, 1996). Freckling (presence of small, flat, brownish spots) of the gums, tongue borders, and lining of the cheeks may be present in dark-skinned persons (Estes, 1998). In addition, the gingiva (gums) in dark-skinned persons may have a blue or variegated appearance (Estes, 1998).

Normal skin should be warm and dry without excessive warmth. Perspiration and oiliness should be minimal. Healthy skin is intact and free of itching, cracking, flaking, or scaling (Thompson & Wilson, 1996). Most non-hairy areas of the skin normally feel smooth and soft to the touch (Estes, 1998; Thompson & Wilson, 1996). Roughness is normal and expected on exposed areas, such as the elbows, knees, soles of the feet, and palms of the hands (Estes, 1998). A number of normal variations of the skin may be present.

The sun-exposed areas of the skin may exhibit slightly darker pigmentation or freckles (Estes, 1998; Thompson & Wilson, 1996). Freckles are commonly found on the face, neck, arms, and back (Thompson & Wilson, 1996).

Moles (also known as **nevi**) range in color from tan to dark brown and may be flat or raised (Thompson & Wilson, 1996). Most moles are harmless, but moles should be checked monthly for the warning signs of skin cancer: Changes in size, color, shape, sensation, surface characteristics, and surrounding skin, and bleeding, require referral for further medical investigation (Estes, 1998; Thompson & Wilson, 1996). **Striae,** commonly called stretch marks, may appear silvery, tan, or pink and result from rapid or prolonged stretching of the skin (Estes, 1998; Thompson & Wilson, 1996). A normal finding after pregnancy, abdominal striae may also be due to abdominal tumors or other causes of abdominal distension, or obesity (Estes, 1998).

Calluses, superficial areas of thick, rough skin, are a result of thickening of the skin due to prolonged pressure (Estes, 1998; Seidel, Ball, Dains, & Benedict, 1999). Calluses occur primarily on the weight-bearing areas of the foot (sole) and on the palmar surface of the hand (Estes, 1998; Seidel et al., 1999). They feel firm or hard to the touch and are usually not painful (Estes, 1998; Seidel et al., 1999).

Birthmarks are usually flat and can be tan, red, or brown (Thompson & Wilson, 1996) (see Figure 18–1).

Promoting Skin Wellness

The three most important things a woman can do to promote the health of her skin are (1) protect it from the dam-

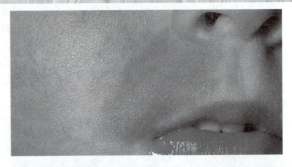
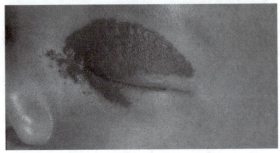

Figure 18–1 Birthmarks: Port-Wine Stain and Strawberry Mark

Source: *Medical-Surgical Nursing: Critical Thinking in Client Care* 2e by Lemone/Burke, Copyright 2000. Reprinted by permission of Pearson Education, Inc., Upper Saddle River, NJ.

aging effects of ultraviolet radiation, (2) refrain from smoking, and (3) keep the skin well hydrated.

Avoiding Sun Damage

The sun emits energy in the form of ultraviolet radiation (UVR) in a broad spectrum of wavelengths. Ultraviolet radiation, which has a shorter wavelength than visible blue or violet light, bears the major responsibility for sunburn and other undesirable phenomena, such as cataracts (U.S. Environmental Protection Agency, 1995). Both ultraviolet A (UVA) and ultraviolet B (UVB) light penetrate the surface of the skin and can cause skin damage, including premature aging of the skin and skin cancer (Cook, 1997; U.S. Environmental Protection Agency, 1995). Ultraviolet C (UVC) light is absorbed by the **ozone layer,** a thin shield in the earth's atmosphere, and does not reach the surface of the earth (Coldiron, 1998; Leber, Perron, & Sinni-McKeehan, 1999). In the future, UVC light may become an important factor in the development of skin disorders as the ozone layer becomes increasingly depleted (Leber et al., 1999). This discussion will focus on the two kinds of ultraviolet light that are currently problematic, UVA and UVB.

UVB, the short-wave UV rays, are partially absorbed by the ozone layer and cause the burning of the outer layer of the skin (Cook, 1997; U.S. Environmental Protection Agency, 1995). UVA, the long-wave UV rays, are not absorbed by the ozone layer, penetrate more deeply, and may weaken the inner connective tissue of the skin (Cook, 1997; U.S. Environmental Protection Agency, 1995). Research data indicate that UVA plays a significant role in photoaging (Coldiron, 1998; Melton, 1998). More information on photoaging appears in the section on skin cancers.

The amount of UV radiation that reaches the earth's surface depends on several factors, including time of day, time of year, latitude, altitude, weather conditions, and ozone depletion (U.S. Environmental Protection Agency, 1995). For example, at noon, when the sun is highest in the sky, the sun's rays travel the shortest distance through the atmosphere, and UVB levels are at their highest. UVB intensity is greatly reduced, however, in the early morning and late afternoon, when these rays pass through the atmosphere more obliquely. Because UVA levels are not sensitive to ozone, UVA intensity levels change in the same manner as visible sunlight during the day.

UV intensity is greatest in the summer months (U.S. Environmental Protection Agency, 1995). UV rays are strongest at the latitude of the equator, as the sun is directly overhead and the ozone layer is thinner in the tropics. As altitude increases, so does UV intensity, due to a decreased atmospheric layer for absorbing the harmful rays. On cloudy days, UV levels are reduced but not completely eliminated; a person can get sunburn on a cloudy day.

The ozone layer protects life on the earth by absorbing some of the sun's harmful UV rays. The ozone layer has been depleted by the presence of substances such as chlorofluorocarbons (CFCs) used in refrigerants, insulating foams, and solvents; pesticides, such as methyl bromide; halons used in fire extinguishers; and methyl chloroform used in industrial processes (U.S. Environmental Protection Agency, 1995). Ozone layer depletion results in increased UV radiation's reaching the earth's surface, increasing the risk that people will experience overexposure. Overexposure can contribute to serious health problems, including skin cancer, cataracts, and immune suppression (U.S. Environmental Protection Agency, 1995). A natural repair process is expected to restore the ozone layer, provided the ozone-depleting substances are phased out and no longer used. In many communities, consumers can get daily information about the UV index in local weather reports on the television and radio.

The **ultraviolet index,** a product of a joint effort among the National Weather Service, the U.S. Environmental Protection Agency, and the Centers for Disease Control and Protection, serves as a useful reminder for consumers about the dangers of UV exposure and the need for sun protection (Coldiron, 1998). The daily ultraviolet index provides a next-day forecast of UVR intensity at midday (noon) for selected cities in the United States (Coldiron, 1998; U.S. Environ-

mental Protection Agency, 1995). The index is numbered on a 0–10+ scale as follows: 0–2, minimal; 3–4, low; 5–6, moderate; 7–9, high; and 10 or higher, very high. The burning risk for a fair-skinned person was used as the basis for this index. The computer model used by the National Weather Service for calculating the UV index takes into account the amount of ozone, cloud cover, latitude, elevation, and time of year (U.S. Environmental Protection Agency, 1995). Although sun protection measures against overexposure should always be taken, safeguards are especially critical when the UV index predicts moderate or higher levels of UVR.

The American Academy of Dermatology and the American Cancer Society recommend three methods for avoiding excessive exposure to the sun: wear protective clothing, apply sunscreen, and stay out of the midday sun (Mayo Foundation for Medical Education, 2000b).

Knowing Your Skin Phototype

A risk classification system has been developed to help individuals estimate their personal risk for sun damage (Fitzpatrick, Johnson, Wolff, Polano, & Suurmond, 1997). Individuals are classified as belonging to one of six **skin phototypes,** or **SPTs,** depending on their answers to certain questions. Each person is asked, "Do you tan easily?" Persons with SPT I or II answer this question by immediately saying, "No," and persons with SPT III or IV answer, "Yes." Persons with SPT I or II are considered "melanocompromised"; that is, they have a limited capacity to tan after exposure to UVR. Persons in the SPT I category sunburn easily with brief exposure (30 minutes) and never tan. A subgroup of SPT I, SPT II persons sunburn easily but have difficulty tanning. Persons in the SPT III category experience some sunburn with brief exposures but eventually develop a marked tan. SPT IV persons tan easily and do not sunburn with brief exposures. Persons with SPT III or IV are considered "melanocompetent." Approximately 25 percent of white-skinned persons in the United States are SPT I or II. Brown-skinned persons are termed SPT V, and those with black skin are termed SPT VI. The SPT classification of various ethnic groups has not yet been determined, but some Asians and Hispanics have SPT I or II (Fitzpatrick et al., 1997).

Prevent Photoaging

Photoaging, or **dermatoheliosis,** is a skin syndrome that results from an excessive and/or prolonged exposure of the skin to UVR in early life (before age 35) (Fitzpatrick et al., 1997). The incidence of photoaging is most prevalent in persons of skin phototypes I to IV. Even persons in category V, however, are at risk for photoaging if they have a history of prolonged exposure to sunlight or UVR from artificial sources. The most susceptible population for the development of dermatoheliosis are persons with SPT I or II (Fitzpatrick et al., 1997).

The repeated exposure to UVR damages and breaks down the supportive **elastin** and **collagen** fibers in the skin. Elastin and collagen are two types of protein that give the skin its strength and elasticity. Another result of UVR exposure is an alteration in the small blood vessels of the dermis, with resultant decreased circulation to the skin (Fitzpatrick et al., 1997).

The cumulative effects of UVR can cause the skin to lose its resilience—resulting in a tough or weathered appearance, wrinkling, mottled pigmentation, and loose and sagging skin (Mayo Foundation for Medical Education, 2000b, 2000c; National Institute on Aging, 2000). Photo-damaged skin also bruises and tears more easily and takes longer to heal (National Institute on Aging, 2000). Exposure to UVR may also cause **solar keratoses** (rough surface growths) and **solar lentigines** (age spots) to develop. People whose skin has photoaged often look older than their chronological age. Persons with photoaging usually have a history of working in outdoor occupations, such as farming, construction work, and lifeguarding, or of frequently engaging in outdoor sports. Often, there is a family history of dermatoheliosis (Fitzpatrick et al., 1997).

Although sun damage may not be evident in a younger person, it will become evident later in life (National Institute on Aging, 2000). The prevention of sun damage must start in childhood, at birth, and continue throughout the life span. It is never too early to begin protecting the skin from the sun. The sun—specifically, UVA and UVB rays—is responsible for 90 percent of the skin damage and deterioration associated with chronological aging (Melton, 1998).

The treatment of photoaging includes a variety of modalities, including topical therapy such as tretinoin (Retin-A) and alpha hydroxy acids. Tretinoin, a derivative of vitamin A, is available by prescription in lotions, gels, and creams in varying concentrations and may reverse some of the connective tissue damage and vascular changes seen in dermatoheliosis (Fitzpatrick et al., 1997). Alpha hydroxy acids (AHA), usually listed as lactic acid or glycolic acid on the label, are found in many over-the-counter lotions and creams. These products produce a mild shedding of the surface of the skin called **exfoliation** (Mayo Foundation for Medical Education, 2000b). The regular use of AHA-containing products has shown improvement in skin texture, softness, skin discolorations, and fine lines (Kneedler, Sky, & Sexton, 1998). Although the manufacturers of these products say fine lines and wrinkles can be reduced, skin irritation and increased sensitivity to sunlight may occur (Mayo Foundation for Medical Education, 2000b). Until the results of an ongoing FDA research study are known, the FDA recommends that individuals use only alpha hydroxy acid products with clearly labeled ingredients, composed of 10 percent or less of these acids, and with a pH of 3.5 or higher (as the pH increases, the acidity of the product decreases) (Mayo Foundation for Medical Education, 2000b).

Surgical techniques include chemical peels, collagen injections, dermabrasion, laser resurfacing, and cosmetic surgery. Higher concentrations of alpha hydroxy acids are used in so-called salon mini-peels or in **chemical peels** (Mayo Foundation for Medical Education, 2000b). Chemical peels can produce cosmetic benefits, including a reduction in fine lines and wrinkles caused by sun damage (Kneedler et al., 1998). **Collagen** injections (also known as **soft tissue augmentation**) can be used to decrease facial lines caused by solar damage, to reduce scars, and to enhance lips (Lasehair, Incorporated, 2000a, 2000b). Purified animal collagen (bovine) or fat from the person's thigh or abdomen (**autologous fat transfer**) is injected beneath the skin to replenish the natural collagen support layer. Fat transfer reduces the potential for allergic reactions. When bovine collagen is used, a preliminary skin test is performed on the forearm to check for sensitivity to the collagen (Lasehair, Incorporated, 2000b). The test involves waiting four weeks for any reaction. The majority of people do not have reactions to this skin test (Lasehair Incorporated, 2000b). After treatment, an immediate difference in the appearance of the skin is noted. Another surgical technique, **dermabrasion,** the actual sanding down of the skin, can be used to help smooth the outer layer of the skin (Mayo Foundation for Medical Education, 2000b). **Laser resurfacing** is a procedure in which the thin outer layer of the skin is vaporized with a carbon dioxide laser (LeRoy, 1997). The laser produces a shrinking of the underlying tissue, resulting in a tightening of the skin, with reduced or eliminated wrinkles (Mayo Foundation for Medical Education, 2000a). A **cosmetic surgical procedure,** such as a blepharoplasty (eye lift) or rhytidectomy (face lift), can be performed to correct the effects of the sun and aging. Women who wish to have healthy, attractive skin are advised to follow the guidelines below:

- Avoid sun exposure early in life; protect children and teenagers, because the majority of an individual's sun exposure occurs before age 20 (U.S. Environmental Protection Agency, 1995).
- Use daily sunscreen on the parts of the body exposed to the sun. The American Academy of Dermatology (2000b) recommends using a sunscreen with at least a *sun protection factor (SPF) of 15*. Sunscreen products are labeled with a rating known as the **sun protection factor,** or SPF. The SPF indicates the length of time a person can stay in the sun before getting sunburned. For example, if a person would normally burn in 20 minutes without sunscreen, the application of a product with an SPF of 15 allows the person to remain in the sun for approximately 20 × 15, or 300, minutes without burning (Cook, 1997).
- Apply sunscreens liberally at least 30 minutes before going outside. The application of sunscreen at least 30 minutes before sun exposure allows adequate absorption by the skin (Cook, 1997). Avoid under-applying sunscreens. Most people skimp on the

amount of sunscreen used, leaving some people with less than adequate coverage (Brink, 1999; Franz, 1999; Hill, 1999). An ounce (a shot glass full) of sunscreen is required to adequately cover the body and most people use about half this amount (Brink, 1999; Cook, 1997; Franz, 1999; Hill, 1999). If only 50 percent of the recommended amount of sunscreen is applied, the individual receives only 50 percent of the SPF (Franz, 1999). For example, Franz (1999) points out that a consumer who applies only 1 mg/sq cm of SPF 30 may actually receive the sun protection of an SPF of 15.

- Reapply sunscreens after swimming or perspiring. The effectiveness of many sunscreens is diminished after swimming, perspiring, or toweling off.
- Do not sunbathe and/or use tanning salons. In 1998, an estimated 50,000 tanning salons existed in the United States and were increasing at an annual rate of 4 percent (Coldiron, 1998). Tanning salons have erroneously advised consumers that UVR does not harm the skin and that tanning booths provide a safe tan (Coldiron, 1998).
- Avoid going out in the sun between the hours of 10 A.M. and 3 P.M. when the UV rays are strongest.
- If you must be in the sun, wear tight-weave, protective clothing, including long sleeves, slacks or trousers, a hat, and maximum sunscreen. A hat protects several areas, including the eyes, ears, face, and back of the neck.
- Watch for the daily UV index and take precautions to protect your skin.
- Check your skin for signs of skin cancer.

Not Smoking

Women who wish to have youthful, attractive skin should not smoke. Research has demonstrated that smokers tend to develop more wrinkles than nonsmokers of the same age, complexion, and sun exposure history (National Institute on Aging, 2000). In addition, people who smoke are more likely than nonsmokers to experience premature wrinkling (Boyd et al., 1999). Smoking causes **elastosis** (nodular, inelastic, sagging skin), a pale and sallow appearance, and deep wrinkles around the lips, and it impairs the skin's ability to heal (Fitzpatrick et al., 1997; Mayo Foundation for Medical Education, 2000b, 2000c). Boyd et al. (1999) have termed the combination of increased wrinkling, gauntness, and discoloration "smoker's face."

Although a number of studies have demonstrated the effect of smoking on skin function, the exact pathogenic mechanisms involved are not clear (Frances, 1992). Smoking probably causes numerous harmful effects through multiple interactive mechanisms (Frances, 1992). One likely mechanism is a genetic sensitivity to cigarette smoke. The evidence for this mechanism is that the amount of wrinkling among family members who smoke seems to vary widely from family to family. Whereas the members of some families seem to be strongly wrinkle-prone, the members of others develop relatively few wrinkles despite heavy smoking and extensive sun exposure (Frances, 1992).

Another likely mechanism is related to smoking's effect on peripheral vascular blood flow. Both tissue perfusion and oxygenation are decreased in smokers as a result of the vasoconstrictive properties of nicotine, together with the increased carbon monoxide levels in smokers' blood (Frances, 1992; Mills, 1993). This overall reduction in blood flow to the skin is probably involved in the premature aging process (Krupsi, 1991).

One mechanism is particular to women: Cigarette smoking induces an increase in the hydroxylation of estradiol, a precursor of estrogen, thereby leading to a relative **hypoestrogenism** (low estrogen levels). Estrogen plays a role in the maintenance of skin thickness and elasticity. Women who smoke experience a degree of skin dryness and atrophy similar to that experienced by menopausal women who are not on hormone replacement therapy (Frances, 1992).

Finally, cigarette smoking may play a role in skin damage through the various effects of free radicals on elastic tissue metabolism and synthesis (Frances, 1992). As one of the most significant exogenous sources of free radicals, cigarette smoke depletes antioxidant supplies and initiates and accelerates carcinogenic transformation. It also damages proteins and lipids, and it alters the activity of critical enzymes, membrane receptors, and transport proteins (Wolf, Wolf, & Ruocco, 1998). Free radicals are known to damage other organs and are thought to be the major culprits in smoking-related skin damage: "The skin is directly and intensely exposed to cigarette smoke and to smoke from exhalation. It is the first tissue that comes into contact with cigarette smoke and, therefore, is exposed to greater concentrations of free radicals than any other organ in the body, except perhaps the lungs" (Wolf et al., 1998, p. 637). More research is needed on the exact ways in which free radicals in cigarette smoke affect the skin.

Maintain Texture and Hydration

There are a number of strategies for maintaining the texture and hydration of the skin. One is to avoid using harsh soaps, which can irritate and dry the skin. Mild, defatted, or glycerin soaps, such as Dove, Tone, Caress, Alpha Keri, Basis, Eucerin, and Neutrogena, are recommended for the face. Mild facial cleaners, such as Cetaphil, Aveeno, and Aquanil, can also be used to clean facial skin and then rinsed off or wiped off with a cotton pad. Antibacterial soaps are harsh and should never be used on the face. They should be strictly reserved for underarms, genital areas, hands, and feet (Mayo Foundation for Medical Education, 2000a).

The use of a humidifier at home may help relieve dry skin problems. Humidifiers add moisture to the air and create a moister environment for the skin (National Institute on Aging, 2000).

Proper bathing can also have a beneficial effect on skin. Hot water is to be avoided because it can strip the natural oils from the skin and is therefore drying. A daily 10-minute tub bath in water no warmer than 90°F, however, is most beneficial. Previously, experts thought frequent bathing was drying to the skin, but daily soaking is currently recommended (Mayo Foundation for Medical Education, 2000a). After bathing, the skin should be gently dried by first brushing away any excess water with the hands and then patting or blotting the skin with a towel—skin should never be vigorously rubbed or stretched. The skin should be left slightly moist in preparation for the application of bath oil or moisturizer, which seals moisture into the skin (Cook, 1997). Moisturizing creams or lotions, such as Curel, Eucerin, Lubriderm, and Moisturel, are recommended (Mayo Foundation for Medical Education, 2000a; National Institute on Aging, 2000). An inexpensive petrolatum jelly, such as Vaseline, can also be used to preserve the natural moisture of the skin (Cook, 1997).

Being Knowledgeable About Sunscreen Products

Both UVA and UVB rays are harmful and can cause skin damage. UVB causes sunburn, but the more abundant UVA penetrates deeper into the skin and damages it (Cook, 1997; U.S. Environmental Protection Agency, 1995). Although nearly all sunscreen products provide some UVB protection, no product currently available totally screens out UVA rays (Cook, 1997). The SPF protection ratings apply only to UVB rays and indicate only the length of time a person can tolerate the sun without burning (Brink, 1999; Cook, 1997; Melton, 1998). Currently, there is no way to estimate the amount of UVA protection provided by a sunscreen (Cook, 1997).

Some of the ingredients in sunscreens provide protection against UVB rays, some provide a degree of protection against UVA rays, and some do both. Para-aminobenzoic acid (PABA) filters only UVB (Cook, 1997). Zinc oxide, titanium dioxide, and avobenzone provide the best protection from UVA, whereas oxybenzone and parasol 1789 partially blocks UVA and blocks UVB rays (Cook, 1997). Consumers should check the labels of sunscreen products carefully to make sure they will provide a measure of protection from both UVA and UVB rays.

A Food and Drug Administration (FDA) ruling on the labeling of sunscreen products went into effect in May 2001 (Brink, 1999). Claims such as "sunblock," "waterproof," and "all-day protection" are no longer allowed on labels because these terms are inaccurate and give consumers a false sense of security (Hill, 1999). The FDA's decision was based on the facts that (1) nothing completely blocks the sun and (2) any topical lotion is washed off with sufficient sweating or swimming (Brink, 1999). Manufacturers will be able to use the words "water resistant" if a sunscreen survives 40 minutes in the water and "very water resistant" if it continues to work after 80 minutes in the water (Brink, 1999). The sun protection factor (SPF) continues to be required on labels, but the labels no longer identify the exact amount of sun protection factor. Instead, the numbering is reduced to three categories: *minimum*—SPF 2 to 11 for minimal protection; *moderate*—SPF 12 to 29 for moderate protection; and *high*—SPF 30 or higher for maximal protection (Brink, 1999; Hill, 1999). Sunscreen products with an SPF greater than 30 are able to list "30+" on the label (Brink, 1999; Hill, 1999). According to the FDA, SPF numbers higher than 30 cannot be listed because methods for testing their effectiveness are lacking (Brink, 1999). The labeling regarding claims of protection against UVA rays did not change (Brink, 1999). If a sunscreen provides partial protection from UVA and protection from UVB rays, the manufacturer can still use the term "broad spectrum."

The FDA ruling has received much criticism for a number of reasons. Both the American Academy of Dermatology (AAD) and the Skin Cancer Foundation (SCF) claim that the new labels provide misleading information about the amount of sun protection actually provided by a particular product (Hill, 1999; Franz, 1999). The AAD maintains that sunscreen products with an SPF of 15 confer only *minimum* protection, not the *moderate* protection they would be labeled as providing under the new rules. Because the "moderate" category includes an SPF of 12, consumers will have to use "high" category sunscreen products to get the amount of protection recommended. The SCF encourages the use of sunscreen products with an SPF above 30 to compensate for the problem of underapplication (Hill, 1999). According to Hill (1999), the FDA disregarded research evidence indicating that an SPF of 15 provides only minimal protection and set the ranges for SPF protection arbitrarily (Hill, 1999). Although the new labels instruct consumers to apply sunscreens liberally, this is no guarantee that people will change their application habits sufficiently to get adequate coverage (Hill, 1999).

Diseases and Problems of the Skin

The common diseases and problems of the skin include acne vulgaris, rosacea, age spots, and several varieties of skin cancer.

Acne Vulgaris

The term **acne** refers to an inflammation of the hair follicle accompanied by one or more of a variety of skin lesions (Reeves & Maibach, 1998). Vulgaris is the Latin word for "common." Common acne is seen most commonly in adolescent females 10 to 17 years old and males 14 to 19, though it can occur initially at age 25 or older (Fitzpatrick et al., 1997). Women ages 20 to 35 tend to have chronic outbreaks of the lower face, particularly the chin area (Reeves &

Maibach, 1998). Acne is less common in Asian Americans and African Americans. Endocrine factors are thought to play a role; acne occurs more frequently and severely in males than in females (Fitzpatrick et al., 1997; Reeves & Maibach, 1998). Factors other than race and gender that may contribute to the occurrence and severity of acne include heredity, emotional stress, the bacterial flora of the skin, the use of cosmetics and moisturizers, and pressure applied to the skin by the hands or objects (Copstead, 2000; Fitzpatrick et al., 1997; Reeves & Maibach, 1998). Both pregnancy and high-estrogen oral contraceptive use decrease the severity of symptoms (Reeves & Maibach, 1998). Sunlight improves acne in many cases, may have no effect in some persons, or may occasionally aggravate acne in very fair-skinned persons (Reeves & Maibach, 1998). Contrary to popular opinion, exacerbations are *not* related to diet, chocolate, fatty foods, junk foods, vitamins, minerals, or anything the person did or did not do (Fitzpatrick et al., 1997; Reeves & Maibach, 1998).

Acne is caused by a combination of increased sebum (oily material) production by the sebaceous glands, hair follicle obstruction, and bacterial colonization and inflammation (Habif, 1996). The sebum produced by the sebaceous glands prevents drying of the skin and hair (Seidel et al., 1999). Sebaceous gland secretion is under the influence of **hormones**—specifically, androgens (Fitzpatrick et al., 1997; Habif, 1996). In predisposed persons, sebum production increases in the sebaceous glands, allowing a microorganism called *Propionibacterium acnes (P. acnes)* to proliferate in the sebum (Fitzpatrick et al., 1997; Habif, 1996). The overproduction of the epithelial cells that line the hair follicle, called hyperkeratosis, causes loose cells to slough off and block the follicular canal (Copstead, 2000; Fitzpatrick et al., 1997; Habif, 1996). The resultant obstruction of the hair follicle produces the blackheads and whiteheads associated with acne. Bacterial colonization with *P. acnes* and other organisms generates substances, such as lipases and proteases, that cause the intense, inflammatory reaction sometimes seen in acne (Fitzpatrick et al., 1997; Habif, 1996). The treatment of acne vulgaris is directed toward interrupting this cycle of events.

SYMPTOMS

An outbreak of acne vulgaris typically includes a variety of lesions, including both open and closed comedones, papules, pustules, papulopustules, nodules, cysts, and scars. **Open comedones** are known as blackheads; **closed comedones** are called whiteheads. A whitehead contains keratin and lipid debris and appears as a firm, white "bump" (Fitzpatrick et al., 1997; Habif, 1996). A blackhead develops if the follicular opening dilates; the black color is a result of the tyrosine in the follicular orifice being oxidized to melanin (Fitzpatrick et al., 1997). These noninflamed lesions are not painful. **Papules** are raised, firm, circumscribed inflamed areas that are less than one centimeter in diameter (Seidel et al., 1999; Thompson & Wilson, 1996). **Pustules** are in-flamed, raised superficial lesions filled with purulent fluid (Seidel et al., 1999). **Nodules** are elevated, firm circumscribed inflamed lesions that occur deeper in the dermal layer than a papule and are approximately 1 to 2 centimeters in diameter (Thompson & Wilson, 1996). **Cysts** are raised, circumscribed, encapsulated, inflamed lesions that can be found in both the skin and the tissues beneath it. Cysts are filled with liquid or semisolid material (Thompson & Wilson, 1996) and can be found on the face, neck, upper arms, chest or back, or buttocks (Fitzpatrick et al., 1997; Habif, 1996). **Scars** are a natural result of the healing of dermal inflammation, whereby fibrous tissue replaces normal skin (Reeves & Maibach, 1998; Seidel et al., 1999). Scarring can also be related to the aggravation of lesions through manipulation, such as picking and squeezing (Reeves & Maibach, 1998).

TREATMENT

Multiple treatment modalities are used in the management of acne vulgaris. A variety of topical and oral agents are used, depending on the stage of the acne lesions (Habif, 1996). Most cases are controlled by a combination of therapies (Habif, 1996; O'Donoghue, 1999). The application of topical agents to the entire acne-prone area is necessary in order to treat existing lesions and to prevent additional lesions from forming (Habif, 1996; Reeves & Maibach, 1998). Generally, topical agents should be applied in a thin layer. Compliance with the treatment regimen is paramount, especially because it may take several weeks for visible improvement to occur (Reeves & Maibach, 1998).

Comedolytic Agents Agents such as retinoids, sulfur products, and acids, are used to treat both open comedones and closed comedones.

Since the 1970s, topical creams containing tretinoin, a retinoid derivative of vitamin A called all-transretinoic acid, have been available (O'Donoghue, 1999). Tretinoin (also known as Retin-A, retinoic acid, and Vitamin A acid) prevents the obstruction of the sebaceous glands by slowing the deposit of epithelial cells in the sebaceous follicles and improving the penetration of other topical medications (O'Donoghue, 1999). Retin-A cream and Retin-A gel are examples of retinoid products that have been available for many years. Newer products, developed in the late 1990s, include Retin-A micro 0.1 percent gel, Differin gel, and Avita cream. Advances have been made that allow the medications to be delivered slowly, in a less irritating manner, thus preventing redness, burning, and drying.

A newer retinoid, isotretinoin (13-cis-retinoic acid, accutane), a derivative of vitamin A, has been called a "magic bullet" in the treatment of severe acne (Webster, 1998). Isotretinoin works by suppressing sebum production, inhibiting comedo formation, and modulating the inflammatory response (Webster, 1998). The advantages of isotretinoin include its anti-inflammatory action and its ability to reduce both the size of the sebaceous glands and the production of sebum (thereby inhibiting the proliferation of *P. acnes*). Isotretinoin confers prolonged remission after therapy is stopped (months to years) and helps lessen scarring (Habif, 1996; O'Donoghue, 1999; Reeves & Maibach, 1998). The disadvantages of isotretinoin are that it can cause the following: birth defects; ulcerated lips; dry mucous membranes; dry, chapped skin; dry nose or eyes; impaired night vision; hair shedding; joint pain and muscle pain; stiffness; tendonitis; increased serum lipids (total cholesterol, high-density lipoproteins, triglycerides); and elevated liver enzyme levels (Fitzpatrick et al., 1997; O'Donoghue, 1999; Reeves & Maibach, 1998; Webster, 1998). The side effects usually occur early in treatment, and (Reeves & Maibach, 1998) improvement can be slow and occur over a period of two to five months (Fitzpatrick et al., 1997). In 1998, the FDA reported isolated cases of depression, psychosis, and a rare occurrence of suicidal thoughts and behaviors associated with isotretinoin therapy. It was noted that stopping the drug may not be sufficient to remedy these adverse affects (Food and Drug Administration, 2000). Due to isotretinoin's ability to cause birth defects, pregnancy should be avoided during treatment (Fitzpatrick et al., 1997; Habif, 1996), and the drug should not be prescribed for any female of childbearing age if the possibility of pregnancy exists (O'Donoghue, 1999). For any person capable of becoming pregnant, the manufacturer of the drug and the FDA recommend initial pregnancy testing, with a repeat pregnancy test in one month and the initiation of oral contraceptives (Reeves & Maibach, 1998). Only after pregnancy testing has been done twice and oral contraceptive therapy started should isotretinoin therapy be initiated (Reeves & Maibach, 1998). Due to isotretinoin's known side effects and an ongoing investigation of additional side effects, the FDA recommends using isotretinoin only for severe cystic or nodular acne that is unresponsive to other therapy (Reeves & Maibach, 1998). Supplemental therapy with vitamin A should be avoided, due to its potential to increase the side effects of isotretinoin (Reeves & Maibach, 1998). Although isotretinoin is teratogenic (able to cause birth defects), it is not mutagenic (able to cause gene mutations). After discontinuing isotretinoin therapy, women can safely get pregnant, but a waiting period of at least one to two months is recommended (Habif, 1996; O'Donoghue, 1999).

Persons on isotretinoin therapy must have monthly blood work to closely monitor lipid levels and liver function. Relapses occur in about 39 percent of cases, with 23 percent requiring oral antibiotics or additional isotretinoin (Habif, 1996). Multiple courses of therapy may be required; however, the response to repeat treatment is consistently successful and seems to be safe (Habif, 1996).

Sulfur products, such as Sulfacet-R lotion, Klaron lotion, and Novacet cream, have a keratolytic (lesion-removing) and mild antibacterial effect (O'Donoghue, 1999). These agents cause a mild drying and peeling of the skin (Habif, 1996).

They are useful in older persons, very young persons, those with sensitive skin, and those allergic to tretinoin or benzoyl peroxide.

Salicylic acid (referred to as **beta-hydroxy acids**), in concentrations of 20 to 30 percent, is currently used topically for chemical peels of the face (O'Donoghue, 1999). Care must be taken to avoid systemic toxicity (known as salicylism), which is characterized by tinnitus (ear ringing), anemia, renal symptoms, cardiac symptoms, and disturbances in acid-base balance. (O'Donoghue, 1999).

Alpha hydroxy acids (AHAs) are used to interrupt the obstruction of the hair follicle. AHAs decrease the cohesion of keratinocytes and prevent plugging (Kneedler et al., 1998). AHAs also dislodge existing comedones and prevent the formation of new ones. They "unroof" (open up) pustules and loosen keratinocytes lining the follicular epithelium (Kneedler et al., 1998). Glycolic acid, in 4 to 6 percent concentrations, is used to produce a facial peel. The topical preparation is left on the skin for one to five minutes and then rinsed thoroughly with water. Glycolic acid has been used very successfully for acne, in combination with salicylic acid and benzoyl peroxide (Kneedler et al., 1998).

Topical Antibacterial Agents Antibacterial agents, such as benzoyl peroxide, azelaic acid, and antibiotics, are used to attack the major bacterial organism *P. acnes* and to interfere with the inflammatory response.

Benzoyl peroxide, an antibacterial agent, effectively treats inflammatory acne by its lipophilic action, meaning that it is absorbed by the fatty cells of the sebaceous glands. Benzoyl peroxide creates an oxygen-rich environment that is incompatible with *P. acnes* proliferation. In addition to its antibacterial action, benzoyl peroxide prevents the plugging of the hair follicle and may suppress sebum production (Reeves & Maibach, 1998). It is available over-the-counter and by prescriptions in gels, creams, and washes in concentrations of 2.5 percent, 5 percent, and 10 percent (Habif, 1996; O'Donoghue, 1999). Water-based gels cause less drying and irritation than products with an alcohol or acetone base (Reeves & Maibach, 1998). Users should be warned that benzoyl peroxide may bleach colored clothing (O'Donoghue, 1999; Reeves & Maibach, 1998). A small percentage of users develop an allergic contact dermatitis (O'Donoghue, 1999; Reeves & Maibach, 1998).

Azelaic acid, used for mild acne, has been shown to be as effective in preventing comedones as tretinoin and has an antibacterial effect comparable to that of benzoyl peroxide (Reeves & Maibach, 1998). This preparation has a mild depigmenting (bleaching) effect, making it potentially useful for the postinflammatory hyperpigmentation that occurs as a result of acne (O'Donoghue, 1999; Reeves & Maibach, 1998).

Topical erythromycin and topical clindamycin have similar antibacterial and anti-inflammatory effects. Both drugs penetrate the hair follicle to reduce the population of *P. ac-*

nes and are effective in treating papulopustular lesions (Reeves & Maibach, 1998). Topical erythromycin, available in gels, solutions, and topical towelettes, has been shown to be very gentle and safe to use during pregnancy (O'-Donoghue, 1999). Available in solutions, gels, and lotions, topical clindamycin in the 1 percent concentration is also nonirritating to most patients (O'Donoghue, 1999). Both the combination of erythromycin with topical benzoyl peroxide (Benzamycin) and the combination of clindamycin with topical benzoyl peroxide are more effective than either agent alone (O'Donoghue, 1999). Although clindamycin does not need to be refrigerated, Benzamycin requires refrigeration, making this a possible drawback (O'Donoghue, 1999). The safe use of topical clindamycin in pregnancy has not been established (Lookingbill et al., 1997).

Combination Topical Therapy Tretinoin (Retin-A, retinoic acid, or Vitamin A acid) can be combined with topical antibiotic agents with or without benzoyl peroxide (O'Donoghue, 1999; Reeves & Maibach, 1998). Usually, topical antibiotics with or without benzoyl peroxide are applied during the day, with tretinoin applied at bedtime (O'Donoghue, 1999; Reeves & Maibach, 1998). The spacing of the application of these agents is due to their chemical incompatibility (Reeves & Maibach, 1998). Combination topical therapy commonly causes irritated, dry skin.

Oral Antibiotics Several oral antibiotics are used in the treatment of acne. However, oral antibiotics are additive therapies and should not be the sole form of treatment (Fitzpatrick et al., 1997).

For several decades, oral tetracycline has been a major therapeutic agent for papular, pustular, and cystic acne (Habif, 1996; O'Donoghue, 1999). Tetracycline is antiinflammatory, antibacterial, and inexpensive (O'Donoghue, 1999). Its disadvantages include the possible reduction of the efficacy of oral contraceptives, possible gastrointestinal intolerance (such as nausea, vomiting, and diarrhea), photosensitivity, and the potential for *Candida albicans* (yeast) superinfections (O'Donoghue, 1999; Reeves & Maibach, 1998). Tetracycline can stain the primary teeth of fetuses and the secondary teeth of children under the age of nine years. The combination of tetracycline and isotretinoin may cause pseudotumor cerebri, a benign intracranial swelling, and the two should never be used together (Fitzpatrick et al., 1997; Habif, 1996). Tetracycline must be taken on an empty stomach. Certain antacids, iron, and dairy products interfere with the gastrointestinal absorption of this drug.

Oral erythromycin has therapeutic actions and advantages comparable to those of oral tetracycline. It also has lipophilic, anti-inflammatory, and antibacterial actions and is inexpensive. The specific antibiotic chosen for treatment depends on several factors, including the person's age, allergy history (past allergic reactions), and previous therapeutic success with the drug (O'Donoghue, 1999). Erythromycin is safe for persons taking oral contraceptives and will not pose a problem if pregnancy occurs during treatment, although discontinuing oral therapy after pregnancy is confirmed is recommended (O'Donoghue, 1999). Photosensitivity is not associated with erythromycin. Erythromycin's disadvantages include possible gastrointestinal intolerance, the potential for *Candida albicans* superinfections, and a potential resistance on the part of the *P. acnes* organism (Habif, 1996; O'Donoghue, 1999). Usually, it is recommended that erythromycin be taken one hour before or two hours after meals.

Minocycline, a tetracycline derivative, has proven effective in pustular acne cases that have been resistant to other medications, such as tetracycline and erythromycin (Habif, 1996; Reeves & Maibach, 1998). The advantages of minocycline (in comparison with tetracycline and erythromycin) include superior absorption from the gastrointestinal tract, and fewer associated instances of gastrointestinal upset, vaginitis, and photosensitivity. Also, minocycline can be taken with food and in conjunction with isotretinoin. Minocycline's disadvantages include its potential for causing dizziness, hyperpigmentation of the gums and skin, a syndrome resembling lupus erythematosis (see Chapter 20) and hepatitis (inflammation of the liver). Minocycline is also more expensive than tetracycline or erythromycin, but, generic forms are now available (Reeves and Maibach, 1998).

Doxycycline is yet another antibiotic used in the management of acne. Its advantages are similar to those of minocycline (O'Donoghue, 1999; Reeves & Maibach, 1998). It is not known to lead to hepatitis or to the development of the lupus erythematosus–like syndrome (O'Donoghue, 1999). The major disadvantages are its higher potential to cause marked photosensitivity and its cost (Habif, 1996; O'Donoghue, 1999).

When other antibiotics have failed, trimethoprim-sulfamethoxazole (Bactrim) is used for resistant pustular acne (Habif, 1996). The advantages of trimethoprim-sulfamethoxazole include its good absorption from the gastrointestinal tract and its value in treating follicular infections caused by bacteria that are hard to eradicate (Habif, 1996; O'Donoghue, 1999). Its disadvantages include sulfur-allergic reactions (rashes, itching and rash, urticaria), and photosensitivity (Habif, 1996; O'Donoghue, 1999).

Hormonal Therapy Oral contraceptives can be useful in suppressing ovarian hypersecretion of androgens, which can trigger acne (Habif, 1996). The exact mechanism of action is not known, but these drugs do suppress endogenous (produced by the body) hormones and may activate a hormone-binding globulin in the blood that assists in reducing hormone levels. Several products useful in treating acne include Ortho Tricyclic, Demulen, Ovucon 35, Modicon, Brevicon, and Ortho-Novum 7/7/7 (Habif, 1996; O'Donoghue, 1999). Persons taking oral contraceptives must consider the benefits and risks of therapy and be monitored for potential side effects (Reeves & Maibach, 1998). Improvement may not be seen for three months (Reeves & Maibach, 1998).

These signs include premenstrual worsening of acne, a pubic hair line that extends upward on the abdomen, hirsutism (excess body hair), male pattern alopecia (hair loss), and acne lesions on the lower face, jawline, and chin (O'Donoghue, 1999). Spironolactone can also be used for persons in whom other acne treatments have failed (Habif, 1996). Most persons with acne, however, do not have an abnormal level of androgen in their blood (Habif, 1996). The drug spironolactone may be used to treat women whose acne is caused by excessively high blood levels of the androgens testosterone and dehydroepiandrosterone (DHEAS). Such women will experience premenstrual worsening of their acne, and other signs of androgen excess, such as a pubic hair line that extends upward on the abdomen, excess body hair, and male pattern hair loss. Spironolactone works in the hair follicles and sebaceous glands (O'Donoghue, 1999).

Systemic corticosteroids—specifically, glucocorticoids, such as dexamethasone or prednisone—can be used in severe, painful flare-ups of nodular acne to suppress the adrenal production of androgens (Habif, 1996; O'Donoghue, 1999; Reeves & Maibach, 1998). They are also used in acne cases that are nonresponsive to oral contraceptives or spironolactone (Habif, 1996). Glucocorticoids are customarily used for short-term therapy (2 to 4 weeks) (O'Donoghue, 1999; Reeves & Maibach, 1998) but may be prescribed for 6 to 12 months (Habif, 1996). Corticosteroids are useful in persons who are unable to take isotretinoin. They are also used along with isotretinoin, and the combination therapy produces improvement more rapidly than the use of isotretinoin alone (O'Donoghue, 1999). Injecting corticosteroids directly into large nodules can also be effective (Reeves & Maibach, 1998).

Laser Resurfacing Laser resurfacing is used in the treatment of acne-scarred or -pitted skin (LeRoy, 1997). In laser resurfacing, a carbon dioxide laser is used to vaporize the top and middle layers of the skin, depending on the condition of the skin (LeRoy, 1997). The laser emits intense light, which penetrates to a depth only about half the thickness of a human hair, thus minimizing the risk of burning (LeRoy, 1997). Laser resurfacing causes a tightening, smoothing, or remolding of the outer layer of the skin by shrinking the skin's collagen strands (LeRoy, 1997). Three days after treatment, the skin appears red and forms a slight crust. The skin is kept moist with topical ointments or semipermeable dressings, and the crust peels in about a week. It takes an additional one to two weeks for the vaporized layers of the skin to regenerate. Additional dressings or ointments are needed during this time. Postoperative skin care includes hydration and protection from UV light (LeRoy, 1997).

Allograft Dermis Residual scars from acne can be treated with a relatively new option called allograft dermis. A new graft material (Alloderm) has been developed from human skin obtained from tissue banks in the United States. The obtained skin is processed to produce an acellular (all the cells are removed) matrix that has the structure of normal human collagen. The advantages include the elimination of a rejection response (due to a lack of cells); a low infection rate; the ability to use the grafts for up to two years after processing, if kept refrigerated; and the ability to customize the graft material to the size and depth of person's scar or skin depression (Besecker & Hart, 1999). After the scarred areas are marked and the face scrubbed with an antiseptic, rehydrated grafts are inserted into "pockets" created by the back-and-forth motion of a needle (Besecker & Hart, 1999). Black-and-blue marks may be visible for a few days and slight swelling at the graft sites may persist for several weeks. Postoperative care includes keeping Steri-strips in place for three days and applying topical antibiotic ointment.

Psychological and Emotional Treatment The cosmetic disfigurement related to acne, especially its facial lesions and scarring, is a major source of psychological and emotional distress (Besecker & Hart, 1999; Fitzpatrick et al., 1997). Mallon and others (1999) reported that persons with severe acne had levels of social, psychological, and emotional problems as great as those reported by persons with chronic disabling disorders, such as asthma, epilepsy, diabetes, back pain, and arthritis. Acne is certainly not a trivial disease and may have a substantial impact on a person's quality of life (Mallon et al., 1999). Each person needs to be individually evaluated regarding her ability to cope with the disease and her need for psychological or psychiatric therapy or intervention (Fitzpatrick et al., 1997). As Reeves and Maibach (1998) note, the myths related to acne occurrence, such as acne's being related to dietary intake, must be destroyed and the misplaced guilt relieved.

Rosacea

Rosacea, pronounced "rose-ay-sha," comes from the Latin word meaning "like roses" (Fitzpatrick et al., 1997). Rosacea is a chronic, acnelike disorder that affects the hair follicles of the face. It is characterized by increased capillary reactivity to heat, with resultant flushing and ultimately telangiectasia (Fitzpatrick et al., 1997). Telangiectasia (pronounced "tell-an-jek-taze-yah") is a permanent dilation of superficial capillaries and small veins which manifests as fine, red lines (Estes, 1998; Thompson & Wilson, 1996). The affected areas blanch with direct pressure (Thompson & Wilson, 1996). Although it was previously called acne rosacea, this disorder is unrelated to true acne but often coexists with it. Acne may have preceded the onset of the rosacea (Fitzpatrick et al., 1997). Rosacea can cause significant cosmetic disfigurement (Fitzpatrick et al., 1997).

Rosacea occurs mostly in fair-skinned adults, especially women ages 30 to 50, with peak incidence between the ages of 40 and 50. Rosacea occurs most frequently in persons of Celtic and southern Italian ancestry, but rarely in brown- or black-skinned persons (Fitzpatrick et al., 1997; Reeves & Maibach, 1998). For some unknown reason, women develop rosacea more often than men, with some cases associated with menopause (American Academy of Dermatology, 2000a). Children are rarely affected by this disorder (Weedon, 1997). Skin changes in rosacea are gradual and develop over prolonged periods of time (American Academy of Dermatology, 2000a; National Rosacea Society, 2000). Rosacea is a chronic disorder characterized by cycles of remissions and exacerbations, and it progresses with a gradual worsening of symptoms (National Rosacea Society, 2000).

The pathogenesis of rosacea is poorly understood (Weedon, 1997), and the exact cause of rosacea is presently unknown (American Academy of Dermatology, 2000a). Rosacea is a multiphasic disease, and various factors are most likely responsible for its stages. The heightened vascular reactivity seen in fair-skinned individuals who blush easily is a major precipitating factor (Webster, 1998). Other factors include frequent blushing, exposure to sunlight (especially in combination with frequent blushing), and alcohol consumption, which dilates blood vessels in the face and elsewhere (Higgins & duVivier, 1999).

Recent interest has focused on *Heliobacter pylori* as a possible causative agent; however, the research results are inconclusive at best. Rebora, Drago, and Parodi (1995) found that 84 percent of the 31 patients with rosacea in their study were *Heliobacter pylori* positive. However, Sharma, Lynn, Kaminski, Vasudeva, and Howden (1998) found that although the patients with rosacea in their study reported more indigestion and antacid use, they were not more likely than the patients without rosacea to be infected with heliobacter (Sharma et al., 1998). Additional large case-control studies are needed before a causal relationship between Heliobacter pylori and rosacea can be established (Rebora et al., 1995).

The development of rosacea was also reported in three persons infected with the human immunodeficiency virus (HIV) (Vin-Christian, Maurer, & Berger, 1994), and those patients responded well to standard therapy. Finally, there has been one case report of a rosacea-like eruption thought to be a result of megadoses of vitamin B-6 and vitamin B-12 (Sherertz, 1991). That causal link is strengthened by the fact that the facial eruption did not respond to usual treatment but improved dramatically after the vitamin supplement was discontinued (Sherertz, 1991). More research on the etiological factors of rosacea is warranted.

SYMPTOMS

Persons with rosacea usually have a long history of flushing in response to heat stimuli in the form of hot liquids, spicy foods, sun exposure, hot baths, or hot weather. They typically also experience flushing after alcohol ingestion and in cold weather (Fitzpatrick et al., 1997; National Rosacea Society, 1998). Although acne may have preceded the onset of rosacea by sev-

---

Box 18–1   Most Common Rosacea Triggers (Percentage of People)

◆ Sun exposure	61 percent
◆ Emotional stress	60 percent
◆ Hot weather	53 percent
◆ Alcohol	45 percent
◆ Spicy foods	43 percent
◆ Exercise	39 percent
◆ Wind	38 percent
◆ Hot baths	37 percent
◆ Cold weather	36 percent
◆ Hot drinks	36 percent
◆ Skin care products	24 percent

Source: Adapted from National Rosacea Society (1998). *Coping with rosacea: Tips on lifestyle management for rosacea sufferers.* Barrington, IL: Author.

---

eral years, rosacea frequently arises without any preceding history of acne or other skin problems (Fitzpatrick et al., 1997). Emotional stress, wind, exercise, and skin care products are other factors that can aggravate flare-ups of rosacea (National Rosacea Society, 1998). Occasionally, an embarrassing or tense moment triggers flushing (American Academy of Dermatology, 2000a). See Box 18–1 for a list of the most common triggers of rosacea flare-ups, based on a National Rosacea Society survey of more than 400 rosacea sufferers.

Rosacea can lead to the development of **rhinophyma,** enlargement of the nose, which is more common in men (Galderma Laboratories, 1997). This disease can also lead to the development of a cushionlike swelling of the forehead; a swelling of the eyelids; a cauliflower-like swelling of the earlobes; and a swelling of the chin (Fitzpatrick et al., 1997). The disfigurement of the nose, forehead, eyelids, ears, and chin are a result of sebaceous gland hyperplasia and lymphedema (Fitzpatrick et al., 1997). Approximately 50 percent of persons with rosacea have vision problems due to eye involvement (American Academy of Dermatology, 2000a). Rosacea can lead to keratitis, which is an inflammation of the cornea, and chronic inflammation of the eyelids (blepharitis), conjunctiva (conjunctivitis), and episclera (episcleritis) (Fitzpatrick et al., 1997).

The National Rosacea Society (1998) has identified three stages of rosacea: early, middle and advanced. The early stage is characterized by intermittent episodes of redness on the cheeks, nose, forehead, or chin. Tiny blood vessels (**telangiectasia**), which blanche under direct pressure, may be visible on the skin's surface (Thompson & Wilson, 1996).

Conjunctivitis (inflammation of the eyelids mucous membranes) may cause the eyes to have a gritty sensation or appear watery or bloodshot. In the middle stage, the facial redness becomes permanent, tiny bumps or pimples may appear, and blood vessels may become more visible. The eyes may be more bloodshot. In the advanced stage, inflammation is more severe, and the nose may become red, bumpy, and swollen due to excessive tissue. In this stage, inflammation of the eyes and surrounding areas may result in loss of vision.

TREATMENT

A cure for rosacea is not available at this time, but compliance with treatments and lifestyle modifications can reduce the symptoms and progression of the disorder (National Rosacea Society, 1998). Treatments including topical medications, oral medications, and surgery to reduce or eliminate symptoms. Early intervention and treatment is a key element in keeping rosacea from worsening and preventing enlargement of the blood vessels or enlargement of the nose (Galderma Laboratories, 1997). A combination of treatments is frequently recommended.

Due to the lack of familiarity with rosacea, many people do not recognize this disorder in its earliest stages. If left untreated, rosacea usually worsens and may be more difficult to treat (American Academy of Dermatology, 2000a). Self-diagnosis and treatment are strongly discouraged, due to possible worsening of the condition by some over-the-counter remedies (American Academy of Dermatology, 2000a).

Topical Therapy   Topical therapies include metronidazole gel, corticosteroid creams, and benzoyl peroxide and erythromycin gels. Metro Gel or cream in 0.75 percent concentration is effective in reducing papules, pustules, and erythema in persons with rosacea (Fitzpatrick et al., 1997). A thin layer of medication is applied to a clean, dry face twice a day, morning and evening. Metronidazole's exact action is not known, but it may have antibacterial and anti-inflammatory effects.

Mild corticosteroid creams, such as hydrocortisone 1 percent, may be used to reduce redness (Reeves & Maibach, 1998). These creams are applied twice daily. Rosacea may be worsened by potent topical corticosteroids (Reeves & Maibach, 1998).

Benzoyl peroxide gel can be effective for the papulopustular component of rosacea (Reeves & Maibach, 1998). (See the section Acne Vulgaris for details on this medication.) Erythromycin gel can also be used topically (Fitzpatrick et al., 1997).

Oral Antibiotics   Tetracycline is started in divided doses until lesions clear and is gradually reduced to a daily dose. Minocycline and doxycycline, usually given twice a day, are alternative antibiotics used in the management of rosacea. Doxycycline has the potential to cause marked photosensitivity. Both minocycline and doxycycline are more expensive than tetracycline. (See the section Acne Vulgaris for information on the advantages and disadvantages of these drugs.)

Oral Isotretinoin   Oral isotretinoin is used in persons with severe cases of rosacea who do not respond to antibiotics (Fitzpatrick et al., 1997). (See the section Acne Vulgaris for detailed information on its use and potential side effects.)

Surgical/Laser Treatment   Dermabrasion can help smooth the outer layer of the skin (Mayo Foundation for Medical Education, 2000b). Excess tissue related to rhynophyma can be removed with a scalpel, with a laser, or through electrosurgery (American Academy of Dermatology, 2000a). Laser therapy can also be used to destroy dilated blood vessels and dramatically reduce redness.

Lifestyle Modifications   Lifestyle modifications can assist persons with rosacea to cope with the disorder (National Rosacea Society, 1998). The following strategies are recommended:

- Wear sunscreen with an SPF of 15 or higher all year round.
- Stay in air-conditioned environments on hot, humid days.
- Cover the cheeks and nose with a scarf in cold weather.
- Use a moisturizer daily during cold weather.
- Use stress-management techniques (see Chapter 7).
- Monitor your reaction to alcoholic beverages and reduce or avoid intake if indicated.
- Avoid common aggravating spices, such as the various kinds of pepper.
- Decrease the temperature in heated beverages and reduce your intake.
- Discover and avoid foods that cause flushing.
- Use warm water and gentle cleansers on the face morning and night.
- Modify bathing routines by avoiding hot water, hot tubs, and saunas.
- Avoid pulling, tugging, rubbing, or scratching the face with the hands or objects, such as sponges, washcloths, and loofahs.
- Apply medication or skin care products to clean, dry skin.
- Modify exercise routines by avoiding heavy exertion or high-intensity workouts that aggravate overheating or flushing.
- Break up exercise workouts into shorter, more frequent sessions—such as 15 minutes twice a day, rather than 30 minutes all at once.
- Avoid overheating while exercising indoors by using a fan or air conditioner or by opening windows for appropriate ventilation.
- Stay cool while exercising by drinking cool liquids, chewing on ice, or spraying cool water on your face.

Age Spots

Age spots, commonly known as "liver spots," are flat, irregularly shaped, pigmented **macules** (flat lesions) that appear on the sun-exposed surfaces of the body (Thompson & Wilson, 1996). The hyperpigmentation is due to aging and accumulated sun damage. The medical terms for them include **lentigo** or **lentigines, lentigo simplex, solar lentigines,** and **senile lentigines.**

Age spots affect more than 90 percent of fair-skinned Euro-American and Asian American adults in middle age (Mayo Foundation for Medical Education, 2000b). Younger individuals may develop age spots in sunny climates. Age spots occur equally among men and women (Fitzpatrick et al., 1997). They are most commonly found on body surface areas having repeated exposure to the sun, especially the face, the backs of the hands, and the back (Mayo Foundation for Medical Education, 2000b; Thompson & Wilson, 1996). They become more numerous with advancing age (Weedon, 1997).

The development of age spots is related to freckling during adolescence and frequent sunburns during adulthood (Weedon, 1997). Although the exact pathogenesis is unknown, chronic exposure to the sun is believed to cause **melanocytes** (cells that produce the skin-darkening pigment, melanin) to proliferate and cause an uneven pigmentation of the skin (Estes, 1998; Fitzpatrick et al., 1997).

Symptoms

Gray, light to dark brown, or black spots are present on sun-exposed areas of the body (Mayo Foundation for Medical Education, 2000b; Weedon, 1997). Flat macules from 3 mm to 3 cm in diameter develop on the face, hands, or back (Fitzpatrick et al., 1997; Mayo Foundation for Medical Education, 2000b; Weedon, 1997). Some age spots are as large as 5 cm (Fitzpatrick et al., 1997). Age spots are frequently multiple and can increase in size over several years (Weedon, 1997). Sun exposure can darken age spots (Mayo Foundation for Medical Education, 2000b). True age spots do not become cancerous (Mayo Foundation for Medical Education, 2000b).

Treatment

Although medical treatment is not needed (Mayo Foundation for Medical Education, 2000b), persons with age spots frequently seek treatment for cosmetic reasons. Several over-the-counter topical medications are available that help fade the hyperpigmented areas, including Porcelana, Nude It Fade Cream, and Esoterica. Over-the-counter creams, called "bleaching agents" by the FDA, contain hydroquinone, which inhibits melanin production in the lower layers of the epidermis (American Pharmaceutical Association, 1996; Pray, 1999), slowly allowing the skin to fade. Skin changes can be seen as soon as three weeks to up to three months. It is generally thought that, if no improvement is seen in three months, treatment should be discontinued (American Pharmaceutical Association, 1996). When the use of hydroquinone products is discontinued, the color usually returns (Reeves & Maibach, 1998). Persons using hydroquinone-containing products should apply them in a thin layer twice a day, avoid getting the cream in the eye, and avoid sun exposure (wear sunscreen, protective clothing, and limit sun exposure) (Pray, 1999). When using hydroquinone, sun exposure is counterproductive, because the sun promotes melanin production (Pray, 1999). The possible disadvantages of hydroquinone include irritation, contact dermatitis, a change in nail color from applying the product to the skin, and transient **leukoderma,** or lighter skin (American Pharmaceutical Association, 1996; Pray, 1999). A more serious adverse reaction called ochronosis was initially reported in South African women who used hydroquinone to lighten their skin tone (Pray, 1999). **Ochronosis** involves an ochre or blue-black discoloration of the skin on the cheeks, forehead, nose, sides of neck, and around the eyes. The prolonged use of hydroquinone for overall lightening of the skin can cause the skin to darken (Pray, 1999). In the United States, cases of ochronosis have been reported in Hispanics and African Americans using over-the-counter products containing the FDA-approved maximum of 2 percent hydroquinone (Pray, 1999). Dark-skinned persons should be cautioned not to use these products for overall lightening of the skin.

Other over-the-counter products, such as Retinol Actif Pur and Plentitude Revitalift moisturizers and face creams, contain a form of retinol (vitamin A) and other ingredients to minimize the effects of the sun. Several lotions and creams by Alpha Hydrox and others contain glycolic acid, a type of alpha hydroxy acid (AHA), which may improve skin discolorations (Kneedler et al., 1998). Many of these products also contain sunscreens. Prescription topical medications, such as tretinoin (Retin-A) in gels, lotions, and creams can be used for age spots. It may take several months for tretinoin to lighten age spots (Reeves & Maibach, 1998).

Chemical peels involve applying acids to burn the outer layer of the skin, causing the skin to peel off and allowing the regeneration of new, smoother evenly pigmented skin (Mayo Foundation for Medical Education, 2000b). The acids used in chemical peels are stronger than those available in topical creams. Trichloroacetic acid and phenol are commonly used acids. Some dermatologists are using concentrated alpha hydroxy acids for chemical peels (Kneedler et al., 1998). The contraindications for chemical peels include recent dermabrasion or other chemical peels; prior radiation; having had a reaction to topical retinoic acid, glycolic acid, or the anticancer drug 5-fluorouracil; current use of oral retinoids, antiplatelet agents, or photosensitizing agents; a history of herpes simplex; pregnancy; and a history of collagen disease or autoimmune disease (Kneedler et al., 1998). After the chemical peel, the skin forms a scab for about 10 days and appears pink for approximately three months. The potential complications of chemical peels include scarring, permanently lighter skin (hypopigmentation), blotchy skin, and an increased susceptibility to sunburn (LeRoy, 1997; Mayo Foundation for Medical Education, 2000b).

Dermabrasion is another technique used to reduce age spots, and wrinkling as well. The skin is literally sanded down with a small, rotating, abrasive wheel (Mayo Foundation for Medical Education, 2000b). The technique causes a scab to form, along with swelling that usually lasts a few weeks.

Laser resurfacing is another effective treatment for age spots and wrinkles. Its advantages include predictable and reproducible results (LeRoy, 1997), as well as suitability for persons who may not be candidates for chemical peels.

Actinic Keratoses

Actinic keratoses, also called **solar** or **senile keratoses,** are premalignant lesions found on the sun-exposed surfaces of the skin (Huether, 1998). The vast majority of lesions occur on the upper limbs, head, and neck (Salasche, 2000). They appear as skin-colored or red, rough patches or elevated bumps (Moy, 2000). The surrounding areas have tiny blood vessels (Huether, 1998).

The prevalence of actinic keratoses is highest in middle-aged to elderly Euro-American persons with a history of significant UVR exposure (Cockerell, 2000; Huether, 1998; Salasche, 2000). Individuals with darker skin have the potential to develop actinic keratoses if they go out in the sun with unprotected skin (Northeast Dermatology Associates, 2000), but they are rare in African Americans. Actinic keratoses are more prevalent in males, especially those who had outdoor recreational or occupational exposure in the early decades of their lives (Salasche, 2000). The occurrence of actinic keratoses increases with age (Salasche, 2000).

A genetic propensity, a history of cumulative sun damage, and immunosuppression increase the likelihood of developing actinic keratoses (Northeast Dermatology Associates, 2000; Salasche, 2000). Fair-skinned persons with light-colored eyes, such as blue or green or hazel, and red or blonde hair are at particular risk. Additional risk-enhancing characteristics possessed by such individuals is that they don't tan well, they sunburn easily, and they tend to develop freckles (Salasche, 2000). Repetitive sun exposure over several decades also increases the risk for actinic keratoses (Salasche, 2000). Immunosuppression due to cancer chemotherapy, acquired immune deficiency syndrome (AIDS), or organ transplantation increases the potential for developing actinic keratoses (Northeast Dermatology Associates, 2000).

Actinic keratoses are formed when the ultraviolet radiation in sunlight causes keratocytes, or skin cells, to change their structure and proliferate. The structural change is manifested primarily as mutations in a specific gene called p53 (Cockerell, 2000). When confined to the top layer of the skin, the new cell clusters are called actinic keratoses; when they extend to the deeper tissues, they are called **squamous cell carcinoma** (Cockerell, 2000). Both actinic keratoses and squamous cell carcinomas represent different stages of the same disease; actinic keratoses represent skin cancer in its earliest stages (Cockerell, 2000). Lesions may remain stable, or they may enlarge and extend into the deeper layers of the skin. As neoplastic cells extend into the deeper layers, they may spread to distant sites. There is no way to predict which actinic keratosis will progress into carcinoma or which individual will develop metastatic cancer (Cockerell, 2000).

The term *actinic keratosis* was originally developed on the basis of the clinical appearance and texture of the lesions; it does not reflect their histopathology or pathobiology. Cockerell (2000) proposes that the term *actinic keratoses* be eliminated and replaced with a more appropriate term, such as *keratinocytic intraepidermal neoplasia (KIN)* or *solar keratotic intraepidermal squamous cell carcinoma*, in order to more accurately describe the underlying pathobiology.

SYMPTOMS

Actinic keratoses manifest as elevated red or skin-colored papules or plaques that are flat-topped and rough (Moy, 2000). Commonly, these scaly areas are found on the sun-exposed areas of the face, back of the hand, or bald scalp, and the scaliness is frequently felt before it is seen. The lesions range from 1 mm to several centimeters in diameter. There can be one or many, and they are sometimes joined together. Broken blood vessels, yellowish discoloration, or blotchy pigmentation may be evident in surrounding areas (Moy, 2000). A progression to thickened, hypertrophic lesions and subsequently to squamous cell carcinoma is possible. Thickened lesions may be indistinguishable from squamous cell carcinoma without a biopsy. Actinic lesions may be tender and may itch or burn. A pigmented actinic keratosis may resemble a scaling age spot (Moy, 2000). **Pinguecula** are actinic keratoses that develop on the conjunctiva of the eye. Actinic keratoses occurring on the lips are known as **actinic chelitis.** The patient may report dry, rough, and scaling lips and may have areas of ulceration or fissures.

TREATMENT

As there is no definite way to distinguish between an actinic keratosis and a squamous cell carcinoma without performing a biopsy, aggressive treatment is recommended (Moy, 2000). **Cryotherapy,** or freezing the lesions with liquid nitrogen by a spray device or cotton-tipped applicator, provides quick, effective treatment (Dinehart, 2000). Healing occurs in one to two weeks. This therapy rarely results in hypopigmentation (the loss of pigment), hyperpigmentation (increased pigment), scarring, textural skin changes, blisters, or infection. The lesions can also be surgically removed, which provides tissue for cellular analysis. If, for some reason, a lesion is not removed, it should continue to be evaluated for progression to squamous cell carcinoma. Individuals who have already developed actinic keratoses must use protective clothing or sunscreen to prevent lesions from developing elsewhere (Huether, 1998).

Topical 5-fluorouracil (such as Fluoroplex, Efudex) is used for multiple actinic keratoses on widespread areas of the body. It selectively destroys lesions with minimal effect on the adjacent normal skin. The medication is applied twice a day for two to four weeks (Dinehart, 2000). Topical 5-fluorouracil causes discomfort, including pain, itching, and burning at the application site. Patients require adequate preparation for the "normal effects," including redness, inflammation, and ulceration (Dinehart, 2000). Direct sunlight should be avoided during treatment in order to prevent intense pain and discomfort from sun exposure (Dinehart, 2000). Persons who have multiple lesions, have a high pain threshold, and are compliant are the best candidates for this treatment. The medication's expense may be a drawback, however.

Masoprocol cream, 10 percent, a newer topical treatment, is used for 28 days. Its common side effects include erythema and flaking, with most reactions reported as mild to moderate (Northeast Dermatology Associates, 2000).

Another newer treatment, Levulan PDT therapy, has been approved for facial and scalp actinic keratoses (American Cancer Society, 2000e). This therapy involves the application of Levulan (5-aminolevulinic acid) to an actinic keratosis lesion, followed 14–18 hours later by photodynamic therapy (PDT) (DUSA Pharmaceuticals, 2000). The drug is applied with a Kerastick™, a pencil-sized device developed by DUSA Pharmaceuticals for applying the appropriate dose. The absorption of Levulan by the rapidly dividing cells of the lesion causes a conversion into a light-sensitive drug activated by a light source. The patient wears protective eyewear, as the lesion is exposed to blue light for approximately 15 minutes. A tingling or burning sensation is experienced during therapy, with the formation of scales or crusts in a few days. This is the first treatment for actinic keratoses that targets only the lesions and not normal skin (Intelligent Network Concepts, 2000).

Curettage and electrosurgery are used to scrape the lesion, and electrocautery—heat applied through an electric needle—controls bleeding at the surgical site.

Skin Cancers

Skin cancer is the most prevalent of all cancers. The American Academy of Dermatology (2000b) has referred to skin cancer as an undeclared epidemic. In 2000, the American Cancer Society (2000a) has estimated that 1.3 million new cases of highly curable basal and squamous cell cancers will be diagnosed. A more deadly form of skin cancer, melanoma, is expected to occur in approximately 47,700 persons. Overall, skin cancer deaths are projected to be between 9,600 and 7,700 from melanoma with another 1,900 from other skin cancers. This is tragic, as the vast majority of skin cancers could be prevented if people would protect their skin from the sun's rays.

RISK FACTORS

The overexposure to sunlight is universally accepted by the medical community as the principal cause of skin cancer—especially sun exposure that results in sunburn and blistering (American Academy of Dermatology, 2000b). Exposure to UVR from tanning lights and booths also places people at greater risk (American Cancer Society, 2000b). Other etiological factors include fair (light-colored) skin, repeated exposure to medical and industrial Xrays, occupational exposure to chemicals (such as coal, arsenic, or insecticides), the presence of scarring from disease processes or burns, and a family history of skin cancer (American Academy of Dermatology, 2000b; American Cancer Society, 2000d). The risk for skin cancer is more than 20 times greater for Euro-Americans than for dark-skinned African Americans due to the UVR protective effect of the skin pigment melanin (American Cancer Society, 2000d). Immunosuppression, such as after organ transplantation, and radiation therapy may also increase the risk (Leber et al., 1999). Smoking doubles the risk of developing squamous cell carcinoma of the skin, but not basal cell carcinoma. The reason for this difference is not clear, but both local and systemic effects are thought to play a role in the process of carcinogenesis (Mills, 1993).

Whereas the development of melanoma is strongly correlated with intermittent, intense exposure to UV radiation, the development of SCC and BCC skin cancers is correlated with chronic, cumulative sun exposure (Lang, 1998; Leber et al., 1999). A history of having suffered three or more blistering or severe sunburns as a child or adolescent (before age 20) increases a person's risk for developing melanoma as an adult (Lang, 1998; Leber et al., 1999). Melanoma occurs more frequently in light-skinned individuals who live close to the equator; the highest incidence is in Queensland, Australia (Lang, 1998; Weedon, 1997). The increased incidence in Queensland is related to the intense solar radiation in that location and the Celtic background of the population (Lang, 1998). Being fair-skinned; having red or blonde hair and blue eyes; having a history of freckling, especially on the upper back; tanning poorly; and sunburning easily increase one's risk of developing melanoma (Lang, 1998). Although the risk is 20 times higher for Euro-Americans than African Americans, persons with darkly pigmented skin *can* develop melanoma, especially on the palms of the hands, on the soles of the feet, under the nails, and inside the mouth, with rare involvement of the internal organs (American Cancer Society, 2000b).

Outdoor summer jobs as a teenager for three or more years and actinic keratoses also increase the risk for melanoma (Leber et al., 1999), as does having numerous nevi (moles), whether atypical or normal in appearance (Lang, 1998; Weedon, 1997).

A familial history of melanoma is another risk factor. Family members of melanoma patients tend to have many large moles, which are frequently atypical in appearance, and tend to develop initial melanomas at a young age and additional melanomas over their lifetimes (Lang, 1998). Another risk factor is a history of exposure to sun-tanning devices.

Approximately one-half of all melanomas occur in persons over the age of 50, but persons in their twenties and thirties can develop it also. It is interesting to note that melanoma is the most common form of skin cancer in the under-30 age group (American Cancer Society, 2000b).

Malignant melanomas develop from a malignant transformation of melanocytes, or pigment cells, present in the epidermis (Leber et al., 1999). Melanomas usually occur on the sun-exposed areas of the body but can also occur in nonexposed areas (Leber et al., 1999). Initially, the tumor cells grow in a radial pattern and are confined to the epidermis and upper dermis. The disease can be cured during this so-called grace period (Fitzpatrick et al., 1997). The radial growth phase is followed by invasive vertical growth, in which cells invade the dermis, with a possible metastatic spread. The exact pathophysiological mechanism involved is not yet understood.

Three skin lesions are considered potential precursors of melanoma: congenital nevomelanocytic nevus (CNN), Clark's melanocytic nevus (CMN), and lentigo maligna (LM). CNN is a benign, pigmented lesion usually present at birth or by early infancy (Fitzpatrick et al., 1997). It is equally prevalent in males and females and occurs in all ethnic groups. These nevi, or growths, can be very small or large enough to cover an entire segment of a person's trunk, head, neck, or extremity. They can be light or dark brown; can be oval, round, or irregular in shape; and can have regular or irregular borders. The skin surface may be distorted in some way, and coarse hair may be present. Regardless of size, all CNN lesions may eventually give rise to malignant melanoma. Although the exact risk is not known, persons with CNN may have an average 6 percent lifetime risk of developing melanoma (American Cancer Society, 2000b).

Another potential precursor of melanoma, Clark's melanocytic nevus is a pigmented lesion with a clearly delineated border. CMN can look like typical moles but can also resemble melanomas. They appear in late childhood, usually prior to the onset of puberty, but new lesions continue to develop over many years throughout a person's lifetime (Fitzpatrick et al., 1997). CMN are known to develop in Euro-Americans, but no data are available on their incidence in African Americans. Japanese Americans are not known to develop CMN. The lifetime risk of developing melanoma for a person with CMN is between 6 and 10 percent, depending on factors such as age, family history, and the number of lesions (American Cancer Society, 2000b).

The skin lesion lentigo maligna is the precursor of the relatively uncommon form of melanoma lentigo, maligna melanoma. LM lesions are flat and irregularly bordered and may be tan, brown, or black. They have a stainlike quality, with striking variations in color. They usually occur as single lesions on sun-exposed areas of the body and are most common in Euro-Americans, especially those with skin photo-

types I, II, and III. They are rare in brown and black-skinned persons (Fitzpatrick et al., 1997). A change in the pigmentation to a darker brown or black, and the development of elevated plaques, signify that the lesion has invaded the dermis and has become a lentigo maligna melanoma. The percentage of lentigo maligna lesions that evolve into lentigo maligna melanoma ranges from 5 to 8 percent (Fitzpatrick et al., 1997).

Squamous cell carcinomas account for 20 percent of all skin malignancies. They are frequently seen in persons with outdoor occupations and in industrial workers exposed to carcinogens (Fitzpatrick et al., 1997). SCC is the second most common form of cancer in Euro-Americans and the most common type of skin cancer in African Americans (Leber et al., 1999). More than two-thirds of all skin cancers in African Americans are SCCs, and they commonly develop on sites of pre-existing inflammation, injury, or trauma (Leber et al., 1999). Men are three times more likely to develop SCCs than women (American Cancer Society, 2000d).

Squamous cell carcinomas arise from keratinocytes in the upper layers of the epidermis. They usually develop from an **actinic keratosis** confined to the epidermis (Fitzpatrick et al., 1997). Actinic keratoses and squamous cell carcinomas represent different stages of the same disease. SCC lesions can either remain stable within the dermis or extend and metastasize to distant sites (Cockerell, 2000). There is no way to predict which precancerous conditions will progress into carcinoma or which individual will develop metastatic cancer.

Basal cell carcinomas make up 75 percent of nonmelanoma skin cancers and are the most common skin cancers. They occur frequently in Euro-Americans and occasionally in black- and brown-skinned persons (Porth, 1998). Men are twice as likely as women to develop BCCs (American Cancer Society, 2000d). While BCCs are more often seen in men after age 40, SCCs occur more frequently in men after the age of 50 (Leber et al., 1999).

Basal cell carcinomas arise from the deepest layer of the epidermis, the basal cell layer (American Cancer Society, 2000d). These growths tend to slowly grow upward and laterally or downward to the junction of the dermal and epidermal layers. BCCs can invade the surrounding tissues, such as the nose, eyelid, or ear, causing severe local destruction, which may require extensive surgical excision. Metastasis to bone or distant sites is rare because tumor invasion of blood or lymph vessels is uncommon (Huether, 1998).

SYMPTOMS

The ways in which malignant melanomas manifest vary according to their type. Melanomas are classified into four major types based on their growth pattern (Leber et al., 1999). Superficial spreading melanoma is the most common, accounting for about 70 percent of all melanomas (Fleischer, Herbert, Feldman, & O'Brian, 2000). They are typically found on the upper backs of men and women and the legs of women. Nodular melanomas account for about 20 percent of melanomas

Figure 18–2   Clark's Levels for Staging the Invasion of a Melanoma

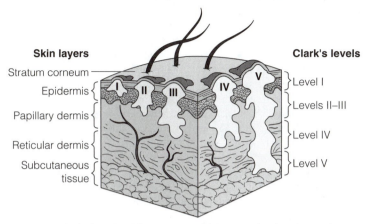

Skin layers / Clark's levels

Stratum corneum — Level I
Epidermis — Levels II–III
Papillary dermis — Level IV
Reticular dermis — Level V
Subcutaneous tissue

Source: *Medical-Surgical Nursing: Critical Thinking in Client Care,* 2e by Lemone/Burke, Copyright 2000. Reprinted by permission of Pearson Education, Inc., Upper Saddle River, NJ.

(Reeves & Maibach, 1998) and commonly occur on men's trunks and women's legs. They enter into an immediate vertical growth phase, grow rapidly, and metastasize within weeks or months (Fleischer et al., 2000). Lentigo maligna melanoma accounts for approximately 5 percent of melanomas. Acral lentiginous melanoma comprises 2 to 10 percent of all melanomas and occurs on the palms, soles, fingers, toes, nailbeds, or cuticles (Skin Cancer Foundation, 2000).

The American Cancer Society has compiled a list of warning signs, known as the ABCDE rule of melanoma, to facilitate the identification of melanomas at an early stage (Fitzpatrick et al., 1997):

A: Asymmetry—One side of the lesion looks different from the other.

B: Border irregularity—The lesion's edges are ragged, notched, or scalloped.

C: Color—The lesion's color is varigated, or nonuniform, or it undergoes a change in color.

D: Diameter—The lesion is more than 6mm wide, or larger than a pencil eraser.

E: Enlargement or elevation—The lesion grows laterally or vertically.

Both squamous cell carcinomas and basil cell carcinomas occur on the sun-exposed skin of the body. SCCs often manifest as slowly growing bumps with a rough surface or as flat, reddish patches in the skin. Elevated SCCs are soft and movable and may be inflamed at the base (Seidel et al., 1999). BCCs manifest as flat, scaly areas, or as small, raised, shiny or waxy areas that bleed easily after a minor injury (American Cancer Society, 2000d). The raised type are pearly or ivory and feel firm to the touch. Irregular blood

vessels or blue, brown, or black discolorations may be visible in them. Some such lesions ulcerate and develop crusts (Huether, 1998).

DIAGNOSIS AND TREATMENT

Biopsy, or the surgical removal of a sample of cells from a suspicious lesion, together with microscopic examination of the specimen are the methods used to differentiate benign from cancerous lesions. Biopsy is also used to determine the thickness of melanomas, which has implications for determining a person's prognosis and treatment options (American Cancer Society, 2000a). The **Clark level of invasion** (see Figure 18–2) reflects the thickness of the lesion in relation to the vertical growth or penetration of the lesion into the skin and subcutaneous tissue. The pathologist judges the level of invasion, rather actually measuring it (American Cancer Society, 2000a). Roman numerals ranging from I to V are assigned, with higher numbers indicative of deeper melanomas (American Cancer Society, 2000a).

In the **Breslow measurement technique**, a microscope and a small ruler called a micrometer, are used to evaluate the thickness of a skin biopsy specimen (American Cancer Society, 2000a). The micrometer measures the distance between the top portion of the skin and the deepest point of tumor penetration (Lang, 1998). The newer Breslow measurement has displaced the Clark level as the first prognostic factor, as it is easier and not dependent on the pathologist's judgment (American Cancer Society, 2000a). Both techniques may still be used, as the Clark's level occasionally rates a melanoma as more advanced than it would be according to the Breslow measurement (American Cancer Society, 2000a). Persons with melanoma lesions less than

0.76 mm thick consistently have excellent prognoses, with 99 percent cure rates, and those with lesions greater than 4 mm have very poor prognoses (Lang, 1998). Survival rates are variable for melanoma lesions whose thickness ranges from 0.76 to 4 mm (Lang, 1998).

Prior to treatment, a comprehensive health history and physical examination will be completed, along with appropriate laboratory tests. A skin biopsy provides important information about the thickness of the lesions. An incisional biopsy involves the removal of only a portion of the tumor; the entire tumor is removed in an excisional biopsy. An excisional biopsy is preferred for any lesion that may be a malignant melanoma (Leber et al., 1999). Other types of biopsies—such as a **shave biopsy** in which the top skin layers are shaved with a surgical blade, and a **punch biopsy,** in which a deeper sample of skin is removed—are not recommended for suspected melanomas, because an accurate measurement of their depth is not possible (American Cancer Society, 2000a).

The preferred treatment for melanoma involves a simple excision of the lesion, with the removal of the surrounding noncancerous tissue, depending on the tumor thickness (American Cancer Society, 2000c; Leber et al., 1999). A scar results, due to the skin edges' being stitched together. Thin melanomas (less than 1 mm thick) have the best chance of being cured with this method (Lang, 1998). Nonmelanoma skin cancers can also be treated with simple excision.

In **Mohs micrographic surgery,** used for both melanoma and nonmelanoma skin cancers, microscopic layers of skin are removed as the tumor's location and margins are carefully mapped by the doctor (American Cancer Society, 2000c). The advantages of Mohs surgery include the maximal preservation of healthy tissue, an ability to assess surgical margins before closing the wound, and better appearance after surgery (American Cancer Society, 2000d; Lang, 1998; Leber et al., 1999). Mohs micrographic surgery is particularly useful for difficult sites, such as the eye, ear, nose, lips, and penis, where the risk of undetected spread and recurrence is high (Leber et al., 1999). The majority of nonmelanoma skin cancers can be completely cured by simple excision or Mohs micrographic surgery (American Cancer Society, 2000b).

If a melanoma lesion is greater than 1 mm thick, a **sentinel node biopsy** is performed. The sentinel node is the first lymph node to which a cancer is likely to spread from its primary site. This procedure involves locating the lymph nodes that drain lymph fluid from the skin at the melanoma site. A blue dye (blue vitriol) or a radioactive chemical (technetium 99) is injected into the melanoma site, allowing either visualization (with the dye) or detection with a Geiger counter (with the radioactive chemical) and subsequent removal (American Cancer Society, 2000c; Leber et al., 1999). If the sentinel node contains melanoma, an appropriate node dissection is done (American Cancer Society, 2000c; Lang, 1998). If the node does not contain melanoma, further surgery can be avoided (American Cancer Society, 2000c). This procedure has promise for the future treatment of melanoma but lacks standardization for its use and universal support for its value (American Cancer Society, 2000c).

When the diagnosis of melanoma is confirmed, a **therapeutic lymph node dissection** can be performed. The lymph nodes closest to the melanoma site are examined and removed if found to be abnormally hard or enlarged. A microscopic examination is performed to see if the melanoma has spread to the lymph nodes. Generally, a lymph node biopsy is performed first, and, if the results indicate evidence of melanoma, then a therapeutic lymph node dissection is done (American Cancer Society, 2000c). The lymph node biopsy may entail a sentinel node biopsy, or, in the case of only a single enlarged node, a fine needle biopsy may be performed. Lymph node dissection is done for nonmelanoma skin cancers if nearby lymph nodes are enlarged (American Cancer Society, 2000d).

Laser surgery may be performed to kill nonmelanoma skin cancer cells (American Cancer Society, 2000d) and is particularly useful for SCC in situ and BCC. Data comparing the results of this method with standard surgical methods of treatment are pending (American Cancer Society, 2000d).

Cryosurgery with liquid nitrogen can be used to kill nonmelanoma skin cancer cells. Blistering and crusting may form, resulting in a wound that takes several weeks to heal (American Cancer Society, 2000d).

Surgery may need to be performed where melanoma has spread to distant organs, such as the brain or lungs. The metastasis of melanoma is generally thought to signal a noncurable disease; however, surgery may still be done to improve a person's quality of life (American Cancer Society, 2000c). When only a few melanoma metastases are visible on computerized tomography (CT) or magnetic resonance imaging (MRI) scans, other lesions that are too small to be detected are likely to be present, accounting for the poor prognosis (American Cancer Society, 2000c). Skin grafting and reconstructive surgery may be performed for large nonmelanoma skin cancers and melanomas when it is not possible to bring the wound edges together (American Cancer Society, 2000d).

Chemotherapy, used to treat melanoma and advanced nonmelanoma skin cancers, involves the administration of anticancer drugs by vein or by mouth to kill cancer cells that have metastasized beyond the skin to lymph nodes and organs. These agents have a number of side effects, depending on the drug given, the dosage given, and the length of treatment (American Cancer Society, 2000c). Many remedies are available for the temporary side effects associated with chemotherapy, such as antiemetic drugs to prevent nausea and vomiting (American Cancer Society, 2000c). Chemotherapy is not as effective in cases of melanoma as it is in some other forms of cancer. It may, however, relieve symptoms and extend survival for a while (American Cancer Society, 2000c). Chemotherapy agents can be used in combination with immunotherapy agents.

Immunotherapy, also called biological therapy, is used to enhance the ability of a person's immune system to more effectively recognize and destroy cancer cells (American Cancer Society, 2000c). In immunotherapy, the **cytokines** interferon-alpha and interleukin-2, are used to boost the immune response in persons with melanoma (American Cancer Society, 2000c). Persons with melanoma who have local regional metastases, a local recurrence, in-transit metastases (nests of tumors found between the primary tumor and the draining lymph node), or primary lesions smaller than 4 mm with clinically negative lymph nodes are candidates for this treatment (Leber et al., 1999). Cytokines have been shown to shrink metastatic melanomas and may prevent the growth of melanoma cells that have broken off a primary site and traveled to body organs and other sites (American Cancer Society, 2000c). Vaccine therapy is a newer modality used to stimulate the body's immune system in similar ways that vaccines act to prevent diseases such as polio and measles (American Cancer Society, 2000c). Weakened melanoma cells, or substances made from them, are used to stimulate the person's immune system to selectively destroy melanoma cells (American Cancer Society, 2000c). Clinical trials continue on the development of a possible melanoma vaccination.

Radiation therapy can be used to kill cancer cells by focusing external beam radiation on the skin tumor or by placing radioactive materials directly in the tumor, which is called **internal** or **implant radiation.** Nonmelanoma skin cancers that have spread to the lymph nodes can also be treated with radiation therapy (American Cancer Society, 2000d). However, because it is possible for subsequent skin cancers to develop at the site of radiation treatment, radiation alone is not recommended as the primary treatment for nonmelanoma skin cancers (Leber et al., 1999). Radiation can be used as an adjuvant therapy after surgery to kill any remaining cancer cells that are still present yet were undetectable during surgery (American Cancer Society, 2000d). Although not commonly used to treat primary melanomas, radiation is frequently used to relieve the symptoms of melanoma metastases to the brain and other body organs, as well as for lesions that cannot be surgically removed (American Cancer Society, 2000c). Radiation is sometimes used as the primary therapy for non-melanoma skin cancer in older persons who cannot tolerate surgery (American Cancer Society, 2000d).

An experimental chemotherapy, **isolated hyperthermic limb perfusion (IHLP),** is used to treat melanomas of the extremities (arms and legs) after the melanomas have been surgically excised and for recurrent or satellite lesions (Lang, 1998). High doses of chemotherapy agents, heated to slightly above normal body temperature, are injected via an artery into the involved limb and prevented from reaching the rest of the body (American Cancer Society, 2000c). IHLP can be used in combination with other modalities.

Controlled studies and testing continue on this investigational treatment.

A number of promising new or experimental treatments are taking place. A list of current clinical trials can be obtained by calling the National Cancer Institute (NCI) Cancer Information Service toll-free at 1-800-4-CANCER or by visiting the NCI's clinical trials website for patients (www.cancertrials.nci.nih.gov) or for healthcare professionals (www.cancernet.nci.nih.gov/prot/protsrch.html) (American Cancer Society, 2000c, 2000d).

Skin Wellness Self-Assessment

How many of the following statements can you respond to with a healthy yes?

1. *I have no abnormal lesions on my skin.*
2. *My skin is not dry, irritated, flaking, or scaling.*
3. *I apply a sunscreen of at least SPF 15 to the exposed parts of my body all year long.*
4. *I avoid sunbathing and tanning booths.*
5. *I limit the amount of time I spend in the sun, especially during the peak hours from 10 A.M. to 3 P.M.*
6. *I periodically examine all my skin surfaces for suspicious lesions.*
7. *I use only mild products to cleanse my face.*
8. *I apply moisturizer after bathing or showering.*
9. *I use facial moisturizers that do not cause blemishes such as blackheads. I look for the word "noncomedogenic" on the label.*
10. *I wear wraparound sunglasses to help prevent fine lines from forming on my skin and to protect my eyes.*

New Directions

Several promising research studies and clinical trials are under way that hold promise for treating and preventing skin disorders. A new technique that involves the injection of a small amount of synthetic collagen into the skin to stimulate the growth of natural collagen is being investigated. This technique may be useful for improving wrinkles but has not yet received FDA approval (Mayo Foundation for Medical Education, 2000b).

New research is evaluating the use of blue and red light wavelengths in the treatment for acne vulgaris. Although more research is needed, the light, which removes harmful UVR, has been shown to decrease visible lesions in treated areas (BBC News, 2000).

New research is being done in an effort to identify the mechanisms by which ultraviolet light alters genes in such a way that actinic keratoses and skin cancers develop. For example, the p16 gene has recently been identified as the gene that causes some types of melanoma to run in families, and studies of p53 suppressor gene mutation have raised the hope that a gene therapy for skin cancers will soon be available (Leffell, 2000).

Advances in gene analysis may pinpoint the genetic causes of skin cancer and may allow the detection of persons at high risk for developing melanoma (Lang, 1998). The p16 gene has recently been identified as the gene that causes some types of melanoma to run in certain families (American Cancer Society, 2000c). Researchers have also recently identified genes that make melanoma skin cancer spread. These findings may provide the groundwork for targeting therapies and preventive strategies for these deadly cancers (*Genes Linked to Spread of Melonoma Identified*, 2000).

QUESTIONS FOR REFLECTION AND DISCUSSION

1. *What are the implications of environmental pollution—specifically, air and water pollution—for the health of the skin?*
2. *What inferences can be made about a person's lifestyle based on a skin assessment?*
3. *Might a woman who understands the effects of UVR on skin still deliberately acquire a deep suntan? Why or why not?*
4. *Of what would an optimal skin care and protection regimen for yourself consist? Consider all pertinent factors.*
5. *Did any of the information in this chapter come as a surprise to you? If so, what and why?*

RESOURCES

Books

Fleischer, A. B., Feldman, S. R., Katz, A. S., & Clayton, B. D. (2000). *20 common problems in dermatology.* New York: McGraw-Hill.

Kenet, B. J. (1999). *How to wash your face: America's leading dermatologist reveals the essential secrets for youthful, radiant skin.* New York: Simon & Schuster.

Organizations

The American Academy of Dermatology, Inc.
P.O. Box 4014
Schaumburg, IL 60168-4014
Web: http://www.AAD.org

Dermatology Nurses' Association
East Holly Ave. Box 56
Pitman, NJ 08071-0056
Phone: 1-800-454-4DNA or 609-256-2300
E-mail: dna@mail.ajj.com

National Rosacea Society
800 South Northwest Highway, Suite 200
Barrington, IL 60010
Web: http://www.rosacea.org

REFERENCES

American Academy of Dermatology. (2000a). *Rosacea* [On-line]. Available: http://www.AAD.org/aadpamphrework/rosacea.html

American Academy of Dermatology. (2000b). *Skin cancer: An undeclared epidemic* [On-line]. Available: http://www.AAD.org/aadpamphrework/skincan.html

American Cancer Society. (2000a). *Melanoma: Prevention and risk factors* [On-line]. Available: http://www3.cancer.org/cancerinfo/main_cont.asp?st=pr&ct=50

American Cancer Society. (2000b). *Melanoma: Treatment* [On-line]. Available: http://www3.cancer.org/cancerinfo/main_cont.asp?st=tr&ct=50

American Cancer Society. (2000c). *Nonmelanoma skin cancer: Overview* [On-line]. Available: http://www3.cancer.org/canceronfo/load_cont.asp?ct=51&doc=43&Language=English

American Cancer Society. (2000d). *Photodynamic therapy* [On-line]. Available: http://www3.cancer.org/cancerinfo/load_cont.asp?ct=51&doc=85&Language=English

American Cancer Society. (2000e). *Slip slop slap!* [On-line]. Available: http://www3.cancer.org/cancerinfo/load_cont.asp?ct=51&doc=90&Language=English

American Pharmaceutical Association. (1996). *Handbook of nonprescription drugs* (11th ed.). Washington, DC: Author.

BBC News. (2000). *BBC news bulletin: Light therapy 'best for acne'* [On-line]. Available: http://www.news.bbc.co.uk/hi/english/health/newsid_838000/838201/htm

Besecker, B., & Hart, C. G. (1999). A new treatment option for acne scars: Allograft dermis. *Dermatology Nursing, 11*(2), 111–114.

Boyd, A. S., Stasko, T., King, L. E., Cameron, G. S., Pearse, A. D., & Gaskell, S. A. (1999). Cigarette smoking-associated elastotic changes in the skin. *Journal of the American Academy of Dermatology, 41,* 23–26.

Brink, S. (1999, June 14). So much for sunblock: FDA sets new guidelines for protection against deadly rays. *U.S. News & World Report,* p. 65.

Cockerell, C. J. (2000). Histopathology of incipient intraepidermal squamous cell carcinoma ("actinic keratosis"). *Journal of the American Academy of Dermatology, 42,* S11–S17.

Coldiron, B. M. (1998). The UV index: A weather report for skin. *Clinics in Dermatology, 16,* 441–446.

Cook, A. R. (1997). Judging the risks: Tips for safer tanning. In A. R. Cook (Ed.) *Health reference series: Vol. 22. Skin disorders sourcebook* (pp. 315–326). Detroit, MI: Omnigraphics.

Copstead, L. C. (2000). Alterations in the integumentary system. In L. C. Copstead & J. L. Banasik (Eds.), *Pathophysiology: Biological and behavioral perspectives* (2nd ed., pp. 1178–1220). Philadelphia: W. B. Saunders.

Dinehart, S. M. (2000). The treatment of actinic keratoses. *Journal of the American Academy of Dermatology, 42,* S25–S28.

DUSA Pharmaceuticals. (2000). *Products and technology: Actinic keratoses—How Levulan PDT for AKs works* [On-line]. Available: http://www.dusapharma.com/html/AK.htm

Estes, M. E. Z. (1998). *Health assessment and physical examination*. Albany, NY: Delmar.

Fitzpatrick, T. B., Johnson, R. A., Wolff, K., Polano, M. K., & Suurmond, D. (1997). *Color atlas and synopsis of clinical dermatology: Common and serious diseases* (3rd ed.). New York: McGraw-Hill.

Fleischer, A. B., Herbert, C. R., Feldman, S. R., & O'Brian, F. (2000). Diagnosis of skin disease by nondermatologists. *American Journal of Managed Care, 6*(10), 1149–1156.

Food and Drug Administration. (2000). *FDA talk paper: Important new safety information about Accutane,* February 25, 1998 [On-line]. Available: http://www.fda.gov/medwatch/safety.htm

Frances, C. (1992). Smoking and the skin. *International Journal of Dermatology, 31,* 779–780.

Franz, R. (1999). AAD concerned about FDA cap on sunscreens. *Dermatology Nursing, 11*(4), 299.

Galderma Laboratories. (1997). *Rosacea: What you should know.* Fort Worth, TX: Author.

Genes linked to spread of melanoma identified. (2000, August 3). *Washington Post,* p. A7.

Habif, T. B. (1996). *Clinical dermatology: A color guide to diagnosis and therapy* (3rd ed.). St. Louis: Mosby-Year Book.

Higgins, E., & duVivier, A. (1999). Alcohol intake and other skin disorders. *Clinics in Dermatology, 17,* 437–441.

Hill, M. J. (1999). What's wrong with this picture? [Editorial]. *Dermatology Nursing, 11*(4), 240.

Huether, S. E. (1998). Structure, function, and disorders of the integument. In K. L. McCance & S. E. Huether (Eds.), *Pathophysiology: The biologic basis for disease in adults and children* (3rd ed., pp. 1517–1554). St. Louis: Mosby-Year Book.

Intelligent Network Concepts. (2000). *New treatment for actinic keratoses approved by the FDA* [On-line]. Available: http://pharminfo.com/pubs/medbrief/mb13_1.html

Kneedler, J. A., Sky, S. S., & Sexton, L. R. (1998). Understanding alpha-hydroxy acids. *Dermatology Nursing, 10*(4), 247–262.

Krupsi, W. C. (1991). The peripheral vascular consequences of smoking. *Annals of Vascular Surgery, 5,* 291–304.

Lang, P. G. (1998). Malignant melanoma. *Medical Clinics of North America, 82,* 1325–1358.

Lasehair, Incorporated. (2000a). *Collagen replacement therapy: Frequently asked questions* [On-line]. Available: http://www.lasehair.net/coll_faq.htm

Lasehair, Incorporated. (2000b). *Collagen replacement therapy: For a softer, smoother look in minutes* [On-line]. Available: http://www.lasehair.net/coll.htm

Leber, K., Perron, V. D., & Sinni-McKeehan, B. (1999). Common skin cancers in the United States: A practical guide for diagnosis and treatment. *Nurse Practitioner Forum, 10*(2), 106–112.

Leffell, D. J. (2000). The scientific basis of skin cancer. *Journal of the American Academy of Dermatology, 42,* S18–S22.

LeRoy, L. (1997). Laser resurfacing: The nurse's role. *Dermatology Nursing, 9*(3), 173–175.

Lookingbill, D. P., Chalker, D. K., Lindholm, J. S., Katz, H. I., Kempers, S. E., Huerter, C. J., Swinehart, J. M., Schelling, D. J., & Klauda, H. C. (1997). Treatment of acne with a combination of clindamycin/benzoyl peroxide gel compared with clindamycin gel, benzoyl peroxide gel and vehicle gel: Combined results of two double-blind investigations. *Journal of the American Academy of Dermatology, 37*(4), 590–595.

Mallon, E., Newton, J. N., Klassen, A., Stewart-Brown, S. L., Ryan, T. J., & Finlay, A. Y. (1999). The quality of life in acne: A comparison with general medical conditions using generic questionnaires. *British Journal of Dermatology, 140*(4), 672–676.

Mayo Foundation for Medical Education. (2000a). *How to care for dry, itching skin. Mayo Clinic health oasis: Reliable information for a healthier life* [On-line]. Available: http://www.mayohealth.org/mayo/9808/htm/skinsb5/htm

Mayo Foundation for Medical Education. (2000b). *Skin care: Keeping your skin healthy at any age. Mayo Clinic health oasis: Reliable information for a healthier life* [On-line]. Available: http://www.mayohealth.org/mayo/9808/htm/skin/htm

Mayo Foundation for Medical Education. (2000c). *Tips for keeping skin healthy. Mayo Clinic health oasis: Reliable information for a healthier life* [On-line]. Available: http://www.mayohealth.org/mayo/9808/htm/skinsb2/htm

Melton, M. (1998, September 14). Deep-fried by the sun: Ultraviolet-A proves to be the culprit in causing the wrinkles and sags of old age. *U.S. News & World Report,* p. 50.

Mills, C. M. (1993). Smoking and skin disease. *International Journal of Dermatology, 32*(12), 864–865.

Moy, R. L. (2000). Clinical presentation of actinic keratoses and squamous carcinoma. *Journal of the American Academy of Dermatology, 42,* S8–S10.

National Institute on Aging. (2000). *Age page: Skin care and aging* [On-line]. Available: http://www.nih.gov/nia/health/pubub/skin.htm

National Rosacea Society. (1998). *Coping with rosacea: Tips on lifestyle management for rosacea sufferers.* Barrington, IL: Author.

National Rosacea Society (2000). *What is rosacea?* [On-line]. Available: http://www.rosacea.org/p2.html

Northeast Dermatology Associates. (2000). *What is actinic keratosis?* [On-line]. Available: http://www.nedermatology.com/skincancer/ak/

O'Donoghue, M. N. (1999). Update on acne therapy. *Dermatology Nursing, 11*(3), 205–208.

Porth, C. M. (1998). *Pathophysiology: Concepts of altered states of health* (5th ed.). Philadelphia: Lippincott-Raven.

Pray, W. S. (1999). *Nonprescription product therapeutics.* Philadelphia: Lippincott-Williams & Wilkins.

Rebora, A., Drago, F., & Parodi, A. (1995). May *Heliobacter pylori* be important for dermatologists? *Dermatology, 191,* 6–8.

Reeves, J. R. T., & Maibach, H. (1998). *Clinical dermatology illustrated: A regional approach* (3rd ed.). Philadelphia: F. A. Davis.

Salasche, S. J. (2000). Epidemiology of actinic keratoses and squamous carcinoma. *Journal of the American Academy of Dermatology, 42,* S4–S7.

Seidel, H. M., Ball, J. W., Dains, J. E., & Benedict, G. W. (1999). *Mosby's guide to physical examination* (4th ed.). St. Louis: Mosby.

Sharma, V. K., Lynn, A., Kaminski, M., Vasudeva, R., & Howden, C. W. (1998). A study of the prevalence of *Heliobacter pylori* infection and other markers of upper gastrointestinal tract disease in patients with rosacea. *American Journal of Gastroenterology, 93*(2), 220–222.

Sherertz, E. F. (1991). Acneform eruption due to "megadose" vitamins B_6 and B_{12}. *Cutis, 48*(2), 119–120.

Thompson, J. M., & Wilson, S. F. (1996). *Health assessment for nursing practice*. St. Louis: Mosby-Year Book.

U.S. Environmental Protection Agency. (1995). *The sun, UV, and you: A guide to the UV index and sun-safe behavior* [EPA Publication No. 430-K-95-005]. Washington, DC: Author.

Vin-Christian, K., Maurer, T. A., & Berger, T. G. (1994). Acne rosacea as a cutaneous manifestation of HIV infection. *Journal of the American Academy of Dermatology, 30*(1), 139–140.

Webster, G. F. (1998). Acne and rosacea. *Medical Clinics of North America, 82*(5), 1145–1154.

Weedon, D. (1997). *Skin pathology*. Edinburgh, Scotland: Churchill Livingstone.

Wolf, R., Wolf, D., & Ruocco, V. (1998). Smoking and the skin, radically speaking. *Clinics in Dermatology, 16,* 633–639.

19

Neurological Wellness and Illness

Lynn S. Warner and Cathy McNew

Objectives

1. *Describe the capabilities of neurologically intact individuals in terms of cognitive, sensory, and motor functioning.*
2. *Identify dietary factors that promote neurological wellness.*
3. *List safety precautions for the prevention of head trauma and spinal cord injury.*
4. *Compare and contrast tension and migraine headaches in terms of risk factors, signs and symptoms, and current treatment.*
5. *Discuss multiple sclerosis in terms of its manifestations and therapies.*
6. *Describe the changes in mental status associated with dementia and Alzheimer's disease and discuss current treatments.*
7. *Compare and contrast the types of seizure disorders in terms of pathology, manifestations, and treatment.*
8. *Discuss Parkinson's disease in terms of its signs and symptoms, its impact on the activities of daily living, and available treatments.*

Introduction

This chapter addresses both neurological wellness and selected neurological illnesses of particular concern to women. The markers of optimal neurological functioning are described and strategies for optimizing neurological wellness are presented. Neurological conditions and diseases that affect the brain, spinal cord, and peripheral nerves of the body, such as headache, multiple sclerosis, dementias, epilepsy, and Parkinson's disease, are discussed in terms of presentation and their impact on the quality of women's lives.

Neurological health problems are characterized by both responses unique to a given individual, and responses commonly experienced by most individuals who have the problem. The diagnosis of neurological problems may require sophisticated technology as well as the knowledge of an experienced neurologist. Treatment plans are often complex and may include medication, surgery, nursing care, and rehabilitative therapies. Recent advances in the treatment of neurological problems include immunological therapies for multiple sclerosis and the aggressive, multidisciplinary treatment of head trauma.

Markers of Neurological Wellness

Persons whose neurological system are intact enjoy cognitive, sensory, and motor functioning that is "normal" in the sense that no deficits are apparent.

Normal Cognition

People who are neurologically well have stable and consistent cognition, or thought processes. They have sufficient memory, problem-solving ability, and judgment to function independently. Difficulty with thought processes can be manifested by changes in alertness and orientation to time, person, and place and by unusual responses to questions or statements. Identifying the cause of a decrease in cognitive ability requires investigation to determine whether an **organic** (physical) or **inorganic** (emotional or spiritual) problem exists. Both organic and inorganic phenomena can cause alterations in thought processes.

Normal Sensory Functioning

A person with an intact, optimally functioning neurological system has sensory abilities that are quite stable in that they change only slowly, with advancing age. Thus, a person's ability to see, to hear, and to feel pain and other sensations should not change suddenly, within minutes or hours, or even relatively rapidly over a period of days, weeks, or months. When organic problems are present in the brain, changes in vision are frequently the first symptoms reported. Blurred vision, double vision, or difficulty with peripheral vision may mean that the occulomotor nerve in the brain has been disrupted or that something is impinging on the optic nerve. Such symptoms can also be caused by a problem in the occipital lobe of the brain, where visual stimuli are inter-

preted. Of course, visual problems may also be related to changes within the eye itself; the difficulty with near vision, called **presbyopia,** that often accompanies aging is not considered a warning sign of neurological impairment.

Numbness, tingling, and difficulty perceiving touch and/or changes in temperature in any part of the body may be symptomatic of a neurological problem, as may loss of **proprioception,** which allows us to sense the position of our extremities in space, even when our eyes are closed. Without intact proprioception, which is dependent on the intact functioning of the neurons, spinal cord, and brain, we would not be able to coordinate our movements.

Normal Motor Functioning

People who are neurologically intact do not suddenly lose muscle strength in any part of the body and they do not suddenly lose their ability to speak clearly or to walk with their customary level of ability. Suddenly developing weakness or paralysis in any muscle group may signal the onset of a significant neurological problem. For example, a lopsided smile, slurring of speech, difficulty in chewing and swallowing, or sudden weakness in one or more extremities may be related to problems in the major nerves within the head that control these functions. Muscle strength is assessed relative to one's normal strength. A reduction in strength that compromises the ability to carry out daily activities is cause for concern.

Involuntary trembling, or **tremors,** and involuntary muscle contractions called **spasms** are also abnormal and usually manifest in the face, neck, or extremities. Problems with balance may be related to muscle weakness in a lower extremity but also to brain dysfunction or an inner ear problem.

Persistent changes in thought processes, vision, hearing, sensation, strength, or balance may reflect the onset of a significant neurological problem. Although such changes are often subtle and inconsistent initially, they typically persist and eventually worsen. Although the affected individual may notice the changes, it is often the case that friends or relatives bring them to her attention. It is crucial that medical attention be sought immediately if a neurological problem is suspected. Information about the individual's previous level of functioning and usual behaviors is invaluable in making a diagnosis.

Promoting Neurological Wellness

A proactive approach to maintaining neurological wellness focuses on nutrition and the prevention of injury. Good general health is required to ensure the health of the neurological system because all body systems are interrelated. For example, the circulatory system provides nourishment and oxygen to the neurons, the functional units of the nervous system. If the blood vessels that provide such nourishment are compromised by the presence of plaques, the functions of the neurons will be affected. The B vitamins are nutrients of particular importance to the nervous system.

Taking in Adequate Amounts of Vitamins and Minerals

Neurological wellness is dependent on an adequate intake of the B vitamins—water-soluble vitamins that play an essential role in cellular metabolism. B vitamins act as coenzymes—that is, facilitators of chemical reactions. They promote protein synthesis and take part in enzyme-releasing reactions and the development of new cells. Some B vitamins function interdependently; for example, folate and vitamin B-12 activate each other. Neurological problems related to B vitamin deficiencies do not typically result from the loss of one B vitamin but, rather, from an insufficient intake of a number of them. A varied diet that includes meat, fish, poultry, eggs, legumes, nuts, milk products, vegetables, fruit, and grain products is the best insurance against B vitamin deficiency.

Adequate blood levels of certain minerals are also necessary for neurological wellness. These include calcium, magnesium, zinc, and sodium. A low blood level of calcium, for example, may result in intermittent spasms of the arms and legs **(tetany),** due to nervous and muscular excitability. Minerals, however, can build up in the body, and excessively high levels can cause neurological dysfunction. For example, a high blood level of calcium may result in **calcium rigor,** an inability of the muscles to relax after contraction.

Preventing Injury

Approximately 512,800 U.S. women experience head injuries each year (*Traumatic Brain Injury,* 1999) and approximately 2,200 experience spinal cord injuries (*Spinal Cord Injury,* 2001). Most such injuries are related to automobile accidents or sustained while engaging in recreational activities. Women also experience head injuries during episodes of domestic violence. Campaigns to prevent these serious traumas promote the use of seat belts and discourage the use of intoxicating substances while driving. They also involve public education regarding the risks of diving into water of unknown depth and the importance of wearing safety helmets while biking, rollerblading, mountain climbing, and so on. Finally, campaigns to prevent head and spinal cord injury focus on encouraging women in abusive relationships to seek counseling and protection.

 Neurological Illnesses and Problems

The neurological problems that commonly afflict women include headaches, multiple sclerosis, cognitive disorders, epilepsy, and Parkinson's disease (Kaplan, 1999).

Headaches

Headaches are characterized by acute or chronic pain felt in various areas of the head. Headache is a common malady experienced by at least three-fourths of the American population, and women suffer from headache more frequently than men (Rosenfeld, 1999). There are two categories of headache: primary headaches, for which no specific cause has been identified, and secondary headaches, which have a known cause. Secondary headaches result from structural changes within the brain, such as tumors and aneurysms (Hickey, 1997). Primary headaches comprise the majority of headaches reported by individuals and there are three main varieties: tension, migraine, and cluster headaches. Cluster headaches occur primarily in men and will not be discussed.

TENSION HEADACHES

Tension headaches are the most common type of headache; they account for more than 75 percent of all headaches (Rosenfeld, 1999). Tension headaches occur more frequently in women (Schwartz, Stewart, Simon, & Lipton, 1998) and are more common in persons age 30 to 39 years. Tension headaches that occur only occasionally are said to be episodic or acute. Headaches that occur frequently are referred to as chronic. Tension headaches are not related to organic disease. Rather, they are caused by stress-related contraction of muscles in the neck and scalp (National Headache Foundation, 1998). The actual pain is thought to be caused by the constriction of small arteries secondary to the muscle contractions (Hickey, 1997; National Headache Foundation, 1998).

Symptoms   Episodic tension headaches cause bilateral pain and may last 30 minutes to 7 days. The pain is often described as a sensation of soreness, weight, and pressure or as the feeling that a viselike band is surrounding the head. Increased sensitivity to light and/or sound may also be present. There is no nausea or increased intensity of the headache with physical activity. Chronic tension headache has the same characteristics as the episodic variety, except for the duration and the resulting disruption in sleep patterns. In order to be considered chronic, tension headaches must last at least 24 hours per episode and occur at least fifteen days per month during a 6-month period (Jenson, 2001).

Diagnosis   An accurate description of the nature of the headaches, including severity, duration, and frequency, can greatly aid a clinician in identifying the type of headache being experienced. Keeping a "headache diary" reflecting associated experiences can also be helpful. A thorough health history will be taken and a physical assessment will be done. **Imaging studies,** such as magnetic resonance imaging (MRI) and computerized tomography (CT) scans, may be needed. CAT scans and MRIs can be thought of as sophisticated, sequential x-rays that reveal far more about body structures than a conventional x-ray. Effective treatment depends on an accurate diagnosis of the type of headache being experienced.

Treatment Episodic tension headaches can be relieved with over-the-counter analgesics such as ibuprofen or acetominophen. Taking measures to decrease stress and promote relaxation is helpful. Preventive measures include a well-balanced diet, aerobic exercise, and stress management (see Chapter 7). Prescription beta-blocking and calcium channel–blocking drugs have proven effective for some individuals. Tricyclic antidepressants such as amitriptyline are frequently effective for chronic tension headaches, as chronic headaches are often associated with sleep disturbances, which may be a sign of depression (National Headache Foundation, 1998). The tricyclics have analgesic as well as antidepressant effects.

MIGRAINE HEADACHES

Migraine headaches are severe, one-sided headaches that are recurrent and debilitating. It is estimated that 23 million people suffer from migraines with a 3 to 1 ratio of female to male sufferers (Hickey, 1997). Female hormone levels seem to influence the frequency and severity of migraines in women who are susceptible to them. Menstrual cycle phase has been found to influence the frequency of headaches in approximately 65 percent of female migraine sufferers (National Headache Foundation, 1998). Taking birth control pills increases headache frequency in 50 percent of women, decreases frequency in 10 percent, and does not affect frequency in 40 percent (Hickey, 1997). Seventy-five to 80 percent of female migraine sufferers who become pregnant report complete cessation of their headaches. Migraine headaches often begin in childhood or young adulthood and may become less frequent as the individual grows older. A number of factors known to trigger migraine headaches in persons prone to them are listed in Box 19–1. Migraine headaches are characterized by throbbing, one-sided pain that is caused by the presence of swollen blood vessels in the affected part of the brain. The swelling is thought to be caused by an inflammatory process to which the individual has a hereditary predisposition (National Headache Foundation, 1998).

Symptoms There are five phases to what is known as the **migraine cycle:** the premonition phase, the aura, the headache phase, the termination of the headache, and the postdrome phase. Approximately 60 percent of all migraine sufferers experience the symptoms that fit into the **premonition phase,** which occur hours or a few days prior to a headache. These include irritability, mental slowness, depression, fatigue, a feeling of being cold, a craving for certain foods, an increase in thirst and urination, a lack of appetite, and an increase or decrease in activity level. The second phase of the migraine cycle, the **aura,** consists of an unusual symp-

---

Box 19–1 Migraine Headache Triggers

Medications, Foods, and Beverages

- Medications that cause swelling of the blood vessels—for example, nitroglycerine, isordil
- Taking excessive amounts of medication for migraines or other headaches
- Caffeine—for example, coffee, tea, cola
- Tyramine in alcoholic beverages—for example, red wine and beer
- Tyramine in foods— for example, aged cheese, pickled foods, canned figs
- Chocolate
- Nitrites in cured meats
- Sulfites in dried fruit and wine
- Monosodium glutamate in meat tenderizers
- Yeast products
- Dairy products

Other Triggering Factors

- Bright lights, sunlight, fluorescent lights, television, and movie viewing
- Excessive noise
- Alterations of sleep-wake cycle
- Hormonal changes associated with menstrual cycle
- Stress
- Fatigue
- Fever

---

tom that warns that a headache is impending. The aura may be experienced in a number of ways: A person who has a **visual aura** sees spots or other such phenomena. Another person might experience a **sensory aura,** such as numbness and tingling of the face or extremities or the inability to move an arm or leg. Still another person might experience a change in her level of alertness. Such symptoms last from a few minutes to an hour. It is thought that the aura is caused by reduced blood flow to the nerves in certain parts of the brain secondary to the constriction of the blood vessels supplying the brain and its surrounding tissues. Only a minority of individuals who have migraines experience auras (Hickey, 1997; National Headache Foundation, 1998). The next phase in the migraine cycle, the **headache phase,** is caused by dilation of the blood vessels. Although the pain is usually lateralized to one side of the head initially, it may later involve both sides as the intensity increases. Nausea frequently accompanies the headache, and a sensitivity to light, sound, and smell may also be experienced. Blurred vision, nasal stuffiness, changes in appetite, abdominal cramps, sensations of heat or cold, tenderness of the scalp and neck muscles, and changes in thought processes are also commonly reported. The headache phase lasts from a few hours to three days. As the intensity of the pain diminishes during the fourth phase, the **termination phase** of the headache, the individual may experience exhaustion, irritability, or depression and may have difficulty concentrating. During the period following the headache, the **postdrome phase,** she may feel refreshed or may continue to have difficulty with depression (Hickey, 1997).

Diagnosis A family history of migraine headaches is helpful in establishing a diagnosis. A physical examination, including a thorough neurological examination, will be done to rule out an organic cause of the headache problem. Imaging studies, such as magnetic resonance imaging (MRI) and computerized tomography (CT) scans, may also be done to detect any structural changes in the brain. Patients may be asked to keep a diary of their headache experiences in order to identify any triggers and to detect the presence of a typical migraine cycle (Hickey, 1997).

Treatment The treatment of migraine headaches includes both nondrug and drug therapies. The nondrug approaches involve avoiding the triggers that have been identified for a given individual. Common dietary triggers are alcohol, aged cheese, chocolate, monosodium glutamate, and additives found in hot dogs and lunchmeat. Changes in lifestyle may be necessary if the frequency and severity of migraine attacks are to be reduced. Consuming a balanced diet, getting regular aerobic exercise and sufficient rest, and managing stress more effectively may be necessary (Hickey, 1997; Khurana, 1999; National Headache Foundation, 1998).

Nonpharmacological therapies are also useful in easing the pain of migraine. Resting in a quiet, dark environment and applying ice packs intermittently to the head may be helpful. Massage, relaxation training (see Chapter 7), acupuncture, and biofeedback (see Chapter 11) have also been reported to be useful in the treatment of migraines. Daily biofeedback sessions have been shown to reduce the frequency and intensity of headaches (National Headache Foundation, 1998).

Drug therapy for migraine headaches includes **prophylactic therapy,** meant to prevent attacks, and **ablative therapy,** aimed at stopping or reducing the severity of the headache once it has occurred. A number of drugs are used in prophylactic therapy. Women who suffer from menstrual migraines often use various combinations of nonsteroidal anti-inflammatory drugs (NSAID), such as ibuprofen, and alpha adrenergic blockers, such as ergotamine, during the phase of their cycle when they are most vulnerable. NSAIDs decrease inflammation and swelling, whereas adrenergic blocking drugs prevent the early vasoconstriction that occurs in the migraine cycle. When cyclic prophylaxis is not sufficient, hormonal therapy comprised of low doses of estrogen and progestin can be used (Maloney, Matthews, Scharbo-Dahaan, & Strickland, 2000).

Box 19–2 Strategies for Getting Maximal Relief from Migraine Headaches

- Be a self-advocate; see a health care provider about your headaches and schedule regular follow-up appointments.
- Educate yourself about migraines so you will know what to communicate to the health care provider. The National Headache Foundation (NHF) is an excellent resource.
- Keep a headache diary that includes past medical history and therapies, and information specifically addressing your headaches—for example, date, length of each migraine, severity, symptoms, triggers, impact on your life, and response to medications. Share this information with your care provider.
- Have reasonable expectations about treatment. Different therapies may need to be tried until a therapeutic regimen is found. A variety of preventative medications may need to be tried before one is found to reduce migraines—for example, nonsteroidal anti-inflammatory drugs (such as ibuprofen) and riboflavin, and prescription medications—for example, beta blockers, calcium channel blockers, valproate, sertraline, and ergotamine.
- Be honest about all current medications and other therapies, including nontraditional therapies.
- Exercise regularly, but warm up gradually.
- Follow a diet low in fat and rich in complex carbohydrates.
- Avoid oral contraceptives, especially if you smoke or have a family history of stroke.

Other drugs traditionally used to prevent migraine attacks include caffeine and Depakote. Caffeine prevents blood vessels from swelling, and Depakote suppresses high-frequency neuronal firing in the brain. Although Depakote is primarily used to prevent seizures, it is also effective in preventing migraine headaches. The FDA has recently approved newer medications, such as sumatriptan (Imitrex), for the prevention of migraines. Sumatripan relieves migraine pain by constricting the blood vessels within the brain and reducing inflammation (National Headache Foundation, 1998). Box 19–2 lists health practices that may limit the impact of migraine headaches. Medication use during pregnancy to prevent and treat migraines needs to be closely monitored. Vasoconstricting medications, such as ergotamine and sumatriptan, are not appropriate during pregnancy because they might compromise the fetal blood supply. Using multiple drugs is contraindicated due to the possibility of adverse effects to the fetus. Fortunately, medications such as meperidine (Demerol) and acetaminophen (sold as Tylenol and other brand names) are effective and can safely be taken during pregnancy under physician or nurse-midwife supervision (Khurana, 1999). Biofeedback, yoga, and Tai chi have all been found to be helpful in lessening the frequency and severity of migraine headaches.

Multiple Sclerosis

Multiple sclerosis (MS) is an unpredictable, chronic neurological disorder that causes disability predominantly in young adults and is two to four times as common in women as in men. The onset of symptoms typically occurs between the ages of 20 and 30. Approximately 1 million people worldwide, and more than 500,000 people within the United States and Canada, have been diagnosed with MS (Holland & Halper, 1999). Individuals with MS are predominantly Caucasians of Northern European ancestry.

The symptoms of MS are due to what is known as the **demyelinization** of the neurons in the brain, spine, and eye. Myelin is a fatty, insulating coating found on the **axons** (the part of the neuron that conducts impulses). Myelin allows rapid and smooth communication among nerve cells. In demyelinization, the myelin sheath becomes degraded, most likely due to an inflammatory process that is **autoimmune**. Figure 19–1 illustrates an axon with its myelin sheath. Repetitive bouts of inflammation result in random patches of demyelinization, with subsequent scarring. Patches of scar tissue, known as *plaques,* also develop. The demyelinization and plaque formation cause impulses to be conducted along the axon in erratic patterns. This interruption in message transmission causes the motor and cognitive problems associated with MS. The precise cause of the inflammatory, autoimmune process that gives rise to MS is unknown, but a number of factors have been implicated, such as environmental pollution, viral infections, and heredity.

An early diagnosis and initiation of aggressive treatment is important in MS. Trapp and his colleagues (1998) recently found that the axon itself, in addition to the myelin sheath, is attacked by the immune system and that permanent neurological problems may result. There are several different types of MS; they are differentiated in Box 19–3.

SYMPTOMS

The symptoms of MS are usually subtle initially. Affected individuals report transient episodes of one or more of the following: blurred vision, numbness and tingling of arms and legs, dizziness, lack of coordination, spasticity, weakness, difficulty moving, fatigue, depression, and difficulties with thought processes. Transient disturbances in bowel, bladder, and sexual functioning may also occur (Lang, 1996). Because the symptoms of MS come and go, they may be regarded as odd annoyances rather than as manifestations of a serious neurological disease (Coyle, 1998).

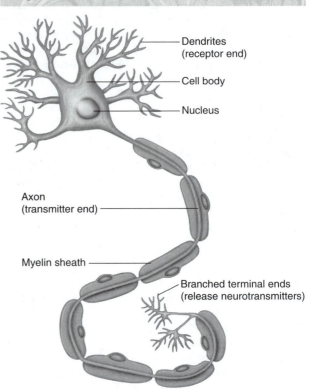

Figure 19–1   Axon and Myelin Sheath

Dendrites (receptor end)

Cell body

Nucleus

Axon (transmitter end)

Myelin sheath

Branched terminal ends (release neurotransmitters)

Source: *Human Diseases: A Systemic Approach* 5e by Mulvihill/ Zelman/Holdaway/Tompary/Turchany, Copyright 2001. Reprinted with permission of Pearson Education, Inc., Upper Saddle River, NJ.

DIAGNOSIS

Symptoms similar to those associated with MS should prompt healthcare providers to conduct a thorough neurological examination. While the initial assessment may suggest the presence of MS, a definitive diagnosis requires both a pattern of recurring symptoms and confirmation that plaques are present in at least two areas of the central nervous system.

Diagnostic imaging, particularly magnetic resonance imaging (MRI), has become the most useful diagnostic tool for the identification of **lesions** (discrete areas in which the neurons are abnormal) in the central nervous system. In an MRI, patients are placed in a magnetic field, which produces clear images of body structures. Plaques can be visualized when they reach approximately 2 mm in size.

Additional diagnostic procedures, such as evoked potential tests and an analysis of spinal fluid, may be necessary. In **evoked potential testing,** electrical impulses from the brain are recorded as the individual looks at various images and listens to a variety of sounds. Deviations from normal may indicate the presence of inflammatory processes that were not imaged by an MRI, possibly because they were not yet large enough to be detected. **Cerebrospinal fluid (CSF),** which is a clear fluid that circulates between the brain and spinal column, may be analyzed for the presence of excessive numbers of white blood cells and certain types of protein, such as myelin basic protein and immunoglobulin G antibodies (*Emerging Therapies,* 1998). A procedure known as **lumbar puncture** (spinal tap) is used to remove CSF from the spinal canal. A fine needle is inserted between the vertebrae and a small amount of fluid is withdrawn.

TREATMENT

Unfortunately, MS is not curable. The primary treatment goals are to alleviate symptoms and impede the disease process in order to maximize the individual's functional status. Some individuals benefit from therapy with **steroid** drugs, such as hydrocortisone and dexamethasone, which can reduce the inflammatory response and the immune system's attack on the myelin. A number of side effects, such as diabetes, weight gain, acne, stomach ulcers, osteoporosis, and hypertension, can result from steroid therapy. Recent advances in the treatment of MS include the use of drugs that dampen the immune response and slow the progression of the disease, such as alpha interferon (Avonex), beta interferon (Beterseron), and copolymer 1 (Copaxone). Avonex is also used to treat high-risk individuals who do not meet the formal criteria for a diagnosis of MS but have had an isolated neurological episode suggestive of demyelination and have had brain lesions detected via MRI (*When the Doctor Suspects MS,* 2001). If steroid and immune-dampening drugs prove ineffective, more toxic immunosuppressive agents, such as methotrexate, may be used. Immunosuppressive agents may

result in changes in menses and, in pregnant women, an increased risk for birth defects (Coyle, 1998; Emerging Therapies, 1998). A balanced diet, rest, and moderate exercise to preserve strength and reduce stress are recommended to promote well-being in MS patients.

Problematic symptoms can be controlled with both medication and nonpharmacological approaches. The drug Baclofen (lioresal), an antispasmotic, is frequently used to control spasticity, as is physical therapy. Exercise, an adequate intake of dietary fiber, and a water intake of at least eight glasses per day are necessary to prevent constipation. Cranberry juice and vitamin C tablets help prevent urinary tract infections. Oxybutynin (Ditropan), a prescription medication that blocks involuntary contraction of the bladder, can be used for urinary frequency.

Women with MS typically report that the disease has a significant emotional impact on themselves and their families. Visible symptoms, such as spasms and an erratic walking pattern, may be embarrassing. Fatigue may limit their participation in homemaking and family activities. MS typically strikes relatively young women who may have demanding multiple roles such as wife, mother, and wage earner. Consequently, there is often concern about maintaining a viable role within the family and community (Jacopini, 2000).

Depression is frequently present during the active phases of MS. The unpredictable pattern of the disease, and its uncertain outcome, may precipitate fear and frustration. Compromised mobility, plus fatigue, bowel and bladder problems, and sexual dysfunction, can contribute to high levels of stress within the family. Medication and counseling can be helpful in reducing the intensity of emotional responses.

Although MS can be a challenging disease, it is by no means a hopeless one. Advances in diagnosis and treatment allow many MS patients to remain relatively independent for years. On average, two-thirds of all persons with MS are still able to walk 20 years after having been diagnosed (*When the Doctor Suspects MS,* 2001). Participating in MS support groups is beneficial for both patients and family members. Patients often need ongoing support in order to cope with the active phases of the disease and to achieve optimal functioning during the dormant ones. Strong family relationships and spirituality have both been associated with a higher quality of life in MS patients.

Cognitive Disorders: Delirium and the Dementias

As noted in the section on neurological wellness, cognitive functioning depends on the ability to acquire, retain, and process information. A decline in cognitive functioning often manifests as a change in behavior and personality, or difficulty in understanding or using language. Approximately 4 million Americans suffer from some kind of cognitive dysfunction. Cognitive dysfunction can result from a variety of discrete and often treatable conditions, such as head injury or hypothryroidism, or from more generalized and irreversible changes in the brain. *Delirium* and *dementia* are two terms used to denote either temporary or permanent decreases in cognitive functioning.

DELIRIUM VERSUS DEMENTIA

Temporary cognitive dysfunction resulting from a known, discrete cause is referred to as **delirium.** Permanent and irreversible cognitive dysfunction related to generalized, irreversible changes in the brain is called **dementia.** In delirium, the ability to focus one's attention is the most notable symptom, whereas, in dementia, problems with memory, particularly recent memory, are the predominant manifestations. Whereas delirium will resolve when the underlying cause is treated or resolves on its own, dementia is permanent and progressive.

Differentiating between delirium and dementia may be difficult. If the symptoms develop quickly and a cause can be identified, delirium is usually the obvious diagnosis. Delirium can be mistaken for dementia, however, if an undetected, treatable problem causes changes in cognitive function to occur more slowly. Delirium can also *lead* to dementia, as in individuals who suffer a head injury and never regain their previous level of cognitive functioning. The complexity increases when considering the numerous types of delirium and dementia (*Delirium and Dementia,* 1999; Forno, Maki, & Kawas, 1998).

Delirium can be caused by primary brain disease or by diseases of the body that also affect the brain. The potential causes of delirium are divided into four categories:

metabolic, toxic, structural, and infectious. Disorders in all four categories alter the transmission of the signals within the brain and affect the arousal mechanisms in the brain stem (*Delirium and Dementia,* 1999). The metabolic causes of delirium, such as severe hypothyroidism, change the environment around the nerve cells by creating an imbalance of electrolytes, hormones, oxygen, or nourishment for the nerve cells. Toxic causes, such as an overdose of narcotics, introduce substances within the brain that impede normal nerve cell function. Box 19–4 lists the metabolic and toxic causes of delirium. The structural lesions that can cause delirium include brain tumors and abscesses and the occlusion and hemorrhage of blood vessels in the brain. Individuals with structural lesions may have neurological changes that reflect an impairment of specific areas of the brain. For example, multiple occlusions of the blood vessels that nourish parts of the left hemisphere of the brain can result in difficulty with language. Imaging studies, such as CT scans and MRIs, are useful in determining the type and location of structural lesions. The infectious causes of delirium include infections within the brain, such as meningitis or encephalitis, and infections elsewhere in the body, such as pneumonia, urinary tract infections, and viral infections. Prompt treatment usually restores the individual's cognitive function (*Delirium and Dementia,* 1999).

As is the case with delirium, the causes of dementia include primary brain pathology as well as systemic changes that affect the brain. The causes of dementia are also categorized as metabolic, toxic, structural, and infectious. Box 19–5 lists the causes of dementia. The distinguishing feature of the dementias is that they are not treatable, at least not presently, and therefore progress slowly but inevitably. The most well-known and feared variety of dementia is Alzheimer's disease.

Box 19–4   Metabolic and Toxic Causes of Delirium

- Chronic low oxygen often associated with chronic obstructive lung disease.
- Acute periods of low blood oxygen levels associated with cardiac arrest and anesthesia accidents.
- Carbon monoxide poisoning.
- Nutritional and vitamin deficiencies—for example, pernicious anemia or pellagra can cause chronic memory problems.
- Liver or kidney failure.
- Exaggerated parathyroid gland activity resulting in high levels of calcium in the blood.
- Severe and frequent low blood sugar levels.
- Repeated bilateral shock therapy for depression.
- Toxins and drug toxicity—for example, metals and alcohol.

Source: Adapted from *Merck Manual of Diagnosis and Therapy,* Edition 17, edited by Mark H. Beers and Robert Berkow. Copyright 1999 by Merck & Co., Inc., Whitehouse Sation, NJ.

Box 19–5   Structural and Disease Related Causes of Dementia

- Multiple interruptions of blood supply within the brain.
- Traumatic brain injury.
- Brain tumors.
- Normal pressure hydrocephalus.
- Infections—for example, meningitis, encephalitis, and AIDS.
- Diffuse disease of the central nervous system— for example, Parkinson's Disease, Huntington's chorea.

Source: Hickey, J.V. (Ed). (1997). *The clinical practice of neurological and neurosurgical nursing.* Philadelphia: Lippincott, Williams & Wilkins.

ALZHEIMER'S DISEASE

Alzheimer's disease (AD) is also one of the more frequently occurring forms of dementia, accounting for more than 50 percent of the dementias in the elderly (*Delirium and Dementia*, 1999). Between the ages of 65 and 74 years, the incidence of AD in females and males is similar (Progress Report on Alzheimer's Disease, 1999). However, because the incidence of Alzheimer's disease increases with age, and because women have a longer life span, approximately two-thirds of all AD patients are women (Forno et al., 1998).

Within the past decade, Alzheimer's disease (AD) has been the focus of considerable research. Genetic research has identified two types of AD: **familial (FAD)** and **sporadic.** FAD accounts for 20 percent and sporadic for 80 percent of all AD patients. Mutations in genes on three chromosomes (21, 14, and 1) occur in approximately 50 percent of familial AD cases and occasionally in sporadic cases. Familial AD typically has an early onset, affecting people from 30 to 65 years of age. Sporadic AD has a later onset, typically developing after 65 years of age. Genetic factors are also present in FAD: The inheritance of the **allele** (alternate form of a gene) apolipoprotein E 4 (APOE 4) on chromosome 19 confers an increased risk, as it promotes the development of **amyloid plaques** in the brain (*Delirium and Dementia*, 1999).

The presence of amyloid plaques is the anatomical hallmark of AD. Amyloid is a cellular protein, which, when present in large deposits, disrupts neuron-to-neuron communication, possibly by causing nerves to lengthen and twist. The presence of tangles of nerves, or **neurofibrils,** is characteristic of AD. Although the development of amyloid plaques and neurofibrils is associated with normal aging, these structures are significantly more prevalent in AD. It has not, however, been definitely proven whether these anatomical changes are the *causes* or the *results* of the Alzheimer's disease process (Progress Report on Alzheimer's Disease, 1999).

The pathophysiology of AD also causes other changes to occur in the brains of afflicted persons. **Neurotransmitters** are substances that facilitate communication between nerve cells. In AD, levels of the neurotransmitter acetylcholine are significantly diminished, which reduces the speed and frequency at which messages are transmitted in the brain. Acetylcholine is essential to the process of forming memories and is commonly used by nerve cells in the brain's hippocampus and cerebral cortex-regions, which are typically devastated by AD. Research also suggests that damage to neurons in AD may be related to oxidative damage secondary to the overproduction of free radicals, which damage genes and thus interfere with protein synthesis. Free radicals have been found in abundance in brain structures damaged by AD. Ultimately, these processes contribute to cell death; Alzheimer's patients who exhibit severe symptoms are often found to have experienced brain infarctions (death of brain tissue). They may also suffer from vascular disease in the arteries that transport oxygen and nourishment to the brain (*Delirium and Dementia*, 1999). Functional imaging studies show microvascular changes and a reduction in glucose use by the nerve cells in the temporal, parietal, and prefrontal cortices (Progress Report on Alzheimer's Disease, 1999).

Research on Alzheimer's disease addresses genetics, infections, vascular diseases, and environmental factors. The risk factors for AD are family history, advancing age, Down syndrome, a history of serious head trauma, and a lower level of education. Possible environmental factors, such as exposure to aluminum, zinc, and viruses, are currently being investigated.

Symptoms The early stages of AD are characterized by subtle, slowly progressive changes in cognitive functioning. The loss of memory for recent events, forgetfulness, confusion, and problems with language and with learning new information may be present and contribute to the personality changes noticed by others. Women in the early stages of AD tend to lose more language function than men. The influences that contribute to this disparity are unknown but may be related to the fact that women typically have more highly developed language centers than men. Because memory is language-dependent, the affects of AD may initially be more noticeable in women (Forno et al., 1998).

During the intermediate stage of AD, individuals completely lose their ability to learn and retain new information. Remote memory may also be lost, and individuals may wander and become lost or injured. Persons suffering from Alzheimer's disease may also become easily agitated or angered. Eventually, during the severe, or **terminal** (leading to death), phase of the disease, afflicted individuals become totally dependent on others. Control over body functions is lost, and nourishment, hygiene, and other necessities must be provided by a caregiver. Alzheimer's patients are at risk for many complications of their disease, which are enumerated in Box 19–6. One of the most significant effects of AD is the overwhelming impact it has on the care provider during all stages.

Diagnosis The onset of noticeable symptoms may stimulate either the person with Alzheimer's disease or a family member or friend to seek assistance from a healthcare provider. The provider will seek to differentiate between normal features of aging and the cognitive changes that herald the onset of AD. For example, depression, a frequent psychiatric problem in the elderly, can cause symptoms similar to those of early-stage AD. Organic problems, such as brain infarction or subdural hematoma (bleeding in the brain), can also mimic symptoms of AD. The diagnosis of early-stage AD can be made only after other possible causes of the decline in cognitive functioning have been excluded. In order to accomplish this, a thorough health history will be taken, and a physical examination will be done, along

Box 19–6 Potential Complications of Alzheimer's Disease

- **Behavioral**
  Hostility   Agitation
  Wandering   Uncooperativeness
- **Psychiatric**
  Depression   Anxiety
  Delusions   Paranoid reactions
  Hallucinations
- **Metabolic**
  Dehydration   Infection
  Drug toxicity
- **Other**
  Falls   Incontinence
  Medication side effects Confusion at dusk
  Constipation   (sundowning)
  Sleep disturbance   Orthostatic hypotension
  Glaucoma   Urinary retention
  Seizures   Movement disorders
                           Worsened confusion

Source: Adapted from *Merck Manual of Diagnosis and Therapy,* Edition 17, edited by Mark H. Beers and Robert Berkow. Copyright 1999 by Merck & Co., Inc., Whitehouse Station, NJ.

Box 19–7 Tests and Procedures Used in Diagnosing Alzheimer's Disease

- A thorough health history and physical examination.
- Laboratory and imaging tests commonly used to exclude other causes of dementia:
  CBC, electrolytes, and other blood tests
  Thyroid function
  Folate and B12 levels
  VDRL test for syphillis
  Urine analysis
  ECG and chest x-ray
  Imaging: CT or MRI
  Assess pupillary response to dilute anticholinergic eye drops (to rule out nervous system malfunction)
- Neuropsychological examination; ongoing assessments of cognitive impairment that clinically confirms diagnosis.
- Definitive diagnosis made only from brain tissue biopsy (not ordinarily performed).

Source: Adapted from *Merck Manual of Diagnosis and Therapy,* Edition 17, edited by Mark H. Beers and Robert Berkow. Copyright 1999 by Merck & Co., Inc., Whitehouse Station, NJ.

with laboratory testing and various neurological imaging studies, including MRI, positron emission tomography (PET), and single photon emission computed tomography (SPECT) scans. The PET scan measures metabolic activity within the brain, and the SPECT scan reveals how well blood perfuses the brain. Box 19–7 lists the tests and procedures used to establish a diagnosis of AD.

In the past, AD was frequently misdiagnosed. The recent identification of markers such as APOE4, which can assist in identifying individuals at risk as well as those with AD, have made the diagnosis of this devastating disorder more certain, although at this time the majority of patients with other dementias have no genetic markers. Recent findings in the field of neuroimaging have also enhanced the accuracy with which AD can be diagnosed. For example, it is now known that the combination of low scores on memory tests and a reduction in the size of the hippocampal area of the brain suggests that AD is present (Progress Report on Alzheimer's Disease, 1999). Box 19–8 lists criteria that support the probable diagnosis of AD.

Treatment   Treatment falls into three areas: (1) preventing the disease, (2) slowing the progression of cognitive decline, and (3) limiting associated negative behaviors, such as forgetting and wandering. Research on the prevention of AD, especially for women, has focused on hormone replacement therapy—namely, estrogen replacement—as well as vitamin E and anti-inflammatory agents, such as steroids and ibupro-

Box 19–8 Criteria for Probable Diagnosis of Alzheimer's Disease

- Dementia established by clinical examination; documented by Mini-Mental State Examination; and confirmed by neuropsychologic tests.
- Deficits in two or more areas of cognition.
- Progressive worsening of memory and other cognitive functions.
- No disturbance in consciousness.
- Onset between ages of 40 and 90 years, most after 65.
- No systemic disorders or brain disease that could be the cause of memory and cognitive deficits.

Source: Adapted from *Merck Manual of Diagnosis and Therapy,* Edition 17, edited by Mark H. Beers and Robert Berkow. Copyright 1999 by Merck & Co., Inc., Whitehouse Station, NJ.

fen. Initially, the administration of estrogen or estrogen compounds was thought to be helpful. However, more recently, some clinicians question the preventive impact that estrogen and vitamin E supplements have for AD (National Institute of Aging, 2000).

Estrogen and vitamin E are prescribed frequently in hopes of slowing the progression of cognitive decline. Three additional medications, tacrine (Cognax), rivastigmine (Exelon), and denepezil hydrochloride (Aricept), act by inhibiting acetylcholinesterace, an enzyme that breaks down the neurotransmitter acetylcholine. Acetylcholine supports cognition, and its levels are reduced in AD. Tacrine, denepezil hydrochloride, and rivastigmine neither stop nor reverse disease progression and are reported to help only some AD patients for periods of time ranging from a few months to a few years (Progress Report on Alzheimer's Disease, 1999). Studies are underway to ascertain whether they are helpful in the prevention of AD.

A number of nonpharmacological practices and therapies can be used to help people with Alzheimer's disease function at the highest possible level. They include frequent orientation reinforcement, music therapy, a bright and cheerful environment, the minimizing of that which is unfamiliar, low-stress activities, and a safe environment for walking. Maintaining consistency regarding caregivers and daily routines may also lessen the frequency of behavioral outbursts.

Interacting with a person who has Alzheimer's disease can be extremely stressful for family members and caregivers, particularly in the later stages of the disease. Witnessing the steady decline into helplessness of a spouse or parent often triggers both sadness and anger, and the overall physical, emotional, and financial burden can be tremendous. It is imperative that a support system be available for counseling, healthcare supervision, financial advising, and respite care. Placement in a healthcare facility is often necessary during the intermediate and terminal phases of AD. A cure is currently not feasible despite considerable research. Hope for a cure rests in genetic research.

Epilepsy

Epilepsy is a chronic neurological disease characterized by recurrent, unprovoked **seizures** (abnormal, involuntary movements, behaviors, or perceptions) that result from altered brain function. A seizure, or even multiple seizures, related to a *temporary* injury or condition is considered an isolated event and does not warrant the diagnosis of epilepsy. The causes of seizures and epilepsy are many and include any disease or illness that causes a disruption of the neurons in the brain. Frequently, the cause is unknown. Neurons can become unstable because of a genetic defect, as in juvenile myoclonic epilepsy; because of a metabolic abnormality such as a low blood glucose level or a high blood alcohol level; or because of abnormal discharges in a focal area of the brain. Such discharges could be caused by a brain tumor, a cerebral vascular accident (stroke), a head injury, or a structural defect in the brain.

Epilepsy affects an estimated 2.5 million people in the United States and 40 million worldwide (National Institute of Neurological Disorders and Strokes [NINDS], 2000).

Approximately 10 percent of the population will experience a seizure at some point, but not all will go on to develop epilepsy (Hauser, Annegers, & Kurland, 1993). Children and the elderly have a greater incidence of seizures. Epilepsy affects 3.4 percent of men and 2.8 percent of women. The higher incidence of epilepsy in men is thought to be related to men's greater risk of sustaining injury to the brain in the form of cerebral palsy, head injury, and cerebrovascular disease (Hauser, Annegers, & Kurland, 1993). Although more men have epilepsy, women who have it face special challenges, as both seizures and exposure to anti-epilepsy drugs (AEDs) can compromise reproductive health.

The majority of individuals with epilepsy are able to control their seizures with medication. The few who cannot, however, find that uncontrolled epilepsy compromises quality of life. The risk of being injured during a seizure or having one in public is a source of anxiety for individuals with uncontrolled epilepsy and their families. Most adults who have epilepsy choose not to disclose their disorder to others because of the perceived stigma (Warner, 1996).

The way in which a seizure is manifested varies according to its type and the part of the brain from which it arises. An individual having a seizure may display an altered level of consciousness and/or experience involuntary movements (convulsions) or the cessation of movement. She may also experience sensory or psychic phenomena or autonomic disturbances; for example, an individual may describe a smell, sound, sight, a sense of déjà vu, or a fluttering sensation from within.

SYMPTOMS

The Commission on Classification and Terminology of the International League Against Epilepsy (1981) classifies seizures into two broad categories: **generalized seizures,** which are bilateral and without a focal origin, and **partial seizures,** which begin in a focal area of the brain. Generalized seizures are further subclassified according to the clinical signs and symptoms they cause. **Typical absence seizures,** formerly referred to as *petit mal seizures,* cause brief episodes of impaired awareness. For example, a person experiencing a typical absence seizure may suddenly stare into space for a brief period and then return to normal behavior with no memory of the event. Another possibility is that a person having an absence seizure may unknowingly carry out a repetitive behavior, such as blinking the eyes several times in rapid succession. Generalized seizures may also manifest as unusual and, in some instances, somewhat spectacular, motor activity. An individual may suddenly lose all muscle tone in a limb or throughout the body and might drop something or fall to the ground. The person might jerk her body suddenly, as people often do as they are falling asleep. The type of generalized seizure most often portrayed in movies, and therefore most familiar to the public, is the **tonic-clonic seizure,** formally known as a *grand mal seizure.* A person experiencing such a seizure will simultaneously lose consciousness, fall to the ground, and exhibit a stiffening of the entire body. The stiffening phase is known as the **tonic phase** of the seizure. The tonic phase is followed by the **clonic phase,** during which the muscles **convulse** (contract and relax) rhythmically. Onlookers can best aid persons experiencing tonic-clonic seizures by preventing them from injuring their head or limbs. It is a myth that persons experiencing tonic-clonic seizures "swallow their tongues," although the tongue may be bitten as the jaws clamp down during the tonic phase of the episode. The person will stop breathing for a few seconds, but respiration will resume spontaneously. The majority of seizures do not manifest as convulsions but, rather, as changes in behavior, which can range from a fleeting loss of awareness lasting a few seconds to repetitive actions lasting a few minutes.

Partial seizures, formerly known as *auras,* are experienced consciously and may occur in isolation or may be a signal that a generalized seizure is imminent. The ways in which partial seizures are experienced depends on the areas of the brain involved. An individual may experience a jerking or stiffening in a certain part of the body or may have a sensory experience that is visual, tactile, auditory, or olfactory (smelled). **Psychic partial seizures** may cause the person to experience a specific perception, memory, or emotion.

DIAGNOSIS

Diagnosing epilepsy involves establishing that seizures are occurring and identifying the cause and any precipitating factors. The diagnostic workup may include a history and physical examination, an electroencephalogram, brain imaging studies, and laboratory studies. A correct diagnosis is crucial; a misdiagnosis of epilepsy may unnecessarily subject the person to expensive laboratory tests and medications that can cause serious side effects. Even more dire consequences are the loss of one's driver's license and possibly employment as well. Such losses can seriously compromise an individual's independence.

An **electroencephalogram (EEG)** is a noninvasive brain-wave study that is similar to an electrocardiogram. It confirms the presence of abnormal electrical activity in the brain and may yield information regarding the type and location of the seizure focus. In some individuals, the EEG may be abnormal only when a seizure is actually occurring. If the EEG is normal or indicates a focal origin of seizure activity, a CAT scan or MRI, may be needed to evaluate cerebral structures. MRIs are preferred over CT scans because of their greater sensitivity for identifying small lesions. In selected cases, radioisotope scanning, such as SPECT or PET scans, may be used to determine whether there is a single epileptic focus, which could be removed surgically, or whether there are multiple foci, which would rule out surgery as a treatment option.

Identifying and managing the factors that precipitate seizures may reduce the frequency with which seizures occur and the amount of medication needed to control them. Seizure precipitants include sleep deprivation, hyperventilation, photosensitivity, anxiety and stress, concurrent illness or fever, fluid or electrolyte imbalances, hormonal changes (such as those during menses), and alcohol or drugs.

TREATMENT

Medical treatment is directed toward using medication to control the abnormal electrical discharges occurring in the brain. In 80 percent of individuals diagnosed with epilepsy, seizures can be controlled by medication. Before the decision to initiate medical treatment is made, however, the probability and risk of recurrent seizures will be weighed against the toxicity and side effects associated with medications. If drug therapy is decided on, treatment will be initiated with the single drug that has shown the best combination of high efficacy for the type of seizure in question and low toxicity/side effect profile (Shorvon, 2000).

Unfortunately, approximately 20 percent of individuals with epilepsy continue to have uncontrolled seizures despite the use of medications. A number of therapies are available to such persons: surgery, vagal nerve stimulation, and a ketogenic diet.

Surgical procedures, such as temporal lobectomy or hemispherectomy, may be an option for individuals who have partial seizures. In a **temporal lobectomy,** the temporal lobe from one side of the brain is removed. In a **hemispherectomy,** the entire right or left side of the brain is removed to decrease the frequency of seizures. Individuals who have certain forms of generalized seizures may have a **palliative** (treats symptoms but not the cause) procedure, known as corpus callosotomy, performed to decrease the severity of the seizures. In **corpus callosotomy,** the corpus callosum, a neuronal "highway" that connects the right and left hemispheres, is severed.

A device known as a **vagal nerve stimulator** was approved in 1997 by the Food and Drug Administration for the treatment of seizures not well controlled by medication. The device, a pulse generator the size of a pocket watch, is surgically placed under the soft tissues of the upper left chest, and electrodes attached to it are wrapped around the left vagus nerve in the neck. The device stimulates the vagus nerve when a seizure is imminent, thus desynchronizing brain activity and aborting the seizure. The device works well for some patients.

Another treatment alternative for stubborn seizure disorders is the **ketogenic diet,** a low-carbohydrate diet that forces the body to burn fat instead of carbohydrates for energy, thereby causing ketones (by-products of fat metabolism) to be produced in the body. The diet seems to work best with children who have certain forms of epilepsy.

IMPLICATIONS FOR WOMEN

Epilepsy has unique implications for women. Ovarian sex steroid hormones alter neuronal excitability and can influence the frequency with which seizures occur. The overall effect of estrogen is to increase neuronal excitability, whereas progesterone reduces excitability. Thirty to 50 percent of women with epilepsy experience **catamenial** (associated with the menstrual cycle) exacerbations of seizure frequency. Seizures can be more frequent just before and during the menstrual flow and at ovulation, corresponding with the rise and fall of estrogen and progesterone levels (Herzog & Klein, 1996). The onset of juvenile myoclonic epilepsy (JME) at puberty may be associated with the substantial increase in sex hormones that occurs at that time. Research investigating the effect of menopause on epilepsy is ongoing, but results to date are inconclusive.

The effects of anti-epilepsy drugs (AEDs) may be somewhat different in women than in men because of women's smaller body size, higher body fat content, lower body water content, and lesser muscle mass. Interactions with endogenous hormones and with therapeutic hormones in the form of oral contraceptives and menopausal hormone replacement therapy may also alter AED efficacy. Conversely, AEDs can alter the effectiveness of other drugs and hormones. For example, the AEDs listed in Box 19–9 cause binding of the hormones in birth control pills, leading to contraceptive failure. In order to ensure contraceptive protection, women on those AEDs must take higher-dose oral contraceptives, which contain more than 50 ug of estradiol. Most oral contraceptive preparations contain only 35 ug of estrogen. Progesterone-only oral contraceptives may also be ineffective in women who are on certain AEDs. Intramuscular medroxyprogesterone (Depo-Provera) has not been evaluated for efficacy in women receiving these AEDs.

The older AEDs, including sodium phenytoin and carbamazepine, are associated with bone disorders, such as osteoporosis, secondary to bone demineralization. The effects of the newer AEDs on bone health have not been evaluated; additional studies are required. Women who take AEDs should supplement their diets with calcium and Vitamin D. The most severe bone abnormalities are seen in women who are receiving multiple AED drugs and those who have been taking AEDs for a long period of time (Morrell, 1998).

Women with epilepsy are also at risk for reduced fertility. Schupf & Ottman (1994) found that women with epilepsy are only 37 percent as likely to become pregnant as women without epilepsy. AEDs may cause abnormalities in basal concentrations of gonadotropins and ovarian sex steroids. In addition, AEDs may increase the risk of developing specific reproductive disturbances, such as polycystic ovary (PCO) disease, a condition in which the presence of multiple cysts interferes with ovarian function. Isojarvi and colleagues (1993) found a higher risk of PCO disease with the use of valproate as compared with carbamazepine, but many experts disagree with the results. A large international study on the incidence of PCO disease in individuals who take valproate or tolamotrigine is underway.

Epilepsy is associated with sexual dysfunction in both men and women. Women with epilepsy report a global **hyposexuality** (decreased libido), which may have physiological or psychological causes. It is thought that electrical discharges in certain parts of the brain, or drug-induced alterations in the sex hormones, interfere with decreased arousal. Impaired so-

Box 19–9   Antiepileptic Drugs That Can Inactivate Oral Contraceptives

- ◆ phenytoin (Dilantin)
- ◆ carbamazepine (Tegretal)
- ◆ phenobarbitol (Luminal)
- ◆ valproic acid (Depakote)
- ◆ primidone (Mysoline)
- ◆ ethosuximide (Zarontin)

Source: Adapted from Table 4, "Effects of Various AEDS on Hormonal Contraception." Morrell MJ, Montouris G, Gidal BE, Zupanc, ML. *Managing Epilepsy in Women Across the Reproductive Cycle: ACME Monograph for Neurologists,* Copyright © 2001. Reproduced with permission from Projects in Knowledge, Inc., Secaucus, New Jersey.

cial development and self-esteem related to the diagnosis of epilepsy may also play a role. Also, both men and women with epilepsy report fearing that they will have a seizure during sexual intercourse. Counseling may be helpful in resolving psychologically induced sexual dysfunction.

Epilepsy is one of the most frequent neurological complications encountered during pregnancy. It affects 0.3 to 0.6 percent of all pregnancies (Norwitz & Repke, 1998). Women who take AEDs are at greater risk for spontaneous abortion, miscarriage, and preterm delivery. These adverse outcomes may be secondary to recurrent tonic-clonic seizures that may be associated with fetal hypoxia (low blood oxygen levels). Epilepsy can also compromise fertility; AED-induced abnormalities in the formation of the endometrium can compromise implantation of the ovum.

Pregnancy can affect the frequency during which seizures occur. Approximately 30 percent of women with epilepsy experience an increased frequency of seizures, and 30 percent experience a decrease. The rest notice no change. Changes in seizure frequency may be related, at least in part, to the effects of pregnancy on AED metabolism. Another factor may be poor medication compliance prompted by the fear that the medication may have an adverse effect on the fetus. Optimizing medical management during pregnancy and informing women about the reasons for changes in their drug regimen may improve compliance. Women need to understand that, when they are pregnant, they need *greater* doses of medication in order to maintain the same serum level. They must also understand that uncontrolled seizures may be dangerous to the fetus. The risk of bearing a child with congenital anomalies in the general population is 2 to 4 percent but is 4 to 8 percent in women with epilepsy, regardless of medication (Morrell, 1997). The possible mechanisms leading to fetal malformation include the effects of maternal seizures and AEDs and genetic predisposition.

Exposure to AEDs during pregnancy is associated with an increased risk of congenital abnormalities in offspring. Major malformations include cleft palate and cleft lip, congenital heart disease, and neural tube defect. Cleft lip and palate are increased by 4.7 percent in children with AED-treated mothers, compared with children of non-AED mothers. The incidence of congenital heart defects is two to four times that of the normal population. Carbamazepine and valproate are associated with neural tube defect at an incidence of 0.5 to 2 percent. Minor abnormalities, which the child may outgrow, can also occur. The risk of birth defects increases significantly when more than one AED drug must be taken (Morrell, 1998).

The United States Public Health Service recommends that all women of childbearing age who are capable of becoming pregnant consume 0.4 mg of folic acid daily for the purpose of reducing the risk of having a child with a neural tube defect. For women who have already had a child with a neural tube defect, the suggested dose is 4 mg per day. Definitive doses of folic acid in women with epilepsy have not been identified, but a dose of 0.8 to 5 mg per day during the reproductive years is recommended.

Neonates whose mothers have epilepsy are at risk for early hemorrhage. It is thought that AEDs interfere with the metabolism of vitamin K, which is essential for sufficient clotting ability. A vitamin K deficit can be avoided by supplementing the mother with 10 mg per day during the last month of pregnancy or by supplying the neonate with vitamin K at birth.

Women with epilepsy are not routinely discouraged from breast-feeding their infants. The concentration of AEDs in breast milk is inversely proportional to the degree to which the AEDs are protein-bound. Highly protein-bound drugs, such as phenytoin and valproate, have a very low concentration in breast milk, whereas drugs with low or no protein binding can be expected to maintain concentrations in the breast milk that are close to the mother's serum level (Morrell, 1998). The benefits of breast-feeding must be weighed against the risks of exposure to the medications. Decisions about breast-feeding should be based on an assessment of the neonate in regard to irritability, poor feeding, or inadequate weight gain.

Living with epilepsy can be extremely challenging for individuals and their family members. Support groups are an excellent source of support, education, and social interaction. The Epilepsy Foundation of America in Landover, Maryland, is an excellent resource for educational materials and referral sources (Warner, 1996).

Parkinson's Disease

Parkinson's disease (PD) is a movement disorder resulting from chronic degenerative changes in an area of the brain known as the substantia nigra. The substantia nigra, an area of the basal ganglia, is located deep within the brain, lateral to the thalamus. The brain cells in the basal ganglia allow us to carry out purposeful movement in a smooth, coordinated manner. In order for that to occur, there must be a fine balance between excitatory and inhibitory neural activity. The prime excitatory neurotransmitter is acetylcholine, and its inhibitory counterpart is dopamine. Dopamine is secreted by the cells of the substantia nigra. Histological examination of brain tissue taken from persons suffering from PD shows neuronal loss in the substantia nigra and the presence of two types of abnormal tissue, Lewy bodies and pale bodies, within the substantia nigra. In PD, Lewy bodies are also present in the basal ganglia, cerebral cortex, brain stem, and spinal cord. Although Lewy bodies are characteristic of PD, they are also seen in Alzheimer's disease and other neurodegenerative diseases.

By the time an individual begins to experience the symptoms of PD, she has lost 80 to 85 percent of the neurons that synthesize dopamine. This drastic decrease in dopamine causes the hypokinetic (slow movement) symptoms characteristic of PD (Aird, 2000).

Approximately 1 million Americans have PD, with women and men affected in equal numbers. PD is the second most common neurodegenerative disease after Alzheimer's. It typically develops after the age of 40 and before the age of 70, but it is most common in people over 55 years of age. However, 10 percent of cases affect individuals under age 40 (Olanow & Koller, 1998). As life expectancy increases, so does the incidence of PD.

Although both inherited and environmental factors have been implicated in the etiology (cause) of PD, no specific cause has been found. Studies have, however, documented an increased incidence of PD in individuals who have a family history of it and in individuals who have been exposed to insecticides and herbicides. Other factors that have been linked to an increased incidence include living in a rural area, drinking well water, and having routinely eaten nuts or seeds in the 10 years prior to diagnosis (Hickey, 1997).

Currently, a number of researchers are focusing on selective oxidative stress secondary to environmental toxicity as a promising contributing factor in PD. It is known that, when cell membranes, including brain cell membranes, are exposed to oxidative metabolic byproducts, such as hydrogen peroxide, superoxide anions, and hydroxy-radicals, membrane disruption and cellular death occur. It is now thought that PD may develop as a result of a combination of genetic predisposition and exposure to an environmental toxin (Jankovic & Stacy, 1999).

SYMPTOMS

The cardinal features of PD can be summed up by the acronym TRAP: tremor, rigidity, akinesia (absence or slowness of movement), and postural instability. Resting tremor (shaking) is present in 70 to 80 percent of cases. It is worsened by stress and generally disappears or decreases with movement. Tremor usually involves the limbs, face, jaw, and tongue. Forearm tremor usually involves a combination of pronation and supination that has been described as "pill rolling." Affected individuals use a variety of methods to conceal tremors, such as holding one hand with the other or sitting on the affected hand.

The rigidity characteristic of PD involves stiffness and a resistance to smooth movement that is equal in all muscle groups and that remains when the extremities are moved passively. If a tremor is also present, most of the rigidity may be broken up by rhythmic "catches" on movement (cogwheel phenomenon).

If akinesia is present, the activities of daily living, such as dressing, feeding, or brushing teeth, will be carried out very slowly. Related features are the **facial mask** (loss of facial expression), **dysarthria** (slurred speech), **dysphagia** (difficulty swallowing), limited ability to swing the arms, and **micrographia** (slow and small handwriting). Drooling of saliva is common due to an inability to swallow it. In more advanced stages of PD, frequent freezing of movement is seen; this manifests as hesitancy in initiating movement or difficulty with turning while walking.

Postural instability (PI) often occurs in the advanced stages of PD. The head tilts forward, and the posture becomes stooped. Walking involves small, slow, shuffling steps. There is a tendency to propel forward or fall backward when standing or walking. Other signs of PD include difficulty in turning in bed and walking in an enclosed space, such as an elevator.

Disturbed sleep and depression are also common in PD, as are difficulties with vision, constipation, seborrhea, and excessive sweating. Slowness of thought, cognitive problems, and dementia may occur later in the disease. The behavioral and psychiatric disorders associated with PD can be more disabling than the motor dysfunction. Depression is estimated to occur in 40 to 60 percent of patients with PD and may be related to the duration of the disease and the amount of interference with activities of daily living. Because it occurs in younger individuals, PD affects family life and career development.

Parkinson's disease can be quite disabling. Individuals with PD lose not only control over their body movements but their independence as well. Most eventually need assistance in carrying out day-to-day activities. Support groups are available to help patients and their families cope with the many problems associated with PD.

DIAGNOSIS

The diagnosis of PD is usually based on the signs and symptoms. Movement disorder specialists consider a good response to dopamine-like drugs to be useful in supporting the diagnosis. The main difficulty in the clinical diagnosis of PD is distinguishing the disease from conditions that mimic it. MRI is crucial in ruling out a stroke and other degenerative disorders.

TREATMENT

The pharmacological treatment of PD is divided into two main categories: symptomatic and protective. **Symptomatic treatment** is used to improve signs and symptoms of the disease. **Protective treatment** interferes with the pathophysiological mechanisms of the disease. The goal of therapy is to reverse the functional disability, although the ablation of all the signs and symptoms is not currently possible, even with the highest doses of medication. Treatment is very individualized, and the patient, as well as the healthcare provider, plays a role in therapeutic decisionmaking. Symptomatic treatment is often not initiated until the symptoms begin to interfere with the activities of daily living, because many of the medications have significant side effects and because tolerance to the medications can develop. Although the mainstay of treatment is medication, the day-to-day management of PD requires a multidisciplinary approach involving occupational, physical, speech, and dietary therapy, as well as nursing care and the use of various other support systems.

Drugs The mainstay of medical treatment for PD is the drug combination levodopa/carbidopa (Sinemet). Levodopa is converted into dopamine in the brain. Because certain enzymes would ordinarily break down levodopa before it reached the brain, carbidopa is administered along with levodopa to block the enzymes and allow more levodopa to reach the brain. As the disease progresses, however, the benefits received from levodopa tend to decrease, whereas its side effects tend to increase. The side effects of levodopa include dose-related alterations in motor functioning and behavioral and psychiatric disorders, including dementia, depression, hallucinations, psychosis, and sleep disturbances. **Orthostatic hypotension** (becoming dizzy while rising to a sitting or standing position) and gastrointestinal side effects can also occur (Herndon, Young, Herndon, & Dole, 2000).

Selegiline (Eldepryl) is another drug used in PD. It selectively inhibits monoamine oxidase, the enzyme that metabolizes dopamine, and it protects brain cells from free radical damage. Selegiline is often used initially in place of levodopa. However, there is considerable controversy over the use of this drug. Recent studies indicate that it is best used to prolong levodopa's symptomatic benefit (Waters, 1998).

Anticholinergic drugs, including benzotropine (Cogentin) and trihexyphenidyl (Artane), are the oldest drugs used in the symptomatic treatment of PD. The anticholinergics are thought to be most effective in decreasing tremor, although they also improve rigidity and slowness. As their name suggests, anticholinergic agents antagonize cholinergic (excitatory) neurons, which normally would have been balanced by the anti-excitatory effects of dopamine. Anticholinergics have numerous side effects that limit their use.

Amantadine (Symmetrel) is an antiviral agent found to have an anti-Parkinson's effect, although the precise mechanism of action is not well understood. It is known that amantadine releases dopamine from peripheral neuronal storage sites in animals, and it might exert a similar effect in humans. Amantadine has a minimal effect on tremors, and the development of tolerance often limits its use. Amantadine is frequently used in patients who are in the later stages of the disease and those who are on maximal doses of levodopa.

High doses of the antioxident vitamin E (tocopherol) are sometimes used in PD. Epidemiological data suggest a correlation between a relatively low vitamin E intake and the onset of PD. Also, some studies suggest that PD patients who receive vitamin supplementation have a more benign clinical course than those who do not (Whitney, Cataldo, & Rolfes, 1998). Although there is controversy regarding the relationship between vitamin E and risk for PD, some investigators have concluded that a high intake of dietary vitamin E may protect against PD. More research is needed in this area.

Another class of drugs used in PD is the dopamine agonists. These include bromocriptine (Parlodel), pergolide (Permax), pramipexole (Mirapex), and ropinirole (Requip). Dopamine agonists bypass failing neuronal pathways and stimulate receptors in the substantia nigra directly. With the exception of levodopa, this category seems to be the most effective class of drugs for PD. The older dopa agonists, bromocriptine and pergolide, are used as adjunctive therapy with levodopa and may allow a reduction in its dose. Unfortunately, these agents are associated with a high incidence of dose-related side effects, including postural hypotension and hallucinations. The newer drugs, pramipexole and ropinirole, can be used by themselves to control general symptoms. They cause fewer side effects than some other drugs because they bind to different dopamine receptors.

The latest category of drugs used to combat PD are the catechol-0-methyl transferase (COMT) inhibitors. COMT breaks down dopamine in the peripheral circulation and in the brain. Inhibiting its action raises dopamine levels and allows them to be sustained for a longer period of time. Two COMT-inhibiting drugs, tolcapone (Tasmar) and entacapone (Comtan), have shown promise in the treatment of PD, although the rate at which they cause side effects remains high. Because tolcapone can cause liver disease, its use requires frequent monitoring of liver function.

Surgical Treatment   The surgical treatment for PD consists of constructive and destructive procedures. **Constructive procedures** implant into the brain new cells that can synthesize dopamine. Transplanting human embryonic mesencephalic tissue into the basal ganglia of PD patients has been demonstrated to improve motor function and to decrease rigidity and slowness of movement. The pattern and degree of symptomatic relief have varied among patients who have had the procedure, and more clinical trials are needed before it can be considered a standard treatment (Hagell, 2000).

Destructive procedures, such as thalamotomy and pallidotomy, are used to stop overactive areas in various parts of the brain from causing motor dysfunction. They have proved extremely effective in treating tremor, rigidity, and drug-induced dyskinesia. The side effects include cerebral **hematomas** (blood collecting in an area of the brain), ischemic cerebrovascular accidents (strokes), and inadvertent damage to the brain. Another surgical method of controlling PD symptoms involves the direct electrical stimulation of the subcortical areas of the basal ganglia. This procedure is thought to work via a variety of mechanisms, depending on the type of stimulation applied and the location of the stimulating electrode (Waters, 1998). With the resurgence of surgical procedures, additional research is required to guide patient selection and assess overall outcomes.

New Directions

The MS Society and the National Institute of Allergy and Infectious Diseases are conducting a $20 million study of gender differences in immune functioning. The knowledge gained from this project may shed light on why women tend to develop autoimmune diseases, such as MS, more often than men and may lead to better treatments for such diseases as well. Clinical trials are being conducted on approximately 70 new drugs and devices intended to help MS patients.

Research on neurodegenerative disorders, particularly AD and PD, focuses mainly on interventions that may limit the degenerative effects of these disorders. Introducing specialized nerve cells developed from embryonic stem cells into the brains or spinal cords of laboratory animals has been found to yield positive results by researchers at the University of Bonn, the National Institutes of Health in Maryland, and the University of Wisconsin–Madison (Brustle et al., 1999). Administration of methylcobalamine, a form of vitamin B-12, has shown some promise in the treatment of PD, AD, and MS. A naturally occurring substance known as coenzyme Q10 has been shown to slow the disruption of neural cellular metabolism in laboratory mice. Because a significant reduction of CoQ10 levels has been noted in Parkinson's patients, coenzyme Q10 may have potential for slowing the progression of the disease (*CoQ10 and the Brain*, 1998). Researchers at the National Institutes of Health are exploring a number of approaches to the treatment of dementia. These include anti-inflammatory agents, such as ibuprofen; estrogen and estrogenic compounds; antioxidants, such as ginkgo biloba; and a compound known as nerve growth factor (*Regenerating Brain Cells*, 1998). An anti-amyloid vaccine has been shown to reduce amyloid deposits (such as those that develop in the brains of patients with Alzheimer's disease) in the brains of mice (Helmuth, 2000). Research into genetic factors associated with neurodegenerative disorders is also underway.

Neurological Wellness Self-Assessment

If the following statements apply to you, your neurological system is probably functioning well.

1. *I do not get frequent headaches.*
2. *I seldom have difficulty keeping my balance.*
3. *I have no unexplained weakness in any of my extremities.*
4. *I have no constant or intermittent sensation of numbness or tingling anywhere in my body.*
5. *My vision never becomes temporarily blurred or dim.*
6. *I have never had a seizure.*
7. *I have never been told I sometimes exhibit unusual behaviors I do not remember.*
8. *I seldom forget important occasions or appointments.*
9. *I do not get lost in familiar places.*
10. *No family member or friend has ever told me I am getting forgetful.*

QUESTIONS FOR REFLECTION AND DISCUSSION

1. *What are some possible reasons that more women than men suffer from headaches?*
2. *Have you known anyone with dementia? If so, what is your attitude toward her or him?*
3. *If you were to be afflicted with MS, what would be the most challenging aspect of the disease for you?*
4. *If you were to be afflicted with epilepsy, what would be the most challenging aspect of the disease for you?*
5. *If you were to be afflicted with Parkinson's disease, what would be the most challenging aspect of it for you?*
6. *What resources for individuals with neurodegenerative disorders are available in your area?*

RESOURCES

Books

Hickey, J. V. (Ed.). (1997). *The clinical practice of neurological and neurosurgical nursing.* Philadelphia: Lippencott.
Kaplan, P. W. (Ed.). (1998). *Neurological diseases in women.* New York: Demos.

Organizations

Alzheimer's Disease Education Referral Center
P.O. Box 8250
Silver Spring, MD 20907-8250
Phone: 1-800-438-4380
http://www.alzheimers.org

Epilepsy Foundation
4051 Garden City Drive
Landover, MD 20785-7220
http://www.efa.org

National Headache Foundation
428 W. St. James Place, 2nd Floor
Chicago, Il 60614
Phone: 1-888-643-5552
http://www.headaches.org

National Multiple Sclerosis Society
733 Third Avenue
New York, NY 10017
http://www.nationalmssociety.org

The Parkinson's Movement Disorder Institute
9940 Talbert Ave., Suite 204
Fountain Valley, CA 92708
Phone: 714-378-5062
http://www.pmdi.org

REFERENCES

Aird, T. (2000). Functional anatomy of the basal ganglia. *Journal of Neuroscience Nursing, 32*(5), 250–253.
Brustle, O., Jones, K. N., Leavesh, R. D., Karran, K., Chanday, K., Westler, O. D., Duran, I. D., & McKay, R. D. (1999). Embryonic stem cell-derived glial precursors: A source of mylelinating. *Science, 285,* 754–756.
Commission on Classification and Terminology of the International League Against Epilepsy. (1981). Proposal for revised clinical and electroencephalographic classification of epileptic seizures. *Epilepsia, 22,* 489–501.
CoQ10 and the brain. (1998). *Life Extension Foundation Collector's Edition, 32,* 38–40.
Coyle, P. K. (1998). Multiple sclerosis. In P. W. Kaplan (Ed.), *Neurological diseases in women* (pp. 251–264). New York: Demos.
Delirium and dementia. (1999). *Merck Manual of Geriatrics.* Available: http://www.merck.com/pubs/mm_geriatrics/90x.htm
Emerging therapies. (1998, February). *Harvard Women's Health Watch,* pp. 4–5.
Forno, G. D., Maki, P. M., & Kawas, C. H. (1998). Alzheimer's disease in women and the role of estrogens. In P. W. Kaplan (Ed.), *Neurological diseases in women* (pp. 161–172). New York: Demos.
Hagell, P. (2000). Restorative neurology in movement disorders. *Journal of Neuroscience Nursing, 32*(5), 256–262.
Hauser, W. A., Annegers, J. F., & Kurland, L. T. (1993). Incidence of epilepsy and unprovoked seizures in Rochester, Minnesota: 1935–1984. *Epilepsia, 34*(3), 453–468.
Helmuth, L. (2000). Alzheimer's Congress: Further progress on beta-amyloid vaccine. *Science, 289,* 5478.
Herndon, L. M., Young, K., Herndon, A. D., & Dole, E. J. (2000). Parkinson's disease revisited. *Journal of Neuroscience Nursing, 32*(4), 216–221.
Herzog, A. G., & Klein, P. (1996) Three patterns of catamenial epilepsy. *Epilepsia, 37,* 83.

Hickey, J. V. (Ed.) (1997). *The clinical practice of neurological and neurosurgical nursing.* Philadelphia: Lippincott, Williams, & Wilkens.

Holland, N., & Halper, J. (1999). Current treatment of multiple sclerosis. *Advance for Nurse Practitioners, 4,* 27–32.

Isojarvi, J. I. T., Laatikainen, T. J., Pakarinen, A. J., Juntunen, K. T. S., & Mullyla, V. V. (1993). Polycystic ovaries and hyperandrogenism in women taking valproate for epilepsy. *New England Journal of Medicine, 329,* 1383–1388.

Jacopini, G. (2000). The experience of disease: Psychosocial aspects of movement disorders. *Journal of Neuroscience Nursing, 32*(5), 263–265.

Jankovic, J., & Stacy, M. (1999). Movement disorders. In C. G. Goetz & E. J. Goetz (Eds.), *Textbook of clinical neurology* (pp. 655–679). Philadelphia: Saunders.

Jensen, R. (2001). Mechanisms of tension-type headache. *Cephalalgia, 21* (7), 786–789.

Kaplan, P. W. (1999). *Neurological diseases in women.* New York: Demos.

Khurana. (1999). Migraines. In P. W. Kaplan (Ed.), *Neurological diseases in women.* (pp. 173–188). New York: Demos.

Lang, A. E. (1996) Movement disorder symptomatology. In W. G. Bradley, R. B. Daroff, G. M. Fenichel, & C. D. Marsden (Eds.), *Neurology in clinical practice, principles of diagnosis and management* (pp. 299–320). New York: Butterworth-Heinemann.

Maloney, F. M., Matthews, K. B., Scharbo-Dehaan, M., & Strickland, O. L. (2000). Caring for the woman with migraine headaches. *The Nurse Practitioner 25*(2), pp. 17–18, 21–22, 24, 27, 28, 30, 33, 36.

Morrell, M. J. (1997). Pregnancy and epilepsy. In R. J. Porter & D. Chadwick (Eds.), *The epilepsies 2* (pp. 320–325). Boston: Butterworth-Heinemann.

Morrell, M. J. (1998). Seizures and epilepsy in women. In P. W. Kaplan (Ed.), *Neurologic diseases in women* (pp. 219–228). New York: Demos.

Morrell, M. J., Montouris, G., Gidal, B. E., & Zupanc, M. L. (2001). Managing epilepsy in women across the reproductive cycle. *ACME Monograph for Neurologists.* Secaucus, NJ: Projects in Knowledge, Inc.

National Headache Foundation. (1998, March). *Migraine.* Chicago, IL: National Headache Foundation.

National Institute of Aging. (2000). [On-line]. Estrogen replacement therapy not effective treatment of Alzheimer's disease in some women. *National Institute of Aging News.* Available: www.alheimers.org/nianews.

National Institute of Neurological Disorders and Strokes (NINDS) Consensus Conference. (2000, March). *Curing Epilepsy: Focus on the Future,* Betheseda, MD.

Norwitz, E. R., & Repke, J. T. (1998). Obstetric issues in women with neurological diseases. In P. W. Kaplan. (Ed.), *Neurologic diseases in women* (pp. 119–134). New York: Demos.

Olanow, C. W., & Koller, W. C. (1998). An algorithm (decision tree) for the management of Parkinson's disease: Treatment guidelines. *Neurology, 50* (Suppl 3), 551–557.

Progress report on Alzheimer's disease. (1999). *Merck Manual of Geriatrics.* [On-line]. Available: http://www.alzheimers.org/pubs/pr99.htm

Regenerating brain cells. (1998). *Life Extension Foundation Collector's Edition 2,* pp. 34–37.

Rosenfeld, I. (1999, February 7). When a nasty headache comes along. *Parade Magazine,* pp. 18, 20, 21.

Schupf, N., & Ottman, R. (1994). Likelihood of pregnancy in individuals with idiopathic/cryptogenic epilepsy: Social and biological influence. *Epilepsia, 35*(4), 750–756.

Schwartz, B. S., Stewart, W. F., Simon, D., & Lipton, R. B. (1998). Epidemiology of tension-type headache. *Journal of the American Medical Association, 249* (5), 381–384.

Shorvon, S. D. (2000). *Handbook of epilepsy treatment.* Malden, MA: Blackwell Science Ltd.

Spinal cord injury. (1999). [On-line]. National Center for Injury Prevention and Control. Available: http://www.cdc.gov/ncip/pub-res/scicongress.htm

Trapp, B. D., et al. (1998). Axonal transaction in the lesions of multiple sclerosis. *New England Journal of Medicine, 338,* 278–285.

Traumatic brain injury. (1999). [On-line]. National Center for Injury Prevention and Control. Available: http://www.cdc.gov/ncipc/pub-res/tbicongress.htm

Warner, L. S. (1996). *The relationship of selected psychosocial and pathysiological variables to depression in epilepsy patients.* Unpublished doctoral dissertation, the Catholic University of America, Washington, DC.

Waters, C. H. (1998). *Diagnosis and management of Parkinson's disease.* Los Angeles: Professional Communications.

When the doctor suspects MS. (2001). *Women's Health Advisor, 5*(5), 4–5.

Whitney, E. N., Cataldo, C. B., & Rolfes, S. R. (1998). *Understanding normal and clinical nutrition* (5th ed.). Belmont, CA: Wadsworth.

Zeidenstein, L. (1998). Alternative therapies for nausea and vomiting of pregnancy. *American Journal of Nurse Midwifery, 43*(5), 392–393.

20

Immunological Wellness and Illness

Eric Doerfler and Joan Davenport

Objectives

1. *Describe the basic components of the human immune system and explain their function.*
2. *List three measures that can be taken to promote immunological wellness.*
3. *Identify possible modes of transmission of HIV disease and AIDS and list two major ways in which the disease affects women differently than men.*
4. *Compare and contrast true allergy with metabolic intolerance.*
5. *Discuss the autoimmune diseases rheumatoid arthritis and lupus in terms of their pathophysiology, symptoms, and treatment.*
6. *Compare and contrast Type 1 and Type 2 diabetes mellitus in terms of their risk factors, pathophysiology, and treatment.*
7. *Identify three complications of diabetes mellitus.*
8. *Identify two possible explanations for the rise in immunological disease in humans.*

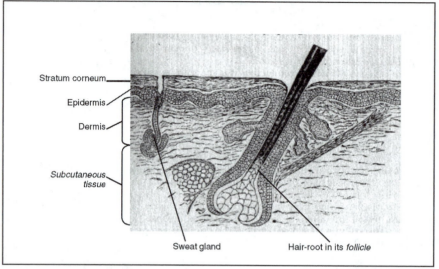

Figure 20–1 Components of Normal Human Skin

Stratum corneum

Epidermis

Dermis

Subcutaneous tissue

Sweat gland

Hair-root in its *follicle*

Source: Reprinted with permission from Gray's Anatomy, Copyright 1974 by Running Press Book Publishers, Philadelphia and London.

Introduction

Nature is alive with all sorts of organisms struggling for survival—sometimes at our expense. Human immunity is a collection of systems designed to protect us from the consequences of that lively competition. Human immunity includes systems as simply understood as our skin to those as complex as the cells within the bloodstream that govern our responses to everything from bacteria to our food. It is a system that must distinguish between what is nourishing and what is deadly, and it is a system that in healthy people is both balanced and dynamic. In this chapter, the markers of a healthy immune system will be described, and the measures that can be taken to support immune competence will be discussed. Immune-related illnesses and problems that commonly affect women, such as AIDS, arthritis, lupus, and Type 1 diabetes, will be addressed in terms of their symptoms, diagnostic procedures, and treatment. Type 2 diabetes and gestational diabetes will also be discussed.

Markers of Immunological Wellness

A healthy, optimally functioning immune system has a number of anatomical and physiological characteristics, such as an intact skin and mucous membrane barrier against infection, adequate numbers of immune cells and antibodies in the blood and bodily fluids, and an intact, healthy lymphatic system. Individuals who enjoy immunological wellness are relatively free of infections and allergy, and they experience rapid healing from wounds and infections.

Intact Skin and Mucous Membranes

The material boundary between the world and what is within us is the skin. The surface of the skin is made up of a tough outer coating of water-resistant cells called the keratin layer. Unbroken, this layer is virtually impenetrable to bacteria and viruses. Beneath it lie the epidermal and dermal layers (see Figure 20–1) which are rich with blood and lymphatic fluid, a clear liquid that supports immune functioning by draining away microscopic wastes. In these deeper layers of the skin, the moist environment allows for the movement of the free cells and chemicals that are also part of the immune system.

Some areas of the body are not protected by skin. The eyes, nose, respiratory tract, vagina, and urethra are all in some measure open to the insults of the outside world. These structures are lined with mucous membranes—nonkeratinized tissues that readily admit and lose moisture. These membranes are lined with cells that secrete mucus—a mixture of water, glycoproteins, and other substances that retard evaporation and provide a more viscous and, thus, more stable environment for the cells and chemicals of the immune system.

The mucous membranes of the mouth, digestive tract, and vagina also include "friendly" bacteria such as the *Lactobacillus* bacterium found in the vagina, which can help control the potentially harmful germs that are also part of the body's ecosystem (Taylor-Robinson, 1999). These benign organisms, which live within or on us, but do not feed off of us, are known as **commensals.** The immune system recognizes the helpful nature of these bacteria and attacks them only if they become too numerous. Although antibiotic therapy has remained the cornerstone of the treatment of vaginal and bowel infections in traditional Western medicine, healthcare providers who prefer a more integrated approach often use ecosystem balancing, which involves the introduction of friendly bacteria, instead of, or in addition to, standard treatments.

Finally, the mucous membranes are rich in antibodies, enzymes, and related substances that in various ways kill, or lyse, bacteria, deactivate, or denature, viruses, and in some cases neutralize harmful chemicals.

Adequate Numbers and Functioning of Immune Factors in the Blood and Other Bodily Fluids

The immune factors include the various types of white blood cells and antibodies.

WHITE BLOOD CELLS

In addition to red blood cells, the blood of a healthy person contains adequate numbers of the various kinds of white blood cells (WBCs), which are the mobile agents of what is known as **cellular** immunity. Beginning as stem cells in the bone marrow, WBCs differentiate into the two major white blood cell types: macrophages and lymphocytes. On maturation, these cells migrate into the general circulation. Macrophages consume and lyse foreign bacteria, virus-infected host cells (for example, a lung-lining cell infected with the influenza virus), and other damaged and foreign material. They are assisted in this by the lymphocytes. During their final stage of maturation, lymphocytes migrate from the marrow to either the blood or the thymus gland, which is located below the thyroid gland, in the upper chest. Lymphocytes that mature in the thymus are called T-lymphocytes, or T-cells; they provide the cellular immunity that controls all other responses in the immune system. Those maturing in the blood and spleen are called B-lymphocytes, or B-cells and are responsible for the manufacture of antibodies and cytokines and, thus, contribute to the other type of immunity, humoral immunity. **Humoral immunity,** gets its name from *humour,* an antiquated word for fluid (Rhodes & Pflanzer, 1992). These lymphocytes and the chemicals they secrete interact to prevent overwhelming infection, as well as to destroy other harmful foreign substances. T-cells are also responsible for the phenomena collectively called allergy. The total WBC numbers, or *counts,* give a general indication of how well a person can respond to bacterial and viral assaults. For example, neutrophils, a type of B-lymphocyte, are among the first cells to

respond to such invasion. In some people undergoing bone-marrow suppressive therapies, such as cancer chemotherapy, and in some exposures to radioactivity, a condition called **neutropenia** develops, in which fewer than about 2,500 neutrophils can be found in a cubic millimeter of blood. Patients with neutropenia suffer frequent fevers and infections, many of which are life-threatening.

ANTIBODIES

Antibodies are protein molecules that are released by B-cells. Their function is to attach themselves to **antigens** (foreign organisms, tissues, and certain chemicals). They are active molecules that can damage foreign entities directly, while also marking them for attack by other components of the immune system. When an antigen enters the body, the B-cells produce antibodies precisely tailored to that antigen. For example, when a person is infected with a new virus, cells known as CD4 T-cells create a "map" of the surface of the invading virus, and "present" this biochemical information to various arms of the immune system. One such arm is the B-cells, which then divide into two cell lines: the larger line is the plasma cells that secrete antibody precisely configured to match the "map" of the virus, and thus specific to it. The smaller cell line is comprised of memory cells, which serve as repositories of biochemical information about the nature of antigens. They will "remember" the surface map of the virus in order that specific antibodies can be speedily manufactured should the body be invaded by it again (Rhodes & Pflanzer, 1992). If the body is capable of mounting a rapid, strong anti-body defense to a particular antigen, the individual is said to be **immune** to it.

The degree of immunity an individual possesses to a specific antigen is expressed in terms of **antibody titer** (levels determined by laboratory analysis). A sufficient titer constitutes proof that the person has developed a relatively high level of immunity to the antigen. Having sufficient antibody titers to organisms to which persons in this country are usually immune is one marker of immunological health. Antibody titers for a wide range of infectious agents can be obtained through laboratory techniques.

Vaccination It was nineteenth-century physician Edward Jenner who observed that, although young women who milked cows as part of their daily chores often caught a mild rash disease called cow pox, they rarely contracted the dreaded disease smallpox. Jenner conceived the idea that something about the cow pox infection was protecting the women from smallpox. He developed a technique for purposely inoculating people with cow pox and found that it did, indeed, protect them from smallpox. Vaccination immunotherapy was born.

Vaccines work by exposing the CD4 (antigen-presenting) cells in the immune system to the germs that cause disease. It is important that only **devitalized,** or killed, versions of these viruses and bacteria are used; alternatively, only the fractions of the proteins that will stimulate reaction in the host without causing disease are used. Sometimes mild fever responses or muscular soreness occurs as a result of vaccination; this reflects the immune system's processing of the vaccine to develop active immunity, or antibodies.

One nuisance that has not been abated by vaccination therapy to date is the common cold. It is difficult to acquire permanent immunity to the common cold for two reasons. First, antibody does not necessarily persist. With time, levels of antibody to most potential antigens decline. Unless the person is re-exposed to a given antigen, immunity is "forgotten" and must be reacquired. The second reason is that there are more than 100 different antigenic subtypes. Thus, even though one may have had a cold only months ago, a different subtype of virus presents the immune system with an antigen for which it may possess no antibody (Garibaldi, 1985). By the time a person begins to produce antibodies to the new virus, she is already sneezing.

The development of vaccines to confer immunity to diseases that kill or cripple was one of the twentieth century's most important medical advances. Controversies regarding the actual impact of vaccination on human health, however, exist. McKeown (1979) has argued that morbidity and mortality related to the dreaded diseases of the 1800s–1900s plummeted, not so much because of vaccination but because the diseases were already in decline due to natural ecological factors and hygiene. Others, such as vaccination opponent Randall Neustaedter, maintain that immunization can actually *cause* health problems, such as environmental allergy, attention deficit disorder, and autism (Neustaedter, 1996). Some of this theorizing is based on the fact that vaccines are cultivated in animal tissue—commonly, eggs or animal brain tissue—which might contain unrecognized viruses that remain active in the vaccine. Although most scientists believe that vaccines have done much more good than harm, the thesis that mass immunization changes our health ecology may deserve further investigation.

CELLULAR AND CHEMICAL COMPONENTS OF THE IMMUNE SYSTEM

The immune system has weapons in its arsenal in addition to B-cells and antibodies. An example of the immune system's response to a cut finger can illustrate the function of some of these other immune components. In this scenario, we will focus on antigenic invasion and the immune response, ignoring **hemostasis,** which stops the bleeding, and **tissue repair,** which closes the wound.

When the outermost layer of protection that the skin provides is breached by, say, a rusty nail, several things begin to occur immediately. The antigenic invaders in this case are the bacteria in the environment—which we cannot evade, no matter how much antibacterial soap we use. As the tissue is rent by the nail, mast cells scattered within are torn open and

release histamine (see Figure 20–2). Histamine causes nearby intact capillaries to become more porous, and a chemical called bradykinin draws macrophages through these porous walls to move out of the capillaries and into the fine tissues near the injury. The fluid portion of the blood leaks out also, accounting for the redness and swelling seen at the edges of such an injury. (Histamine is also partially responsible for the itch one feels as the cut heals.) Other chemicals are released into the wounded area as well. For example, the protein complex complement serves as a kind of "candy coating" to encourage macrophages in the more voracious consumption of bacteria and debris. Interleukins are chemical signalers that increase local immune activity, bring distant cells to a certain site, grow greater numbers of certain immune cells, and perform various other regulatory tasks that help to maintain balance while all of this occurs. The constellation of changes that occurs in response to an injury constitute what is known as the **inflammatory response.**

People with properly functioning immune systems do not suffer *excessively* from minor viral and bacterial infections. Exposures to a wide range of bacteria and viruses over time cause the immune system to store the knowledge of how to respond quickly to invaders. Under normal circumstances, immune competence increases as an organism matures. This explains why children typically get more viral infections than adults.

The body's ability to respond rapidly and strongly to foreign tissue, such as infectious organisms, can be tested by means of a series of injections containing the noninfectious proteins of various bacteria. Typically, several injections are made, among them saline (0.9 percent sterile salt water). Saline, which causes no reaction in the body, is given for the purpose of discovering or ruling out false positive reactions due to **nocebo,** a negative version of the placebo effect (see Chapter 27). If the signs of inflammation arise after the saline injection, in a conscious person, the individual's belief that a reaction should occur is likely responsible for the swelling and redness, rather than a true immune response. Should this happen, interpreting whatever reactions occur when the protein preparations are injected will be more difficult, because belief will be operating also. When a person fails to mount a reaction to injected antigens, **anergy,** or a failed immune response, has been demonstrated. Thus, anergy testing is one means of evaluating immune responses. Table 20–1 provides a brief description of all the components of the immune system.

Although the presence of sufficient numbers of immune cells and sufficient levels of immune system chemicals is still considered to be the classic marker of immunological wellness, information uncovered by the field of **psychoneuroimmunology** (see Chapter 27) suggests that the exact nature of the factors that determine whether or when a person will become ill, and whether and how she will recover, remains a mystery. It seems likely, however, that the solution

Figure 20–2   Immune System Activated by an Injury

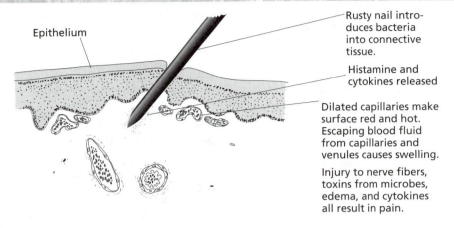

Epithelium

Rusty nail intro-
duces bacteria
into connective
tissue.

Histamine and
cytokines released

Dilated capillaries make
surface red and hot.
Escaping blood fluid
from capillaries and
venules causes swelling.

Injury to nerve fibers,
toxins from microbes,
edema, and cytokines
all result in pain.

Immediate tissue response

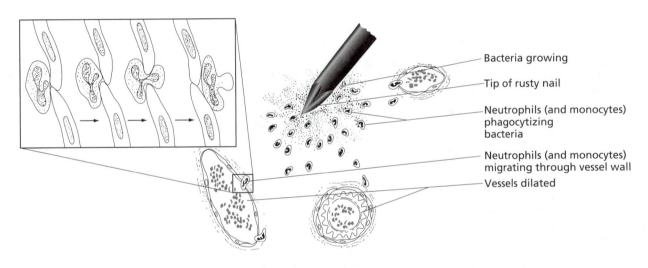

Bacteria growing

Tip of rusty nail

Neutrophils (and monocytes)
phagocytizing
bacteria

Neutrophils (and monocytes)
migrating through vessel wall

Vessels dilated

Specific cell response

Source: Tortura, G. J., & Anagnostakos, N. P. (1981). *Principles of anatomy and physiology,* 3e. Harper & Row Publishers. This material is used by permission of John Wiley & Sons, Inc.

to this mystery lies at the junction of the psyche, the nervous system, and the immune system.

An Intact and Functioning Lymphatic System

An individual with a healthy immune system must have an intact lymphatic system. The term *lymphatic system* refers to a bodywide network of small drainage vessels called **lymphatics,** through which lymph flows (see Figure 20–3). The fluid portion of the lymph is interstitial fluid that has been absorbed into the lymphatic system. Lymph also contains protein and other substances, which are ultimately returned to the blood for recycling. Although the lymphatic system plays an important role in the functioning of the cardiovascular system, it is also a major component of the immune system. B-lymphocytes proliferate in the lymph nodes; T-lymphocytes migrate in and out of them, searching for foreign tissue. Certain areas of the nodes are lined with bacteria-destroying macrophages. When the lymphatic system is functioning adequately, it helps rid the body of cancer cells and various infectious agents. Lymphatic tissue is found in the spleen, thymus gland, and tonsils, as well as in the form of Peyer's patches in the intestines (Marieb, 1989). Only

TABLE 20–1   Major components and processes of the immune system.

Antibodies	Chemicals, created by B-cells, that are designed by the body's immune system to coat antigenic invaders, thereby deactivating them, or at least making them more attractive to cells that will consume and destroy them
Antigen	A molecule or cluster of molecules of any substance that can elicit a reaction from the immune system; it must join with a carrier molecule in the body (called a **hapten**) in order to do this
Basophils	A WBCs designed to prevent infestations with parasites (protozoans, worms, and so on)
Complement	A complex, sequential cascade system of proteins that interact to create an environment that enhances the actions of other components of the immune system; kills cells directly, helps release histamine from mast cells, helps the "leakage" of blood serum into damaged or infected tissues, and draws immune cells to the site of those tissues
Cytokines	Chemicals that literally make cells move, including interferons, interleukins, complement, histamine, and bradykinin; attract cells to sites of infection or cancer, help immune cells flourish and grow when needed, and adjust the types of cells that are grown
Eosinophils	WBCs designed to prevent infestations with parasites; implicated in allergy and allergic reactions
Interferons	Cytokines that directly deactivate viruses; they are partly responsible for the fevers and achiness felt during viral infections; also inhibit tumor growth
Interleukins	Include a number of cytokines produced by monocytes; they promote growth of T-cells, mast cells, and some antibodies, and have other actions
Killer (CD8) cells	Cells that track host (body) cells that have become infected with bacteria or viruses and must be eliminated
Macrophages	These "large eaters" are monocytes that have become larger in order to *phagocytize* (engulph) their targets
Monocytes	The second line of defense behind the neurophils; WBCs that phagocytize bacteria, remove injured or dead body cells and foreign particles, and produce interferon
Phagocytosis	The process in which specialized cells can surround and consume antigens, such as bacteria; literally means "to eat the cell"
Stem cells	The orginal WBC grown in bone marrow; stem cells are immature; as they mature, they *differentiate* into all other cell types

in recent years has an understanding of the complexity of lymphatic system functioning begun to emerge.

Promoting Immunological Wellness

Promoting immunological wellness involves maintaining good hygiene, consuming a healthy diet, using herbal supplements wisely, avoiding the toxins found in mind- or mood-altering substances and in various environmental contaminants, and exercising sensibly.

Maintaining Good Hygiene

There is much wisdom in the venerable parental command "Wash your hands." Hygiene is a fundamental necessity for

the maintenance of good health. It was 19th-century physician Ignaz Semmelweis who observed that women in childbirth who were attended by midwives suffered far less often from what was then called childbed fever, but is now known to have been a generalized staphylococcal infection, than women attended by student physicians. This was because many of the student physicians went right from the pathology lab (where they dissected corpses) or from the ward to the childbed—often with blood or tissue on their aprons. The subsequent discovery of microorganisms confirmed that the physicians had been unwittingly spreading fatal infections to their maternity patients. Many of the organisms responsible for the plagues that once raged across Europe and the Americas, and that now cause epidemics in poorer nations, are disseminated to populations by the means of open sewers. Indeed, the use of sanitary sewers to carry away human waste has been associated with declines in many bacterial diseases. Outbreaks of food-borne ill-

Figure 20–3   Lymphatic System

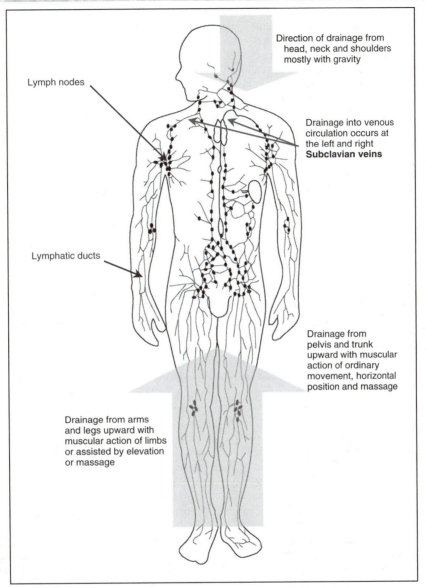

Direction of drainage from head, neck and shoulders mostly with gravity

Lymph nodes

Drainage into venous circulation occurs at the left and right **Subclavian veins**

Lymphatic ducts

Drainage from pelvis and trunk upward with muscular action of ordinary movement, horizontal position and massage

Drainage from arms and legs upward with muscular action of limbs or assisted by elevation or massage

nesses, such as hepatitis A and infections caused by the organism *Campylobacter,* are often traced to food handlers who fail to wash their hands after defecation. Taking simple measures to keep food, water, and oneself reasonably clean go a long way toward reducing the burden on the immune system (Ford, 1993).

It should not be inferred, however, that *total* insulation from microorganisms and mild infections is desirable. Various microbial occupants of the skin, vaginal tract, and other areas may contribute to overall microecological bal-ance. Indeed, studies suggest that occasional mild infections or exposure to environmental microorganisms as a child may strengthen long-term immunity and may prevent, or mitigate the potential for, the development of allergic diseases, such as asthma (Holgate, 1999). Far worse, our overuse of antibiotics is causing resistant strains of bacteria to emerge and proliferate. This phenomenon is already posing a threat to healthcare providers' ability to treat serious, resistant infections (Brook & Gober, 1996; Kaye, Fraimow, & Abrutyn, 2000).

Consuming a Healthy Diet

A comprehensive review of the literature on the various effects of diet on immunity is beyond the scope of this book. However, a few generalizations can be made. As seems to be the case with hygiene, a balanced approach may be best regarding diet. A diet that includes a variety of vegetables, fruits, and whole grains that are fresh or at least well preserved, plus plenty of pure water, will provide the immune system with everything it needs to maintain itself (see Chapter 3). Although meats, fish, and dairy products consumed in moderate quantities, as well as small amounts of oils and fats, and sugars are not harmful, meats and milk may increase the challenge presented to our immune systems.

Many nonorganically produced meats and milk products contain very small amounts of antibiotics, which are fed to cattle and chickens in order to curtail infections. Over time, exposure to this antibiotic source is thought to lead to the emergence of antibiotic-resistant bacterial strains in humans. As bacteria in the environment come in contact with low levels of antibiotics, they can undergo genetic changes that lower their susceptability to those antibiotics. With continued exposure to antibiotics in living systems, the emergent resistant strains of those bacteria live on, whereas the remaining wild-type bacteria die off, leading to an enlarging reservoir of resistant bacteria in the environment (Threlfall, Ward, Frost, & Willshaw, 2000).

Although studies have clearly shown that dietary deficiencies can lead to poor immune function, it is not known whether supplementing the diet with antioxidants, minerals, herbs, and the like enhances immune function. In fact, there is some suggestion that a modest restriction of overall caloric intake, consistent with the practices of some Eastern ascetics, may actually enhance immune function, as long as the basic nutritional requirements are met (Good & Lorenz, 1992).

Some vitamins, however, are used in relatively large doses to accomplish **short-term** therapeutic goals related to immunity. For example, supplementation with at least 1,000 mg of vitamin C per day may shorten the duration of a cold and lessen its symptoms, providing it is begun immediately when the first symptoms are detected. There is, however, little good evidence that vitamin C supplementation can *prevent* colds (Hemila & Douglas, 1999).

Scientists have also begun to investigate the role nutritional antioxidants, such as beta-carotene and tocopherol (vitamin E), play in neutralizing free radicals, a potential source of immune system harm (ATBC Cancer Prevention Study Group, 1994; Hercberg et al.,1998). Free radicals are electrically charged molecules that contain extra oxygen. They are produced in the body during normal exposure to a variety of toxicants—air pollution, for example—and during normal metabolism (Rhodes & Pflanzer, 1992). Free radicals damage genetic material in cells, which compromises the functioning of various sensitive tissues. Free radicals, such as superoxide, being highly charged, can damage a cell's DNA and lead to the abnormal, unchecked growth of a cell-line that is cancerous. Although the body contains enzymes, such as superoxide dismutase, glutathione peroxidase, and catalase, which capture and neutralize free radicals (Mates, Perez-Gomez, & Nunez de Castro, 1999), excessive exposure to free radical–generating toxins may overwhelm the body's endogenous defenses. Consequently, taking supplemental antioxidants has been suggested as a way of enhancing the body's ability to scavenge and eliminate free radicals. The results of studies testing this hypothesis have been mixed (Frieling, Schaumberg, Kupper, Muntwyler, & Hennekens, 2000; Garewal et al., 1999; Klaunig & Kamendulis, 1999; Lee, Cook, Manson, Buring, & Hennekens, 1999; Wang & Russell, 1999). The efficacy of antioxidant supplementation in preventing cancer, coronary heart disease, and other diseases related to free radical damage has yet to be established.

Using Herbal Supplements Wisely

The traditions of both Eastern and Western medical systems include the use of herbal medicines that enhance the activity of the immune system. A few of the herbs that can be safely used for this purpose are listed in Table 20–2.

Some herbal immune system boosters are best used as "simples"—that is, as single agents added to the daily diet, while others are customarily taken in combination with other agents. An example of a simple herb is *echinacea*. Echinacea works best when taken alone, and it should be noted that it loses its effectiveness if taken for longer than eight weeks (Bergner, 1997; Rehman et al., 1999). Other immuno-stimulating herbs are better used in synergistic (more powerful used in concert) combinations, as some of their constituents can be harmful if taken singly, in sufficient dosage to be effective. Chinese medicine works on this principle, with several herbs used in each formula to balance out their harmful features and enhance their useful ones (Beinfield & Korngold, 1995).

It is important to avoid the long-term use of immune-enhancing and other herbal supplements without professional guidance. Some herbs are contraindicated for some people; others are commonly misused (see Chapter 11). Although *goldenseal* is thought by many to be an herbal antibiotic, this is not quite correct. Berberine, the best-known component of goldenseal does appear to have some antibacterial properties, but berberine may not always find its way into affected tissues. Goldenseal does seem to enhance the activity of antibodies on mucous membranes and is often used by herbalists and naturopathic physicians in cases of sinus infection or diarrhea. However, the overuse of goldenseal, or the inappropriately timed use, may actually *weaken* mucosal immunity by burning out the mechanism by which it enhances that activity (Rehman et al., 1999). The popular notion that goldenseal alters the results of forensics tests for drug abuse is false. Novelist Uri Lloyd created the idea to advance the plot of his novel *Stringtown on the Pike* (Bergner 1996). Moreover, this difficult to cultivate herb is being harvested nearly to extinction. Goldenseal is best used

TABLE 20–2   Herbs for immune system self-care.

Common Name	Botanical Name	Use/Action
Astragalus (herb)	*Astragalus membranaceous*	Western studies appear to support its use in Chinese medicine to boost antitumor and antiviral immunity (Chu, Wong, & Mavligit, 1988).
Echinacea (herb)	*Echinacea spp.*	It boosts the activity of monocytes and "killer" T-lymphocytes against virus-infected cells, and it builds the number of these cells (Sun, Currier, & Miller, 1999).
Goldenseal (herb)	*Hydrastis canadensis*	It is antimicrobial (Skidmore-Roth, 2001) and seems to increase available immunoglobulins in mucus tissue (Rehman etal., 1999)
Shiitake (mushroom)	*Lentinus edodes*	It was found to inhibit the formation of dental cavities by interfering with plaque (Shouji, Takada, Fukushima, & Hirasawa, 2000).
Stinging nettle (herb)	*Urtica dioica*	It traditionally has been used to reduce seasonal pollen allergy symptoms. Studies of *U. dioica* do show immunological activity, but the research is not yet conclusive.

only on the advice of an herbalist or a healthcare provider familiar with its proper use.

Avoiding Mind- or Mood-Altering Substances That Compromise Immunity

The practice of using mind- or mood-altering substances—such as alcohol, tobacco, or marijuana—for pleasure and even religious reasons has a long history and is likely to continue, despite the Western world's "war on drugs." It must be remembered, however, that all of these agents are toxic to a certain extent and become more so when used frequently and in large amounts. Cannabis, alcohol, cocaine, and so on can increase oxidant loads, obstruct the work of the white blood cells lining the lungs, and decrease nutrient supplies to the tissues (Caiaffa et al., 1994; Pillai & Watson, 1990).

Of all the mind- or mood altering substances, *tobacco* may pose the most serious threat to the overall health of the nation. The many people who smoke it use quantities sufficient to cause grievous long-term damage to the structures related to immunity in the lungs and vascular system. This can lead to frequent lung infections, as well as poor recovery from infectious disease.

An exhaustive review of how each of the many available mind- or mood-altering substances impacts the immune system is beyond the scope of this chapter. However, the key points to remember are as follows:

1. *Drug-delivery systems (such as cigarette or marijuana smoke) compromise immunity, and that effect increases with the frequency and heaviness of use.*
2. *The drugs themselves can compromise immunity. An example is the increase in HIV levels seen in infected individuals who use cocaine (Peterson et al., 1991).*
3. *Habitual drug use can lead to behaviors, such as skipping meals, that have a negative impact on immune health.*

The safest approach is simply to not use such substances at all. For those who do use them, however, concern for the immune system as well as other systems of the body calls for a degree of moderation and some attention to safety.

Avoiding Environmental Toxins

Toxins that can either depress immune functioning or inappropriately stimulate the immune system of susceptible individuals are to be found both in the home and in the wider environment. In the home, for example, dust, dust mites, pollen, dander, and similar agents can all create problems for persons with asthma. Indeed, even exposure to perfumes, candle smoke, off-gassing from clothes dryers, detergents, and the like can cause symptoms in some individuals, and those symptoms can involve multiple body systems. Some popular authors take a very stringent approach to preventing these problems, advocating air filtration, water filtration, (or the use of bottled water), and the use of so-called hypoallergenic soaps and cosmetics. Although these measures may be appropriate for some individuals, there are few data supporting their more general use.

In the wider environment, the concern is about industrial pollutants and the presence in the biosphere of highly concentrated toxic agents. The fact that such toxins alter the immune system has been demonstrated in numerous human and animal studies. Low lymphocyte and neutrophil counts, decreased immunity to bacteria and tumor cells, and a host of other effects have been associated with exposure to asbestos, benzene, magnetic fields, and other industrial hazards and contaminants (Lisiewicz, 1993). Schierhorn, Zhang, Matthias, and Kunkel (1999) showed that ozone and nitrous oxide lead to inflammation in the respiratory tract and that asthma can be aggravated by this. McMurry, Lochmiller, McBee, and Qualls (1999) demonstrated general immunotoxicity in wild rats living in an abandoned oil refinery. Stiller-Winkler, Idel, Leng, Spix, and Dolgner (1996) observed higher levels of immunologically reactive proteins in women living in areas with heavy industrial pollution. What has yet to be definitively determined is *the level of exposure* that will produce adverse effects in humans. Nevertheless, women who work in industries that expose them to solvents, heavy metals, and so on are strongly advised to educate themselves about possible contaminants and to use appropriate protective gear.

Exercising Sensibly

Exercise, although beneficial overall, nevertheless places oxidative stress on the body, and oxidative stress has implications for immune functioning. Although there are few data on the overall effect of exercise on immunity, some discrete effects have been identified. For example, there is some evidence that vigorous exercising during an episode of fever may have negative effects, including fatigue and slowed recovery (Simon, 1991). Exercise in the absence of fever, however, has been associated with an increase in the leukocyte (white blood cell) count. This immune response to exertion may have developed as an adaptive response early in human evolution, when vigorous exertion was connected to life-threatening events; fighting wild animals in close combat would have involved an increased risk of infection from bites and the like (Simon, 1991). Interestingly, drugs that block the action of adrenaline also block exertion-induced increases in white blood cell production, suggesting that excitation in the adrenaline circuit is a key element in this phenomenon. The results of studies on the effects of exercise on antibody secretion are mixed, with levels rising in unconditioned exercisers and actually falling a bit (temporarily) in conditioned athletes. However, there doesn't seem to be any functional significance to this difference, as increased rates of infection in athletes have not been observed (Simon, 1991).

The overall functional impact of exercise on immunity is uncertain. In general, people feel better and have lower rates of cardiovascular and other disease when they exercise regularly. Thus far, however, exercise has not been shown to confer protection against infection.

Immunological Illnesses

In this section, several illnesses stemming from either the underfunctioning of the immune system (AIDS) or the overfunctioning of the immune system (allergy, autoimmune

syndromes) are addressed. The disorders that afflict women in the greatest numbers will be addressed in detail.

Acquired Immune Deficiency Syndromes

The term *acquired immune deficiency syndromes* can refer to any exogenously induced condition that involves the chronic depression of immune system functioning. Significant acquired immune underfunctioning has two major causes: toxicity due to drug therapy and infection with the human immunodeficiency virus (HIV). It is the latter, however, that is popularly known as acquired immune deficiency syndrome—AIDS. In the remainder of this section, the popular term *AIDS* will be used to refer to the disease entity that eventually results from infection with HIV. Congenital immune deficiency diseases also exist. They usually involve genetic errors, which lead to the absence of one or more key immune system components, such as certain antibody classes. They are uncommon and will not be further discussed in this chapter.

DRUG-INDUCED IMMUNE DEFICIENCY

Although infection with HIV is the most common cause of dangerously decreased immune function, the second most common cause is therapy with drugs that suppress the immune system. The suppression of the immune response is a goal in the treatment of autoimmune diseases and an undesirable side effect of many cancer treatments. Certain drugs used in chemotherapy cause immune suppression, as does radiation therapy. Patients whose levels of neutrophils (also called granulocytes) and macrophages decrease as a result of cancer therapy are often candidates for treatment with **granulocyte-stimulating factors** or **granulocyte-macrophage stimulating factors (GCSF or G-MCSF),** which can reduce the risk of overwhelming infection by increasing counts of available WBCs (Wujick, 1993).

HIV AND AIDS

Acquired immune deficiency syndrome (AIDS) is caused by the human immunodeficiency virus (HIV). HIV infection causes the progressive deterioration of the immune system, which can eventually result in the development of other life-threatening infections. HIV belongs to a class of viruses, the retroviruses, that gets its name from the way it copies its crude genetic information into a human host's more sophisticated genetic coding. HIV directly infects a variety of lymphocyte known as the CD4-type. The CD4 designation has to do with the type of molecular coding found on the surface of this type of lymphocyte: "CD" means "cluster differentiation," and "4" indicates it is the fourth type out of 73 known types. The CD4 coding is primarily found on T-lymphocytes known as "helper cells" and monocytes/macrophages. In HIV infection, the virus enters the host's CD4 lymphocytes and copies its genetic code into the host's DNA. As infected host cells divide and reproduce in response to infections and to meet normal replacement needs, new HIV is grown also. New lymphocytes that are produced may die because of the effects of the virus they now produce, or they may be attacked by other elements of the host's immune system. As the major coordinators of the immune system, the CD4 T-lymphocytes reproduce rapidly, and this makes them vulnerable to HIV, which replicates quickly within its host cells. While relatively few viruses may have entered the body during the initial infection, their numbers can exceed a million viruses per mL of serum in a short period of time. Two to six weeks after the initial infection, the immune system rallies to resist the infection, and viral levels decrease to a baseline that can range from a few hundred copies of virus per mL to a few hundred thousand (Clark et al., 1991). With the passage of time, however, CD4 T-cell counts fall and the host's ability to repel infections and destroy abnormal tissue is severely compromised.

The level of virus in the blood reliably predicts how soon sickness from immune damage will occur (Mellors, 1996). Information about viral levels (**viral load assays**), in addition to CD4 counts, are used to track the rate at which immune destruction is occurring and to predict how long infected persons will live. People who are known to be infected with HIV are not considered to have AIDS as a disease entity until their CD4 count goes below 200 (normal is 500–1,900 cells per mL), or they develop one or more AIDS-defining conditions. **AIDS-defining conditions** are infections and cancers that commonly afflict HIV-positive persons. They include pneumonia from *Pneumocystis carinii*, a common environmental pathogen that AIDS victims lose their ability to destroy; mycobacterial disease, from a common bacterium that generally goes unnoticed; generalized *yeast infections;* and meningitis and other brain infections. Other AIDS-defining infections include serious gastrointestinal infection with organisms such as *microsporidiosis.* The AIDS-defining cancers include Kaposi's sarcoma, a tumor of vascular tissue, and lymphoma, a tumor of the lymphatic system. Although these conditions are usually aborted early by a competent immune system, they persist and become very severe if the immune system is incompetent. Because they respond poorly to antibiotics and anticancer therapies, they are often chronic and frequently lethal. The rates at which HIV infection progresses to AIDS are similar in men and women (Junghans, 1999). Death occurs from a combination of general debility—as the body cannibalizes its own proteins to fight off infection—and the ravages of the infections or cancers themselves.

Transmission Considered to be the most common immune deficiency illness in the world, HIV disease is spread through exposure to infected blood and bodily fluids. Sufficient HIV to transmit infection is found in the blood, semen and pre-ejaculate, and vaginal fluids. It is also present in spinal, amniotic, and synovial fluids, which are generally encountered only by healthcare workers. More than 800,000

Americans have been afflicted by HIV disease (Jones et al., 1999). Adult and adolescent females account for about 18 percent of that total—about 150,000 individuals in all. Heterosexual transmission accounts for two-thirds of the infections among women. *HIV is more easily transmitted from male to female than female to male;* in a northern Californian population, Padian, Shiboski, Glass, and Vittinghoff (1997) demonstrated an increased efficiency of transmission from male to female by a ratio of 8:1. This is thought to be because women are more likely than men to sustain minor abrasions to their genital mucosa during penetrative sex. Anal sex is considered to confer the most risk, followed by vaginal sex and then oral sex, but relative risks are poorly delineated (Quayle, 2000). Nonpenetrative sex has not been linked with HIV transmission.

Because infection with HIV usually leads to chronic illness and eventual death, it is imperative that it be avoided. Women must work together to improve access to, and use of, disease prevention technologies, such as male and female condoms (see Chapter 17). Unequal power relationships with men prevent many women from insisting on condom use. Some individuals avoid condoms because of the common human desire for maximal intimacy.

HIV is also frequently spread among drug abusers who share needles, with nearly a third of new cases occurring via this route. Although avoiding intravenous drug use entirely is ideal, women who do inject themselves with drugs must at least refrain from sharing needles. Some cities in Europe have experimented with needle-exchange programs, in which users exchange their old syringes for sterile ones. Presumably, this reduces transmission by reducing trafficking in unsterile syringes.

HIV infections from blood transfusions, transplants, and blood products are now exceedingly rare in the West. Blood and blood products have been routinely screened for HIV and other infections since 1984. Healthcare providers, who are at risk for getting contaminated by patient blood in the mucous membranes of their eyes or in openings in their skin, do occasionally become infected. Most providers make a considerable effort to protect themselves.

Symptoms The symptoms of HIV infection, known as **primary HIV syndrome,** or **PHIVS**—occur in about 80 to 90 per cent of newly infected people, usually 14 to 28 days after the exposure. They include fever, swollen lymph nodes, sore throat, rash, and body aches. All occur at a level associated with the flu or other minor viral illness (Tindall et al., 1988). It is important that women who develop such flulike symptoms after a recent potential exposure to HIV, such as unprotected sex with a new partner, consult a healthcare provider. Newly developed therapies allow some newly infected persons to avoid higher levels of chronic infection with HIV if they are treated early and aggressively (Lori, 1999).

Once infection has become chronic, there are often no symptoms for several years, depending on the aggressiveness of the viral strain involved and the host's immune status. The virus and the host's immune system may reach a point of balance, which may last for many years. Even with CD4 counts above 500, however, some individuals experience persistently swollen lymph nodes, candidal vaginitis, malaise and achiness, or, rarely, neurological problems. As counts decline below 500, bacterial pneumonias and oral candidal infections often develop, and there is an increased risk that certain cancers will develop. In women, there is an increased risk of cervical cancer heralded by an abnormal Pap test (Assad et al., 1998). The U.S. Centers for Disease Control and Prevention recommends a baseline Pap test for HIV-positive women, followed by another at six months, and then annually thereafter if the first two are benign. Many individuals, however, have CD4 counts approaching 200 for years without any significant symptoms. Often, in the untested individual, the first sign of HIV infection is a life-threatening **opportunistic infection** (such as pneumocystic pneumonia), so-named because the germ takes advantage of the opportunity afforded by the diminished immunity.

Diagnosis   The usual test for HIV infection is the **HIV antibody test,** which reveals the presence of antibodies to HIV. This test, however, cannot yield a positive result until the host's immune system has had time to manufacture antibodies against HIV in detectable amounts (**seroconversion),** which typically does not occur for 6 to 12 weeks. In situations in which PHIVS is suspected, the direct measurement of viral burden in the blood (viral load assays) may be indicated. Although not considered diagnostic for HIV infection, such assays enable clinicians to intervene and possibly prevent a high viral baseline level from developing. Mellors (1996) showed that higher baseline virus levels are associated with more rapid advancement to clinical AIDS. Viral load assays have revolutionized the management of HIV disease. They enable clinicians to glimpse the level of viral activity against the immune system and to check a patient's response to antiviral medications.

Treatment   Prior to 1995, the treatments for HIV were few and largely ineffective. The drug azidothymidine, or AZT, (now called zidovudine) typically extended life for only a couple of years. Antibiotic therapy staved off some infections, but only for a while. In 1996, however, the discovery of a class of antiviral agents called **protease inhibitors** launched a revolution in AIDS therapy. What is known as **combination therapy,** the use of multiple antiviral agents, has changed the face of HIV disease and of virology itself. Combination therapy has proved more effective than single agent therapy in reducing the levels of virus in the bloodstream, thus preventing CD4 cells from being killed off and preserving immunity. The reason combination therapy works so well is that it thwarts a phenomenon known as **mutation,** or genetic adaptation. HIV is very capable of making genetic adaptations that confer resistance to antiviral drugs.

Combination therapy presents HIV with several agents with differing mechanisms, thus requiring the HIV to develop many genetic mutations in order to resist the drugs. As long as the drugs are taken properly, the probability that a given population of HIV can successfully mutate against all of the drugs in a regimen is low (Balzarini, 1999).

The initial step in managing HIV disease currently is to obtain a baseline level of viral burden at a time when the immune system and the virus are still in balance. Establishing a baseline enables clinicians to track the patient's response to medication. If a medication is effective, the serum viral burden will decline to undetectable levels within a maximum of 24 weeks, and ideally within 2 weeks. The term *undetectable level* does not mean that all HIV has been eradicated from the blood. It means only that *the most sensitive test available cannot demonstrate viral particles in the blood.* This difference is important; many patients mistakenly believe that a laboratory finding of undetectable levels means they are free of HIV, and this is not the case. Virus invariably remains—hiding in lymph nodes, the spleen, the nervous system, the gonads, and other areas of the body. Recently, it has been suggested that patients need to be on chemotherapy for HIV for 50–60 years in order to rid the body completely of the virus (Finzi, 1999). The guidelines for treating HIV are summarized in Box 20–1.

Not everyone needs medication immediately on diagnosis. The U.S. Department of Health and Human Services has outlined guidelines for the treatment of HIV in individuals who meet various criteria pertaining to symptoms, viral load and CD4 count. Some authorities favor earlier, more aggressive treatment, whereas others advocate watchful waiting, as long as patients are without symptoms and their CD4 counts remain high. There are advantages and disadvantages to both approaches: Early treatment may preserve the functioning of the immune system, but the drugs that are effective against HIV are inherently toxic. Watchful waiting spares the body toxicity but may allow the immune system to deteriorate. Meanwhile, researchers are working to develop less toxic drugs. At this time, chemotherapy with toxic agents is the only proven therapy against the progression of HIV infection to AIDS and death (U.S. Department of Health and Human Services/Henry J. Kaiser Family Foundation, 2000). Box 20–2 lists recommendations regarding self-care for HIV-positive persons.

In addition to conventional therapies, there are many **alternative** approaches to battling HIV and its consequences. Alternatives to treatment with drugs known to be toxic are very attractive to HIV-infected persons. However, although antiviral drugs are toxic, their benefit has been irrefutably demonstrated; as more individuals in the Western Hemisphere than ever are being spared advancement to clinical AIDS and its lethal infections (Jones et al., 1999). Asians and Africans, unfortunately, are dying in greater numbers than ever, as a lack of financial resources prevents them from purchasing the drugs that might save them. No

Box 20–1   How HIV Treatment Decisions Are Made

Treatment decisions are based on *the readiness of the patient to take medications* and are made in the context of the patient's CD4 lymphocyte count and the burden of HIV in the bloodstream.

Clinical Category	CD4 and Viral Load (VL)	Recommendation
Symptomatic	Any value	Treat
Asymptomatic	CD4 < 500 or VL > 20,000	Offer treatment; base on estimate of disease-free survival and willingness to accept therapy
Asymptomatic	CD4 > 500 and VL < 20,000	May treat, but many experts would delay therapy

Antiretrovirals are designed to suppress the growth of HIV. A combination of these from three categories are chosen (1) to maximally suppress the virus, (2) to minimize toxicity to the patient, and (3) to keep the regimen as simple as feasible.

Nucleoside Analogs	Nonnucleoside Reverse Transcriptase Inhibitors	Protease Inhibitors
Substitute for the building blocks of DNA as the virus attempts to write its genetic code into the host DNA; side effects include nausea, vomiting, anemia, nerve pain, muscle damage, pancreatitis, and liver damage	Directly inhibit the enzyme *reverse transcriptase,* which helps the virus write its code into the host DNA, can cause rashes, sometimes serious; efavirenz may cause temporary mental symptoms, including vivid dreams; nevirapine may cause liver damage	Inhibit the enzyme *protease,* which slices the newly formed viral proteins into useable components for assembly into a new viral particle; most cause some gastrointestinal discomfort; daily dosages are usually quite high, leading to "pill fatigue"; have been suspected of causing diabetes and problems with cholesterol

Source: U.S. Department of Health and Human Services/Henry J. Kaiser Foundation (2000). Guidelines for the use of antiretroviral agents in HIV-infected adults and adolescents. Wilmington, DE: DuPont.

alternative therapies have been empirically demonstrated to definitively halt the virulent replication of HIV, although some do seem to be beneficial. Massage therapy has been found to increase CD4 counts in some patients (Ironson et al., 1996). The nutrient N-acetyl cysteine (NAC), a precursor of glutathione, has been shown to help suppress HIV growth (Simon, Moog, & Obert, 1994; Sprietsma, 1999); although no large-scale clinical trials have been done, it may be a helpful supplement for infected persons. Many HIV-positive individuals use alternative therapies in conjunction with more traditional therapy. Women who are HIV-positive may wish to familiarize themselves with the literature on this, so that they can collaborate with their healthcare workers in developing a complementary therapy strategy that may enhance their ability to deal with the effects of HIV disease and the effects of toxic medications.

One factor that fuels rumors of the efficacy of various alternative approaches is *variability* in both the virulence of

the constantly evolving strains of HIV and individuals' inherent ability to resist the virus. Recent advances in immunology suggest that the immune systems of some people are able to severely limit the ability of the virus to grow and cause disease (Clerici et al., 1999; Michael, 1999). This phenomenon may explain some of the "miracle cures" seemingly brought about by various herbs and other alternative approaches.

Allergy

Allergy occurs when the immune system treats a common environmental contaminant as an antigen and creates an inflammatory response, either local or generalized. This reaction forms the basis of allergy, or **allergic hypersensitivity.** Dusts, pollens, animal danders, chemical vapors, and drugs can all trigger this response. At best, this phenomenon causes discomfort as histamines, kinins, and other chemicals

Box 20–2   Self-Care for HIV-Positive Individuals

Rest

Adequate sleep is important to everyone (see Chapter 6). HIV-positive individuals should attempt to keep their sleep schedule as regular as possible, generally going to bed and arising at roughly the same times. This makes staying on a proper medication schedule easier, because some antiviral drugs are taken at bedtime, and others are taken on an empty stomach.

Diet

A balanced diet can be supplemented with B complex vitamins, often helpful to those who suffer (or wish to avoid) nerve pain from medications such as stavudine or didanosine. Also, N-acetyl cysteine, or "NAC," 500 mg twice a day, can replete glutathione stores, necessary for proper immune health. Taking a daily vitamin with minerals, including iron for menstruating women, helps keep the body saturated with necessary nutrients, which can be depleted by stress and drug therapy, as well as by chronic infection.

Herbs

St. John's wort *(Hypericum perforatum)*, a popular alternative antidepressant should not be used by HIV-positive persons because its main constituent, hypericin, can interact unfavorably with protease inhibitors, reducing their effectiveness. Herbs such as valerian *(Valeriana officinalis)*, passionflower *(Passiflora incarnata)*, and scullcap *(Scutellaria lateriflora)* can be used for problems with sleep, as well as for anxiety or nervousness. The evidence on the use of echinacea *(Echinacea spp.)* is mixed. It doesn't seem to cause harm, and there's limited evidence it may help the immune system. HIV-positive persons should consult a professional before taking herbal remedies.

Preventive Care

Adequate dental care is very important, especially for those with lower CD4 counts, as dental abscess can be a serious problem in the immunocompromised. Pap tests need to be done more frequently only initially. Two or three negative tests within 12 to 18 months in a woman with an adequate CD4 count means she can then have them done annually, although some authorities feel that all HIV-positive women should have Pap tests every 6 months.

Sexual Health

Condoms should be used even by couples in which both individuals are HIV-positive. Recent evidence shows that not only can a new viral strain "superinfect" an existing infection but drug-resistant strains can be passed between partners who have had dissimilar antiviral drug exposures. Female condoms are one means of taking control of one's sexual activity when confronted with a male partner who will not wear a male condom. Condoms also help prevent sexually transmitted diseases (STDs), which, by inflaming mucus tissues, make the passage of HIV into a new host easier.

Interacting with the Healthcare System

HIV-positive persons should take care to note new or strange symptoms, and to write them down, so they may be easily recalled during an office visit. It is imperative that HIV-positive patients feel comfortable with their provider and that the provider allows sufficient time for communication. Moreover, HIV-positive persons should consult only providers who have expertise in treating HIV-related diseases. It has been shown that people living with HIV live longer if seen by providers, whether infectious disease physicians, family physicians, nurse practitioners, or physician assistants, who see many HIV patients.

---

are released; at worst, it can cause incapacitation or even death. Asthma (see Chapter 13) is now recognized as an allergic inflammatory disease. Four types of hypersensitivity reactions are recognized (see Table 20–3).

A true allergy can be documented by measurable immune responses, such as increases in eosinophils in a complete blood count or by the discovery of the stigmata of allergic reactions, the **immune complexes** noted in Table 20–3. Hay fever (allergic rhinitis) is a problem for about 25 to 30 percent of the population, making it perhaps the most commonly recognized form of allergy in the United States (Jones, Carney, & Davis, 1998). **Intolerance** to various substances can be caused by mechanisms other than true allergy.

Intolerance to certain foods, for example, can be caused by enzyme defects, simple irritation, or toxins in the food.

Diagnosis

The presence of true allergy can be established only by appropriate testing. This can involve the injection of small amounts of the suspected products under the skin to check for reactions. The diameter of the skin reactions is measured and recorded. Positive reactions of a certain minimum size are considered diagnostic for allergy to that substance. Test injections typically include proteins from various grass pollens, mold spores, dairy proteins, dust mites, and other sources.

TABLE 20–3   Types of hypersensitivity.

Classification	Primary Immune System Activity	Examples of Disorders in the Class
Type I	Antigens and antibodies form complexes on mast cells and basophils; histamine and related substances are released to cause symptoms.	Hay fever, hives, allergy, anaphylactic shock (extremely low blood pressure due to an allergic reaction)
Type II	Antibodies react with host cell-surface molecules; the resulting complex attracts killer cells (CD8 cells) to destroy the tissue.	Hemolytic (blood-destroying) anemias, transfusion reactions, organ transplant rejection
Type III	Antibodies react with host cell-surface molecules or exogenous antigens; these immune complexes are deposited in various tissues and attract WBCs that secrete tissue-destroying enzymes. This causes inflammation.	Systemic lupus, rheumatoid arthritis, streptococcal kidney inflammation, drug reactions
Type IV	T-lymphocytes act directly in response to an antigen. The reaction is said to be "delayed" as it occurs more slowly than in other types of hypersensitivity.	Contact dermatitis, some types of drug sensitivity (this reaction that is used in anergy testing)

TREATMENT

The treatment of allergy involves three primary approaches. The first is avoidance, with the idea that avoiding contact with the offending substance will reduce allergic symptoms. The second approach is to curtail production of the substances that cause inflammation and symptoms. Treatment with antihistamines is by far the most common means of doing this. Some antihistaminic drugs are available over-the-counter, whereas others are available by prescription only. The choice of antihistamine for therapy depends on such factors as the severity of the allergy, side effects, and cost. The third—and relatively new—approach to the treatment of allergy is the use of intranasal steroids, which, when inhaled on a regular basis, reduce the inflammation that results from the release of histamine.

Anaphylaxis is the term used to describe a severe, life-threatening allergic response to a substance. Anaphylaxis is characterized by marked swelling, which can involve the airway and compromise breathing. It also involves a severe drop in blood pressure and can lead to cardiopulmonary arrest if emergency medical treatment with oxygen, intravenous fluids, adrenaline (epinephrine), and antihistamines is not provided.

Autoimmune Diseases

In autoimmune disease, an individual's immune system attacks tissues within her own body. At least two dozen major illnesses resulting from this poorly understood phenomenon have been identified. All the autoimmune diseases have some features in common—most notably, inflammation. Some autoimmune diseases are easily diagnosed via laboratory testing; these are called **seropositive diseases.** Others called **seronegative diseases,** produce no markers in serum and often elude precise diagnosis.

RHEUMATOID ARTHRITIS

Rheumatoid arthritis (RA) is perhaps the best known of the seropositive autoimmune diseases. In RA, for reasons that are as yet unknown, the immune system causes inflammation of the linings of the joints, and this leads to progressive damage, deformity, pain, and limited use (Mahat, 1998). The incidence of RA in women is about 1 percent, which is three times the rate in men. RA usually develops when an individual is 40 to 50 years old, but it can develop at any time, including during childhood. Rheumatoid arthritis is found everywhere in the world. Studies of twins have found that a genetic tendency for RA runs in families. Some cases arise after a viral or bacterial infection, but the reason for this is not known. Although the exact cause of RA is unknown, recent research has yielded more information about how RA affects joints and other body tissues. The earliest occurring lesions in RA include injury to microscopic blood vessels and a thickening of the tissue (the **synovium**) that lines the **joint capsule.** Increased numbers of T-lymphocytes, particularly CD4 cells and cytotoxic CD8 varieties, are found in affected joints. Levels of Interleukin-1 (IL-1) and another compound called tumor necrosis factor alpha (TNF-alpha), are high during the inflammatory phase of the disease and are believed to be involved in the destruction of bone that leads to the deformities seen in advanced RA. Interestingly, people with RA who develop HIV disease can experience an improvement in their RA symptoms (Lapadula et al., 1997), due to suppression of the immune response. Although most RA-related debility is due to the destruction of joints, **extra-articular manifestations** can occur as the disease progresses: Nodules may appear beneath the skin, and pain and collapsing joint architecture lead to restricted movement, which in turn leads to muscular deconditioning and atrophy in the affected parts of the body. In a small number of cases, inflammation of blood vessels occurs also (Grassi, De Angelis, Lamanna, & Cervini, 1998).

Symptoms At its onset, rheumatoid arthritis typically causes fatigue, generalized weakness, anorexia, and vague musculoskeletal symptoms followed by symmetrical **polyarthritis,** or multiple joint inflammations. The most commonly affected bony structures are the "knuckle" joints and the large middle joints in the fingers (Peck, 1998). The wrist, elbow, knee, foot, and cervical spinal joints may also be involved. Often, the initial symptoms are more severe than later ones and include joint swelling as well as pain, fever, and perhaps swelling of the lymph nodes **(lymphadenopathy)** and the spleen **(splenomegaly).** If the fever is higher than 38°–39°C, a concurrent infection may be present (Grassi et al., 1998).

Diagnosis Although there is no test that definitively diagnoses RA, antibodies called **rheumatoid factors (RF)** are found in the blood in about 75 percent of cases. The presence of RF in the blood, however, does not always mean that a person has rheumatoid arthritis. RF are found in the blood of up to 5 percent of persons who have no symptoms of RA, most commonly in those who have recently received a vaccination or who have an active infection or another seropositive autoimmune disease (Mahat, 1998). RA is usually diagnosed on the basis of a combination of symptoms, laboratory tests for generalized inflammation, and elevated RF, although low or absent RF does not rule out RA. An X ray or magnetic resonance imaging (MRI) can be used to gauge the extent of joint involvement. Women of childbearing age with RA should be tested for the presence of compound's known as **antiphospholipids** (also known as anticardiolipins), because these have been implicated in miscarriages, strokes, and other problems in women with RA (Peck, 1998).

Treatment Aspirin, often in prodigious dosages, has been the cornerstone of traditional therapy for early stage RA since the late nineteenth century. More recently, nonsteroidal anti-inflammatory drugs (NSAIDs) have assumed a leading role in mitigating both the pain and the inflammation of RA (Peck, 1998). These agents include the prototypical drug ibuprofen, as well as newer agents, such as oxaprozin and nabumetone, which reduce the number of daily doses needed. A class of NSAIDs called **cyclooxygenase-II inhibitors,** such as celecoxib and rofacoxib, require dosing only once a day and are less likely than other NSAIDs to cause gastric ulcers (see Chapter 15).

Currently, the management of RA also involves treatment aimed at preventing joint destruction (Pincus, O'Dell, & Kremer, 1999). **Antimetabolic drugs,** which interrupt critical metabolic processes in cells, and **immunomodulating agents** which alter the functions of the immune system,

are used reduce inflammation. Methotrexate is a commonly prescribed antimetabolite that can cause RA to go into **remission**—that is, to subside temporarily. Its side effects include anemia and low WBC counts, nausea, vomiting, and abdominal pain. These effects can be minimized by the concurrent use of the nutrient folic acid and the drug leucovorin. Immunomodulators include cyclosporine—used to suppress immunity—and infliximab and etanercept—used to block TNF-alpha (Cornell, 1997). The immunomodulators are newer disease-modifying agents that are less toxic than some of the older drugs and that effectively decrease the rate at which pathological changes in joints occur. These features mean improved comfort and function for individuals with RA.

Although rest has been advocated for patients with RA (Hakkinen et al., 1999; Klepper 1999; Van den Ende, Vliet Vlieland, Munneke, & Hazes, 1998), exercise has also been found to be of benefit to people living with RA. Hakkinen et al. (1999) found increases in muscle strength among RA patients who exercised, and Bell, Lineker, Wilkins, Goldsmith, and Badley (1998) found no deleterious effects and many positive ones—including reduced pain, better overall function, and improvements in sense of well-being—with exercise and physical therapy. Dance-exercise therapy has also been used with positive effects in RA patients (Noreau, Moffet, Drolet, & Parent, 1997). Walking, swimming, dancing, and other well-tolerated activities are generally safe and beneficial for RA sufferers; however, those who have marked debility or joint deformity should consult a physiatrist, a physical therapist, or another experienced professional before embarking on an exercise program (Neuberger et al., 1997).

Although no alternative therapy has been shown in clinical trials to definitively reverse RA, several have been shown to reduce the symptoms and improve function. Because food allergy has been implicated in some individuals' exacerbations of arthritic symptoms (Darlington & Ramsey, 1993; Van de Laar & Van der Korst, 1992; Van de Laar et al., 1992), testing for food allergy may be of some benefit. An elimination diet can be used to ferret out food intolerances that are not truly allergic. Each of the following foods, in turn, is eliminated from the diet for two months: (1) milk and milk products, (2) all sugar except fruits, (3) citrus, and (4) all vegetables from the nightshade family (tomatoes, potatoes, eggplant, peppers, paprika, chili). At the end of each trial, any improvement in symptoms are noted and recorded. The foods associated with increased symptomatology are then omitted from the diet. In order to avoid nutrient deficiencies, elimination diets should be undertaken in partnership with a healthcare professional knowledgeable regarding proper nutrition.

The results of studies on the efficacy of acupuncture as a treatment for RA have been mixed, with more trials showing at least some positive effect on symptoms (Bhatt-Sanders, 1985). In a small number of studies (Andrade, Ferraz, Atra, Castro, & Silva, 1991; Gibson, Gibson, MacNeill, & Buchanan, 1980), homeopathy was found to be somewhat effective in reducing RA symptoms. Glucosamine, a popular dietary supplement found to be helpful in osteoarthritis, has not yet been evaluated as a treatment for RA. The use of dietary supplementation with fatty acids is detailed in the following section.

LUPUS AND RELATED RHEUMATOID DISEASES

The term *lupus* encompasses a small collection of diseases related to immune hyperactivity. This section will focus on one of them, systemic lupus erythematosus (SLE), because it is a significant health problem for women. Eighty-five percent of the half-million people in the United States with SLE are female. A still higher incidence occurs in African Americans, who are often afflicted with a more severe degree of disease (Bertino & Lu, 1993).

In SLE, the immune system ultimately attacks the body's own DNA, the basic material of genetic coding. Immune complexes, the molecular clusters of antibodies and antigen that form when antibodies are produced against the person's own molecules, such as cell-surface proteins, cause direct cell damage or interfere with cellular functions. SLE can damage many different tissues in the body, including the skeletal system, blood, heart, blood vessels, nerves, lungs, kidneys, digestive tract, and eyes. Systemic lupus can be fatal, and the most common serious event capable of precipitating death from SLE is kidney damage (Bergner, 1998). The fetuses of pregnant women with SLE are often harmed, and miscarriage is not uncommon. Despite all this, the early prognosis for SLE is fairly good, with a 10-year survival of up to 90 percent (McCowan,

1998). Although no specific genes that cause SLE have been identified, there are some indications that inherited characteristics may confer vulnerability to it.

Symptoms SLE is called "the great imitator" because its symptoms can resemble those of many other diseases. Its initial manifestation can involve symptoms in almost any system of the body, including fatigue, nausea and anorexia, weight loss, generalized pain or anemia, and skin photosensitivity. Joint pain, however, is far and away the most common symptom—as in the case of RA—and affects 90 percent of people with SLE. The less common symptoms include mental dysfunction, pneumonia, pleurisy, and facial rash (McCowan, 1998). SLE-related nephritis (kidney inflammation and scarring) also occurs in most individuals with SLE (Austin & Balow, 1999).

Diagnosis SLE is diagnosed more on the basis of clinical criteria than by laboratory testing. Although individuals with SLE may have abnormal laboratory values, suggestive of inflammation, such as an elevated erythrocyte sedimentation rate (ESR) and/or C-reactive protein (CRP) level, they may also show no abnormalities on laboratory testing. The **antinuclear antibody (ANA) test,** customarily done when SLE is suspected, is not specific for SLE, but high titers point to the diagnosis and are present in 95 percent of cases (Bertino & Lu, 1993). Tests for the presence of anti-double-stranded DNA and Smith antibodies are specific for SLE but are positive in only 30 to 60 percent of affected persons (McCowan, 1998). Table 20–4 lists the

TABLE 20–4 Diagnostic criteria for SLE.

Criterion	Definition
1. Facial rash	Skin redness, flat or raised, over the cheekbones, tending to spare the folds at the corners of the nose
2. Discoid rash on body	Red, raised patches with scaling and blocked follicles; scarring can occur in older lesions
3. Photosensitivity	Skin rash as a result of unusual reaction to sunlight, as diagnosed by patient history or physician observation
4. Oral ulcers	Oral or nasopharyngeal ulceration, usually painless, observed by physician
5. Arthritis	Nonerosive arthritis (in which the bone is not broken down) involving two or more peripheral joints, characterized by tenderness, swelling, or effusion (excess fluid in the joint)
6. Serositis	Inflammation of the lining of the lung or the heart
7. Kidney disorder	Persistent excessive protein in the urine or evidence of cellular breakdown in the kidneys ("casts" in the urine)
8. Neurological disorder	Seizures or psychosis, in the absence of offending drugs or known metabolic problems
9. Blood disorder	Anemia from fragile red cells with excess reticulocytes (immature red cells), or WBC counts less than $4,000/mm^3$ total on two or more occasions, or low lymphocyte counts less than $1,500/mm^3$ on two or more occasions, or low platelet counts (less than $100,000/mm^3$) in the absence of offending drugs
10. Immunological disorder	Positive results on various lab tests related to the immune system
11. Antinuclear antibody	An abnormal level of antinuclear antibody in the blood at any point in time and in the absence of drugs known to be associated with "drug-induced lupus" syndrome.

Source: Tan, E. M., et al. (1982). *Arthritis & Rheumatism, 25,* 1271–7. Reprinted by permission of Wiley-Liss, Inc., a subsidiary of John Wiley & Sons, Inc.

criteria for the diagnosis of SLE. A person is considered to have SLE if any 4 or more of the 11 criteria are present, serially or simultaneously, during any interval of observation.

Treatment Systemic lupus is a remitting-relapsing disease. That is to say, its symptoms alternately flare and disappear over time. In many cases, flares are mild, and only nonprescription strength-ibuprofen is required to control joint pain and muscle aches. When flares are very severe and debilitating, however, aggressive therapy is required to induce remission.

Therapy with potent steroids, such as prednisone or methylprednisolone, has been the mainstay of anti-inflammatory therapy in SLE for decades. Unfortunately, steroid drugs have side effects, including elevated blood pressure and blood sugar levels. They can also alter the function of the adrenal glands and decrease bone density. Antimalarial drugs, such as hydroxychloroquine, have also been successful in reducing symptoms (Wang et al., 1999). The antimalarials' most well-known side effect is damage to the retina. Although that occurs fairly infrequently, regular visits to an ophthalmologist are nonetheless still considered obligatory for patients on such agents (Wang et al., 1999). However, the basic pathophysiology in SLE is the hyperactivation of immunity; thus, immunosuppressive drugs have a long history of use in SLE. Immunosuppressive drugs are reserved for serious SLE flares, particularly when the disease is attacking vital organs, such as the kidneys. They are not used to prevent long-term damage, as they are in rheumatoid arthritis, because that strategy has not proven effective in SLE.

Although many people with SLE use various nontraditional therapies, such as massage therapy, therapeutic touch (TT), transcendental meditation (TM), faith-based approaches, and the like (see Chapter 11), to ease the milder symptoms of their disease, there have been few formal studies of their effectiveness. The efficacy of some popular dietary supplements, however, is supported by both anecdotal reports and clinical trials. For example, a fish oil–derived supplement called **eicosapentaenoic acid (EPA)** has been shown to decrease the symptoms in SLE patients (Walton et al. 1991). Popular authors, such as Andrew Weil (1990) and Michael Murray and John Pizzorno (1998), recommend limiting the intake of series-2 prostaglandins found in saturated fats (as in butter and other animal fats) and adding fish, fish oils, or other sources of EPA (such as black currant oil or flaxseed oil) to the diet. The suggested dosage is at least 500 mg of EPA or linolenic acid, a precursor of EPA, per day. Black currant oil at a dosage of 500 mg per day is recommended, as black currant oil contains linolenic acid. Weil also acknowledges the power of suggestion, as discussed in Chapter 11: "Do not stay in treatment with . . . doctors who make you feel hopeless about your condition. The suggestions of practitioners . . . can be powerful influences on your . . . health" (1990, p. 307).

People who suffer from diseases of the immune system should not take herbal remedies without the guidance of a provider well versed in the use of herbs and other natural products. Herbs such as echinacea, astragalus, ginseng, lomatium, ligusticum (also known as osha), and Oregon grape (Mahonia), as well as certain mushrooms (shiitake, maitake, and reishi), have measurable effects on immunity that can *increase* inflammatory symptoms (Bongiovanni, 2000).

Dihydroepiandrosterone (DHEA) is a hormone precursor that is available as a food supplement. It is commonly taken by athletes, AIDS patients, and others seeking to increase lean body mass. Although there is little evidence that supports its efficacy as a muscle builder, there is some evidence that people with SLE tend to be deficient in DHEA. Moreover, in a population of SLE patients taking 200 mg/day for a six-month period, supplementation with DHEA resulted in the maintenance of bone density. The subjects in the study were all on steroid therapy, which normally decreases bone density (Van Vollenhoven, Park, Genovese, West, & McGuire, 1999). Loss of bone density is a problem for patients on long-term steroid therapy for RA, SLE, and other related diseases.

Persons who have SLE must take care to use sunscreen and proper sun shading to protect themselves from sunlight. The rashes and other aggravations related to SLE are directly linked to excessive sun exposure (McCowan, 1998); in general, SLE patients have a low tolerance for sun exposure.

OTHER DISORDERS OF IMMUNITY

Disorders of immunity cover a wide range. For effective self-care and wellness, women ought to be aware that investigation into the role of immune dysregulation in human disease is an emerging field, with many diseases that had been poorly understood now being linked to immune system hypo- or hyperactivity. Hypoactivity of the immune system, of course, largely manifests as either infection or cancer. The symptoms related to weakened immunity are readily detected by healthcare providers, who then take steps to treat the underlying problem, as well as its consequential infection or cancer.

Hyperactivity of the immune system, however, presents a different sort of problem: how to decrease immunity sufficiently to suppress symptoms but not so much that the body is predisposed to cancer and other hypoimmune disorders. Diseases related to the hyperfunctioning of the immune system include vasculitis, temporal arteritis, mixed connective tissue disease, and some diseases of the thyroid gland.

Vasculitis inflames blood vessels in various regions of the body, causing disease in nearby tissue. For example, **temporal arteritis,** which can cause immediate blindness, is a form of vasculitis specific to the temporal artery in the head. The disorder known as **mixed connective-tissue disease** is similar to SLE, but immune complexes are properly cleared and pulmonary, rather than renal involvement is more common. Several diseases of the thyroid gland are now known to result from immune dysregulation. In **Grave's disease,** immunoglobulins bind to thyroid cells and stimulate thyroid hormone production. In some types of **primary hypothyroidism,** the thyroid gland's ability to produce hormone is weakened by circulating auto-antibodies specific to that tissue. Why this happens is not known. Thyroid disorders are discussed in Chapter 24.

Some putative disorders of immunity are highly controversial. The existence of food allergies not detectable by conventional testing, but causing weakness, malaise, depression, and a host of other variable symptoms, is supported by some, mostly alternative, practitioners but is scoffed at by other, mostly traditional health professionals. Similarly divergent opinions pertain to sick building syndrome, in which symptoms are seen as related to the chemicals in construction materials and ventilation problems. Persons diagnosed as having environmental allergies are believed to be allergic to many substances in the indoor and outdoor environment. Low-grade, systemic infection with "yeast," or the organism *Candida albicans,* is thought to cause a variety of symptoms from recurring, intractable vaginal infections to fatigue, depression, and headaches. Finally, a host of symptoms has been attributed to the presence of parasitic worms in the gastrointestinal tract. A subculture of individuals who believe themselves to be suffering from one or more of these conditions has become established, and many of those belonging to it are women. The prevalence of these conditions among women likely reflects society's view of women as prone to illness (see Chapter 1) and women's greater likelihood of pursuing evaluation and treatment for symptoms, in comparison with men.

There are several factors women who think they might be suffering from one or more of these conditions might consider. First, new diseases are still being discovered and catalogued. That a diagnosis elicits controversy or even derision in some quarters does not mean that it will not ultimately be found to be legitimate. Only in recent years has the link between the *Helicobacter pylori* organism and stomach ulcers become apparent, based on the discoveries of an Australian physician who was at first scorned and derided for his contention that ulcers should be treated with antibiotics. Conversely, however, history books are rife with accounts of medical fads ultimately proven to have had no basis in fact; the nineteenth-century epidemic of hysteria (see Chapter 1) is a case in point, and there are many others. Like their antecedents, well-meaning clinicians of today apply a range of controversial therapies to conditions that are poorly understood, and this is a legitimate, if frustrating, part of the process of making advances in human health. However, like their antecedents, some unscrupulous contemporary providers foist useless treatments on patients with imaginary diseases.

Consumers who wish to explore the possibility that they have one of the syndromes discussed in this section, would do well to bring an open-minded approach, balanced by a degree skepticism, to a study of the available literature. Although the Internet is a rich source of information, it can be difficult for nonhealth professionals to separate fact from fiction. A genuine partnership with a knowledgeable and experienced clinician is the safest context in which to experiment with unusual methods of diagnosis and treatment.

Box 20–3 Major Risk Factors for Diabetes Mellitus

♦ Family history of diabetes (parents or siblings with diabetes)
♦ Obesity (greater than 20 percent over desired body weight or a body mass index [BMI] greater than 27 kg/m^2)
♦ African-American ethnicity
♦ Age over 44 years
♦ Previously identified impaired fasting glucose or impaired glucose tolerance
♦ Hypertension (blood pressure greater than or equal to 140/90)
♦ HDL cholesterol level less than or equal to 35 mg/dl
♦ Triglyceride level greater than or less than 250 mg/dl
♦ History of gestational diabetes or delivery of babies over 9 pounds

Source: American Diabetes Association. (1998). Report of the expert committee on the diagnosis and classification of diabetes mellitus. *Diabetes Care, 21*(Suppl 1), S5–S19.

Diabetes

Diabetes, known medically as diabetes mellitus (DM), is an all too common disease and a major health problem for those who have it. One form (Type 1) is considered to be an autoimmune disease. The other form (Type 2), while not generally considered to be autoimmune in nature, will be addressed here for the sake of expediency.

Diabetes is the most common endocrine disease in the world (Gavin, 1999). The World Health Organization (WHO) predicts that diabetes will affect more than 300 million persons worldwide in the twenty-first century (King, 1998). The term *diabetes* is used to refer to several related disorders that cause **hyperglycemia,** the presence of higher than normal levels of glucose in the blood.

According to current estimates by the American Diabetes Association (ADA), 16 million people in the United States have DM and one-third of these have not yet been diagnosed (American Diabetes Association, 1997). Diabetes is now the seventh leading cause of death in this country. Its incidence increases with age and is somewhat higher in women (Frizzell, 2000). The major risk factors for diabetes are listed in Box 20–3.

There are four categories of diabetes: Type 1 DM, Type 2 DM, gestational (related to pregnancy) diabetes, and other specific types. Type 1 DM used to be known as juvenile diabetes and as insulin-dependent diabetes mellitus (IDDM), and Type 2 DM was known as noninsulin-dependent diabetes mellitus (NIDDM). Those terms are no longer used, as it is now felt that classifying a disease on the basis of treatment rather than cause is confusing.

Type 1 DM is considered in most cases to be an autoimmune disease. In some situations, however, no autoimmune pathology leading to the development of diabetes can be identified; these cases are classified Type 1 idiopathic. The term **idiopathic** means that no cause has been identified. Type 2 DM is the most prevalent form of diabetes. It involves insulin resistance and an associated defect in insulin secretion; although it is not currently considered to be autoimmune. Gestational diabetes is glucose intolerance that develops or is recognized during pregnancy (American Diabetes Association, 2001).

INSULIN AND CARBOHYDRATE METABOLISM

Insulin regulates carbohydrate metabolism. The major function of insulin is to facilitate the movement of glucose into the individual cells of the body, where it is metabolized as an energy source. Insulin also fosters certain metabolic processes that decrease the amount of glucose in the blood.

Insulin is secreted by beta cells in an area of the pancreas known as the **islets of Langerhans.** It is synthesized from a precursor called **proinsulin** (Cleveland, 1999). Neurotransmitters, gastrointestinal and pancreatic hormones, and the nutrients in digestion all influence the rate at which insulin is produced by the pancreas. Insulin secretion is normally exquisitely fine-tuned by the body in order to maintain a relatively stable serum glucose concentration that varies only slightly, whether an individual is fasting, as during sleep, or eating regularly.

Insulin accomplishes this task by fostering processes that decrease blood glucose levels and by acting on muscle cell membranes in a way that causes the membranes to allow glucose to enter the cells. Insulin is *not* needed, however, for glucose to cross the cell membranes of certain kinds of cells: red blood cells, the cells that make up the kidney epithelium, and the cells in nerve, brain, intestinal, liver, and retinal tissues.

The insulin-mediated processes that decrease blood glucose levels are **glycogenesis,** the conversion of glucose into **glycogen** (a stored form of glucose) and the conversion of glucose into fat, which is stored as adipose tissue. Insulin also suppresses **glycogenolysis,** the conversion of glycogen back into glucose, and **gluconeogenesis,** the manufacture of glucose from raw materials in fats and proteins. Thus, resistance to insulin causes the production of too much glucose and prevents muscle cells from using it for energy (Cleveland, 1999).

In order for just the right amount of blood glucose to be moved into the cells for energy production, dietary intake, insulin production, and metabolism must be very well balanced. If this balance is not maintained, abnormally high glucose levels will be present in the serum, and the individual cells will not be able to avail themselves of normal, glucose-driven metabolic pathways.

When the body's ability to maintain normal blood glucose levels and to use glucose for energy properly is lost, two types of problems occur. The first is that the individual cells are unable to function normally; they do not have the fuel to perform their specific functions. Second, the elevated levels of glucose circulating throughout the vascular system stress the body in ways specific to the involved organs. This stress results in the complications of diabetes, which include myocardial infarction, vision loss, amputations, kidney failure, and neurological impairment.

TYPE 1 DIABETES MELLITUS

Type 1 DM accounts for approximately 10 percent of all cases of DM worldwide. It is more common in some societies than others. The rate of Type 1 DM is reported as higher for whites than for nonwhites; whites are affected 1.5 to 2 times more often than nonwhites. The peak age at onset is 11 to 13, but girls may be slightly older than boys at diagnosis. There is *no* gender difference in rates of Type 1 DM (Huether & Tomky, 1998). Individuals who have an unusual form of Type 1 DM known as *ideopathic DM* make up a small subgroup of Type 1 diabetics, and most of are of Asian or African descent (American Diabetes Association, 1997). Although ideopathic Type 1 DM is not an autoimmune disease, it does seem to be strongly heritable.

In both autoimmune and idiopathic Type 1 DM, the pathophysiological defect lies in the destruction of the pancreatic beta cells. When beta cells are destroyed, little or no insulin is secreted, and hyperglycemia results. Type 1 DM associated with an immune-related destruction of the beta cells has genetic predispositions and seems to be related to environmental factors still not fully understood. Patients with immune-mediated Type 1 DM are prone to other autoimmune disorders, such as Grave's disease and Hashimoto's thyroiditis (see Chapter 21) (American Diabetes Association, 1997).

TYPE 2 DIABETES MELLITUS

Unlike those with Type 1 DM, individuals with Type 2 do not necessarily have impaired production of insulin. Rather, in Type 2 DM there is a *cellular resistance* to the action of the insulin and a relative, but not absolute, insulin deficiency (American Diabetes Association, 1997). Autoimmune destruction of beta cells is *not* a factor. The specific cause of Type 2 DM is unknown, but obesity is very strongly linked to Type 2 DM. Obesity itself is considered the major risk factor in the disease's onset, and obesity alone causes some degree of insulin resistance. After 5 to 10 years of secreting large amounts of insulin to compensate for increasing insulin resistance, obese individuals' beta cell function finally reaches its limits, and insulin production becomes insufficient to regulate blood sugar levels. At this stage, overt Type 2 diabetes mellitus develops, and blood glucose levels become abnormal (DeFronzo, 1999).

The association between **central abdominal obesity** and diabetes has been studied since the early 1960s. Intra-abdominal fat is seen as the primary fat store responsible for the insulin resistance seen in Type 2 DM (Brunzell & Hokanson, 1999). Fortunately, many women tend to accumulate excess adipose tissue in the thighs and hips, but, when there is an increased central or abdominal fat accumulation, the risk for insulin resistance increases. Exercise or calorie restriction resulting in a *loss* of intra-abdominal adipose reduces the insulin resistance seen in this group of individuals.

There are four primary abnormalities in Type 2 DM: impaired insulin secretion, increased glucose production, decreased muscle uptake of glucose, and the overproduction of free fatty acids by fat cells (DeFronzo, 1999). Impaired insulin secretion occurs when the beta cells become worn out by the demands of insulin resistance. Increased glucose production occurs when insufficient insulin is produced to suppress glycogenolysis and gluconeogenesis. In addition, the scarcity of insulin prevents adequate levels of glucose from entering muscle cells. Finally, in Type 2 DM, the fat cell possesses a defect in glucose uptake, and insulin is unable to suppress **lipolysis,** the breakdown of lipids, resulting in the overproduction of free fatty acids, which in turn stimulate gluconeogenesis.

GESTATIONAL DIABETES

Gestational diabetes mellitus (GDM) is considered a complication of pregnancy and is a factor in 4 percent of all pregnancies (American Diabetes Association, 2000). A risk assessment for GDM is a recommended component of the first prenatal visit. The factors placing women in a high-risk, moderate-risk, or low-risk category and the recommended screening procedures are included in Table 20–5. Gestational diabetes is detected in the same ways as are other forms of diabetes.

The maternal risk associated with gestational diabetes includes the subsequent development of Type 2 DM, with all its attendant potential complications. Fifty to 60 percent of women who have gestational diabetes will convert to Type 2 DM within five years. The risk to the fetus includes an excessively high birth weight and the potentially life-threatening complication of fetal hypoglycemia.

DIAGNOSIS

There are three tests generally used to diagnose DM of all types: the fasting glucose level; the casual, or random, glucose level; and the glucose tolerance test. All three are based on the amount of glucose in the serum portion of a blood sample. It is important to understand that the amount of glucose present in the blood fluctuates over the course of a day. There will be relatively more sugar present in the blood following the ingestion of a meal, particularly a high-carbohydrate meal, than after a period of fasting. A person is considered to be fasting if she has been without caloric intake for eight hours or more, and a normal fasting glucose level is considered to be less than 126 mg/dl. A fasting glucose level greater than 126 mg/dl is suggestive of diabetes. The amount of sugar present in the blood of a person who has eaten recently is called a random, or casual, glucose level. A normal casual glucose level is not greater than 200 mg/dl, and a level greater than 200 mg/dl in the presence of the early symptoms of diabetes (see Box 20–4) suggests that the disease is present. The third test used in the diagnosis of diabetes is the glucose tolerance test (GTT). During a GTT, a dose of glucose is taken orally, and subsequent periodic glucose levels are determined. Positive results on each of these tests should be confirmed by repeat testing on a different day (American Diabetes Association, 1997).

Individuals with Type 1 DM are usually *not* obese at diagnosis, but the presence of obesity does not rule out the diagnosis. Most people with Type 1 DM, however, are thin.

TABLE 20–5	Risk factors and screening recommendations for gestational diabetes.	
Category	**Associated Factors**	**Recommended Screening**
High-risk	Marked obesity, prior history of GDM, glycosuria, or strong family history of DM	Immediately and, if normal, again at 24–28 weeks of gestation: Fasting plasma glucose If normal, follow up with oral glucose tolerance test

Box 20–4   Early Symptoms of Diabetes

- Polyuria (increased urination)
- Polydipsia (increased thirst)
- Polyphagia (increased appetite)
- Fatigue
- Weakness
- Sudden vision changes
- Tingling or numbness in hands and feet
- Dry skin
- Nonhealing sores
- Recurrent infections, including vulvovaginitis in women

TREATMENT

Diabetes is a chronic, life-long disease. It is treated through a combination of diet, exercise, drug therapy, frequent monitoring of blood sugar levels, and stress management. A person with diabetes must make the management of her disease a daily priority. The first step in learning to manage diabetes is acquiring the appropriate education.

Education   Education about the nature of diabetes as a disorder begins when the disease is first diagnosed. Early diabetes education is usually conducted on a one-to-one basis and often involves members of the patient's family and significant others. Education will continue over time and will build on the individual's experience and previous knowledge. Once a diabetic person has mastered the rudiments of coping with the disease, additional education is often provided in group settings, so that the participants can share their knowledge and experience with others. Professionals from various disciplines, such as medicine, nursing, dietetics, pharmacy, psychology, and social work, participate in diabetic education.

Nutritional Therapy   A new diabetic learns about the basic carbohydrate, protein, and fat components of food and the correct distribution of these components in the diet. Managing the *carbohydrate* component of the diet properly is especially important, because glucose is produced mainly through carbohydrate metabolism. The ADA recommends that adult diabetics consume 45–60 g of carbohydrate at each of the three main daily meals. The diabetic is taught to count carbohydrates carefully and that each serving of starch, milk, or fruit contains approximately 15 g of carbohydrate. Concentrated sweets in the form of candy and icings must be severely limited, but there are many sugar-free treats available commercially. In addition to learning to plan meals and count carbohydrates, diabetic persons—particularly Type 2 diabetics—must learn to control their weight in order to reduce the level of insulin resistance in the body. Fatty tissue, particularly in the form of central or abdominal obesity, is known to give rise to insulin resistance.

Exercise   Exercise is very important for diabetics, because it lowers insulin resistance and promotes cardiovascular health. Prior to beginning any exercise program, however, diabetic individuals must undergo a thorough health assessment. This is because problems such as coronary atherosclerosis (see Chapter 12) often go undetected in this population until a catastrophic event, such as a heart attack, occurs. The neurological impairment that diabetes causes can damage the sensory nerves of the cardiac system, so that a diabetic person may feel little or no chest pain, even though her heart is not getting enough oxygen. In the absence of cardiac abnormalities, diabetics are advised to exercise three to five times each week for 20 to 30 minutes, and they must measure their blood glucose level before beginning each exercise session. This is because vigorous exercise can actually increase the amount of glucose in the blood. Activity should be postponed if the blood glucose is greater than 300 mg/dl or if ketones are present in the urine of a Type 1 diabetic. If the blood glucose level is less than 100 mg/dl, a snack should be eaten before the exercise begins. A general rule of thumb for snacking is that 15 g of carbohydrate should be eaten for every 30 minutes of exercise that is planned.

Pharmacological Interventions   Drug treatment for DM is currently limited to insulin administered **parenterally**—by injection—or non-insulin oral agents that work in a variety of ways. As Type 1 diabetics cannot manufacture sufficient insulin, they must take that hormone as their primary form of drug therapy. Because insulin would be destroyed by the gastric acid in the stomach if it were taken orally, it must be administered by injection. Some Type 2 diabetics can control their disease with diet and exercise alone. Others must also take drugs to boost insulin production in their failing pancreases and/or drugs that make the cells more sensitive to insulin. Some Type 2 diabetics even need to take insulin. The treatment of gestational DM includes nutritional therapy, calorie restriction to reduce hyperglycemia and triglyceride levels in obese women, moderate exercise, and insulin if other measures do not satisfactorily lower serum glucose levels. Oral antidiabetic agents are *not* used during pregnancy (American Diabetes Association, 2000).

In the past, the insulin used in DM therapy came from porcine or bovine pancreatic tissue. Today, however, most is synthesized through recombinant DNA technology and is bioidentical to human insulin. These new insulins are a great boon to diabetics, because the insulins obtained from the tissues of pigs and cows sometimes caused an allergic reaction (Cleveland, 1999). Insulins vary as to how long they take to begin working in the body, how long they take to reach their peak effect, and how long their effects last. Many diabetics must take both short-acting and longer-acting forms in order to achieve maximum blood sugar control. They can inject them at different times or mix the two forms together in the same syringe for a single injection. Premixed insulin products that contain both short- and long-acting forms are also available. The insulin preparations commonly available in the United States are listed in Table 20–6. Regular, or short-acting, insulin is the only type that can be administered either intravenously or **subcutaneously** (under the skin). All the other types can be administered only by subcutaneous injection.

Diabetics who need or desire precise blood sugar control often use **insulin pumps.** An insulin pump is a device about the size of a beeper that can be worn on a belt or elsewhere outside the body. It is connected to a catheter inserted beneath the patient's skin. It holds a daily supply of insulin and can be programmed to release it frequently in small amounts on whatever schedule the diabetic person deems suitable in light of the day's eating and activity plan. The use

TABLE 20–6 Types of insulin available in the United States.

Insulin	Onset	Duration
Very short-acting: Humalog	15 minutes	4 hours
Short-acting: Regular	30 minutes	3–6 hours
Intermediate-acting: NPH	2–4 hours	10–18 hours
Long-acting: Ultralente	6–10 hours	18–20 hours
Premixed: 70/30 (70% NPH/30% Regular)	30 minutes	12–18 hours
50/50 (50% NPH/50% Regular)	30 minutes	12–18 hours
75/25 (75% NPH/ 20% Humalog)	15 minutes	12–18 hours

creasing the liver's production of glucose and reducing cellular resistance to insulin (Cleveland, 1999). Drugs in the alpha-glucosidase inhibitor group reduce glucose absorption in the small intestine by inhibiting the enzyme for which they are named; this reduces after-meal glucose levels. There are several different drugs in each of these groups; healthcare providers choose from among them, taking into consideration such factors as the patient's lifestyle, history of compliance, and disease severity and the drug's cost. Oral agents are not prescribed for Type 1 diabetics. Table 20–7 lists the oral agents according to their classification and provides more detailed information about one drug in each group.

Chromium picolinate, an essential trace element that plays a role in the metabolism of insulin, is marketed as a dietary supplement and may decrease insulin resistance in Type 2 diabetic individuals. Chromium increases the number of insulin receptors on insulin-sensitive tissues, and chromium deficiency is known to contribute to insulin resistance (Mathuna, 2001). Plasma chromium levels have been found to be 40 percent lower, and urinary excretion rates three times higher, in diabetics than in nondiabetic individuals (Morris, 1999). The results of clinical trials conducted to determine whether supplementation with chromium enhances insulin sensitivity and glucose tolerance have been mixed, and it has been suggested that supplementation may be efficacious only in diabetics who are chromium *deficient* (Mathuna, 2001). Chromium is found in foods such as brewer's yeast, wheat germ, cheese, liver, peanut butter, chicken, and spinach. A diet high in complex carbohydrates, but not

of an insulin pump can obviate the undesirable fluctuations in insulin levels that occur when insulin is injected in relatively large amounts only a few times a day (Schultz, 2000).

Many Type 2 diabetics need oral antidiabetic agents in order to maintain normal blood glucose levels. A number of such agents are available. Drugs in the sulfonylurea, biguanide, and thiazolidinediones groups work by both de-

TABLE 20–7 Examples of oral antidiabetic agents.

Type	Sample Drug (Generic and Brand Names)	Actions
Second-generation sulfonylureas	Glipizide (Glucotrol)	Stimulates the pancreas to make more insulin
Third-generation sulfonylureas	Glimepiride (Amaryl)	Stimulates the pancreas to make more insulin
Meglitinides	Regaglinide (Prandin)	Stimulates the pancreas to release more insulin
Biguanides	Metformin (Glucophage)	Decreases liver production of glucose and breaks insulin resistance
Alpha-glucosidase	Acarbose (Precose)	Inhibits enzyme in small intestine to reduce after-meal glucose levels
Thiazolidinediones	Rosiglitazone (Avandia)	Breaks insulin resistance and decreases liver production of glucose
Combination agents	Glyburide and Metformin (Glucovance)	Stimulates pancreas to make more insulin, decreases liver production of glucose, and reduces insulin resistance

simple sugars, enhances its absorption, whereas taking antacids hinders it. Chromium picolinate, the form most often used in dietary supplements, is generally considered to be safe; however, little information is available about its long-term effects (Mathuna, 2001).

Alpha lipoic acid (ALA), a chemical produced naturally in the body as part of the cycle of energy production (Krebs cycle) may be efficacious in the prevention and treatment of nerve damage caused by diabetes. ALA is a powerful antioxidant that has been found to retard free radical damage to small blood vessels and nerves in diabetic rats. As diabetic humans have been found to have significantly lower levels of antioxidants in their bodies than nondiabetic individuals, researchers speculate that supplementation with ALA, and other antioxidants, may retard the onset of complications in diabetic individuals, and perhaps the onset of the disease itself (Nardino, 2000). The studies conducted to date on the use of ALA in diabetics have been small and some have been methodologically flawed; however, a large clinical trial involving medical centers in North America and Europe is underway to investigate the usefulness of ALA in the prevention and treatment of diabetic neuropathy. ALA is approved for the treatment of diabetic neuropathy in Germany and is available as a food supplement in the United States. In the trials in which it has been found to be effective, dosages of 600 mg/day or more were used, and few side effects were documented. Because ALA has a **hypoglycemic** (blood sugar-lowering) effect, individuals who elect to try it should inform their healthcare providers and monitor their blood sugar levels more frequently.

Monitoring The ADA recommends that a number of assessments be performed periodically on diabetic persons in order to determine their level of diabetic control and to monitor complications and medication side effects. One of the most important of these tests is the **hemoglobin A1C** (glycosylated hemoglobin) test, which reflects whether blood glucose levels have been running normal or high over the past two months. Hemoglobin, like all cells and tissues in the body, becomes glycosylated, or coated with glucose, when glucose levels in the body are excessively high. Over time, glycosylation damages cells and tissues. Many of the complications of diabetes affecting not only the blood vessels and the heart but also the eyes, kidneys, and nerves occur because of this process. Because hemoglobin is carried on red blood cells (RBCs), the degree to which the hemoglobin becomes glycosylated depends on how much glucose is present within the red blood cells, which live for approximately 120 days in the body. Assessing the degree to which the hemoglobin has become glycosylated provides a pretty good estimation of whether the individual has been able to maintain acceptable glucose levels over most of the life span of the RBCs in the blood sample. In contrast to a serum glucose reading, which reflects only the level that existed *at the time the blood sample was drawn*, the hemoglobin A1C test

TABLE 20–8	Tests used in monitoring DM.
Test	**Frequency**
Fasting glucose	Every three to six months
Hemoglobin A1C	At diagnosis, then quarterly until the goal is met, then as needed
Creatinine	Before starting some oral medications
Microalbumin	Yearly
Lipid profile	Yearly
EKG	For baseline
Blood pressure	Every visit

provides information about the average level of glucose control over a period of months. The tests and the frequency with which they are carried out are listed in Table 20–8.

In addition to having tests ordered by a physician or another healthcare provider, diabetic patients are expected to keep a daily diary of food intake, glucose levels, activity, and illnesses. This diary is useful when the individual's condition changes and alterations in therapy become necessary. Diabetic individuals must also monitor their own serum blood glucose levels frequently. Self-monitoring provides direct and immediate feedback about their food choices, the benefits of exercise, and the efficacy of medications. Many varieties of home glucose meters are available.

Stress Management Managing stress is an important part of managing diabetes. Both physical and emotional stress elevate serum glucose levels. This is because stress stimulates the sympathetic nervous system, causing the fight-or-flight mechanism to come into play. As part of this mechanism, glucose is produced from glycogen stores, and from fats and protein, to prepare the body for action. Diabetic individuals are assessed for physical stressors, such as the presence of concurrent additional diseases, as well as for causes of emotional stress. Physical disorders are addressed, and education in stress-reduction techniques is offered. Psychological counseling may be recommended. The individual is encouraged to participate in health-maintenance behaviors, such as getting an annual flu shot and attending promptly to injuries and infections.

COMPLICATIONS OF DIABETES

The complications of diabetes are very widespread. The most common *short-term* complications are hypoglycemia, diabetic ketoacidosis, and hyperglycemic hyperosmolar nonketosis. The *long-term* complications include damage to various organs and structures of the body. Chronically elevated blood glucose levels damage all organs and cause their level of function to deteriorate. This damage is differentiated as **macrovascular** (large blood vessel) **disease, microvascular** (small blood vessel) **disease,** and **neuropathy** (damage to nerves).

Box 20–5 Signs and Symptoms of Hypoglycemia

- Shaking
- Tachycardia (fast heart rate)
- Diaphoresis (sweating)
- Anxiety
- Dizziness
- Hunger
- Impaired vision
- Weakness and fatigue
- Headache
- Irritability

Box 20–6 Signs and Symptoms of Severe Hyperglycemia

- Extreme thirst
- Increased urination
- Dry skin
- Hunger
- Blurred vision
- Drowsiness
- Nausea

Hypoglycemia The term *hypoglycemia* refers to an abnormally low blood sugar level. Mild to moderate hypoglycemia can cause symptoms such as physical weakness, sweating, a rapid heart rate, and the inability to think clearly. Severe hypoglycemia can cause unconsciousness, seizures, and even death. Hypoglycemia can develop under a number of circumstances. An inadequate food intake, too much insulin or oral antidiabetic medication, or extra exercise without a balancing snack can cause blood sugar levels to become dangerously low. Hypoglycemia often has a sudden onset and can progress to **insulin shock** (very low blood pressure and unconsciousness) if not treated. The neurological complications of diabetes can also mitigate the individual's experience of hypoglycemia, causing it to be recognized late in the course of the problem or not at all. The symptoms of hypoglycemia are listed in Box 20–5.

Diabetic Ketoacidosis Diabetic ketoacidosis (DKA) is a life-threatening complication with a mortality rate as high as 19 percent (Grinslade & Buck, 1999). Whereas persons with Type 1 DM are prone to DKA, Type 2 diabetics develop it only infrequently. Ketoacidosis develops when the body is almost completely unable to metabolize glucose as an energy source because there is no insulin in the blood to "unlock" the cells and allow glucose to enter. The signs that serum glucose levels are becoming dangerously high are excessive urination and marked sensations of hunger and thirst. Other signs are listed in Box 20–6. When there is no glucose in the cells to support metabolism, the body mistakenly assumes that there is not enough glucose available, and it activates several mechanisms designed to increase the amount of glucose in the blood. The hormone glucagon is released from alpha cells in the pancreas; glucagon stimulates glycogenolysis, the conversion of glycogen to glucose, gluconeogenesis, the synthesis of glucose from proteins and fat, and the process of lipolysis. Lipolysis is a process by which stored fats are broken down into fatty acids, which can be further broken down and used as fuel by the body. When there is insufficient glu-

cose in cells, however, the use of fatty acids for fuel yields metabolites known as ketone bodies. Ketone bodies are potent organic acids; when produced in quantity, they cause the body to become relatively too acidic, and the serious condition known as **acidosis** results. Initially, the body attempts to combat the acidosis through compensatory respiratory measures called **Kussmaul respirations.** These deep, rapid respiratory efforts increase the exhalation of carbon dioxide, which forms carbonic acid when dissolved in water, in an attempt to excrete acids. This compensatory mechanism is inefficient, however, and does not keep up with the acids produced through ketone production.

Acidosis is life-threatening in itself, but diabetic ketoacidosis also causes severe dehydration. The large amount of glucose in the blood increases its **osmolarity,** or concentration. The body senses this thickening blood and moves water out of the tissues and into the bloodstream to dilute it. This triggers excessive urination, and the body's tissues rapidly dehydrate. The balance of the various electrolytes in the blood, such as sodium and potassium, is disturbed, often to a life-threatening degree. By the time an individual in this condition reaches a medical facility, she has an obviously altered mental status and may even be comatose. Neurological, cardiac and respiratory functioning is impaired (Grinslade & Buck, 1999). Occasionally, persons who had not been previously diagnosed as having Type 1 DM will develop DKA as their initial symptom (Huether & Tomky, 1998).

Treating DKA involves replacing fluid intravenously, correcting electrolyte imbalances, and lowering serum glucose levels with insulin administration. Once the individual has been stabilized, the treatment is aimed at identifying and treating the underlying cause of the episode of DKA. Infection is the most common event resulting in DKA, with the failure to administer adequate amounts of insulin as the second most common cause of DKA.

Hyperglycemic Hyperosmolar Nonketosis Hyperglycemic hyperosmolar nonketosis (HHNK) is somewhat similar to diabetic ketoacidosis, but it affects individuals with *Type 2 DM,* rather than those with Type 1. When the blood glucose level becomes severely elevated, Type 2 diabetics exhibit the signs of hyperglycemia but do not have the increased level of ketones in their blood. Therefore, they do not develop acidosis. Although the amount of insulin produced by Type 2 diabetics is insufficient for normal metabolism, enough is produced to prevent the ketosis seen in DKA. Events that precipitate HHNK include pneumonia, stroke, and some medications, such as steroids, diuretics, and drugs used to control seizures (Frizzell, 2000).

Macrovascular Disease Macrovascular disease affects the blood vessels that are larger than capillaries. Diabetes can cause atherosclerotic plaques to develop in these vessels. This complication is more prevalent in patients with Type 2 DM, and the degree of the atherosclerotic changes seems unrelated to the severity of the DM. Persistently elevated serum glucose levels cause smooth muscle cells within the walls of the arteries to proliferate. This muscle proliferation results in the development of the fibrous plaques characteristic of atherosclerosis. The resulting vessel narrowing causes decreased blood flow and organ damage.

Some lipoprotein abnormalities are also thought to contribute to the macrovascular changes associated with diabetes. Some studies have identified aberrations in high-density lipoproteins, low-density lipoproteins, and triglyceride levels (see Chapter 12). The most consistent finding in diabetics is elevated triglyceride levels (Steiner, 1999). Elevated triglyceride levels in individuals with DM are associated with a greater risk of atherosclerosis. The heart, brain, and peripheral tissues are most susceptible to the ravages of macrovascular disease.

As the inside diameter of the coronary arteries narrows with fibrous plaque, the risk of myocardial infarction (MI) increases. Myocardial ischemia, chest pain, and damage to the heart muscle or valves may result. Diabetes is a known independent risk factor for several forms of **coronary heart disease** (Grundy et al., 1999).

Moreover, diabetic persons who have coronary artery disease have a poorer prognosis than do nondiabetic persons. In their meta-analysis of the literature on women and men with diabetes and coronary heart disease, Lee, Cheung, Cape, and Zinman (2000) reported that women who have both coronary heart disease and diabetes have a greater risk of dying than men who have both diseases. Diabetic individuals *without* a previous history of MI are known to be at the same risk of dying as nondiabetic individuals *with* a history of MI. Therefore, diabetics without known cornonary heart disease should be vigilantly assessed and followed medically. An additional reason for doing so is the neuropathy associated with DM. Diabetic patients with myocardial ischemia may not experience the expected chest pain.

Diabetic individuals are also prone to developing **heart failure.** This is because the protein in the heart muscle becomes glycosylated and gradually loses its ability to contract sufficiently (Grundy et al., 1999). Diabetes also increases the risk that the carotid arteries in the neck will become partially occluded by plaque and that irreversible brain damage will result. Persons who do not have diabetes are more likely to experience only transient symptoms from carotid artery atherosclerosis (Grundy et al., 1999). The mortality from stroke, or cerebral vascular accident (CVA), has been found to be as much as three times greater in diabetics than in persons who do not have diabetes.

Peripheral blood flow is also diminished in the person with DM. This is because plaque makes the arteries in the extremities, particularly the legs, *narrow* and because the presence of large amounts of sugar in the blood tends to make it *thicker.* Those two factors, narrow vessels and thick blood, can cause blood clots, or **thrombi,** to develop. Once a clot forms, it can block the blood flow to the extremity. When this happens, tissue beyond the clot starts to die from a lack of the oxygen normally carried in blood. As progressive tissue death occurs, the extremity becomes **gangrenous**—that is, blackened and hard—usually beginning at the toes and spreading upward. Once that occurs, the amputation of all or part of the limb is necessary.

Microvascular Disease The term *microvascular disease* refers to progressive thickening of the walls of the capillaries, the smallest blood vessels in the body. This thickening occurs as a result of the accumulation of fructose, sorbitol, and the end-products of glycosylation. These sugars interfere with cell wall metabolism (Frizzell, 2000) and cause the capillary membranes to become too thick to allow oxygen to diffuse readily from the capillary blood into tissue cells. Eventually, the tissues become less and less functional and finally start to die. When this occurs in the extremities, skin changes become noticeable and progress to small, patchy areas of gangrene.

Unfortunately, microvascular changes do not occur only in the extremities; they also affect the eyes, the kidneys, and the nerves. Small blood vessels in the retina of the eye bleed or break off, leading to retinal ischemia (lack of oxygen) and eventual blindness. The risk of **retinopathy,** or disease of the retina, in a diabetic is 25 times that in the nondiabetic population. Diabetic retinopathy develops more quickly in those with Type 2 disease than those with Type 1, but most individuals who have diabetes mellitus display some degree of retinopathy (Huether & Tomky, 1998). Often, a concern about diabetes is first raised by an eye doctor during a routine eye examination or when a person seeks care because of a change in vision.

The **kidneys** are also very vulnerable to microvascular changes; diabetes is the leading cause of end-stage renal disease in the Unites States (Frizzel, 2000). Glomerular function is altered in diabetic individuals, causing protein to appear in the urine and hypertension and progressive renal insufficiency to develop. The kidneys play a vital role in the control of blood pressure; as kidney disease progresses, blood pressure goes up. Glomerular changes occur *early* in the course of the disease, often before overt signs of DM appear (Huether & Tomky, 1998).

Neuropathy Neuropathy occurs as a result of altered cellular metabolism in diabetic individuals. Impaired blood flow to the nerves results in a loss of myelin, the protective and insulating covering that allows electrical impulses to be conducted rapidly across nerve fibers (Frizzell, 2000). This results in a variety of problems; one of the most important is a decrease in the ability to feel pain and other physical sensations. This occurs primarily in the hands and feet, and it leads to injury and the development of diabetic ulcers. Diabetic persons may also lose their ability to feel pain related to cardiac ischemia; they often do not experience the warning sign of angina. Neuropathy can also cause urinary incontinence and sexual impotence. Gastric problems associated with diabetes complications include delayed emptying of the stomach, constipation, nausea, diarrhea, and bowel incontinence (McCloud & Mishler, 1999). Neuropathy is thought to be *the most frequently occurring complication* of diabetes and has similar prevalence rates for Type 1 and Type 2 DM (Huether & Tomky, 1998).

Immunological Wellness Self-Assessment

Use your answers to the questions below to gauge your level of immunological wellness.

1. *Am I habitually engaging in behaviors that may compromise immunity (smoking, using recreational drugs, missing sleep)?*
2. *Am I getting more than two or three colds a year? If so, what am I doing that might be compromising my immunity or excessively exposing me to viruses?*
3. *Am I engaging in sex with unfamiliar or nonmonogamous partners without using a barrier, such as a condom? Am I sharing needles with which to inject heroin and/or cocaine?*
4. *Does my diet contain adequate amounts of fresh, whole foods? If not, have I added a multivitamin to my daily diet?*
5. *Do I give myself time to recover from occasional minor illnesses, or do I always try to push past such "inconveniences"?*
6. *Am I knowledgeable about the proper use of any immune-enhancing dietary supplements I am taking? Am I aware of the contraindications to their use?*
7. *If I choose to be vaccinated against various diseases, am I keeping my vaccinations up to date?*
8. *Do I have my blood sugar level checked as part of my periodic health checkup?*

New Directions

Immunotherapy is an exciting and promising field of research. It addresses the therapeutic approaches used to adjust the immune system in order to treat or prevent disease. Discrete disciplines within the immunotherapy field include biotherapy, psychoneuroimmunology (discussed in Chapter 27), and certain applications of gene therapy and genetic engineering. Immunotherapy also includes the use of vaccination as therapy, as opposed to prevention, in certain situations in which an attempt is made to modify existing disease.

Recombinant DNA technology is used to manufacture relatively large amounts of bioactive substances that have a therapeutic application. Recombinant DNA technology involves the deliberate recombination of natural genetic blueprints (DNA strands) within cell cultures to create new blueprints, or genetic codes, which can then direct the manufacture of the desired substance within those cell cultures. Substances produced in large amounts via recombinant DNA technology include GCSF and GM-CSF; interferon (to treat viral infections, such as hepatitis C); blood growth factors, such as erythropoietin (used in anemia); and interleukin-2, which may increase CD4 counts in HIV disease. A similar approach in cancer therapy involves the creation of *genetically engineered viruses and bacteria,* which may be able to carry anticancer agents directly to tumor cells, because they will carry immunological coding that targets only those cells. This may avoid the terrible toxicities endured when nontumor cells are unavoidably exposed to the nonspecific cancer drugs now available.

The use of vaccines as therapy in HIV infection is now being investigated. In order to understand the role that vaccines play, it is necessary to recall the discussion and illustration of immune system activation. In order to mount a defense against HIV, the immune system must read and copy the antigenic signature on HIV and HIV-infected cells. Only then can CD4 cells convey the nature of the antigen to the other branches of the immune system, so that they will recognize and fight cells that contain it (Brander & Walker, 1999). However, in AIDS patients with advanced disease, the CD4 cells that have copied the virus's unique antigenic signature may have been killed. When such patients are responding well to treatment, they have no HIV in their blood, so, even when their CD4 counts rise, the cells have no source of HIV from which to read and copy antigen to be presented to the remaining branches of the system. This is a problem, because drug therapy for HIV does not cure the disease; it merely suppresses the virus. An HIV vaccine, which would contain the antigenic markers of HIV but not active virus, could be used to teach the reemerging CD4 cell population how to "see" HIV again—and, thus, how to present antigen to the remaining T- and B-lymphocytes.

An intermittent approach to HIV therapy is being investigated as a more appropriate treatment for individuals able to mount some degree of immune response to the virus. Jozviak, Doerfler, and Woodward (1999) observed that several AIDS patients on long-term antiviral therapy seemed to develop an immune response to HIV when their treatments were repeatedly interrupted. In those patients, the virus sometimes did not rebloom to its former baseline level and grew more slowly overall. This phenomenon may represent an "autovaccination" effect that leads to immune responsiveness. For such individuals, intermittent, rather than continuous, drug therapy may prove to be the better way of controlling this disease over decades; the drugs will help the immune system recover, and the immune system will help the drugs suppress HIV.

New research on the treatment of autoimmune disease is also being done. Tumor necrosis factor alpha seems to be a major culprit in the destruction of cartilage in RA and in the organ damage seen in SLE. TNF-alpha-blocking agents are being tested that may provide therapy that is more specific and less toxic.

New treatment options for diabetes are also on the horizon. One is the transplantation of pancreatic beta cells from donor organs to Type 1 diabetics. The transplanted beta cells produce insulin, and blood glucose levels are maintained at normal levels without the need for medication (Sweeney & Lapp, 2000). This therapy is not widely available, however, because the need for pancreatic cells far exceeds the available organs available for transplantation. Another drawback to this procedure is that, because of the risk that their bodies may reject the transplanted cells, patients receiving them must take drugs to suppress their immune systems. Two new drug therapies currently being investigated are a long-acting insulin, which may stabilize blood sugar for 24 hours, and a form of insulin that can be taken via inhalation rather than injection. Such an innovation would reduce the need for both injections and pancreatic beta cell transplantation (Schultz, 2000). The experimental inhaled insulin has a more rapid onset of action than the long-acting insulin, but both products provide a similar level of glucose control (Danner, 2000).

QUESTIONS FOR REFLECTION AND DISCUSSION

1. *Identify the ways in which social policies affect the spread, treatment, and so on, of infectious diseases.*
2. *What roles might political and social activism play in the prevention and treatment of infectious disease?*
3. *Discuss steps women can take to maintain immuneological wellness.*
4. *At one time, infectious diseases were the scourge of humankind; now, especially in industrialized societies, hyperimmune diseases are emergent. How might technological advancements change the types of disease from which people suffer?*
5. *Discuss the relationship between the Western world's ecological balance and human health?*

RESOURCES

Books

Brower, M., & Leon, W. (1999). *The consumer's guide to effective environmental choices.* Three Rivers Press.

Hiser, E. (1999). *The other diabetes: Living and eating well with type 2 diabetes.* William Morrow.

Murray, M., & Pizzorno, J. (1998) *Encyclopedia of natural medicine.* Prima Health.

Pincus, T. (1999). Gretchen Henkel & John Kliprel (Eds.) *The Arthritis Foundation's guide to good living with rheumatoid arthritis.* Longstreet Press.

Wallace, D. J. (2000). *The lupus book: A guide for patients and their families.* Oxford University Press.

Weil, A. (1988). *Health and healing.* Boston: Houghton Mifflin.

Whitaker, J. M., & Arthur, M. C. (1994). *Reversing diabetes.* Warner Books.

Organizations

The Allergy and Asthma Network
2751 Prosperity Ave., Suite 150
Fairfax, VA 22031-4397
Phone: 1-800-878-4403
Web: www.aanma.org

The American Autoimmune-Related Diseases Association
22100 Gratiot Ave.
E. Detroit, MI 48021
Phone: 818-776-3900
Web: www.aarda.org

The American Diabetes Association
1660 Duke St.
Alexandria, VA 22314
Phone: 703-549-1500
Web: www.diabetes.org

The Lupus Foundation of America
1300 Piccard Dr., Suite 200
Rockville, MD 24032
Phone: 1-800-558-0121
Web: www.lupus.org/lupus

Websites

Journal of the American Medical Association. HIV/AIDS Resource Center: www.ama-assn.org/special/hiv

REFERENCES

American Diabetes Association. (1997). Report of the expert committee on the diagnosis and classification of diabetes mellitus. *Diabetes Care, 20*(7), 1183–1197.

American Diabetes Association. (2000). Gestational diabetes mellitus: Definition, detection, and diagnosis. *Diabetes Care, 23*(1), 77.

American Diabetes Association. (2001). Standards of medical care for patients with diabetes mellitus. *Diabetes Care, 24,* 33.

Andrade, L. E., Ferraz, M. B., Atra, E., Castro, A., & Silva, M. S. (1991). A randomized controlled trial to evaluate the effectiveness of homeopathy in rheumatoid arthritis. *Scandanavian Journal of Rheumatology, 20*(3), 204–208.

Assad, L. S., Riester, K., Fruchter, R. G., Palefsky, J., Burk, R. D., Burns, D., Miotti, P., Jordan, C., Muderspach, L. I., Anastos, K., & Greenblatt, R. (1998). *HIV RNA level is a risk factor for abnormal cervical cytology.* Fifth Conference on Retroviruses and Opportunistic Infections, February 2–8, 1998, Chicago, IL. Abstract No. 716.

ATBC Cancer Prevention Study Group. (1994). The alpha-tocopherol, beta-carotene lung cancer prevention study: Design, methods, participant characteristics, and compliance. *Annals of Epidemiology, 4*(1), 1–10.

Austin, H. A., & Balow, J. E. (1999). Natural history and treatment of lupus nephritis. *Seminars in Nephrology, 19*(1), 2–11.

Balzarini, J. (1999). Suppression of resistance to drugs targeted to human immunodeficiency virus reverse transcriptase by combination therapy. *Biochemical Pharmacology, 58*(1), 1–27. Available: http://rheumatology.medscape.com/Medscape/CNO/1999/ACR/ACR-06.html

Beinfield, H., & Korngold, E. (1995). Chinese traditional medicine: An introductory overview. *Alternative Therapies in Health and Medicine, 1*(1), 44–52.

Bell, M. J., Lineker, S. C., Wilkins, A. L., Goldsmith, C. H., & Badley, E. M. (1998). A randomized controlled trial to evaluate the efficacy of community based physical therapy in the treatment of people with rheumatoid arthritis. *Journal of Rheumatology, 25*(2), 231–237.

Bergner, P. (1996). Goldenseal and the common cold: The antibiotic myth. *Medical Herbalism, 8*(4), 1, 4–6.

Bergner, P. (1997). Contraindications for echinacea? *Medical Herbalism, 9*(1), 1, 11–14.

Bergner, P. (1998). Adverse effects anecdotes. *Medical Herbalism, 10*(4), 15.

Bertino, L. S., & Lu, L. (1993). The bite of a wolf: Systemic lupus erythematosis. *Rehabilitation Nursing, 39*, 50–57.

Bhatt-Sanders, D. (1985). Acupuncture for rheumatoid arthritis: An analysis of the literature. *Seminars in Arthritis and Rheumatology, 14*(4), 225–231

Bongiovanni, B. (2000). *Lupus—Complementary approaches.* [Online]. Available: http://wellweb.com/ALTERN/diseases/lupus.htm

Brander, C., & Walker, B. D. (1999). T lymphocyte responses in HIV-1 infection: Implications for vaccine development. *Current Opinion in Immunology, 11*(4), 451–459.

Brook, I., & Gober, A. E. (1996). Prophylaxis with amoxicillin or sulfisoxazole for otitis media: Effect on the recovery of penicillin-resistant bacteria from children. *Clinics in Infectious Disease, 22*(1), 143–145.

Brunzell, J., & Hokanson, J. (1999). Dyslipidemia of central obesity and insulin resistance. *Diabetes Care, 22*, C10–C12.

Caiaffa, W. T., Vlahov, D., Graham, N. M., Astemborski, J., Solomon, L., Nelson, K. E., & Munoz, A. (1994). Drug smoking, pneumocystis carinii pneumonia, and immunosuppression increase risk of bacterial pneumonia in human immunodeficiency virus–seropositive injection drug users. *American Journal of Respiratory and Critical Care Medicine, 150*(6 Pt 1), 1493–1498.

Chu, D. T., Wong, W. L., & Mavligit, G. M. (1988). Immunotherapy with Chinese medicinal herbs. II: Reversal of cyclophosphamide-induced immune suppression by administration of fractionated astragalus membranaceus in vivo. *Journal of Clinical Laboratory Immunology, 25*(3), 125–129.

Clark, S. J., Saag, M. S., Decker, W. D., Campbell-Hill, S., Roberson, J. L., Veldkamp, P. J., Kappes, J. C., Hahn, B. H., & Shaw, G. M. (1991). High titers of cytopathic virus in plasma of patients with symptomatic primary HIV-1 infection. *New England Journal of Medicine, 324*(14), 954–960.

Clerici, M., Salvi, A., Trabattoni, D., Lo Caputo, S., Semplici, F., Biasin, M., Ble, C., Meacci, F., Romeo, C., Piconi, S., Mazzotta, F., Villa, M. L., & Mazzoli, S. A. (1999). Role for mucosal immunity in resistance to HIV infection. *Immunology Letter, 66*(1–3), 21–25.

Cleveland, L. (1999). Drugs affecting blood glucose levels. In L. Cleveland, D. Aschenbrenner, S. Venable, & J. Yensen (Eds.), *Nursing management in drug therapy* (pp. 677–706). Philadelphia: Lippincott.

Cornell, S. (1997). New directions in rheumatoid arthritis. *Advance for Nurse Practitioners, 5*(3), 61–64.

Darlington, L. G., & Ramsey, N. W. (1993). Review of dietary therapy for rheumatoid arthritis. *British Journal of Rheumatology, 32*(6), 507–514.

DeFronzo, R. (1999). Pathophysiology of type 2 diabetes: The role of insulin resistance. *Consultant, suppl.* S8–S16.

Finzi, D. (1999). Latent infection of CD4+ T cells provides a mechanism for lifelong persistence of HIV-1, even in patients on effective combination therapy. *Nature Medicine, 5*(5), 512–517.

Ford, R. B. (1993). Role of infectious agents in respiratory disease. *Veterinary Clinics of North America: Small Animal Practice, 23*(1), 17–35.

Frieling, U. M., Schaumberg, D. A., Kupper, T. S., Muntwyler, J., & Hennekens, C. H. (2000). A randomized, 12-year primary-prevention trial of beta carotene supplementation for nonmelanoma skin cancer in the physicians' health study. *Archives of Dermatology, 136*(2), 179–184.

Frizzell, J. P. (2000). Altered endocrine function. In B. Bullock & R. Henze, (Eds.), *Focus on pathophysiology* (pp. 669–718). Philadelphia: Lippincott.

Garewal, H. S., Katz, R. V., Meyskens, F., Pitcock, J., Morse, D., Friedman, S., Peng, Y., Pendrys, D. G., Mayne, S., Alberts, D., Kiersch, T., & Graver, E. (1999). Beta-carotene produces sustained remissions in patients with oral leukoplakia: Results of a multicenter prospective trial. *Archives in Otolaryngology and Head and Neck Surgery, 125*(12), 1305–1310.

Garibaldi, R. A. (1985). Epidemiology of community-acquired respiratory tract infections in adults. *American Journal of Medicine, 78*(6b), 32–37.

Gavin, J. R. (1999). New developments in diabetes management: Role of second generation thiazolidinedione insulin sensitizers. *Consultant, Supp. no.* S7.

Gibson, R. G., Gibson, S. L., MacNeill, A. D., & Buchanan, W. W. (1980). Homoeopathic therapy in rheumatoid arthritis: Evaluation by double-blind clinical therapeutic trial. *British Journal of Clinical Pharmacology, 9*(5), 453–459.

Good, R. A., & Lorenz, E. (1992). Nutrition and cellular immunity. *International Journal of Immunopharmacology, 14*(3), 361–366.

Grassi, W., De Angelis, R., Lamanna, G., & Cervini, C. (1998). The clinical features of rheumatoid arthritis. *European Journal of Radiology,* (Suppl 1), S18–S24.

Grinslade, S., & Buck, E. (1999). Diabetic ketoacidosis: Implications for the medical-surgical nurse. *MedSurg Nursing, 8*(1), 37.

Grundy, S., Banjamin, I., Burke, G., Chait, A., Eckel, R., Howard, B., Mitch, W., Smith, S., & Sowers, J. (1999). Diabetes and cardiovascular disease: A statement for healthcare professionals from the American Heart Association. *Circulation, 100,* 1134–1146.

Hakkinen, A., Sokka, T., Kotaniemi, A., Kautiainen, H., Jappinen, I., Laitinen, L., & Hannonen, P. (1999). Dynamic strength training in patients with early rheumatoid arthritis increases muscle strength but not bone mineral density. *Journal of Rheumatology, 26*(6), 1257–1263.

Hemila, H., & Douglas, R. M. (1999). Vitamin C and acute respiratory infections. *International Journal of Tuberculosis and Lung Diseases, 3*(9), 756–761.

Hercberg, S., Galan, P., Preziosi, P., Roussel, A. M., Arnaud, J., Richard, M. J., Malvy, D., Paul-Dauphin, A., Briancon, S., & Favier, A. (1998). Background and rationale behind the SU.VI.MAX Study, a prevention trial using nutritional doses of a combination of antioxidant vitamins and minerals to reduce cardiovascular diseases and cancers. SUpplementation en VItamines et Mineraux AntioXydants Study. *International Journal for Vitamin and Nutritional Research, 68*(1), 3–20.

Holgate, S. (1999). The epidemic of allergy and asthma. *Nature, 402*(Suppl 6760), b3–b4.

Huether S. E., & Tomky, D. (1998). Alterations of hormonal regulation. In K. McCance & S. Huether (Eds.), *Pathophysiology: The biologic basis for disease in adults and children* (3rd ed., pp. 656–706). St. Louis: Mosby.

Ironson, G., Field, T., Scafidi, F., Hashimoto, M., Kumar, M., Kumar, A., Price, A., Gooncalves, A., Burman, I., Tetenman, C., & Patarca, R. (1996). Massage therapy is associated with enhancement of the immune system's cytotoxic capacity. *International Journal of Neuroscience, 84*(1), 34–38.

Jones, J. L., Hanson, D. L., Dworkin, M. S., Alderton, D. L., Fleming, P. L., Kaplan, J. E., & Ward, J. (1999). Surveillance for AIDS-defining opportunistic illnesses, 1992–1997. Morbidity and Mortality Weekly Report *(MMWR), 48*(SS-2), 1–22.

Jones, N. S., Carney, A. S., & Davis, A. (1998). The prevalence of allergic rhinosinusitis: A review. *Journal of Laryngology and Otology, 112*(11), 1019–1030.

Jozviak, J. L., Doerfler, R. E., & Woodward, W. C. (1999). *Intermittent antiretroviral therapy (ART) can induce reduction of viral rebound during ART-interruption.* Seventh European Conference on Clinical Aspects and Treatment of HIV-Infection, October 23–27, Lisbon, Portugal. Abstract No. 236.

Junghans, C. (1999). Uniform risk of clinical progression despite differences in utilization of highly active antiretroviral therapy: Swiss HIV Cohort Study. *AIDS, 13*(18), 2547–2554.

Kaye, K. S., Fraimow, H. S., & Abrutyn, E. (2000). Pathogens resistant to antimicrobial agents: Epidemiology, molecular mechanisms, and clinical management. *Infectious Disease Clinics of North America, 14*(2), 293–319.

King, H. (1998). Global burden of diabetes mellitus, 1995–2025: Prevalence, numerical estimates and projections. *Diabetes Care, 21,* 1414–1431.

Klaunig, J. E., & Kamendulis, L. M. (1999). Mechanisms of cancer chemoprevention in hepatic carcinogenesis: Modulation of focal lesion growth in mice. *Toxicological Sciences, 52*(2 Suppl), 101–106.

Klepper, S. E. (1999). Effects of an eight-week physical conditioning program on disease signs and symptoms in children with chronic arthritis. *Arthritis Care Research, 12*(1), 52–60.

Lapadula, G., Iannone, F., Zuccaro, C., Covelli, M., Grattagliano, V., & Pipitone, V. (1997). Recovery of erosive rheumatoid arthritis after human immuno deficiency virus-1 infection and hemiplegia. *Journal of Rheumatology, 24*(4), 747–751.

Lee, I. M., Cook, N. R., Manson, J. E., Buring, J. E., & Hennekens, C. H. (1999). Beta-carotene supplementation and incidence of cancer and cardiovascular disease: The Women's Health Study. *Journal of the National Cancer Institute, 91*(24), 210–216.

Lee, W., Cheung, A., Cape, D., & Zinman, B. (2000). Impact of diabetes on coronary artery disease in women and men. *Diabetes Care, 23*(7), 962.

Lisiewicz, J. (1993). Immunotoxic and hematotoxic effects of occupational exposures. *Folia Medica of Cracou, 34*(1–4), 29–47.

Lori, F. (1999). Treatment of human immunodeficiency virus infection with hydroxyurea, didanosine, and a protease inhibitor before seroconversion is associated with normalized immune parameters and limited viral reservoir. *Journal of Infectious Diseases, 180*(6), 1827–1832.

Marieb, E. (1989). *Human anatomy and physiology.* Redwood City, California: The Benjamin Cummings Publishing Company.

Mahat, G. (1998). Rheumatoid arthritis. *American Journal of Nursing (AJN), 98*(12), 42–43.

Mates, J. M., Perez-Gomez, C., & Nunez de Castro, I. (1999). Antioxidant enzymes and human diseases. *Clinical Biochemistry, 32*(8), 595–603.

Mathuna, D. (2001). Chromium supplementation for the treatment of type 2 diabetes. *Alternative Medicine Alert, 3*(4), 40–43.

McCloud, M., & Mishler, M. (1999). Interventions for clients with diabetes. In D. Ignatavicius, M. L. Workman, & M. Mishler (Eds.), Medical-surgical nursing across the health care continuum (3rd ed., pp. 1635–1686). Philadelphia: W.B. Saunders.

McCowan, C. B. (1998). Systemic lupus erythematosis. *Journal of the American Academy of Nurse Practitioners, 10*(5), 225–231.

McKeown, T. (1979). *The role of medicine: Dream, dirage or nemesis?* Princeton, NJ: Princeton University Press.

McMurry, S. T., Lochmiller, R. L., McBee, K., & Qualls, C. W. (1999). Indicators of immunotoxicity in populations of cotton rats *(Sigmodon hispidus)* inhabiting an abandoned oil refinery. *Ecotoxicology and Environmental Safety, 42*(3), 223–235.

Mellors, J. W. (1996). *Prognostic value of viral load determinations*. Third Conference on Retroviruses and Opportunistic Infections, February 1, 1996, Washington, D.C. Abstract No. 174.

Michael, N. L. (1999). Host genetic influences on HIV-1 pathogenesis. *Current Opinion in Immunology, 11*(4), 466–474.

Morris, B. (1999). Chromium action and glucose homeostasis. *Journal of Trace Element Experimental Medicine, 12*, 61–70.

Murray, M., & Pizzorno, J. (1998). *Encyclopedia of natural medicine*. Rockin, CA: Prima Health.

Nardino, R. (2000). Alpha-lipoic acid for the prevention and treatment of diabetic neuropathy. *Alternative Medicine Alert, 3*(7), 74–76.

Neuberger, G. B., Press, A. N., Lindsley, H. B., Hinton, R., Cagle, P. E., Carlson, K., Scott, S., Dahl, J., & Kramer, B. (1997). Effects of exercise on fatigue, aerobic fitness, and disease activity measures in persons with rheumatoid arthritis. *Research in Nursing and Health, 20*(3), 195–204.

Neustaedter, R. (1996). *The vaccine guide: Making an informed choice*. Berkeley CA: North Atlantic Books.

Noreau, L., Moffet, H., Drolet, M., & Parent, E. (1997). Dance-based exercise program in rheumatoid arthritis: Feasibility in individuals with American College of Rheumatology functional class III disease. *American Journal of Physical Medicine and Rehabilitation, 76*(2), 109–113.

Padian, N. S., Shiboski, S. C., Glass, S. O., & Vittinghoff, E. (1997). Heterosexual transmission of human immunodeficiency virus (HIV) in northern California: Results from a ten-year study. *American Journal of Epidemiology, 146*(4), 350–357.

Peck, B. (1998). Rheumatoid arthritis: Early intervention can change outcomes. *Advance for Nurse Practitioners, 6*(7), 34–38, 41.

Peterson, P. K., Gekker, G., Chao, C. C., Schut, R., Molitor, T. W., & Balfour, H. H. (1991). Cocaine potentiates HIV-1 replication in human peripheral blood mononuclear cell cocultures. Involvement of transforming growth factor-beta. *Journal of Immunology, 146*(1), 81–84.

Pillai, R. M., & Watson, R. R. (1990). In vitro immunotoxicology and immunopharmacology: Studies on drugs of abuse. *Toxicology Letter, 53*(3), 269–283.

Pincus, T., O'Dell, J. R., & Kremer, J. M. (1999). Combination therapy with multiple disease-modifying antirheumatic drugs in rheumatoid arthritis: A preventive strategy. *Annals of Internal Medicine, 131*(10), 768–774.

Quayle, A. (2000). *Mucous membrane susceptibility to HIV infection*. [On-line]. Available: www.medscape.com/SCP/IIU/1994/v07.n06/u438.lawrence/u438.lawrence.html#Mucous

Rehman, J., Dillow, J. M., Carter, S. M., Chou, J., Le, B., & Maisel, A. S. (1999). Increased production of antigen-specific immunoglobulins G and M following in vivo treatment with the medicinal plants *Echinacea angustifolia* and *Hydrastis canadensis*. *Immunology Letter, 68*(2–3), 391–395.

Rhodes, R., & Pflanzer, R. (1992). *Human physiology*. Fort Worth, TX: Saunders College Publishing.

Schierhorn, K., Zhang, M., Matthias, C., & Kunkel, G. (1999). Influence of ozone and nitrogen dioxide on histamine and interleukin formation in a human nasal mucosa culture system. *American Journal Respiratory Cell and Molecular Biology, 20*(5), 1013–1019.

Schultz, S. (2000, September). Living with diabetes is getting easier—and a cure could be on the way. *U.S. News & World Report*, 74.

Shouji, N., Takada, K., Fukushima, K., & Hirasawa, M. (2000). Anticaries effect of a component from shiitake (an edible mushroom). *Caries Research, 34*(1), 94–98.

Simon, G., Moog, C., & Obert, G. (1994). Effects of glutathione precursors on human immunodeficiency virus replication. *Chemico-biological Interactions, 91*(2–3), 217–224.

Simon, H. B. (1991). Exercise and human immune function. In R. Ader, D. L. Felten, & N. Cohen (Eds.), *Psychoneuroimmunology* (pp. 869–895). San Diego: Academic Press.

Skidmore-Roth, L. (2001). *Mosby's handbook of herbs and natural supplements*. St. Louis, MO: Mosby.

Sprietsma, J. E. (1999). Cysteine, glutathione (GSH) and zinc and copper ions together are effective, natural, intracellular inhibitors of (AIDS) viruses. *Medical Hypotheses, 52*(6), 529–538.

Steiner, G. (1999). Risk factors for macrovascular disease in type 2 diabetes. *Diabetes Care, 22*, C6–C9.

Stiller-Winkler, R., Idel, H., Leng, G., Spix, C., & Dolgner, R. (1996). Influence of air pollution on humoral immune response. *Journal of Clinical Epidemiology, 49*(5), 537

Sun, L. Z., Currier, N. L., & Miller, S. C. (1999). The American coneflower: A prophylactic role involving nonspecific immunity. *Journal of Alternative and Complementary Medicine, 5*(5), 437–446.

Sweeney, R., & Lapp, T. (2000). NIH announces trials of insulin-transplant therapy. *American Family Physician, 62*(8), 1757.

Taylor-Robinson, D. (1999). The future of bacterial vaginosis-related research. *International Journal of Gynecology and Obstetrics, 67*(Suppl 1), S35–S38.

Threlfall, E. J., Ward, L. R., Frost, J. A., & Willshaw, G. A. (2000). Spread of resistance from food animals to man—the UK experience. *Acta Veterinaria Scandinavica Supplementum, 93*, 63–68, discussion 68–4.

Tindall, B., Barker, S., Donovan, B., Barnes, T., Roberts, J., Kronenberg, C., Gold, J., Penny, R., & Cooper, D. (1988). Characterization of the acute clinical illness associated with human immunodeficiency virus infection. *Archives of Internal Medicine, 148*(4), 945–949.

U.S. Department of Health and Human Services/Henry J. Kaiser Family Foundation. (2000). *Guidelines for the use of antiretroviral agents in HIV-infected adults and adolescents*. Wilmington, DE: DuPont.

Van de Laar, M. A., Aalbers, M., Bruins, F. G., Van Dinther-Janssen, A. C., Van der Korst, J. K., & Meijer, C. J. (1992). Food intolerance in rheumatoid arthritis. II: Clinical and histological aspects. *Annals of the Rheumatic Diseases, 51*(3), 303–306.

Van de Laar, M. A., & Van der Korst, J. K. (1992). Food intolerance in rheumatoid arthritis. I: A double blind, controlled trial of the clinical effects of elimination of milk allergens and azo dyes. *Annals of the Rheumatic Diseases, 51*(3), 298–302.

Van den Ende, C. H., Vliet Vlieland, T. P., Munneke, M., & Hazes, J. M. (1998). Dynamic exercise therapy in rheumatoid arthritis: A systematic review. *British Journal of Rheumatology, 37*(6), 677–687.

Van Vollenhoven, R. F., Park, J. L., Genovese, M. C., West, J. P., & McGuire, J. L. (1999). A double-blind, placebo-controlled, clinical trial of dehydroepiandrosterone in severe systemic lupus erythematosus. *Lupus, 8*(3), 181–187.

Walton, A. J., Snaith, M. L., Locniskar, M., Cumberland, A. G., Morrow, W. J., & Isenberg, D. A. (1991). Dietary fish oil and the severity of symptoms in patients with systemic lupus erythematosus. *Annals of the Rheumatic Diseases, 50*(7), 463–466.

Wang, C., Fortin, P. R., Li, Y., Panaritis, T., Gans, M., & Esdaile, J. M. (1999). Discontinuation of antimalarial drugs in systemic lupus erythematosus. *Journal of Rheumatology, 26*(4), 808–815.

Wang, X. D., & Russell, R. M. (1999). Procarcinogenic and anti-carcinogenic effects of beta-carotene. *Nutrition Reviews, 57*(9 Pt 1), 263–272.

Weil, A. (1990). *Natural health natural medicine.* Boston: Houghton Mifflin.

Wujick, D. (1993). Infection control in oncology patients. *Nursing Clinics of North America, 28*(3), 639–650.

21

Thyroid Wellness and Illness

Lorraine W. Bock

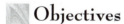

Objectives

1. *Briefly describe the thyroid's function.*
2. *Identify three hormones involved in thyroid function.*
3. *Compare and contrast the symptoms of hypothyroidism and hyperthyroidism.*
4. *Discuss thyroid nodule evaluation and treatment options.*
5. *Discuss the implications of thyroid dysfunction for reproduction in women.*
6. *Discuss the possible links between thyroid malfunction and other chronic illnesses.*

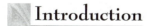

Introduction

The thyroid—a small, butterfly-shaped organ located in the front of the neck—is the primary organ responsible for controlling the metabolic rate of the entire body. The thyroid gland is formed by two triangular pieces of tissue called the lateral lobes, which are located just below the larynx (the voicebox) on either side of the trachea (the windpipe) and are joined together by a small, elongated piece of tissue called the isthmus. The organ is estimated to weigh between 10 and 20 grams (Andreoli, Bennett, Carpenter, & Plum, 1997). It is responsible for secreting two primary hormones—**T3**, or **triiodothyronin**, and **T4**, or **thyroxine.** These hormones regulate the body's use of energy, support growth, and help regulate body temperature. The thyroid gland is controlled by the anterior pituitary gland, which is nestled deep inside the brain. The pituitary gland produces **thyroid stimulating hormone (TSH),** which in turn stimulates the thyroid gland to produce 100 percent of the circulating T4 and about 20 percent of the circulating T3. The rest of the circulating T3 is made through the conversion of T4 by removing iodine (deiodination) and occurs primarily in the liver and the kidneys (Thyroid Physiology, 1999a, http). A hormonal feedback system involving the hypothalamus determines the amount of TSH produced by the anterior pituitary. This entire controlling mechanism is known as the **hypothalamic-pituitary-thyroid axis.**

Three important plasma proteins—thyroxine-binding globulin (TBG), transthyretine (thyroxine-binding prealbumin), and albumin—mediate thyroid functioning by binding

TABLE 21–1 Effects of thyroid hormone levels on the body.

Body Function	Increased T3 or T4	Decreased T3 or T4
Basal metabolic rate	Increased	Decreased
Heart rate	Increased	Decreased
Blood pressure	Increased	Decreased
Pulse rate	Increased	Decreased
Respiratory rate	Increased	Decreased
Digestion	Increased (diarrhea)	Decreased (constipation)
Hair	Soft, fine	Dry, dull, brittle
Skin	Moist, pink	Dry, sallow
Muscles	Fine tremors, inflammation	Weak
Thought processes	Rapid	Slowed
Memory	Good	Impaired
Emotional expression	Exaggerated	Dulled
Deep tendon reflexes	Hyperactive	Hypoactive
Hearing and vision	Acute	Dulled
Fertility	Normal	Impaired

with some T3 and T4 molecules after they are released into the circulation, thus rendering them inactive. Only the unbound, or free, thyroid hormones actually bind to the thyroid receptor sites in the tissues and effect metabolism and system functioning.

In this chapter, the markers of thyroid health will be identified and strategies for promoting thyroid health will be presented. The patterns of thyroid malfunction common in women will be described and discussed in terms of pathophysiology, signs and symptoms, diagnosis, and treatment. The consequences of thyroid malfunctioning concomitant with other conditions common in women will also be addressed, as will the controversial thyroid condition known as Wilson's syndrome.

Markers of Thyroid Wellness

The thyroid hormones have an effect on virtually all of the body systems. When the thyroid gland is functioning properly, the body as a whole runs smoothly. The thyroid gland effects significantly the basal metabolic rate, the cardiovascular and respiratory systems, digestion, the skin, musculoskeletal function, the central nervous system, and reproduction and fertility. When an individual's thyroid gland is functioning normally (assuming her diet and caloric intake are optimal, and there is no pathology elsewhere in the body) her skin will be smooth, will be reasonably moist, and will appear to be normal in color, not sallow. Her hair will be reasonably shiny and healthy, and her nails will not be unusually brittle. Her digestive system will function well, and there will be no constipation or diarrhea. Her muscle strength will be normal in terms of her age and

level of conditioning, and she will not suffer from muscle cramping. Her energy level will not seem unusual; she will appear neither lethargic nor excessively stimulated. Her perception of her body temperature will not seem unusual, in that she will not chronically complain of being either too hot or too cold when others in the same area appear to be comfortable. Her body weight will be normal for her height and build; she will not appear to be overweight. Her cognition will not appear to have changed for the worse; there will be no unusual forgetfulness or "fuzzy" thinking. There will be no decline in mood and no outright depression. Her reproductive system will function normally, and her fertility will not be impaired. Table 21–1 summarizes the effects of thyroid hormone levels on body functions and characteristics.

Promoting Thyroid Wellness

An adequate intake of **iodine** is essential for the synthesis of thyroid hormone. The recommended daily requirement of iodine is 150 micrograms per day (Price & Wilson, 1997). In the United States, foods are enriched with iodine in order to minimize the likelihood of deficiency. Some have deemed the North American diet perfect for optimal thyroid gland functioning (Etiology of Hypothyroidism, 1999b, http).

As is the case with many substances, however, excessive amounts of iodine in the diet can be harmful. Therefore, persons with known thyroid disease must use caution when ingesting nutritional supplements, especially those containing seaweed and kelp, as these are known to contain large amounts of iodine (Nutrition and Prevention for Graves Disease, 2000d, http).

Avoiding or breaking the smoking habit is another way to promote optimal thyroid functioning. Smoking as a hazard to many body systems has been well documented, and the thyroid can be included in the list of body organs and systems negatively affected by cigarette smoking. In research studies done on twins, both the smoking habit and the amount of tobacco consumed were found to be associated with thyroid disease. Smoking was most strongly associated with autoimmune thyroid diseases, such as Graves' disease (Basic Facts about Graves Disease, 2000a, http).

For some women, screening tests for thyroid dysfunction are indicated as a strategy for promoting thyroid wellness. Because hypothyroidism has been linked with coronary heart disease, all women over the age of 50 should have a thyroid function test annually (Thyroid Hormone Resistance, 1999c, http).

Thyroid Illnesses and Problems

Thyroid dysfunction is common in women and usually falls into one of three categories: **hypothyroidism,** or underfunctioning of the gland; **hyperthyroidism,** or overfunctioning of the gland; and the presence of **thyroid nodules,** which are abnormal growths within the thyroid gland itself.

Hypothyroidism

The most common of all malfunctions of the thyroid gland is hypothyroidism, a condition in which insufficient amounts of thyroid hormones are produced. The etiologies of this problem are varied, but the symptoms, consequences, and treatments are similar, regardless of the cause. The risk factors associated with hypothyroidism are listed in Box 21–1.

Hashimoto's thyroiditis is recognized as the most common cause of hypothyroidism in the United States and is categorized as a chronic autoimmune disorder in which the thyroid is gradually destroyed. It is associated with abnormalities in the T- and B-cells in the lymphatic system and the presence of microsomal thyroglobulin antibodies in the blood. Hashimoto's thyroiditis is an inherited condition and has been linked to other autoimmune diseases, such as rheumatoid arthritis. The incidence varies from 0.3 to 5 cases per 1,000 individuals, and the disease is twice as common in women than men (Etiology of Hypothyroidism, 1999b, http). Hypothyroidism is most common in midlife; it has been estimated that up to 24 perent of women develop the disease by the time they reach age 65 (*Hypothyroidism,* 2000). The precise circumstances that cause Hashimoto's thyroiditis to manifest remain a mystery.

Box 21–1   *Risk Factors Associated with Hypothyroidism*

- Age > 60
- Female sex
- Use of certain medications
- Family history of thyroid disease
- Personal history of previously resolved thyroid disease
- Goiter
- History of thyroid nodules
- History of radiation treatments to the head and neck
- Previous diagnosis of a nonthyroid autoimmune disease

SYMPTOMS

Hypothyroidism slows metabolism and has a dampening effect on many processes in the body. Depending on the severity of the problem, individuals whose thyroid glands are underfunctioning may have either obvious symptoms or symptoms that are more subtle. Persons with obvious disease often present with an enlarged, firm thyroid gland (see Figure 21–1), also known as a goiter; a slow pulse and high blood pressure; dull, fragile hair; thick, brittle nails; dry, scaly, yellowish skin; and nonpitting edema of the face, hands, and lower legs. They also complain of constipation, weight gain, cold intolerance, cramping in the extremities, changes in menstruation, difficulty concentrating, and depression. Persons with more subtle symptoms may have a thyroid gland that is only slightly enlarged; such people complain of a tendency to put on weight easily and to retain fluid, tiredness, and a poor memory (O'Sullivan, 1998).

DIAGNOSIS

The diagnosis of hypothyroidism is based on laboratory tests that reveal a normal or elevated TSH, decreased serum T3 and T4 levels, elevated titers of thyroglobulin and thyroid peroxidase antibodies, and irregular patterns of radioactive nucleotide uptake on scanning. If thyroid cancer is suspected, an ultrasound of the thyroid may be performed. Hashimoto's thyroiditis is a progressive disease, and, if TSH levels are normal initially, the levels should be monitored at least annually to detect elevations.

TREATMENT

The treatment of hypothyroidism consists of careful monitoring of the gland's size and supplementation with thyroid hormone to normalize TSH levels. Less than 5 percent of patients are likely to have a spontaneous recovery from chronic autoimmune hypothyroidism. Because the range of normal TSH values is so wide, and because hypothyroidism

Figure 21–1   Enlarged Thyroid

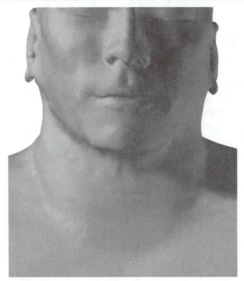

Normal anterior view of neck

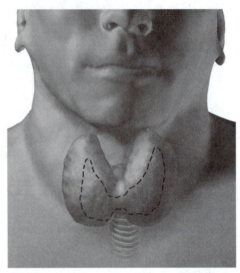

View of neck with goiter, normal thyroid size is indicated by dashed line

Source: *Human Diseases: A Systematic Approach,* 5e by Mulvihill/Zelman/Holdaway/Tompary/Turchany, Copyright 2001. Reprinted by permission of Pearson Education, Inc. Upper Saddle River, NJ.

is now seen as a risk factor for cardiovascular disease, treating mildly symptomatic women with high-normal TSH levels is now being advocated by some physicians (Hypothyroidism, 2000), who feel that there may be considerable interpersonal variation in what constitutes normal TSH levels. Hypothyroidism can also develop after certain viral infections, childbirth, surgery, or radiation therapy. It is especially common after radi-

ation for Hodgkins and non-Hodgkins lymphoma. There are also a number of drugs that can cause hypothyroidism. Those most likely to damage the thyroid gland are lithium, used in the management of psychiatric disorders, and amiodarone, used in the treatment of life-threatening cardiac rhythm disorders. Iodine-containing dyes used in radiological testing can also adversely affect the thyroid gland. Other drugs that can injure the thyroid gland include dopamine, phenytoin (Dilantin), rifampin, steroids, and the cytokines (Clinical Management of Hypothyroidism, 1999a, http).

During the treatment of hypothyroidism with supplemental thyroid, hormone levels are usually checked every 6 weeks until they stabilize, because it usually takes that long for levels to stabilize at a given dosage. After stabilization occurs, routine testing is done every 6 to 12 months. The onset of thyroid-related symptoms necessitate a return to more frequent testing.

Certain foods and dietary supplements are known to interfere with the absorption of thyroid hormones and with thyroid functioning itself. Women who are taking thyroid hormones must take care not to take calcium or iron supplements at the same time, because both of these substances can interfere with the absorption of thyroid hormone. Fiber-rich foods can do the same thing, and it is recommended that thyroid medication be taken one hour before, or two hours after, eating. Finally, soy protein can both depress thyroid function and interfere with the absorption of levothyroxine. Women with a family history of hypothyroidism, or who are on thyroid medication, may wish to limit their consumption of soy products (Hypothyroidism, 2000).

Hyperthyroidism

The overproduction of thyroid hormone, or hyperthyroidism, is less common than hypothyroidism but still remains one of the most commonly diagnosed thyroid disorders. Hyperthyroidism is said to be present when the levels of T3 and/or T4 in the bloodstream are elevated. Hyperthyroidism can be caused by an intrinsic medical condition or by oversupplementation with thyroid hormone. So-called diet doctors often use thyroid hormone to facilitate weight loss, resulting in potentially life-threatening complications and long-term side effects.

Intrinsic hyperthyroidism is called Graves' disease. Like Hashimoto's thyroiditis, **Graves' Disease** is a chronic autoimmune disorder. Graves' disease is five times more common in women than in men (O'Sullivan, 1998). In Graves' disease, the thyroid is attacked by antibodies called thyroid stimulation immunoglobulins (TSI). These immunoglobulins trick the thyroid gland into believing it is receiving a strong message from the pituitary gland, and it works harder to produce and release more T3 and T4. The extra thyroid hormone in the blood accelerates the metabolic rate of every body system and causes the symptoms enumerated in Box 21–2 (Basic Facts about Graves' Disease, 2000a, http).

SYMPTOMS

Some symptoms of hyperthyroidism are the exact *opposites* of those associated with hypothyroidism. These include weight loss in spite of increased appetite, a rapid heart rate, heat intolerance, insomnia, irritability, and agitation. Paradoxically, hyperthyroidism can also cause some of the *same* symptoms as hypothyroidism—namely, goiter, thinning of the hair, hypertension, fatigue, and difficulty concentrating. A goiter results when TSI stimulation of the thyroid causes it to enlarge, as well as to produce excessive amounts of hormone. Other symptoms of hyperthyroidism include hyperresponsive deep tendon reflexes, fine muscle tremors, diarrhea, and sweating. Persons suffering from Graves' disease that is not treated early also develop **exophthalmia,** or bulging eyes, caused by an increase in fatty tissue and muscle in the orbits. Hyperthyroidism is diagnosed on the basis of the same blood tests used to diagnose hypothyroidism.

TREATMENT

The treatment of Graves' disease is aimed at controlling the excessive production of thyroid hormone. This is done by administering **antithyroid drugs** or by **surgery.** The most commonly used antithyroid medication is propylthiouracil, which blocks the synthesis of thyroid hormones by interfering with thyroid peroxidase and blocking the conversion of some of the T4 to T3. An alternative is using If I-131, which is radioactive iodine, to shrink the thyroid. Patients who choose this therapy can expect to see a return to normal thyroid functioning within six weeks to three months. The final treatment option is the surgical removal of all or part of the thyroid gland. Patients who choose surgery are treated with antithyroid drugs preoperatively to reduce the size of the gland.

The choice of treatment for hyperthyroidism depends on many factors, including the size of the gland, the patient's reproductive status, cost, the ease of treatment, and the expected side effects. Regardless of the treatment chosen, long-term monitoring of thyroid function is required.

Another, less common cause of hyperthyroidism is the uncontrolled leakage of stored thyroid hormone from the thyroid gland into the bloodstream due to structural damage to the gland. This is usually a temporary and self-limiting condition that requires careful monitoring and occasionally the use of medication to control the symptoms. The absence of the symptoms necessary for the diagnosis of Graves' disease favors the diagnosis of hormone leakage (All about Hyperthyroidism, 2000, http).

Regardless of its underlying cause, hyperthyroidism can worsen suddenly and cause life-threatening cardiovascular symptoms. This uncommon occurrence is known as **thyroid storm.** This dangerous outpouring of thyroid hormone can be precipitated by surgery, radioactive iodine therapy, or severe physiological stress. Patients develop flushing, rapid heartbeat, a dysrhythmia known as atrial fibrillation, and cardiac failure. The classic diagnostic symptom is a fever out of proportion with the rest of the symptoms. The treatment is symptomatic and aimed at preserving life until circulating thyroid hormone levels can be reduced.

Thyroid Nodules

As is the case with other thyroid disorders, thyroid nodules are more common in women than men. Thyroid nodules are cystic or solid lumps that usually develop in the lateral lobes of the thyroid gland. They can be benign, or they can be malignant (McCaffrey, 2000). It is estimated that about 10 percent of the population have thyroid nodules that can be palpated on physical examination of the neck. Researchers also estimate that an additional 30 percent of the population have one or more nonpalpable nodules in the thyroid gland. Most thyroid nodules in adults are benign; those that are malignant can be treated successfully with surgery, radiation, and chemotherapy (Living with Thyroid Nodules and Goiter, 2000e, http).

It is important to determine the nature of the nodules that appear on the thyroid gland, because some forms can lead to an increase in thyroid hormone production, and some can be malignant. The first step in diagnosing the nature of a nodule is performing an ultrasound to determine its exact location and consistency, so that a sample of the tissue can be removed by FNA (fine needle aspiration) and examined by a pathologist. Occasionally, the FNA will produce a specimen that cannot be adequately examined, and a traditional surgical biopsy is recommended (Oertal, 1996). The treatment of benign thyroid nodules is based on the symptoms and blood tests and often consists of monitoring the thyroid hormone levels and examining the gland every six months. Thyroid cancers are rare (Like Gore, 4 out of 10 People Develop Thyroid Nodules, 2000b, http).

Wilson's Syndrome

Wilson's syndrome, a controversial form of hypothyroidism, is named after E. Denis Wilson, MD, who identified the syndrome in the early 1990s. According to Dr. Wilson, the syndrome bearing his name is characterized by the inability of the body to convert T4 into the more active T3. In Wilson's syndrome, traditional thyroid monitoring tests often yield normal results, and taking thyroid hormone (T4) does not alter the symptoms (Cathcart, 1995). Dr. Wilson's publication *Wilson's Syndrome: The Miracle of Feeling Well* lists more than 40 symptoms that, when combined with a consistently low basal body temperature, contribute to the diagnosis of Wilson's syndrome. Many of these symptoms are the same as those associated with other forms of hypothyroidism. The symptoms unique to Wilson's syndrome include decreased wound healing, decreased sex drive, food cravings, tinnitus, hypoglycemia, and headaches. Dr. Wilson also associates Wilson's syndrome with irritable bowel syndrome, psoriasis, and halitosis. The treatment of Wilson's syndrome involves supplementing the individual with T3 instead of the more commonly used T4.

The American Thyroid Association (ATA) adamantly opposes Dr. Wilson's research and has published a position statement regarding his theories. According to the ATA, Dr. Wilson's research data are flawed, and the symptoms he lists are imprecise. The ATA also maintains that scientific research does not uphold the superiority of T3 over T4 as a thyroid supplement and that supplementation with T3 can be dangerous to the cardiovascular system (American Thyroid Association, 2000). However, improper supplementation with T4 has also been shown to produce adverse cardiovascular effects.

Thyroid Disease and Female Reproduction

Thyroid disease has implications during pregnancy and may affect fertility as well. It has been theorized that malfunctioning of the thyroid may be the underlying problem that causes some women to be unable to conceive a pregnancy or carry one to term (Autoimmune Thyroid Disease and Miscarriage, 2000b). However, although research has established that autoimmune disorders do play a part in infertility and many of the common thyroid disorders involve autoimmunity, no definitive relationship between autoimmune thyroid disease and infertility or miscarriage has been established.

Although the effect of thyroid disorders on fertility is still unclear, two distinct thyroid disorders that can arise during pregnancy have been identified. One is transient hyperthyroidism of hyperemesis gravidarium, and the other is postpartum thyroiditis.

Transient hyperthyroidism of hyperemesis gravidarium involves an increased production of thyroid hormones in early pregnancy. It is thought to be a trigger for hyperemesis gravidarium, which is severe, protracted nausea and vomiting during pregnancy. The disorder usually resolves by the eighteenth week of pregnancy, and it is not treated unless hyperemesis develops (Transient Hyperthyroidism of Hyperemesis Gravidarium, 2000b, http).

Postpartum thyroiditis (PPT), or inflammation of the thyroid subsequent to delivery, is an autoimmune disorder that affects between 1.1 and 16.7 percent of women worldwide. In the United States, it is estimated to affect between 6 and 8 percent of postpartum women (What Is the Prevalence of Post Partum Thyroiditis?, 2000c, http). About one-fifth of the women diagnosed with PPT will develop permanent hypothyroidism within five years after delivery. PPT sometimes goes unrecognized, because its symptoms—fatigue, depression, and anxiety—mimic those commonly associated with the normal postpartum period. New mothers are often tired, worried, and somewhat depressed, and women who complain of these symptoms are rarely screened

for thyroid disorders. The treatment is based on the presenting symptoms and the results of laboratory testing.

Controversy exists as to whether thyroid disease screening should be offered routinely to women after childbirth. The advocates favor screening all women, especially those at high risk for thyroid malfunction. The opponents of mass screening question its cost-effectiveness.

Thyroid Wellness Self-Assessment

Ask yourself the following questions and consider your answers in light of the information in this chapter.

1. *Am I having more difficulty controlling my weight than I used to?*
2. *Has my hair become somewhat dull and dry, my nails brittle, and my skin drier and more sallow?*
3. *Do I seem to be frequently too hot or too cold, regardless of how others around me are experiencing the temperature?*
4. *Do I suffer from excessive fatigue, feel somewhat depressed, and feel that I am not always thinking clearly?*
5. *Do I suffer from leg or foot cramps?*
6. *Have I been losing weight without dieting, feeling jittery, and having difficulty sleeping?*
7. *Have I noticed a visible thickening of my neck and/or difficulty swallowing?*
8. *Am I having difficulty recovering from a recent severe viral infection?*
9. *Do I have a family history of thyroid disease?*
10. *Am I suffering from postpartum fatigue, depression, or other symptoms?*
11. *Have I noticed a recent change in my elimination pattern?*
12. *If I am age 30 or older, and answered yes to any of the previous questions, have I had a screening test for thyroid dysfunction?*

New Directions

Most current thyroid-related studies are focusing on ways in which thyroid functioning affects various health problems. Recent studies on the relationship between hypothyroidism and homocysteine levels suggest that patients with low levels of circulating thyroid hormone have elevated levels of homocysteine and that normalizing thyroid hormone levels decreases homocysteine (Thyroid Deficiency and Heart Disease, 1999e, http). Because homocysteine level is currently seen as a marker for coronary heart disease, hypothyroidism is considered to be a risk factor for coronary heart disease as well (Thyroid Deficiency and Heart Disease, 1999e, http).

Additional research has shown a link among hypothyroidism, aortic atherosclerosis (plaque in the aorta, a large artery), and myocardial infarction, especially in postmenopausal women. Although the mechanism by which hypothyroidism fosters atherosclerosis is not fully understood, it is believed to be related to serum thyroid antibodies and thyroid peroxidase (Thyroid Deficiency and Heart Disease, 1999e, http). More research is needed to clarify exact relationships in both heart disease and vascular disease.

Another exciting area of thyroid research concerns sleep disorders. Although it is widely accepted that patients with symptomatic hypothyroidism have a high incidence of sleep apnea, studies to date have had too few participants to demonstrate clinical links between thyroid disease and sleep disturbances to justify definitive recommendations (Thyroid Testing and Thyroid Hormone Replacement in Patients with Sleep-Disordered Breathing, 1999f, http). Research into the relationship between thyroid dysfunction and sleep disorders is ongoing.

QUESTIONS FOR REFLECTION AND DISCUSSION

1. *You notice that a friend has started sleeping more, her skin and hair seem dry and brittle, and she complains of constipation. Would you intervene in this situation, and, if so, how?*
2. *Your overweight friend has started regular visits with a local diet doctor. She is losing weight rapidly and has "more energy than ever before." You realize that one of the medications she has been started on is T4. How would you approach her with your concerns?*
3. *How would you advise a friend anticipating a pregnancy who confides to you that she has a history of hypothyroidism?*
4. *If someone you knew were diagnosed with a thyroid nodule, how would you support and educate her?*
5. *Do you think routine screening for thyroid dysfunction should be offered to women? If yes, which women and why?*

RESOURCES

Books

Wood, L., Cooper, D. S., & Ridgway, E. C. (1995). *Your thyroid: A home reference.* Ballentine.

Organizations

The American Thyroid Association
Townhouse Office Park
55 Old Nyack Turnpike, Suite 611
Nanuet, NY 10954
Web: http://www.thyroid.org/

Thyroid Foundation of America
Ruth Sleeper Hall
40 Parkman St.
Boston, MA 02114-2698
Phone: 1-800-832-8321
Web: http://clark.net/pub/tfa/

The Thyroid Society
7515 South Main St., Suite 545
Houston, TX 77030
Phone: 1-800-THYROID
Web: http://www.the-thyroid-society.org/thyroid.html

REFERENCES

American Thyroid Association. (2000). *Statement on Wilson's syndrome* [On-line]. Available: http://www.thyroid.org/annone/wilson.htm

Andreoli, T., Bennett, J., Carpenter, C., & Plum, F. (1997). *Cecil essentials of medicine* (4th ed.). Philadelphia: W. B. Saunders.

Cathcart, R. F. (1995). *Symptoms of Wilson's syndrome* [On-line]. Available: http://www.mall-net.com/cathcart/wilsons.html

Dr.Koop.com. (2000, December 21). *All about hyperthyroidism* [On-line]. Available: http://www.drkoop.com/conditions/hyperthyroidism/library/hyperthyroidism_all_about.html

Dr.Koop.com. (2000a, December 21). *Basic facts about Graves disease* [On-line]. Available: http://www.drkoop.com/conditions/graves_disease/library/graves_disease_basics.html

Dr.Koop.com. (2000b, December 17). *Like Gore 4 out of 10 people develop thyroid nodules* [On-line]. Available: http://www.drkoop.com/news/dartmouth/december/tipper_surgery.html

Dr.Koop.com. (2000c, December 17). *Living with thyroid nodules and goiter* [On-line]. Available: http://www.drkoop.com/news/dartmouth/december/thryoid_nodules.html

Dr.Koop.com. (2000d, December 17). *Nutrition and prevention for Graves disease* [On-line]. Available: http://www.drkoop.com/conditions/graves_disease/library/graves_disease_nutrition.html

Hypothyroidism. (2000). *Women's Health Advisor, 4*(11), 3, 7.

McCaffrey, T. V. (2000). *Ten best readings on thyroid cancer* [On-line]. Available: http://www.medscape.com/moffitt/CancerControl/2000/v07.n03/cc0703.../cc0703.06.mcca.htm

Medscape. (1999a). *Diabetes & endocrinology clinical management volume 2—Clinical management of hypothyroidism* [On-line]. Available: http://www.medscape/endocrinology/ClinicalMgmt/CM.v02/CM.v02-06.html

Medscape. (1999b). *Diabetes & endocrinology clinical management volume 2—Etiology of hypothyroidism* [On-line]. Available: http://www.medscape/endocrinology/ClinicalMgmt/CM.v02/CM.v02-09.html

Medscape. (1999c). *Diabetes & endocrinology clinical management volume 2—Thyroid hormone resistance* [On-line]. Available: http://www.medscape/endocrinology/ClinicalMgmt/CM.v02/CM.v02-11.html

Medscape. (1999d). *Diabetes & endocrinology clinical management volume 2—Thyroid physiology* [On-line]. Available:

http://www.medscape/endocrinology/ClinicalMgmt/CM.v02/CM.v02-11.html

Medscape. (1999e). *Thyroid deficiency and heart disease* [On-line]. Available: http://www.medscape.com/MJP/NDA/1999/v23.n12/nda2312.o5.html

Medscape. (1999f). *Thyroid testing and thyroid hormone replacement in patients with sleep-disordered breathing* [On-line]. Available: http://www.medscape.com/medquest/ENT/1999/v78.n10/ent7810.0.../ent7810.02.mick-01.htm

Medscape. (2000b). *Diabetes & endocrinology—Autoimmune thyroid disease and miscarriage* [On-line]. Available: http://www.medscape/endocrinology/journal/2000/v02.n02/c.../ca-mde0203.htm

Medscape. (2000b). *Transient hyperthyroidism of hyperemesis gravidarium: A sheep in wolf's clothing* [On-line]. Available: http://www.medscape.com/ABFP/JABFP/2000/v13.n01/fpl301.05.caff/fpl1301.05.caff-01.html

Medscape. (2000c). *What is the prevalence of postpartum thyroiditis?* [On-line]. Available: http://www.medscape.com/medscape/features/question/2000/02.2000/q749.html

Oertal, Y. C. (1996). Fine-needle aspiration and the diagnosis of thyroid cancer. *Endocrinology Metabolic Clinics of North America, 25,* 69–91.

O'Sullivan, S. (1998). Nursing management of adults with thyroid or parathyroid disorders. In P. Beare & J. Meyers (Eds.), *Adult health nursing,* (pp. 1382–1405). St. Louis: Mosby.

Price, S. A., & Wilson, L. M. (1997). Pathophysiology: Clinical concepts of disease processes (5th ed.). St. Louis: Mosby-Year Book.

Wilson, E. D. (1996). *Wilson's syndrome: The miracle of feeling well.* Orlando, FL: Cornerstone.

22

Sexual Wellness and Illness

Elva J. S. Winter

Objectives

1. *Discuss how women's sexuality relates to culture, physical and emotional health, and rest and relaxation.*
2. *Identify at least five ways to overcome sexual shame and inhibition.*
3. *Describe women's sexual response cycle and the changes associated with aging.*
4. *Discuss women's sexual dysfunctions in terms of their causes and treatments.*
5. *Discuss the incidence, symptoms, and treatments of sexually transmitted diseases.*

Introduction

There is no universally accepted definition of human sexuality or, in particular, women's sexuality. Different cultures ascribe different meanings to sexual behaviors and practices. For example, practices such as polygamy (men having more than one woman as wife at the same time), gender cross-dressing, homosexuality, marriage between family members, and penis piercing are acceptable and even valued in some societies but not in others. Historically, rules about sexual behaviors have been embedded in and upheld by cultural units, such as families, schools, religion, and the media. Within the cultural units of a society, an individual member of that society learns its rules about sexual behavior—that is, what is considered right and what is considered wrong (Suggs & Miracle, 1993).

Current academic and scientific thought considers human sexuality to be a biopsychosocial phenomenon composed of dimensions of gender and history (see Box 22–1). Of those dimensions, gender roles, in particular, profoundly influence the expression of women's sexuality. For example, in April 1999, the Supreme Court of Zimbabwe made a unanimous decision that "adult females are inherently inferior to males and have a status akin to that of teenager," citing the "nature of African society" as its basis (Laumann, Paik, & Rosen, 1999). Thus, how women in Zimbabwe express their sexuality is different from how women in more enlightened countries express their sexuality because of the roles that women are expected to assume.

An individual's sexuality is influenced by biology, personal characteristics, and culture. A woman's thoughts, self-image, values, emotions, and spirituality, as well as her erotic feelings, partners, environment, choices, and actions, all affect her sexuality. Additionally, many women have negative sexual experiences, which later inhibit their full expression of their sexuality.

A particular woman's sexual health should be viewed within her personal, her historical, and her cultural contexts. For example, sexual wellness for women in more primitive parts of the world primarily has to do with freedom from genital diseases and healthful childbirth conditions. In more advanced societies, a woman's self-awareness and actualization of her sexual potential, freedom from genital diseases, and healthful childbirth conditions are central tenets of sexual wellness.

Markers of Sexual Wellness

The one and only marker of sexual wellness is a sexual response that is satifactory to the woman in question. Sexual wellness is entirely subjective, and cannot be determined on the basis of external criteria.

Box 22–1 Components of Human Sexuality: The Biopsychosocial Dimensions of Gender Plus History

- *Sex*—Having female or male anatomy and physiology
- *Gender identity*—Sense of oneself as being female or male
- *Gender roles*—How one behaves to demonstrate that one is female or male
- *Gender orientation*—One's attraction, erotically, to one's own gender or to the other gender (homosexuality or heterosexuality)
- *Historicity*—One's present placement in time in a society, plus the influences of one's cultural heritage

---

Sexual Response that is Satisfactory to the Woman

Factors related to sexual response include the erogenous zones, the sexual response cycle, the pubocoxygeous muscle, variability in arousal and orgasmic response, and frequency and kinds of sexual expression. Aging also affects the nature of sexual response.

THE EROGENOUS ZONES

Erogenous zones are the areas of the body especially sensitive to touch because they are richly endowed with nerve receptors. Touching those areas stimulates a person erotically—that is, it brings about sexual arousal.

The erogenous zones include the mouth, lips, tongue, ears, breasts, nipples, neck, armpits, fingers, palms of hands, abdomen, navel, inner thighs, anus, soles of feet, and toes (Allgeier & Allgeier, 1991; Rathus, Nevid, & Fichner-Rathus, 1993). Theoretically, however, all of the skin is an erogenous zone because all of the skin is innervated. As Montagu (1986) notes, "in no other relationship is the skin so totally involved as in sexual intercourse. . . . Touch is the true language of sex" (p. 204). Spinal cord–injured people whose genital sensation has been destroyed have shown that body areas not usually considered to be erogenous can become eroticized. In fact, through touch of those areas, and fantasy, those so injured can even experience orgasm, thus demonstrating that genital stimulation is not always necessary for orgasm.

SEXUAL RESPONSE CYCLE

Masters and Johnson (1966) identified a four-stage sexual response cycle of **excitement, plateau, orgasm,** and **resolution.** Kaplan (1977) suggested that a stage of **desire** to initiate or to be responsive to sexual stimulation precedes the stage of excitement. **Reed's erotic stimulus pathway (ESP) model of sexual response,** described by Stayton (1992), includes the sexual response cycle stages identified by Masters and Johnson and by Kaplan. Women can easily identify with the ESP model because of its holism. Its stages, as applied to women, are discussed in the following sections.

ESP Phase 1: Seduction   A woman seduces herself into being interested sexually in another person, and vice versa. There is concurrent self-generated *desire* for sexual activity as she responds to real or fantasized sensory stimuli.

ESP Phase 2: Sensation   The woman is absorbed in sensations of seeing, hearing, smelling, tasting, and touching, and, as she continues cognitively to label the sensory stimulations as erotic and exciting, she becomes aroused or excited. During *excitement,* vasocongestion engorges the pelvis, the labia majora, the labia minora, the vagina, and the clitoris, causing the clitoris to enlarge and become erect, darkening the color of the labia minora, and initiating vaginal lubrication with clear fluid oozing from the vaginal walls. The upper two-thirds of the vagina lengthens and expands. Nipple erection occurs and the breasts increase in size. Skin flush on the face, neck, and chest can occur. The woman experiences increases in heart rate, respiration, blood pressure, and muscle tension.

The highest level of arousal in the Sensation Phase is plateau. At *plateau,* the uterus and upper two-thirds of the vagina rise within the pelvic cavity. The lower one-third of the vagina has narrowed because of the swelling of the tissues around it. The narrowed lower vagina is known as the **orgasmic platform.** The clitoris is more sensitive and retracts behind the clitoral hood, a fold of skin, for protection. Heavier, faster breathing, and faster heart rate, and higher blood pressure occur. Generalized muscle contractions can occur, and the skin flush may spread to the abdomen, thighs, and back.

ESP Phase 3: Surrender   The woman surrenders to the experience of heightened sensation. Respiratory rate, heart rate, blood pressure, and sex flush peak. Generalized body muscle contractions can occur. *Orgasm occurs for many, but not all, women.* Female orgasm was described by Kolodny, Masters, and Johnson (1979) as "simultaneous rhythmic contractions of the uterus, the orgasmic platform, and the rectal sphincter, beginning at 0.8 second intervals and then diminishing in intensity, duration and regularity" (p. 15). Researchers (Singer, 1973) have speculated about the presence of different kinds of orgasm—vulval, uterine, blended, and ejaculatory orgasms (which are addressed in the section on the G-spot and female ejaculation). Previously, however, Masters and Johnson (1966) had noted that a woman's physiological response is the same, whether the source of stimulation is clitoral or vagi-

nal. Whether or not a woman experiences orgasm in the Surrender Phase, her experience of heightened sensation is generally pleasurable.

ESP Phase 4: Reflection   A woman cognitively and subjectively reflects on what she has experienced. Physiologically, a *resolution* of tissues and structures to the pre-arousal condition occurs. Vasocongestion gradually diminishes, causing genital tissues and structures to resume their pre-aroused color, size, and placement. Breasts and nipples return to their pre-aroused state. Breathing, heart rate, and blood pressure return to normal. Sex flush disappears, and the muscles relax. Sweating occurs in some women (Allgeier & Allgeier, 1991; McCammon, Knox, & Schnacht, 1993).

THE G SPOT AND FEMALE EJACULATION

The Grafenberg spot, or **G spot,** so-named by Perry and Whipple (1981) to honor Ernest Grafenberg, the gynecologist who first reported it in 1950, is a felt, but not seen, area of sensitivity on the front wall of the vagina about one to two inches inside the vaginal opening. Perry and Whipple (1981) suggest that the G spot swells when rubbed and can be stimulated to orgasmic response, resulting in ejaculation of fluid for some women. That a G spot exists has been both refuted (Alzate & Lodono, 1984; Masters, Johnson, & Kolodny, 1989) and supported (Darling, Davidson, & Conway-Welch, 1990; Ladas, Whipple, & Perry, 1982). In general, some women are aware of having a G spot area of sensitivity, and some are not.

Three types of ejaculation can occur for some women at orgasm, in addition to what may be ejaculation from prostate-type tissue located around the G spot (Heinman & LoPiccolo, 1988). Those three types of ejaculation are (1) fluid from the glands around the urethra, which fill with fluid during sexual arousal; (2) vaginal lubricating fluid expelled by women who produce a large amount of fluid; and (3) residual urine expelled from the urethra during muscular orgasmic contractions. Some women who experience ejaculation are more aware of the ejaculation than are others; however, most are not aware of the source of the ejaculate.

PUBOCOCCYGEUS MUSCLE

The **pubococcygeus (PC) muscle** is one of the pelvic floor muscles that surround the vagina, anus, and urethra. Pelvic floor muscles contract involuntarily during orgasm. Kegel (1952) developed a set of exercises for women to strengthen the PC muscle after childbirth and believed that sexual pleasure can be enhanced by strengthening the muscle. Although that theory has not been widely substantiated, it is known that having a strong PC muscle can prevent the stress incontinence that many women experience after having borne children. Heinman and LoPiccolo (1988) believe that women develop a sense of control and connection with their genitals when they practice Kegel exercises.

Women can locate their PC muscles in two ways. One way is to insert two fingers into the vagina and then to contract the muscles around the finger. The other way is to stop the flow of urine during midstream by contracting the muscles around the vagina. The technique for performing Kegel exercises is described in Chapter 16.

VARIABILITY IN AROUSAL AND ORGASMIC RESPONSE

Women seem to have their highest number of orgasms between the ages of 20 and 40 years and have more orgasms toward age 40 than age 20 (Reinisch, 1990). Reasons could be that women become more easily orgasmic over a period of time of responding, because of learning, or because with age and experience they feel more secure and less inhibited in sexual relating, or that as they grow older and are with older male partners they may experience longer periods of arousal (Reinisch, 1990).

About 10 percent of all women have never experienced orgasm by any method of stimulation. About 50 to 75 percent of women who do have orgasms do not have them when penile-vaginal thrusting is the only kind of stimulation. About the same percentage require *direct clitoral stimulation* to have orgasm (Reinisch, 1990).

Kinsey, Pomeroy, Martin, and Gebhard (1953), investigating the percentage of marital sexual intercourse that results in orgasm, found that 36 to 44 percent of the women studied had orgasm during some but not all of their marital intercourse. About one-third of those women had orgasm only a small part of the time, one-third of the women about half the time, and one-third of the women a large part of the time but not 100 percent of the time. In that study, 14 percent of the women who experienced multiple orgasms had two or three orgasms in a sexual encounter. Some women, however, found further touching and stimulation irritating after they experienced one orgasm (Reinisch, 1990).

What is necessary to a particular woman's experience of sexual pleasure and orgasm is the right kind of stimulation, in the right places, for the right duration of time for her. For most women, that stimulation almost always involves, but is not limited to, stimulation of the clitoris, because of its large and sensitive nerve supply. Women's ability to be totally absorbed in the moment, and to enjoy sexual imagery and fantasy, also is associated with peak arousal and meaningful sexual experience (Scantling & Browder, 1993).

It seems, then, that most women can be assured that their arousal response is normal even though it may not fit a textbook description of response or mirror the response of another woman. A heterosexual woman should understand that her male partner's arousal response likely is faster than her own and that the male response, too, is normal. When women affirm the individuality and normality of their own

responses, they set the stage for being active rather than reactive sexual participants and thereby increase their sexual health by assuming responsibility for their own sexual actions and pleasure.

Frequency and Kinds of Sexual Expression

"Insistence on one normative pattern of female sexuality . . . is folly" (Stimpson & Person, 1980, p. 3). *Female sexualities* is a more appropriate term, as women's reports about their sexual behaviors corroborate (Reinisch, 1990; Scantling & Browder, 1993; Taylor & Surnall, 1993). Although people are born as sexual organisms, becoming sexual humans is a process undergone by living in relationships and in societies. Consistent with her human growth and values at any point in time, a woman may choose to express her sexuality in numerous nongenital or genital ways. A woman who is celibate is still a sexual person—just one not expressing herself, genitally, with another.

As women free themselves from the social scripting of gender role expectations and learn about who they are as unique women, they begin to act sexually in ways consistent with their self-formulated beliefs and values. Thus, over the course of a lifetime, one woman may experience masturbation, celibacy, homosexuality, and heterosexuality, whereas another woman may experience only heterosexuality, and another, only homosexuality. Within each of those contexts, what those women do genitally or nongenitally to express their sexuality is a measure of their self-awareness, personal growth, and values at various points in time. Their self-assertion and values determine with whom they share themselves sexually, how frequently they do so, and in which activities they engage.

Aging and Sexuality

At about age 50 menopause occurs, and estrogen production decreases in women until about age 60. Masters and Johnson (1966) noted the *physiological effects of decreased estrogen* (see Box 22–2).

The physical changes associated with decreased estrogen do not cause women to become asexual. When women's attitudes are positive, they learn ways to compensate, so as to maintain active sexual expression. For example, hormone replacement therapy, vaginally applied estrogen cream, water-soluble lubricants inserted into the vagina, and the use of saliva during intercourse can alleviate vaginal dryness.

The degree to which older people are sexually active is debatable. Reinisch (1990) noted that one-fourth of older women and men who are alone give up active sexual expression and depend on social friendships for companionship. Seagraves and Seagraves (1995) reviewed the literature and concluded that there is a gradual decline in sexual interest

Box 22–2 *Physiological Effects of Decreased Estrogen at Menopause*

- The vaginal walls thin and become pink, rather than being thick and red.
- The vagina shortens and narrows because elasticity decreases.
- The amount and rate of vaginal lubrication decrease, and painful vaginal intercourse can result. An exception is that some women who remain sexually active one or two times per week do not decrease lubrication.
- The uterus and cervix decrease in size.
- Fibrous tissue replaces some glandular breast tissue.
- Sex flush and nipple erection during sexual arousal decrease.
- Bartholin's gland secretion diminishes.
- Vaginal contractions during intercourse are less intense and occur over a shorter period.
- Uterine cramping may occur during intercourse.
- Women may need to urinate after intercourse.
- More direct tactile stimulation is needed for vaso-congestion and arousal to occur.

Source: Masters, W. H., & Johnson, V. E. (1966). *Human Sexual Response*. Boston: Little Brown and Company.

and activity with age. However, Brecher (Brecher & The Editors of Consumer Reports Books, 1984) and Cross (1993) present older women and men as interested in sexual expression. The view of diminishing yet active sexual interest is confirmed by a 1999 survey by the American Association of Retired Persons (AARP) and *Modern Maturity* magazine of 1,384 persons over the age of 45 years, 788 of them women (Jacoby, 1999).

In the AARP/*Modern Maturity* survey, 91 percent of the women ages 40 to 59 said they would not want to be denied sexual relations, whereas 65 percent of the women over 75 said they would be content without sexual relations. About half of the persons ages 45 to 59 said they have sexual relations at least once a week. Twenty-four percent of the women ages 60 to 74 reported having sexual intercourse at least once a week. Sixty-one percent of the women rated their sexual relationship with a partner as extremely satisfying or very satisfying. The older women with partners saw them as both physically attractive and romantic. About 33 percent of the women under age 60 acknowledged having masturbated in recent months, whereas less than 10 percent of the women age 75 and older did. The survey revealed, also, a diminishing expression of sexuality in women as they age and become partnerless, even to the degree of their not receiving touching (Jacoby, 1999).

Older women must address the changes in their physiological sexual functioning because of age and the changes due to illness or injuries. Alterations in their physical appearance and abilities create questions of finding and being sexually attractive to a partner. However, sexual relating does occur for women despite these obstacles. Rehabilitation therapists and sexual counselors can help women gain knowledge and skills to enhance their sexual functioning.

The medications used to treat illness can affect sexual functioning, For example, some drugs used to treat elevated blood pressure can cause decreased sexual interest, decreased vaginal lubrication, delayed orgasm, or an inability to experience orgasm (McCammon et al., 1993). Some antidepressant drugs can inhibit orgasm, and some anti-anxiety drugs can inhibit sexual interest and orgasm (Montejo, Llorca, Izquierdo, & Rico-Villademoros, 2001; Saks, 2000). Taking some steroids, androgens, or testosterone can increase or decrease sexual desire (Rogers, 1990). Women who take maintenance medications of any kind should discuss the possible sexual side effects with their healthcare providers, so as to increase the likelihood of maintaining their sexual response.

Promoting Sexual Wellness

Women can promote their sexual wellness by becoming knowledgeable about sexuality, providing for privacy and relaxation during sexual experiences, cultivating trust and intimacy in the context of sexual relationships, and overcoming sexual shame and inhibition.

Developing Self-Knowledge

Having an authentic knowledge and understanding of oneself is crucial to sexual wellness. Sexual relationships are built on personal relationships, and knowing oneself can only enhance one's ability to relate to others. Thus, women who are in touch with their *own* values, goals, desires, and preferences are more likely to enter into fulfilling sexual relationships than women who rely on *others* to tell them what they "should" want, believe, and feel. Whereas some women find it relatively easy to know themselves, others have more difficulty. In their landmark book *Women's Ways of Knowing*, Belenky, Clinchy, Goldberger, and Tarule (1986) described the various ways in which the women they had interviewed approached knowledge and knowing. The ways ranged from being silent and having no opinions on subjects, thus accepting the authority and opinions of others, to analyzing and synthesizing their own objective observations and subjective experience, thus creating knowledge on their own. A *silent woman* who accepts external authority is unaware that she can take steps to learn about her sexuality and that she can change how she expresses her sexuality. The woman who *analyzes and synthesizes* from her own observations and experiences expresses her sexuality from an active, rather than a passive, perspective, constantly learns more about herself, and, in a sense, recreates herself. She keeps integrating the physical, emotional, and sexual dimensions of herself and becomes healthier.

Women who have difficulty in thinking for themselves can learn to move *away* from accepting the opinions of others and to move *toward* formulating their own opinions. Doing so is more a developed skill than an inherent talent. Women who increase their ability to think for and know themselves become more competent to address and resolve past and present emotional and relationship issues, thus increasing their potential for satisfying sexual relationships.

As the quality of a given woman's thinking improves over time, with maturation, experience, education, and deliberate effort, the expression of her sexuality will likely change. For example, a woman's *motivation* for engaging in sexual activity might be altered. Women engage in sex for many reasons, which include but are not limited to power, fun, pleasure, exploration, novelty, validation, intimacy, competition, safety, love, and affection. The set of reasons that underlies a woman's pattern of sexual behavior will change over time, as her knowledge and understanding of herself increase. The *nature* of a woman's sexual expression may also change along with her knowledge of herself; she may become more assertive in seeking that which pleases and fulfills her.

The world is perceived through the senses of hearing, seeing, tasting, smelling, and touching. Then, human brains process and organize those perceptions into experiences. Sexual experiences also occur this way. Through the senses, people become receptive to sexual attraction, arousal, and action- or rejection of the same. For example, hearing a particular voice tone, type of music, or certain words can be sexually inviting and arousing, or it can produce tension and intimidation.

Another important aspect of a woman's self-knowledge is awareness of which sensory experiences are and are not erotic for her. People are more likely to respond sexually when they see what *they* consider to be an attractive or erotic face or form than when they view one that they do not find attractive or erotic. Similarly, certain tastes (such as saltiness or sweetness) and smells (such as musk or heavy perfume) can be pleasing or displeasing, enticing or repelling, to a given individual. Individuals also vary in the degree to which they find elements of touch (temperature, pressure, and pain) to be comfortable, pleasurable, or sexually arousing.

The way in which humans organize perceptions into experiences with sexual meaning is, to some degree, learned within one's culture. Thus, a heterosexual American woman is likely to allow the touch of another woman to be experienced as pleasant or comfortable, but not as erotic, because her culture devalues homosexuality. Similarly, an Asian woman will more likely respond sexually to the familiar music of her culture than to Native American

rhythms. Being aware of how one's culture and social history have helped shape one's sexuality is another important part of self-knowledge. Developing sensory/sensual/sexual self-awareness is the central thesis of a number of programs that have been developed to foster women's sexual growth (Barbach, 1975; Heinman & LoPiccolo, 1988).

Providing for Privacy and Relaxation

A woman must have both privacy and relaxation in order to freely explore her sexuality. Privacy is space and time wherein one does not fear interruption. Relaxation is a state in which one is feeling rested and free of social restraint and anxiety. The combination of privacy and relaxation provides the best opportunity for a woman to explore her body, and identify the sensory stimuli she experiences as sexually enjoyable. Privately relaxed and safe, a woman can focus on what she is hearing, seeing, tasting, smelling, and touching, as well as focus on her own responses to those stimuli.

Cultivating Trust and Intimacy in the Context of Sexual Relationships

Not all of the sexual interactions between people are intimate encounters. Intimacy within human relationships, however, is valued by many persons, and many people find intimacy within sexual relating to be important. *Trust* is the foundation of intimacy. Gordon and Snyder (1989) hold that trusting one's partner not to respond with hurt or attack while disclosing one's deepest, most important thoughts and feelings is central to intimacy. In intimate relationships, there is a give and take between the partners that tolerates the various moods and emotions of each, the pleasing and irritating habits, anger, and arguments. According to this view, intimacy thrives through commitment, mutual caring, listening, and attention to the needs of oneself and of one's partner.

Schnarch (1991), on the other hand, believes that the *trust of oneself* is more essential to intimacy than is the trust of one's partner. Schnarch (1991) maintains that, when one discloses deep thoughts and feelings to a partner, the partner's affirmation is less important than is the discloser's ability to tolerate the partner's response. According to Schnarch (1991), intimate relationships provide an opportunity for each partner's continuous self-confrontation, self-knowledge, and self-validation, as well as increased knowledge of the partner. The growth of both partners is possible to the degree that each one personally has developed the ability to disclose vulnerabilities and to engage with another without expecting or requiring an affirming response.

Sexual relationships wherein there is trust of oneself and of one's partner present opportunities for intimate sexual sharing. To many women, intimate sexual sharing is more desirable than superficial, nontrusting sexual exchange, because there is more depth, meaning, and fullness in their relationship with a partner. Some women find that intimate sexual experiences facilitate their spiritual growth, as well (Feuerstein, 1989; Scantling & Browder, 1993; Taylor & Surnall, 1993). Overall, the way in which trust, intimacy, and spirituality interrelate for the individual women is well worth studying as women address their sexuality and sexual health.

Overcoming Sexual Shame and Inhibition

People learn to be sexual, and they acquire attitudes about sexuality within their particular culture, social system, and life events. Some women enter adulthood feeling shame, low self-esteem, and sexual inhibition. These attitudes generally are the result of sociocultural attitudes and life events that devalue and objectify girls and women and their sexuality. Women who have been victimized by incest or rape have been humiliated, and they, especially, are likely to experience subsequent shame and low self-esteem. However, women who have been treated as sex objects or property within their cultures and women survivors of incest or rape all have been abused. Consequently, their attitudes relating to sexuality often include powerlessness, anger, rage, fear, shame, guilt, and mistrust of themselves, of others, and of sexuality. Those women may be unclear about personal boundaries, since they were not respected as individuals. As well, they may be ignorant or unsure about the pleasure of touch. Remaining in such a condition is not conducive to women's sexual health. However, neither women's cultures nor their individual oppressors will repair the damage done to them. Therefore, the women themselves must strive to overcome the injury of having learned negative sexual attitudes and sexual inhibitions.

There are several actions women can take to heal themselves and to create a sexually healthful present. First, they can address with themselves, family, friends, or counselors the facts of their lives that seem to have caused their negative emotions and attitudes of shame, fear, and powerlessness regarding themselves and their sexuality. At the same time, they can read and can converse with knowledgeable others to identify broader sociocultural values that contributed to their situation. Dealing with their emotions while doing cognitive investigation should help them comprehend the sociocultural unjustness of their being adult women of shame and sexual inhibition and should help them decide not to let their past or others in the past control them now or in the future.

Of primary importance in that decision is the need to decide to let the past be the past—not to forget it but to let go of the unhealthful emotions generated by the past that influence women's present sexual relating. Of equal importance are decisions to give themselves now what they needed or wanted during their youth in order to generate self-worth. Such gifts include respecting themselves; learning

self-assertion, including how to state their point of view and to be heard; practicing decision making, possibly by becoming a part of groups where decisions are made regularly; acquiring skills to increase their competence in various areas, such as sports; and increasing their ways of thinking beyond conditioned thoughts and responses by identifying distortions in their thinking and correcting them. Additional gifts are reclaiming their childhood curiosity and ability to play by participating in creative endeavors, such as art and games; valuing their bodies by investigating their sensory responses and learning to be comfortable with them, especially touch; developing personal boundaries and an awareness of others' boundaries; and creating concrete, realistic goals in stepwise fashion about their sexual wants and behaviors (Bass & Davis, 1988; Maltz, 1991; Maltz & Holman, 1987).

Women can overcome shame, sexual inhibition, and other negative sexual learnings over time as they begin to take responsibility for themselves sexually and as they choose to relate to others who assume such responsibility. Studying an academic human sexuality textbook, taking a human sexuality course, and reading books about women and sexuality are all ways to take responsibility. Reading books about healing from sexual abuse can be enlightening and empowering for any woman, even if she does not consider herself to have been abused.

Women's Sexual Illnesses and Problems

The sexual illnesses and problems with which women must sometimes contend include sexual dysfunctions that occur in the desire phase of the sexual response cycle, the excitement phase, and the orgasmic phase.

Sexual Dysfunctions

The term *sexual dysfunction* means that a phase of the sexual response cycle is not functioning as it has in the past or as it could. For women, there can be dysfunctions of the desire phase (within the Seduction Phase of the ESP), of the excitement phase (within the Sensation Phase of the ESP), and of the orgasmic phase (within the Surrender Phase of the ESP).

The *DSM-IV TM* (American Psychiatric Association, 1994) characterizes a sexual dysfunction as either *lifelong,* meaning that it has always been present, or *acquired,* meaning that the dysfunction appears after a time of normal functioning. As well, dysfunctions can be *situational,* meaning that they occur only at particular times, or they can be *generalized,* meaning that they occur all the time, in all sexual encounters.

It is important to understand how women's sexual dysfunctions are manifested. However, it is just as important to comprehend that women's sexual dysfunctions occur not just because of organic factors but also because of social, economic, and political forces. A society's gender and ethnic role expectations of women, the realities of living with or without enough money and power, and access to information and services figure mightily into whether or not a woman functions healthfully or is dysfunctional, including her sexual functioning. With that point in mind, women are cautioned not to be seduced into having their complex sexual functioning medicalized and co-opted by economic profit seekers, such as drug-manufacturing companies (Loe, 2000). Drugs may be indicated as treatment sometimes but usually are not the only healing measure indicated for women's sexual dysfunctions.

DESIRE PHASE DISORDERS

The desire phase disorders include hypoactive sexual disorder, sexual aversion disorder, and sexual addiction.

Hypoactive Sexual Desire Disorder Lack of sexual desire is common among women, beginning as early as in a woman's midtwenties and increasing with age (Davis, 2000; Laumann, Paik, & Rosen, 1999). Davis (2000) notes that androgenic hormones seem to be important in women's having sexual desire, that low levels of androgen correspond with women's diminished sexual desire, and that androgen levels in women begin declining in their midtwenties.

Naming a phenomenon hypoactive sexual desire means that someone has made a judgment that people ought to experience sexual desire, yet there is no agreement as to what a normal level of desire is. It is reasonable that different people experience different degrees of sexual desire and that, within a couple, the individual levels differ as well. Often, the partner with less desire is labeled to have a desire disorder, when, in fact, there just is an *unevenness of desire* in the relationship, and neither partner is ill.

The *DSM-IV TM* notes that, if a woman has little or no sexual desire and sexual fantasy and is distressed or experiences interpersonal problems because of her level of desire, a diagnosis of hypoactive sexual desire can be made. A woman in such a condition, with or without sexual counseling, can examine various factors to assess their impact on her level of desire. Those factors include, but are not limited to, fatigue, illness, depression, boredom, issues of partner cleanliness, and timing of sexual interactions. The woman also can explore how her daily stress, family and work responsibilities, and relationship satisfaction and dynamics, such as anger with her partner, are affecting her sexual desire. Finally, gender roles and attitudes she has learned about sexuality, as well as past traumatic sexual events, may also be affecting her sexual desire.

The psychosocial treatment of hypoactive sexual desire that relates to those factors just cited obviously involves addressing and resolving the accompanying issues, so that the woman is freer to allow herself to experience desire. McCarthy (1995) notes that women can do the work associated with personal issues, as well as the work needed to nurture sexual

desire, by becoming better educated about sexuality and sexual activities. They can work by themselves, with a partner, or with a competent therapist. For example, a woman with a full-time job plus full-time home and childcare responsibilities whose spouse refuses to share the home and parenting responsibilities equally cannot be expected to experience sexual desire spontaneously. Such a woman, working alone, can choose to engage a baby-sitter or friend on a midweek evening to attend to the children and house while she pampers herself and rests, preparing to share sexually with her spouse later. However, the same woman can choose to work with her husband and a therapist to try to achieve more equitable sharing of the home and childrearing activities, anticipating that such achievement will result in an increased sexual desire.

A possible physical basis for women's lack of sexual desire should be entertained, too. It has been demonstrated that treating postmenopausal women with estrogen-androgen therapy, in contrast to estrogen therapy alone, increases sexual desire (Davis, 2000; Sarrel, Dobay, & Wijta, 1998; Studd, Colins, & Chakravarti, 1977). Davis (2000) suggests that the role of androgens in female sexual desire has not been well researched. A possible future finding may be that diminishing levels of circulating androgens in women is the primary cause of their lack of desire. Women with low sexual desire can initiate a discussion with their healthcare providers about the most recent research findings and a possible physiological treatment for their condition.

Sexual Aversion Disorder The *DSM-IV TM* criteria for sexual aversion are an aversion to and an active avoidance of genital contact with another person. The affected person experiences personal or interpersonal distress because of the problem. Such a woman may experience moderate or severe anxiety, such as sweating or palpitations, when thinking about or when placed in sexual situations. The cause of the fear associated with sexual aversion usually is having learned negative attitudes and facts about sexuality and, often, having experienced past sexual trauma.

A sexually avoidant woman can conquer her aversion. It is possible to learn accurate facts about sexuality, to replace negative attitudes with positive ones, to learn how a past sexual trauma led to the present sexual aversion, and to learn anxiety-reducing techniques. She can seek out that learning on her own, or she can work with a competent sexual counselor to gain insight and to learn new behaviors.

Sexual Addiction Excessive sexual desire that results in compulsive or addictive sexual actions is called sexual addiction. Change from those behaviors is possible. A woman experiencing compulsive, addictive sexual behaviors is best advised to seek treatment from competent professionals who specialize in sexual addiction. The regular participation in sexual addictions support groups often is part of the treatment.

EXCITEMENT PHASE DISORDER: FEMALE SEXUAL AROUSAL DISORDER

An inability to relax and to become sexually aroused enough to experience vaginal swelling and lubrication is an occasional problem for most women. However, according to the *DSM-IV TM,* the diagnosis of female sexual arousal disorder is made for women who experience sexual arousal disorder recurrently or who persistently have inadequate vaginal swelling and lubrication, and the situation, as well, causes them personal or interpersonal distress.

Arousal disorder can be related to low sexual desire and an altered ability to be comfortable in sexual sharing. Thus, a woman with sexual arousal disorder should explore first what might be interfering with her sexual desire and her comfort in sexual interaction and should resolve those issues. The resolution of issues usually results in increased personal comfort and openness to experiencing sexual desire. Anxiety in sexual interactions then diminishes, and there is an increased ability to relax and to become sexually aroused. The decreased vaginal lubrication that occurs with age is not called sexual arousal disorder and can be aided by using water-soluble lubricants, such as KY jelly, Silken and Astroglide, or liquids, such as KY liquid and Replens.

ORGASMIC PHASE DISORDER: FEMALE ORGASMIC DISORDER

The *DSM-IV TM* describes female orgasmic disorder as a delay in orgasm or the absence of orgasm after a period of adequate sexual excitement. The delay or absence is persistent or recurrent, and the situation causes the woman personal or interpersonal distress. A woman who never has experienced orgasm can be said to be anorgasmic or pre-orgasmic. As with female sexual arousal disorder, the woman should begin addressing her concern by examining the elements that relate to her sexual desire and comfort with sexuality, generally, and then specifically with a partner.

A label of **pre-orgasmia** suggests that a woman can learn to be orgasmic, and, in fact, the sexual growth programs of Barbach (1975) and Heinman and LoPiccolo (1988) are designed to facilitate that happening. In those programs, a woman becomes aware of her sexual knowledge and attitudes, as well as her own sexual response. She learns to stimulate herself to orgasm, perhaps with the use of a vibrator or fantasy, and then learns to communicate with a partner about her sexual response and to transfer her new orgasmic ability into the partnered situation.

Penile-vaginal intercourse usually stimulates a man effectively. However, penile-vaginal intercourse often does not provide the right kind of stimulation in the right places for the right amount of time for some women to be orgasmic. A woman's sexual arousal response to touch incorporates her whole body and, in particular, the more highly innervated areas of her breasts, pubic area, clitoris, vagina, and anal area. The amount, kinds, and places of stimulation all figure into her eventual arousal to orgasm. The clitoris, especially, must be stimulated adequately, and that is not always possible with a penis in the vagina. A woman who is orgasmic or who becomes orgasmic may or may not experience orgasm with penile-vaginal intercourse. In either case, her response is normal. Pressure put on a woman by herself or by a partner to experience orgasm, or multiple orgasms, is ineffective. A pressured woman cannot relax. For orgasm to occur, a woman must be physiologically relaxed and willing to engage in sexual activity.

SEXUAL PAIN DISORDERS

The sexual pain disorders include dyspareunia and vaginismus.

Dyspareunia Genital pain that accompanies sexual intercourse is called **dyspareunia.** It can occur before, during, or after sexual intercourse and can be mild, severe, dull, or sharp. To be diagnosed as dyspareunia, the situation must cause the woman pain plus personal or interpersonal discomfort (American Psychiatric Association, 1994). The primary physical characteristics of dyspareunia are lack of vaginal lubrication; vaginal irritation or inflammation from sexually transmitted diseases or other vaginal or pelvic infections; and sensitivity to powders, perfumes, soaps, lotions, douches, or contraceptives.

Women who have had an episiotomy or a vaginal tear while giving birth may develop scar tissue, which results in pain that is aggravated by vaginal intercourse. Laser and other removal of genital warts can result in a kind of chronic sensitivity of nerve endings, which is experienced as pain. The malplacement of abdominal or pelvic organs or diseases in those organs, especially of the uterus and ovaries, can produce pain when the pressure and movements of vaginal intercourse are experienced.

Dyspareunia also can be caused by psychological factors, which interfere with a woman's ability to relax and to engage willingly and actively in sexual intercourse. Such factors include incorrect sexual knowledge, negative sexual attitudes, relationship issues, and past traumatic sexual events.

The treatment of dyspareunia consists of identifying and addressing the cause. Thus, water-soluble lubricants can be used if decreased lubrication is a problem. Discontinuing the use of particular irritating products may be necessary, as may the medical or surgical treatment of correctable conditions. For relationship problems and related issues, counseling is indicated. The woman and her partner may need to limit or discontinue vaginal intercourse and focus on other sexual behaviors that can be equally pleasurable.

Vaginismus The *DSM-IV TM* (American Psychiatric Association, 1994) defines vaginismus as "recurrent or persistent involuntary spasm of the musculature of the outer third of the vagina that interferes with sexual intercourse . . . causing marked distress or interpersonal difficulty" (p. 515). The spasm prevents the entry of anything into the vagina. Thus, a penis cannot pass through the spasm; for some women, neither can a vaginal speculum for a gynecological examination. A woman with vaginismus often does experience sexual arousal, including lubrication and orgasm.

Vaginismus is not a common condition. Its cause usually is psychological and has to do with a trauma the woman experienced, such as rape, painful gynecological examinations, or abortion. A simple illustration is of a woman who, as a child during innocent peer sex play, had her vaginal area poked with sticks for an "examination." That child grew to be a woman who experienced vaginismus in attempted coitus. Additionally, some medical or surgical circumstances, such as vaginal surgery, can initiate vaginismus.

The treatment of vaginismus is relaxation training to aid the woman in decreasing anxiety and the gradual insertion of graduated sizes of dilators into the vagina once relaxation is learned. The dilators can be supplied by a physician or can be the woman's fingers, but they always are well lubricated and never forced into the vagina, and the woman herself inserts them. Once the woman can contain a particular-sized dilator for a period of 10 to 15 minutes, she is ready to learn to contain the next size. Eventually, as her fear diminishes and her ability to vaginally contain a penis-like object increases, the woman is able to transfer her learning into a sexual situation to accommodate a partner's fingers or penis without spasm.

The inadequacy of the *DSM-IV TM* nomenclature for dyspareunia and vaginismus has been addressed by Pukall, Reissing, Binik, Khalife, and Abbott (2000). In their work with women who have sexual pain, they find it more appropriate to have women use the pain classification system of the International Association of the Study of Pain (Merskey & Bogduk, 1994; Wesselmann, Burnett, & Heinberg, 1997) to chart their progress. They maintain that focusing on the description of the pain syndromes experienced by women rather than on the fact that the pain inhibits the women's sexual relating, as does the *DSM-IV TM*, increases the possibilities of arriving at appropriate and successful treatment. Pukall et al. (2000) further suggest classifying dyspareunia and vaginismus as **urogenital pain** rather than as sexual pain.

Sexually Transmitted Diseases and Problems

About one in five persons in the United States has a sexually transmitted disease (STD). A newer term is sexually transmitted infection (STI). This section discusses the most common sexually transmitted diseases that women experience. Women should know that both the incubation time and the signs and symptoms of these diseases are different for men. Sexually active women should seek knowledge of those differences in order to avoid contracting disease via heterosexual relations.

Good sources for that information are Planned Parenthood Federation of America, Sex Information and Education Council of the United States (SIECUS), and the American Social Health Association (ASHA). The diseases addressed in this chapter include trichomoniasis, chlamydia, gonorrhea, syphilis, human papillomavirus, cytomegalovirus, chancroid, genital herpes, hepatitis A, and hepatitis B. The problems include infestations with pubic lice and with the mite that causes scabies. Infection with the HIV virus is addressed in Chapter 20.

TRICHOMONIASIS

Trichomoniasis is a common vaginal infection caused by the protozoan *Trichomonas vaginalis*. It is transmitted through sexual intercourse. About 6 million women and their partners are infected every year. A diagnosis is made microscopically by observing the protozoan moving in a smear of vaginal secretions placed on a slide which has been moistened with saline (Youngkin & Davis, 1997). An increased number of white blood cells also may be present in the wet mount.

There is no definite incubation period before the symptoms appear. A woman with the disease can be asymptomatic, even if the infection has been present for years. The symptoms consist of an off-white, yellow, or greenish purulent discharge that may be bubbly and foul-smelling. The vagina may feel itchy or irritated, and the vagina and labia may be swollen. There may be pain on urination or during sexual intercourse. A vaginal speculum examination may show a cervical mucosa dotted with petechiae (small, flat red dots), a phenomenon called *strawberry cervix* (Youngkin & Davis, 1997).

For treatment, the Centers for Disease Control and Prevention (CDC) (1998) recommends a single oral dose of Metronidazole for the infected person and for all sexual partners concurrently. If the symptoms persist, oral Metronidazole is prescribed for seven days. If the symptoms still persist, other dosage regimens of retronidazole are used. Persons being treated must abstain from drinking **alcohol** while taking Metronidazole, and for two days following the last dose, or flushing and vomiting can occur. They should **abstain from sexual intercourse** until their treatment and that of their partners is completed. No follow-up is necessary if the symptoms resolve with treatment.

CHLAMYDIA TRACHOMATIS

Chlamydia is the most common sexually transmitted bacterial infection in the United States. Its occurence does not have to be reported to the CDC; however, the CDC estimates that about 4 million acute infections occur each year. The number of cases that are reported to the CDC has increased every year since at least 1995. The highest incidence of chlamydia is in teens and young adults from the ages of 15 to 25. It is most prevalent in lower socioeconomic groups and large urban populations. The bacteria are intracellular, and the infected woman experiences tissue damage from an inflammatory cellular immune response. Bacteria can infect the vagina, the anus, and the oral cavity of adults. A pregnant woman infected with chlamydia can transmit the disease to her newborn as the baby passes through the birth canal, causing eye infections and pneumonia in the infant.

A diagnosis can be made from cultures of the discharge from around the cervix, which will be found upon microscopic examination to contain many epithelial cells. Special lab tests (ligase chain reaction assay and polymerhase chain reaction assay) identify 10 to 20 percent more cases than do cultures (Handsfield, 1996). Sometimes urine tests can identify chlamydia.

The incubation period from the time of exposure to the exhibition of symptoms is from one to three weeks. However, *most women have no symptoms*. Those who do may experience abnormal vaginal discharge, pelvic pain or pressure, burning on urination, urinary frequency or urgency, vaginal bleeding after intercourse, or fever. An objective examination of the cervix may show reddening around the cervical opening and bleeding of the area when it is touched lightly with a swab (Youngkin & Davis, 1997).

The treatment recommended by the CDC (1998) is a single oral dose of azithromycin, or seven-day oral treatment with erythromycin, dfloxacin, or doxycycline. Pregnant women should be treated according to the most recent CDC guidelines.

Infected persons should **abstain from sexual intercourse** for seven days after a single-dose treatment, or until a seven day treatment has been completed. Additionally, they should abstain until all sexual partners have been treated and cured. The sexual partners of an infected person should be tested and treated if they have had sexual contact with the infected person within 60 days preceding the onset of her symptoms or diagnosis, or if they have been the infected person's most recent sexual partner, even if it was more than 60 days before the onset of the symptoms or diagnosis.

The disease may present no signs and symptoms, or very subtle ones, thus delaying diagnosis, and there is a high reinfection rate. Therefore, the disease can progress to result in pelvic inflammatory disease (see chapter 17), tubal infertility, and ectopic pregnancy.

The CDC (1998) recommends screening sexually active adolescents during yearly physical exams even if they do not have symptoms. It also recommends screening women ages 20 to 24 if they have new or multiple sexual partners or if they do not use barrier forms of birth control, and it recommends testing pregnant women. It is also wise to test for other STDs in a person who has chlamydia.

GONORRHEA

The CDC estimates that 600,000 new infections of gonorrhea occur yearly, although the incidence has decreased overall over the past 20 years. The number of cases reported to the CDC decreased from 690,169 in 1990 to 345,087 in 1998. The highest incidence is in persons under the age of 24 who live in high-density urban populations (and in many rural areas) and who have multiple sexual partners and unprotected sexual intercourse. One woman for every 1.2 men contracts gonorrhea. Direct contact with infected mucous membranes by vaginal or anal intercourse, or oral sex, especially fellatio (oral stimulation of the penis), is necessary for the transmission of the infecting organism, *Neisseria gonorrhoeae diploccus bacterium*.

A diagnosis is made by culturing smears of secretions from the cervix, urethra, rectum, and pharynx. Typically an examination of the culture shows the gonorrhoeae organism within neutrophils, but, in 50 percent of the smears from a female cervix or rectum, they are not found. Culture seems to identify the organism with about 80 to 90 percent accuracy in symptomatic women. Special ligase chain reaction and polymerhase chain reaction assays are also used and can be used to screen voided urine samples (CDC, 1998).

The incubation period in women is 2 to 10 days. Many women have no symptoms, even though the infection is present in the endocervix, rectum, urethra, or pharynx. Women with early symptoms may have a green or yellow-green vaginal or rectal discharge, pain or burning on urination, vaginal bleeding between periods, or rectal burning or itching. About 20 to 40 percent of all infected women have infections that are persistent and **subclinical** (causing no obvious symptoms).

A vaginal examination with a speculum may be normal but often shows pus, bleeding, or swelling within the cervix. An examination of the rectum with an anoscope may show reddening and swelling of the anal mucous membrane, pus, or bleeding. Pharyngeal (throat) symptoms are rare (Youngkin & Davis, 1997).

Infected women who go untreated for the infection may develop complications later and may experience fever, back pain, abdominal pain, lymph node swelling and tenderness, sore throat, or pain in the upper abdomen and shoulders. The complications include fallopian tube scarring, ectopic pregnancy, and bacteremia, the presence of bacteria in the blood, with resulting arthritis and dermatitis. Infected pregnant women may experience premature membrane rupture, premature labor, or postpartum endometriosis. Pregnant women can pass on the infection through infected secretions to their newborns, resulting in blindness or meningitis of the newborns (CDC, 1998).

The *Neisseria gonorrhoeae organism* has evolved through the years to become resistant to many antibiotics. At present, the CDC (1998) treatment regimen recommendation for uncomplicated gonococcal infections of the cervix, rectum, and urethra is treatment with antibiotics. A single intramuscular dose of the antibiotic ceftriaxone; a single oral dose of cefixime, ciprofloxacin, or ofloxacin plus azithromycin; or a seven-day oral administration of doxycycline may be given. The CDC (1998) recommended regimen for the treatment of uncomplicated pharyngeal gonococcal infecton is the same but excludes the single oral dose of cefixime. Recommendations for treatment of pregnant women and of newborns can be found through the CDC (1998).

Infected persons who are treated do not have to return for follow-up unless their symptoms persist. The sexual partners of the infected person should be treated if they had sexual contact within 60 days of the time the infected person developed symptoms or was diagnosed. If the infected person developed symptoms over 60 days after having had sexual intercourse, then the last partner with whom she had relations should be treated. Infected persons should *not* have sexual intercourse during treatment and until symptoms have been eliminated in themselves and their partners (CDC, 1998).

SYPHILIS

Syphilis is caused by the *Treponema pallidum,* a spirochete bacterium that slowly replicates itself in the body. Syphilis is transmitted through direct sexual contact with an infected person who has the disease. The first stage of the disease is known as **primary syphilis.** If primary syphilis goes untreated, the individual will develop **secondary syphilis** within a month or two. After about 10 years, **tertiary syphilis** will develop. Syphilis can also be transmitted prenatally from the mother to the developing fetus. After the discovery and use of penicillin to treat syphilis, its incidence declined. The number of cases reported to the CDC has decreased each year since 1990, with about 50,000 cases reported that year and about 7,100 reported in 1998. The number of reported cases of syphilis in all stages has declined yearly as well, to about 46,500 in 1997 (CDC, 1998).

A diagnosis is made through an examination of serous fluid in the lesions present in primary or secondary syphilis. The examination is done with dark-field microscopy or fluorescent antibody tests and the *treponema pallidum* identified. Special blood tests, the Venereal Disease Research Laboratory (VDRL) test and the rapid plasma antigen (RIPR) test, can make a positive identification of the infection three to six weeks after the infection and continue to do so through all stages of the disease (Youngkin & Davis, 1997).

The incubation period for syphilis is three to six weeks. After that, **chancre**—a rounded, painless lesion with some serous discharge—appears, indicating the presence of **primary syphilis.** In women, it usually appears on the labia or vaginal entrance, but it also can be located in the rectum, mouth, or vagina. Enlarged lymph nodes can be felt in the area of chancre presentation. In three to six weeks, the chancre and enlarged lymph nodes resolve. Because lesions often are hidden or have a nontypical appearance, they often are missed and a diagnosis is not made (Youngkin & Davis, 1997).

Secondary syphilis occurs about one to two months after the resolution of the chancre. A generalized skin rash, which usually involves the palms of the hands and soles of the feet, appears. Painless ulcers on the mucous membranes, genital or anal warts, enlarged lymph nodes, alopecia (hair loss), fever, tiredness, or headache may occur. Those symp-

toms resolve in one to three months, but there may be latent secondary symptoms manifested for up to four years after the primary phase (CDC, 1998).

Tertiary syphilis develops about 10 or more years after infection. Ulcerative lesions of the skin, liver, or bones are typical. The central nervous system and cardiovascular system can be compromised, with the development of phenomena such as meningitis, dementia, and arteritis.

The CDC (1998) notes that the preferred drug of treatment in all stages of syphilis is parenterally administered penicillin G. The CDC suggests that, when infected persons are allergic to penicillin, they should be desensitized and then treated. The CDC recommends that anyone who has been sexually exposed to a person in any stage of syphilis should be evaluated, tested for the disease, and treated according to the varied guidelines it presents.

HUMAN PAPILLOMAVIRUS INFECTION

Human papillomavirus (HPV) infection is the most common viral sexually transmitted disease, with about 3 million cases occurring yearly in the United States. Most infections are unrecognized, subclinical, and asymptomatic. HPV is a slow-growing virus of a family of more than 60 strains, more than 20 of which can infect the genitals, and persons can be infected with more than one type. Types 6 and 11 cause visible warts. Types 16, 18, 31, 33, and 35 may or may not cause visible warts but definitely are associated with squamous cell cancer of the external genitalia, anus, vagina, and cervix. HPV is spread by direct contact in oral, vaginal, or anal intercourse. Pregnant women can pass the virus to developing fetuses, who develop warts in their throats (Youngkin & Davis, 1997).

The diagnosis of HPV begins with a visual examination to identify obvious lesions. When acetic acid solution is applied to the genitals, previously unseen infected tissue turns white and then can be examined with microscopic lenses. A Pap smear can show a pattern of cells that suggests the presence of HPV. Microscopic examination of cells from lesions can identify the virus strain.

The incubation period is from one to six months or longer. The symptoms are painless bumps or warts commonly appearing on the labia, vagina, urethra, cervix, or anus. Single warts can be flesh-colored or pink, and dry. Close multiple warts may have a cauliflower-like appearance. The warts may not be bothersome at all but may itch, become ulcerated, or be painful, and the woman may experience bleeding with intercourse, vaginal discharge, or a bad odor from them (Youngkin & Davis, 1997).

Treatment does not destroy the HPV; it merely eradicates the obvious lesions. The CDC (1998) advises that treatment should be based on what the infected person wants, the available resources, and the expertise of the healthcare provider. It suggests that no one treatment is better than any other when the treatment goal is the removal of visible lesions. The treatment modalities include medicative creams, solutions, or gels that the infected person applies repeatedly over a period of months and others that clinicians apply for more immediate removal, as well as removal by surgery and laser therapy. CDC (1998) states that the treatment modality should be changed if the warts have not greatly improved after three healthcare provider treatments and disappeared after six treatments. Unfortunately, treatment by surgical removal can result in chronic pain syndromes (CDC, 1998).

Follow-up after the removal of the warts is not necessary, but the HPV-infected person should be alert for recurrences and seek treatment if desired. Sexual partners should be counseled that *the HPV-infected person may be contagious in the absence of obvious lesions* and that using condoms can reduce the risk of transmission. Because many cases of HPV infection are subclinical, sexual partners already may be infected and should be advised to be assessed for the presence of HPV and other STDs.

CYTOMEGALOVIRUS INFECTION

Approximately 60 to 70 percent of people have been infected with cytomegalovirus but likely do not know it, because it occurs asymptomatically or with flulike symptoms. The virus is spread via contact with bodily fluids, such as saliva, tears, urine, genital secretions, and breast milk. Women most likely to have contracted cytomegalovirus seem to be older, be of lower socioeconomic status, have had several pregnancies, or have had a larger number of sexual partners. The danger of cytomegalovirus is the transmission of it to a fetus or an infant through the placenta, vagina, or breast milk. Some infants born with the disease have few problems, but others have serious effects, such as mental retardation, especially if the mother transmitted it during the first trimester of pregnancy (Youngkin & Davis, 1997).

The diagnosis of cytomegalovirus is made with blood antibody tests. One specific antibody test can determine whether or not the person was infected within the past 60 days.

Cytomegalovirus can neither be prevented, nor cured. Pregnant women who suspect they may have contracted cytomegalovirus or who have flulike symptoms can be tested for its presence; if the test is positive, they should discuss the implications for fetal and infant transmission with their healthcare providers (CDC, 1998).

CHANCROID

Chancroid is caused by the *Haemophilus ducreyi*, a bacillus, through vaginal or anal intercourse with an infected person. The bacillus causes ulcerative lesions on the genitalia. The CDC reports that chancroid is endemic in some parts of the United States but occurs only in outbreaks in other areas. Cases reported to the CDC have decreased regularly since 1990. In 1990, the number of cases reported to the CDC was about 4,200; in 1997, it was 243.

A diagnosis is made by examining a culture from the lesions and identifying *Haemophilus ducreyi*; however, the

sensitivity, the rate at which existing disease is detected, is about 80 percent. A probable diagnosis can be made in a person with painful genital ulcers and painful lymph nodes who tests negative for syphilis and herpes simplex virus (HSV) (Youngkin & Davis, 1997).

The symptoms of chancroid for women are chancroid ulcers on the external genitalia or around the anus. The ulcers are painful and may be accompanied by tender or painful inguinal (groin) lymph nodes, which at times may contain pus. Other symptoms are painful urination, painful intercourse, pain on having bowel movements, and vaginal discharge.

The CDC (1998) recommends treatment with a one-time oral dose of azithromycin, a one-time intramuscular dose of ceftriaxone, a 3-day oral treatment with ciprofloxacin, or a 7-day treatment with erythromycin. Ulcers should improve within 3 days of treatment, although healing overall may take over 2 weeks, depending on the size and number of ulcers. The sexual partners should be treated if they had sexual contact with the infected person within 10 days of symptom presentation, even if they themselves do not have symptoms.

GENITAL HERPES SIMPLEX VIRUS INFECTION

About 25 percent of the U.S. population is infected with genital herpes simplex virus (HSV), which reflects a 30 percent increase over the past 20 years. There are two types of herpes simplex virus—HSV1 and HSV2. Both types cause painful, ulcerative lesions primarily in the oral and genital area, but lesions can appear on any skin or mucous membrane surface. HSV is transmitted through kissing and sexual contact with an infected person, with or without symptoms. *Many persons do not know that they are infected.* However, they still can transmit the virus to another. Such transmission occurs because the virus resides within certain nerves in an infected person's body and travels along them to the skin or mucous membrane surface, to be shed in skin cells from those spots. HSV can be transmitted from pregnant mother to fetus, as well (Youngkin & Davis, 1997).

A diagnosis is made by culturing the virus from lesions or secretions. HSV2 seems more associated with recurrent genital HSV than does HSV1.

The incubation period for primary HSV (the initial episode) is about 3 to 21 days, usually 3 to 10 days. The symptoms for women are lesions on the labia, on the anal area, on the vaginal entrance, or around the mouth. The lesions are painful, contain fluid, break open, weep, and then dry and crust. With genital lesions, lymph nodes in the groin may swell and be painful. The woman may have chills, fever, painful urination, tiredness, headache, or vaginal discharge. The symptoms reach a peak about 5 days after they begin and then resolve over 2 to 3 weeks (Youngkin & Davis, 1997).

There usually are recurrent HSV outbreaks after the initial infection. About four episodes per year is average for women. The number and severity of recurrences seem to decrease over time. A few days prior to a recurrent episode, some women experience a tingling or pain where lesions will develop. Most recurrent episodes resolve in 7 to 10 days.

There is no agent that can entirely prevent or eradicate HSV or eliminate its transmission by asymptomatic cell shedding. To lessen the severity of initial episodes, and decrease the frequency of recurrent ones, the CDC recommends oral dosing with various antiviral agents, such as acylovir, famciclovir, or valacyclovir. Intravenous dosing may be necessary if severe complications, such as meningitis, develop (CDC, 1998).

Infected persons should abstain from sexual activity at times when they feel lesions about to occur and when lesions are present. They should use condoms with all new or non-infected partners. Sexual partners who have symptoms should be evaluated, treated, and educated about HSV. Pregnant women who know they have HSV should inform their healthcare providers to learn about the risks to the fetus or infant and to plan.

Comfort measures during outbreaks include powdering the lesions with dry cornstarch, wearing loose clothes, soaking in tepid or warm water, urinating in water if urination is painful, and air drying the lesions or blowing air from fans or cool hair dryers over them (Youngkin & Davis, 1997).

HEPATITIS A

Hepatitis A is a viral inflammation of the liver caused by infection with the hepatitis A virus (HAV). The virus reproduces itself in the liver and is shed in the feces. Viral contamination from feces is highest from two weeks before symptoms develop until one week after. HAV is transmitted via any practice that causes contaminated feces from one person to reach the oral area of another person. Touching infected clothes or linens, using the household items of an infected person, and ingesting contaminated water or food or raw shellfish are common routes of transmission. Sexual activity involving contact with anal material or fluid can also cause infection. Contracting HAV confers immunity from contracting it again. The annual number of cases reported to the CDC from 1990 to 1997 fluctuated between about 24,000 and 31,000. About 22,000 cases were reported in 1998. About 33 percent of the U.S. population has had HAV (CDC, 1998).

The diagnosis is confirmed by blood test, which identifies antibodies to hepatitis A antigen. The incubation period is three to four weeks. Adults with symptoms may be tired and have anorexia, a low-grade fever, nausea or vomiting, upper abdominal pain, or jaundice. The symptoms last about a week. Infected persons do not develop chronic liver disease or become carriers of HAV.

The treatment consists of resting, washing hands well after toileting, not preparing food for others, and avoiding ingesting alcohol and medications that are metabolized by the liver. An occasional acute severe infection requires hospitalization for supportive hydration and care.

Good personal hygiene overall helps prevent its transmission. Immune globulin (IG) which contains antibodies to HAV (see Chapter 20) can be administered intramuscularly to uninfected persons planning to be in situations where HAV is present in order to create a three- to six-month period of immunity, with 85 percent effectiveness. Inactivated hepatitis A vaccine can be administered in a series for long-term immunity, with 94 to 100 percent effectiveness (CDC, 1998).

HEPATITIS B

Hepatitis B is a viral liver disease caused by infection with the hepatitis B virus (HBV). HBV is present in the blood of infected persons and can be transmitted to others through sexual intercourse and the sharing of IV needles. One can acquire HBV infection from a contaminated blood transfusion. A mother with HBV can transmit it to her newborn at birth. About 240,000 new HBV infections occur in the United States yearly, and about 30 to 60 percent of them are sexually transmitted. There are about 1 million carriers of HBV in the United States. HBV is much more contagious than HAV (CDC, 1998).

A diagnosis is made by a blood test that determines the presence of antibodies to HBV antigen. Specific tests identify whether the infection is active, chronic, or infectious.

Infected persons can be asymptomatic. When present, the symptoms include nausea, vomiting, tiredness, anorexia, muscle aches, diarrhea, and jaundice. Infected persons can experience mild disease, chronic liver disease, or eventual liver cancer, liver failure, and death. Infected persons can be asymptomatic carriers of the disease (CDC, 1998).

Supportive treatment for the symptoms is needed. The treatment with antiviral agents that interfere with the replication of the virus is being explored. Lamivudine has been eliminating the infection in some persons. The sexual partners of infected persons should be treated with hepatitis B immune globulin to confer temporary, immediate immunity. The CDC (1998) recommends that various categories of persons be vaccinated against HBV to reduce transmission. Those categories include (1) sexually active homosexual and bisexual men and (2) sexually active heterosexual women or men who have recently been diagnosed with another STD, have had more than one sexual partner in the past six months, have been treated in an STD clinic, or are prostitutes. Women may want to review all the CDC-recommended categories to assess their personal vulnerability to becoming infected.

HIV, the virus that causes acquired immune deficiency syndrome (AIDS) is addressed more comprehensively in Chapter 20. The virus is present in blood, vaginal secretions, and the semen of infected persons.

PARASITE INFECTIONS: PEDICULOSIS PUBIS AND SCABIES

Pediculosis pubis is infestation with the insects commonly known as pubic lice or *crabs*. Lice are transmitted by sexual and other direct contact. Pubic lice can also infect beards, eyelashes, and armpits. Lice can be seen moving on hairs, and the white eggs of lice, **nits,** can be seen attached to hairs. Itching is the strongest symptom. The infected person may also see the lice or nits, or she may notice bites on the surrounding skin. Various nonprescription remedies are available for treatment; the directions should be followed carefully. Prescription medications include Permethrin (a cream rinse), Lindane (a shampoo), and pyrethrins with piperonylbutoxide, which is applied to the skin. Toxicity, such as seizure or anemia from prescribed medications, however, can occur, because the medicine is absorbed through the skin. Infected persons should be treated until the lice and nits are gone. Clothes and bedding should be washed in hot water and machine-dried in heat or left alone for 72 hours to allow the parasites to die. The infected person's sexual partners of the past month should also be treated.

Scabies is caused by the mite *Sarcoptes scabiei*. Adults acquire scabies through sexual transmission or other personal contact with an infected person. Itching is the chief symptom. Treatment is with prescription medications, such as Permethrin, Lindane, or a sulfur-containing cream, until the itching subsides or until no live mites are observed. Clothes and bedding should be washed and dried as for the treatment of lice, and the infected person's sexual partners of the past month, as well as persons living in the same household or sharing personal space with the infected person, should be treated.

Sexual Wellness Self-Assessment

Use the following questions to evaluate your sexual wellness.

1. *Am I aware of my erogenous zones and my physical sexual response?*
2. *Do I practice Kegel exercises?*
3. *Am I content with my orgasmic ability?*
4. *Am I prepared to address the changes in my sexuality that are associated with aging?*
5. *Do I form my own opinions about my sexual expression?*
6. *Do I exercise regularly?*
7. *Do I create an atmosphere of privacy and relaxation within which to experience sexual pleasure?*
8. *Am I addressing any issues of self-esteem, shame, or inhibition I may have?*
9. *Am I addressing any specific sexual dysfunctions I have?*
10. *Am I able to be intimate with another person?*
11. *Do I protect myself from STDs and seek treatment for infections as needed?*
12. *Am I continuously learning about my own sexuality?*

New Directions

Many areas of women's sexuality need to be researched. There is a need for reliable research into the psychophysiological assessment of female sexual dysfunctions and then the development of standardized criteria and procedures for evaluating women's sexual function and dysfunctions (Meston, 2000). Research is needed to illuminate the major issue in treating women's sexual dysfunctions, which is making accurate comprehensive diagnoses of the problems and then using appropriate treatments, including drugs and psychotherapy measures (Berman & Berman, 2000a). The pathology of women's sexual pain disorders also needs to be researched (Pukall et al., 2000). Further understanding of the sexual side effects of psychotropic drugs on women is needed (Saks, 2000), and the ways in which androgens influence women's sexual interest is of fundamental research importance (Davis, 2000). The recognition of the inadequacy of research about how abdominal, pelvic, and genital surgery affect women's sexual function is just surfacing (Lefkowitz & McCullough, 2000). There has been minimal research into the specific etiologies of women's sexual dysfunctions and neurological diseases, such as multiple sclerosis, stroke, peripheral nerve disease, and epilepsy, yet sexual dysfunction is a common complication of those diseases (Kalayjian & Morrell, 2000).

Women's sexual dysfunction medical treatments that have arisen out of recent research include the development of Viagra for women (sildenafil), as well as topical prostaglandin creams, to stimulate blood flow to the genital area—and to the clitoris, in particular—to increase lubrication and sensation (Berman & Berman, 2000b; *Female Sexual Dysfunction Drug,* 1998). A testosterone patch to increase women's sexual pleasure and orgasm after menopause is being investigated (Berman & Berman, 2000a; *Testosterone Patch,* 2000), and a clitoral vacuum device, the EROS-CTD, approved by the FDA in May 2000, is intended to increase blood flow and subsequent lubrication and sensation (Berman & Berman, 2000a; *Urometrics,* 2000).

Two additional topics of women's sexuality recently researched are female adolescent sexual desire (Tolman, 2000) and anorexia nervosa and sexual behavior in women (Ghizzani & Montomoli, 2000). Recent sexuality conference topics have included the newly recognized patterns in sexual response, female ejaculation, the sexuality of breast cancer survivors, sexual issues of minority women, sexual desire, women as sexual aggressors and victims, orgasm faking, women and condom use, and use of the female condom. Positive contributions that the world's religions might make on women's sexuality and sexual health is being researched internationally.

Future sexually transmitted disease research includes developing microbicides for women. Microbicides would be applied as vaginal foams, gels, films, creams, or suppositories and would prevent infection by killing the causative organisms of HIV and other STDs or would prevent the organism's replication after infection (Suiter, 2000).

Questions for Reflection and Discussion

1. How would your expression of your sexuality be different if you were of the opposite gender?
2. How might you express your sexuality differently if you had been born and reared in a foreign culture?
3. Do you agree or disagree with this statement: Sexual interactions between people who are dating are no more spontaneous than are those between married people. Explain your answer.
4. Who should be responsible for addressing and resolving a sexual dysfunction? Support your answer.
5. How can someone overcome homophobia?
6. What sexual benefits are there to growing older?
7. How would you decide whether or not an Internet source that supplies sexual information is a credible one?

Resources

Journals

The Kinsey Institute for Research in Sex, Gender, and Reproduction, Inc., publishes on-line an extensive list of reputable sexology journals (www.indiana.edu/~kinsey). A few standard journals that should be available in academic libraries are *Archives of Sexual Behavior; Journal of Homosexuality; Journal of Lesbian Studies; Journal of Psychology and Human Sexuality; Journal of Sex and Marital Therapy; Journal of Sex Education and Therapy; Journal of Sex Research; Medical Aspects of Human Sexuality; Sex Roles: A Journal of Research; Sexual Addiction and Compulsivity; Sexuality and Culture; Sexuality and Disability;* and *SIECUS Reports.*

Organizations

American Association of Sex Educators, Counselors, and Therapists (AASECT)
P.O. Box 238
Mount Vernon, IA 52314-0238
Fax: 319-895-6203
Web: www.aasect.org

American Social Health Association (ASHA)
P.O. Box 13827
Research Triangle Park, NC 27709-3827
Phone: 919-361-8400
Web: www.ashastd.org

Centers for Disease Control and Prevention (CDC)
U.S. Department of Health and Human Services
1600 Clifton Rd.
Atlanta, GA 30333
Phone: 404-639-3311
Web: www.cdc.gov

CDC National AIDS hot line
Phone: 1-800-342-2437

The Kinsey Institute for Research in Sex, Gender, and Reproduction, Inc.
Morrison 313, Indiana University
Bloomington, IN 47401
Phone: 812-855-7686
Web: www.indiana.edu/~kinsey

National Herpes Hot Line
Phone: 919-361-8488

National Women's Health Network
514 10th St., NW, Suite 400
Washington, DC 20004
Phone: 202-628-7814
Web: www.womenshealthnetwork.org

Planned Parenthood Federation of America
810 7th Ave.
New York, NY 10019
Phone: 1-800-829-7732
Web: www.plannedparenthood.org

Sex Information and Education Council of the United States (SIECUS)
130 West 42nd St., Suite 350
New York, NY 10036-7802
Phone: 212-819-9770
Web: www.siecus.org

The Society for the Scientific Study of Sexuality (SSSS)
P.O. Box 208
Mount Vernon, IA 52314-0238
Phone: 319-895-8407
Web: www.ssc.wisc.edu/ssss

Websites

American Board of Sexology: www.sexologist.org

Gay/lesbian civil rights organizations: www.hatewatch.org/mongay.html

Herpes Resource Center: www.ashastd.org/herpes/hrc

National Gay and Lesbian Task Force: www.ngltf.org

Parents, Family, and Friends of Lesbians and Gays (PFLAG): www.pflag.org

Rape, Abuse, Incest National Network (RAIN): www.rainn.org

SIECUS Life Behaviors of a Sexually Healthy Adult: www.siecus.org/pubs/cnct/cnctOO03.html

The National Council on Sexual Addiction and Compulsivity: www.ncsac.org

References

Allgeier, E. R., & Allgeier, A. R. (1991). *Sexual interactions.* Boston, MA: D. C. Heath.

Alzate, H., & Lodono, M. L. (1984). Vaginal erotic sensitivity. *Journal of Sex and Marital Therapy, 10,* 49–56.

American Psychiatric Association. (1994). *Diagnostic and statistical manual of mental disorders* (4th ed.). Washington, DC: Author.

Barbach, L. G. (1975). *For yourself: The fullfillment of female sexuality.* New York: Doubleday.

Bass, E., & Davis, L. (1988). *The courage to heal: A guide for women survivors of child sexual abuse.* New York: Harper & Row.

Belenky, M. F., Clinchy, B. M., Goldberger, N. R., & Tarule, J. M. (1986). *Women's ways of knowing: The development of self, voice, and mind.* New York: Basic Books.

Berman, L., & Berman, J. (2000a). *Non-pharmaceutical treatments/therapies for female sexual dysfunction* [On-line]. Available: http://www.womenssexualhealth.com

Berman, L. A., & Berman, J. R. (2000b). Viagra and beyond: Where sex educators and therapists fit in from a multidisciplinary perspective. *Journal of Sex Education and Therapy, 25*(1), 17–24.

Brecher, E. M., & The Editors of Consumer Reports Books. (1984). *Love, sex, and aging: A Consumer's Union report.* Boston: Little, Brown.

Centers for Disease Control and Prevention (CDC). (1998). *Guidelines for treatment of sexually transmitted diseases.* Bethesda, MD: CDC.

Cross, R. (1993). What doctors and others need to know: Six facts on human sexuality and aging. *SIECUS Reports, 21*(5), 7–9.

Darling, C. A., Davidson, J. K., & Conway-Welch, C. (1990). Female ejaculation: Perceived origins, the Grafenberg spot/area, and sexual responsiveness. *Archives of Sexual Behavior, 19*, 29–47.

Davis, S. (2000). Testosterone and sexual desire in women. *Journal of Sex Education and Therapy, 25*(1), 25–32.

Female sexual dysfunction drug [On-line]. (1998). Available: http://www.pharmacology.about.com/health/pharmacology/library

Feuerstein, G. (Ed.). (1989). *Enlightened sexuality: Essays on body-positive spirituality.* Los Angeles, CA: Crossing Press.

Ghizzani, A., & Montomoli, M. (2000). Anorexia nervosa and sexuality in women: A review. *Journal of Sex Education and Therapy, 25*(1), 80–88.

Gordon, S., & Snyder, C. W. (1989). *Personal issues in human sexuality: A guidebook for better sexual health.* Boston: Allyn & Bacon.

Handsfield, H. H. (1996). *A practical guide to sexually transmitted diseases.* Minneapolis: McGraw-Hill Healthcare Information Group.

Heinman, J. R., & LoPiccolo, J. (1988). *Becoming orgasmic: A sexual and personal growth program for women.* Upper Saddle River, NJ: Prentice-Hall.

Jacoby, S. (1999, September–October). Great sex: What's age got to do with it? *Modern Maturity,* 43–45, 74.

Kalayjian, L. A., & Morrell, M. J. (2000). Female sexuality and neurological disease. *Journal of Sex Education and Therapy, 25*(1), 89–95.

Kaplan, H. S. (1977). *Disorders of sexual desire.* New York: Simon & Schuster.

Kegel, A. H. (1952). Sexual functions of the pubococcygeus muscle. *Western Journal of Surgery, 60,* 521–524.

Kinsey, A. C., Pomeroy, W. B., Martin, C. E., & Gebhard, P. H. (1953). *Sexual behavior in the human female.* Philadelphia: W. B. Saunders.

Kolodny, R. C., Masters, W. H., & Johnson, V. E. (1979). *Textbook of sexual medicine.* Boston: Little, Brown.

Ladas, A. K., Whipple, B., & Perry, J. D. (1982). *The G spot and other recent discoveries about human sexuality.* New York: Holt, Rinehart & Winston.

Laumann, E., Paik, A., & Rosen, R. (1999). Sexual dysfunction in the United States: Prevalence and predictors. *Journal of the American Medical Association, 281,* 537–544.

Lefkowitz, G. K., & McCullough, A. R. (2000). Influence of abdominal, pelvic, and genital surgery on sexual function in women. *Journal of Sex Education and Therapy, 25*(1), 45–48.

Loe, M. (2000). Female sexual dysfunction: For women or for sale? *The Network News: National Women's Health Network, 25*(1), 1, 6.

Maltz, W. (1991). *The sexual healing journey: A guide for survivors of sexual abuse.* New York: HarperCollins.

Maltz, W., & Holman, B. (1987). *Incest and sexuality: A guide to understanding and healing.* Lexington, MA: Lexington Books.

Masters, W. H., & Johnson, V. E. (1966). *Human sexual response.* Boston: Little, Brown.

Masters, W. H., Johnson, V. E., & Kolodny, R. C. (1989). *Human sexuality* (4th ed.). New York: HarperCollins.

McCammon, S., Knox, D., & Schacht, C. (1993). *Choices in sexuality.* Minneapolis, MN: West.

McCarthy, B. (1995). Bridges to sexual desire. *Journal of Sex Education and Therapy, 21*(2), 132–141.

Merskey, H., & Bogduk, N. (1994). *Classification of chronic pain* (2nd ed.). Washington, DC: IASP Press.

Meston, C. (2000). The psychophysiological assessment of female sexual function. *Journal of Sex Education and Therapy, 25*(1), 6–16.

Montagu, A. (1986). *The human significance of the skin.* New York: Harper & Row.

Montejo, A. L., Llorca, G., Izquierdo, J. A., & Rico-Villademoros, F. (2001). Incidence of sexual dysfunction associated with antidepressant agents: A prospective multicenter study of 1022 outpatients. *Journal of Clinical Psychiatry, 62* (Suppl. 3), 10–21.

Perry, J. D., & Whipple, B. (1981). Pelvic muscle strength of female ejaculation: Evidence in support of a new theory of orgasm. *Journal of Sex Research, 17,* 22–39.

Pukall, C. F., Reissing, E. D., Binik, Y. M., Khalife, S., & Abbott, F. V. (2000). New clinical and research perspectives on the sexual pain disorders. *Journal of Sex Education and Therapy, 25*(1), 36–44.

Rathus, S. A., Nevid, J. S., & Fichner-Rathus, L. (1993). *Human sexuality in a world of diversity.* Boston: Allyn & Bacon.

Reinisch, J. M., with Beasley, R. (1990). *The Kinsey Institute new report on sex: What you must know to be sexually literate.* New York: St. Martin's Press.

Rogers, A. (1990). Drugs and disturbed sexual functioning. In C. I. Fogel & D. Lauver (Eds.), *Sexual health promotion* (pp. 485–497). Philadelphia: W.B. Saunders.

Saks, B. R. (2000). Sex receptors: Mechanisms of drug action via biochemical receptors on sexual response of women. *Journal of Sex Education and Therapy, 25*(1), 33–35.

Sarrel, P., Dobay, B., & Wijta, B. (1998). Estrogen and estrogen-androgen replacement in postmenopausal women dissatisfied with estrogen-only therapy: Sexual behavior and neuroendocrine response. *Journal of Reproductive Medicine, 43,* 847–856.

Scantling, S., & Browder, S. (1993). *Ordinary women, extraordinary sex: Every woman's guide to pleasure and beyond.* New York: Dutton.

Schnarch, D. M. (1991). *Constructing the sexual crucible: An integration of sexual and marital therapy.* New York: W.W. Norton.

Seagraves, R., & Seagraves, K. (1995). Sexuality and aging. *Journal of Sex Education and Therapy, 21*(2), 88–102.

Singer, I. (1973). *The goals of human sexuality.* New York: W.W. Norton.

Stayton, W. R. (1992). A theology of pleasure. *SIECUS Report, 20*(4), 9–15.

Stimpson, C. R., & Person, E. S. (Eds.). (1980). *Women, sex, and sexuality.* Chicago: The University of Chicago Press.

Studd, J. W. W., Colins, W. P., & Chakravarti, S. (1977). Estradiol and testosterone implants in the treatment of psychosexual problems in postmenopausal women. *British Journal of Obstetrics and Gynecology, 84,* 314–315.

Suggs, D. N., & Miracle, A. W. (1993). *Culture and human sexuality: A reader.* Modesto, CA: Brooks/Cole, Wadsworth.

Suiter, E. (2000). Waging war on STDs—And drugmaker apathy—With microbicides. *The Network News: National Women's Health Network, 25*(2), 1, 4.

Taylor, D., & Surnall, A. C. (Eds.). (1993). *The time of our lives: Women write on sex after 40.* Pasadena, CA: Crossing Press.

Testosterone patch [Online]. (2000). Available: http://www.personalmd.com

Tolman, D. L. (2000). Object lessons: Romance, violation, and female adolescent sexual desire. *Journal of Sex Education and Therapy, 25*(1), 70–79.

Urometrics [Online]. (2000). Available: http://www.urometrics.com

Wesselmann, U., Burnett, A. L., & Heinberg, L. J. (1997). The urogenital and rectal pain syndromes. *Pain, 73,* 269–294.

Youngkin, E. Q., & Davis, M. S. (1997). *Women's health: A primary care clinical guide.* Norwalk, CT: Appleton & Lange.

23

Pregnancy and Childbearing

Lynn Bradley, Marilyn J. Horan, and Patricia Molloy

CHAPTER OUTLINE

Objectives

1. *Discuss the importance of preconception screenings and guidelines.*
2. *Describe the stages of normal prenatal development.*
3. *Explore the normal processes associated with pregnancy, labor, delivery, and the postpartum period.*
4. *Compare and contrast the normal discomforts associated with pregnancy and the warning signs of the complications that can occur.*
5. *Identify the factors that should be considered when a person or couple prepare a birth plan.*
6. *Explain some of the disorders and/or complications that can occur during the childbearing cycle.*
7. *Identify the safety considerations in newborn care and feeding.*
8. *Discuss the options available to a woman experiencing an unplanned pregnancy.*

Introduction

Every woman who wishes to be, or is about to become, a biological mother hopes that her pregnancy will culminate in the birth of a healthy baby. By becoming informed about ways to promote a healthy pregnancy and to prepare for delivery and the responsibilities of motherhood, a woman can increase the likelihood that this wish will come true. A baby's health is influenced by genetic, biological, nutritional, and environmental factors from preconception to birth. Although genetics cannot be changed, nutritional and many environmental factors can. With appropriate information and guidance, women can take steps to maintain or improve their physical, psychological, and spiritual health in the period known as preconception, as well as throughout pregnancy and during labor, delivery and the postpartum period. Healthcare providers can be sources of support and guidance, as well as technical intervention, to help maximize a woman's chances of giving birth to a healthy baby.

Choosing a Healthcare Provider

Choosing a healthcare provider to guide a woman and her family through pregnancy is an important personal decision. The provider is responsible for assisting throughout pregnancy and delivery, facilitating care after delivery, and helping families adjust successfully to the changes accompanying the arrival of a new baby. Many women consult providers *in advance* of conception, to ensure a healthy pregnancy from the very beginning. Today, the focus of most practitioners has expanded beyond the mother to include the childbearing *family* as a whole. Healthcare providers recognize that, when one member of the family system is affected by pregnancy and birth, all the other members are also affected, and the family structure changes. It is important that women and their families feel comfortable and confident in their choice of provider. The right provider will promote the best possible pregnancy outcome by offering guidance on a wide range of issues and decisions related to pregnancy, as well as technical expertise and support.

Factors in Choosing a Provider

Many factors can influence a woman's or family's choice of a maternity care provider. The factors pertaining to the individual or family include the availability of financial resources, individual behaviors and beliefs concerning healthcare, and access to transportation. Other factors are the relative availability of maternal services, problems related to underfunding of services, understaffing and overcrowding in public clinics, and lack of coordination and bureaucratic obstacles related to the provision of health services to needy individuals. Fortunately, the trend is toward better care for American women: In 1987, the U.S. attorney general's *Healthy People 2000 Progress Review* found that only 76 percent of American women received prenatal care in the first trimester of pregnancy; in 1996, 82 percent of women were receiving such care. These gains included percentage increases among traditionally medically underserved groups, such as African Americans, Hispanics, and Native Americans.

Providers of Obstetrical Care

A number of different providers offer obstetrical healthcare. These include obstetricians/gynecologists, family practice physicians, and certified nurse-midwives.

An *obstetrician/gynecologist (ob/gyn)* is a licensed physician with specific training and certification in women's health and obstetrical (pregnancy) care. Many ob/gyns belong to group practices and have a traditional Western medical approach, emphasizing modern technology and research. They almost always conduct deliveries in hospitals. These physicians are competent to provide maternity care under all circumstances, and their advanced skills and training are invaluable in the care of women who either have complications or are at high risk for them.

Family physicians' training prepares them to provide care throughout a *normal* pregnancy and delivery. Family physicians care for the entire family and, therefore, can provide continuity from obstetrical to pediatric care.

Certified nurse-midwives (CNMs) and *certified midwives (CMs)* are advanced practice nurses (see Chapter 9) who care for pregnant women and their families. They are registered nurses (RNs) who have graduated from an advanced education program accredited by the American College of Nurse-Midwives (ACNM) and have passed a rigorous national certification exam. The services that nurse-midwives provide to *healthy* women and their babies include prenatal care, care during labor and delivery, postpartum care, well women gynecology and normal newborn care, and preconception care, counseling, and education in health maintenance and disease prevention. Certified nurse-midwives are prepared to address many common gynecological and obstetrical health problems. However, should major difficulties develop, they will collaborate with, or recommend referral to, a physician. The scope of practice of nurse-midwives differs from state to state. Many women and their families have been attracted to midwifery care because nurse-midwives traditionally offer individualized, family-centered care. Nurse-midwives have also historically supported alternatives to hospital births, including birthing centers and home births.

Preparation for Conception

There are many steps a woman can take to increase her chance of conceiving and carrying a healthy baby. An important one is to schedule an appointment with a healthcare provider for preconception counseling or to request that preconception counseling be included in the annual gynecological exam (Reynolds, 1998). The preconception visit will include an assessment of any risk factors that may be present and instruction regarding optimal diet, substances to avoid, and the like. The risk assessment, which involves eliciting relevant information about both prospective parents and a physical examination of the prospective mother, will identify any factors that might compromise the pregnancy. It will also identify any health problems in the woman and provide an opportunity to correct them in order to prevent a poor pregnancy outcome. Counseling regarding optimal diet and other aspects of lifestyle will promote a healthy pregnancy and fetus.

Risk Assessment

The preconception risk assessment should include a complete medical history, including the woman's social and family history. Current nutritional practices and possible environmental exposure to toxins (see Chapter 5) should be explored. The health history of the man who will father the child should be discussed as well, if possible. The biological father's age, medical history, current physical health, use of social or street drugs, family history of genetic disorders, and history of exposure to environmental toxins are of prime importance.

Of particular importance in the medical histories of both intended parents are chronic diseases, such as hypertension, diabetes, seizures, tuberculosis, thyroid disorder, and mental illness. Managing these conditions properly during pregnancy is of prime importance in ensuring optimal fetal development. The healthcare provider will also need to know about any prescription or over-the-counter (OTC) medications the intended mother is taking. This includes herbs and other kinds of dietary supplements (see Chapter 11). Pregnant women should *not* use nonsteroidal anti-inflammatory drugs (NSAIDs) to treat pain or fever without first consulting a physician or midwife. Maternal use of NSAIDs such as aspirin, ibuprofen (Motrin, Advil), and naproxin (Aleve) has been associated with the development of persistent pulmonary hypertension of the newborn, a serious lung disorder (Alano, Ngougmna, Ostrea, & Kondur, 2001). Exposure to lead, mercury, pesticides, organic solvents, and/or a contaminated water supply in the workplace or home should be reported to the provider.

The provider will ask the woman about her menstrual pattern and the date of her last menstrual period and will inquire whether there have been any gynecological problems, such as endometriosis, or reproductive tract surgery, such as previous cesarean sections or removal of a uterine fibroid. She will also inquire about any prior pregnancies that resulted in therapeutic abortion, miscarriage, premature labor and delivery, or birth defects.

The provider will also want to know about the woman's social history. Included in this area is information about relationships, nutrition, and drug use or abuse. The provider will ask about the woman's significant relationships and inquire about emotional support or the lack of it, as well as problems with domestic violence. The provider will also ask about the woman's current eating patterns, including diet and food preferences, vitamin and mineral supplementation, special diets (such as vegetarianism), and any history of eating disorders. The woman will also be asked about her past and present patterns of smoking, drinking, and using other drugs, such as cocaine or marijuana. It is important that woman be candid about this, because all drugs impact a developing fetus.

Physical and Gynecological Exams

A general physical exam will be performed, focusing on the thyroid, heart, lungs, and abdomen. A breast and pelvic exam will also be performed, and a Pap test will be done. Screening for sexually transmitted diseases (STDs), including gonorrhea, chlamydia, yeast infections, bacterial vaginosis, and herpes will also be carried out. The provider will also order a variety of laboratory tests to screen for such problems as anemia, hepatitis, tuberculosis, and some hereditary diseases.

Preconception Lifestyle Guidelines

Women who intend to conceive are given instructions on a variety of topics, including immunizations, various drugs they may be taking, diet, food supplements, and environmental toxins.

Immunizations are of major concern in pregnancy because of their effect on the growing fetus. Most American women of childbearing age will have received all necessary immunizations—rubella (German measles), varicella (chicken pox), and hepatitis B—well before a pregnancy is planned. In general, all vaccines are best avoided during pregnancy unless the risk of exposure is greater than the possible risk of vaccination. If a woman of childbearing age has been immunized with rubella varicella, or hepatitis B vaccine, it is best to wait three months before trying to conceive. Live viruses, such as measles, mumps, rubella, varicella, and live polio virus, are contraindicated during pregnancy, because they can cause fetal infection (Holzman, 1998). However, in some instances, it is necessary for women to receive certain vaccines during pregnancy, especially if there is a significant risk of exposure to infectious agents. Healthcare providers have guidelines as to which vaccines may be administered.

The method of contraception a woman has been using in the past can affect conception. Birth control pills can alter the hormonal levels that affect pregnancy and should be discontinued at least one month prior to an attempted conception. Women who use other methods of birth control, such as an IUD, Norplant, or Depo-Provera injections, should

also wait at least one menstrual cycle before attempting conception (Olds, London, & Ladewig, 2000).

Any medications a woman is taking have the potential to wreak havoc with a pregnancy. Over-the-counter medications, even aspirin, should be avoided. Women should check with a healthcare provider about both over-the-counter and prescription drugs that may seem indispensable. The risk of birth defects associated with various medications is based on fetal susceptibility. Timing is an important variable: During the first two weeks after conception, a drug may have no effect, but, at 5 to 10 weeks' gestation, there may be effects on developing organs. Beyond 8 weeks, substances could cause a reduction in overall fetal growth.

Women who plan to become pregnant should be sure they are consuming a healthy diet (see Chapter 3), because nutrition before conception is critical to the prevention of many birth defects. Although there is little research on how specific foods affect fertility, there is strong evidence that reversing the effects of general malnutrition improves conception rates (Somer, 1995).

Being at one's optimum body weight is preferable when entering a pregnancy, because being 10 percent or more underweight or 20 percent or more overweight can lead to complications during pregnancy. Both conditions can also affect the menstrual cycle and, therefore, fertility. Dieting by reducing calorie intake should occur *before,* not during, pregnancy (Somer, 1995).

A multivitamin and mineral supplement containing the B vitamin folic acid (0.4 milligrams) should be taken daily to prevent neural tube defects, defects in the embryonic structure forming the brain and spinal column. This supplement should be added to the diet at least one month prior to attempting conception.

Many women of childbearing age use herbs on a daily basis for various reasons and need to be aware of their effect on pregnancy and/or a fetus prior to conception. Women who use herbs should be aware that, although herbs have been used traditionally for many years for a variety of conditions, not all constituents of herbs have been identified or scientifically studied. It is best to check with a healthcare professional before using any herbs or herbal preparations, especially prior to and during pregnancy. Commonly used herbs that should be avoided both during the two months prior to conception and during pregnancy include the following: *laxative herbs,* such as flaxseed, aloe vera, senna, castor oil, catnip, and dong quai; *steroidlike herbs,* such as licorice, ginseng, and hops; *diuretic herbs,* such as buchu, horse tail, and juniper berries; and *antihistaminic herbs,* such as osha, ma huang, and ephedra. Herbal agents that promote menstruation (emmenagogues), such as angelica root, lemon balm leaves, dong quai, feverfew, goldenseal root, hyssop leaves, mugwort, rose flowers, wood sorel, wormwood, and yarrow, should be completely avoided while trying to conceive and during pregnancy (Weed, 1986). Some *cooking herbs* that can cause miscarriage should be avoided during the first trimester and used only in small amounts during the remainder of the pregnancy; these include basil, caraway seeds, celery seeds, ginger, fresh horseradish, savory, marjoram, nutmeg, rosemary, saffron, sage, parsley, tarragon, thyme, and watercress. *Herbs used to facilitate labor* should be used only under the guidance of a qualified healthcare professional. Many herbal teas should be used sparingly during pregnancy, because the composition and safety of many remain unknown. Teas believed to be safe include red raspberry leaf, nettle, peppermint, chamomile, wild yam, bilberry, and echinacea (Tierra, 1998).

Federally required testing of food additives before they are approved for use generally assures safety in the United States. Some additives on the market, however, are still questionable. Although the research is not conclusive, women should probably avoid *aspartame* (NutraSweet) preconception and during pregnancy, as some research has linked it to mental handicaps in infants and health problems in adults. Other additives that can adversely affect maternal and fetal health include *butylated hydroxytoluene (BHT)* and *monosodium glutamate (MSG)*. The consumption of BHT by animal mothers has been linked to behavioral problems in their young (Verrilli & Mueser, 1998).

Caffeine consumption should be limited to two servings or less a day. Excessive caffeine use has been linked to infertility (Stanton & Gary, 1995). Consuming more than six cups of coffee a day can cause miscarriage, according to a study conducted by a group of researchers from the National Institute of Child Health and Human Development and the University of Utah (Johnson, 1999). There is no safe level of *alcohol* intake during pregnancy, despite common wisdom to the contrary. Alcohol consumption increases the risk of miscarriage, stillbirth, and death in early infancy (Somer, 1995).

Women who intend to conceive, as well as women who are pregnant, must do all they can to avoid general environmental contaminants (see Chapter 5). If at all possible, women should discontinue *smoking* prior to pregnancy. If mothers are unable to quit smoking, reducing the number of cigarettes to 10 or fewer a day can reduce the risk of bearing a low birth weight infant. Another environmental factor to be considered is *heat*. Heat is considered a teratogen, a substance that has negative effects on the development of a fetus. Tub water cannot be hotter than 100°F without risk, and hot tubs and saunas should be avoided. Women who are pregnant, or trying to become pregnant, should not change cat litter boxes because of the risk of toxoplasmosis, a disease caused by infectious organisms sometimes present in cat feces.

Conception

Each month, the body of a woman of childbearing age prepares for pregnancy. Approximately 2 weeks after menstruation (in a 28-day cycle), ovulation takes place. **Ovulation** is the process in which a mature egg or ovum, is released and travels down the fallopian tubes, propelled by tiny hairs, or cilia, to the uterus. The ovum is usually fertilized within 24 hours of being expelled from the ovary. During this time, the estrogen secreted by the ovaries stimulates the lining of the uterus to thicken with blood and nutrients that could support and maintain a fertilized egg. If fertilization does not take place, the uterine lining is shed during menstruation, and the process begins again.

Conception begins when a male germ cell—a sperm, or spermatazoan—penetrates an ovum and forms a **zygote.** The ovum and the spermatazoan each contribute half of the genetic material necessary to create a human being. The new human cell has 23 pairs of chromosomes in its nucleus—half contributed by the mother and half by the father. Twenty-two pairs of the chromosomes are identical in males and females and are known as **autosomes.** In the remaining pair of chromosomes, called the **sex chromosomes,** there is a difference between the female and the male. The female sex chromosome pair contains identical chromosomes (XX), but the male sex chromosome pair contains two different chromosomes (XY). The chromosomes carry **genes,** the basic units of inheritance (Olds et al., 2000). Fertilization is complete when the sperm and the egg nucleus join together to make a set of 46 chromosomes.

Once fertilization is complete, the zygote travels to the uterine cavity, and **implantation** (establishment of a uterine blood supply for the zygote) occurs within 5 to 9 days. Conception and subsequent implantation occur within approximately 17 days of intercourse.

Infertility

The term *infertility* refers to the inability to conceive after 12 months or more of unprotected intercourse (Somer, 1995). Couples experiencing infertility should seek medical advice if trying to conceive. Age is a strong driver in the likelihood of infertility, which occurs in only 1 percent of teenagers but in up to 25 percent of couples in their mid- to late thirties. According to some estimates, 50 percent of couples in their forties are infertile (Somer, 1995). Conception rates drop off rapidly as women age beyond 40. Other aspects of the health history and medical status of prospective mothers and fathers can affect fertility; endometriosis in the woman and low sperm count in the man are particularly problematic. A discussion of the many interventions of which infertile individuals or couples can avail themselves is beyond the scope of this chapter.

Pregnancy Tests

The detection of hormones particular to pregnancy, especially **human chorionic gonadotropin (HCG),** is the mechanism by which most pregnancy tests work. Tests for HCG can be done on either urine or serum (blood). Serum HCG can be performed as early as one week after implantation, when HCG levels can be as low as 25 mIU/mL.

HCG levels double approximately every two days with normal pregnancy.

Although the serum HCG test is the most accurate pregnancy test, there are many commercially available urine pregnancy tests that are accurate, although some tests have a high rate of **false negatives.** A false negative test is said to have occurred when the test reads negative when the woman is actually pregnant. False negatives can occur in home pregnancy tests if lipids (blood fats) are elevated, if immunoglobulin levels (proteins acting as antibodies) are high, and if serum protein is low. False positive tests are very rare but can occur if HCG comes from another source, such as a tumor of the pancreas, ovary, or breast. Pregnancy tests should be repeated by a healthcare provider when only a home test was used.

Pregnancy

The duration of pregnancy is approximately 40 weeks from the time the ovum is fertilized. This equates to 9 calendar months or approximately 266 to 280 calendar days. If a pregnancy continues past 42 weeks, labor is usually induced, because mortality and morbidity rates increase rapidly after 42 weeks. The **expected delivery date (EDD)** (formerly EDC for expected date of confinement) is usually calculated (assuming a 28-day menstrual cycle) using **Naegele's Rule.** This rule adds 7 days to the first day of the last menstrual period, subtracts 3 months from that date, and then adds 1 year. For example, if the first day of the last menstrual period was July 4, 2002, the EDD would be April 11, 2003. Only a few women will deliver precisely on their due date. However, Naegele's Rule is still the most accurate method of estimation: most women will deliver plus or minus 5 days from their calculated EDD. The factors negatively impacting the reliability of this calculation include having a history of irregular menses, conceiving while breast-feeding, ovulating although amenorrheic, and conceiving before the regular menses cycle is established or after discontinuing oral contraceptives.

The approximately 40-week period before delivery is referred to as the **antepartal period** or **antepartum.** It is divided into three trimesters, or three three-month periods. The first trimester begins with the first week of pregnancy and ends at the twelfth, lasting a total of 12 weeks. The second trimester begins at 13 weeks, ends at 27 weeks, and lasts 15 weeks. The third trimester begins at 28 weeks, ends at 40 weeks, and lasts 13 weeks.

Signs of Pregnancy

The hormonal changes that occur during pregnancy cause physical changes, which can be detected by the woman herself or a healthcare provider who examines her. These signs are classified according to the following categories: pre-

sumptive, probable, and positive. When **presumptive signs** occur, the woman can be reasonably certain that she is pregnant. Presumptive signs include the following: amenorrhea (the cessation of the menstrual cycle); morning sickness (including nausea and vomiting); frequent urination; breast tenderness and fullness; darker pigmentation of the nipples; quickening (the mother's perception of fetal movement); Chadwick's sign (blue discoloration of the vagina); striae (stretch marks or lines on the skin); and fatigue.

With the appearance of **probable signs,** the woman can be even more certain that she is pregnant. Probable signs include enlargement of the abdomen; a fetal outline distinguishable by abdominal palpation; changes in the size and consistency of the uterus (Hegar's sign); softening of the cervix (Goodell's sign); Braxton-Hicks contractions (mild uterine contractions that occur intermittently during pregnancy); and a positive pregnancy test.

The absolutely **positive signs** of pregnancy are the presence of fetal heart sounds; fetal movements felt by an examiner; and an X ray or ultrasound that outlines the fetal skeleton.

Certain terms are commonly used to describe a woman's pregnancy history. The term **nulligravida** refers to a woman who has never been pregnant. A **nullipara** is a woman who has not sustained pregnancy to the age of viability, which in the United States is considered 20 weeks. A **primipara** is a woman who is in the middle of her first pregnancy. A **multipara** is a woman who has carried two or more pregnancies to the stage of viability. The term **gravida** refers to the number of pregnancies, regardless of outcome: gravida 4 means a woman has had four pregnancies. **Parity** refers to the number of pregnancies the woman has experienced that reached the stage of viability. Thus, a woman who is described as gravida 2 para 1 has given birth to one child and is pregnant for a second time. A **full-term pregnancy** is a pregnancy that lasts at least 36 weeks or results in the birth of a 2,500 gram infant. A **preterm** infant is one born between 28 and 36 weeks or at a weight of 100–2,499 grams. The term **abortion** is used to refer to both the spontaneous end of a pregnancy, also called miscarriage, and induced terminations. The term is also used to refer to a fetus born dead before 20 weeks of pregnancy and weighing less than 500 grams. **Ectopic pregnancies** are nonviable pregnancies that implant in sites other than the uterus (such as in the fallopian tubes).

Stages of Fetal Development

The first 14 days after conception is referred to as the **pre-embryonic period** (Olds et al., 2000). During this period, there is rapid cellular growth and differentiation of the zygote. The **placenta,** an organ formed within the uterus to support the embryo throughout pregnancy, also begins to develop. At this time, HCG, which is produced by the placenta during pregnancy, is secreted and can be detected in the maternal serum as early as the eighth day after ovulation.

Box 23-1 Fetal Milestones

Month 1

♦ Head, body, arms, and leg formation
♦ Heart beats on day 25
♦ One-quarter inch long, with a tail
♦ Called a fetus after the fifth week

Month 2

♦ Internal organs formed
♦ Spine and major joints able to move
♦ Length 1 inch
♦ Fetal heart tones heard with a special stethoscope as early as 8 weeks

Month 3

♦ Sex organs develop; fingers, toes, soft nails, eyes, nose, ears, and mouth visible
♦ Weighs 1 ounce; four inches long

Month 4

♦ Strong heartbeat
♦ Body parts fully formed; kicks, swallows, moves, sleeps
♦ Six and one-half to 7 inches long; weighs 4 to 5 ounces

Month 5

♦ Rapid growth
♦ Quickening—mother feeling strong fetal movements
♦ Eight to 12 inches long; weighs ½ to 1 pound

Month 6

♦ Fetal parts can be felt on exam; organs well developed
♦ Soft, fine hair over body
♦ Skin clear and wrinkled
♦ Twelve to 14 inches long; weighs 1½ pounds

Month 7

♦ Kicks, stretches, sucks thumb, coughs, hiccups, and opens and closes eyes
♦ Fifteen inches long; weighs 2½ pounds
♦ Forty-five percent chance of survival if born prematurely at 26 weeks and 60 percent (with specialized care) at 28 weeks

Month 8

♦ Periods of waking and sleeping
♦ Rapid brain growth
♦ Lungs not fully developed
♦ Seventy percent chance of survival (with specialized care) if born at this point

Month 9

♦ Lungs mature at 36 weeks
♦ Fetus plump; arms and legs filling out
♦ Mature; chance of survival 90 percent if born at this point

Month 10

♦ Lungs completely developed
♦ Fetal head usually rotates to vertex position (head first)
♦ Nineteen to 21 inches long; weighs 6 to 9 pounds
♦ Most babies born at approximately 40 weeks.

Source: *Maternity Nursing: Care of the Childbearing Family*, 3e by Sherwen/Scoloveno/Weingarten, Copyright 1999. Reprinted with permission of Pearson Education, Inc., Upper Saddle River, NJ.

After implantation, groups of cells in the zygote, known as the **embryonic disc,** differentiate into three layers: the **ectoderm,** or outer layer of cells; the **mesoderm,** the middle layer; and the **endoderm,** the internal layer. The ectoderm eventually gives rise to the hair, skin, nails, nervous tissue, mammary glands, ears, and nasal cavities. The mesoderm becomes the bones, muscles, cartilage, teeth, ligaments, tendons, kidneys, ureters, and gonads. The endoderm produces the epitheleum of the digestive, respiratory, and urinary tracts, as well as the thyroid and liver (Olds et al., 2000). The **amnion,** a membrane that forms over the dorsal (spinal surface) part of the embryo, arises from the ectoderm, and ultimately surrounds the entire embryo, like a bubble that expands as the embryo grows. This bubble eventually fills with amniotic fluid—the bag of waters. The pre-embryonic period is followed by the **embryonic period,** which lasts through the eighth week of pregnancy. During this period, **organogenesis,** the development of all organs and tissues, takes place. Growth of the fetus occurs in a **cephalocaudal pattern,** with the head developing before the extremities.

The **fetal period** begins at the end of the eighth week after fertilization, and it ends at delivery of the newborn. During this period, the fetus grows and matures into the newborn. The rate at which the fetus grows is astronomical; an incipient new human consists of 2 cells at conception and 10 trillion cells by the time she is born. During each month of this fetal period, the fetus attains a new milestone in growth and development (see Box 23–1).

Figure 23–1   Amniocentesis

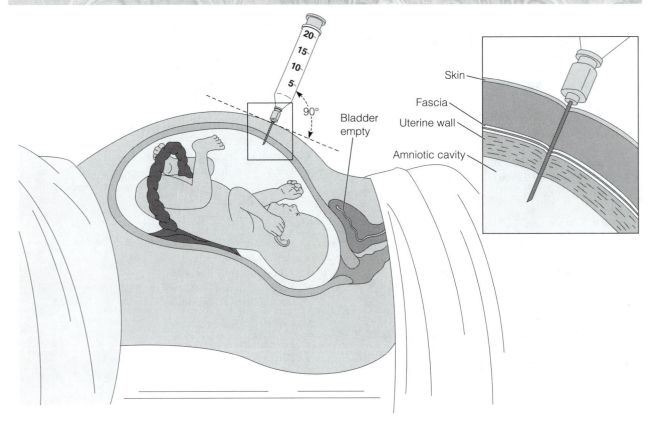

Source: *Maternal Newborn Nursing: A Family and Community-based Approach* 6e by Olds/London/Ladewig, Copyright 2000. Reprinted wtih permission of Pearson Education, Inc., Upper Saddle River, NJ.

Prenatal Screening

Couples with known genetic diseases in their families may benefit from genetic counseling. In early pregnancy, a number of tests can determine whether there are any genetic abnormalities in the fetus. These tests include amniocentesis, chorionic villus sampling (CVS), cordocentesis, alpha feto-protein screening (MSAFP), and embryoscopy.

AMNIOCENTESIS

In amniocentesis, a small amount of amniotic fluid is extracted from the amniotic sac through a needle inserted into the pregnant mother's abdomen (see Figure 23–1). This procedure is usually done between 15 and 18 weeks of gestation. The fluid that is extracted is tested for genetic defects or neural tube defects. Amniocentesis can also be performed later in pregnancy to determine if the fetal lungs are mature enough for an early delivery, if necessary, for maternal well-being.

CHORIONIC VILLUS SAMPLING (CVS)

Chorionic villus sampling is a procedure that is performed in the first trimester of pregnancy, at 9 to 12 weeks of gestation. It is commonly used to screen for genetic abnormalities when the mother is older or has borne previous children with genetic aberrations. Couples usually receive genetic counseling prior to the procedure and sign a consent form. The health-care provider obtains fetal cells to determine if any chromosomal abnormalities are present. Real-time ultrasound is used to guide a long, thin catheter into the uterus through the vagina to obtain a sample of the chorionic villi which are tiny, finger-like projections embedded in the uterine lining. (see Figure 23–2). The procedure takes approximately 20–25 minutes, and confirmed test results are available in 5–10 days. An advantage of chorionic villus sampling is it can be done earlier in pregnancy than amniocentesis. A disadvantage is that it may cause fetal limb defects, especially if the test is performed earlier than 10 weeks of gestation. The risk of miscarriage is 3 in 200, or about three times the risk of amniocentesis.

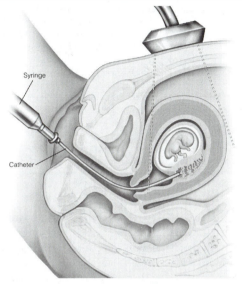

Figure 23–2 Chorionic Villus Sampling Using Cervical Approach

Syringe

Catheter

Source: *Maternity Nursing: Care of the Childbearing Family*, 3e by Sherwen/Scoloveno/Weingarten, Copyright 1999. Reprinted with permission of Pearson Education, Inc., Upper Saddle River, NJ.

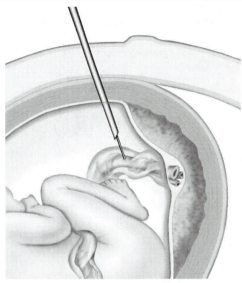

Figure 23–3 Cordocentesis

Source: *Maternity Nursing: Care of the Childbearing Family*, 3e by Sherwen/Scoloveno/Weingarten, Copyright 1999. Reprinted with permission of Pearson Education, Inc., Upper Saddle River, NJ.

CORDOCENTESIS

Cordocentesis, also referred to as **percutaneous umbilical blood sampling (PUBS),** is a method of obtaining a blood sample from the fetus in utero to screen for abnormalities. As with CVS, couples that undergo this procedure sign a consent and receive genetic counseling with an explanation of the risks and benefits of cordocentesis. The blood sample is obtained by passing a needle through the pregnant woman's abdominal wall and into the umbilical cord (see Figure 23–3). This process can also be used to give the fetus a blood transfusion. This is a highly specialized procedure and can carry risks to the fetus such as the inadvertent puncture of an organ.

ALPHA FETOPROTEIN SCREENING

Alpha fetoprotein is a substance produced by the fetus that is also found in the mother's blood. High levels may indicate a neural tube defect or other abnormal conditions; low levels may indicate Down's syndrome or other abnormalities. Maternal serum is collected between 16 and 18 weeks of pregnancy, and the level of alpha fetoprotein is measured relative to a standard level. Two other tests are sometimes done along with the AFP: The HCG level may be determined, along with the unconjugated estriol (a form of estrogen)

level. Together, these tests are known as the **triple screen.** The triple screen assists in identifying fetuses with Down's syndrome, also called **trisomy 21.**

EMBRYOSCOPY

Embryoscopy is a fairly new experimental method used to visualize and sample fetal blood and tissue, as well as to perform intrauterine fetal surgery. The procedure is guided by ultrasound and is usually done via a miniature scope inserted into the mother's abdomen. Embryoscopy can be done as early as six weeks of gestation. There is a risk of fetal death when this procedure is performed.

Major Maternal Physiological Changes During Pregnancy

During pregnancy, many changes occur in the mother's body to accommodate the growth and maintenance of the fetus. These changes are gradual, and they begin in the first trimester.

In *early pregnancy*, the mother's body undergoes both structural and hormonal changes. An important structural change is the formation of the **placenta** by the third month. The placenta supplies nutrients to the fetus throughout

TABLE 23–1   Major hormones of pregnancy.

Hormone	Functions During Pregnancy
Estrogen: A steroid hormone produced early in pregnancy by the ovary; later, the placenta produces most of this hormone	Softens tissues, assists with growth of the uterus and breasts, increases sodium and water retention, is measured in blood or urine
Progesterone: A steroid hormone produced early in pregnancy by the ovary and later mostly by the placenta	Helps relax smooth muscle and decrease smooth muscle tone, decreases gastrointestinal motility, increases basal body temperature, increases water absorption, increases smooth muscle cells
Human chronic gonadotropin (HCG): A hormone produced by the placenta in the second week of pregnancy	Maintains the corpus luteum of early pregnancy, is the basis of early pregnancy testing in blood and urine, level gradually rises until 10 weeks of pregnancy and then falls to low levels at 20 weeks
Human placental lactogen (HPL): A hormone produced by the placenta, secreted by chorionic villi	Is involved in the growth of the fetus, placenta, and breasts; assists in maintaining a constant supply of glucose and protein for the fetus

pregnancy. It is a fetal organ comprised of the chorionic villi. The fetus and placenta are connected by means of an **umbilical cord,** which contains two arteries and one vein. The developing placenta secretes the hormone human chorionic gonadotropin (HCG) for the first three to four months of pregnancy. HCG maintains the **corpus luteum,** glandular tissue in the ovary, which secretes the hormones estrogen and progesterone. The corpus luteum maintains the pregnancy until the placenta becomes mature and begins to secrete estrogen and progesterone on its own. Levels of HCG rise steadily from conception onward. Table 23–1 outlines the major hormones of pregnancy and the functions of these hormones.

Changes also occur in the mother's cardiovascular system. The mother's red blood cell count and total blood volume increase during pregnancy, beginning at the tenth week. Ultimately, the number of red blood cells increases by 25 percent, and, by the thirty-fourth week, blood volume is 30 to 50 percent higher than it was prior to the pregnancy. These changes are necessary to accommodate the increased requirements of oxygen and nutrients for the growing uterus and fetus. The greater number of red blood cells produced, and the fact that the fetus depletes the mother's iron supply, creates a greater need for *iron* in pregnancy—especially late in pregnancy. Pregnant women require iron supplements throughout pregnancy, especially if they are iron-deficient (anemic). *Cardiac output* increases by 33 percent during pregnancy and peaks at 28 weeks' gestation. With the blood volume increasing to meet the needs of the growing fetus, the heart has to pump more blood through the aorta during pregnancy. The *pulse rate* increases by eight beats per minute to accommodate the increased blood volume and output. *Blood pressure* decreases slightly during the first and second trimesters due to a decrease in peripheral vascular resistance.

Changes in the *respiratory system* occur also. Gas exchange is improved in the lungs, and there is an increased movement of the diaphragm and flaring of the ribs. This increases the tidal movement of air, making respiration more efficient and decreasing the concentration of carbon dioxide in the mother's blood. These alterations allow better oxygen transport to, and carbon dioxide removal from, fetal circulation. **Dyspnea** or shortness of breath, results from pressure exerted on the diaphragm and lungs by the growing fetus.

The *gastrointestinal system* undergoes changes during pregnancy. There is a decrease in the amount of hydrochloric acid produced by the stomach, and gastric emptying is slowed. These changes promote better absorption of nutrients from the stomach and the gastrointestinal tract, so that the fetus is optimally nourished. With the growth of the uterus, there is an increase in appetite and thirst. In late pregnancy, the pressure of the uterus decreases the capacity for a large meal.

Renal (kidney) blood flow increases during pregnancy. The glomerular filtration rate, the rate at which the kidneys filter substances from the blood, increases to accommodate the growing fetus. Urination is frequent in early and late pregnancy, due to the pressure the enlarging uterus places on the bladder. In addition, there is relaxation of the bladder due to hormonal changes during pregnancy. This change promotes the incomplete emptying of the bladder and urinary tract infections in some women.

During pregnancy, the *connective tissues* become more relaxed and elastic, and the joints become more flexible in order to prepare the mother's pelvis for delivery. These changes are caused by the increased production of **relaxin,** a hormone secreted by the placenta during late pregnancy. Relaxin also causes blood vessels in the pelvis, skin, and muscles to dilate.

Changes in *breast tissue* also occur during pregnancy. Breast tenderness and fullness are caused by estrogen. The breasts enlarge and may become lumpy and more sensitive.

The **areola,** the ring of tissue surrounding the nipple, becomes darker, and the **Montgomery's tubercles,** the rounded protuberances on the areola, become more pronounced. Veins may be more pronounced as well, and nipples may be sensitive and erect. **Colostrum,** a yellowish, antibody-rich fluid produced before true breast milk is available, may be intermittently secreted from the breasts after the twelfth week.

During pregnancy, hormonal shifts and the associated *emotional changes* can contribute to mood swings, mixed feelings about pregnancy, and food cravings.

Maternity Care

Maternity care involves monitoring the growth and well-being of the fetus and the health of the mother. The mother should make regular visits to her healthcare provider, and tests and other evaluations should be done at various stages of the pregnancy in order to detect any developing problems. The mother is provided with information about breast care, diet, and exercise, and she is assisted, if necessary, in planning to care for her baby. Mothers are also encouraged to discuss any emotional problems they may be having and are apprised of the warning signs that a problem with the pregnancy may be developing.

PRENATAL HEALTHCARE VISITS

At an initial prenatal visit to a healthcare provider, a risk assessment will be done, the EDD will be established, initial laboratory work will begin, and counseling will be offered on topics such as nutrition and weight gain, exercise, sexual activity, alcohol, drugs, smoking, and diseases (such as AIDS/HIV) that can affect the mother and fetus. Prenatal visits should be made monthly through the first 28 weeks, then every 2 weeks until 36 weeks, weekly until 40 weeks, and finally twice weekly until delivery. Typically, 15 visits are made over the course of a pregnancy. At each visit, the mother's blood pressure will be taken, her weight measured to confirm the healthy development of the fetus, and her urine analyzed for glucose and protein. If abnormal urine tests are obtained, the woman will be asked to fast and then have the tests repeated.

At 16–20 weeks' gestation, an ultrasound test (see section on Fetal Assessment) may be performed, although this test will become less accurate as time goes on. At weeks 24–28, a blood test will be done to check for gestational diabetes, although this screening may be performed earlier in the pregnancy if the mother is at high risk. About the same time, an antibody titer will be performed to determine whether there is Rh incompatibility (a situation in which the mother's immune system attacks the fetus's red blood cells) between the mother and fetus. The provider will also palpate the mother's abdomen to determine the position of the fetus in the uterus.

In a woman's first pregnancy, fetal movement can be felt at 20 weeks, but this sensation can be confused with gas. Mothers will be asked to begin doing **fetal kick counts** at about 28 weeks' gestation, or when fetal movement is felt consistently, as a means of tracking the health of the fetus. A minimum of 10 movements should occur over a two-hour period. Movements should be tracked at a consistent time each day, such as after eating or walking. At weeks 32–36, an STD (sexually transmitted disease) screen for gonorrhea, chlamydia, syphilis, and group B strep will likely be repeated, so that, if the mother is infected, she can be treated prior to delivery. This is especially important if a woman is having symptoms, such as a fever or vaginal discharge, or if she has a partner with symptoms. If a mother has a history of genital herpes, she should be examined for the presence of lesions, because herpes can be transmitted to an infant in the birth canal during delivery. If a woman has lesions at the time of labor, delivery by cesarean section is recommended. Expectant mothers should continue to report fetal kick counts during the third trimester. If the pregnancy extends past 40 weeks, a **nonstress test (NST)** (see section on Fetal Assessment) should be performed twice weekly to determine whether and how much the fetus's heart rate increases when the fetus moves.

As delivery grows nearer, the mother's healthcare provider will give her information about the signs and symptoms of labor, as well as the options for pain control during delivery. A tour of an obstetrics floor at a hospital or birthing center should also be considered at this time. The mother should also attend childbirth classes. A labor coach should also be selected if the mother desires a labor companion.

The options of breast-feeding and bottle-feeding will also be discussed at this point in the pregnancy. Mothers who intend to breast-feed will be taught the methods of preparing their nipples in advance of birth. Concepts related to infant care will also be introduced, including **bonding,** the attachment of the child to its parents through physical contact. Bonding will be described in terms of when it occurs and the importance of parenting and the involvement of the baby's father. Infants' sleeping patterns and how to negotiate night feedings will be reviewed. Information about supportive resources, such as the La Leche League (breast feeding) and local community groups that deal with baby care and parenting, will be offered.

FETAL ASSESSMENT

A number of tests are usually done to assess fetal well-being as a pregnancy progresses. These tests include ultrasound, the nonstress test, the contraction stress test, and the biophysical profile.

Ultrasound testing uses high-frequency sound waves to assess fetal and maternal well-being. It can provide information about fetal age, size, position, and heartbeat, as well as the amount of amniotic fluid present, and it can identify some placental and fetal abnormalities, as well as the presence of multiple fetuses. There are many other uses of this technology, and it can be done any time during pregnancy. Ultrasound is a relatively safe procedure, it has been used for 25 years, and it can be done several times during pregnancy without known adverse effects. There are two types of ultrasound procedures: transabdominal ultrasound and transvaginal ultrasound. **Transabdominal ultrasound** is a low-risk, painless procedure done while the pregnant woman has a full bladder, so that the fetus will be pushed higher into the abdomen for a clearer test result. The woman lies on her back, and a small amount of gel is applied to her abdomen. A transducer, a hand-held device that emits ultrasound waves, is moved slowly over her abdomen, and images of the fetus are seen on a monitor. Pictures of the fetus can be taken for later comparisons. This approach is usually used in the second and third trimesters of pregnancy. **Transvaginal ultrasound,** in which a small, lubricated transducer probe is inserted into the woman's vagina, is usually performed in the first trimester of pregnancy, as it allows a better view of small structures, such as the embryo or a possible ectopic pregnancy.

In a **nonstress test,** a monitor and an ultrasound transducer are also used. The fetal heart rate normally increases to a certain level immediately after each movement of the fetus. If it does, the test is deemed *a normal reactive test,* meaning the fetus is healthy. If the heart doesn't accelerate with fetal movement, the test is considered *a nonreactive,* or abnormal, test.

A **contraction stress test** is performed if the NST results are abnormal. It reflects the quality of placental functioning and fetal status. Uterine contractions are induced to determine how the fetal heart will react to the stress of labor. If the pregnant woman is not experiencing frequent, spontaneous contractions, they are encouraged by nipple stimulation with hot towels or breast massage. Breast stimulation causes the release of the hormone oxytocin from the anterior pituitary gland, which in turn stimulates uterine contractions. If nipple stimulation fails, **pitocin,** a drug that induces contractions, is administered to the mother intravenously in order to produce sufficient contractions for the test.

A **biophysical profile (BPP)** uses real-time ultrasound as a tool to assess fetal well-being. This scanning is a noninvasive test that assesses five key fetal biophysical parameters: fetal heart rate reactivity, fetal breathing movements, fetal body movements, fetal tone, and amniotic fluid volume. Each parameter is scored according to certain criteria, and the scores are totaled. A perfect total score of 10 represents a fetus that is not compromised. A score of 7 or less is indicative of a fetus that may be compromised. In many cases, it is necessary to repeat this test up to three times a week.

BREAST CARE

Breast care becomes particularly important during the third trimester. Most women should consider switching to a maternity or nursing bra that is wider in width and cup size in order to support the enlarged breasts. Nipple care is also important, especially for mothers who intend to nurse. Harsh soaps and detergents should not be used on the nipples because they can be irritating. Mothers who plan to breast-feed can toughen their nipples by allowing them to air-dry after showering, letting them rub against clothing each day, and rubbing them with terrycloth towels. Masse cream can be applied, and hydrous lanolin is particularly helpful if the nipples are fissured (have broken skin). Rolling the nipples between the fingers is helpful, especially if they are inverted. Rolling promotes the early expression of colostrum. Towel drying and nipple pulling can help bring out inverted nipples, which may pose a problem if the mother intends to breast-feed.

Guidelines for Nutrition and Weight Gain

One of the most important things a pregnant woman can do in order to ensure her own health and that of her fetus is to nourish herself optimally without gaining an excessive amount of weight.

NUTRITION

An appropriate diet must be consumed throughout pregnancy for both the fetus's development and the mother's health and stamina. Prior to pregnancy, a woman close to ideal body weight should be consuming about 2,000 calories daily in recommended servings from the basic groups of the USDA Food Guide Pyramid (see Chapter 3). During pregnancy, a woman will have to add about 100 calories to her normal diet during the first trimester and 300 calories daily thereafter, in order to accommodate the growing fetus (Kolasa & Weismiller, 1995). It is recommended that these calories come from one additional serving from the milk group and another from the meat and meat alternative group (Somer, 1995). The meat and meat alternative group is recommended because of its wealth of protein, which will accommodate the increase in blood volume of the mother and the growth of the fetus. However, many women in the United States already consume adequate protein, although their intake of fruits, vegetables, and dairy products is inadequate. In that case, more of those foods should be consumed (Kolasa & Weismiller, 1995). In the milk group, vitamin D–fortified low-fat or nonfat milk is particularly a good choice, because it is the single best dietary source of calcium and vitamin D (Somer, 1995), which are needed to build the fetus's bones as well as to maintain those of the mother. By the second trimester, a woman should be consuming one quart of milk, or the equivalent, per day in order to assure adequate calcium intake. Fats, especially saturated fats, should be limited, as should foods laden with sugar. Pregnant women should avoid highly processed food and junk foods, as should everyone.

Pregnant vegetarians who eat eggs, milk, and other protein sources daily may need to make only minimal changes in their usual diet (Kolasa & Weismiller, 1995). Eggs and milk are both sources of complete protein, and either can be combined with incomplete protein sources to provide needed amino acids. Vegans, who eat no animal products whatsoever, will need a nutritional supplement during pregnancy or may consider temporarily adding foods such as eggs, dairy products, and fish to their diet. Otherwise, an absolute commitment to obtaining all essential nutrients from the diet is required. The recommended foods for pregnant vegans include whole grains, beans, green and yellow vegetables, soy milk, tofu, and tempeh (Verilli & Mueser, 1998). Pregnant women must be sure to take in adequate amounts of vitamins and minerals. Guidelines are available from healthcare providers. Although women should not exceed the recommended guidelines, because the overconsumption of even essential vitamins and minerals can have negative effects, they must be certain to meet them. An inadequate intake of various micronutrients can compromise fetal development. For example, a calcium intake that is inadequate or poorly absorbed may result in suboptimal bone development in the fetus. Also, the fetus may leech calcium from the mother's bones, and it may take years to replenish her supply (Somer, 1995). Vitamin D, protein, phosphorus, and magnesium are also needed for proper fetal bone formation (Somer, 1995). If the maternal diet does not contain at least 0.4 mg of folic acid during the first trimester, neural tube defects may be present in the fetus. Iron, along with copper and vitamin B-6, is essential for the proper oxygenation of the fetus (Somer, 1995). Iron needs double in pregnancy; 30–60 mg of elemental iron should be consumed daily. If a mother is anemic, this level should be raised to 60 mg twice a day for at least six weeks.

Although food is the best source of nutrients, it is difficult for many pregnant women to eat enough of the proper foods to obtain all the essential nutrients. Therefore, nutritional supplements will usually be prescribed in order to assure that adequate resources are available for fetal development.

WEIGHT GAIN

The approximate total weight gain over the course of a pregnancy should be 25 to 35 pounds for mothers who are already at their ideal weight. If underweight, a mother should be encouraged to gain the number of pounds she needs to reach her ideal weight plus an additional 25–35 pounds. Being 10 percent or more below ideal body weight is not desirable during pregnancy, as the fetus may be compromised. Mothers who are overweight to start with should gain no more than 15 to 25 pounds. An additional 5 pounds should be gained if the mother is an adolescent, smokes, or has multiple gestation (in this case, 15 to 20 pounds per fetus are added).

During each prenatal visit, the mother's weight is recorded, and gains should follow a recommended pattern. The recommended pattern of weight gain for women of ideal prepregnancy weight during the first trimester is 2 to 4 pounds (0.90 to 1.80 kg). After the first trimester, mothers should be gaining about 4 pounds per month, or 1 pound (0.45 kg) per week for the second and third trimesters, for a

TABLE 23–2	Distribution of weight gained during pregnancy.
Source	**Weight (Pounds)**
Infant	7.50
Placenta	1.50
Amniotic fluid	2.00
Breast tissue	1.00
Uterus	2.50
Blood	3.50
Other fluid	2.75
Other	3.25

Source: Copyright © 1998 by Verilli and Mueser From: While Waiting, 2nd edition by Verilli and Mueser. Reprinted with permission of St. Martin's Press, LLC.

total of 29 pounds (13.18 kg) (Sherwen, Scoloveno, & Weingarten, 1995).

Pregnancy is *not* the time to diet, even for overweight women, because an adequate intake of calories and nutrients is so important. If the recommended diet is followed throughout pregnancy, women will not put on significant extra weight in the form of body fat.

The approximate distribution of the weight gained during an average pregnancy is shown in Table 23–2. The weight of the infant, placenta, and amniotic fluid is lost at delivery. Excess weight gained during pregnancy should be lost gradually during the postpartum period.

Excercise During Pregnancy

When a woman is pregnant, she must balance the benefits of exercising with the associated risks and must make allowances for the physiological changes she is undergoing (Carlson & Parrish, 1998). Newly pregnant women who customarily exercise should review their routines with their healthcare providers during the early prenatal visits. Activities such as walking and running are usually safe during the first two trimesters. Other beneficial exercises include strength training, which may reduce the likelihood that lower back pain will develop, water sports, and other exercises that do not put stress on the joints (Carlson & Parrish, 1998).

After the first trimester, a pregnant woman should seek to keep her heart rate under 140 beats per minute while exercising. She should work out no more than four times per week, and each session should last no longer than 15–20 minutes. She should terminate an exercise session if she feels fatigue or discomfort (Carlson & Parrish, 1998).

After the first trimester, exercises done in the *supine position*, lying on the back, should last no more than four seconds at a time. This is because the weight of the uterus on the vena cava, a large vein, might impede blood flow in the mother and compromise the fetus's oxygen supply. After the first trimester, sports that require agility, balance, and strength should be avoided because of the risk of musculoskeletal injury. Exercises that involve bouncing are controversial and may best be avoided, as should sports that require quick twisting and turning or that are associated with high rates of injury. No new strenuous exercises should be taken up. During the third trimester, mobility will be restricted and women will no longer be able to engage in many of their customary activities (Carlson & Parrish, 1998).

Exercises designed to prepare the body for labor and delivery can be done during pregnancy. Instructions on how to do pelvic floor exercises, Kegel exercises, the pelvic rock, leg lifts, and ankle rolling are available from healthcare providers and childbirth education instructors.

Planning for Birth and Childcare

The birth of a child is a major event in the life of any person or couple. A **birth plan** is a tool that expectant parents can use to explore their childbirth and childcare options and choose those most important to them. The process of preparing the birth plan can also enhance communication between the pregnant woman and her partner, if applicable, and between the couple and the healthcare provider. The topics and options that are explored during the preparation of the birth plan include the following: choice of birth setting; the nature of the partner's participation in the process; what technological devices will be used; whether older children, other relatives, or friends will be present; whether music, soft lighting, and the like are desired; who will cut the umbilical cord; how the baby will be fed; how long the mother will remain in the hospital/birthing center after birth; and what arrangements will be made for caring for the baby after birth.

A woman expecting to bring a child home after delivery must be fully aware of how dependent on her that child will be. Women should not hesitate to look to their partners, family members, and other resources for support—including help with the household chores after delivery. Healthcare providers should be able to provide information on options for community support, if needed. The place where the baby will sleep must be identified, and needed baby furniture and clothing must be acquired. Mothers who plan to work outside their homes after the baby is born must also make plans for childcare.

Sex During Pregnancy

Sex does not have to end when pregnancy begins. The common perception that pregnant women are no longer sexual beings has more to do with societal perceptions than physi-

ology. Many pregnant women wonder whether the sexual feelings they have while pregnant are normal and whether having sex will put their babies at risk. Fantasies about sex during pregnancy are normal and common to most, if not all, pregnant women. In most cases, intercourse during pregnancy will not harm a fetus. However, there are certain conditions under which healthcare providers will advise pregnant women not to have sex: If a woman has had more than one spontaneous abortion (miscarriage), intercourse may prove a risk for her pregnancy. This is also true if a woman is showing signs of threatened miscarriage in either her first or third trimester. If there is leakage of fluid or bleeding from the vagina at any time, intercourse should not be attempted and the healthcare provider should be notified. If intercourse causes pain, it should be suspended and a provider consulted.

Protecting the fetus from toxins to which it may be exposed as a result of intercourse is also a consideration. If a male partner works in an environment in which toxins are known to concentrate in sperm, a condom should be worn (Boston Women's Health Collective, 1998). Although having sex during pregnancy usually causes no harm, it is not mandatory. The most important thing is for partners to talk over their options, such as sexual activity with or without vaginal intercourse, and to make decisions that they both find comfortable and satisfying.

Attitudes and Emotions

In the first trimester, a woman may feel ambivalent about her pregnancy, or she may be shocked to find herself pregnant. Such feelings are normal; they usually dissipate by the end of the first trimester and are replaced by acceptance (Rubin, 1984). Some mothers have trouble accepting changes in the appearance of their bodies. Negative feeling can also be reinforced by a partner's attitudes. It is important for couples to talk these feelings through and to seek out information and counseling through a maternal healthcare provider and other professionals. Problematic attitudes toward pregnancy on the part of family, friends, or society in general should be discussed with professionals.

The emotional changes seen during pregnancy include mood instability, resentment, and sometimes euphoria. These changes are likely to be the byproducts of physiological, especially hormonal, changes (O'Brien, 2000). Lifestyle changes and the mother's advancing pregnancy may affect both partners' emotions (see Table 23–3). Depression may occur during pregnancy, and requires treatment if severe or prolonged.

Signs of Impending Miscarriage

It is not uncommon for women to miscarry a pregnancy, particularly a first pregnancy, during the first trimester. The

TABLE 23-3   Family changes during the childbearing cycle.

Family Component	Changes During Childbearing
Structure	First pregnancy involves shift from stable (wife-husband) dyad to a volatile (mother-father-child) triangle. Subsequent pregnancies involve development of several complex, shifting triangular structures. Family members must occasionally cope with being the "isolate" the individual left out when two members of a triangle temporarily form a dyad in a triangle. Stress and tension may increase. Additional subsystems must be established: mother-child; father-child; sibling; grandparent-grandchild.
Power	Patterns often alter; egalitarian power patterns often become more "traditional," with father as decision maker. Fetus and newborn may become very powerful in family system, producing major changes in parents' behavior and family patterns.
Boundaries	Mother's boundary incorporates another human, the embryo-fetus within; mother becomes a "protective" container for fetus, progressively closing in and focusing her attention inward. Father's boundary must expand to give support and become empathetic with mother. Family boundary must become highly permeable to selected input—for example, healthcare and education.
Affect (feelings)	Stress arising from structural change may alter feeling tone in family system. Danger signs are perception of hidden anger and hostility; pervasive depression; and apathy; unresponsiveness, or "flat" emotion.
Intergenerational patterns and roles	Parents' parents must "move up" a generation to become grandparents. Each member of the family system (both nuclear and extended) must assume new roles—whether it is a first or subsequent pregnancy.
Communication patterns	Family members must learn to communicate as a triangle. One member needs to learn to tolerate being a temporary outsider, or "isolate," left out of communications, because only two people can communicate at one time.
Cultural background and rituals	Family members from different cultural backgrounds may have different values concerning pregnancy and childbearing, may perceive new roles differently, and may have different practices and rituals for this event. Differences can produce family conflict and stress.

Source: *Maternity Nursing: Care of the Childbearing Family* 3e by Sherwen/Scoloveno/Weingarten, Copyright 1999. Reprinted by permission of Pearson Education, Inc., Upper Saddle River, NJ.

symptoms of miscarriage are abdominal pain and vaginal bleeding. Having a single miscarriage does not mean a woman cannot sustain a healthy pregnancy later. The warning signs of trouble with pregnancy during the second trimester include the leakage of fluid or blood from the vagina, unusual vaginal discharge, abdominal pain, generalized edema, severe headaches, visual disturbances, and dizziness. *Should any of these symptoms appear, medical care should be sought immediately.*

During the third trimester, additional warning signs include the absence of fetal movement in a 12-hour period and painful urination. The signs of early labor, such as low pelvic pressure or rhythmic low back pain, especially in addition to abdominal pain, cramps, or contractions, should be reported to a healthcare provider immediately.

Minor Problems

The profound physiological and anatomical changes associated with the pregnant state bring with them a host of minor, but uncomfortable and annoying, problems—such as nausea and vomiting, constipation, heartburn, hemorrhoids, round ligament and back pain, fatigue, urinary frequency and burning, edema, leg cramps, changes in pigmentation, stretch marks, varicose veins, dyspnea, flatus (intestinal gas), hair loss, and cravings, among other discomforts.

NAUSEA AND VOMITING

Many pregnant women experience nausea and vomiting. A woman can be nauseated but not vomit at all, or she can be both nauseated and vomit some or all of the time. These symptoms are normal and, unless severe and long-lasting, do not harm either the pregnant woman or her baby. Usually, nausea and vomiting occur early in pregnancy, during the first three to four months, and is commonly referred to as **morning sickness.** However, some women have these symptoms beyond the first trimester and at various times of the day. Some experience them throughout their pregnancies.

The hormonal changes that occur during the first trimester of pregnancy, such as increased levels of estrogen, cause nausea and vomiting by stimulating the vomiting center in the brain stem and decreasing motility in the stomach and intestines. They also alter the digestion of sugar. Viral or bacterial infections can also contribute to nausea and vomiting, as can emotional disturbances.

Morning sickness can often be minimized via dietary changes. Reducing fat intake and avoiding foods high in refined sugar, such as cakes, candy, cookies and soda, can be helpful, as can eating more complex carbohydrates, such as cereals, crackers, and breads. If nausea and vomiting occur, meals should be smaller and more frequent; six smaller meals spread out throughout the day and evening are recommended. Eating on awakening can also help—dry crackers can be kept at bedside. Another strategy is not drinking fluids for 30 minutes before and after meals. Consuming lots of water may also lessen symptoms, as may eating a protein snack of hard-boiled eggs, cottage cheese, or cheese before going to bed. Taking no more than 50 mg of vitamin B-6 three times a day has been shown to enhance liver activity, which can diminish nausea (Zeidenstein, 1998). However, this practice should not be discontinued abruptly, because withdrawal from pyridoxal-5-phosphate (the active form of vitamin B-6) can have negative result in mothers or babies. Vitamin B-6 should be taken in dosages no higher than 20 mg a day after birth because exceeding this amount can reduce milk production. Other supplements helpful in easing morning sickness include vitamins B-12, C, and E and extra magnesium and potassium (Somer, 1995). Safe herbal teas, such as goldenseal, peppermint, spearmint, and raspberry leaf, should also help mitigate symptoms (Somer, 1995). Deep breathing and relaxing can also help with nausea. Recently, a wristband was developed that applies pressure to the wrist to help control the nausea and vomiting of pregnancy by stimulating a pressure point in the wrist (Evans et al., 1993). In severe cases, healthcare providers can prescribe antinausea medication.

CONSTIPATION

Constipation can be a problem throughout pregnancy, especially in the third trimester, because of decreased GI motility. Constipation can also be a problem following delivery. See Chapter 15 for general information about preventing and treating constipation. Stool softeners and other laxative preparations should be used only if necessary and with a healthcare provider's approval.

HEARTBURN

Heartburn is a common, benign problem that normally dissipates after birth. Many women get heartburn after meals or when bending or lying down. Although heartburn can occur at any time during a pregnancy, it is most common in the third trimester, when the enlarged uterus compresses the stomach. The resulting decrease in gastric motility and gastric acid secretion delays digestion and leads to fullness, indigestion, and heartburn. Hormonal influences also promote heartburn; progesterone relaxes the gastroesophageal sphincter, which allows an upward movement of gastric contents, which irritate the lower esophagus.

Some general strategies for preventing and treating heartburn are outlined in Chapter 15. Pregnant women should eat smaller but more frequent meals and limit fluids with meals, in order to prevent heartburn. Bicarbonate of soda and other medicines should not be taken because of possible risks to the fetus. Safe, natural remedies that can relieve heartburn and are safe for pregnant women include peppermint or chamomile tea, raw papaya or papaya juice, slippery elm bark powder in capsules as needed, almonds, cashews, and filberts (Frye, 1998). There are no known documented or dangerous side effects to using these foods or herbs during pregnancy (Gagnon, 1993). When heartburn is experienced, drinking a large glass or two of plain water will help dilute the acid, and drinking three to four ounces of milk may temporarily relieve discomfort. Lying on the right side will also drain the acid away from the esophagus. Lying on the right side 30 minutes before meals may also help. If none of these measures reduces discomfort, a healthcare provider should be consulted, and she may prescribe safe antacids.

HEMORRHOIDS

Hemorrhoids are varicose veins inside and/or outside the anal opening. Hemorrhoids can develop during pregnancy because of the pressure the enlarged womb exerts on the lower intestine and rectum—especially during the last trimester. In addition, the normal hormonal changes of pregnancy relax smooth muscle tissue, which enables hemorrhoidal veins to swell and protrude outside the anus. If a woman has hemorrhoids prior to pregnancy, they may itch and bleed more during pregnancy. Preventing constipation (see Chapter 15) helps minimize the possibility that hemorrhoids will develop, because straining to pass hard stools dilates veins. If hemorrhoids are already present, laying a cold compress soaked with witch hazel on the area for 15 to 20 minutes may provide relief. Ice packs applied to the anal area may also relieve discomfort. External hemorrhoids can be gently pushed inside the rectum with a finger that has been lubricated with petroleum jelly. Placing petroleum jelly inside the rectum just prior to a bowel movement may make it easier to pass a stool. Ointments available from the drug store may reduce the inflammation of hemorrhoids, but, because all topical drugs are absorbed through the skin, healthcare providers should be consulted about which preparations are safe to use when pregnant. Hemorrhoids are usually most troublesome right after delivery. As a rule, they should disappear within two weeks of giving birth. A healthcare provider can be consulted, if necessary.

ROUND LIGAMENT AND BACK PAIN

Both pelvic structures called the round ligaments and the muscles and nerves in the mother's back can give rise to pain during pregnancy. The round ligaments are fibrous cords that support the front and sides of the uterus and undergo considerable enlargement during pregnancy. This expansion comes in response to the considerable amount of tension placed on these ligaments as the uterus grows, rises out of the pelvis, and tilts forward. Tension on the ligaments can produce sharp, shooting pelvic pains, which usually occur in the second half of pregnancy, especially during the third trimester. These pains can become more frequent as pregnancy progresses. They are most likely to be felt when making a quick movement, getting up from a chair or bed, or after sexual intercourse. Poor posture may also contribute. Round ligament pain goes away after birth.

Backache during pregnancy is caused by strain on the muscles and ligaments that support the back. The weight of the fetus changes the mother's center of gravity, which strains the lower back. Hormones soften groin muscles, which results in more strain being placed on the abdomen and back. Pain in the upper back usually results from the tilt of the mother's head, neck, and enlarging breasts. Back pain is most often a problem for multiparous (having experienced more than one pregnancy) women, though it can afflict any mother with poor abdominal muscle tone and posture. As pregnancy advances, episodes of back pain are likely to become more frequent. Performing exercises that strengthen the back may prevent discomfort. Mothers can obtain information about helpful exercises and additional strategies for minimizing and soothing back pain from their healthcare providers.

FATIGUE

Fatigue most often occurs in the first and third trimesters of pregnancy. It also is perhaps the most common complaint in the period following childbirth (Somer, 1995). Fatigue is caused by physiological changes, including changing hormone levels and increasing weight, which can negatively affect sleep and add to the effort of getting through the day. Emotional changes that fuel sleeplessness can also contribute to fatigue.

To combat fatigue, pregnant women must set aside enough hours for sleep, including, if possible, naps during the day. Caffeine should be avoided, and fluids should be consumed well before bedtime in order to avoid interrupting sleep with the need to urinate. Iron-rich foods are most important, as well as combining carbohydrate- and protein-rich foods to regulate energy and blood sugar levels (Somer, 1995). Warm milk before bed can also aid sleep, because milk contains the amino acid tryptophan, which is the raw material for serotonin, a chemical in the brain that has a calming effect. In addition to milk, other dietary sources of tryptophan are bananas, cottage cheese, and turkey (*The Physician's Desk Reference: A Family Guide to Natural Medicine and Healing Therapies*, 1999). Getting regular exercise should also help in avoiding fatigue. Women with unyielding fatigue should be screened for depression and referrals for follow-up made when appropriate (Sherwen, Scoloveno, & Weingarten, 1999). See Chapter 6 for more information about sleep and problems with sleep.

URINARY FREQUENCY AND BURNING

Urinary frequency—the need to urinate very often—can continue throughout pregnancy. Even in the first trimester, pressure exerted on the bladder by the developing fetus can precipitate the need to urinate. By the third trimester, this pressure becomes more extreme, and the movement of the fetus to a lower position in the pelvis during the last month of pregnancy further increases the need to urinate frequently. There is little that pregnant women can do to avoid urinary frequency. Fluid intake should definitely *not* be reduced, as this creates dehydration and actually makes frequency worse; the concentrated urine irritates the bladder and causes the sensation of needing to urinate.

Pregnant women should be aware of the signs and symptoms of urinary infection and, if such signs are present, should contact their healthcare providers as soon as possible, so that any infection can be treated promptly. They should also observe hygiene-related and other practices that prevent urinary tract infection (see Chapter 16). Dysuria, difficult or painful urination, which occurs in the third trimester can be a sign of difficulty with the pregnancy and is a reason to seek immediate medical care.

SWELLING

Swelling (edema) is a result of the normal physiological increase in tissue fluids caused by the increased blood volume and hormone levels of pregnancy. Normal swelling occurs in the second and third trimesters of pregnancy—usually below the waistline. *Dependent* edema is said to exist when fluid accumulates in the legs and feet throughout the day due to gravity; pregnant women often complain that their shoes are too tight. Edema can also be *generalized*, appearing in the face, hands, and feet. Generalized edema can become severe and problematic. A pregnant woman who awakens with generalized swelling and experiences dizziness, blurred vision, headaches, upper abdominal pain, or nausea should seek medical care immediately.

The techniques for the relief of dependent edema include elevating the feet and legs and wearing support panty hose, particularly when standing for long periods during the day. Also effective are changing position often, avoiding long car rides, and not standing in one position for a long time.

Lying on the left side, whenever possible, to keep the weight of the fetus off the large vein that returns blood to the heart, and rocking from the ball of the foot to the toes to stimulate leg circulation, also help. Foods high in *sodium,* such as lunch meats, potato chips, and other highly processed or prepared foods, should be avoided, because they promote water retention. However, even if swelling is occurring, pregnant women need to make sure they take in enough fluid and salt to make up for possible losses through perspiration, especially during the summer months.

LEG CRAMPS

Leg cramps are a common problem during the second and third trimesters, because uterine pressure impedes blood flow to and from the legs. Diet can also play a role if the woman is not consuming enough of certain minerals such as calcium. The sudden stretching of leg muscles can also cause cramps (Frye, 1998). If leg cramps are persistent, they should be mentioned to a healthcare provider because of the possibility that **phlebitis,** an inflammation of the veins, is present. This possibility should be investigated before repeatedly massaging cramped muscles, for the following reason: If phlebitis is present, a blood clot may have formed in the involved vein. Massage might dislodge the clot, causing it to travel upward in the venous system and through the heart until it finally obstructs an artery in the lung. The resulting **pulmonary embolism** can be life-threatening.

If leg cramps are related to deficiencies in minerals such as calcium, magnesium, or sodium, the condition can be remedied by eating more foods rich in those nutrients (see Chapter 3). If the mother is already consuming the amount of dietary calcium recommended, an increased phosphorus intake may be causing the calcium to be excreted and a higher calcium intake may be needed. This possibility should be discussed with a healthcare provider. Carbonated soft drinks are a common source of excess phosphorus in the diet.

Wearing support panty hose will increase circulation to the feet and lessen the possibility of cramping. Switching from high heels to flats during the day can be a trigger for cramps and should be avoided. Muscle-relaxing techniques, such as stretching, may also be useful in preventing leg cramps, because they improve blood flow to the extremities (Sherwen et al., 1999). The stretch should be gentle and constant, with no jerking.

CHANGES IN PIGMENTATION

Darkening of the skin during pregnancy is caused by an increase in the production of ovarian and pituitary hormones that affect **melanocytes,** the cells within the skin that produce the pigment melanin. The areas that can darken, typically beginning in the second trimester, include the areola, the midline of the abdomen, the armpits, the perineum, and the face. The dark line that sometimes extends down the center of the abdomen is called the **linea nigra.** A darkening

of patches of skin on the face is known as **chloasma.** Hyperpigmentation usually returns to normal after pregnancy.

Protecting the face from sunlight can minimize chloasma. Women can safely use zinc oxide on the face to block out the sun's rays while they are outside. Strong commercial products should not be used to bleach out hyperpigmented areas during pregnancy, but applying lemon wedges to the face is safe and may lighten the skin.

STRETCH MARKS

Starting in the second trimester, **striae gravidarium,** abdominal stretch marks, develop because of increases in the hormones *relaxin* and *estrogen.* Both hormones promote tissue absorption of water, which in turn relaxes the skin's collagen fibers. The relaxed collagen fibers separate easily, causing stretch marks to appear. Unfortunately, there is not much that can be done to alleviate stretch marks. The discoloration that accompanies the marks will become less noticeable and fade after delivery, even though the stretch marks themselves will remain. If the skin is also dry, moisturizing lotions or cocoa butter can be used.

VARICOSE VEINS

Varicose veins develop when blood pools in the extremities due to hormonal influences and interference with circulation during pregnancy or because of hereditary abnormalities in vein structure. During the second trimester of pregnancy, the hormone *progesterone* relaxes the vein walls, making it difficult for blood to return to the heart from the extremities. Also, the enlarged uterus exerts pressure on the abdominal veins, thereby reducing blood return from the lower limbs and exacerbating pooling.

Pregnant women should avoid round garters, knee-high stockings, and tight waist bands, because their tourniquet-like effect impedes venous return to the heart. Standing with the knees locked should also be avoided, because it causes muscle contractions in the legs that prevent proper venous return. Wearing elastic support panty hose and putting them on while lying down improves blood flow in the veins, as do changing positions frequently during the day, avoiding prolonged standing or sitting, and elevating the legs and hips with the knees flexed and supported by pillows. Walking also helps, as the rhythmic contractions of the calf muscles "milk" the blood back up to the heart.

SHORTNESS OF BREATH

Shortness of breath, known medically as **dyspnea**, can occur during pregnancy because the growth of the fetus and uterus prevents complete lung expansion. This symptom appears later in pregnancy and is usually mild. Adjusting body position to allow maximal expansion of the chest and avoiding large meals largely prevent dyspnea. Some women can breathe better if they sleep with the head of their bed raised on blocks or with pillows behind their back. Healthcare practitioners can instruct women experiencing this symptom on *abdominal breathing,* in which the abdomen, not the chest, rises and falls with each breath. If symptoms are not relieved or worsen, women should seek medical attention immediately.

GAS

Intestinal gas, or **flatus,** is most commonly a problem in the third trimester. Increased amounts of intestinal gas are formed during pregnancy because the enlarged uterus compresses the bowel. This compression delays the passage of food through the intestines, thus allowing more time for gas to be formed by bacteria in the colon. The presence of excess gas, plus the decrease in intestinal tone caused by the muscle-relaxing effects of progesterone, can lead to abdominal distention.

To decrease flatus, pregnant women should avoid gas-forming foods, such as beans, cabbage, and onions, as well as foods that contain a lot of white sugar. Adding bran and roughage to the diet will also decrease gas, as will increasing fluid intake, exercising, and using comforting herbal teas, such as chamomile (Gagnon, 1993). Eating four or five small meals a day rather than three large meals should also provide some relief.

HAIR LOSS

Some women experience hair loss during pregnancy; occasionally, up to 40 percent of a given woman's hair has fallen out by the time the child is delivered. Although hair loss is not a well-understood phenomenon, it is thought to be related to hormonal changes (Somer, 1995). A healthy lifestyle—consuming a healthy, nutrient-rich diet and getting enough rest—may prevent or curtail hair loss but is not guaranteed to do so. When hair loss occurs, there is nothing to do but let this symptom run its course. Mothers should be reassured that their hair will grow back.

CRAVINGS

Cravings for certain foods and beverages are common during pregnancy. Such cravings, which are likely to begin during the first trimester, do not appear to reflect a true physiological need. Foods with a high sodium or sugar content are the ones often craved (Frye, 1998).

Sometimes, women crave substances that do not fall into the category of food. A craving for something such as starch, laundry detergent, clay, dirt, ice, or wax is known as **pica.** Pica is more widespread than is believed by many healthcare professionals (Kolasa & Weismiller, 1995). The desire to consume nonnutritive substances may indicate a severe dietary deficiency of minerals or vitamins, particularly iron.

Women experiencing food cravings should be steered toward healthy foods rather than junk food, both to assure healthy nutrition and avoid undue weight gain. Women experiencing pica should be cautioned about eating nonfood products, because this behavior can adversely affect their own nu-

trition and well-being, as well as that of their baby. Nutritional counseling is important in such cases, and testing for parasites or poisoning may be indicated (Sherwen et al., 1999).

OTHER DISCOMFORTS OF PREGNANCY

Other, less common but not unusual, discomforts can arise during pregnancy (Sherwen et al., 1999). These include headache, cramping, dizziness, urinary incontinence, heavy vaginal discharge, bleeding from the nose or gums, excessive salivation, experiences of bad tastes and smells, food intolerances, upper body aches, Braxton-Hicks (transitory uterine) contractions, aching joints, carpel tunnel syndrome, and **supine hypotension syndrome,** which is the low blood pressure that can occur when the pregnant woman lies on her back. Healthcare providers should be consulted if any of these symptoms become unmanageable, and *no medications, even over-the-counter drugs (such as aspirin), should be used without consultation.* Some general measures that will help with some of these complaints include ample rest, a good diet, good dental care, and the use of relaxation techniques.

Complications of Pregnancy

Serious **complications,** or adverse developments during pregnancy, occur infrequently, but, when they do occur, they threaten the health or life of the fetus, and perhaps of the mother as well. Maternal death due to complications related to pregnancy or birth is rare, but the risk for African American women is three to four times that of Euro-American women, and the risk for Hispanic, Asian, and American Indian women, although lower than that of African American women, is still higher than that of Euro-American women (Pregnancy-related deaths among black, Hispanic, Asian/Pacific Islander, and American Indian/ Alaska Native Women—United States, 1991–1997, 2001). The complications of pregnancy include Rh incompatibility (in which the mother's immune system attacks the fetus's red blood cells), placental problems, excessive vomiting, and hypertension.

RH-NEGATIVE MOTHERS

Blood tests done early in pregnancy can determine whether a mother has Rh-negative (without the Rh factor) blood. If she does, and her fetus has Rh-positive blood (blood that contains the Rh factor), her immune system will become sensitized to the foreign Rh antigen and will start to build up antibodies, which will attack the Rh-positive blood of the child. The number of antibodies produced the first time an Rh-negative woman carries an Rh-positive child is usually not sufficient to harm the fetus, but, in future pregnancies with Rh-positive fetuses, the antibody response can severely compromise or kill the child. To avoid this scenario, Rh-negative mothers who are carrying Rh-positive babies are given an injection of **Rh immune globulin (RhoGam)** within 72 hours of delivery. This prevents potentially fatal damage to future Rh-positive fetuses. Rh-negative mothers with Rh-positive babies must receive RhoGam even if the first pregnancy ends in miscarriage or abortion. In a small number of cases, antibodies that will attack the fetus are produced, anyway. An injection of RhoGam at 28 weeks is recommended in these cases, followed by another dose after delivery. Receiving RhoGam is safe for both mothers and their babies (Verilli & Mueser, 1998).

PLACENTAL PROBLEMS

Because the placenta is a highly vascular organ, any alteration in its placement or attachment can result in serious hemmorhage, with great risk for the mother and fetus. Often, there is no indication of a problem until bleeding and/or pain occur. The two placental problems that develop most frequently are placenta previa and abruptio placentae.

Placenta Previa   In placenta previa, the placenta implants in the lower segment of the uterus instead of higher up. As it grows, it ends up near or covering the inside of the cervix (see Figure 23–4). Women at risk for developing this disorder include those with a large placenta, uterine scarring, or prior surgery of the reproductive tract, as well as those who are 35 years of age or older. The key symptom of placenta previa is *painless* vaginal bleeding in the second or third trimester as a result of the placenta's separating from the uterine wall as the cervix begins to dilate. Unless the placenta is completely separated from the uterine wall, delivery is postponed until at least 36 weeks' gestation, when the fetus is more mature. If separation is complete, cesarean section is the delivery method of choice unless the placenta is only slightly out of place and will move up in the uterus during labor. In such a case vaginal delivery may be preferred, because the fetal head will put pressure on the bleeding area during labor.

Abruptio Placenta   Abruptio placenta is the *premature separation* of a normally implanted placenta. It usually occurs after 20 weeks' gestation. There are three major types of abruptio placenta: *marginal,* in which the edge separates, causing external bleeding; *central,* in which the placenta separates in the middle, causing concealed hemmorhage; and *complete,* in which the placenta separates entirely, causing external and internal bleeding.

   The key symptoms with this disorder are *pain* and *bleeding.* With a small area of separation, there is a small amount of bleeding, mild pain, and, in most cases, a healthy fetus. On the other hand, if the area of separation is large, there is usually heavy bleeding, severe abdominal pain, and a boardlike feel to the mother's abdomen. She will quickly go into shock from the heavy bleeding, and the fetus will exhibit signs of distress

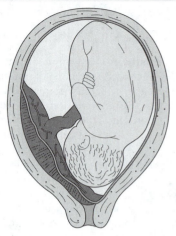

Figure 23–4   Placenta Previa

Source: *Maternal-Newborn Nursing: A Family and Community-based Approach* 6e–Clinical Handbook by Olds/London/Ladewig, Copyright 2000. Reprinted with permission of Pearson Education, Inc., Upper Saddle River, NJ.

from a lack of oxygen. The goals of treatment are to control the bleeding and deliver a healthy fetus in the shortest amount of time via a cesarean section. However, if the bleeding occurs when the mother is in active labor and delivery is imminent, a vaginal delivery may be considered.

EXCESSIVE VOMITING

Nausea and vomiting from the sixth through the twelfth weeks (first trimester) of pregnancy is common and not serious. However, in **hyperemesis gravidarum,** excessive nausea and vomiting of pregnancy, the problem goes well beyond normal, lasting four to eight weeks or longer. The mother vomits several times each day, and is unable to retain food or fluids. Left unchecked, this results in dehydration, weight loss, stomach pain, and heartburn, putting the fetus at risk for fetal growth retardation because of the mother's poor nutrition. There are many theories, both physical and psychological, as to the cause of excessive vomiting: (1) an endocrine imbalance related to increased amounts of estrogen; (2) the presence of pieces of the placenta in the maternal circulation; and (3) maternal stress, leading to the mother's rejecting the pregnancy and "vomiting the child." The actual cause is unknown.

   The early treatment of hyperemesis is aimed at preventing significant maternal weight loss and fetal growth retardation. If the problem is severe, the mother is hospitalized, put on a restricted intake of food and fluids until the vomiting stops, and started on intravenous fluids with vitamins. She gradually begins frequent small feedings, avoiding greasy foods and foods that provoke the symptoms. Counseling may be offered to rule out any psychological factors that may be causing the problem.

HYPERTENSIVE DISORDERS

Blood pressure elevation in pregnancy and the complications related to it are *the major contributors to illness and/or death in both mother and fetus*. Hypertension is believed to be present in about 7 percent of all pregnancies. Hypertension can be problematic for mothers who were hypertensive prior to pregnancy, or it can arise as a result of the pregnancy (**pre-eclampsia**). Also, pre-existing hypertension can be exacerbated (worsened) by the pregnancy. Pre-eclampsia most commonly occurs during the third trimester and is diagnosed by the presence of severe edema, elevation in blood pressure, and/or the presence of protein in the urine (proteinuria). If untreated, pre-eclampsia can progress to true eclampsia, producing life-threatening seizures in the mother. In another type of hypertension, which occurs only in the second half of pregnancy, during labor, or within 48 hours of delivery, blood pressure is elevated, but there is no protein in the urine.

The cause of the hypertensive disorders that arise during pregnancy is still unknown, and many different theories regarding it exist. The risk factors include extremes of maternal age, family history, first pregnancy, and a history of pre-eclampsia and/or hypertension. Mothers who are hypertensive during pregnancy are closely monitored. They may be put on bed rest and their kidney and liver function monitored. Salt in the diet will be restricted. Fetal assessment will include a biweekly nonstress test and biophysical profile, and mothers will be asked to do frequent and careful fetal kick counts. Calcium supplements and low-dose aspirin have been used in some cases, but their role in prevention is not yet clear. Research in this area continues.

Labor and Delivery

Labor and delivery can be likened to a journey into the unknown. Labor is a unique experience for each woman, and subsequent labors may be different for the same woman. Labor is generally easier for women who are physically fit, have maintained good prenatal care, have a good support system in place, and are well educated about how to help make their labor more comfortable.

Preliminary Signs of Labor

There are six occurrences just prior to the onset of labor that signal the pregnant woman that the time for delivery is nearing. These include lightening (the mother's abdomen feels less heavy), weight loss, a burst of energy, stronger Braxton-Hicks contractions, a bloody show (discharge from the vagina), and rupture of membranes. Even when all of these symptoms occur, it is often very difficult for the mother to determine if she is truly in labor.

As suggested by the word *lightening*, the pregnant woman's abdomen suddenly feels less heavy as the fetus drops lower in her pelvis in preparation for birth. Breathing becomes easier, but additional pressure is placed on the bladder. In a woman expecting her first child, lightening occurs about two weeks prior to the onset of labor; in subsequent pregnancies, however, it may not occur until labor is well underway. *Weight loss* occurs when hormone levels change a few days prior to the onset of labor. The body retains less fluid, and the mother may lose as much as three pounds. Some mothers become alarmed by this occurrence and fear that the fetus has stopped growing or died. Also just prior to the onset of labor, the woman may find herself full of *energy*, with a desire to prepare her home for the baby's arrival. Carrying out these preparations is known popularly as *nesting*. The energy burst is related to a surge in the hormone adrenaline. It is intended to provide the mother's body with enough energy for the work of labor. It is wise, however, for mothers to resist the temptation to do too much, lest they use up all of their stored energy and become quickly exhausted once labor begins.

The *Braxton-Hicks* contractions that have been occurring periodically throughout the pregnancy become stronger as the onset of labor approaches, but they are usually not strong enough to make the mother think she is in true labor. As the cervix begins to dilate from pressure put on it by the baby's head, the blood-tinged mucus that has plugged the cervix to protect the uterus throughout pregnancy is released. At times, this mucus is quite bloody, making it difficult for the mother to determine whether she is experiencing a *bloody show* or a potentially dangerous bleeding episode. The amniotic sac ruptures prior to the onset of labor in about 12 percent of women. In the remainder of women, it ruptures well after labor has begun, either spontaneously or when a healthcare provider performs an **amniotomy,** which is the artificial rupture of the membrane (see Figure 23–5). If the membranes should rupture at home, it is important that the mother inspect the fluid for *color,* which is normally clear with specks of white and fetal hair in it; *odor*—there normally is none; and *amount*—normally a large amount. The mother should also make sure there is *fetal movement* following the rupture of the membranes. This is an indication that the fetus is not in danger. Once the mother's water breaks, she should call her healthcare provider and go to the hospital to be examined, even if she is not experiencing any contractions. Once the water breaks, there is a 24-hour window during which the baby should be delivered; after this, the danger of infection in the mother and the fetus increases.

It is often difficult for the mother to determine if she is really in labor, especially if this is her first experience with the process (see Table 23–4). It is important however, that the mother not hesitate to contact her healthcare provider even if she is uncertain.

Figure 23-5   Amniotomy

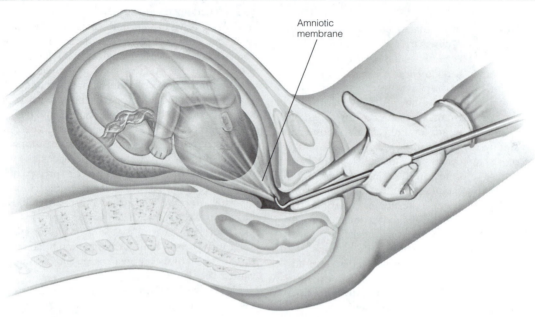

Amniotic
membrane

Source: *Nursing Care of the Childbearing Family* 2e by Sherwen/Scoloveno/Weingarten, Copyright 1995. Reprinted wtih permission of Pearson Education, Inc., Upper Saddle River, NJ.

TABLE 23-4   Comparison of true and false labor.

True Labor	False Labor
Contractions are at regular intervals.	Contractions are irregular.
Intervals between contractions gradually shorten.	There is usually no change.
Contractions increase in duration and intensity.	There is usually no change.
Discomfort begins in back and radiates around to abdomen.	Discomfort is usually in abdomen.
Intensity usually increases with walking.	Walking has no effect on or lessens contractions.
Cervical dilatation and effacement are progressive.	There is no change.

Source: *Maternal Newborn Nursing: A Family and Community-based Approach* 6e–Clinical Handbook by Olds/London/Ladewig, Copyright 2000. Reprinted with permission of Pearson Education, Inc., Upper Saddle River, NJ.

Stages of Labor

There are four *stages* of labor, with three distinct *phases* within the first stage. Even a mother who experiences a pre-cipitous (fast) labor and delivery goes through all of the stages, although very quickly. The four stages of labor are the dilatation stage, the expulsive stage, the placental stage, and the restorative stage.

DILATATION STAGE

The first stage of labor begins with the first *true contraction* and ends with full *dilation* (opening) of the cervix. The combined pressure from the fetus and the amniotic fluid helps this process occur. Initially, the contractions experienced in this stage are far apart and fairly comfortable. At the end of the stage, however, they become more forceful, frequent, and uncomfortable. There are three distinct phases of this first stage of labor: the latent phase, the active phase, and the transition phase.

Latent Phase   This phase begins with the onset of regular contractions and is fairly comfortable for the mother. She is very sociable and excited, usually walking around, but still exhibiting some anxiety. She experiences her contractions as a low backache with cramps similar to menstrual cramps. During the normal 12- to 14-hour duration of this phase, the cervix (uterine opening) dilates to 3–4 centimeters and becomes completely **effaced,** or thinned out (see Figure 23–6). The latent phase is sometimes referred to as the *warm-up* phase of labor.

Active Phase   *Active* is an appropriate word for this phase because of the increasing speed at which labor progresses.

Figure 23–6   Effacement of the Cervix

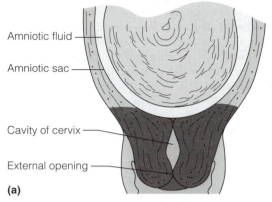

Amniotic fluid

Amniotic sac

Cavity of cervix

External opening

(a)

At the beginning of labor, there is no cervical effacement or dilation. the fetal head is cushioned by amniotic fluid.

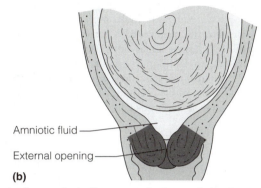

Amniotic fluid

External opening

(b)

Beginning cervical effacement: As the cervix begins to efface, more amniotic fluid collects below the fetal head.

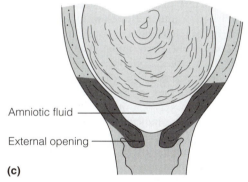

Amniotic fluid

External opening

(c)

Cervix is about one-half effaced and slightly dilated. The increasing amount of amniotic fluid below the fetal head exerts hydrostatic pressure on the cervix.

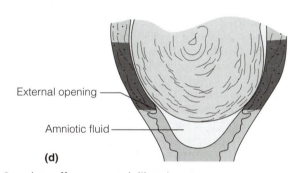

External opening

Amniotic fluid

(d)

Complete effacement and dilatation occurs.

Source: *Maternal Newborn Nursing: A Family and Community-based Approach* 6e–Clinical Handbook by Olds/London/Ladewig, Copyright 2000. Reprinted with permission of Pearson Education, Inc., Upper Saddle River, NJ.

This phase can last from a few minutes to as long as six hours; during it, the cervix dilates from 4 centimeters to 8 centimeters as the fetus descends farther in the pelvis, the contractions become more frequent, and discomfort intensifies. The mother becomes more serious and inwardly focused, no longer initiating interactions with those around her. She begins to use the relaxation techniques learned in childbirth education classes as she becomes more uncomfortable. Both she and her coach should be either at, or traveling to, the hospital or birthing center in this phase. This is an ideal time for the mother to request an epidural anesthetic so that she will be more comfortable and be able to work with the contractions. Her membranes rupture during this phase if they have not already done so.

The Transition Phase   This is the shortest but most intense of the phases, lasting anywhere from 15 minutes to 2 hours. It begins when the cervix is dilated to a diameter of 8 centimeters, when contractions become much stronger and closer together. Some mothers liken this phase of their labor to an out-of-body experience because of the very intense feelings they encounter. Some women are overwhelmed by the intensity of their contractions and feel out of control and scared; they want to give up and go home. Nausea, vomiting, shivering, and shaking often occur. The mother may suddenly become very irritable with those around her, often not wanting to be touched or spoken to. It is important that this not be taken personally; nor should the mother attempt to censor herself, as this is a normal occurrence in this phase and will pass with the beginning of the second stage. As the cervix gets closer to full (10 centimeters) dilation, the mother experiences an uncontrollable urge to *push*, as well as strong *rectal pressure*. This is an indication that the fetal head is almost through the cervix, and the mother is about to enter the second stage of labor. Many healthcare providers attempt to prevent the mother from pushing at this time for fear that the cervix, which may not yet be fully dilated, will bruise and swell, thus prolonging labor. However, the latest research shows that the mother should *not* be prevented from pushing but, rather, should be encouraged to bear down when she feels the urge (Petersen & Besuner, 1997).

EXPULSIVE STAGE

The mother actually delivers the child during the expulsion stage, which begins when the cervix becomes fully dilated. During the expulsive stage, the mother typically feels that she is back in control and that her energy has been renewed—even though the contractions are longer, more frequent, and even more intense. She may experience a great feeling of euphoria, as she will soon see the face of her newborn. With each contraction, the mother has an involuntary urge to contract her abdominal muscles and push, to deliver the fetus. The expulsive stage can last from a very few minutes to as long as three hours. It ends with the delivery of the baby.

Recent research has shown that many nurses and other healthcare providers strongly encourage the mother to push intensely with each contraction by holding her breath and bearing down for as long as she can. Their rationale is the need to shorten the second stage of labor in order to prevent extended pressure on the fetal head and umbilical cord, both of which can cause problems for the fetus. However, this sustained, strenuous, style of pushing has been shown to *interfere with oxygen exchange* between the mother and the fetus, putting the fetus at an even greater risk. The newest protocols from The Association of Women's Health and Newborn Nursing (AOWHNN) recommend that healthcare providers discourage prolonged maternal breath holding and, rather, support the mother's involuntary bearing-down efforts, as in the first stage (Petersen & Besuner, 1997).

PLACENTAL STAGE

The placental stage begins after the baby has been delivered. During this stage, the contractions, which temporarily cease at delivery, begin again in order to shrink the size of the uterus and allow the placenta to deliver. The mother may receive a dose of Pitocin (oxytocin), a medication used to contract the uterus, to help deliver the placenta and prevent excessive bleeding. However, a woman's body produces an endogenous (natural) form of oxytocin during the process of breast-feeding, so many women choose to put the newborn to breast immediately after delivery in order to contract the uterus and hasten the separation and delivery of the placenta.

RESTORATIVE STAGE

Not often recognized as a stage of labor, **restoration** is a critical period for new family bonding. It is also an ideal time to begin breast-feeding, as the newborn is usually alert and will suck well. This stage lasts from 1 to 4 hours following delivery, when the mother's body begins to stabilize following the hard work of labor and the loss of the products of conception. She feels exhausted but excited and often experiences a shaking chill, which lasts approximately 20 minutes, although she does not complain of feeling cold. The shaking is caused by the body's production of adrenaline plus its reaction to the loss of the heat from both the fetus and the placenta. The new mother will be watched closely during this stage for any unusual bleeding, changes in blood pressure, or a full bladder, which can cause the uterus to relax, with resultant bleeding.

Monitoring of the Fetus During Labor

The intense nature of labor requires that the fetus be watched closely for any signs of stress, as indicated by changes in its heart rate and rhythm. Often, in early labor, the fetal heart is assessed with the use of a fetoscope or an ultrasonic doppler. These are simple, hand-held devices that are used by the healthcare provider.

As labor progresses, an **electronic fetal monitor (EFM)** may be attached to the mother. It will record her contractions and the reaction of the fetal heartbeat to these contractions, giving an indication of how the fetus is reacting to the stress of labor (see Figure 23–7). Mothers who are at high risk, receiving Pitocin and/or epidural anesthesia, or who develop a problem with labor will almost certainly be attached to a monitor.

There are two different methods of electronic fetal monitoring: external and internal. In *external* monitoring, two doppler devices are strapped to the mother's abdomen, one to monitor the fetus and one to assess the contractions. This method can be used continually but can also be used intermittently to allow the mother to walk around, returning periodically to be monitored for a short period of time (see Figure 23–7).

Internal monitoring involves placing a fetal electrode on the baby via the mother's vagina in order to record the heart tones (see Figure 23–8). If the healthcare provider wishes to also monitor the mother's contractions more accurately, an intrauterine pressure catheter will also be placed inside the uterus.

Internal monitoring is the method of choice if the mother is receiving Pitocin or has developed a problem during labor. Once a mother is connected to this internal monitor, however, she is no longer able to walk around. In recent years, however, a telemetric method of monitoring has been developed: A small box that transmits signals via radio waves is strapped to the mother's thigh and connected to the in-

Figure 23–7   Electronic Fetal Monitoring

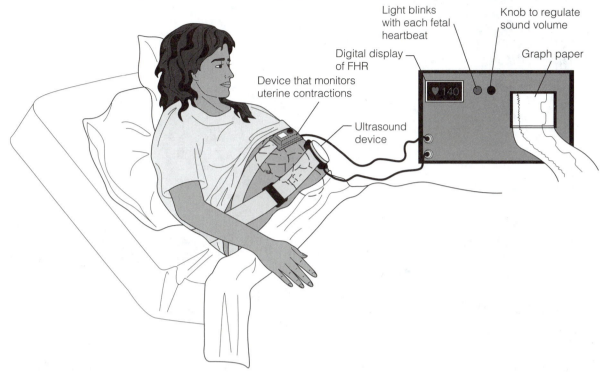

Source: *Maternal Newborn Nursing: A Family and Community-based Approach* 6e–Clinical Handbook by Olds/London/Ladewig, 2000. Reprinted with permission of Pearson Education, Inc., Upper Saddle River, NJ.

ternal monitor leads. This allows vital information about the mother and fetus to be sent to a central monitor at the nurse's station while the mother remains ambulatory.

Pain Control

The pain of childbirth is not the result of pathology but, rather, is a normal and functional occurrence with a limited duration. A certain amount of pain during labor alerts both the mother and the healthcare provider to what is occurring. Pain during labor is caused by the contraction of the uterus, the pressure of the fetus on the perineum, and the stretching of the cervix as it dilates and thins. Other factors can also heighten or lessen the pain of labor. The amount of knowledge the woman has about what is happening to her body, her level of fear or anxiety, her past experiences with pain, her culture, and the amount of support she has all influence the degree to which labor is experienced as painful. The simple fact is that most women *fear* labor, and that fear causes *tension*, which in turn increases pain. Therefore, the goal of any type of pain relief chosen by the mother in labor is to decrease fear and tension, thereby limiting the pain experience. Although there are a number of methods available today, only the most commonly used ones are discussed in this section.

ANALGESICS

Analgesics are medications that are used to promote the mother's comfort and allow her to rest between contractions. Several types of drugs are used as analgesics during labor. *Tranquilizers* help decrease tension and apprehension, as well as relieve any nausea or vomiting. It is important to remember, however, that they do not relieve the pain of labor. *Narcotics* decrease the mother's perception of pain but can also prolong the labor if given too early: Narcotics cause the contractions to decrease in intensity and sometimes stop. Conversely, if given too late (too close to delivery), a narcotic can result in a decreasing fetal heart rate and cause the newborn to be very sleepy at birth. Both of these analgesia options can be used at lower doses in combination with other pain relief options, such as regional anesthetics, to increase the mother's comfort even further.

It is vital that a woman who is offered medication during labor be knowledgeable about the effect that medication

Figure 23–8   Technique for Internal Fetal Monitoring

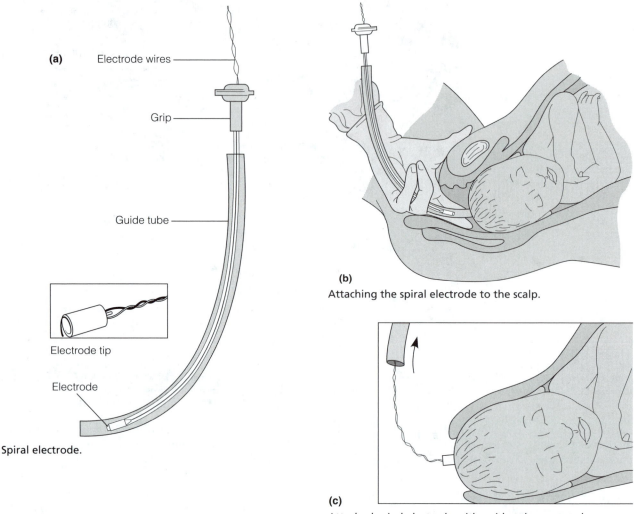

(a) Electrode wires

Grip

Guide tube

Electrode tip

Electrode

Spiral electrode.

(b) Attaching the spiral electrode to the scalp.

(c) Attached spiral electrode with guide tube removed.

Source: *Maternal Newborn Nursing: A Family and Community-based Approach* 6e–Clinical Handbook by Olds/London/Ladewig, Copyright 2000. Reprinted by permission of Pearson Education, Inc., Upper Saddle River, NJ.

will have on her body, as well as on her fetus. Women must ask how the medication will be administered, the expected effects, the implications for the baby, and any safety considerations, such as whether the mother must remain in bed.

REGIONAL ANESTHETICS

Regional anaesthetics involve the injection of a local anesthetic into an area near a nerve (nerve block) to cause temporary loss of sensation to the area. The three most common types of regional anesthetic blocks used in childbirth are the pudendal, local, and epidural. If a woman must have a cesarean birth, she will need more comprehensive anesthesia in the form of a spinal block.

Pudendal Block   In pudendal block, an injection of an anesthetic is administered into the nerves around the perineum during the second stage of labor, providing pain relief in the upper two-thirds of the vagina and the entire perineum. This helps minimize perineal discomfort due to pushing and provides anesthesia for an episiotomy and/or forceps delivery.

Local Block   Local anesthesia works only on the area into which it is actually injected and is used primarily in women who undergo **episiotomy** (an incision that enlarges the vaginal opening). Just prior to delivery, a numbing drug is injected into the lower perineum, between the vagina and rectum, so that the episiotomy incision will not be painful.

Epidural Block   In epidural block, an anesthetic drug is injected into the spinal canal, near the spinal cord. This is done via a catheter placed between the vertebrae in the mother's lower back during the first stage of labor. It causes numbness in the abdomen, in the pelvic and perineal areas, and in the lower legs. Epidural block is currently the most popular and safest method of pain relief available to laboring women. It relieves the pain caused by the contractions, perineal pressure, episiotomy, and forceps delivery. Epidurals allow mothers to remain relaxed and alert during labor. A "light" version is now available that allows mothers to retain sensation in their legs and to walk during labor.

If there is a need for a cesarean section, the mother will require an injection of an anesthetic into her spinal fluid to provide anesthesia from the nipple line down to the feet.

NONDRUG INTERVENTIONS FOR PAIN

Some mothers wish to forego medications or anesthesia in labor for fear of the effect on their body or their fetus. A number of drug-free options are available to these women, all of which encourage the use of a support person or coach to stay with the mother in labor. One of the most common is *Lamaze childbirth education*, in which the mother and her partner learn relaxation and breathing techniques to help her relax and deal with the pain of labor. Although many women use this technique exclusively without any medications, the Lamaze program does allow the use of medications and anesthesia along with the relaxation techniques.

Other techniques not specific to labor or Lamaze include *imagery* to take the mother's mind off of the pain and *accupressure* to alleviate tension. Techniques such as *therapeutic touch, biofeedback,* and *hypnosis,* can also be used (Brucker, 1984). The sensations produced by massage may compete with pain messages from the brain, or the mother may choose to walk with her coach, which distracts her from the pain and which may accelerate labor.

During the natural childbirth era of the 1960s, the importance of having a caring person with the laboring woman began to be recognized. Research studies have shown that the presence of a support person during the entire labor can decrease the length of labor, the need for pain medication, the rate of complications, and the rate of c-section deliveries (Klaus, Kennell, & Klaus, 1993). The coach helps the mother relax throughout the labor and provides emotional support. The labor coach is usually someone very close to the mother, such as the baby's father or the mother's own mother, sister, or best friend. The coach can also help communicate the mother's needs and desires to the nursing staff.

In addition to the birth partner, some expectant parents choose to hire a **doula,** a woman trained to provide continuous physical, emotional, and educational support to the couple before, during, and after childbirth (Klaus et al., 1993). The doula is nurturing, helpful, and objective. She is there to provide emotional support and comfort measures. Her role is not to interfere with the relationship between the mother and her birth partner but, rather, to spare the birth partner the pressure of handling the labor alone. Neither does the doula interfere with the role of the nurse; she works *with* the nursing staff to expand the care being given. Klaus and colleagues have called this kind of birth assistance "mothering the mother." Studies have shown significant benefits to women who choose the added assistance of a doula. In comparison with mothers who did not have a doula present during labor, doula-assisted mothers were found to spend more time with their newborns and to be more affectionate toward them. They also showed less anxiety and fewer signs of depression and had higher self-esteem at six weeks after birth (Klaus et al., 1993).

Operative Obstetrics

There are two common surgical procedures that may be used when the healthcare provider determines that the mother needs some assistance with the delivery of her baby: episiotomy and cesarean section.

EPISIOTOMY

In the past, episiotomies were routinely done on women delivering their first babies; in the late 1980s, it was the number one surgical procedure in the country, second only to cutting the umbilical cord (Pritchard, MacDonald, & Gant, 1985). Recent research, however, shows that there is little evidence to support the routine use of episiotomy; in fact, it has been shown to increase the occurrence of bleeding, lacerations, and pain, among other adverse effects. Nurse-midwives and family practice physicians have been shown to be less likely than obstetricians to perform episiotomies. The former are more likely to stretch the perineum by gently massaging it and applying warm compresses. They also typically deliver the fetal head more slowly (Maier & Malone, 1997). It is, therefore, imperative that childbearing women discuss with their providers the advantages and disadvantages of episiotomies, as well as the risk factors that will predispose them to the need for this surgical procedure.

CESAREAN SECTION

When a maternal or fetal complication that prevents a vaginal delivery exists, the fetus will need to be delivered through an abdominal and uterine incision. This intervention is considered major abdominal surgery.

In 1988, the rate of cesarean section deliveries in the United States rose to a high of 24.7 percent of all deliveries (Sachs, 1999). A study by the Agency for Healthcare Research and Quality revealed that up to 24 percent of these surgical deliveries had been done because the diagnosis "failure to progress" was made very early in labor. That such a diagnosis was frequently being made so early in labor, when cervical dilatation was minimal, was viewed with concern by women's advocates and some healthcare providers as well. They based their concern on the recommendation of the American College of Obstetricians and Gynecologists (ACOG) that cervical dilatation be at 4 cm or greater before a diagnosis of failure to progress is made (American College of Obstetricians and Gynecologists, 2000). A number of theories to account for the high rate of cesarean sections performed in this country during the 1980s have been put forth: Some have argued that obstetricians may have disagreed with or misunderstood the ACOG guidelines, or they may have just felt more comfortable performing the section early in labor. Women's advocates have suggested that some physicians have been practicing "defensive medicine" for fear of having a bad outcome, had they allowed the mother to labor longer (Gifford et al., 1999). No doubt at least partly in response to negative publicity, the rate of cesarean deliveries fell each year between 1989 and 1996 (Young, 2001).

In the past, the rule of thumb was once a section, always a section—meaning that, if the mother had one c-section, every subsequent delivery would have to be a c-section. The reasoning behind this adage was the belief that a uterus with a scar can rupture during the course of the next labor. This, however, is now known to be untrue. Statistics show that 86 percent of all c-sections are done via a **low segment incision,** or bikini cut. This segment of the uterus holds little chance of rupture in subsequent labors, so the current feeling is that these women should be given the opportunity to deliver vaginally (Enkin, Keirse, & Neilson, 2000).

When a mother who has had a cesarean birth chooses to deliver vaginally with a subsequent pregnancy, she is said to be having a **vaginal birth after cesarean** or **VBAC.** In order for vaginal delivery to be permitted, there must be no pregnancy or labor complications, there must be no history of uterine rupture, and the mother must be fully informed about her decision. It is important for her to know that each labor following a cesarean is considered a "trial labor," with multiple precautions taken should a repeat cesarean be warranted.

Whereas the cesarean rate declined during the early and mid 1990s, it is now increasing. Some obstetricians even argue that women should have the option of choosing a cesarean delivery as a means of avoiding the discomfort of labor and possible damage to pelvic tissues during vaginal delivery (Harrer, 2000). However, according to the American College of Obstetricians and Gynecologists (ACOG), current research indicates that vaginal delivery is *not* a significant cause of urinary incontinence (see Chapter 16) and uterine prolapse (downward displacement of the uterus due to relaxation of pelvic tissues), and there is therefore *no* justification for substituting cesaeran delivery for a normal vaginal birth (American College of Obsetricans & Gynecologists, 2000). Moreover, in comparison with vaginal birth, cesarean delivery is associated with a high risk of **morbidity** (illness) for both infants and mothers. A 7-year, retrospective study of nearly 30,000 births found that pulmonary hypertension, a serious lung disorder, occurs almost five times as often in infants delivered by cesarean than in infants delivered vaginally (Levine, Ghai, Barton, & Strom, 2001). Mothers who deliver via cesarean are more likely to be rehospitalized than mothers who deliver vaginally because of complications, such as surgical wound infection, uterine infection, blood clots, and pulmonary embolism (Lydon-Rochelle, Holt, Martin, & Easterling, 2000).

The National Women's Health Network (www.women shealthnetwork.org), a watchdog organization that scrutinizes the healthcare provided to women, maintains that childbrith is fundamentally a normal process that only occasionally requires an extreme form of medical intervention, such as cesarean delivery. It warns that obstetricians who are biased against natural birth and in favor of cesarean delivery may slant the information they give to women by exaggerating the frequency with which pelvic tissue damage is associated with vaginal delivery (Young, 2001).

Complications of Labor and Delivery

In most cases, childbirth is a normal, healthy process for the mother and her fetus. However, in about one-fourth of all pregnancies, a deviation from normal presents a threat to maternal and/or fetal well-being. Because there are quite a number of possible complications, we will discuss in this chapter only the two that occur most commonly: dystocia (abnormal labor) and abnormal fetal presentation.

DYSTOCIA

Dystocia is said to exist when the process of labor deviates from normal. Labor can become abnormal when there is a disturbance of any factor that helps the uterus contract and the cervix efface and dilate. When the uterus becomes dysfunctional, it may either never fully relax, putting both the mother and fetus in danger during labor, or relax too much, causing inefficient contractions. Still another dysfunction can occur when the uterus contracts so frequently and intensely that a very rapid delivery will occur. These three types of dystocia are known technically as hypertonic uterine dysfunction, hypotonic uterine dysfunction, and precipitous labor.

Hypertonic Uterine Dysfunction When the uterus never fully relaxes between contractions, the mother and fetus are put at risk because of decreased blood flow through the placenta. There is decreased oxygen flow to the fetus and exhaustion on the part of the mother, who experiences frequent, intense, and painful contractions that have little effect on the cervix. This often happens early in labor and causes the mother to become discouraged by the increasing pain and relative lack of progress in the labor. If the healthcare provider determines that the fetus is in a normal position and that the amniotic membrane is still intact, the mother will be given a sedative, which will allow her to rest and stop the abnormal activity of the uterus. In most cases, the mother will awaken and begin a normal labor.

Hypotonic Uterine Dysfunction This abnormality is the result of contractions that are of poor quality and lack the intensity needed to dilate and efface the cervix. In contrast to hypertonic dysfunction, hypotonic dysfunction occurs in active labor, usually when the cervix is dilated to 4 centimeters or more. This dysfunction is often referred to as *secondary uterine inertia,* because the labor begins normally and then the frequency and intensity of contractions decrease. The contractions in this type of labor are not effective enough to be painful. This type of dysfunction is a common occurrence when the uterus is overdistended with a twin pregnancy or a very large fetus. It can also occur when pain medication is given too early in the labor process and with any regional anesthesia. The major risk with this complication is bleeding after delivery, when the uterus is unable to shrink down and clamp off blood vessels.

Prior to beginning the treatment for a hypotonic dysfunction, the healthcare provider will ascertain that the fetus is in a proper position, the mother's pelvis is adequate size, and the mother is in the active stage of labor. If all these conditions are present, the healthcare provider will rupture the amniotic sac, insert an internal fetal and uterine monitor, and watch the labor closely. Often, there is a need for **augmentation** or stimulation, of labor, using the drug Pitocin to help the uterus contract effectively. If neither of these interventions is successful, a c-section may be warranted.

Precipitous Labor This type of labor is one that is completed in less than 3 hours. The mother experiences five contractions or more over a 10-minute period, which she describes as "intense." Women who experience this type of labor and delivery have perineal soft tissues that stretch readily, allowing the fetus to pass through the pelvis quickly and easily. Complications in the mother are rare with a pre-

cipitous labor, but her anxiety level is much higher than usual because of the intensity of the contractions. Often, this type of labor ends in the mother giving birth without assistance, so the mother will need assurance that she will not be left alone for the delivery. The fetus, on the other hand, may experience a lack of oxygen due to the intensity of the mother's contractions or head trauma if the birth outlet does not stretch easily.

ABNORMAL FETAL PRESENTATION

Even a slight variation of the position (presentation) of the fetus can adversely affect the labor. The variation can affect the contractions and/or the descent of the fetus through the mother's pelvis. As there are a number of adverse presentations, we will discuss only two of the most common: occiput posterior and breech.

Occiput Posterior In occiput posterior, the fetus is positioned so that it will be born facing upward instead of downward, as is normal. Also referred to as a posterior head, occiput posterior occurs in only 10 percent of laboring women. It is often caused by a narrowing of the mother's pelvis, which prevents the fetus from rotating its head in the usual manner. Occiput posterior can occur in, and prolong, both the first and second stages of labor, with the mother experiencing severe back pain, because the back of the fetal head is pressing on her sacrum (lower back) and coccyx (tail bone). Comfort measures during this type of labor include using counterpressure on the sacrum and coccyx, giving the mother backrubs, and/or turning her from side to side—which may, at the same time, help rotate the fetal head.

Breech This abnormal presentation—with the lower part of the fetus behind the cervix and the head in the upper portion of the uterus—occurs in about 3.5 percent of births. The reason has to do with the fact that the fetal head is usually found in the area of the uterus in which there is the most room. If the mother has a low-implanted placenta, the fetal head will be in the upper part of the uterus. The types of breech presentations are determined by the positioning of the fetal legs (see Figure 23.9). In a **frank breech presentation,** the buttocks are behind the cervix, with the legs extended up toward the face. In a **full,** or complete, **breech,** the fetus sits crossed-legged above the cervix. In a **footling,** or incomplete, **breech** presentation, one or both legs are extended behind the cervix.

In past years, any type of a breech presentation was an automatic indication for a c-section unless the baby was small and the mother had a large pelvis. Now, one-third to one-half of all breech presentations are delivered vaginally, with each occurrence treated individually and labor watched very closely. No matter what method of delivery is

Figure 23–9   Breech Presentation

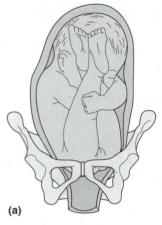

(a)

Frank breech.

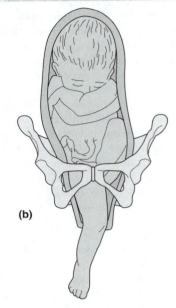

(b)

Incomplete (footling) breech.

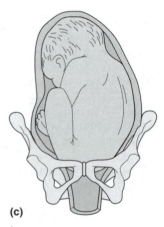

(c)

Complete breech.

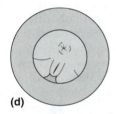

(d)

On Vaginal examination, the nurse may feel the anal sphincter, (d) the tissue of the fetal buttocks feels soft.

Source: *Maternal Newborn Nursing: A Family and Community-based Approach* 6e–Clinical Handbook by Olds/London/Ladewig, Copyright 2000. Reprinted with permission of Pearson Education, Inc., Upper Saddle River, NJ.

chosen, however, the risk for maternal and fetal trauma is still higher due to the abnormal presentation.

The Postpartum Period

During the postpartum period, the uterus gradually shrinks back to its normal size (uterine involution), the episiotomy wound (if present) heals, the new family bonds, and breastfeeding or bottle-feeding becomes established. Most women feel they have largely recovered from childbirth within two weeks of delivery. New mothers face the daunting challenges of learning to care for their newborns and adjusting their lives to accommodate motherhood.

Following delivery, depression and other emotions may be fueled by factors such as changes in sexual relationships between partners and a perception that too much attention is going to the new baby. Postpartum "blues" are common, and usually last from three to eight days after delivery. Depression, or excessive sadness, can occur both during pregnancy and after birth. Fatigue can cause or contribute to this. It is important, too, for new mothers to get at least eight hours of sleep a day, particularly soon after the birth. Partners should be involved in childcare to the greatest degree possible, and it is important to use communication to negotiate baby care, responsibilities, and to communicate each partner's needs. Unnecessary household chores should be eliminated if they add to stress after birth.

Because childbearing is treated by society as a joyful experience, the woman who feels depression instead of joy usually suffers in silence, reluctant to share her true feelings with her family and/or her healthcare provider. She may feel that, if she admits to depression and doubts about her ability to mother, both will be used against her—perhaps even to the point of removing her child from the home. Mothers who feel overwhelmed and sad should consider joining a support group, such as a local parenting group, or obtain counseling. If sadness persists for any member of the family, clinical depression needs to be considered and ruled out or treated.

Uterine Involution

It is essential that the uterus contract after delivery in order to seal off the blood vessels torn during delivery. If this does not occur, excessive bleeding may occur. In first births, this process may not be painful, but, in subsequent ones, it causes cramps known as **afterpains.** If the uterus is larger than it should be, and there is still bleeding and cramping, **endometritis,** an infection of the lining of the uterus, may be the cause. Nurses palpate the uterus frequently (to determine whether it is contracting) in the hours after birth and massage it, if necessary, to induce it to contract. They distinguish normal bleeding from excessive bleeding by counting the number of pads used to absorb the flow. They also note the color and consistency of the flow as it changes over time. By the tenth day after birth, the uterus should no longer be palpable.

The general term for discharge from the uterus after birth is **lochia.** Immediately following delivery, lochia is bright red and consists mostly of blood. As the uterus contracts and becomes smaller, bleeding slows and eventually stops. Within three days, lochia changes to a brownish mix of blood and mucus and then to a yellowish-whitish discharge made up of microorganisms and cell fragments. Lochia should cease by the tenth day postdelivery (*Bantam Medical Dictionary,* 1996).

Changing pads frequently and avoiding the use of tampons decrease the possibility that irritation and/or infection will develop. Infections can develop in the uterus (in 2 to 8 percent of pregnant women) or in the urinary tract or breast (Sherwen et al., 1995). A temperature of 100. 4°F or above in a mother following delivery may indicate the presence of infection. Most infections respond to broad-spectrum antibiotics within 36 hours.

Episiotomy Care

The proper care of the episiotomy wound, as well as any hemorrhoids that may be present, is important. Doing Kegel exercises and warming the area for 15 minutes at a time with a gooseneck lamp positioned 12 inches from the perineum can help the healing process. Flushing the perineum with warm water and applying witch hazel compresses, ice packs, and benzocaine sprays are methods of promoting healing and reducing discomfort. Sitz baths, which should be offered at the hospital, along with an explanation of how to take similar baths at home, also relieve perineal discomfort.

Breast-feeding

Breast-feeding is encouraged because of the benefits for both babies and mothers. There is consensus in the medical community that breast milk contributes to the development of a strong immune system (Michaels, 2000) and is the best source of nutrition for the growing baby. Breast-feeding also protects an infant from juvenile-onset diabetes and may assist in avoiding other illnesses, such as sudden infant death syndrome (SIDS), obesity, coronary heart disease, and lymphoma later in life. Breast milk stimulates the growth of positive bacteria in the infant's digestive tract, reducing the incidence of stomach upset, diarrhea, and colic. Research also suggests that nursing benefits mothers as well, through helping the uterus retract, helping the mother lose weight, and lowering her risk of developing breast cancer and osteoporosis (Somer, 1995). Although the benefits are well documented, currently only slightly more than half of American women choose to breast-feed initially, and two-thirds of those quit in the first six months, despite the recommendation from the American Academy of Pediatrics that infants be nursed exclusively during their first six months and then continue to receive breast milk, along with their other food, at least until their first birthday (Michaels, 2000). The decision not to breast-feed initially, or to stop after a few weeks or months, can be due to many factors, including the belief that nursing is not successful, discomfort during nursing, and the logistical difficulties of nursing.

Not all women should choose to nurse their babies. Women who have conditions or diseases, such as AIDS, that can be passed through breast milk, and women with continuing substance-abuse problems, should not breast-feed (Sherwen et al., 1999).

Breastfeeding is not an innate skill in human mothers. Instruction is needed and can be obtained in prenatal classes, from obstetricians, or from maternity nurses. **Maintaining an adequate milk** supply is the key to success in breastfeeding. Mothers' anxieties about producing enough milk are usually unfounded, but signs of inadequate milk supply include a baby who is not content after feeding, a drop in the number of wet diapers, and the baby's failure to gain weight. A number of techniques can be used to improve milk production, such as nursing or pumping more frequently, and allowing the baby to nuzzle at the breast. Michaels (2000) suggests that taking two or three capsules daily of fenugreek seed, which is available at most health food stores, may improve milk production.

When the mother's milk first comes in, **engorgement,** the painful filling of the breasts with milk, can occur; the breasts become markedly enlarged, hard, and painful. Engorgement can be alleviated through early nursing of the infant or, if this does not suffice, the use of a breast pump or even manual expression of the milk from the breasts. Warm-to-hot showers encourage release of the milk from the breasts, as does heat from lightbulb kept 12–18 inches away from the breasts. A supportive bra should be worn. Healthcare providers should provide information on these options.

Nipple care as described relative to the third trimester in the section on pregnancy should continue after breast-feeding has started. One way of minimizing nipple tenderness is to use only one breast during each feeding and alternate them. The proper positioning of the baby is also important; specific instructions are available from obstetricians & midwives. Nursing the baby in short, frequent sessions rather than longer, infrequent ones will cut down on nipple soreness and increase the milk supply. Although nipple tenderness may be a problem at first, breast-feeding should not be uncomfortable after the first week or two, if all is well. If discomfort persists, **thrush,** a type of yeast infection, may be present and the healthcare provider will prescribe an antifungal agent (Michaels, 2000). *Plugged milk ducts,* appearing as lumps in the breast, can also cause pain and can be caused by missed feedings, inadequate food or fluid intake, a tight-fitting bra, or exhaustion. To relieve this condition, mothers can nurse more frequently, apply warm compresses to the sore area, and massage the breast while nursing. Drinking more fluids and snacking regularly on high-protein foods may be helpful, as may taking *lecithin,* a natural compound that contains choline, inositol, phosphorus, and various fatty acids (*Physician's Desk Reference,* 1999). Getting more rest may be helpful as well (Michaels, 2000). **Mastitis,** or inflammation of the breast, causes symptoms that include soreness, redness, aching, and fever. If fever is present, the healthcare provider should be contacted, and antibiotics will most often be prescribed. Continuing to breast-feed or pump milk may also help (Michaels, 2000).

LOGISTICS

Working mothers face a particular challenge with the logistics of breast-feeding, but women at home may also be challenged by the need to juggle nursing demands with those of running a household and/or caring for other children. Using breast pumps is key to providing flexibility; milk can be expressed and saved for use at other times. If a private setting in which to pump is available, a high-quality automatic cycling double pump (rented or purchased) will allow the most milk to be expressed in the shortest time. Otherwise, a small, lightweight manual pump that can easily be taken into a bathroom stall may be a better choice, even though only one breast can be pumped at a time. Community resources for the support of nursing mothers are listed in the Re-

sources section at the end of this chapter. Local parenting groups can also provide assistance.

NUTRITION AND EXERCISE

Women who are breast-feeding require 500 to 700 more calories per day than they did when they were pregnant (Somer, 1995). Like pregnant women, nursing mothers must be conscientious regarding their diets. They must drink at least six 8-ounce glasses of water a day, in addition to other beverages. Alcohol intake should be limited: no more than 2 to 2 1/2 ounces of liquor, 8 ounces of wine, or two cans of beer should be consumed in any one day; nor should they have more than one serving of a caffeinated beverage (Kolasa & Weismiller, 1995).

Breast-feeding women who follow a strict vegetarian diet are likely to produce milk that is low in vitamin B-12 and should consume supplements or vitamin B-12–fortified foods. Babies fed vitamin B-12–deficient milk are at risk of developing nerve problems, anemia, and metabolic disorders (Somer, 1995).

Exercising after childbirth may help avoid postpartum blues and promote feelings of well-being: limited research suggests that women who return to exercising have higher fitness levels and produce more mlk (Somer, 1995). When breast-feeding, women must consume enough calories for both nursing and exercising. Nursing should be done before exercising to avoid the discomfort of engorged breasts. After birth, routine exercises can be started as early as one week postpartum, but waiting six weeks is recommended (Carlson & Parrish, 1998). In either case, jarring and bouncing moments should be avoided in this early period (Somer, 1995). In addition, exercise should be resumed gradually, beginning with Kegel exercises (see Chapter 16) on the first day postpartum. By the beginning of the second week, the mother should have progressed to abdominal, buttock, and thigh-toning exercises.

During the postpartum period, many physiological changes must take place; it may take as long as 12 weeks for the abdominal wall and joints to return to their prepregnancy state. Whether a woman had a vaginal or cesarean delivery will effect the amount of time her body takes to return to normal (Carlson & Parrish, 1998).

Bottle-feeding

If breast-feeding is not desired, a tight-fitting bra should be worn, ice packs placed on the breast, and analgesics taken if needed. The healthcare provider should be consulted about appropriate formula choices to replace breast milk. Mothers who do not breast-feed can expect the return of their menses within six to eight weeks.

Sex and Birth Control

After birth, waiting about two weeks before attempting intercourse is recommended. This is not only because of discomfort a woman may feel if her body has not recovered enough from the birthing process, which may include an episiotomy, but also because of the danger of infection.

Sexual dissatisfaction may occur after birth for a variety of reasons. Either parent may feel resentment about a baby in relation to the spouse. A partner who stays at home and is the primary caregiver may resent the other partner's freedom, whereas the parent who works outside the home may resent and feel distant from the primary caregiver, who now seems to care only about the baby. Given these possible scenarios, it is very important that partners work to communicate their needs, make time for just each other, and maintain intimacy in their relationship.

Finally, contrary to some beliefs, it is possible for a woman to get pregnant again soon after giving birth—even if she is breast-feeding. Therefore, contraception must be used as soon as intercourse resumes. The recommended form of contraception is foam and condoms until a woman's first postpartum checkup, at which time another method may be approved. Acceptable forms of contraception vary, depending on whether a woman breast-feeds. Although women may begin using most forms of birth control four weeks after birth, oral contraceptives are not appropriate for women who are breast-feeding, because the hormones will be passed to the baby in the milk. Women who are not breast-feeding may begin using oral contraceptives as soon as two weeks postdelivery, though they should not be started sooner than that because of the risk of blood clots. Norplant can be inserted immediately postpartum even if breast-feeding, but a woman must wait six weeks to have a diaphragm fitted or to have an IUD inserted. Tubal ligation (tying the fallopian tubes) can be done immediately postpartum or after waiting six weeks.

Education Regarding Care of the Newborn

It is important that parents see and touch their newborns as soon as possible after birth. This supports the process of bonding. New parents have a great deal to learn about how to care for their babies. For example, all parents must be taught how to position their babies safely in the crib or bassinet: Babies who have just been fed should be positioned *on their right sides, with a rolled blanket at their backs* so that, if they burp up milk or formula, it will run out of the mouth, where it cannot be inhaled into the trachea. This position will also assist with digestion. Later, they should be repositioned on their backs, with blankets and covers well away from the face. Infants who have not recently been fed are placed on their backs for sleeping. The American Academy of Pediatrics (1996) recommends that infants not be put on their stomachs for the first few months of life, because the prone position has been associated with an increased incidence of sudden infant death syndrome. Other issues related to safety that should be addressed include the prevention of

injuries in the home, the mandatory use of car seats placed in the back of the automobile, and the dangers of leaving children unattended in cars.

Parents should be apprised of typical infant sleeping patterns and with bowel patterns, including the appearance of **meconium,** the first stools of a newborn, and the normal amount and color of subsequent stools. Parents must also learn about abnormalities, such as diarrhea and bloody stools, as well as how to choose diapers, keep the baby clean, treat diaper rash, and care for the umbilical cords of newborns.

All new mothers should be made aware of the importance of taking their babies back to providers for checkups and immununizations, beginning with the six-week well baby checkup. New mothers should have a phone number to call if questions or emergencies come up.

The Circumcision Controversy

For parents who give birth to a boy, the issue of whether to have the newborn circumcised arises. Male infants have traditionally been circumcised for a number of years, either for medical or religious reasons.

Although the medical benefits of the procedure are known to be better hygiene and decreased incidence of both sexually transmitted diseases and urinary tract infections, there are also complications that go along with the procedure, such as bleeding, infection, and inflammation of the penis (VanRyzin, 2000). In addition, neonatal pain control studies have shown that infants who have been circumcised without some form of pain control show a greater pain response at four- and six-month vaccinations, providing evidence that the pain of the circumcision has lasting effects on the child. For this reason, researchers are recommending that a nerve block of the pelvis be done even on premature infants who are to be circumcised (Olds et al., 2000). The American Academy of Pediatrics' (1999) policy on circumcision recommends *against* the procedure but suggests that, if it is done, analgesics be used to decrease the newborn's pain. Some critics today call the procedure barbaric and medically unnecessary: "Opponents question whether it is acceptable for parents to consent to removal of part of their son's anatomy solely to conform to socially acceptable aesthetic critera" (VanRyzin, 2000, p. 232).

Unplanned Pregnancy

Even a much desired and expected pregnancy can be physically and emotionally stressful. An unplanned, unwelcome one can be devastating, especially for women who lack resources and/or are not in a stable relationship. Many women who find themselves unexpectedly pregnant find it difficult to know whom to talk to, what to do, or where to go for help. Today, a woman who finds herself pregnant has a number of options.

Answering the following questions can help her choose from among them (Iowa Women's Health Center, 1999):

- How do I feel about the pregnancy?
- How does the father feel about the pregnancy?
- Do I want to become a parent at this time in my life?
- Am I ready to care for a baby 24/7?
- Where will we live?
- Will I raise the child alone?
- Who will support or help me?
- Can I provide for this baby financially?

A number of agencies and organizations will assist women who are facing an unwanted pregnancy at little or no cost. They include the following.

- Crisis pregnancy centers—Counselors will generally speak only with the pregnant woman. Live-in facilities may be available.
- A family planning clinic, such as Planned Parenthood
- An adoption agency
- The county health department or department of social services—Welfare or food stamp workers will guide the woman to the correct department
- Mental health centers/family services agencies

In general, a woman experiencing an unplanned pregnancy has three choices: to bear and *parent* the baby, to bear the baby and put it up for *adoption,* or to *terminate* the pregnancy. It is important that a woman think beyond her first reaction to the pregnancy and weigh all of her available options before making one of the most important decisions of her life. Making a choice that she will feel good about over the long term will take time, thought, and patience. Also, women who fully explore their options and make their own decisions generally have fewer regrets and negative emotional consequences (Gladney Center for Adoption, 1999).

Adoption

Making the decision to place for adoption an infant she is not equipped to rear is a courageous act of love on the part of a mother. The process of adoption can be confidential or open. In a *confidential adoption,* the birth and adoptive parents do not know one another. The adoptive parents have only background information on the birth parents. The birth parent(s) may lose all contact with the child for life, although more states are taking the controversial steps of opening adoption records, so that biological parents and their adult children can find each other if both are willing.

An *open adoption,* on the other hand, is one in which the birth and adoptive parents have some degree of knowledge of one another. Depending on the type of open adoption, the birth mother may simply read about the possible adoptive couples and pick one, or both sets of parents may meet

and interact before the baby's birth. The birth mother may even maintain some level of contact with the baby after it is born. The type of adoption the mother chooses is entirely up to her.

Abortion

Unwanted pregnancy, together with an inability to provide for the child, is the primary reason that women have abortions. However, the decision to terminate a pregnancy is a very complex one that is influenced by such factors as personal beliefs and values, experience, and the amount of support available from significant others. The most salient factor is often the impact bearing a child would have on the woman's life. Women who are considering abortion are given counseling to assist them in deciding whether to go through with the procedure. Tests are done to confirm the pregnancy, and the woman is educated as to the type of procedure she will have, depending on whether she is in the first or second trimester of her pregnancy. There are two procedures commonly used for the termination of pregnancy: vacuum suction curettage and dilatation and extraction (D&E). In both procedures, a large catheter attached to suction is used to remove the uterine contents. The **vacuum suction procedure** is used to terminate first-trimester pregnancies. It is used up to and including the sixteenth week. The **dilatation and extraction procedure** is used to terminate pregnancies in the second trimester, from the sixteenth through the twentieth weeks of pregnancy. The cervix is first dilated; then suction is used to remove the uterine contents.

An oral medication called **RU486** is currently available for the very early termination of pregnancy. This medication was under clinical trial in the United States in the late 1990s, and the FDA gave approval for its use in September 2000. If given within 48 hours of a missed menstrual period, it is very effective. However, the safety of the drug is controversial, and the cost is that of a surgical abortion.

Sources of Community Support

Whether the woman experiencing an unplanned pregnancy chooses to keep her baby, terminate the pregnancy, or give her newborn up for adoption, there are numerous organizations to which she can turn for guidance. The following is a partial list:

Planned Parenthood (www.plannedparenthood.org)
A national organization that deals with all reproductive health issues
220 19th St. NW, Washington, DC 20036

Parents Without Partners (www.ParentsWithoutPartners.org)
An international organization providing education, support, and social activities related to bring up children alone
7910 Woodmont Ave., Washington, DC 20014

Single Mothers by Choice (www.parentsplace.com/family/
    singleparent/gen)
Provides information and support to single moms and those
contemplating a pregnancy
P.O. Box 1642, Gracie Square Station, New York, NY 10028
    (212-988-0993)

National Right to Life Committee (www.nrlc.org)
Provides information about abortion alternatives
419 7th St. NW, Washington, DC 20045 (202-626-8800)

National Abortion Rights Action League (www.naral.org)
A reproductive choice advocate and political arm of the prochoice
movement
1156 15th St., Suite 700, Washington, DC 20005

New Directions

Promising new advances in healthcare for pregnant women
and their children are on the horizon. Examples of these innovations are to be found in the categories of AIDS treatment during childbirth and fetal assessment.

A major issue in childbirth is the danger that a pregnant
woman with AIDS will pass the disease to her baby during
delivery or later, during breast-feeding. Recently, it has been
discovered that giving the mother two standard antiviral
medications, AZT and 3TC, beginning with the onset of labor and continuing the medication regime in both the
mother and newborn for one week following delivery, decreases by 11 percent the chance that HIV will be passed to
the newborn. The medications protect the newborn from
exposure to AIDS-contaminated blood and secretions, as
well as from HIV in breast milk (Haney, 1999).

A new tool for fetal assessment, 3-D ultrasound, is being used increasingly in hospitals. It provides a true three-
dimensional picture of the fetus, with a surface view of the
fetal organs and face. It also yields more accurate information about fetal weight and length.

Another new fetal assessment modality, pulse oximetry,
is now being used to assess fetal arterial oxygen saturation.
Oxygen saturation reflects fetal health or distress more than
do the changes registered on an electronic fetal heart rate
monitor, which are sometimes misleading. In fetal pulse
oximetry, an oximetry catheter is inserted through the
vagina and applied to the surface of the fetal head. This innovation has the potential for decreasing the number of unnecessary cesarean sections done because of false positive
readings on electronic heart rate monitor strips.

Finally, a new test has been developed to determine fetal Rh status as early as the 14th week of pregnancy. By the
second trimester, the mother's blood carries enough fetal
DNA to allow the determination of the fetal Rh factor
through an analysis of the mother's blood. As research in the
area of fetal DNA continues, the probability of being able to
test for other genetic diseases via maternal blood increases.

QUESTIONS FOR REFLECTION AND DISCUSSION

1. *What factors would be most important to you in
   choosing a provider of obstetrical care? Would you
   consider a nurse-midwife? Why or why not?*
2. *What are the pros and cons of electronic monitoring and
   other technologies used during labor?*
3. *What factors would enter into your choice of measures to
   control pain during labor and delivery?*
4. *Do you think you would choose to breast-feed a child?
   Why or why not?*
5. *Would you have your male newborn circumcised? Why or
   why not?*

RESOURCES

Books

Truth, Lies and the Unexpected on the Journey to Motherhood
    (2001), by Naomi Wolf-Doubleday.

For a free comprehensive mail-order catalog of books, call
the following:

ASPO (Lamaze Childbirth Education): 1-800-368-8404
Birth and Life Bookstore: 1-800-443-9942
International Childbirth Education Association: 1-800-624-4934

Videotapes

American College of Obstetricians and Gynecologists (ACOG)
1-800-762-2264
www.acog.org

"Pregnancy and Postnatal Exercise Program"
Injoy Productions
1-800-326-2082
www.injoyvideos.com

"Special Delivery"(birthing options/three labors and births)
"Giving Birth: Challenges and Choices" (c-section/epidurals/
    home birth)
"Baby to Be: The Video Guide to Pregnancy"
"Special Women: How a Labor Assistant Makes Birth Safer" (doulas)
"Pregnant, Single, and Prepared" (for single moms)
"Everymom's Prenatal Exercise and Relaxation Video"
"Breastfeeding: Better Beginnings"
"The Adoption Option" (video and resource book)

Organizations

Coping with Overall Pregnancy/Parenting Experience (COPE)
37 Clarendon St.
Boston, MA 02116
Phone: 617-357-5588

Cesarian/Support Education and Concern (C/SEC)
22 Forest Rd.
Framingham, MA 01701
Phone: 508-877-8266

International Lactation Consultant Association
201 Brown Ave.
Evanston, Il 60202-3601
Phone: 708-260-8874

La Leche League
1400 North Michigan Rd.
Schaumburg, IL 60173
Phone: 1-800-525-3243

National Adoption Information Clearinghouse (NAIC)
11426 Rockville Pike, Suite 410
Rockville, MD 20852
Phone: 301-231-6512

Parenthood After Thirty
451 Vermont Ave.
Berkeley, CA 94707
Phone: 415-524-6635

Postpartum Support International
927 N. Kellog Ave.
Santa Barbara, CA 93111
Phone: 805-967-7636

Single Parent Resource Center
141 W. 28th St., Suite 302
New York, NY 10001
Phone: 212-947-0221

Maternity Support Garment Vendors

Each of these companies provides elastic belly slings that
support from below and crisscross in the back:

Moore Products ("Loving Lift")
P.O. Box 647
Belmont, CA 94002-0617
Phone: 415-592-8174

Trennaventions ("Action Lift" and "Baby Hugger")
RR1, Box 253 D
Derry, PA 15627-9740
Phone: 412-694-5283

Websites

All About Pregnancy
www.about.com/pregnancy- A commercial site with extensive
    links to other commercial sites, as well as to educational sites
    sponsored by recognized institutions.

Childbirth
www.childbirth.org-A private site run by nurse midwives, doulas
    and childbirth educators. Provides information on many
    topics related to pregnancy and childbirth.

La Leche League International
www.lalecheleague.org-A site devoted to promoting breast feeding and
    providing assistance to mothers who wish to nurse their babies.

National Association of Childbearing Centers
www.birthcenters.org-Contains information on locating birthing
    centers, midwives and doulas, as well as links to related sites.

The authors would like to thank Elizabeth Carmody, N. Clair
Fancher and Susan Nogueira for their assistance in the preparation
of this chapter.

REFERENCES

Alano, M. A., Ngougmna, E., Ostrea, E. M., & Kondur, G. G. (2001). Analysis of nonsteroidal anti-inflammatory drugs in meconium and its relation to persistent pulmonary hypertension of the newborn. *Pediatrics, 107*(3), 519–523.

American Academy of Pediatrics. (1996). Task force on infant positioning: Positioning and sudden infant death syndrome (SIDS) update. *Pediatrics, 98*(6), 1216–1218.

American Academy of Pediatrics. (1999). Task force on circumcision: Circumcision policy statement. *Pediatrics, 103*(3), 93.

American College of Obstetricians and Gynecologists. (2000). *Evaluation of caesarian delivery.* Washington, DC: Author.

Bantam medical dictionary (2nd ed.). (1996). New York: Bantam Books.

Boston Women's Health Collective (Eds). (1998). *Our bodies, ourselves: For the new Century.* New York: Touchstone.

Brucker, M. (1984). Non-pharmacological methods for relieving pain and discomfort in pregnancy. *Maternal Child Nursing Journal, 9,* 390–394.

Carlson, B., & Parrish, D. (1998). Exercise during pregnancy: What to tell your patients. *Women's Health in Primary Care, 1*(2), 171–179.

Enkin, M., Keirse, M. J., & Neilson, J. (2000). *A guide to effective care in pregnancy & childbirth* (3rd ed.). Oxford: Oxford University Press.

Evans, A., et al. (1993). Supression of pregnancy-induced nausea and vomiting with sensory afferent stimulation. *Journal of Reproductive Medicine, 18*(8), 603–606.

Frye, A. (1998). *Holistic midwifery: A comprehensive textbook for midwives in homebirth practice* (2nd ed.). Portland, OR: Labrys Press.

Gagnon, D. O. (1993). *Liquid herbal drops in everyday usage.* Santa Fe: Botanical Research and Education Institute.

Gifford, S. G., Morton, S. C., Fiske, M., Keesey, J., Keeler, E., & Kahu, K. (1995). Lack of progress in labor as a reason for caesarian. *Obstetrics and Gynecology, 95*(4), 589–595.

Gladney Center for Adoption. (1999). *Choices: A decision making guide for unplanned pregnancy* [On-line]. Available: http://www.gladney.org/html/pregnant/decision.htm

Haney, D. (1999). *Childbirth AIDS treatment works* [On-line]. Available: http://www.infobeat.com/stories/cgi/story.cgi?id=2558288297-f09

Harer, W. B. (2000). Patient choice cesarean. *A COG Clinical Review, 5*(2), 1, 13–16.

Holzman, G. B. (Ed.). (1998). *Precis: An update in obstetrics and gynecology.* American College of Obstetrics and Gynecology. (ACOG).

Iowa Women's Health Center (IWHC). (1999). *Facing an unplanned pregnancy* [On-line]. Available: http://obgyn.uihc.uiowa.edu/Patinfo/Prenatal/pregqstn.htm

Johnson, L. (1999, November 24). *Caffeine/miscarriage risk studied* [On-line]. Available: http://www.infobeat.com/stories

Klaus, M. H., Kennell, J. H., & Klaus, P. H. (1993). *Mothering the mother.* Menlo Park, CA: Merloyd Lawrence Books.

Kolasa, K. M., & Weismiller, M. D. (1995, July). Nutrition during pregnancy. *American Family Physicians,* p. 209.

Levine, E. M., Ghai, V., Barton, J. J., & Strom, C. M. (2001). Mode of delivery and risk of respiratory diseases in newborns. *Obstetrics and Gynecology, 97*(3), 439–442.

Lydon-Rochelle, M., Holt, V. L., Martin, D. P., & Easterling, T. R. (2000). Association between method of delivery and maternal rehospitalization. *Journal of the American Medical Association, 283*, 2411–2416.

Maier, J. S., & Malone, J. A. (1997). Nurse advocacy for selective versus routine episiotomy. *Journal of Gynecological and Neonatal Nursing, 26*(2), 155–161.

Michaels, D. L. (2000, December/January). Breastfeeding: Beyond the basics. *Parenting,* pp. 175–181.

O'Brien, L. P. (2000, December/January). Ten pregnancy myths. *Parenting,* p. 130.

Olds, S. B., London, M. L., & Ladewig, P. A. (2000). *Maternal-newborn nursing: A family and community-based approach* (6th ed.). Upper Saddle River, NJ: Prentice Hall Health.

Petersen, L., & Besuner, P. (1997). Pushing techniques during labor: Issues and controversies. *Journal of Gynecological and Neonatal Nursing, 26*(6), 719–725.

The physician's desk reference: A family guide to natural medicines and healing therapies. (1999). New York: Random House.

Pregnancy-related deaths among black, Hispanic, Asian/Pacific Islander and American Indian/Alaska Native women— United States, 1991–1997. (2001). *Mortality and Morbidity Weekly Report (MMWR), 50*(18), 361–364. Washington, DC: Centers for Disease Control.

Pritchard, J. A., MacDonald, P. C., & Gant, N. F. (1985). *Williams obstetrics* (17th ed.). New York: Appleton-Century-Crofts.

Reynolds, H. D. (1998). Preconception care: An integral part of primary care for women. *Journal of Nurse Midwifery, 43*(6), 34–36.

Rubin, R. (1984). *Maternal identity and maternal experience.* New York: Springer.

Sachs, M. (1999). Risks of cesarean section. *New England Journal of Medicine, 340*, 54–57.

Scoloveno, M. A. (1999). *Clinical companion for maternity nursing: Care of the childbearing family* (3rd ed.). Stamford, CT: Appleton-Lange.

Sherwen, L. N., Scoloveno, M. A., & Weingarten, C. T. (1995). *Nursing care of the childbearing family* (2nd ed.). Norwalk, CT: Appleton-Lange.

Sherwen, L. N., Scoloveno, M. A., & Weingarten, C. T. (1999). *Maternity nursing: Care of the childbearing family* (3rd ed.). Norwalk, CT: Appleton-Lange.

Somer, E. (1995). *Nutrition for a healthy pregnancy.* New York: Henry Holt.

Stanton, C. K., & Gary, R. H. (1995). Effects of caffeine consumption on delayed conception. *American Journal of Epidemiology, 142*(12), 1322–1329.

Tierra, M. (1998). *Planetary herbology.* Twin Lakes, WI: Lotus Press.

VanRyzin, L. (2000). The circumcision debate. *American Journal of Nursing, 100*(7), 24a–b.

Verilli, G. E., & Mueser, A. M. (1998). *While waiting* (2nd ed.). New York: St. Martin's Griffin.

Weed, S. (1986). *The wise woman herbal for the childbearing years.* Woodstock, NY: Ash Tree.

Young, D. (2001). Maternal Choice and Elective Cesarean. *The Network News,* July/August 1, 4–5.

Zeidenstein, L. (1998). Alternative therapies for nausea and vomiting of pregnancy. *American Journal of Nurse Midwifery, 43*(5), 392–393.

24

Menopause

Lorraine W. Bock and Marian C. Condon

Objectives

1. *Define the terms used to describe the time frames, symptoms, and therapies associated with menopause.*
2. *Discuss the ways in which the menopausal transition can affect women's self-concept, focus, and behaviors.*
3. *Describe the alterations in hormone production associated with menopause.*
4. *Identify the physiological changes and symptoms associated with midlife hormone shifts.*
5. *Discuss the pros and cons of various hormone treatments for menopausal symptoms.*
6. *Compare and contrast the bio-identical and nonbio-identical hormones used in ERT and HRT.*
7. *Identify self-care options for managing menopausal symptoms, including the use of herbs and alterations in lifestyle.*

Introduction

It is estimated that the postmenopausal years comprise one-third to one-half of American women's lives. Most women will have as many postreproductive years as they had reproductive ones (Faloon, 1998; Sheehy, 1993). Approximately 10 to 15 percent of women sail through menopause, known in medical circles as the **climacteric,** with no or few troublesome symptoms. A similar percentage experience debilitating symptoms, which decrease their quality of life significantly. The great majority, 70 to 80 percent of women in this culture, experience only temporary discomforts, such as hot flashes, difficulty sleeping, and mood swings (Hales, 1999). Over half of the women who responded to a poll conducted by the North American Menopause Society viewed the menopausal transition as a positive phase in their lives (McQuaide, 1997).

The term *menopause* was coined in the early 1800s by French physician Gardanne to describe the constellation of physical changes that coincide with the end of menstruation (Lock, 1998). In the past, menopause was seen as a *natural* event, problematic only because it heralded the end of fertility and was sometimes accompanied by troublesome but temporary symptoms. Findings from biomedical research conducted over recent decades, however, have led many to suggest that menopause is an *unnatural* consequence of the extension of the human life span and a phenomenon that can have long-term, negative implications for health with which the body is ill equipped to deal. Unfortunately, research on menopause began in earnest only relatively recently, as women acquired more status and power in society. Similarly, menopause was a taboo subject, rarely mentioned even by women themselves not long ago. Now, menopause is openly discussed, and its benefits as well as the problems it can bring are being identified. In recent years, the term *perimenopause* has been used to describe the 2 to 10 years over which the hormone shifts that will result in the permanent cessation of menstruation occur.

Whether natural or unnatural, menopause is a significant transition that affects women physically, psychologically, and socially, in ways that can be viewed as either positive or negative. Women and their healthcare providers can now choose from a number of therapies designed to relieve temporary menopausal discomfort and/or prevent future menopause-related health problems. Unfortunately, however, the body of existing research is insufficient to provide clear guidelines as to which interventions are best. The situation is further complicated by the fact that the information in the hundreds of articles, books, and pamphlets that have been published on the subject of menopause is often extremely complicated, inaccurate, outdated, or incomplete. This chapter is intended to provide clear, current, and balanced information about what is known about menopause, the ways in which it affects women and women's health, and the various treatments that are available for problems that develop.

Terminology

Premenopause, perimenopause, menopause, and *postmenopause* are all terms used to describe the phases of a woman's reproductive cycle. Often used interchangeably, the terms can be confusing and sometimes even misleading. Medically, the terms have distinct meanings and describe unique phases of female reproduction. *Premenopause* is the term used to define the period during which a predictable pattern of hormone secretion occurs in the body. Hormones are produced and released in a regular, rhythmic pattern, and menstruation occurs approximately every 28 to 30 days. Normally, adult women are capable of becoming pregnant during the premenopausal years.

Perimenopause is defined as the period of time during which hormone secretion begins to decline as a prelude to menopause. A woman is born with a finite number of ovarian follicles that have the potential to mature and produce an ovum, or egg. During each month, one, or sometimes more, follicles ripen and produce an egg. This process gives rise to the rise and fall of various hormones during the menstrual cycle (see Chapter 17). When the number of remaining follicles capable of maturing in a woman's ovaries declines to a certain level, her menstrual cycles begin to become irregular, and her hormone levels begin to shift in a manner that can cause symptoms such as irregular periods, hot flashes, night sweating, and alteration in libido. This can occur at any age but typically begins in the early to mid forties. Perimenopause can last anywhere from 2 to 10 years (Shapiro, 2001).

Eventually, the ovaries become devoid of functional follicles, and menstrual cycling will cease permanently. A woman who has gone 6 to 12 months without experiencing a menstrual period is considered to have reached *menopause*. The median age at which women in the United States reach menopause is 51.3 years, with a range of from 47 to 55 years of age. Women who have little body fat, smoke cigarettes, are malnourished, or are of non-European ancestry tend to reach menopause up to 4 years earlier than women who do not have any of those characteristics, and women who have had an ovary removed enter menopause sooner than women who have not. The age at which a woman began to menstruate does not predict the age at which she will reach menopause (McKinlay, Brambilla, & Posner, 1992). Unfortunately, although symptoms such as hot flashes and difficulty sleeping typically have abated by the time true menopause occurs, the side effects of hormone depletion, such as bone loss, vaginal atrophy, and coronary heart disease, can begin to develop. Whether these developments are due mainly to hormone depletion or to a less than ideal lifestyle, however, is still being debated.

Surgical menopause is the term used to define the estrogen loss caused by the removal of the ovaries before hormone production would naturally begin to change. Surgical menopause causes an abrupt interruption in estrogen production and can have severe side effects. *Premature menopause* is diagnosed when estrogen production declines due to ovarian failure not caused by outside influences, prior to age 40 (*What Is Menopause?* 2000).

The term used to refer to the years after menopause is *postmenopause*. Women usually experience few symptoms during this period.

The term *hormone replacement therapy (HRT)* refers to the use of a combination of hormones, such as estrogen, progesterone, and sometimes testosterone, to combat the symptoms related to the decline of hormone levels in the body. A similar term, *estrogen replacement therapy (ERT)*, is frequently used interchangeably with HRT, but this is inaccurate; ERT properly refers only to the use of *estrogens* in hormone replacement.

Other terms commonly used in the discussion of menopause describe specific symptoms. For example, *hot flashes,* or *hot flushes,* are sensations of heat that arise in a part of the body, such as the face, or the entire body. They come on suddenly, can vary in intensity from mild to severe, last less than two minutes, and are sometimes accompanied by sweating. The exact physiological mechanism by which hot flashes occur is not known, but physiologists suspect that declining levels of estrogen and rising levels of Follicle Stimulating Hormone (FSH) cause the thermoregulatory center in the hypothalamus, and the mechanisms that cause arteries to expand and contract, to become unstable (Longscope, Crawford, & McKinlay, 1996). *Night sweats* are periods of profuse sweating that accompany hot flashes that occur at night. They often cause considerable discomfort and can interrupt sleep.

Menopause: A Natural Process or a Deficiency Disease?

Whether menopause is a natural part of the female reproductive cycle has been debated for many years. Prior to 1930, the year in which the first female hormone (estrone) was isolated and its chemical structure determined, the medical community had seen menopause as a natural and inevitable, although turbulent, event that signaled the end of the reproductive years. After that time, however, physicians began to use synthesized hormones to treat the symptoms of menopause and to conceptualize menopause as a *deficiency disease*. The rate at which menopause became medicalized accelerated in 1966, with the publication of the book "Feminine Forever," in which Dr. Robert Wilson, a gynecologist practicing in New York, argued that estrogen could promote bone and cardiovascular health and preserve youthful vigor and appearance (Shapiro, 2001). Many who see menopause as an inherently pathological state of hormone deficiency argue that it is a function of modern women's unnaturally long lives. According to this view, prior to the agricultural age, the human life span was relatively short, and it was natural for most women to die before they reached menopause. Proponents of the hormone deficiency theory maintain that women started having appreciable numbers of postmenopausal years only after improvements in the food supply, living conditions, and medical care rendered human life less nasty, brutish, and short. This theory holds that menopause is a socially constructed, age-related, hormone deficiency disease that produces symptoms and increases the risk of illness.

There is, of course, an opposing view. Sociobiologist Sarah Blaffer-Hrdy (1999), reports that it is *not* necessarily natural for all female animals to die shortly after menopause. She points out that, although most female animals do live only a year or two past the end of their fertility, it is common for pilot whales and elephants, as well as humans, to live for decades after they have quit reproducing. Blaffer-Hrdy cites anthropological research that suggests it is natural for female humans to live past menopause and that doing so is *not* a relatively new phenomenon related to the advance of civiliza-

tion. Studies of surviving hunter-gatherer populations that live much as our remote human ancestors did reveal that, although about half the population (females included) die before the age of 15, the survivors have a good chance of reaching old age. Also, the infants' chances of survival are enhanced if the grandmothers are available to assist the mothers in childrearing; thus, according to this theory, it is *biologically adaptive* for women to live past menopause.

In support of their position, those who see menopause as a natural transition point out that many women have lived to a ripe old age without ERT or HRT and that 25 percent of the women in this country experience only mild menopausal symptoms that require no treatment. Northrup (2001) argues that the body is capable of providing sufficient hormones to maintain health even after ovarian function declines, by manufacturing them in the adrenals, fat cells, skin, and so on. She maintains that the negative physical changes associated with menopause in this culture are related more to *stress* than to lowered hormone levels per se. Chronic stress can exaggerate women's response to the normal hormonal shifts associated with female physiology by overtaxing the adrenal glands and impairing their ability to produce substances such as epinephrine and cortisol, which allow us to maintain our energy and positive mood when stress is present. Many modern women experience excessive levels of stress in their lives, due to factors such as too many responsibilities, insufficient autonomy, too few supportive relationships, a poor diet, and lack of exercise. Interestingly, women who suffer from PMS are known to be more likely to experience a difficult menopause than are women who do not suffer from it (Arpels, 1996). In their study of almost 300 menopausal women, Dennerstein and her colleagues (2001) found that the best predictor of positive mood state *during* menopause is positive mood state *prior* to menopause.

Although the age at which women *enter menopause* is constant across cultures (Hales, 1999), the degree to which women *experience symptoms* is not. For example, Japanese women do not generally complain of hot flashes and mood swings (Lock, 1998). That their diet is high in soy, which contains phytoestrogens, may be a factor, but it is also true that traditional Japanese women are reluctant to discuss matters pertaining to sex and reproduction. The Lusi people of Papua New Guinea have no word for middle age or menopause. A woman who has passed her reproductive years is referred to as a *Tamparonga*, or "big woman"—a title of honor and respect (Hales, 1999). Studies of women in cultures more like our own also suggest that the degree to which menopause is perceived as problematic may be related more to the overall quality of women's lives than to changing hormone levels. Dennerstein, Dudley, Guthrie and Barrett-Connor (2000) studied factors that influenced life satisfaction in a group of middle-aged Australian women. The women were queried about their degree of satisfaction with various aspects of their lives before and after menopause. Most of the women were satisfied with their lives, and satisfaction was found to be *unrelated* to menopausal status, hormone levels, or HRT. Factors positively related to satisfaction with life were feelings for partner and exercise. The factors that affected their satisfaction negatively were daily hassles, interpersonal stress, depressive symptoms, and current smoking. Even in the United States, women overwhelmingly report that their energy, self-esteem, and overall happiness greatly *increase* after menopause (Hales, 1999).

Finally, those who see menopause as a normal transition rather than a deficiency state point out that perceiving women's reproductive organs and hormones as pathological is nothing new. A host of physical and mental problems—most notably, hysteria—have been attributed to women's unique physiology since the time of the Ancient Greeks (see Chapter 1). Physicians of the Victorian era, a time during which women were valued primarily for their ability to please men sexually and to reproduce, characterized menopause as the "gateway to old age through which a woman passes at the peril of her life" (Sheehy, 1993, p. 44).

Hormone Production in the Body

Estrogen is the term used to describe three closely related hormones manufactured in women's bodies—estrone, estriol, and estradiol (also known as 17beta-estradiol). All three forms of estrogen are synthesized from cholesterol, primarily in the ovaries. Estradiol is the most potent of the three forms of estrogen. During a woman's fertile years, its major duties in the body are to stimulate growth in the uterus and breasts, to foster the maturation of egg-bearing follicles in the ovaries, and to stimulate maternal behavior. Estrone and estriol are weaker estrogens, with estriol the weakest of all. Prior to menopause, estriol comprises 90 percent of the estrogen in a woman's body; estradiol, 7 percent and estrone, 3 percent (Low Dog, Riley, & Carter, 2001). After menopause, estrone becomes the predominant estrogen, although the ovaries and the other hormone-producing sites (the adrenal glands and fat cells) continue to manufacture small amounts of estradiol, and progesterone can be converted to estrogen (Northrup, 2001).

Estrogen production is controlled by a complicated sequence of hormone secretion and conversion. These hormones come primarily from the hypothalmus and anterior pituitary gland and include gonadotropin-releasing hormone (GnRH), follicle-stimulating hormone (FSH), and luteinizing hormone (LH). These hormones act on the corpus luteum, the small crater left behind when an ovum is released from a follicle, of the ovary which releases estrogen, and on the ovarian theca cells, which convert androgens (hormones associated with maleness but present in small amounts in women's bodies) to estrogen (McCance & Huether, 1998). The estrogens are involved in many processes in the body, such as the development of reproductive organs, long bone closure after puberty, the maintenance of bone density, the regulation of the menstrual cycle, and various other metabolic functions.

Because estradiol, the most potent estrogen, is produced primarily in the ovaries, the overall estrogenic effect in the body declines as ovarian function deteriorates with age. The notion that the ovaries fail *completely* at menopause, however, is incorrect. Although the ovaries do stop producing eggs, they continue to produce androgens, which can be converted into estrogen-like hormones. Estrone is also produced by adipose (fat) tissue, which is why women with more ample figures often have fewer symptoms related to estrogen loss than do their leaner sisters (Wright & Morgenthaler, 1997).

Progesterone, the second most prevalent female hormone after estrogen, is also necessary for the regulation of the female reproductive cycle. Like estrogen, progesterone is synthesized via an enzymatic conversion of cholesterol in the ovaries, and it is secreted directly by the corpus luteum. Progesterone production is controlled mainly by the secretion of LH from the anterior pituitary gland (McCance & Huether, 1998).

During the childbearing years, progesterone stimulates the uterine lining to thicken with blood-rich tissue to support an embryo. It also relaxes the uterine muscles, thus discouraging the premature expulsion of the embryo. If pregnancy does not occur, progesterone levels drop rapidly, and the uterine lining is shed as menstrual blood. Progesterone also has a sedating and anti-anxiety effect that promotes restful sleep (Northrup, 2001). Progesterone levels also decline during perimenopause and usually decline earlier and more rapidly than estrogen levels (Shapiro, 2001).

Although androgens such as testosterone are primarily considered male hormones, women also produce them in small amounts. Like the other sex hormones, androgens are synthesized from cholesterol in the ovaries and the adrenal cortices, and they are precursors of some female hormones. In women, testosterone is produced mainly in the adrenal glands; along with other androgens, it promotes long bone growth, the production of hair in the axilla and pubic areas, and the activation of the sweat glands (because of this function, testosterone is often implicated in cases of acne).

Testosterone is also the principal hormone that supports the female libido (Berman & Berman, 2001). Serum testosterone levels also decline somewhat during perimenopause and menopause, but then they stabilize in subsequent years. About 50 percent of perimenopausal and postmenopausal women experience a decrease in their desire for sex. Women who undergo the surgical removal of their ovaries, however, experience a precipitous drop in testosterone, and most notice that their desire for sex and response to sexual stimulation declines significantly (Shapiro, 2001). The estrogen contained in HRT can cause testosterone levels to drop even more, because estrogen contains a substance called **steroid binding globulin,** which binds to testosterone and makes it unavailable to the body (Berman & Berman, 2001).

Physical and Other Changes Associated with Perimenopause

Perimenopause is often characterized by phenomena such as irregular menstrual periods, premenstrual bloating and mood swings, an unusually heavy or long-lasting menstrual flow, warm flushes or hot flashes, difficulty sleeping, decreased libido, and a phenomenon known as *brain fog,* or *cotton head*—a decline in the ability to concentrate and remember. Approximately 75 percent of perimenopausal women in this culture have symptoms severe enough to cause them to turn to hormone therapy or alternative sources of relief (Northrup, 2001). The median age at which the symptoms of perimenopause start to manifest is 47.5 years (Hales, 1999). Although the preponderant medical opinion is that perimenopausal symptoms are due to fluxuating estrogen levels, an alternative theory holds that they are due more to the relative lack of progesterone in relation to estrogen. This circumstance is referred to as **estrogen dominance** (Lark, 2000). Proponents of the estrogen dominance theory (Lee, 1999) maintain that relative progesterone deficiency causes water retention, breast tenderness, a decreased sex drive, a craving for sweets and other carbohydrates, and irregular or heavy menstrual periods, whereas true estrogen deficiency causes hot flashes, vaginal dryness, headaches, mental confusion, and recurring urinary tract infections. Both estrogen deficiency and progesterone deficiency are believed to cause depression and mood swings (Northrup, 1998).

A decrease in libido is common during perimenopause. In one study (Sarrel & Whitehead, 1985), 86 percent of the participants reported being less interested in sex and less responsive to it during perimenopause than they had been before. Whereas progesterone levels may play a role, testosterone is believed to be the hormone *most* responsible for sexual drive and responsiveness in women (Berman & Berman, 2001). Of course, depression, anxiety, painful intercourse due to vaginal dryness, and relationship problems with the sexual partner can be factors as well. Estrogen levels, too, can influence sexual response. Estrogen deprivation can lower a woman's sensitivity to touch (Sarrel, 1990). Also, estrogen has a *vasodilating* effect, which allows sufficient blood to engorge the clitoris during sexual stimulation. Women have been shown to experience an *increase* in their sexual responsiveness once their estrogen levels have been restored, even if they are not also receiving testosterone (Sarrel, 1982).

Although mood swings are common during perimenopause, the more serious problem of clinical depression also develops in some women. First-time episodes of clinical depression peak between the ages of 45 and 49, as well as between 25 and 29 (Hales, 1999). Mood swings and depression may be related to a combination of hormonal shifts and life experiences. Hormonal shifts during menopause may stimulate the brain in such a way that suppressed memories,

emotions, unresolved issues, resentments, and the like are brought back into consciousness (Northrup, 2001). Women enter perimenopause at a time when they may also be experiencing a number of stressors common to women at midlife. Children may be leaving home to attend college, pursue a career, marry, and so on, and women who suddenly find themselves alone with their spouses may find themselves renegotiating or re-evaluating the relationship. Aging parents may require a lot of care and attention, and new and unsettling health problems, such as hypertension, overweight, or high cholesterol, may develop. Finally, age-related changes in physical appearance are distressing to many women in this culture, where youth and beauty is highly prized, especially in women.

As ovarian function winds down and estrogen levels drop, the intervals between menstrual periods lengthen. True menopause is said to have arrived when a woman has been without a menstrual period for six months to one year. Hot flashes may continue to occur for one or two years postmenopause. It is imperative that women continue to use birth control until one year after the menstrual cycle appears to have stopped for good (Northrup, 2001).

Physical Changes Associated with Menopause

The systemic bodily changes associated with menopause are related to the decreasing levels of estrogen in the body, and possibly progesterone and testosterone as well. Estrogen is known to have an impact on multiple body systems and organs, including, but not limited to, the bones, heart, blood vessels, skin, genitourinary tract, and brain.

Bones

The bones of the body, despite their hard and solid appearance, are really dynamic structures that are constantly being broken down and then remodeled. A woman's bone mass reaches peak density when she is in her midthirties, and then it begins to slowly decline. After menopause, bone density can decrease at rates approaching 1 to 1.5 percent per year. The decline in bone integrity associated with menopause is thought to be related to declining levels of estrogen and progesterone, although other factors are known to influence bone integrity (see Chapter 14). Estrogen is known to mediate vitamin D formation and to stimulate bone-building cells, and both estrogen and progesterone are thought to contribute to bone strength in other ways that have not yet been clearly demonstrated (Wright & Morgenthaler, 1997).

By whatever mechanism, the reduction in estrogen production following menopause has been proven to contribute to the development of osteoporosis, and scientific studies have shown that the use of ERT following menopause lowers the risk of osteoporosis and the debilitating consequences of it. Most researchers agree that ERT started at any time following the cessation of estrogen production is beneficial to bone density but that ERT started *immediately* following menopause prevents almost 100 percent of potential bone loss (Wright & Morgenthaler, 1997). The nonbioidentical (chemically distinct from the progesterone produced by the body) forms of oral progesterone often given to postmenopausal women along with estrogen neither enhance nor decrease the bone-building effects of estrogen and have *no* bone-preserving effect when administered by themselves. At this time, there are not enough data to say whether supplementation with bio-identical oral progesterone will have an effect on bone (Low Dog et al., 2001).

Heart and Blood Vessels

Estrogen is known to have a number of salutary effects on the cardiovascular system (see Chapter 12). Therefore, until quite recently, it was commonly accepted that estrogen, and estrogen-progestin combinations as well, are cardioprotective, even though women were given estrogen alone in most of the supporting studies. Women who took ERT or HRT were assumed to be significantly reducing their risk of heart attack. Recent studies designed to probe the relationship between hormones and cardiovascular health, however, have yielded results that challenge those assumptions and raise new questions about the ways in which various kinds of estrogen and progesterone-like compounds affect cardiovascular risk factors and cardiac morbidity and mortality.

The first study to cast doubt on the theory that HRT is cardioprotective was **the Heart and Estrogen/Progestin Replacement Study (HERS).** In that study, (Hully et al., 1998) a large prospective study of the relationship between HRT and cardiovascular health, postmenopausal women with preexisting coronary heart disease who were started on full doses of HRT had an *increased incidence* of cardiovascular events, especially during the first year of treatment. The next was the **Estrogen Replacement and Atherosclerosis (ERA)** study, a major clinical trial involving over 2000 women and conducted over 4 years (Herrington et al., 2000). In that study, women with pre-existing coronary artery disease were given ERT, HRT, or a placebo. After several years, there was no difference in the amount of plaque in the arteries of the women in the three groups. Neither the use of ERT nor the use of HRT slowed the progression of plaque development, even though both decreased blood levels of LDL cholesterol and increased blood levels of HDL cholesterol. The ERA study called into question the assumption that estrogen's beneficial effects on cardiac *risk factors* translate into *better clinical outcomes,* such as less plaque in arteries. The results of the HERS and ERA trials stimulated researchers to investigate the ways in which ERT and HRT affected the cardiovascular status of *healthy* women. Consequently, a large clinical trial involving over 16,000 healthy post-menopausal women was conducted as part of the **Women's Health Initiative.** Its preliminary results indicated that while ERT (which may only be given safely to women who have had a hysterectomy) *may* confer a degree of protection against coronary heart disease, HRT *does not.* In fact, HRT was found to slightly *increase* women's chances of developing coronary heart disease, as well as their risk of stroke, blood clots and cancer (Writing Group for the Women's Health Initiative Investigators, 2002).

It should be noted that *non-bioidentical* hormones (see page 509) were used in all the studies in which hormones have been found to have an adverse effect on women's health. For example, *conjugated equine estrogens* and *medroxyprogesterone* were used in the WHI study. This raised the issue of whether the use of bioidentical hormones, particularly bioidentical progesterone, would have yielded a different result. The effects of *all* of the various forms of non-bioidentical hormones should also be determined. More research that addresses these issues is needed.

Skin

As women age, the skin's elasticity, pigmentation, and thickness diminish. These changes result in wrinkling, an increased risk of injury, and a decreased ability to ward off infection. The skin becomes more vulnerable to irritation, and the ability of its sensory nerves to sense pain and changes in temperature is lessened (McCance & Heuther, 1998). The results of a few relatively small studies suggest that ERT or HRT seems to delay wrinkling in nonsmoking Euro-American women, but not in Euro-American women who smoke. ERT or HRT has not been shown to affect wrinkling in African American women, whether they smoke or not (National Women's Health Network, 2000). ERT or HRT may also slightly increase the skin's ability to heal from injury. It must be noted, however, that no large, blinded, randomized trials on estrogen's effect on the skin have been completed to date.

Genitourinary Tract

Estrogen promotes tissue elasticity and lubrication, and the tissues of the external genitalia, vagina, urethra, and bladder have a large number of estrogen receptors (Barton, 2000). When estrogen production in the body declines, the incidence of problems such as vaginal dryness, some forms of urinary incontinence, urinary tract infections, and dyspareunia (pain during sexual intercourse) increases. As estrogen levels decline, the vagina shortens and narrows, and its walls become thinner, paler, and less elastic; the mucus-producing glands atrophy, causing decreased lubrication. A premenopausal woman has a vaginal pH of around 4.0, whereas a postmenopausal woman has a vaginal pH of approximately 6.09 (Low Dog et al., 2001); this relatively more basic vaginal environment is less hospitable to the friendly bacteria (lactobacilli) that inhabit the vagina and keep infectious bacteria at bay. Consequently, postmenopausal women are more susceptible to vaginal and urinary tract infections. Estrogen supplementation, particularly estrogen applied topically to the vagina, has been shown to ameliorate all of these symptoms for most women, especially when used in combination with other interventions, such as water-soluble vaginal lubricants, pelvic floor exercises (Kegels), and bladder training programs (National Women's Health Network, 2000; Northrup, 1999c). Postmenopausal women should avoid douching, because it rinses away lubricating fluids and the healthy organisms that live in the vagina.

Brain

Estrogen is thought to play a role in maintaining a positive mood and memory, as well. One way that estrogen enhances memory is by enhancing nerve impulse conduction in the hippocampus, an area of the brain that is important for memory. In addition, all ovarian hormones bind to the midbrain areas that regulate mood (Northrup, 1999a). The estrogen produced in women's bodies is known to have significant mood-enhancing effects, and ovarian progesterone decreases anxiety and fosters sleep. Therefore, it is not surprising that estrogen and progesterone depletion is thought to be implicated in menopause-related moodiness and depression. Depression is known to be more prevalent in women who undergo surgical, as opposed to natural, menopause, most likely because surgery causes an *abrupt* disruption of hormone production in the body (National Women's Health Network, 2000). Contrary to popular opinion, studies that follow premenopausal women through menopause do *not* suggest that menopause is associated with an increase in psychological or psychiatric problems (Shapiro, 2001). The nineteenth-century view that menopause frequently causes nervous irritability and hysteria (see Chapter 1) is not supported by modern science. Severe problems with hot flashes that lead to sleeplessness, however, can lead to symptoms associated with sleep deprivation (see Chapter 6), and hot flashes that interfere with sleep, but not menopause per se, are known to be associated with depression (Bosworth et al., 2001).

Estrogen loss is also thought to be a factor in the onset of the type of dementia known as Alzheimer's disease (see Chapter 19). The presence of adequate amounts of estrogen is known to promote the growth of the nerve endings that form the synapses through which nerve cells communicate with each other and to promote the presence of growth factors that support nerve cell development. In animal studies, estrogen has been found to increase levels of the neurotransmitter acetylcholine (Alzheimer's Disease, 1999). A relatively small but intriguing body of evidence suggests that maintaining youthful estrogen levels may prevent or delay the onset of Alzheimer's. Unfortunately, none of the studies clarifies the amount of hormone needed to stave off the disease, although higher doses seem to be most effective (Alzheimer's Disease, 1999).

The completed studies investigating potential linkages between estrogen supplementation and enhanced mood and mental functioning are small and have yielded conflicting results. Moreover, some have been flawed by small sample sizes, a short duration, and/or lack of control for intervening variables such as income, educational background, and social status (Freinkel, 2000; National Women's Health Network, 2000).

Interestingly, research suggests that the incidence of depression and memory loss among women in China, a culture in which the elderly are traditionally paid great respect, is significantly *lower* than among women in the United States, where aging is viewed negatively and older women are disdained. It has been suggested that changing our societal attitudes toward aging would be more effective than drug therapy in maintaining mental capacity in older women (Weissman & Olfson, 1995).

Postmenopausal Zest

Not all the changes associated with the menopausal transition are negative. Anthropologist Margaret Mead famously coined the term **postmenopausal zest** to describe the surge of energy and purpose that postmenopausal women typically experience. Women who spend their reproductive years focused on their families often neglect themselves; all their energy goes into caring for others, which usually involves working outside the home as well as in it. Many lose sight of their own desires, dreams, and aspirations because of the many compromises family life requires. By the time women have completed the menopausal transition, however, their children have likely left home, and they have the time, energy, and often the means to pursue their own dreams and desires. Many women in their forties, fifties, and beyond go back to school, enter the business world, or take on ambitious public service projects. Many women who have risen to national prominence did so during the second half of their lives. Political leaders such as Margaret Thatcher, Golda Meir, and Indira Gandhi did not take the helm of their countries until they had reached midlife, and most of the women in the U.S. Congress are in their fifties or older. The great feminist leader Elizabeth Cady Stanton, who continued her activities well into her sixties, wrote of the sense of liberation that she experienced when she had finally left childbearing and childrearing behind.

According to Northrup (2001), there are *biological* as well as *social* reasons for women's midlife enhanced drive and sense of purpose. She maintains that, when women are in their reproductive years, estrogen is their dominant hormone. In addition to fostering nurturing behavior, estrogen fosters compliance and receptivity, possibly because, when human beings were evolving, women stood a better chance of raising their young successfully if they adopted a "go with the flow" stance regarding their powerful male protectors. At the completion of the menopausal transition, however, estrogen levels are *lower,* and testosterone levels are considerably *higher.* Testosterone fuels both aggression and drive. According to Northrup, postmenopausal women, equipped with both the wisdom of their years and a new mix of hormones, are well prepared to follow their dreams wherever they lead. Although Northrup's theory is appealing, it must be remembered that hormonal predilections are either reinforced or opposed by the environment (Blaffer-Hrdy, 1999). Societal restrictions on women's roles and activities, which are diminishing, have enhanced whatever muting effect estrogen has on female assertiveness. It will be interesting to see whether younger women prove to be as energetic and adventurous as their elders, once gender roles have become less well defined and responsibility for childcare is shared more equitably.

Hormone Level Testing

There are many methods of determining whether hormonal shifts related to menopause are occurring in women. The most frequently used method of determining whether the ovaries are beginning to shut down is measuring blood levels of follicle-stimulating hormone (FSH) and leutenizing hormone (LH). When ovarian function begins to wane, the levels of these hormones rise, as the pituitary gland secretes more of them in an effort to stimulate the flagging ovaries. FSH and LH blood levels can be checked throughout perimenopause as a way of monitoring the progression toward ovarian shut down. Blood levels of estrogen and progesterone can also be monitored (McCance & Heuther, 1998).

Measuring the amount of hormones in *saliva* is a newer, and some say more informative, method of determining the levels of various hormones in the body. The amount of hormone in saliva reflects the amount of unbound hormone available to cells in the body. Bound hormone is chemically attached to other molecules and is not active in tissues. Blood tests measure both bound and unbound hormone and do not reflect as accurately the true amount of hormones that is available to the tissues (Northrup, 1998). This noninvasive, painless method of quantifying hormones is rapidly gaining popularity among healthcare providers and consumers. Consumers can even order saliva-collecting kits directly from certain laboratories (see the Resources section

at the end of this chapter), submit the sample through the mail, and receive both a written report and a telephone consultation regarding the results.

Therapies for Problems Associated with Perimenopause and Menopause

The treatment modalities used to control the symptoms associated with perimenopause and menopause and to prevent problems that can arise as a consequence of estrogen loss can be divided into three main categories: hormonal treatments, hormonelike treatments, and nonhormonal treatments. Several types of hormones and hormone combinations, hormonelike substances, plant-based substances, and vitamins are used. Hormones can be either *bio-identical,* which means chemically indistinguishable from the natural hormones produced in the body, or *nonbio-identical,* i.e., similar to, but not exactly the same as, natural hormones. Nonbio-identical hormones are also known as *synthetic hormones,* although this is somewhat misleading, because bio-identical hormones are also synthesized in laboratories. Selective estrogen receptor modulators are synthetic, hormonelike compounds that produce some of the same effects as natural hormones, but not all of them, and are used to prevent some of the consequences of hormone depletion. Phytoestrogens, estrogen-like substances found in plants, herbs, and some vitamins, are used to ameliorate the symptoms of perimenopause and menopause. The elements that make up a healthy lifestyle—such as regular exercise; weight control; avoidance of smoking; low to moderate alcohol use; and a low-fat, low-cholesterol diet—are also important if health is to be maintained during the menopausal years (Finn, 2000; Rajki & Adams, 2000).

Hormonal Treatments

Estrogen and progesterone are the two hormones most commonly prescribed for women in perimenopause and menopause. Testosterone is sometimes prescribed to revive a flagging libido. The functions of estrogen and progesterone in the body are summarized in Table 24–1.

ESTROGENS

Both bio-identical and estrogens (see Figure 24–1) come in many nonbio-identical formulations, including pills, patches, creams, vaginal suppositories, and injections. The hormone most frequently used in ERT and the estrogen portion of HRT is **ethinyl estradiol.** It is synthesized from **equilin,** an equine estrogen extracted from the urine of pregnant mares, and it is not chemically identical to any of the natural estrogens (Wright & Morgenthaler, 1997). By far the most well-known and

TABLE 24–1 Comparison of the functions of estrogen and progesterone.

Estrogen	Progesterone
Prepares endometrium for pregnancy	Maintains endometrial readiness for pregnancy
Causes breast stimulation	Protects against fibrocystic breasts
Increases body fat	Helps use fat for energy
Increases blood clotting	Normalizes blood clotting
Causes salt and fluid retention	Is a natural diuretic
Can contribute to depression and headaches	Is a natural antidepressant
Interferes with thyroid hormone action	Facilitates thyroid hormone action
Decreases sex drive	Restores sex drive
Impairs blood sugar control	Normalizes blood sugar
Increases risk for cancer	Decreases risk for cancer

Figure 24–1 Chemical Structures of Estrogen Molecules

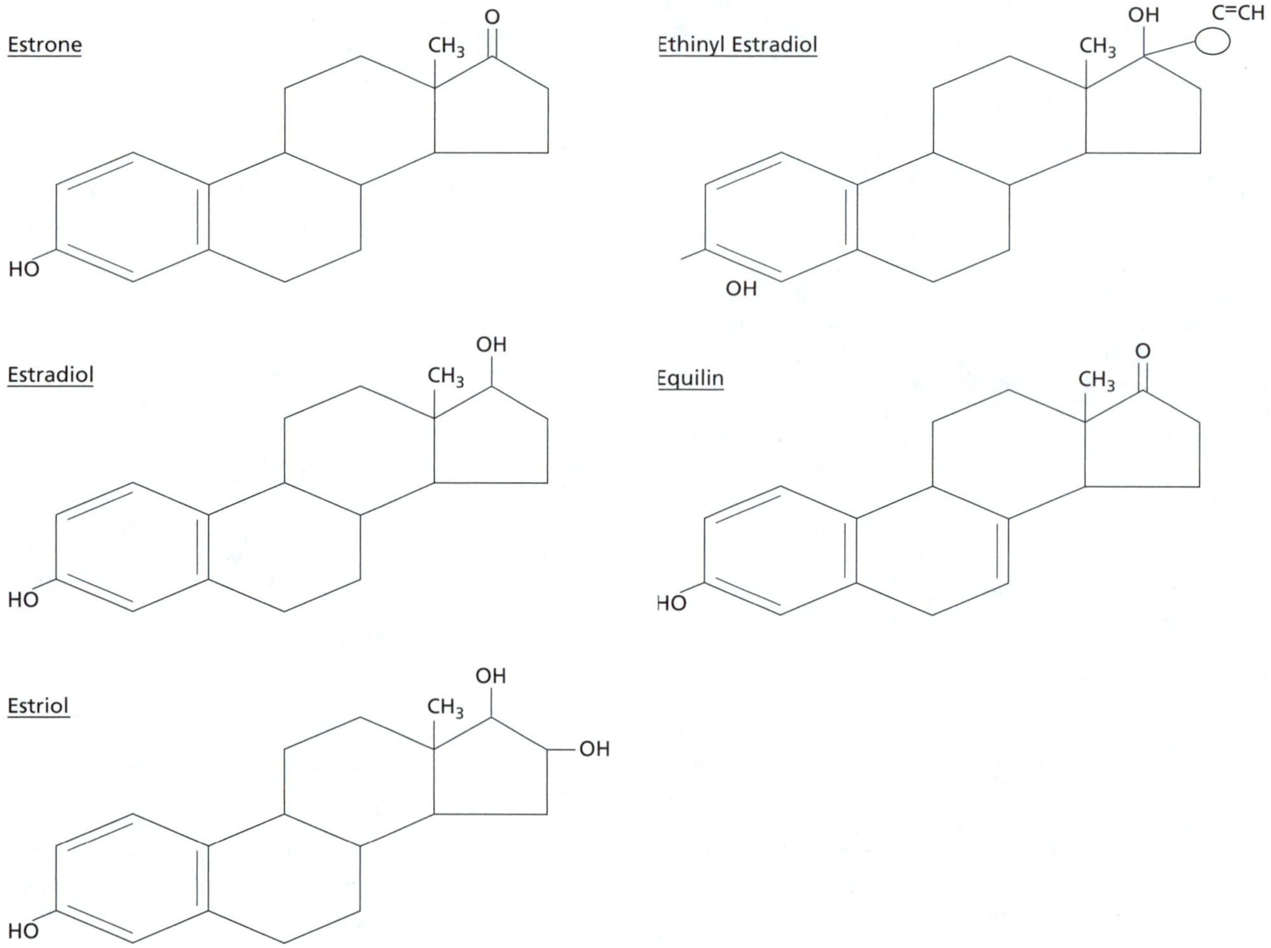
Estrone
O
CH_3
HO
Ethinyl Estradiol
OH
C=CH
CH_3
OH
Estradiol
OH
CH_3
HO
Equilin
O
CH_3
HO
Estriol
OH
CH_3
OH
HO

Box 24–1 Bio-Identical and Nonbio-Identical Estrogen and Progesterone Preparations

- ◆ Oral Estrogen Preparations
  Cenestin—nonbio-identical
  Estinyl—nonbio-identical
  Estrace—bio-identical
  Estratab/Menest—nonbio-identical
  Ogen—nonbio-identical
  Ortho-Est—nonbio-identical
  Premarin—bio-identical
  Tri-Est—bio-identical

- ◆ Estrogen Transdermal Patches
  Climara—bio-identical
  Esclim—bio-identical
  Estraderm—bio-identical
  Vivelle—bio-identical

- ◆ Estrogen Vaginal Rings
  Estring—bio-identical

- ◆ Estrogen Vaginal Creams
  Estriol—bio-identical
  Estrace Cream—bio-identical
  Ogen Cream—nonbio-identical
  Ortho Dienestrol—nonbio-identical
  Premarin Vaginal Cream—nonbio-identical

- ◆ Oral Progesterone Preparations
  Aygestin—nonbio-identical
  Provera—nonbio-identical
  Amen—nonbio-identical
  Prometrium—bio-identical

- ◆ Progesterone Vaginal Creams
  Crinone—bio-identical

- ◆ Combination Estrogen/Progesterone Products
  Prempro—oral-nonbio-identical
  FemHRT—oral-nonbio-identical
  Ortho-Prefest—oral-bio-identical estrogen plus nonbio-identical progesterone
  Combi-Patch—skin patch-bio-identical estrogen plus nonbio-identical progesterone

Box 24–2 Possible Unpleasant Side Effects of Estrogen Supplementation

- ◆ Return of menstrual bleeding
- ◆ Breast tenderness
- ◆ Fluid retention
- ◆ Weight gain
- ◆ Headaches
- ◆ Nausea and vomiting
- ◆ High blood pressure
- ◆ Gall stones
- ◆ Blood clots

rally occurring estrogens, they are not metabolized in the body in exactly the same way. They tend to be longer lasting and to exert a more potent estrogenic effect than the natural hormones and the bio-identical hormones (Wright & Morgenthaler, 1997). The more potent forms of estrogen are a double-edged sword; the greater the estrogenic effect on the body, the greater the positive effect on lipid levels and bone, but it is also more likely that unpleasant and dangerous side effects will result (Ramsey, Ross, & Fischer, 1999; Wright & Morgenthaler, 1997). Many women who originally agree to nonbio-identical estrogen replacement therapy stop treatment after a short period of time due to side effects such as excessive bleeding, breast tenderness, and nausea. Administering synthetic estrogens in lower doses often minimizes the side effects while still providing the desired effects. Box 24–2 lists some possible unpleasant side effects of estrogen supplementation.

Bio-identical estrogens are chemically identical to one of the three types of estrogen found in the female body: estriol, estradiol, and estrone. Tri-Est, a commercial formulation that contains bio-identical versions of the three types of estrogen in varying proportions, is designed to be a copy of nature (Wright & Morgenthaler, 1997). Because estradiol is the strongest of the three natural estrogens, it is compounded to comprise only about 10 to 20 percent of the total estrogen in Tri-Est. Estrone, the second most potent of the three estrogens, also comprises 10 to 20 percent of a Tri-Est compound. The remaining 60 to 80 percent is made up of estriol, the weakest—and therefore the least risky—of the three natural estrogens. Most healthcare providers who prescribe Tri-Est start with these percentages and gradually increase the percentage of estradiol if the symptoms are not relieved. Bi-Est, a bio-identical compound made up of two of the three natural estrogens, is made up of 20 percent estradiol and 80 percent estriol. It is often prescribed for women who are experiencing intolerable menopausal symptoms but who are at high risk for breast cancer (Wright & Morgenthaler, 1997). It has been theorized that estriol exerts a protective effect against

widely prescribed brand of ethinyl estradial estrogen is Premarin. Most of the other estrogens, bio-identical and nonbio-identical alike, are synthesized from materials found in plants, such as wild yam and soy (Northrup, 1999b). Box 24–1 lists the various synthetic estrogens available.

The problem with the nonbio-identical estrogens is that, because they are not chemically equivalent to the three natu-

breast cancer because of the results of animal studies; however, it is premature to make that claim in humans. Nor should it be assumed that women who take only estriol do not need the uterine-protective effects of progesterone; a recent longitudinal study conducted in Sweden found that women who had taken oral estriol for five years had a *higher* risk of developing endometrial hyperplasia and endometrial cancer than women who had taken no hormones (Weiderpass et al., 1999).

Both synthetic and bio-identical estrogen preparations are available for *topical* application in the vagina. These products maintain the integrity of vaginal and urethral tissues but do not cause blood levels of estrogen to rise. Consequently, they are useful for treating vaginal dryness and tenderness and for preventing frequent urinary tract infections from developing, but they do not protect the bones or the heart (Shapiro, 2001).

A major reason that many women elect not to take ERT or HRT is a fear of cancer (HRT and the Fear of Breast Cancer, 2000). Both the natural and the nonbio-identical forms of estrogen are known to raise the risk for both breast and uterine cancer. Estrogen has been described as a weak carcinogen capable of causing low-frequency gene mutations to occur in estrogen-sensitive tissues (Liehr, 2000), and it is known to cause tissue proliferation in the uterus and breasts. Women who are exposed to the body's own estrogens for longer periods of time—for example, those who begin menstruating earlier or experience menopause later—have a relatively higher incidence of breast cancer. Although the addition of progesterone to HRT protects women against uterine cancer, the degree to which estrogen therapy for menopause raises women's risk for breast cancer is unclear. Although some data sets are contradictory, there is reason to believe that taking estrogen for more than 5 years increases the risk of breast cancer slightly. After conducting a meta-analysis of 51 epidemiological studies involving 160,000 women, the Collaborative Group on Hormone Factors in Breast Cancer (1997) concluded that taking hormones for 15 years confers a risk 1.25 times the risk of nonusers. That means that 57 women out of 1,000 who take hormones will get breast cancer, as opposed to approximately 45 out of 1,000 women who do *not* take hormones. Some studies suggest that adding a progestin to the hormone regimen increases the risk even more. A recent study found that, although ERT was associated with only a 6 percent increase in risk compared with nonusers, HRT (with progestin) was associated with a 24 percent increase (Ross, Paganini-Hill, & Wan, 2000). Women who drink alcohol and take HRT, particularly oral HRT, may be at an increased risk for breast cancer, because alcohol affects liver cells in a manner that increases serum estrogen concentrations (Enger, Ross, Paganini-Hill, Longnecker, & Bernstein, 1999).

PROGESTERONE AND THE PROGESTINS

Progesterone is the second most prevalent sex hormone in women. Like estrogen, it is synthesized from cholesterol, and its production declines with ovarian failure at menopause.

Progesterone also comes in bio-identical and nonbio-identical forms. The bio-identical form is known as **micronized** (finely ground) **progesterone.** Micronization is necessary because progesterone in natural form is destroyed by stomach acids. Micronized particles, however, can be dissolved in oil and will then withstand the acid environment of the stomach. Nonbio-identical forms of progesterone are known as **progestins.** Both forms are available in pills, in creams, and by injection.

Women who still have their uterus and wish to take estrogen to quell menopausal symptoms or to prevent coronary artery disease or osteoporosis must take some form of progesterone in order to oppose estrogen's tendency to cause **endometrial hyperplasia,** the thickening of the lining of the uterus, and possibly endometrial cancer. The form of progesterone most commonly prescribed for this purpose is the progestin medroxyprogesterone acetate, marketed as Provera. Other progestins, such as norethindrone, norgestrel, and norgestimate, may also be prescribed. Progestins can be taken in two patterns, depending on whether monthly bleeding is acceptable to the woman. If the progestin is taken cyclically, for only 10–12 days out of each month (at a usual dose of 10 milligrams), cyclic menstrual bleeding will occur in most women. This is because the function of progesterone is to maintain the lining of the uterus to accommodate a pregnancy; if progesterone is withdrawn, the lining will be shed and a menstrual period will result. Many menopausal women, however, are reluctant to return to regular cycling after having been without periods for a number of months. If that is the case, Provera can be taken *daily* at dosages between 2.5 and 5 milligrams (Nurse Practitioner's Prescribing Reference, 2001).

The progestins are known to have several *negative* physiological effects. They reduce estrogen's ability to dilate the coronary arteries, as well as its ability to raise HDL, the good cholesterol. The progestins also cause LDL, the bad cholesterol, to contribute to plaque formation (Shapiro, 2001).

A bio-identical form of oral progesterone, Prometrium, is also commercially available with a physician's prescription. Prometrium is micronized progesterone (derived from yams) in capsule form. Bio-identical progesterone is also available in cream form. Progesterone creams are rubbed onto the skin in areas of high absorption, such as the inner thighs or wrists, and some women rub them directly onto the external genitalia. Rubbing 2 percent bio-identical progesterone cream into the skin daily controls hot flashes in about 85 percent of menopausal women (Leonetti et al., 1999). Although low-dose progesterone creams are sold without a prescription, usually in stores that sell natural products, creams that contain higher doses require a prescription and are not available commercially; they must be made up in compounding pharmacies.

Although progesterone creams will alleviate hot flashes in many women, they will *not* prevent endometrial hyperplasia in women who take ERT. In a randomized clinical trial, even progesterone creams containing much more progesterone than is found in over-the-counter preparations failed to protect the endometrium from the stimulating effects of estrogen (Wren, McFarland, & Edwards, 1999).

Some researchers believe that natural progesterone (not the progestins) has a cancer-preventive effect on the body and that even women who have had hysterectomies should receive progesterone supplementation (Wright & Morgenthaler, 1997; Sutherland, 2000). Natural progesterone does *not* interfere with the positive cardiovascular effects of estrogen; it does not constrict arteries, lower HDL, or foster the deposit of LDL in arterial plaque (Shapiro, 2001). In the Postmenopausal Estrogen/Progestin Interventions (PEPI) trial, HRT with estrogen and oral micronized progesterone had a superior cardioprotective effect to HRT with estrogen and a synthetic progestin. In a study published in the *Journal of the American College of Cardiology,* natural progesterone was found to lengthen the time a cohort of menopausal women already on estrogen were able to exercise without experiencing a shortage of blood flow to their hearts. The women were placed on estrogen and a progestin, which is known to counteract estrogen's vasodilating effect on the heart. After they were switched to natural progesterone, however, they were able to exercise longer without developing an inadequate blood flow to the heart (Rosano et al., 2000). Another study tested the effects of Prometrium in women who had been on HRT with Progestin, and were switched to HRT with micronized progesterone. While on Prometrium, the women reported that their quality of life was better than when they were on a progestin. They experienced an improvement in the rate and severity of their hot flashes, an improvement in depression and mood swings, and an improvement in somatic symptoms, such as fluid retention and headaches. Overall 80 percent reported overall satisfaction with Prometrium. (Fitzpatrick, Pace, & Wiita, 2000).

Women who are allergic to peanuts, who suffer from liver disease or breast cancer, or who are pregnant should not take Prometrium. Prometrium can also cause breast tenderness, dizziness, abdominal bloating, and vaginal discharge, particularly if the dosage is too high. Prometrium is also best taken at night, as it supports sleep (Montplaisir, Lorrain, Denesle, & Petit, 2001).

TESTOSTERONE

Abundant evidence suggests that testosterone improves libido in women. Excessive doses should be avoided, as testosterone can have a negative effect on the lipid profile (Shapiro, 2001). Testosterone can be administered by injection, orally, or topically. It is most commonly supplied to women in the form of Estratest—Premarin plus the *synthetic* testosterone methyltestosterone. Testosterone preparations containing the bio-identical testosterone forms pure testosterone, testosterone propionate or testosterone ethanotate can be obtained by prescription from compounding pharmacies. Applying testosterone topically, as a cream, skin patch, gel, or sublingual spray, bypasses the liver and obviates the possibility of liver damage. Creams and gels applied to the clitoris and inner labia help build up thinning genital tissue. Generally, libido problems respond best to *oral* preparations (Berman & Berman, 2001).

COMBINATION PREPARATIONS

There are several commercially available products that combine nonbio-identical estrogen and progesterone into one product. Combination preparations are generally reserved for women who have retained their uteri and have chosen to take HRT. PremPro and PremPhase are probably the best known of these products. Each tablet contains both conjugated equine estrogens and progestin. PremPro tablets contain consistent amounts of both hormones and are taken daily. Women who take PremPro usually do not have menstrual periods. PremPhase comprises a mix of estrogen-only and estrogen-progestin tablets supplied in a sequential dispenser; a pill is taken daily. Most women taking PremPhase have a regular monthly menstrual cycle. Other oral products, such as Ortho-Prefest, FemHRT, and Activella, are also available, as is a skin patch (Combipatch), which also contains both nonbio-identical estrogen and progesterone. Estratest, a commercial product that delivers the nonbio-identical estrogen (Premarin) and testosterone together in one tablet, is yet another product available to women. It comes in two strengths and is usually given to women who wish to enhance their libido.

It is possible to obtain bio-identical combination hormone products from a compounding pharmacist.

SELECTIVE ESTROGEN RECEPTOR MODULATORS

As their name suggests, the selective estrogen receptor modulators (SERMs) selectively stimulate estrogen receptors in the body. They are estrogen-like drugs that have some, but not all, of the effects of actual estrogen. **Raloxifene** was the first SERM to be developed and remains the most widely used. Formulated by the Eli Lilly company and marketed as Evista, the drug is FDA-approved for the treatment and possible prevention of osteoporosis in postmenopausal women who are not eligible for ERT or HRT. Although raloxifene has the same bone-preserving action on the body as estrogen, it does not prevent hot flashes. It also does *not* appear to stimulate breast or uterine tissue, and its potential for actually inhibiting the development of breast cancer is being evaluated in several studies (Jordan, Gapstur, & Morrow, 2001). The results of preliminary studies suggest, that unlike estrogen, raloxifine does *not* confer protection against cardiovascular disease (Goldberg & Goldberg, 2001). Northrup (2001) cautions that such drugs are very new and that little is known about their long-term effects on women's bodies.

Nonhormonal Treatments

Many women who experience the troublesome symptoms of perimenopause and menopause do not wish to take hormones for one reason or another. Such women often look to nonhormonal treatments to reduce their discomfort. Most effective nonhormonal agents contain phytoestrogens, which compete with the endogenous estrogens (estrogens produced by the body) for binding sites on the cells in various parts of the body. Therefore, they *block* the effects of natural estrogens while exerting their own slightly different estrogenic effect, which is typically not as strong as that of the estrogens produced in the body (Ramsey et al., 1999). Phytoestrogens are found in soybeans, apples, carrots, oats, red clover, and many other food sources. Promensil is a popular nonhormonal treatment for menopause that contains phytoestrogens. It is derived from red clover, and its efficacy has been evaluated in a number of short-term studies. Although the data are preliminary, they suggest that Promensil is safe and is effective for some women (Levlin & Baker, 1999). Many women also use soy products and soy isoflavone concentrates to lessen menopausal symptoms and enhance their overall health (see Chapter 11). Preliminary evidence suggests that phytoestrogens have a *positive* effect both on the breasts and on lipid profiles (Shapiro, 2001). More research is needed in this important area.

A number of herbs have been traditionally used to ease the symptoms associated with perimenopause and menopause. Black cohosh is one of the best known and most frequently used. Although to date black cohosh has not been shown to provide any protection from cardiovascular disease or osteoporosis, it has been demonstrated to be a safe herb that can lessen or abolish hot flashes and ease insomnia, anxiety, and depression (Tillem, 2000). Another herb, Siberian ginseng, has been found to promote the thickening of the vaginal and urethral tissues, which can reduce the discomforts of intercourse during menopause and can assist in the control of urinary incontinence (Sutherland, 2000). Chaste tree fruit (chasteberry) has been used to help alleviate irregularities of the menstrual cycle and severe premenstrual symptoms (Ramsey et al., 1999; Wright & Morganthaler, 1997). A product called Estroven contains a variety of herbs and is currently recommended for short-term use to help ward off hot flashes (Wright & Morgenthaler, 1997).

Herbs and plant substances that do not contain phytoestrogens are also sometimes used to quell various symptoms related to menopause. Valerian root is often recommended as a sleep aid and for the treatment of anxiety (Levlin & Baker, 1999). Lemon balm, passion flower, and kava kava have also been explored for the reduction of nervousness, stress, and sleep disorders (Ramsey et al., 1999). Black cohosh, chasteberry, red clover, soy, and other herbs and substances traditionally used to treat the symptoms related to perimenopause and menopause are discussed more fully in Chapter 11. Because herbs and other plant-based products can interact with prescription medications, woman should consult their healthcare providers before using such products.

A number of lubricant products can help alleviate the problem of discomfort during sexual intercourse due to vaginal dryness. Astroglide, Lubrin, Replens, and K-Y Jelly are all water-soluble lubricants that will not cause the rubber in condoms to disintegrate the way oil-based lubricants do. Astroglide and Replens have the added advantage of being mildly *acidic,* which can help prevent bacterial vaginal infections (Ask the Experts, 2000).

Journaling, or keeping a diary of one's thoughts and concerns, can help women who have spent the first half of their adult lives primarily in the service of others to get in touch with their own deepest feelings and aspirations. Northrup (2001) suggests that the hormonal shifts of perimenopause and menopause make deeply repressed psychic and emotional material more accessible. Another practice that can be very helpful to midlife women is meditation. Meditation (discussed in Chapter 11) is another way to bring repressed material into consciousness. It is also deeply relaxing and is an effective method of stress management.

Promoting Wellness During and After Menopause

Women who reach the age at which the symptoms and health problems related to menopause begin to arise must make decisions about what steps to take to increase their comfort level and to protect their bodies. Making such decisions can be difficult, however, given that the available information about hormones, SERMS, herbs, and the like is contradictory and incomplete. How is a woman facing menopause to decide whether and what kinds of HRT, SERMs, or herbs are indicated for her? For now, the answer to that question is that decisions should be made in consultation with a knowledgeable healthcare provider and should be based on the symptoms present, the woman's individual risk factor profile, and an evaluation of the pros and cons of the various treatment options. One possible approach is to use hormone therapy for a short time to ease the menopausal transition and then begin it again at age 60 or 65, when the risks of developing osteoporosis and dementia become substantial (Angier, 1999). New trials that should clarify the effects of various hormones on the cardiovascular system, such as the 12-year, 160,000-woman Women's Health Initiative, are underway. When the results are in, women and their providers should have a firmer base of information on which to make decisions about HRT, at least with synthetic hormones, and other menopause-related issues. Unfortunately, bio-identical hormones are not being studied in the Women's Health Initiative trial.

Women of menopausal age can also promote wellness by undergoing certain health screening tests regularly. The American Cancer Society recommends annual mammography and Pap smears after the age of 50. Blood cholesterol levels and levels of thyroid hormone should also be monitored yearly, and stool should be tested for the presence of occult (hidden) blood.

New Directions

More research is needed in almost every area relating to menopause. Recent research on estrogen and cardiovascular disease has called into question whether HRT or ERT is appropriate for women with established coronary heart disease. This issue must be resolved. More information is also needed on how estrogen affects the cardiovascular systems of women who do not have pre-existing coronary heart disease (HRT and Heart Disease, 2000). More research on estrogen types, dosages, treatment duration, and delivery devices is needed to determine what is optimum for women of all ages, ethnicities, and health status (Wright & Morganthaler, 1997).

Although there is little doubt that all estrogens have the potential to fuel breast cancer, the relative safety of bio-identical estrogens vs. synthetic estrogens has not been established. Questions also remain as to the effects of progesterone and the progestins on breast health. Recent studies suggest that bio-identical progesterone may exert a protective effect on breast health, whereas the progestins endanger it, but the evidence is preliminary (HRT and Heart Disease, 2000). Another question that must be answered through research is whether estrogen dominance, as opposed to estrogen deficiency, most commonly plays a role in perimenopausal symptoms.

The hormone dehydroepiandrosterone (DHEA) is being investigated as a possible treatment for menopausal problems related to hormone deficiency. DHEA is made by the adrenal glands and is thought to stimulate hormone-producing cells in women. DHEA levels are known to peak at around age 30 and then steadily decline. Low levels of DHEA have been found in women suffering from osteoporosis and immune diseases and have been associated with a higher risk for breast cancer and heart failure. DHEA may be an appropriate treatment for women who cannot take estrogen due to vaginal bleeding, as DHEA does not cause this problem. Some have suggested that it may prove to be a beneficial addition to HRT therapy with estrogen and progesterone (Richinni, 1998). Research into the potential benefits of this hormone is underway.

QUESTIONS FOR REFLECTION AND DISCUSSION

1. *What is your attitude toward menopause? To what degree are you looking forward to it or dreading it? Why?*
2. *What familial and personal factors should be considered when making a decision about HRT or ERT?*
3. *A friend approaches you, asking questions about hormones, herbs, and natural menopause. What would you tell her regarding each of the topics?*
4. *If you were directing research in any of the areas relating to menopause, what areas do you feel warrant the most attention at this time?*
5. *What lifestyle modifications can a woman use to ease her transition to menopause?*

RESOURCES

Books

Northrup, C. (1998). *Women's bodies, women's wisdom; Creating Physical and Emotional Health and Healing.* Bantam Books.

Northrup, C. (2001). *The wisdom of menopause.* Bantam Books.

Organizations

American Menopause Foundation
350 Fifth Ave., Suite 2822
New York, NY 10118
Phone: 212-714-2398

Great Smokies Diagnostic Laboratory
63 Zillicoa
Asheville, NC 28801-1074
Phone: 1-800-522-4762

The North American Menopause Society
P.O. Box 94
Cleveland, OH 94527
Phone: 404-442-7550
Web: www.menopause.org

REFERENCES

Alzheimer's disease. (1999, May). *Women's Health Advisor,* pp. 1, 3.

Andreoli, T., Bennett, J., Carpenter, C., & Plum, F. (1997). *Cecil essentials of medicine* (4th ed.). Philadelphia: W. B. Saunders.

Angier, N. (1999). *Woman: An intimate geography.* New York: Anchor Books.

Arpels, J. C. (1996). The female brain hypoestrogenic continuum from PMS to menopause: A hypothesis and review of supporting data. *Journal of Reproductive Medicine, 41*(9), 633–639.

Ask the experts. (2000). *University of California, Berkeley Wellness Letter, 16*(9), 7.

Barton, S. (Ed.). (2000). *Clinical evidence* (4th issue). London: BMJ.

Berman, J., & Berman, L. (2001). *For women only: A revolutionary guide to overcoming sexual dysfunction and reclaiming your life.* New York: Henry Holt & Company.

Blaffer-Hrdy, S. (1999). *Mother nature.* New York: Pantheon.

Bosworth, H. B., Bastian, L. A., Kuchibhata, M. N., Steffens, D. C., McBride, C. M., Skinner, C. S., Rimer, B. K., & Sieger, I. C. (2001). Depressive symptoms, menopausal status, and climacteric symptoms in women at midlife. *Psychosomatic Medicine, 63*(4), 603–608.

Collaborative Group on Hormone Factors in Breast Cancer. (1997). Breast cancer and hormone replacements: Collaborative reanalysis of the data from 51 epidemiological studies of

52,705 women with breast cancer and 108,411 women without breast cancer. *Lancet, 350,* 1047–1059.

Current medical news. (2000, October 30). *Patient Care,* pp. 9–10.

Dennerstein, L. (2000). *5th European Congress on menopause* [On-line]. Available: *http://womenshealth.medscape.com/Medscape. . .v05.n04. wh0719.denn/pnt-wh0719.denn.html*

Dennerstein, L., Lehert, P., Dudley, E., & Guthrie, J. (2001). Factors contributing to positive mood during the menopausal transition. *Journal of Nervous and Mental Disease, 189*(2), 84–89.

Enger, S. M., Ross, R. K., Paganini-Hill, A., Longnecker, M. P., & Bernstein, L. (1999). Alcohol consumption and breast cancer: Estrogen and progesterone receptor status. *British Journal of Cancer, 79,* 1308–1314.

Faloon, W. (1998, April). Menopause: Stopping the Symptoms Before They Stop You. *Life Extension,* pp. 7–13.

Finn, S. C. (2000). Nutrition issues for women. *Advance for Nurse Practitioners, 8*(11), pp. 46–55.

Freinkel, S. (2000, June). The hormone debate heats up. *Health,* pp. 112–118.

Fitzpatrick, L. A., Pace, C., & Wiita, B. (2000). Comparison of regimens containing oral micronized progesterone or medroxyprogesterone acetate on quality of life in post-menopausal women: A cross sectional survey. *Journal of Women's Health and Gender Based Medicine, 9*(4), 381–387.

Goldberg, I., & Goldberg, H. (2001, February 21). *Effect of a selective estrogen, raloxifene, on lipoprotein* [On-line]. Available: *http://www.womenshealth.medscape. com/HOL/articles/2000/02/hol06/ho106.htm*

Hales, D. (1999). *Just like a woman.* New York: Bantam Books.

Herrington, D. M., Reboussin, D. M., Brosnihan, K. B., Sharp, P. C., Shumaker, S. A., Snyder, T. E., Furberg, C. D., Kowalchuk, G. J., Stuckey, T. D., Rogers, W. J., Givens, D. H., Waters, D. (2000). Effects of estrogen replacement on the progression of coronary-artery atherosclerosis. *New England Journal of Medicine 343*(8), 522–529.

HRT and the fear of breast cancer. (2000, July). *Women's Health Advisor,* pp. 3.

HRT and heart disease: More controversy. (2000, June). *Health News: Heart Watch,* pp. 1–2.

Hulley, S., Grady, D., Bush, T., Furberg, C., Herrington, D., Riggs, B., Vittinghoff, E. (1998). Randomized trial of estrogen plus progestin for secondary prevention of coronary heart disease in postmenopausal women. *Journal of the American Medical Association 280*(7), 605–613.

Jordan, V. C., Gapstur, S., & Morrow, M. (2001). Selective estrogen receptor modulation and reduction in risk of breast cancer, osteoporosis, and coronary heart disease. *Journal of the National Cancer Institute, 93*(19), 1449–1457.

Lark, S. (2000, March). Undoing estrogen dominance. *The Lark Letter,* pp. 2–3

Lee, J. (1999). *What your doctor may not tell you about premenopause.* New York: Warner Books.

Leonetti, H., et al. (1999). Transdermal progesterone cream for vasomotor symptoms and postmenopausal bone loss. *Obstetrics and Gynecology, 94,* 225–228.

Levlin, T., & Baker, D. (1999). *Natural remedies for menopausal symptoms.* Document prepared for subscribers of the *Pharmacist's & Prescriber's Letter.*

Liehr, J. G. (2000). Is estradiol a genotoxic mutagenic carcinogen? *Endocrinology Review, 21,* 40–54.

Lock, E. (1998). Anomalous women and political strategies for aging societies. In S. Sherwin (Ed.), *The politics of women's health: Exploring agency and autonomy* (pp. 178–204). Philadelphia: Temple University Press.

Longscope, C., Crawford, S., & McKinlay, S. (1996). Endogenous estrogens: Relationship between estrone, estradiol, non-protein bound estradiol and hot flashes and lipids. *Menopause, 3,* 77–84.

Low Dog, T., Riley, D., & Carter, T. (2001). An integrative approach to menopause. *Alternative Therapies, 7*(4), 45–55.

McKinlay, S. M., Brambilla, D. J., & Posner, J. G. (1992). The normal menopausal transition. *Maturitas, 14,* 103–116.

McQuaide, S. (1997, February). Baby boom women say mid-life stereotypes are not the norm. *Fordham University Media Report to Women,* p. 5.

Montplaisir, J., Lorrain, J., Denesle, R., & Petit, D. (2001). Sleep in menopause: Differential effects of two forms of hormone replacement. *Menopause, 8*(1), 10–16.

National Women's Health Network. (2000). *Taking hormones and women's health.* Washington, D.C.: National Women's Health Network

Northrup, C. (1998). *The hormone report.* Potomac, MD: Phillips.

Northrup, C. (1999a). Estrogen and your brain: What every woman needs to know. *Health Wisdom for Women,* p. 2.

Northrup, C. (1999b). Is hormone replacement ever really natural? *Health Wisdom for Women,* pp. 1–6.

Northrup, C. (1999c). Menopause and sexual dysfunction: Is estrogen the problem? *Health Wisdom for Women,* pp. 6–8.

Northrup, C. (2001). *The wisdom of menopause.* New York: Bantam Books.

Nurse practitioner's prescribing reference. (Spring 2001). pp. 233–42. New York: Prescribing Reference.

Rajki, M., & Adams, K. (2000). Get moving! A mantra for peri-menopausal women. *Advance for Nurse Practitioners,* pp. 53–59.

Ramsey, L., Ross, B., & Fischer, R. (1999, May). Phytoestrogens and the management of menopause. *Advance for Nurse Practitioners,* pp. 25–30.

Richinni, W. (1998). Cutting through the hype: Hormone replacement therapy with DHEA. *Advance for Nurse Practitioners, 6*(11), 73–74.

Rosano, G. M., Webb, C. M., Chierchia, S., Morgani, G. L., Gabraele, M., Sarrel, P. M., De Ziegler, D., and Collins, P. (2000). Natural progesterone, but not medroxyprogesterone acetate, enhances the beneficial effects of estrogen an exercised-induced myocardial ischemia in postmenopausal women. *Journal of the American College of Cardiology, 36*(7), 2154–2159.

Ross, R., Paganini-Hill, A., & Wan, P. (2000). Effect of hormone replacement therapy on breast cancer risk: Estrogen versus estrogen plus progestin. *Journal of the National Cancer Institute, 92,* 328–333.

Sarrel, P. (1982). Sex problems after menopause: A study of fifty couples treated in a sex counseling programme. *Maturitas, 4,* 231–239.

Sarrel, P. (1990). Sexuality and menopause. *Obstetrics and Gynecology, 75,* 26S.

Sarrel, P., & Whitehead, M. L. (1985). Sex and menopause: Defining the issues. *Maturitas, 7,* 217–224.

Shapiro, S. (2001). *Addressing post-menopausal estrogen deficiency: A position paper of the American Council on Science and Health* [On-line]. Available: *http://www.medscape.com/ Medscape/General/Medicine/journal/2001/v03.n01/ mgm0126.shap*

Sheehy, G. (1993). *Menopause: The silent passage.* New York: Pocket Books.

Study explores estrogen treatment [On-line]. (2000). Available: *http://www.nlm.nih.gov.medlineplus.html*

Sutherland, E. (2000). *A naturopathic approach to menopause with Elizabeth Sutherland* [On-line]. Available: *http://www.my.webmd.com/content/article/1700.50686*

Tillem, J. (2000, February). Black cohosh for the treatment of perimenopausal symptoms. *Alternative Medicine Alert,* pp. 17–18.

Walsh, B. W., Paul, S., Wild, R. A., Dean, R. A., Tracy, R. P., Cox, D. A., & Anderson, P. W. (2000). The effects of hormone replacement therapy and raloxifene on c-reactive protein and homocysteine in healthy post-menopausal women. *Journal of Clinical Endocrinology and Metabolism, 85*(1), 214–218.

Weiderpass, E., Baron, J. A., Adami, H. O., Magnusson, C., Lindgren, A., Bergstrom, R., Correia, N., & Persson, I. (1999). Low potency estrogen and risk of endometrial cancer: A case-controlled study. *Lancet, 353,* 1824–1828.

Wenger, N. K. (2000). Hormonal and nonhormonal therapies for the postmenopausal woman: What is the evidence for cardio-protection? *American Journal of Cardiology, 9*(4), 204–209.

Weissman, M., & Olfson, M. (1995). Depression in women: Implications for healthcare research. *Science, 269*(5225), 799–801.

What is menopause? [On-line]. (2000). Available: *http://www.midlife-passages.com/page33.html*

Wren, B. G., McFarland, K., & Edwards, L. (1999). Micronized transdermal progestrone and endometrial response. *Lancet, 354,* 1447–1448.

Wright, J. V., & Morgenthaler, J. (1997). *Natural hormone replacement for women over 45.* Los Angeles, CA: SMART.

Writing Group for the Women's Health Initiative Investigators. (2002). Risks and benefits of estrogen plus progestin on healthy post-menopausal women: Principal results from the Women's Health Initiative randomized, controlled clinical trial. *Journal of the American Medical Association, 288*(3), 366–388.

25

Violence

Joanne M. Hessmiller and Linda E. Ledray

CHAPTER OUTLINE

Objectives

1. Describe and critically evaluate the current theories of intimate violence causation and intervention.
2. List 10 indicators that intimate violence is present or likely to develop in a relationship.
3. Identify the warning signs of potential lethality and ways of helping someone who is at risk.
4. Identify the ways to prevent intimate violence.
5. Identify the resources present in communities to assist victims of intimate violence, as well as gaps in these resources.
6. Discuss the psychological, spiritual, and physical impact of intimate violence and rape.
7. Identify the factors that increase the likelihood of long-term trauma following a sexual assault.
8. Identify common deficiencies in the medical response to sexual assault victims.
9. Describe the role of the sexual assault nurse examiner.

Introduction

In this chapter, two forms of violence commonly perpetrated against women—intimate (domestic) violence and rape—will be addressed. Both forms of violence are considered in terms of their impact on women's physical, mental, and spiritual health. Interventions known to be helpful are described and their impact evaluated. Strategies for eradicating conditions in our culture and communities that foster violence are considered. The terms *violence* and *abuse* are used interchangeably in this chapter.

Intimate Violence

The term **intimate,** or **domestic, violence** refers to violent or abusive acts that occur within the context of an intimate relationship. People related by marriage and adults who are in a sexual and/or domestic partnership in which they share the same household are considered intimates. Spouse or partner violence in which injury is sustained is not confined to heterosexual relationships; it occurs in same-sex relationships as well, at rates similar to those within the heterosexual population (Lettelier, 1994; Renzetti, 1992). Nevertheless, in terms of sheer numbers, it is overwhelmingly perpetrated by men against their female partners (Tjaden & Thoennes, 2000). Therefore, in this chapter, the noun *woman* and the pronoun *she* is used when referring to survivors of intimate violence, and the noun *man* and the pronoun *he* is used when referring to perpetrators of intimate violence.

Despite Tolstoy's often cited statement (in his book *Anna Karenina*) that, whereas happy families all resemble one another, unhappy families are unique in their misery, many unhappy families *do* resemble one another in terms of the violence that is a reality for the women and children in them. Ignored until relatively recently, the scope and impact of intimate violence and other forms of abuse against women, both in the United States and in other parts of the world, is finally being discussed. This is, in large part, due to the efforts of the battered women's movement and to the publicity surrounding now infamous cases of criminal spousal assault, such as the one involving O. J. and Nicole Brown Simpson.

Prevalence, Incidence, and Demographics

It is difficult to know how widespread intimate violence is. For one thing, both perpetrators and victims alike are often reluctant to talk about the violence in their lives because of shame. For another, victims are often intimidated by their partners into not reporting incidents of violence to authorities. It is also difficult to gauge the prevalence of less severe forms of abuse, as it is likely that only the more severe assaults are reported and ultimately reflected in criminal statistics. Therefore, it is important to understand that statistics may not reflect the full magnitude of the problem, but only the tip of the iceberg.

Because there is often no official reporting on *emotional* abuse and the less severe forms of physical abuse, it is much harder to know the frequency with which they occur. This is a serious problem, as these forms of abuse are widely understood to be just as damaging as more obvious physical violence. Many battered women speak of the hidden yet very open wounds of emotional and psychological abuse and how difficult it is to recover from these assaults on the heart and soul.

It is important to look at both the incidence rates and prevalence rates of intimate violence in order to gauge the magnitude of this problem. **Prevalence rates** tell us the number of people who have been victims of intimate violence within a certain period, whereas **incidence rates** tell us the number of occurrences of intimate violence within a given period of time. According to the most recent National Violence Against Women (NVAW) survey, which includes information about the experience of both men and women, the experience of being physically assaulted and/or raped is widespread among women. The survey estimated the prevalence of assault (the number of women who have been assaulted in the United States) at approximately 1,300,000. The average number of assaults per victim (incidence) was estimated to be 3.4 (Tjaden & Thoennes, 2000).

The prevalence rates of reported rape and physical assault differed significantly among women from different ethnic groups. Native American women were most likely to report rape and physical assault, whereas Asian and Pacific Islander women were least likely to report this. Latinas were less likely to report sexual assault than were non-Latinas. It cannot be concluded, however, that these crimes happen more or less often among women of different ethnicities; the only thing known for sure is that the *reporting* rate differs. More research into the reasons for the different reporting rates among the ethnic groups is needed (Tjaden & Thoennes, 2000).

In most incidences of violence against women, the perpetrator is a *male intimate*. According to the NVAW survey, a current or former intimate partner was responsible for 76 percent of the crimes against the women who were raped and/or physically assaulted. The men, on the other hand, were assaulted most often by a nonintimate; only 18 percent of the men surveyed reported having been assaulted by an intimate. According to the survey, the women who lived with female intimate partners were far less likely to be assaulted (11 percent) than were the women who were married or lived with a male partner (30.4 percent). The men in gay relationships were more likely to be assaulted by their male partners (15 percent) than were the men living in heterosexual relationships (7.7 percent) (Tjaden & Thoennes, 1998).

Forms of Intimate Violence

The various forms of intimate violence and abuse can be organized into three major categories: physical, sexual, and emotional/psychological. The term *physical abuse* refers to actions intended to inflict physical harm. These behaviors include throwing objects, pushing, grabbing, shoving, slapping, kicking, biting, hitting with a fist or an object, choking, or using a weapon, such as a knife or gun. The reality, and even the *threat,* of repeated physical violence enables a batterer to maintain power and control in a relationship, even when he is not using violence.

The term *sexual abuse* refers to both rape, which involves forced or coerced vaginal, oral, or anal penetration, and other forced or coerced sexual acts that do not include penetration. Rape and sexual abuse are discussed in the second half of this chapter.

Emotional/psychological abuse has historically received the least attention in the literature, perhaps because of the difficulty in defining it. In addition, it is difficult to separate physical and psychological violence, because physically violent acts typically have psychological consequences and vice versa (Crowell & Burgess, 1996). Follingstad, Rutledge, Berg, House, and Pollek (1990) have identified four categories of emotional/psychological abuse: verbal abuse, isolation, extreme jealousy, and verbal threats.

Verbal abuse includes ridiculing, name calling, and other forms of verbal harassment that undermine a person's sense of self-worth. More subtle forms of verbal abuse are sometimes disguised as humor. *Isolation* involves actions designed to separate a woman from her networks of support, as well as from the resources she needs to be self-sufficient. The abuser may forbid the woman to see friends and family and otherwise restrict her activities. Economic abuse is a tactic to achieve the isolation. This form of abuse involves denying the woman access to money, taking her money, or severely restricting the manner in which she can use it. It can also include disrupting her employment in some way—for example, by constantly calling her at work, preventing her from getting to work, or putting her in jeopardy of losing her job in some other way. *Extreme jealousy* is often a psychological form of sexual abuse. Women are often repeatedly and unjustly accused of infidelity, and their social contacts and movements are controlled. In some cases, women are stalked, even after they have left the abusive relationship. *Verbal threats* are threats of harm, including violence directed at the woman and her family, children, or friends.

Causes of Abuse

"I can't believe he hit me again—he promised that he would stop it after the last time I had to go to the hospital."

"He says that he just gets so angry that he can't control himself and loses control."

"He's such a nice guy; what does she do to make him so mad?"

These statements reflect the many questions and theories about the *causation* of intimate violence. The gruesome accounts of intimate violence that appear so frequently in the national media prompt the question, How could anyone hurt another person in these ways, let alone someone he *loves*? The need to understand this phenomenon in order to eradicate it has led to the formulation of a number of theories of intimate violence causality. These theories fall into five major categories: biogenic, psychogenic, relational, sociogenic, and integrated.

Biogenic theories suggest that a biological trait or feature is responsible for an individual's use of violence in an intimate relationship. These theories include those based on evolutionary biology (Green, 1999; Silverstein, 1999), physiological and neurophysiological traits (Jacobson & Gottman, 1998; Mirsky & Siegel, 1994), and the use of mind-altering substances (Leonard, 1993). In their research on the impact of physical trauma, Rosenbaum and Hoge (1989) found that 61 percent of the abusers in their sample had a history of a head injury. Jacobson and Gottman (1998) found that 20 percent of male spouse abusers demonstrate less physiological arousal than nonabusive men when involved in a quarrel with their spouses. Based on the information gleaned from research based on biogenic theories, a number of researchers (such as Holtzworth-Munroe and Stuart [1999] and Saunders [1992]) have worked to develop a typology of abusive men, so that more effective interventions can be developed.

Psychogenic theories suggest that an aspect of perpetrators' psychological nature leads them to use violence in intimate relationships. A number of studies have found a high incidence of psychopathology and personality disorders among men who assault their intimate partners (Dutton, 1995; Hamberger & Hastings, 1991). Dutton (1994) sees psychological explanations as the key to understanding why some men abuse their partners frequently, others do so infrequently in response to stressors, but many never do it at all. It seems unlikely, however, that psychopathology alone is the cause of intimate violence. According to Bandura's self-efficacy theory (Bandura, 1997), people become aware of various behaviors through observation and subsequently assess which they are likely to be able to carry out successfully to meet their particular goals. It is possible to explain the deviations described by Dutton (1994) on the basis of men's self-evaluations of their ability to engage in intimate violence and their willingness to accept the likely consequences of that action.

The diversity of both the physical and psychological characteristics identified to date in abusive men suggests that neither biological nor intrapsychic pathology accounts fully for intimate violence. Moreover, it remains unclear as to whether a given characteristic, such as substance abuse, is the *cause* of violence or a *response* to engaging in it or is even a strategy to disavow responsibility for criminal behavior.

Relational theories suggest that the cause of intimate violence lies in an aspect of the relationship between the perpetrator and the victim. Some such theories have been vigorously criticized as victim-blaming (Bograd, 1988; Harway & Hansen, 1993). However, it is clear from the literature that most perpetrators batter in the context of their intimate relationships, that most couples in violent relationships stay together, and that even placing full responsibility for the violence on the perpetrator does not change the need to understand the dynamics of the relationship (Anderson & Schlossberg, 1999). One of the major limitations of relational theories in understanding intimate violence is the assumption that behavioral choices are made in response to a *specific* relationship. Indeed, many batterers have a history of abusing multiple women.

Sociogenic theories examine the role of social and cultural phenomena, such as gender role socialization, misogyny (the hatred or dislike of women), sexism, male-centered language, and women-stigmatizing language, in perpetuating intimate violence. Male-centered language is language that assumes male gender, such as when *fireman* is used instead of the more inclusive term *firefighter*. An example of woman-stigmatizing language is the lack of a male synonym for words such as *slut* and *whore*. Sociogenic theories locate the cause of intimate violence within the *belief systems* of the dominant culture and of specific subcultures. For example, feminist theorists see violence against women as an expression and instrument of a patriarchal value system that is institutionalized both formally and informally in policies and practices in most of the world (Marin & Russo, 1999).

A weakness in the proposition that sociogenic theories best explain the use of violence in intimate relationships is the documented *inconsistency* in patterns of violence among men. As Dutton (1994) pointed out, men can be frequently violent, infrequently violent, or never violent. People interpret their experience of socialization in different ways, and they make choices about which aspects of their culture they will embrace and which they will reject.

Integrated theories, developed more recently, weave together the aforementioned major theories of intimate violence. The idea that many different levels of influence, including individual biology, psychology, and the social and cultural factors, drive an individual's decision to use violence in an intimate relationship is becoming more widely accepted. Examples of these integrated theories include the work of McKenry, Julian, and Gavazzi (1995) and Harway and O'Neil (1999). Harway and O'Neil developed what they have labeled the revised multivariate model. This model is comprised of seven factor-categories that influence men's potential for violence against women:

1. *Macrosocietal—all the conditions and values in the larger society that predispose men to violence.*

2. *Relational—the interpersonal patterns within intimate relationships that appear to predispose one to violence.*
3. *Biological—the entire human physiological, genetic, and hormonal conditions that have the potential to result in violence.*
4. *Psychological—the intrapsychic processes, conscious or unconscious, developed through the course of development that may influence an individual to commit a violent act.*
5. *Social—the values and beliefs internalized by an individual as a result of acculturation and gender role socialization.*

Implicit in the O'Neil-Harway model is the assumption that the psychosocial factors that drive abuse and violence do so in an interacting and complex manner; a given factor may be embedded in one or more other factors, and factors may exert an intensifying or dampening effect on one another.

It is likely that work in the area of integrated theories will one day yield a more complete explanation of the causality of intimate violence and enable the development of successful interventions.

For the most part, the general public sees intimate violence as a function of pathology in individuals and/or their relationships. One of the most entrenched *myths* about intimate violence is that its roots lie solely in individual and relational pathology, rather than in *societal* attitudes and values as well. Some authorities believe that the tenacity of this myth has been aided by the language social science researchers use to describe intimate violence. Jones (1994) writes:

> *Domestic violence is one of those gray phrases, beloved of bureaucracy, designed to give people a way of talking about a topic without seeing what is really going on. Like repatriation or ethnic cleansing, it is a euphemistic abstraction that keeps us at a dispassionate distance, far removed from the repugnant spectacle of human beings in pain. We used to speak of wife beating—words that brought to mind a picture of terrifying action. . . . [Then] . . . professionals in mental health and justice, equipped with professional vocabularies, took up problems of spouse abuse, conjugal violence, and marital aggression , and a great renaming took place, a renaming that veiled once again the sexism that a grass roots women's movement had worked to uncover. (p. 82)*

Academic language strips accounts of violence against women of their *gendered* context and locates them within individual and relationship pathology. The importance of gender role socialization and institutionalized sexism is veiled, as is the *trauma-generating* nature (Bloom, 1997) of a society that accepts violence both as a legitimate way to solve problems and as entertainment. The American tendency to deny societal factors in the causation of intimate violence has been noted by the eminent Scottish sociologists Dobash and Dobash (1992), who do research in the area of intimate violence. They ask, "Why is the United States a therapeutic society in which almost all social, economic and even political problems are seen as personal troubles requiring therapy, and how does this affect movements for social change?" (p. 216). We must struggle to understand and articulate an understanding of the complexity of intimate violence that does not blame the victim and that holds perpetrators accountable for their behavior while working for change at the micro and macro levels of society.

Intimate Violence and Women's Health

Regardless of the form it takes, violence has a negative effect on women's physical, psychological, and spiritual health.

PHYSICAL CONSEQUENCES

Women assaulted by intimates are far more likely than men assaulted by intimates to be *injured*. Using a definition of physical assault that included behaviors from hitting and slapping to using a gun, the most recent report on the prevalence and incidence of physical assault found that 41.5 percent of the women but only 19.9 percent of the men who were physically assaulted by an intimate partner were injured in the most recent physical assault (Tjaden & Thoennes, 2000). The physical injuries from battering can range from relatively minor bruising to injuries requiring hospitalization, major surgery, or death (Berrios & Grady, 1991; Federal Bureau of Investigation, 1993), and women are more likely to be *killed* than men; 75 percent of the 1,800 persons murdered by their intimates in 1996 were female (U.S. Department of Justice, 1998).

Sexual abuse is common in violent relationships and includes a myriad of forced and coerced sexual activities, which can occur concurrent with or after physical abuse. Battered women frequently report that they must respond positively to their partners' sexual overtures or run an elevated risk of physical, sexual, or psychological abuse (Walker, 1994).

The frequency with which women suffer physical abuse during *pregnancy* is deeply troubling. McFarlane, Parker, Soeken, and Bullock (1992) found that 17 percent of women suffer physical or sexual abuse during pregnancy and that *homicide is the leading cause of death among pregnant women.* In a recent study of 651 autopsy reports on pregnant women filed in District of Columbia from 1988 to 1996, it was found that 38 percent of the deaths were due to homicide. The victims were more likely to have been killed early in the pregnancy, which made it difficult for authorities to identify the pregnancy and link it with the homicide (Krulewitch, Pierr-Louis, de Leon-gomez, Guy, & Green, 2001). The frequency with which pregnant women are battered raises the question of how the news of the pregnancy affects perpetrators and what it means to them. It is known that a woman with an unintended pregnancy is 2.5 times more likely to experience physical abuse than is a woman with an intended pregnancy (Goodwin, Gazmarian, Johnson, Gilbert, & Saltzman, 2000).

Abused women suffer the effects of chronic stress in addition to the direct effects of violence. Chronic stress can have disastrous consequences for women's health; the chemicals that are released within the body in response to stress create problems, which range from interference with memory processes to organ damage. They also cause immune system dysfunction, leaving the woman vulnerable to opportunistic infections (Bloom, 1997).

PSYCHOLOGICAL AND EMOTIONAL CONSEQUENCES

Women who have suffered both psychological and physical abuse often report that the psychological violence was *worse* than the physical, as it left invisible wounds that were far harder to heal and often disrupted their lives profoundly, even after they had left the abusive relationship.

People who have lived through intimate partner violence often have a variety of psychological symptoms that are similar to those exhibited by survivors of other kinds of trauma, such as natural disasters and criminal assaults at the hands of strangers. Such symptoms include shock, hyperarousal, confusion, memory problems, and withdrawal, to name just a few (Bloom, 1997). As it is well documented that even a *single* traumatic event can produce these and other symptoms, the finding that ongoing and repetitive violence is extremely damaging to psychological health (Follingstad et al., 1990) is not surprising. Walker (1994) notes, "Each successive instance of violence from a loved and trusted partner is magnified by the memory of previous incidents. Thus, many battered women may spend the rest of their lives both fearing additional abuse and seeking to prevent a recurrence" (p. 58).

Battered women live with the constant threat of violence and with complete unpredictability in their lives. They are also led to believe that they have no alternatives to remaining in the abusive relationship; abusers often intentionally isolate their partners by interfering with their other relationships and by blocking their access to money and even transportation. Such experiences leave battered women feeling shattered, ashamed, guilty, anxious, disconnected, alienated, hopeless, and helpless. Many turn to substance abuse or develop thoughts of suicide (Bloom, 1997; Herman, 1992). It is not unusual for battered women to contemplate suicide as not only a means of escaping physical and psychological pain but also as a means of exercising what they perceive to be the only aspect of their lives that they can still control: whether they live or die (Walker, 1994).

It would be difficult to overestimate the impact battering and other forms of abuse have on women's psyches. Herman (1992) notes the direct parallels between the methods terrorists use to inflict torture (Amnesty International, 1973) and the methods that batterers use to control their partners.

SPIRITUAL CONSEQUENCES

The experience of being a victim of intimate violence has spiritual, as well as physical and psychological, consequences. Such suffering often raises ultimate questions in battered women's minds regarding the *meaning* of the violence and often the meaning of their lives in general (Fortune, 1991). These ultimate questions can be expressed in many different ways. People of faith typically ask how a loving God, or whatever they conceive as a higher power, can allow them to suffer abuse at the hands of the ones they were led to marry or enter into an intimate relationship with.

Fortune (1991) has found through her extensive experience of ministering to people who have suffered intimate violence that religion can be either a *roadblock* or a *resource,* depending on how intimate violence is handled. Religion can be a roadblock if a religious community uses tradition and narrow interpretations of scripture to support the abuser in his violence. Such communities often blame the woman for the violence in the relationship and insist that she remain in the relationship and behave more submissively. Conversely, religion can be a major resource to a survivor when clergy and congregations, aware of the dynamics of intimate violence and abuse, use their knowledge of scripture and tradition to demonstrate that these do *not* support violence and abuse. Congregations can be a major resource for abused persons; they can offer material, emotional, and spiritual support and help them end the violence in their lives. In addition, faith communities can take an active role in prevention by ensuring that domestic violence is addressed in sermons, as well as in religious education programs for adolescent and adult congregants.

Dynamics of Intimate Violence

One of the most frustrating questions asked of battered women and their advocates is, Why do they stay? The fact that this is the question that is asked reveals much about our society. First and foremost, it exposes the societal tendency to *blame victims* for the oppression they have suffered. Second, it reveals *ignorance* regarding the choices that battered women make to end the violence in their lives and the lives of their children. It is critical to work to understand these choices in order to intervene effectively at any level.

As a society, we must ask ourselves why attention is focused on the actions (or inaction) of a *survivor,* not on the actions (or inaction) of the *perpetrators* of domestic violence. To focus on the victim is a subtle way of making her responsible for the violence she has endured. The following are more appropriate, and useful, questions: Why do men abuse, batter, and sometimes literally torture their partners? Why do people and systems within our society condone and sometimes even encourage violence against women? Why does our society fail to hold men accountable for the violence they inflict on the ones they love?

When a battered woman chooses to remain with her partner, those outside the relationship often have difficulty understanding her choice. However, an understanding of the nature and basic dynamics of abusive relationships makes it possible to understand battered women's behaviors as legitimate responses to intimate violence and to view them as the best experts on their lives.

Women who are battered are often told by their abusers that they will be subjected to *further violence* and even *death* if they act to stop the abuse by trying to leave or by contacting authorities. Unfortunately, women *are* most likely to be murdered when trying to report abuse or to leave their relationships (Browne, 1987). Women may also be given reason to fear for the safety of their *children* if they try to leave. The behavior of women who choose to stay can be understood as logical, given their circumstances.

Another factor in battered women's decision to stay is that they often want the violence and abuse, but not *the relationship,* to end. Women can want to preserve the relationship for many reasons, including the love they have for their partners, their religious commitments, and their sense of duty to their children. A very potent factor is that many battered women do not see an *alternative* to their current situation. Many women who have endured emotional and psychological abuse over a period of time internalize the invalidating messages they have received and come to believe themselves incapable of taking care of themselves. Moreover, abusers typically cut their victims off from all possible sources of strength and support, such as a job and relationships with family and friends.

Yet another factor is that some women are fearful of losing custody of their children, should the relationship end. In many cases, they have been told that, if they leave, they will not see their children again. Tragically, this has happened to some women; custody cases tend to be expensive, and many women cannot afford to retain an attorney to advocate for their interests.

The truth about women who have been battered is that most *do* eventually act to end the violence in their lives. Many seek assistance from shelters, which are typically full and have long waiting lists. Others seek help from friends, family members, clergy, and private counselors.

Community Interventions for Intimate Violence

If the epidemic of intimate violence in our communities is to be stemmed, citizens who are not affected by the problem must be willing to work alongside, or on behalf of, those who are. The problem of violence must be clearly defined, in terms of causality, scope, and the nature of the resources that will be necessary to solve it. The cultural beliefs that support the problem must be undermined, and the beliefs that support change must be substituted. Community services that allow individuals to escape or heal violent relationships must be available and accessible to all.

Interventions aimed at preventing or ameliorating the problem of intimate violence can be designed at the primary, secondary, or tertiary levels. At the *primary level,* the goal is to identify and modify the social conditions that create and sustain a social problem. At the *secondary level,* interventions are focused on identifying people at risk for harm and modifying conditions so as to reduce their risk. Interventions at the *tertiary level* are designed to assist individuals already experiencing harm in abusive relationships. Most intimate violence interventions in the United States are tertiary-level interventions.

PRIMARY INTERVENTION

Primary prevention efforts—efforts aimed at changing the *culture* in order to create and sustain conditions that ensure the safety of women and girls—are the least developed interventions. Primary efforts typically meet with considerable social, economic, and political resistance, as they call for fundamental changes in relationships and institutions, and they threaten the structures of privilege on which many in power depend, even when they are unaware of them. In addition, primary prevention efforts can be extremely difficult to fund, due to their complexity, their need for greater resources, and the difficulties encountered in trying to evaluate the success of so broad an effort.

Nevertheless, interventions at this level of prevention are finally being developed. The Transforming Communities Project, which has sponsored many secondary and primary interventions, is an example of such an effort. Another example of a primary intervention is the establishment of the Marin Abused Women's Services (MAWS) of Marin County, California. MAWS is a domestic violence intervention program that began in 1977 to offer a range of services to women who have been abused. It has continued to developed innovative programs in the service of its mission and has increased its focus on the prevention of intimate violence (Rath, 1999). A fundamental goal in each of MAWS' domestic violence prevention projects is to provide opportunities for all the people in the community to become involved in prevention activities at any level of intervention. In 1991, the organization asked itself the following questions (Rath, 1999): "What will it take to move beyond responding to and recovering from violence against women to preventing it from occurring at all? How can we identify and transform the norms and behaviors that perpetuate men's violence against women and girls? How can communities effectively mobilize to change deeply ingrained attitudes and beliefs?" (p. 6). After considering these questions, MAWS developed a new organization, called Transforming Communities: Creating Safety and Justice for Women and Girls, in 1992. This organization is founded on a gender-based analysis of intimate violence and a commitment to developing interventions at the secondary and primary levels. This new organization has developed a number of advocacy projects, many of which are ongoing. These projects include, among others, the establishment of a violence-free apartment complex in a low-income community, a batterer intervention program, and the Novato Community Demonstration Project, which attempts to transform the culture of the city of Novato, California, in ways that will reduce incidences of intimate violence. The core units of the organization are its Community Action Teams (CATs). CATs are independent, self-governing community organizations that remain connected to the project through their commitment to the goals of building a social movement. CATs choose their own projects, and the parent organization provides training, support, and technical assistance. A CAT is usually comprised of three to eight people, who meet regularly to plan together and receive any specialized training that may be needed.

Both adult and teen CATs have implemented many creative programs to end intimate violence in their community (Rath, 1999). One adult CAT enhanced legal advocacy for battered women through a court-watch and letter-writing campaign. Another succeeded in establishing a training program for city personnel that improved the manner in which emergency protection orders also known as **protection from abuse** (PFA) orders (which forbid abusers to approach victims) were used. Other, current adult CAT projects have included providing information in markets and malls to increase citizen awareness regarding the prevention of domestic violence, a campaign called "Color My Home Violence Free: A Community Paint In" and a "Sisterhood Empowerment Club," formed at a local college to provide information on issues important to young women. A CAT-sponsored "Break the Silence/Protest the Violence" event, a funeral procession for a county woman who was murdered by her husband, was covered locally and by *Time* magazine. A campaign called "This Offends Me" drew attention to the connections between sexist advertising and violence against women and girls, and area merchants were given postcards asking them not to sell offensive products. The CAT also engaged in a wide range of activities, which were covered by the media, including issuing public challenges to major corporations that had sponsored advertising that was degrading or potentially dangerous to women and girls (Rath, 1999). A partnership between the CAT and a local newspaper led to 18 articles written by CAT members being published by the paper. The CAT also produced a 23-minute educational videotape on ways of preventing intimate violence plus a manual designed to help people organize other CATs. This tremendously productive CAT also conducted participatory research on the relationship between domestic violence and homelessness and established a support group at a local women's shelter.

One teen CAT worked to educate peers within local high schools by producing assemblies focused on the prevention of intimate violence for students. It also authored a script on teen dating violence, which was made into a nationally distributed 20-minute film, and established an Internet chat room on dating violence (www.theinsite.com). The CAT also sponsored an art project for young children that focused on personal safety and created a "Silent Witness" display for a large shopping mall. "Silent Witness" projects featured displays of life-size cutouts of women's bodies, each of which represents a woman or girl killed by intimate violence.

A number of lessons can be learned from the success of the Transforming Communities project. One is that it is advantageous for groups involved in grassroots efforts to be associated with an established organization that enjoys a very good reputation in the community. The reputation of MAWS gave the Transforming Communities project immediate credibility and gained those associated with it access to community leaders. Also, MAWS' strong resource base made it a certainty that the Transforming Communities project would have the materials it needed. It should also be noted that obtaining input from the community was critically important in all phases of the project (Rath, 1999).

SECONDARY INTERVENTION

Secondary intervention focuses on identifying persons at risk, and reducing that risk. It is now widely recognized that *coordinated community response systems* are more likely than isolated entities to be successful in reducing the incidence of intimate violence in a community (Hart, 1995; Shepard & Pence, 1999). Communities throughout the country have developed domestic violence task forces, the members of which work together to examine gaps in services, seek funding for programs, and engage in dialogue to make certain that offenders are held accountable and that survivors receive adequate protection and access to services. Some communities, such as York County and Philadelphia in Pennsylvania, engage in collaborative reviews of domestic violence fatalities, so that services can be improved and future fatalities prevented.

TERTIARY INTERVENTION

Programs serving battered women typically provide a range of services, including options/empowerment counseling (although not usually psychological counseling), emergency shelter, and legal advocacy. Many programs also offer transitional housing, because the time a woman can remain in a shelter is generally very limited. In options/empowerment counseling, staff members engage battered women in empowering dialogues, in which they are helped to assess their situation and make decisions about the future. Participation in options/empowerment counseling, and in the support groups that are typically available at shelters, is vital to a battered woman's safety. These processes validate her experience, and they help her assess the lethality potential of her abusive partner and develop a safety plan.

Women who have been battered typically also need to assess the relative costs and benefits of pursuing legal action against their partners. The Pennsylvania Protection from Abuse Act (1976, 1993 Amended), like similar legislation in states across the country, enables people who can demonstrate that they have been abused by intimates to secure a range of remedies via *civil* procedures. A women can also press *criminal charges* against her partner if his abuse fits the definitions of actions prohibited by the state criminal code and other related laws.

Legal advocacy programs for battered women have been central in assisting women to evaluate their options and to use the law in their best interests. These programs have also been very effective in advocating for systems reform.

Help is also available for *abusers,* in the form of programs that offer psychoeducational groups focused on stopping abuse. A variety of models of intervention are used, and the programs work closely with the court system in receiving and providing information regarding client compliance with court orders. Intervention programs for abusive men have long been controversial among advocates for battered women, however. Some have questioned the effectiveness of such programs and see them as a danger to women who may remain in their relationships due to their partners' involvement. Programs for abusive men are also seen by some as draining resources that would otherwise be used to provide shelter and other services for women and children (Hessmiller, 1998).

The effort to end intimate violence has focused mostly, but not exclusively, on interventions for individuals.

This "band-aid" approach has done little to eradicate the roots of the problem of violence against women. The existence of tertiary level programs such as the Transforming Communities Project suggests that the movement that began with a call for cultural change mandated by the results of a clear analysis of the implications of gender in our society is beginning to return to that fundamental mission. Preventive interventions at the secondary level, which are intended to change not just individuals but also systems are becoming more common. Also becoming more common are programs whose goal is primary prevention—cutting off intimate violence at its cultural roots by changing the gender role socialization of girls and boys and identifying, questioning, and dismantling the structures of male privilege.

Sexual Assault

Violence against women in the form of sexual assault has a significant and highly negative impact on the emotional and physical health of victims and affects a considerable number of women. Although obtaining accurate and consistent estimates of the incidence of rape has been problematic due to the significant *underreporting* of this crime (Koss & Harvey, 1991). In the most rigorous survey to date, 24 percent of a sample of 6,159 college age women reported having been the victim of a sexual assault or an attempted sexual assault, even as early as the age of 14 years. Only 9 percent, however, had reported their assault to the police (Koss, Gidycz, & Wisniewski, 1987).

Considering the frequency with which women experience sexual assault, it is unfortunate that, until fairly recently, training specific to the needs of sexual assault victims was not included in the basic or advanced education of physicians. Even today, when training is provided, it is typically minimal, taking only one or two hours.

The injuries associated with sexual assault are manifested physically, psychologically, emotionally, and spiritually. The physical problems include both genital and nongenital trauma, sexually transmitted diseases (STDs), and pregnancy. The psychological/emotional impact, which can last for years, is manifested by anxiety, fear, depression, suicidal thoughts, self-blame, shame, and post-traumatic stress disorder (PTSD). Psychospiritual trauma in which an individual's faith in the goodness and justice of God, a hopeless power, the universal, and so on, is shattered, can give rise to problems such as sexual dysfunction, substance abuse, and a long-term decline in physical health.

Short-Term Physical Injuries and Other Problems

Studies indicate that significant physical injury resulting from sexual assault is rare—3 to 5 percent across studies—with less than 1 percent of victims needing hospitalization. Even minor injury usually occurs in only about one-third of the reported rapes. When they do occur, injuries are more common in stranger rapes, and rapes committed in the context of intimate violence, than in date rapes (rape committed during or immediately after a date) or acquaintance rapes (rape committed by a person known to the victim) (Bownes, O'Gorman, & Saters, 1991; Cartwright, Moore, Anderson, & Brown, 1986; Kilpatrick, Edmunds, & Seymour, 1992; Ledray, 1999; Marchbanks, Lui, & Mercy, 1990).

Genital Trauma

Most genital trauma inflicted during a sexual assault is *internal* and consists of abrasions, bruises, and tears (Frank, 1996; Slaughter & Brown, 1992). It can often be seen only with a *colposcope*, an instrument used to magnify tissues in the genital tract. These minor injuries are related to the tightened pelvic muscles, lack of pelvic tilt, and absence of lubrication during the forced penetration. Minor injuries usually heal completely within 48 to 72 hours. When more serious injuries are sustained, they are usually associated with complaints of vaginal pain, discomfort, or bleeding (Cartwright, Moore, Anderson, & Brown, 1986; Geist, 1988; Tintinalli, Hoelzer, & Michigan, 1985). Because rape victims often fear vaginal trauma (Ledray, 1999), it is important that they seek a medical examination and that the extent of the trauma, or the lack of trauma, is explained to them.

Sexually Transmitted Diseases

Although in one study (Ledray, 1991), 36 percent of the rape victims seen in an emergency department stated that their primary reason for coming was concern about having contracted a sexually transmitted disease (STD), the actual risk of that happening is rather low. The Centers for Disease Control and Prevention (CDC) estimates rape victims' risk of contracting gonorrhea at 6 to 12 percent, chlamydia at 4 to 17 percent, syphilis at 0.5 to 3 percent, and HIV at 1 percent (Centers for Disease Control and Prevention, 1998). The actual risk of contracting an STD in a given community, however, varies according to the sociological makeup of that community.

From a forensic and clinical perspective, treating sexual assault victims for STDs *prophylactically*, for the purpose of prevention, is preferable to testing them first and then treating any diseases that are found. Establishing the presence of STD through culturing is both very expensive and time-consuming for the victim. Victims who are initially tested for STDs must return two or three times for additional testing, and, unfortunately, most do not return (Blair & Warner, 1992; Tintinalli et al., 1985). For these reasons, most clinicians recommend prophylactic treatment (CDC, 1998; Frank, 1996; Ledray, 1999).

Since the early 1980s, HIV has been a concern for rape survivors, even though the actual risk still appears to be very low. In a study of 412 Midwest rape victims with vaginal or rectal penetration who were tested for HIV at three months' postrape and again at six months' postrape, it was found that not one had developed an HIV infection (Ledray, 1999). The first rape-related case in which seroconversion (from HIV-negative to HIV-positive) occurred in 1989 (Murphy, Harris, & Forester, 1989). Subsequently, Claydon et al. (1991) reported four more cases in which researchers believe a rape resulted in a subsequent HIV seroconversion. Because it is known that 95 percent of individuals who are going to seroconvert will do so by three months after exposure (see Chapter 20) and 100 percent will do so by six months, the authors of the Claydon et al. (1991) study did not recommend routine HIV testing or prophylactic care. Claydon et al. did note, however, that the assault victims in the study, or their partners, expressed concern about possible exposure to HIV either immediately or within two weeks of the assault. Based on that finding, they recommend that a medical professional provide *all* rape victims with information about their relative risk, testing procedures, and safe sex options.

The issue of how to best deal with HIV infection as a possible consequence of sexual assault is a complicated and controversial one (Blair & Warner, 1992). If the offender is HIV-infected, the probability of a rape victim's contracting HIV from a sexual assault depends on the type of sexual intercourse (anal, vaginal, or oral), the presence of trauma in the involved orifice, the exposure to ejaculate, the viral load of the ejaculate, and the presence of other STDs (CDC, 1998). In most instances, it is impossible to determine the HIV status of the offender in a timely fashion, and offenders may even misrepresent their HIV status to their victims. In the study done by Claydon et al. (1991), two of the assailants had told their victims that they were HIV-positive. However, when apprehended and tested, only one was found to be HIV-positive (Ledray, 1999). The actual risk of the offender's being HIV-infected varies from community to community.

Because there are no good data on the actual risk of HIV infection, the CDC does not make a recommendation regarding the appropriateness of offering postexposure antiviral therapy after sexual assault. The decision to offer prophylactic treatment should be based on the nature of the assault, combined with the HIV prevalence in the specific geographic area (CDC, 1998). A rape is considered *high-risk* if it involved rectal contact, or vaginal contact resulting in vaginal tears, or vaginal contact in the presence of pre-existing vaginal STDs that have caused ulcerations or open sores that disrupt the integrity of the vaginal mucosa. The rape is also considered high-risk if the victim has some reason to know or suspect that the assailant was an IV drug user, HIV-positive, or bisexual. The risks and options, including the impact of the drug regimen, should be explained to the victim, so that she can make an educated decision (Ledray, 1999).

PREGNANCY

The risk of pregnancy from a rape is the same as the risk of pregnancy from any one-time sexual encounter: 2 to 4 percent (Yuzpe, Smith, & Rademaker, 1982). Most sexual assault nurse examiner (SANE) programs (see Section on SANE/SART programs) and medical facilities offer emergency pregnancy preventive care to women at risk of becoming pregnant, provided they have been seen within 72 hours of the rape. After that time, the drugs used to prevent pregnancy are no longer effective. One SANE program operating at a Catholic hospital went so far as to get special permission from the diocese to administer the oral contraceptive *Ovral* (Frank, 1996). The National Conference of Catholic Bishops has agreed that "a female who has been raped should be able to defend herself against a potential conception from the sexual assault. If, after appropriate testing, there is no evidence that conception has already occurred, she may be treated with medication that would prevent ovulation, or fertilization" (National Conference of Catholic Bishops, 1995, p. 16). Sometimes referred to as "the morning-after pill," oral contraceptives such as Ovral and Lovral are used for emergency contraception (see Chapter 17).

Psychological and Spiritual Problems

One of the first longitudinal studies of the psychological impact of rape was completed by a nurse, Ann Burgess, and a social worker, Lynn Holmstrom (Burgess & Holmstrom, 1974). This team followed 92 sexual assault victims from the initial emergency room visit through the following year to evaluate the impact of rape over time and the effectiveness of crisis intervention. Burgess and Holmstrom's work resulted in the coining of the term **rape trauma syndrome,** which is still used today to describe the emotional aftermath of rape especially in legal writing.

There is considerable agreement among researchers that rape victims experience more *psychological distress* than do victims of other crimes. Although anxiety, fear, depression, and symptoms of post-traumatic stress disorder (PTSD) are the most frequently recognized and documented reactions to sexual assault (Burgess & Holmstrom, 1974; Calhoun, Atkeson, & Resick, 1982; Frazier, 2000; Kilpatrick & Veronen, 1984; Ledray, 1994; Resick & Schnicke, 1990), suicidal thoughts, self-blame, and shame can also be identified.

ANXIETY

Anxiety is frequently recognized and documented in the literature as an *immediate reaction* to a sexual assault (Abel & Rouleau, 1995; Burgess & Holmstrom, 1974; Calhoun et al., 1982; Kilpatrick & Veronen, 1984; Ledray, 1994; Resick & Schnicke, 1990). The persistence of anxiety over a longer term is not as well established. Most researchers use self-report measures, such as the Multiple Affect Adjective Check List (MAACL), to establish the presence of anxiety in rape victims. Only a few studies have used more objective instruments to establish that sexual assault victims meet *DSM-IV R (Diagnostic Manual of the American Psychiatric Association)* criteria for long-term anxiety-related disorders. One such study (Frank & Anderson, 1987), found that 82 percent of the rape victims in the study met the *DSM* criteria for generalized anxiety disorder (GAD), compared with 32 percent of the nonvictims. Although other controlled studies have also documented long-term anxiety in victims of sexual assault (Gidycz, Coble, Latham, & Layman, 1993; Gidycz & Koss, 1991; Gold, Milan, Mayall, & Johnson, 1994; Santiago, McCall-Perez, Gorcey, & Beigel, 1985), others have failed to substantiate this finding (Frazier & Schauben, 1994; Riggs, Kilpatrick, & Resnick, 1992; Winfield, George, Swartz, & Blazer, 1990).

Nightmares are also a very common problem following sexual assault. In a study comparing 488 rape victims with 110 nonvictims (Krakow, Tandberg, Barey, & Scriggins, 1995), the rape victims were found to have more nightmares, with 26 percent reporting having numerous nightmares and 53 percent reporting fewer nightmares. The researchers concluded that the nightmares were associated with greater general distress and heightened anxiety. Studies also suggest that rape victims are more likely than control subjects to meet the criteria for *panic disorder* several years after the rape (Burnam et al., 1988; Winfield et al., 1990).

FEAR

Fear tends to be a persistent and long-term problem after sexual assault. Because fear is subjective, it is generally evaluated using self-report measures. Fear of *death* is the most common fear *during* the assault and continued generalized fear after the assault is very common (Dupre, Hampton, Morrison, & Meeks, 1993; Ledray, 1994). Although evidence of the duration and type of fear varies, up to 83 percent of victims report some type of lingering fear following a sexual assault (Frazier, 2000; Nadelson, Notman, Zackson, & Gornick, 1982). Fear after a rape can be specifically related to the factors associated with the sexual assault, or it can be widely generalized to include fear of all men (Ledray, 1994).

As might be expected, rape victims tend to be generally fearful and hyperalert to potential danger following the assault. During the acute stage of recovery from rape, which lasts approximately one year, rape victims are consistently found to be more fearful overall than are noncrime victims (Calhoun et al., 1982; Kilpatrick, Resnick, & Veronen, 1981). Rape victims also tend to be *more* fearful than victims of crimes other than rape (Wirtz & Harrell, 1987). Up to 80 percent of rape victims report being generally fearful, afraid of violence, or afraid of being alone. Nearly as many (75 percent), report a fear of being indoors, outdoors, or in a crowd, and 70 percent report a fear of death (Becker, Skinner, Abel, & Cichon, 1986). Although fear of retaliation by the assailant is common (Ledray, 1984), it is mostly unfounded; except in rapes committed in the context of domestic violence, assailants rarely retaliate against victims who report having been raped (Ledray, 1994).

Studies assessing the *long-term* presence of fear found that the degree of fear experienced by rape victims surpasses that experienced by nonvictims for as long as 46 years postrape (Resnick, Jordan, Girelli, Hunter, & Marhoefer-Dvorak, 1988; Santiago et al., 1985; Wirtz & Harrell, 1987).

Girelli, Resnick, Marhoefer-Dvorak, and Hutter (1986) found that the degree of fear of injury or fear of death experienced during a rape is a more significant predictor of severe postrape fear and anxiety than is the degree of violence that occurred. Thus, it is important to recognize that the *threat* of violence alone can be psychologically devastating (Goodman, Koss, & Russo, 1993).

DEPRESSION

Rape victims have consistently been found to be more depressed than individuals in nonvictim control groups (Burge, 1988; Cohen & Roth, 1987; Ellis, Atkeson, & Calhoun, 1981; Gidycz & Koss, 1989; Gidycz & Koss, 1991; Riggs et al., 1992; Santiago et al., 1985) and more depressed than victims of other crimes (Frazier & Schauben, 1994). Studies that evaluate the level of depression in rape victims typically find that, when rape victims are compared with nonvictim control groups, the results consistently show that depression is most prominent during the first two months after a rape has occurred (Atkeson, Calhoun, Resick, & Ellis, 1982; Kilpatrick, Veronen, & Resick, 1979; Kilpatrick, Resnick, & Veronen, 1981). During this period, rape victims are often mildly depressed (Becker, Skinner, Abel, & Cichon, 1986; Frazier & Burnett, 1994; Ledray 1984) to moderately depressed (Cluss, Boughton, Frank, Stewart, & West, 1983; Frank & Stewart, 1984; Frazier, Harlow, Schauben, & Byrne, 1993; Ledray, 1984; Moss, Frank, & Anderson, 1990).

The depressive effects of rape can continue past the two-month mark. In some studies, 75 to 80 percent of the rape victims reported feeling mildly to severely depressed

six months after being raped (Kimerling & Calhoun, 1994; Norris & Feldman-Summers, 1981). In others, the rape victims continued to be mildly depressed even one year after the assault (Koss, Dinero, Seibel & Cox, 1988; Mackey et al., 1992). Depression is one of the most commonly documented *long-term* responses to rape (Abel & Rouleau, 1995; Atkeson, et al., 1982; Frazier, 2000; Kilpatrick & Veronen, 1984; Ledray, 1994).

Rape victims are also significantly more likely than nonvictims to suffer a *major depression*. In one study, it was found that 38 percent of the individuals who had sought assistance at a rape crisis center met the diagnostic criteria for major depression at six months postassault. The incidence of major depression in the group of matched control subjects in the study was only 6 percent (Frank & Anderson, 1987). Another study (Golding, 1994) reported similar results, with 33 percent of the rape victims meeting the criteria for major depression six months postrape, compared with 11 percent of the controls.

SUICIDAL IDEATION

Whereas completed suicides following a rape are relatively rare, *suicidal ideation*—thoughts of commiting suicide—and *suicide attempts* are not. Up to 20 percent of rape victims attempt suicide (Kilpatrick, Veronen, & Best, 1985), and many more rape victims (33 percent to 50 percent) report having considered suicide at some point after the rape (Ellis et al., 1981; Resick et al., 1988). During the immediate postrape period, rape victims are nine times more likely than nonvictims to attempt suicide (Kilpatrick, Saunders, Veronen, Best, & Von, 1987).

SELF-BLAME

Self-blame is a common response in rape victims (Ledray, 1994; MacFarlane & Hawley, 1993). It was once thought that some self-blame might actually be beneficial to rape victims, as it would foster the sense that what happens to them in the future can be controlled. The reasoning behind this theory was, that if victims believed that their actions had contributed to the rape event, they could believe that a change in their behavior would protect them from another rape. More recent research, however, suggests that self-blame is associated only with the sense that one could have controlled the *past;* it does not confer a belief that what happens in the *future* can be controlled. Self-blame is a *negative* response that is associated with higher levels of depression and poor adjustment postrape (Frazier, 1990).

POST-TRAUMATIC STRESS DISORDER

Post-traumatic stress disorder (PTSD) was first recognized as a diagnosis by the American Psychiatric Association in 1980. Therefore, it has been considered only in rape-impact studies designed after 1980. Rape trauma syndrome (RTS), often described as a specific type of PTSD (Frazier, 2000), is also used in rape-impact studies. The basic elements of a PTSD diagnosis include

- Exposure to a traumatic event
- Reexperiencing of the trauma, such as flashbacks and intrusive memories
- Symptoms of avoidance and numbing, such as attempts to avoid thoughts or situations that remind the survivor of the traumatic event, an inability to recall certain aspects of the traumatic event, and disconnection from others
- Symptoms of increased arousal, such as an exaggerated startle response, feelings of being easily irritated, a constant fear of danger, and a physiological response when exposed to similar events

The symptoms must be present for at least one month and must cause clinically significant distress or impairment (American Psychiatric Association, 1994).

The rate at which PTSD is found to occur in rape victims varies greatly from study to study, depending on the criteria used to define *sexual assault*. When sexual assault victims who have experienced *less severe forms* of sexual assault are included in the studies, the rate for PTSD is low (Winfield et al., 1990). When victims who have experienced *more severe forms* of assault are studied, however, high rates of PTSD are found (Breslau, Davis, Andreski, & Peterson, 1991). Women who report a sexual assault to the police or other authorities report higher PTSD rates than women who are sexually assaulted but do not repeat the assault (Rothbaum, Foa, & Riggs, 1992).

In an extensive review of the literature on the impact of rape, Frazier (1990) found that 75 to 94 percent of the rape victims met the criteria for PTSD at 2 weeks postrape; 60 to 73 percent met the PTSD criteria at 1 to 2 months postrape; 47 to 70 percent met the criteria at 3 to 6 months; and approximately 50 to 60 percent continued to meet the criteria at 12 months postrape and beyond (Foa & Riggs, 1995; Kramer & Green, 1991; Resnick, Yehuda, Pitman, & Foy, 1995; Rothbaum, Foa, & Riggs, 1992; Santello & Leitenberg, 1993). According to Freedy, Resnick, Kilpatrick, Dansky, & Tidwell (1994), the most common symptoms at 6 months postrape are *hypervigilance* (79 percent) and an *exaggerated startle response* (83 percent). PTSD prevalence rates for sexual assault victims several years after the rape are consistently reported to be from 12 to 17 percent (Frazier, 1990; Kessler, Sonnega, Bromet, Hughes, & Nelson, 1995; Kilpatrick et al., 1987).

Factors Associated with Higher Levels of Postrape Trauma

Estimates of the percentages of rape victims who experience *long-term, severe, psychological trauma* vary from 25 percent (Goodman et al., 1993) to 60 percent (Mackey et al., 1992).

The long-term symptoms include depression, anxiety, a loss of sense of safety in the world, PTSD, substance abuse, and an increased sense of vulnerability. Many of these victims look normal to an observer and may even be able to hide their feelings from family and friends, until the symptoms are triggered or intensified by a related stressor (Kilpatrick, et al. 1981; Ledray, 1994).

Pre-assault, assault, and postassault factors all play a role in recovery, although studies of these factors sometimes produce conflicting results (Resick, 1993). The factors associated with more severe and prolonged postrape trauma include prior sexual victimization, the use of avoidant coping strategies, self-blame, prior mental health history (especially of depression), and a history of substance abuse (Frazier, 1990; Ruch, Amedeo, Leon, & Gartrell, 1991). The degree of social support provided by friends and family following the sexual assault and the avoidance of such support are also significant factors (Resick, 1993). Kilpatrick et al. (1989) report that the *fear of death or severe physical harm* increases the risk of PTSD, even if no actual physical injury is sustained during the assault. It is important that rape counselors consider these factors when making initial referrals for follow-up and when making attempts to contact the survivor for follow-up. Early intervention may impact long-term functioning, because distress manifesting as early as two weeks postrape has been found to be associated with long-term distress (Rothbaum et al., 1992).

Problems Related to a Combination of Psychological, Spiritual, and Physical Injuries

A number of problems that can be seen as involving the mind, the spirit, and the body are commonly faced by rape victims. Among these are sexual dysfunction, substance abuse, and a long-term decline in physical health.

SEXUAL DYSFUNCTION

Not surprisingly, studies have found that sexual dysfunction is a common reaction to sexual assault and that it often becomes a *chronic* problem. The symptoms of sexual dysfunction, such as avoidance, loss of interest in sex, loss of pleasure from sex, painful intercourse, and an actual fear of sex, are mentioned repeatedly in the literature (Abel & Rouleau, 1995; Becker et al., 1986; Burgess & Holmstrom, 1979; Chapman, 1989; Frazier, 1997; Kimerling & Calhoun, 1994; Koss, 1993; Ledray, 1994, 1999). It is important to note that, although rape victims may become sexually active again within months of the assault, they may not be able to actually enjoy sex for years; celibacy may be a coping strategy.

SUBSTANCE ABUSE

In a survey of 6,159 college students who had been involved in a sexual assault, Koss (1988) found that 73 percent of the assailants and 55 percent of the victims had been using alcohol or other drugs prior to the incident. Although rape victims may indeed be more vulnerable to being raped as a result of substance abuse, which leads to intoxication and an increased vulnerability (Ledray, 1999), it is important to recognize that rape also can *result* in substance abuse, possibly as an attempt to dull the memory and to avoid thinking about the rape (Goodman et al., 1993; Koss, 1993; Ledray, 1994). In a national sample of 3,006 survivors of rape, the rates of both alcohol and drug use were found to have significantly increased after a sexual assault, even in women with no prior substance use or abuse history (Kilpatrick, Acierno, Resnick, Saunders, & Best, 1997).

Long-Term Decline in Physical Health

There is convincing evidence that sexual assault has a significant and chronic impact on general health for many years. The resultant stress appears to suppress the immune system, thereby increasing susceptibility to disease, and to trigger an increased sensitivity to subtle symptoms and a heightened concern about health (Cohen & Williamson, 1991). Sexual assault victims may also interpret emotional reactions to the assault as physical disease symptoms (Koss, Woodruff, & Koss, 1990), or they may engage in injurious health behaviors, such as increased substance use and eating disorders (Felitti, 1991; Golding, 1994). Increased sexual activity with multiple partners, which sometimes follows rape, especially in a formerly inactive adolescent, can also result in increased exposure to disease (Ledray, 1994).

Victims of sexual assault are more likely to seek medical care than psychological care, because medical care is less stigmatizing and because they perceive the physical symptoms as more salient than the symptoms of psychological distress (Kimerling & Calhoun, 1994). Kimerling and Calhoun found that, in a sample of 115 sexual assault victims, 73 percent had sought out medical services during the first year after a sexual assault, whereas only 19 percent had sought mental health services of any kind. Those who had obtained medical services were most likely to report gynecological problems and sexual dysfunction. Poor *social support* was found to be associated with the higher use of medical services, and higher levels of social support were associated with better actual physical health and better perceived health.

All forms of violent assault have been found to impact health negatively, even after the victim has recovered from the acute injuries incurred during the assault. *Sexual* assault has a more negative effect on health status than assault without a sexual component. In their study of 2,291 victims of nonsexual and sexual assault, Koss et al. (1990) found that, by the end of the first year following the assault, 92 percent of the victims had sought medical care, and, by the end of the second year, 100 percent had sought care. Overall, the sexual assault victims, who made up 23 percent of the sample, sought medical care at a statistically higher rate than did the victims of crime that did not involve sexual assault.

Koss, Woodruff, and Koss (1981) found that the *severity of victimization* is a more powerful predictor of total yearly visits to a physician and outpatient costs than is age, ethnicity, self-reported symptoms, or actual injury. They found that rape victims are twice as likely to seek the help of a physician than are nonvictims; in that study, the visits increased 56 percent in the victim groups, compared with 2 percent in the nonvictim groups.

There is evidence suggesting that the psychological and spiritual trauma associated with sexual assault is related to the long-term decline in physical health often seen in victims of assault, particularly sexual assault. Leserman et al. (1997) studied the health status of victims of physical assault 10 years after the assault had taken place. They charted physical health status in the 99 sexual assault victims and the 68 victims of life-threatening, nonsexual physical abuse. The investigators found that an overall *poorer* physical health status was associated with sexual assault, especially when the victim had incurred physical injury during the assault, had been was attacked by multiple perpetrators, or had had her life threatened during the assault. In a similar vein, Golding (1994) found that women with a history of sexual assault were more likely to have a *severe chronic disease,* such as diabetes, arthritis, trouble walking, paralysis, or fainting, as well as functional limitations (27 percent, vs. 16 percent of the nonrape victims). The rape victims were also more likely to complain of six or more medically unexplained physical symptoms (29 percent, vs. 16 percent of the nonrape victims). The increased incidence of overall explained and unexplained physical symptoms in the rape victims was 60 percent, compared with 36 percent in the nonrape victims.

In a study by Walker et al., (1995), the women with chronic pelvic pain were significantly more likely than the women with no pelvic pain to be victims of sexual abuse. The chronic pain groups were also more likely to be depressed and to have substance-abuse problems, phobias, and sexual dysfunction. Only 1 out of 10 patients were found to have an *organic* condition, even though 11 percent of the primary care visits were related to the chronic pelvic pain, at an average cost of $1,816 per patient.

There is evidence in the literature that obtaining *psychotherapy* after a sexual assault has a positive effect on physical as well as psychological health, although not all studies support this relationship. Waigandt and Miller (1986) compared a group of rape victims who had successfully reorganized (come to terms with what had happened), a group of rape victims who were still psychologically disorganized five years postrape, and a group of nonvictims. They found that both groups of rape victims made 35 percent more visits per year to a medical doctor than the nonvictims; however, the disorganized victims made even *more* visits and perceived their health as *worse* than the organized victims perceived theirs. Moreover, the reorganized victims reported more physical symptoms than the disorganized victims, primarily the pelvic-related disorders dysmenorrhea and incontinence. The disorganized victims also exhibited twice the number of negative health behaviors, such as smoking, excessive alcohol use, and overeating.

The literature is not unanimous in supporting a relationship between psychotherapy and improved physical health in victims of sexual assault; Kimerling and Calhoun (1994) did not find that victims who had sought out psychological services visited providers of physical health care less frequently than victims who had not. More research in this area is needed.

Disclosing, or failing to disclose, that a rape occurred at some point in her history can significantly impact a woman's health. The former was demonstrated in the case study of a 49-year-old woman who experienced intermittent, severe, long-standing hypertension for which no etiology could be found. After a routine health visit to check her blood pressure (BP), she disclosed that she had been having nightmares and was beginning to recall being raped by her sister's boyfriend when she was 14 years old. Immediately after the disclosure, her BP went from 240/150 to 150/105. The next morning, she reported having had a good night's sleep, with no more nightmares, and her BP was a normal 120/85 (Mann & Delon, 1995).

Rape victims who do *not* report and get help in dealing with their assault can suffer ill health for protracted periods of time. Felitti (1991) charted the health status of both a sample of 131 medical patients who had a history of sexual abuse to a group of matched controls who did not, over time. The majority of the assault victims (90 percent) had never before disclosed the abuse. Felitti (1991) found the sexual assault victims, decades later, to be significantly more depressed (83 percent) and experiencing physical symptoms of depression, such as despondency, chronic fatigue, sleep disturbance, and frequent crying spells. Sixty percent had gained more than 50 pounds, and 35 percent had gained more than 100 pounds. Chronic, unexplained headaches were common (45 percent), as were recurrent gastrointestinal disturbances (64 percent). Another study of 100 women concluded that women with a history of sexual abuse are 60 percent more likely to have unexplained pelvic pain and/or abnormal bleeding and are more likely to have gynecological surgery than are women without a sexual assault history (Chapman, 1989). Chapman found that sexual abuse victims have five times the number of hysterectomies and three times the number of pelvic and gynecological surgeries than nonvictims and cautions that unexplained pain in women with a history of sexual abuse may not be removed by a surgical procedure when pain alone is the criterion for the procedure.

SANE and SART Programs

Sexual assault nurse examiners (SANEs) are registered nurses who provide specialized care and services to rape victims, usu-

ally as part of a sexual assault response/resource team (SART). SANE and SART programs were initially developed at the instigation of professional nurses who recognized the inadequacy of the services that were being provided to sexual abuse victims by medical caregivers in emergency departments (EDs) (Burgess & Holmstrom, 1974; Ledray & Chaignot, 1980).

Prior to the development of SANE programs, rape victims who went to EDs for care often had to wait as long as 12 hours in a busy public area, because their wounds were seen as less serious than those of other trauma victims and critically ill persons (Holloway & Swan, 1993; Sandrick, 1996; Speck & Aiken, 1995). In addition, rape victims were often not allowed to eat, drink, or urinate while they waited, for fear of destroying evidence (Thomas & Zachritz, 1993). Doctors and nurses were often not sufficiently trained to do medical-legal exams, and many were lacking in the ability to testify as expert witnesses (Lynch, 1993). Even hospital staff members who were well trained initially often did not complete a sufficient number of exams to maintain an acceptable level of proficiency (Lenehan, 1991; Tobias, 1990; Yorker, 1996), and the documentation of evidence could be rushed, inadequate, or incomplete (Frank, 1996). Moreover, although rape victims' medical needs were met, their emotional needs were overlooked all too often (Speck & Aiken, 1995). Sometimes, victims were even *blamed* for the rape by the ED staff (Kiffe, 1996).

Typically, before SANE programs existed, the rape survivor was faced with a time-consuming, cumbersome succession of examiners, some with only a few hours of orientation to their duties and little experience. Often, the only physician available to do the vaginal exam after the rape was *male* (Lenehan, 1991). Although approximately half of rape victims were unconcerned with the sex of the examiner, this was extremely problematic for the other half. Even many of the male victims preferred to be examined by a woman, as they, too, were probably raped by a man and experienced the same generalized fear and anger toward men that the female victims experienced (Ledray, 1996).

There are many anecdotal and published reports of physicians having been reluctant to conduct the examinations necessary in rape cases. Their reluctance may have been due to many factors, including a lack of experience and training in forensic evidence collection (Bell, 1995; Lynch, 1993; Speck & Aiken, 1995), and the time-consuming nature of the evidentiary exam in a busy ED, with many other medically urgent patients (DiNitto, Martin, Norton, & Maxwell, 1986; Frank, 1996). An additional factor is the knowledge that completing the exam renders practitioners vulnerable to being subpoenaed to testify in court, where they might be questioned by a hostile defense attorney (DiNitto et al., 1986; Frank, 1996; Thomas & Zachritz, 1993; Speck & Aiken, 1995). Whatever their reasons, many physicians flatly refused to do rape examinations (DiNitto et al., 1986). Kettleson (1995) reports that a rape victim was sent home from a hospital without having an evidentiary exam completed because no physician could be found to conduct it.

Because of such problems, rape crisis centers (RCCs) began having advocates available to meet sexual assault victims at the emergency department and advocate for them during the medical exam, much as they advocate for them during the police interview. The development of SANE and SART programs has further rectified these problems in the communities in which they are available. The First Sexual Assault Nurse Examiner programs were established in Memphis, Tennessee, in 1976 (Speck & Aiken, 1995); Minneapolis, Minnesota, in 1977 (Ledray & Chaignot, 1980; Ledray, 1996) and Amarillo, Texas, in 1979 (Antognoli-Toland, 1985).

SANEs are on call to specified emergency departments, medical clinics, community agencies, and independent SANE facilities. Their function is to complete a medical-legal examination of the rape victim, to collect evidence, and to provide support and crisis intervention. SANEs usually function as part of a Sexual Assault Response Team. SARTs can vary greatly in makeup but are often composed of a SANE, a rape crisis advocate, a law enforcement officer, and a prosecutor.

Police or medical facility personnel page the SANE whenever a sexual assault or an attempted sexual assault victim reports to the police or goes to the medical facility within 72 hours of the assault, which is the window of opportunity for the recovery of biological evidence. Typically, SANEs arrive at the medical facility within one hour after having been paged. The medical-legal exam the SANE conducts has five essential components (Ledray, 1998b):

1. *The documentation and care of injuries*
2. *The collection of medical-legal evidence*
3. *An evaluation of risk and the prophylactic treatment of sexually transmitted diseases*
4. *An evaluation of risk and emergency pregnancy interception*
5. *Crisis intervention*

When the SANE arrives, she begins by completing a limited medical interview in order to determine which areas of the victim's body to examine for evidence and potential injuries. She then collects any clothing that may harbor potential evidence (such as hair or fibers), and completes the medical-legal examination. If there was a vaginal assault, she completes a vaginal examination. If a colposcope is available, she takes pictures of any genital injuries. The colposcope magnifies injuries for better visualization and documentation. Because this is a very expensive piece of equipment, not all SANE and SART programs have one available at every examination site. Thorough exams can be completed without a colposcope, though.

Once the medical legal-evidentiary exam is completed, the SANE refers the victim back to the medical staff for care if there are any injuries requiring treatment. Medical treatment is always delayed, when injuries are not life-threatening, so that evidence that would otherwise be lost can be collected first. If there are no injuries requiring additional treatment, the victim is discharged by the SANE. If a police report has been made, a law enforcement officer may be called to provide the victim with safe transportation home, to collect additional evidence, or to complete an interview with the victim. If a rape-crisis advocate is present, she also provides support and crisis intervention and may arrange transportation home for the victim or help her find safe housing, if needed.

Although SANE program development was slow initially, with only three programs operating by the end of the 1970s, development is progressing rapidly today (Ledray, 1996). When the *Sexual Assault Nurse Examiner Development and Operation Guide* was published in 1999 by The Office for Victims of Crime (OVC), 116 SANE programs were identified (Ledray, 1998a). Currently, there are more than 300 SANE programs, and their numbers are growing rapidly.

A flurry of attention was directed to the SANE model in 1994, when the Ford Foundation and John F. Kennedy School of Government at Harvard University named the Tulsa SANE program the winner of their Innovations in State and Local Government Award (Yorker, 1996). In many ways, SANE programs represent a return to the original Rape Crisis Center goal of stopping rape. This time, however, the method is different, and it is coming from within the system, with the goal of collecting better forensic evidence in order to better prosecute offenders. The SANE concept represents an effective model for providing better evidence collection and a more sensitive initial medical response to rape victims (Ledray, 1998b).

In 1992, 72 individuals from 31 programs across the United States and Canada came together in Minneapolis for the first time at a meeting hosted by the Sexual Assault Resource Service, a Minneapolis-based SANE program, and the University of Minnesota School of Nursing. It was at that meeting that the International Association of Forensic Nurses (IAFN) was formed (Ledray, 1996). The American Nurses' Association (ANA) first recognized forensic nursing as a new specialty in 1995 (Lynch, 1993). SANE is now seen as a subspecialty of forensic nursing. At the 1996 IAFN meeting in Kansas City, Kansas, Geri Marullo, the executive director of ANA, predicted that within 10 years the Joint Commission on the Accreditation of Hospitals (JCAHO) would require every hospital to have a specially trained nurse available (Marullo, 1996).

New Directions

The challenge for tomorrow is two-fold: to provide for women more tertiary protection against intimate violence and to see that every healthcare institution has a Sexual Assault Nurse Examiner (SANE) program that works with a Sexual Assault Response Team (SART). This level of care can no longer be optional for women. Effectively dealing with suspected drug-facilitated sexual assault and HIV are also areas of growing concern, which can best be addressed through an up-to-date SANE-SART model.

Questions for Reflection and Discussion

1. *Regarding battered women, how would you respond to the question, Why doesn't she just leave?*
2. *How would you help a friend or family member who is being abused?*
3. *What is the best approach to preventing intimate violence—at what level of intervention and why?*
4. *What activity would you like to suggest for a community action team in your community?*
5. *What role do you feel a rape victim's presexual assault level of functioning plays in her recovery?*
6. *What factors do you believe increase the likelihood of long-term trauma after a rape?*
7. *Would you expect the response of a male rape victim to be the same as or different from that of a female victim? Why or why not?*
8. *Do you think the public tends to respond differently to the rape of a man than to the rape of a woman? If so, in what way and why?*

Resources

Books

Ledray, L. E. (1994). *Recovering from rape*. New York: Henry Holt & Company.

Dugan, M., & Hock, R. (2000). *It's my life now: starting over after an abusive relationship or domestic violence*. Routledge.

Wilson, K. (1997). *When violence begins at home: a comprehensive guide to understanding and ending domestic abuse*. Hunter House.

Other

National domestic violence hotline—staffed 24-hours a day.
Phone: 1-800-799-7233

Department of Justice, Office for Victims of Crime
810 7th Street N.W.
Washington, DC 20531
Phone: 1-800-394-2255

Websites

Minnesota center against violence and abuse (www.minicava.umn.edu) a comprehensive site sponsored by the University of Minnesota

References

Abel, G., & Rouleau, J. (1995). Sexual abuses. *The Psychiatric Clinics of North America, 18*(1), 139–153.

American Psychiatric Association (1994). Diagnostic and statistical manual of mental disorders (4th ed.). Washington, DC: Author.

Amnesty International. (1973). *Report on torture*. London: Duckworth/Amnesty International.

Anderson, S. A., & Schlossberg, M. C. (1999). Systems perspectives on battering: The importance of context and pattern. In M. Harway & J. M. O'Neil (Eds.), *What causes men's violence against women?* (pp. 346–367). Thousand Oaks, CA: Sage.

Antognoli-Toland, P. (1985). Comprehensive program for examination of sexual assault victims by nurses: A hospital-based project in Texas. *Journal of Emergency Nursing, 11*(3), 132–136.

Atkeson, B., Calhoun, K. S., Resick, P. A., & Ellis, E. (1982). Victims of rape: Repeated assessment of depressive symptoms. *Journal of Consulting and Clinical Psychology, 50,* 96–102.

Bandura, A. (1997). *Self-efficacy: The exercise of control.* New York: Freeman.

Becker, J., Skinner, L., Abel, G., & Cichon, J. (1986) Level of post-assault sexual functioning in rape and incest victims. *Archives of Sexual Behavior, 15*(1), 37–49.

Bell, K. (1995, July, August, September). Tulsa Sexual Assault Nurse Examiners Program. *The Oklahoma Nurse*, p. 16.

Berrios, D. C., & Grady, D. (1991). Domestic violence: Risk factors and outcomes. *Western Journal of Medicine,* 155, 133–135.

Blair, T., & Warner, C. (1992). Sexual assault. *Topics in Emergency Medicine, 14*(4), 58–77.

Bloom, S. (1997). *Creating sanctuary.* New York: Routledge.

Bograd, M. (1988). Power, gender and the family: Feminist perspectives on family systems theory. In K. Yllo & M. Bograd (Eds.), *Feminist perspectives on wife abuse* (pp. 211–220). Newbury Park, CA: Sage Publications.

Bownes, I., O'Gorman, E., & Saters, A. (1991). A rape comparison of stranger and acquaintance assaults. *Medical Science Law, 31*(2), 102–109.

Breslau, N., Davis, G., Andreski, P., & Peterson, E. (1991). Traumatic events and post-traumatic stress disorder in an urban population of young adults. *Archives of General Psychiatry, 48,* 216–222.

Browne, A. (1987). *Battered women who kill.* New York: Free Press.

Burge, S. (1988). PTSD in victims of rape. *Journal of Traumatic Stress, 1*(2), 193–210.

Burgess, A., & Holmstrom, L. (1974). Rape trauma syndrome. *American Journal of Psychiatry, 131*(9), 981–985.

Burgess, A., & Holmstrom, L. (1979). Adaptive strategies and recovery from rape. *American Journal of Psychiatry, 136,* 1278–1282.

Burnam, M. S., Stein, J. A., Golding, J. M., Siegel, J. M., Sorenson, S. B., Forsythe, A. B., & Telles, C. A. (1988). Sexual assault and mental disorders in a community population. *Journal of Consulting and Clinical Psychology, 147,* 843–850.

Calhoun, K., Atkeson, B., & Resick, P. (1982). A longitudinal examination of fear reactions in victims of rape. *Journal of Counseling Psychology, 29,* 655–661.

Cartwright, P. S., Moore, R. A., Anderson, J. R., & Brown, D. H. (1986). Genital injury and implied consent to alleged rape. *Journal of Reproductive Medicine, 31*(11), 1043–1044.

Centers for Disease Control and Prevention (CDC). (1998). Sexually transmitted diseases treatment guidelines. *Morbidity and Mortality Weekly Report, 42,* 1–102.

Chapman, D. (1989). A longitudinal study of sexuality and gyne-cologic health in abused women. *Journal of the American Osteopathic Association, 89*(5), 619–624.

Claydon, E., Murphy, S., Osborne, E., Kitchen, V., Smith, J., & Harris, J. (1991). Rape and HIV. *International Journal of STD and AIDS, 2,* 200–201.

Cluss, P., Boughton, J., Frank, L., Stewart, B., & West, D. (1983). The rape victim: Psychological correlates of participation in the legal system. *Criminal Justice and Behavior, 10,* 342–357.

Cohen, L. J., & Roth, S. (1987). The psychological aftermath of rape: Long-term effects and individual differences in recovery. *Journal of Social and Clinical Psychology, 5,* 525–534.

Cohen, S., & Williamson, G. (1991). Stress and infectious disease in humans. *Psychological Bulletin, 109,* 5–24.

Crowell, N., & Burgess, A. (1996). *Understanding violence against women.* Washington, DC: National Academy Press.

DiNitto, D., Martin, P. Y., Norton, D. B., & Maxwell, S. M. (1986). After rape: Who should examine rape survivors? *American Journal of Nursing, 86*(5), 538–540.

Dobash, R. E., & Dobash, R. P. (1992). *Women, violence and social change.* New York: Routledge.

Dupre, A., Hampton, H., Morrison, H., & Meeks, R. (1993). Sexual assault. *Obstetrics and Gynecological Survey, 28*(9), 640–648.

Dutton, D. G. (1994). Patriarchy and wife assault: The ecological fallacy. *Violence and Victims, 9*(2), 167–192.

Dutton, D. G. (1995). *The domestic assault of women: Psychological and criminal justice perspectives* (2nd ed). Vancouver: UBC Press.

Ellis, E., Atkeson, B., & Calhoun, K. (1981). An assessment of long-term reactions to rape. *Journal of Abnormal Psychology, 90,* 263–266.

Federal Bureau of Investigation. (1993). *Uniform crime reports for the United States.* Washington, DC: U.S. Department of Justice.

Felitti, V. (1991). Long-term medical consequences of incest, rape, and molestation. *Southern Medical Journal, 84*(3), 328–331.

Foa, E. B., & Riggs, D. S. (1995). Posttraumatic stress disorder following assault: Theoretical considerations and empirical findings. *Current Directions, 4,* 61–65.

Follingstad, D. R., Rutledge, L. L., Berg, B. J., House, E. S, & Pollek, D. S. (1990). The role of emotional abuse in physi-cally abusive relationships. *Journal of Family Violence, 6,* 81–95.

Fortune, M. (1991). *Violence in the family: A workshop curriculum for clergy and other helpers.* Cleveland: Plilgrim Press.

Frank, C. (1996, December). The new way to catch rapists. *Redbook,* pp. 34–36.

Frank, E., & Stewart, B. D. (1984). Depressive symptoms in rape victims: A revisit. *Journal of Affective Disorders, 7,* 77–85.

Frank, E., & Anderson, P. (1987). Psychiatric disorders in rape victims: Past history and current symptomatology. *Compre-hensive Psychiatry, 28,* 77–82.

Frazier, P. (1990). Victim attributions and post-rape trauma. *Journal of Personality and Social Psychology, 59*(2), 298–304.

Frazier, P., Harlow, T., Schauben, L., & Byrne, C. (1993). *Predic-tors of postrape trauma.* Paper presented at the 1993 meeting of the American Psychological Association, Toronto.

Frazier, P., & Schauben, L. (1994). Causal attributions and recovery from rape and other stressful life events. *Journal of Social and Clinical Psychology, 3,* 1–14.

Frazier, P. (2000). The scientific status of research on rape trauma syndrome. In D. L. Faigmna, D. H. Kaye, M. J. Sakes, & J. Sanders (Eds.), *Modern scientific evidence: The law and science of expert testimony* (Vol. 1, 112–126). St. Paul: West.

Frazier, P., & Burnett, J. (1994). Immediate coping strategies among rape victims. *Journal of Counseling and Development, 72*(4), 633–639.

Freedy, J. R., Resnick, H. S., Kilpatrick, D. G., Dansky, B. S., & Tidwell, R. P. (1994). The psychological adjustment of recent crime victims in the criminal justice system. *Journal of Interpersonal Violence, 9,* 450–468.

Geist, R. F. (1988). Sexually related trauma. *Emergency Medicine Clinics of North America, 299,* 21–24.

Gidycz, C., & Koss, M. (1989). The impact of adolescent sexual victimization: Standardized measures of anxiety, depression, and behavioral deviancy. *Violence and Victims, 4,* 139–149.

Gidycz, C. A., Coble, C. N., Latham, L., & Layman, M. J. (1993). Relation of a sexual assault experience in adulthood to prior victimization experiences: A prospective analysis. *Psychology of Women Quarterly, 17,* 151–168.

Gidycz, C., & Koss, M. (1991). Predictors of long-term sexual assault trauma among a national sample of victimized college women. *Violence and Victims, 3,* 175–190.

Girelli, S., Resnick, P., Marhoefer-Dvorak, S., & Hutter, C. (1986). Subjective distress and violence during rape: Their effects on long-term fear. *Violence and Victims, 1*(1), 35–46.

Gold, S., Milan, L., Mayall, A., & Johnson, A. (1994). A cross-validation study of the trauma symptom checklist. *Journal of Interpersonal Violence, 9,* 12–26.

Golding, J. (1994). Sexual assault history and physical health in randomly selected Los Angeles women. *Health Psychology, 13*(2), 130–138.

Goodman, L., Koss, M., & Russo, N. (1993). *Violence against women: Physical, mental and health effects.* Cambridge, MA: Cambridge University Press.

Goodwin, M. M., Gazmararian, J. A., Johnson, C. H., Gilbert, B. C., & Saltzman, L. E. (2000). Pregnancy intendedness and physical abuse around the time of pregnancy: Findings from the Pregnancy Assessment Monitoring System, 1996–1997. *Maternal and Child Health Journal, 4*(2), 85–92.

Green, A. F. (1999). Biological perspectives on violence against women. In M. Haarway & J. M. O'Neil (Eds.), *What causes men's violence against women?* Thousand Oaks, CA: Sage.

Hamberger, K. L., & Hastings, J. E. (1991). Personality correlates of men who batter and nonviolent men: Some continuities and discontinuities. *Journal of Family Violence, 6*(2), 131–145.

Hart, B. J. (1995). *Coordinated community approaches to domestic violence.* Paper presented at the Strategic Planning Workshop on Violence Against Women, National Institute of Justice, Washington, DC. Battered Women's Justice Project, Pennsylvania Coalition Against Domestic Violence, Harrisburg, PA.

Harway, M., & Hansen, M. (1993). An overview of domestic violence. In M. Hansen & M. Harway (Eds.), *Battering and family therapy: A feminist perspective.* Newbury Park, CA: Sage.

Harway, M., & O'Neil, J. M. (Eds.). (1999). *What causes men's violence against women?* Thousand Oaks, CA: Sage.

Herman, J. L. (1992). *Trauma and recovery.* New York: Basic Books.

Hessmiller, J. (1998). For our own good: The meaning of batterer intervention programs for women who have been abused—A Heideggerian hermeneutic inquiry. Doctoral dissertation, University of Michigan, Ann Arbor.

Holloway, M., & Swan, A. (1993). A & E management of sexual assault. *Nursing Standard, 7*(45), 31–35.

Holtzworth-Munroe, A., & Stuart, G. L. (1999). Abusive typologies of male batterers: Three subtypes and the differences among them. *Psychological Bulletin, 116*(3), 476–497.

Jacobson, N. S., & Gottman, J. M. (1998). *When men batter women.* New York: Simon & Schuster.

Jones, A. (1994). *Next time she'll be dead: Battering and how to stop it.* Boston: Beacon Press.

Kessler, R., Sonnega, A., Bromet, E., Hughes, M., & Nelson, C. (1995). Posttraumatic stress disorder in the National Comorbidity Survey. *Archives of General Psychiatry, 52,* 1048–1060.

Kettleson, D. (1995, June). Nurses trained to take evidence. *Unit News/District News,* p. 1.

Kiffe, B. (1996, August). *Perceptions: Responsibility attributions of rape victims.* Unpublished doctoral dissertation, Augsburg College MSW, Minneapolis, MN.

Kilpatrick, D., Veronen, L., & Resick R. (1979). Assessment of the aftermath of rape: Changing patterns of fear. *Journal of Behavioral Assessment 1,* 133–148.

Kilpatrick D., Resnick, R., & Veronen, L. (1981). Effects of a rape experience: A longitudinal study. *Journal of Social Issues, 37,* 1050–1121.

Kilpatrick, D., & Veronen, L. (1984). *Treatment of fear and anxiety in victims of rape.* (Final report, grant No. R01NG29602). Rockville, MD: National Institute of Mental Health.

Kilpatrick, D. G., Veronen, L. J., & Best, C. L. (1985). Factors predicting psychological distress among rape victims. In C.R. Figley (Ed.), *Trauma and its wake* (pp. 467–472). New York: Brunner/Mazel.

Kilpatrick, D., Saunders, B., Veronen, L., Best, C., & Von, J. (1987). Criminal victimization: Lifetime prevalance, reporting to police, and psychological impact. *Crime Delinquency, 33,* 479–489.

Kilpatrick, D. G., Saunders, B. E., Amick-McMullan, A., Best, C. L., Veronen, L. J., & Resnick H. S. (1989). Victim and crime factors associated with the development of crime-related posttraumatic stress disorder. *Behavior Therapy, 20,* 199–214.

Kilpatrick, D., Edmunds, C., & Seymour, A. (1992). *Rape in America: A report to the nation.* Arlington, VA: National Victim Center.

Kilpatrick, D., Acierno, R., Resnick, H., Saunders, B., & Best, C. (1997). A 2-year longitudinal analysis of the relationship between violent assault and substance use in women. *Journal of Consulting and Clinical Psychology, 65*(5), 834–847.

Kimerling, R., & Calhoun, S. (1994). Somatic symptoms, social support, and treatment seeking among sexual assault victims. *Journal of Consulting and Clinical Psychology. 62*(2), 333–340.

Koss, M., Gidycz, A., & Wisniewski, C. (1987). The scope of rape: Incidence and prevalence of sexual aggression and victimization in a national sample of higher education students. *Journal of Consulting and Clinical Psychology, 55*(2), 162–170.

Koss, M. P. (1988). Hidden rape: Sexual aggression and victimization in a national sample of students in higher education. In A. W. Burgess (Ed.), *Rape and sexual assault* (pp. 3–25). New York: Garland.

Koss, M., Dinero, T., Seibel, C., & Cox, S. (1988). Stranger and acquaintance rape. Are there differences in the victim's experience? *Psychology of Women Quarterly, 12,* 1–24.

Koss, M., Woodruff, W., & Koss, P. (1990). Relationship of criminal victimization to health perceptions among women medical patients. *Journal of Consulting and Clinical Psychology, 58*(2), 147–152.

Koss, M., & Harvey, M. (1991). *The rape victim: Clinical and community interventions* (2nd ed.). Newbury Park, CA: Sage.

Koss, M. (1993). Rape. Scope, impact, interventions, and public policy. *American Psychologist, 48*(10), 1062–1069.

Krakow, B., Tandberg, D., Barey, M., & Scriggins, L. (1995). Nightmares and sleep disturbance in sexually assaulted women. *Dreaming, 5*(3), 199–206.

Kramer, T., & Green, T. (1991). Post-traumatic stress disorder as an early response to sexual assault. *Journal of Interpersonal Violence, 5,* 229–246.

Krulewitch, C. J., Pierr-Louis, M. L., de Leon-gomez, R., Guy, R., & Green, R. (2001). Hidden from view: Violent deaths among pregnant women in the District of Columbia, 1988–1996. *Journal of Midwifery and Women's Health, 46*(1), 4–10.

Ledray, L., & Chaignot, M. J. (1980). Services to sexual assault victims in Hennepin County. *Evaluation and Change,* Special Issue, Minneapolis Medical Research Foundation.

Ledray, L. (1984). Victims of incest. *American Journal of Nursing, 84*(8), 1010–1014.

Ledray, L. (1991). Sexual assault and sexually transmitted disease: The issues and concerns. In A. Burgess (Ed.), *Rape and sexual assault III: A research handbook* (pp. 181–193). New York & London: Garland.

Ledray, L. (1994). *Recovering from rape* (2nd ed.). New York: Henry Holt.

Ledray, L. (1996, March). The sexual assault resource service: A new model of care. *Minnesota Medicine: A Journal of Clinical and Health Affairs, 79*(3), 22–23.

Ledray, L. (1998a). The SANE nurse in the emergency department. *Management Update, 5*(3), 42–45.

Ledray, L. (1998b). Sexual assault: Clinical issues. SANE development and operation guide. *Journal of Emergency Nursing, 24*(2), 197–198.

Ledray, L. (1999). Sexual assault: Clinical issues. IAFN sixth annual scientific assembly highlights. *Journal of Emergency Nursing, 25*(1), 34–38.

Lenehan, G. P. (1991). A SANE way to care for rape victims. *Journal of Emergency Nursing, 17*(1), 46–49.

Leonard, K. E. (1993). Drinking patterns and intoxication in marital violence: Review, critique and future directions for research. *Alcohol and interpersonal violence.* Rockville, MD: National Institute on Alcohol Abuse and Alcoholism, NIH Pub. No. 93–3496.

Leserman, J., Zhiming, L., Drossman, D., Toomey, T., Nachman, G., & Glogau, L. (1997). Impact of sexual and physical abuse dimensions on health status: Development of an abuse severity schedule. *Somatic Medicine, 59,* 152–160.

Lettelier, P. (1994). Gay and bisexual male domestic violence victimization: Challenges to feminist theory and responses to violence. *Violence and Victims, 9*(2), 95–106.

Lynch, V. A. (1993). Forensic nursing: Diversity in education and practice. *Journal of Psychosocial Nursing, 132*(3), 42–46.

MacFarlane, E., & Hawley, P. (1993, June). Sexual assault: Coping with crisis. *The Canadian Nurse,* pp. 21–24.

Mackey, T., Sereika, S., Weissfeld, L., Hacker, S., Zehder, J., & Heard, S. (1992). Factors associated with long-term depressive symptoms of sexual assault victims. *Archives of Psychiatric Nursing, 6*(1), 10–25.

Mann, S., & Delon, M. (1995). Improved hypertension control after disclosure of decades old trauma. *Psychosomatic Medicine, 57,* 501–505.

Marchbanks, P., Lui, K. J. & Mercy, J. (1990). Risk of injury from resisting rape. *American Journal of Epidemiology, 132*(3), 540–549.

Marin, A., & Russo, N. F. (1999). Feminist perspectives on male violence against women. In M. Harway & J. M. O'Neil (Eds.), *What causes men's violence against women?* (pp. 249–255). Thousand Oaks, CA: Sage.

Marullo, G. (1996). *The Future and the forensic nurse: New dimensions for the 21st century.* Presentation at the fourth annual Scientific Assembly of Forensic Nurses, Kansas City, MO.

McFarlane, J., Parker, B., Soeken, K., & Bullock, L. (1992). Assessing for abuse during pregnancy. Severity and frequency of injuries and associated entry into prenatal care. *Journal of the American Medical Association, 267*(23), 3176–3178.

McKenry, P. C., Julian, T. W., & Gavazzi, S. M. (1995). Toward a biopsychosocial model of domestic violence. *Journal of Marriage and the Family, 57,* 307–320.

Mirsky, A. F., & Siegel, A. (1994). The neurobiology of violence and aggression. In A. J. Reiss, K. A. Miczek, & J. Roth (Eds.), *Understanding and preventing violence: Vol, 2, Biochemical influences* (pp. 294–301) Washington, DC: National Academy press.

Moss, M., Frank, E., & Anderson, B. (1990). The effects of marital status and partner support on rape trauma. *American Journal of Orthopsychiatry, 69*(3), 379–391.

Murphy, S., Harris, V., & Forester, S. (1989). Rape and subsequent seroconversion to HIV, *British Medical Journal, 299,* 718.

Nadelson, C., Notman, M., Zackson, H., & Gornick, J. (1982). A follow-up study of rape victims. *American Journal of Psychiatry, 139,* 1266–1270.

National Conference of Catholic Bishops. (1995). *Ethical and Religious Directives for Catholic Health Care Services,* 14–17.

Norris, J., & Feldman-Summers, S. (1981). Factors related to the psychological impact of rape on the victim. *Journal of Abnormal Psychology, 139,* 1266–1270.

Rath, C. (1999). *Transforming communities: A model for organizing.* Harrisburg, PA: The National Resource Center on Domestic Violence.

Renzetti, C. (1992). *Violent betrayal: Partner abuse in lesbian relationships.* Newbury Park, CA: Sage.

Resick, P. (1993). The psychological impact of rape. *Journal of Interpersonal Violence, 8*(2), 223–255.

Resick, P., & Schnicke, M. (1990). Treating symptoms in adult victims of sexual assault. *Journal of Interpersonal Violence, 5*(4), 488–506.

Resnick, H., Kilpatrick, D., Dansky, B., Saunders, B., & Best, C. (1993). Prevalence of civilian trauma and PTSD in a representative national sample of women. *Journal of Consulting and Clinical Psychology, 61*(6), 984–991.

Resnick, H., Yehuda, R., Pitman, R., & Foy, D. (1995). Effect of previous trauma on acute plasma cortisol level following rape. *American Journal of Psychiatry, 152,* 1675–1677.

Resnick, P., Jordan, C., Girelli, S., Hunter, C., & Marhoefer-Dvorak, S. (1988). A comparative outcome study of behavioral group therapy for sexual assault survivors. *Behavior Therapy, 19,* 385–401.

Riggs, D., Kilpatrick, D., & Resnick, H. (1992). Long-term psychological distress associated with marital rape and aggravated assault: A comparison to other crime victims. *Journal of Family Violence, 7,* 283–296.

Rosenbaum, A., & Hoge, S. K. (1989). Head injury and marital aggression. *American Journal of Psychiatry, 146,* 1048–1051.

Rothbaum, B., Foa, E., & Riggs, D. (1992). A prospective study of PTSD in rape victims. *Journal of Traumatic Stress, 5*(3), 455–475.

Ruch, L., Amedeo, S., Leon, J., & Gartrell, J. (1991). Repeated sexual victimization and trauma change during the acute phase of the sexual assault trauma syndrome. *Health and Women, 17*(1), 1–19.

Sandrick, K. J. (1996, June). Inside track: Medicine and law: Tightening the chain of evidence. *Hospitals & Health Networks,* p. 14.

Santello, M., & Leitenberg, H. (1993). Sexual aggression by an acquaintance: Methods of coping and later psychological adjustment. *Violence and Victims, 8*(2), 91–104.

Santiago, J., McCall-Perez, F., Gorcey, M., & Beigel, A. (1985). Long-term psychological effects of rape in 35 rape victims. *American Journal of Psychiatry, 142,* 1338–1340.

Saunders, D. (1992). A typology of men who batter. *American Journal of Orthopsychiatry, 62,* 264–275.

Schechter, S. (1982). *Women and male violence.* Boston: South End.

Shepard, M., & Pence, E. (1999). *Coordinating community responses to domestic violence: Lessons from Duluth and beyond.* Thousand Oaks, CA: Sage.

Silverstein, L. B. (1999). The evolutionary origins of male violence against women. In M. Harway & J. M. O'Neil (Eds.), *What causes men's violence against women?* (pp. 240–248). Thousand Oaks, CA: Sage.

Slaughter, L., & Brown, C. (1992, January). Colposcopy to establish physical findings in rape victims. *American Journal of Obstetrics & Gynecology, 166*(1), 19–23.

Speck, P., & Aiken, M. (1995, April). Focus: Twenty years of community nursing service. *Tennessee Nurse,* pp. 15–18.

Straus, M., & Gelles, R. G. *Physical violence in American families: Risk factors and adaptations to violence in 8,145 families.* New Brunswick, NJ: Transaction.

Thomas, M., & Zachritz, H. (1993). Tulsa Sexual Assault Nurse Examiners (SANE) program. *Journal of Oklahoma State Medical Association, 86,* 284–286.

Tintinalli, J., Hoelzer, M., & Michigan, J. (1985). Clinical findings and legal resolution in sexual assault. *Annals of Emergency Medicine, 14*(5), 447–453.

Tjaden, P., & Thoennes, N. (1998). *Prevalence, incidence and consequences of violence against women: Findings from the national violence against women survey.* Washington, DC: National Institute of Justice & Center for Disease Control and Prevention.

Tjaden, P., & Thoennes, N. (2000). *Full report of the prevalence, incidence and consequences of violence against women: Findings from the national violence against women survey.* Washington, DC: National Institute of Justice & Center for Disease Control and Prevention.

Tobias, G. (1990). Rape examinations by GPs. *The Practitioner, 234,* 874–877.

Walker, L. (1994). *Abused women and survivor therapy: A practical guide for the psychotherapist.* Washington, DC: American Psychological Association Press.

Walker, E., Katon, W., Hansom, J., Harrop-Griffith, J., Holm, L., Jones, M., Hickok, L., & Russo, J. (1995). Psychiatric diagnoses and sexual victimization in women with chronic pelvic pain. *Psychosomatics, 6*(6), 531–540.

Waigandt, C., & Miller, D. (1986). Maladaptive responses during the reorganization phase of rape trauma syndrome. *Response, 1*(2), 36–40.

Winfield, I., George, L. K., Swartz, M., & Blazer, D. G. (1990). Sexual assault and psychiatric disorders among a community sample of women. *American Journal of Psychiatry, 147,* 335–341.

Wirtz, P., & Harrell, A. (1987). The effects of threatening versus nonthreatening previous life events on levels of fear in rape victims. *Violence and Victims, 12*(2), 89–98.

Yllo, K. (1988). Political and methodological debates in wife abuse research. In K. Yllo & M. Bograd (Eds.), *Feminist perspectives on wife abuse.* Newbury Park, CA: Sage.

Yorker, B. C. (1996). Nurses in Georgia care for survivors of sexual assault. *Georgia Nursing, 56*(1), 5–6.

Yuzpe, A., Smith, R., & Rademaker, C. (1982). A multicenter clinical investigation employing ethinyl estradiol combined with dl-norgestrel as a postcoital contraceptive agent. *Fertility and Sterility, 37*(4), 51–56.

U.S. Department of Justice. (1998). *Violence by intimates: Analysis of data on crimes by current of former spouses, boyfriends and girlfriends.* Washington, DC: U.S. Department of Justice.

SECTION V

Emotional and Spiritual Health

26

Psychological/Emotional Wellness and Illness

Jennifer Stoops and Nancy Mann

Objectives

1. *Identify the sociocultural factors that contribute to the development of psychological/emotional disorders in women.*
2. *Discuss selected depressive disorders, eating disorders, and anxiety disorders in terms of symptoms, diagnosis, and treatment.*
3. *Discuss the efficacy of some traditional and nontraditional treatments for psychological/emotional disorders.*

Introduction

This chapter addresses psychological/emotional wellness and illness. The markers that are associated with mental/emotional wellness are described and sociocultural factors that affect women's mental/emotional well being are explored. Selected forms of three psychological/emotional disorders that afflict women more frequently than men are explored: depressive disorders, eating disorders, and anxiety disorders. The nature and criteria for diagnosis of the selected illnesses are described, and the theories regarding their causation are discussed.

Markers of Psychological/ Emotional Wellness

From a clinical point of view, the markers of psychological/ emotional wellness are characteristics and qualities related to three broad categories: thought patterns/perceptions, mood/feelings, and empathy/conscience. Persons considered to be clinically well are free from **psychosis** (the perception of things or circumstances not considered "real" by others), **obsessions** (unwarranted preoccupations), **compulsions** (the seemingly irrational need to perform some act repeatedly), **mood disorders** (either depression or unusual, sustained elation), unwarranted **anxiety** or fear, and **personality disorders** (ingrained, inflexible patterns that cause distress or impair functioning). Although overall basic satisfaction with life, or happiness, is not a requirement for "well" status in the clinical sense, it is a highly desirable characteristic sought by many and is an important factor in the quality of life. As such, it will be discussed briefly in this chapter.

Thought Patterns and Perceptions

Persons who are considered psychologically well are generally accurate in their perception of external reality. They are not **psychotic,** which is to say they do not hallucinate, (see, hear, or feel phenomena that are not real), and they do not hold beliefs that are sufficiently unrealistic and bizarre to be considered **delusions.** Psychologically well individuals are also reasonably realistic in their appraisal of others' attitudes toward them; they do not display a pattern of frequently perceiving ill will or threat where none exists—that is, they are not **paranoid.** Finally, psychologically well persons have thought patterns that are reasonably fluid and appropriate to the environment and circumstance; they are not plagued by obsessions, which are often troubling, recurring thoughts on a particular subject, or compulsions—behaviors carried out frequently for no outwardly apparent reason.

Mood/Feelings

It is normal to have a range of emotional responses to life situations. However, there is a range of feelings and expressions of mood states that is outside of the normal for a psychologically well individual. A **mood** is a pervasive feeling, which alters a person's view of the world. In a **mood disorder,** an individual has a sustained period of time in which the abnormal feelings exist, and the feelings are associated with other symptoms that interfere with the person's functioning in a variety of life arenas, such as social, occupational, and relational. For example, whereas an individual who is faced with adverse circumstances, such as the loss of a loved one, the loss of a job, or a recent diagnosis of a significant illness, may experience a period of sadness, such a brief, temporary response of sadness to a situation does not qualify as a mood disorder. However, the presence of an abnormal mood that interferes with functioning in life constitutes a mood disorder.

The terms *dysphoria, elevated mood,* and *euphoria* are used to describe three significant points along the mood continuum. **Dysphoria** is a transient mood state characterized by irritability or sadness. An **elevated mood** is a mood that is more cheerful than normal, but not pathological. The term **euphoria** refers to an abnormal, usually transient mood characterized by an exaggerated sense of well-being and the sense that the individual can do everything with no limitations. Two other terms, *euthymia* and *dysthymia,* are used to describe mood states that are persistent and typical for the person under discussion. **Euthymia** is a normal range of moods without the variations of dysphoria or euphoria. **Dysthymia,** however, means that the individual suffers from a pervasive feeling of low-level depression or sadness. Because the mood disorders within the depressive range are more common in women, the section Psychological/Emotional Illnesses and Problems will focus on those.

Anxiety/Fear

While everyone experiences anxiety and fear from time to time, persons who suffer from **anxiety disorders** are markedly and frequently fearful and anxious, for reasons that others are likely to consider unimportant or fanciful. There are a number of anxiety disorders, and they are described in some detail in the section on Psychological/Emotional Illnesses and Problems.

Personality

Human beings have a wide range of features as part of their personalities. They may exhibit a tendency to be happy or morose, outgoing or shy, generous or stingy, compassionate or judgmental, flexible or rigid, confident or unsure, ethical or unscrupulous, suspicious or trusting—the list is long. However, an individual can demonstrate a tendency toward any of those characteristics and still be considered to have normal character. However, if certain characteristics become very marked, and highly resistant to attempts to change them, the person is said to be suffering from a **personality disorder.** Two of the better-known personality disorders are **paranoid personality disorder** and **antisocial personality disorder.** Individuals who are *paranoid* have a persistent and unjustified belief that other persons, organizations, and so on mean them harm. *Antisocial* persons have an underdeveloped conscience and behave in ways that are harmful to others without feeling empathy or remorse.

Promoting Psychological/ Emotional Wellness

Like physical wellness, psychological/emotional wellness exists on a continuum. Whereas some individuals are blessed with robust psychological/emotional health, others are less well without being obviously ill. Psychological/emotional health is influenced by many factors, one of which is *physical health*. For example, people who must cope with chronic illnesses are known to be at risk for depression. Therefore, one way to promote psychological/emotional wellness is to follow the guidelines for promoting physical wellness contained in other chapters of this book.

Learning to *manage stress* is another method of promoting good psychological/emotional health. The particular stressors that affect contemporary women, and ways of coping with or eliminating them, are discussed in Chapter 7.

Yet another way to promote psychological/emotional health is to cultivate supportive *relationships* with other people. Social support, which is a function of relationships with others, is known to be related positively to mental health. Chapter 8 contains information on cultivating and preserving relationships with friends and romantic partners.

A wide range of other variables are known to influence psychological/emotional health. These include the degree to which one is able to confide in others and forgive others, whether one has a tendency to be angry and judgmental, and whether one feels connected to something transcendent. The aforementioned variables, and others, are addressed in Chapter 27.

Attending to physical health, cultivating supportive relationships, managing stress and taking steps to recognize and overcome negative personal traits all promote psychological/emotional health. However, individuals who are unhappy and dissatisfied with their lives should not hesitate to consult a mental health professional. Psychotherapy can help individuals make changes in their lives that promote psychological/emotional wellness.

Psychological/Emotional Illnesses and Problems

The illnesses and problems addressed in this section include depressive disorders, anxiety disorders, and eating disorders. The forms of depressive disorders to be addressed include major depression, dysthymic disorder, premenstrual dysphoric disorder and postpartum depression. The anxiety disorders addressed are panic disorder, agoraphobia, social phobia, post-traumatic stress disorder, and generalized anxiety disorder. The eating disorders addressed are anorexia nervosa and bulimia nervosa.

Depressive Disorders

Of the several types of depression that commonly afflict women, two, premenstrual dysphoric disorder and postpartum depression, are found *only* in women, whereas two other forms, major depression and dysthymic disorder, occur *more frequently* in women than in men. All four of these forms of depression are classified as mood disorders in the 4th edition of the *Diagnostic and Statistical Manual of Mental Disorders* (*DSM-IV*), published by the American Psychiatric Association (1994).

Depression is all too common in women. The frequency with which depression is diagnosed in women *increased* during each decade of the twentieth century (Maxmen & Ward, 1995). Major community-based studies have demonstrated that women are twice as likely as men to have an episode of depression (Blazer, 2000), and this gender difference begins as early as the age of 10 for girls and continues through midlife (Kornstein & Wojcik, 2000). It is estimated that, currently, 20 percent of women will experience a major depression in their lifetimes, compared with only 10 percent of men (Maxmen & Ward, 1995). Women are at greatest risk during their childbearing years, between ages 25 and 44 (Wisner, Peindl, Gigliotti, & Hanusa, 1999). However, even in the elderly, women's risk of depression is two to three times that of men (Evans et al., 1999). The reasons for the gender discrepancy are not clearly understood. Although being female is not known to be a risk factor for depression per se (Blazer, 2000), a combination of gender-related differences, including biological, social, economic, and cultural factors may contribute to the higher prevalence (Bhati & Bhati, 1999).

Depression has serious psychological and functional consequences for individuals and their families, as well as social and economic consequences for society (Gullette & Blumenthal, 1996). Studies have shown that persons who have a mood disorder in addition to medical illnesses have a death rate up to 150 percent that of medically ill persons without a mood disorder (Angst, Angst, & Stassen, 1999). The effect of depression on physical functioning has been described as comparable to that of other chronic medical illnesses, such as coronary heart disease. Other studies have demonstrated that depression can affect the quality of life in families, bonding between mother and child, response to treatment in cancer, and recovery from heart attack. Depression is also the single greatest risk factor for suicide. Depression is a *recurring* disease, and, with each recurrence, there is a risk of suicide (Angst et al., 1999).

GENERAL FACTORS THAT MAY CONTRIBUTE TO DEPRESSION

Because several illnesses fall under the general category *depression*, it is difficult to identify one specific cause for these disorders. Currently, the etiology of depression is thought to lie in a combination of at least three key elements: (1) biological factors, (2), psychological factors, and (3) stress (Stahl,

1996). Although most cases of depression are now thought to involve some degree of biological vulnerability, the degree to which the various psychosocial factors contribute to the development of depression, and the ways in which they might interact to foster it, is unclear (Stahl, 1996).

Biological Factors Biological factors thought to play a role in depression include neurotransmitters, the hypothalamus, and hormones. The classic biological hypothesis of depression relates to the body's **neurotransmitters**—the chemicals necessary for the transmission of neuronal impulses from one cell to another. The classic neurotransmitters include serotonin (5HT), dopamine (DA), norepinephrine (NE), epinephrine (E), and acetylcholine (ACh). Initially, researchers believed that the biological cause for depression is a *deficiency* of one or more of these neurotransmitters in the brain. Therefore, it seemed reasonable to believe that depression can be alleviated by replacing the deficient neurotransmitter; this theory was the basis of the development of the first anti-depressants (Stahl, 1996). However, it was found that, when the neurotransmitter was replaced through the administration of an antidepressant drug, symptom relief did not occur for many days or weeks. This suggested that there is more to depression than simply insufficient amounts of a given neurotransmitter. The most recent hypothesis suggests that depression is not due to the amounts of available neurotransmitters but, rather, to the neurotransmitter's ability to *stimulate* the target neuron (Stahl, 2000).

Regardless of the exact nature of the problem, it is a virtual certainty that depression is a function of an abnormality in the way neurotransmitters are produced, stored, broken down, received, or blocked by the receptors (Stahl, 2000). Other aspects of brain function, however, such as the functioning of discrete structures, hormonal activity, blood flow, and brain metabolism, may also be involved in the pathophysiology of depression (American Psychiatric Association, 1994).

The **hypothalamus,** which governs the endocrine system either directly or indirectly, has also been implicated in depression; individuals who suffer from depression have disturbances in sleep and appetite, which are regulated by the hypothalamus (Dilts, 2001). Neurotransmitter deficits may be related to the disinhibitory effect of the hypothalamic-pituitary-adrenal axis (HPA) in the brain, which is characterized by an increased production of steroid hormones, such as cortisol (Akiskal, 2000). The HPA is a self-regulating feedback mechanism involving the hypothalamus, the pituitary gland, and the adrenal glands. CT scans have shown enlargement of the pituitary and adrenal glands in individuals with depression (Akiskal, 2000). Elevated corticotropin releasing factor (CRF), involved in the mechanism to stimulate cortisol release, has been found in the cerebrospinal fluid of individuals who have depression (Dilts, 2001). This feedback mechanism has been implicated in stress response, anxiety disorders, and depressive disorders (Akiskal, 2000).

Women experience hormonal shifts related to their reproductive cycle, which may also affect the development and course of depression (Kornstein & Wojcik, 2000). These shifts occur during the premenstrual phase of the menstrual cycle, the postpartum period, and the perimenopausal period. There is not yet a clear understanding of the mechanisms by which a woman's hormones affect her mood. However, it is thought that some women are oversensitive to the shifting levels of hormones, such as estrogen, progesterone, cortisol, prolactin, and beta endorphin, which occur at different times in the reproductive cycle (Suri & Burt, 1997). The ovarian hormones (estrogen and progesterone) influence the production, release, and uptake of neurotransmitters in the brain, as well as the blood flow to the brain (Sarrel, 1999). Animal studies have shown that estrogen and progesterone alter the activity of the neurotransmitter serotonin (Steiner, 1996). Moreover, there is some evidence that the hormonal effects on serotonin may be related to the etiology of the form of intermittent depression known as premenstrual dysphoric disorder (Steiner, 1996).

Hormonal shifts have also been implicated in postpartum depression, the form of depression that occurs after childbirth. During pregnancy, a woman's levels of estrogen and progesterone rise steadily, then fall rapidly at delivery, reaching prepregnancy levels by the fifth day following delivery (Hendrick, Altshuler, & Suri, 1998). Estradiol, a biologically active form of estrogen produced by the placenta, rises significantly during pregnancy and declines abruptly after delivery (Hendrick et al., 1998). Because estrogen is known to affect serotonin, it has been theorized that postpartum depression is triggered by the fall in estrogen levels. Clinical research, however, has not supported this theory to date. The hormone progesterone also falls abruptly following delivery, but, as is the case with estrogen, there is insufficient clinical evidence to link declining levels of progesterone to the onset of depressive symptoms in the postpartum period (Hendrick et al., 1998).

Many studies have addressed the question of whether the incidence of depression rises in women during menopause, but the results have been inconclusive (Warren & Kulak, 1998). However, studies do suggest that, if a woman has a history of depression or another mood disorder, the perimenopausal period may be a time of increased vulnerabilty to depression, presumably due to hormonal influences (Greendale, Lee, & Arriola, 1999).

Thyroid hormones are also thought to be biological contributors to changes in mood. Individuals with low levels of thyroid hormones may exhibit symptoms of depression. Since women experience thyroid disorders much more commonly than men (see Chapter 21), a thorough evaluation of thyroid function should be done for any woman experiencing depressive symptoms. The correction of a thyroid problem may be all that is needed to alleviate mood symptoms for some women. Because there may be other contributors to the development of the depression, however, many women still require other forms of treatment.

Psychological Factors   A number of theories linking various psychological processes and traits to a vulnerability to depression have been developed. The classical psychological view of depression is the **psychodynamic theory,** which was proposed by Freud and expanded by Abraham (Gabbard, 2000). According to this theory, depression is a function of four dynamics: (1) a predisposition to depression caused by a *disturbed infant-mother attachment* in the first year of life; (2) a link to a real or an imagined *object loss;* (3) the development of a *defense mechanism* to cope with the distress related to object loss; and (4) *conflicting feelings* (loss of love and hate) toward the object, with a resultant feeling of self-directed anger. In essence, this theory examines interpersonal relationships, recurring patterns of conflict, and the meaning of actions and experiences. Psychodynamic theory also stresses the importance of developing mature, rather than immature, *coping strategies.* According to this theory, dysthymic disorder (low-level, chronic depression) results from a failure to have made an adequate transition from adolescence to young adulthood and the resulting suboptimal personality development (Peis & Shader, 1994). *Trauma in childhood* is also seen as a factor that can cause an individual to retain immature coping skills into adulthood (Romans, Martin, Morris, & Herbison, 1999). Karen Horney, who began as a follower of Freud and Abraham, differed with the male psychodynamic theorists in that she believed that women are more prone to psychiatric disorders, particularly depression, because of the *cultural standards that devalue women in society* (Paris, 1994). Horney's was one of the first feminist psychological approaches to the psychodynamics of psychiatric disorders.

Whereas the psychodynamic theory of depression focuses on *past* events, the **cognitive** theory of depression focuses on the *present.* In his cognitive theory of depression, Beck (1964) described depression as a result of *negative thinking,* including the expectation of negative experiences in the future, negative views of self, and negative views of the world. According to cognitive theory, depressed individuals generate negative thoughts automatically. Such thoughts are then *reinforced* by the individual's inability to make positive meaning out of environmental information, particularly information related to interpersonal relationships (Agras & Wilson, 2000). In therapy, the cognitive therapist focuses on correcting the faulty thinking. It is debatable, however, whether the faulty thinking in depression is a consequence or a cause of depression (Maxmen & Ward, 1995).

Another psychological theory of depression, the **interpersonal theory,** is based on the work from what is known as the interpersonal school of psychiatry. In the 1950s, interpersonal theorists applied the concept of *adaptation* to psychiatric disorders, including depression (Klerman, Weissman, Rounsaville, & Chevron, 1996). According to interpersonal theory, problems in interpersonal relationships may both *predispose* a person to psychiatric disorders and *precipitate* such disorders. Conversely, the psychiatric disorder may precipitate interpersonal problems (Klerman et al., 1996).

Women who are depressed often have significant problems in their interpersonal relationships, particularly in role functioning. However, whether these interpersonal difficulties are the cause or the result of depression is debated (Briscoe & Smith, 1973).

Although all individuals evolve and grow in the context of relationships, relationships are believed by some to be more central to the formation of women's sense of self than men's, because men are socialized to be autonomous and competitive, whereas women are socialized to be relationally oriented and cooperative (Rosenblatt, 1995). That relationships are more important to women than they are to men is supported by the fact that, although gender role stereotypes have broken down to an unprecedented degree in the modern world, men are still more likely to become depressed over job-related problems, whereas women are more likely to develop a depression due to an unhappy marriage (Kornstein & Wojcik, 2000). It may be that, because of the importance women assign to relationships, a woman who is unhappy in her marriage may question her ability to establish and maintain relationships—and doubt her own self-worth as a result. She may blame herself for marital conflict or the breakup of her marriage, believing that it is *her* responsibility to make certain that the relationship is successful.

Female persons may face relational challenges that make them more vulnerable for depression throughout their life cycle, beginning in childhood. Girls who lose their mothers prior to the age of 11 are known to be at increased risk for depression as adults (Peis & Shader, 1994). The relationship with one's mother is an important one for everyone, but particularly so for girls, as the mother provides the primary gender role model (Rosenblatt, 1995). The loss of this important relationship at such an early age may cause hidden psychological damage, the symptoms of which will emerge later, when the woman reaches key milestones in her life.

Relational losses *later* in life may also trigger depression in vulnerable women. Many women lose relationships through divorce, others through widowhood. Because women tend to outlive men, they are more likely than men to live out the last years of their lives without a primary relationship.

Stress   Stress may cause, or contribute to, alterations in the neurotransmitter system that have been associated with depression. Animal research has demonstrated that stress, particularly unremitting, inescapable stress, can cause structural changes in the brain (Dilts, 2001; Thase, 2000). Therefore, it is possible that events experienced as stressful cause neurochemical imbalances that contribute to depression in human beings. Stressors that occur in *childhood*, while the brain is in the formative stages, may be particularly likely to alter brain structure and neurochemical balance (Akiskal, 2000). The fact that people with diseases such as coronary heart disease, diabetes, and cancer develop depression at a higher rate than people not so afflicted (Dilts, 2001) may be related to the stressful nature of those diseases.

Sociocultural Factors Pertaining to Women

A number of sociocultural factors are thought to contribute to depression in women, possibly because of the stress they induce. Some of these factors may also at least partially explain women's higher rates of depression in comparison with men. Because of the historic power imbalance between males and females (see Chapter 1), women are more likely than men to be subjected to physical, emotional, and sexual *abuse* at the hands of persons with whom they are in a relationship. Also, because women have taken on new roles in society without abandoning the more traditional ones, they are more likely than men to suffer from *role overload*. Depression is also more common in *poorer* women and *older* women. Societal views about the importance of *beauty* for women, and what constitutes it, may also contribute to depression in women, because depression frequently accompanies eating disorders.

Violence and Abuse All forms of violence and abuse can have long-term consequences for women. For example, women who have been abused have an increased hypothalamic-pituitary-adrenal responsiveness to stress, in comparison with women who have not been abused. They react more strongly to the everyday, unavoidable stresses of life. Women who were sexually abused during childhood tend to use more immature coping skills and have lower self-esteem than women who were not abused, and they are more likely to develop psychological/emotional problems, including depression, in adolescence and adulthood (Romans et al., 1999). Childhood abuse that does not include a sexual component is also a risk factor for manifesting a psychological/emotional disorder as an adult.

Although it is a certainty that a history of childhood abuse makes individual women more vulnerable to depression, it is less clear that childhood abuse factors into the higher rate of depression in women overall. Although it has been asserted that girls experience more abuse overall than boys (Dennerstein, 2001) there is also evidence that girls may simply be more likely to *report* having been abused (Romans, Martin, & Mullen, 1996). However, it is possible that, because women's identities and self-esteem are tied to their relationships, women are more susceptible than men to the psychological consequences of abuse at the hands of a family member or an intimate.

Adult women do tend to be victims of severe domestic violence and abuse more often than men (see Chapter 25), and that may contribute to the greater incidence of depression in women. It also seems likely that abuse at the hands of a person with whom a woman has a sexual or romantic relationship may be especially harmful to women because of their greater relational orientation.

Psychological trauma related to sexual assault is also known to set the stage for depression and other mental illnesses. Women are raped more frequently than men, and this type of stress certainly strikes at the core of a woman's sense of self. Being forced to have unwanted sexual contact may diminish a woman's sense of control over her body, herself, and her emotions (Romans, Martin, Morris, & Herbison, 1999)

Women's Roles in Society Women tend to occupy more roles in society than men, particularly in early and middle adulthood. Many women simultaneously occupy the role of wage earner, spouse, mother, and caretaker to aging parents. Although filling multiple roles can provide a woman with personal satisfaction, doing so may also make her more vulnerable to depression if she feels she is not able to meet all the responsibilities of and to live up to the societal expectations associated with each role.

Three types of role-related problems have been linked with the development of depression: experiencing *role overload*, having roles that are perceived as *noxious*, and having *too few* roles (Nolen-Hoeksema, 1987). Role overload is said to be present when the multiple roles a contemporary woman is expected to assume cause her to become stressed due to the obligations inherent in multiple roles. Whether a role is noxious is a subjective appraisal on the part of the woman; whereas many women enjoy working outside their homes, others do not. However, women who carry out roles that are assigned a relatively low value in society may develop poor self-esteem and have little motivation to perform the role (Repetti & Crosby, 1984). Although it is likely that women who have a problem with having too few roles are in the minority, those who have no meaningful work may feel useless and superfluous. Women who have been primarily mothers and homemakers may become depressed when their children leave home. The societal role expectation that women will bear children provides fertile ground for the development of depression in women who cannot do so. For instance, women undergoing infertility treatments approach each treatment cycle with great hope and are set up for disappointment if a successful pregnancy does not result (Lukse & Vass, 1999).

Socioeconomic Status Low socioeconomic status individuals have a higher incidence of depression than do wealthier individuals, and more women than men, particularly women who belong to ethnic minorities, are poor (see Chapter 2). Women's lower overall socioeconomic status is related to the societal factors addressed in some detail in Chapters 1 and 2.

Age Elderly women are particularly likely to be poor, and to have substandard nutrition and housing as a result, because, until recently, most women worked as homemakers and did not build up retirement accounts of their own. The factors known to be most closely related to depression in elderly women—poor health, bereavement, and caregiver burden (Jenkins, Westlake, & Salloway, 1996)—are also related to societal factors. Because women live longer than men by an average of seven years (Jenkins et al., 1996), they are

TABLE 26–1 Medical conditions and medications associated with increased risk for depression.

Medical Condition	Medications
♦ Cancer	♦ Antihypertensive agents (blood pressure pills)
♦ Inflammatory bowel disease	♦ Oral contraceptives (birth control pills)
♦ Nutritional disorders: vitamin B-12 deficiency	♦ Steroids, such as Prednisone
♦ Endocrine disorders: diabetes, hypothyroidism	♦ Sedatives, such as Valium, Xanax, and Ativan
♦ Central nervous system diseases: Parkinson's, strokes, Alzheimer's Disease, Multiple Sclerosis, and Epilepsy	♦ Histamine 2 blockers, such as Cimetidine and Ranitidine
♦ Chronic pain disorders	♦ Anti-cancer drugs
♦ Chronic infections: TB, HIV/AIDS, herpes zoster, hepatitis	♦ Alcohol
♦ Connective tissue diseases: Arthritis, Fibromyalgia	♦ Opiates, such as Morphine and related agents
♦ Heart disease: MI, heart failure	♦ Amphetamine or cocaine withdrawal
♦ Chronic lung disease: Emphysema	

Source: Adapted from Kornstein, S. G., & Wojcik, B. A. (2000). Gender effects in the treatement of depression. *Psychiatric Clinics of North America: Annual of Drug Therapy, 7,* 23–57; Montano, C. B. (1994). Recognition and treatment of depression in a primary care setting. *Journal of Clinical Psychiatry (Supplement), 55*(12), 18–34; Rouchell, A.M., Pounds, R., & Tierney, J. G. (1996). Depression. In J. R. Rundell & M. G. Wise (Eds.), *Textbook of consultation-liaison psychiatry* (pp. 311–345). Washington, D.C.: American Psychiatric Press, Inc.

more likely than men to be widowed, to suffer from chronic illnesses, and to have to care for ailing spouses.

RISK FACTORS FOR DEPRESSION

The risk factors associated with depression can be categorized as biological, historical, and psychosocial. The risk factors are closely associated with the various etiological factors already discussed.

Biological Risk Factors The biological risk factors include genetic influences (Kendler & Prescott, 1999), which are still poorly understood; hormonal fluctuations; and numerous medical conditions. It is noteworthy that 24 to 46 percent of nonpsychiatrically hospitalized patients have a coexisting mood disorder (Montano, 1994). Depression that develops as a consequence of a medical condition should not be considered a normal response to the illness but, rather, should be viewed and treated as a complication of the illness. The presence of gynecological cancers increase the risk of depression, as women are faced with the challenges of coping with a potentially life-threatening disease, managing the side effects of treatment, and accepting the changes in their appearance and sexual function (Thompson & Shear, 1998). Some medications used to treat medical conditions can also be associated with an increased risk for depression. Table 26–1 lists the medical conditions and medications associated with an increased risk for depression.

Historical Risk Factors The historical risk factors for depression include a family or personal history of having a psychiatric disorder, particularly a mood disorder (Peis & Shader,

1994). For example, having a history of major depression increases a woman's risk of developing postpartum depression (PPD) from 10 to 25 percent and increases her chance of a recurrence of PPD to 50 percent (Suri & Burt, 1997).

Psychosocial Risk Factors The psychosocial risk factors include the following: being unmarried or widowed, being or having been abused or tortured, being socially isolated, having a low socioeconomic status, having poor living conditions, and being a member of an oppressed minority (Kaelber, Moul, & Farmer, 1995). The salience (the predictive power regarding depression) of individual risk factors is often difficult to judge, because more than one is usually present in a given individual. Women tend to have more psychosocial risk factors than men. For example, women have experienced more societal oppression than men, have lower self-esteem overall, and have fewer personal and social resources (Nyamathi, Keenan, & Bayley, 1998).

SYMPTOMS OF DEPRESSIVE DISORDERS

Although the forms of depression have many features in common (see Table 26–2), they differ somewhat from each other in terms of severity and symptom pattern. Major depression, dysthymic disorder, premenstrual dysphoric disorder, and postpartum depression have distinct characteristics and criteria for diagnosis.

Although the general symptoms of depression are the same for women and men, there are a few gender differences in how the symptoms are experienced. For example, men tend to experience a loss of sleep and weight loss, whereas women experience an increase in appetite and weight gain

TABLE 26–2   Basic symptoms of depression.

Vegetative (Biological)	Cognitive	Behavioral	Impulse Control	Physical (Somatic)
Change in sleep	Hopelessness	Low energy	Suicidal or homicidal thoughts	Headaches
Change in appetite	Decreased self-esteem	Lack of motivation		Muscle aches
Change in weight	Negativity	Withdrawal		Stomachaches
Loss of interest in sexual activity	Inappropriate guilt	Slowed movements		
	Poor memory or concentration			

Source: Reprinted with permission from the *Diagnostic and Statistical Manual of Mental Disorders, Fourth Edition, Text Revision.* Copyright 2000. American Psychiatric Association; and Stahl, S. M. (1996). *Essential psychopharmacology: Neuroscientific basis and clinical applications.* Cambridge: Cambridge University Press. Reprinted with permission of Cambridge University Press.

(Kornstein & Wojcik, 2000). Women are also more likely to complain of a depressed mood and may have more associated anxiety and physical symptoms. Overall, depressed women tend to report more symptoms and to have longer episodes, with more distress.

Men and women present with different **comorbidities** (coexisting conditions). When men experience a depression, there may be associated alcohol or drug use, which usually preceded the onset of the depressive symptoms (Kornstein & Wojcik, 2000). In contrast, associated alcohol use in women tends to begin *after* the onset of depression. In a recent study of the Baltimore cohort of the National Mental Health Epidemiologic Catchment Area Project, the risk for heavy drinking in women with a history of a depressive disorder was found to be twice that of the women with no history of depression (Dixit & Crum, 2000). Women may also have more anxiety and eating disorders, as well as more thyroid disorders and migraine headaches associated with depression (Kornstein & Wojcik, 2000). The onset of depression in women is often associated with a particular phase of the reproductive cycle—that is, premenstrual, postpartum, or perimenopausal. Depression can also be triggered by the manipulation of women's hormones, whether for contraception, hormone replacement, or infertility treatment (Kornstein & Wojcik, 2000). Moreover, potential treatment options can be limited by pregnancy and/or the woman's desire to breastfeed.

Symptoms of Major Depression   The World Health Organization is predicting that major depression will be the second most costly medical illness worldwide by the year 2010 (Boland & Keller, 1999). The estimated annual economic cost related to major depression in the United States exceeds $53 billion (Boland & Keller, 1999). Approximately half of all episodes of depression will not be diagnosed, and, of those that are diagnosed, many will not be treated adequately (Dilts, 2001).

Major depression is much more than merely an occasional sad mood or blue day. It is a combination of physical, psychological, cognitive, and behavioral symptoms, which can influence all aspects of a person's life. Major depression is characterized by the presence of a predominantly depressed mood, or a loss of interest in usual activities, over a period of at least two weeks (American Psychiatric Association, 2000). In some individuals, particularly men, the mood symptom may manifest as *irritability* rather than as a depressed mood. In order to establish a diagnosis of major depression, four other symptoms must be present in addition to **anhedonia,** the technical term for the inability to experience pleasure or joy (American Psychiatric Association, 2000). The additional four symptoms include the following: a change in sleep habits, appetite, weight, or sex drive; fatigue or loss of energy; feelings of worthlessness or unwarranted guilt; an inability to concentrate or make decisions; and recurrent thoughts of death or suicide (American Psychiatric Association, 2000). Major depression typically has a gradual onset and, when untreated, can last four months or longer (American Psychiatric Association, 2000).

At times, depression can be severe enough to cause psychotic symptoms, such as delusions and hallucinations. For example, a depressed person may believe that people do not want to be around her or are making fun of her behind her back. This type of delusion is consistent with the diminished self-esteem often associated with depression. At times, a person may experience hallucinations, particularly hearing voices when no one is there. For example, a woman may hear the voice of her deceased abusive father saying to her, "See, I told you that you were no good; you never have been and you never will be!" The hallucinations can become so intense that suicide is seen as the only way to eliminate the misery.

The most worrisome symptom associated with depression is a *lack of impulse control.* With the inability to control impulses, an individual may act on destructive ideas, such as thoughts of suicide, homicide, or infanticide. Each year, approximately 16,000 people die in the United States annually due to suicide; 70 percent of these have a depressive illness

(Stahl, 1996). A careful evaluation of suicidal or homicidal thoughts, plans, and intentions, is crucial in order to prevent this tragedy.

Symptoms of Dysthymic Disorder Dysthymic disorder (or dysthymia) is a *chronic* form of depression in which the symptoms are less severe than those of major depression, but are longer lasting. Symptoms must have persisted for two years before a diagnosis can be established (American Psychiatric Association, 2000). In addition to having a chronically depressed mood, an individual with dysthymic disorder experiences at least two of the other symptoms of depression but to a lesser degree than in major depression. Often, the symptoms of dysthymia have persisted for so long that the individual does not recognize that she has an illness; rather, she believes that her long-term depressed mood is just a part of "who she is" (American Psychiatric Association, 2000).

Individuals who experience both dysthymic disorder *and* a major depressive episode are sometimes referred to as having a "double depression." According to a five-year study on dysthymic disorder, nearly all the patients studied eventually developed a major depression superimposed on their more mild but chronic depressive symptoms (Klein, Schwartz, Rose, & Leader, 2000).

Symptoms of Premenstrual Dysphoric Disorder Premenstrual dysphoric disorder (PMDD) is an episodic depression that develops during the premenstrual phase of a woman's cycle. A key diagnostic feature of PMDD is that there must be mood symptoms that are severe enough to lead to some degree of functional impairment (Yonkers & Davis, 2000). In addition to *severity,* another factor crucial to the diagnosis of PMDD is *timing.* In PMDD, the depressive symptoms occur only during a woman's premenstrual period (Kornstein & Wojcik, 2000). If the mood symptoms occur at other times, the woman may have an underlying mood disorder that worsens with her cycle.

Women in their late twenties or early thirties seem to be most vulnerable to PMDD (Steiner, 1996). Typically, women report that symptoms vary with each cycle. Many report that their symptoms worsen with age until relieved by the onset of menopause (American Psychiatric Association, 1994). The most predominant symptoms tend to be anger and irritability, depressed mood, anxiety or tension, loss of energy and interest, and eating problems (Gehlart, Chang, & Hartlage, 1999). Women experiencing this disorder may also have some of the physical and vegetative symptoms associated with major depression, as well as the physical symptoms associated with the premenstrual period, such as weight gain, headaches, and joint pain, but these symptoms dissipate once menses begins (American Psychiatric Association, 1994). Premenstrual dysphoric disorder shares many of the symptoms of other mood disorders and anxiety disorders. It is important that PMDD be differentiated from those to ensure that the most appropriate treatment options are considered. Of note, a history of physical and psychological complaints associated with the premenstrual period is a significant predictor of problems in the perimenopausal experience (Morse, Dudley, Guthrie, & Dennerstein, 1998).

Although critics of the *premenstrual dysphoric disorder* label oppose the idea that phenomena associated with a normal female biological process are classified as a psychiatric disorder (Rosenthal, 2000), to fail to acknowledge the existence of this disorder would be a disservice to the small minority of women who would benefit from appropriate treatment. It is critical, however, that PMDD be clearly differentiated from the less severe *premenstrual syndrome (PMS).* According to the American Psychiatric Association (1994), approximately 75 percent of women report minor or isolated premenstrual changes, and another 20 percent or so report having premenstrual syndrome; however, only 3 to 5 percent of women experience symptoms severe enough to be called premenstrual dysphoric disorder. Nevertheless, recent years have brought an avalanche of magazine and television advertisements for psychotropic drugs approved by the FDA for the treatment of PMDD. These ads warn women (and the public in general) that what they thought was PMS may indeed be PMDD, thus reinforcing the historical stereotype of women as unfit for public office and other responsible positions because of monthly instability.

Symptoms of Postpartum Depression Postpartum depression (PPD) is a *major* depression that begins within 4 weeks after childbirth (American Psychiatric Association, 1994). However, much of the research and reporting about this disorder has applied the term "postpartum onset" to *any* depression that occurs in the first 6 weeks after delivery (Hendrick et al., 1998). This accounts for the wide variability in the reported rates of postpartum depression from 12 to 60 percent. Approximately 70 percent of women will experience typical "baby blues" during the first 10 days after delivery (American Psychiatric Association, 1994). Baby blues should be distinguished from PPD, which is more severe, persistent, and disabling.

Women who are experiencing PPD have many of the same symptoms as those of a major depression. However, there is a key difference; although it is normal for a new mother to be concerned about the health and well-being of her infant, women with PPD tend to have *excessive* anxiety and tend to worry or obsess about the infant's health (Suri & Burt, 1997).

At its worst, PPD can be associated with *psychotic* features. Postpartum mood disorders with psychotic episodes occur in 1 to 2 women per 1,000 births (Suri & Burt, 1997). Generally, the onset of psychotic features occurs within the first two to three days after delivery. Psychotic features, such as having command hallucinations telling the mother to harm or kill the infant or delusions that the infant is possessed, may lead to infanticide (American Psychiatric Association, 2000). Although the incidence is rare, this risk of infanticide or suicide by the mother underscores the importance of women's receiving appropriate evaluation during the prenatal and postpartum periods. The identification of even a low-level depression in a postpartum woman is vital, so as to not impair the mother's ability to interact with her infant.

Postpartum depression in a mother can have significant negative consequences for her infant if it goes untreated. When evaluated at three months postpartum, depressed mothers have been found to be more likely than nondepressed mothers to express *feelings of dislike* or *indifference* toward their babies (Suri & Burt, 1997). As mothers disengage from their infants, they are less responsive to the infants' social signals, and a lack of maternal responsiveness may have long-lasting effects on the infants' personality development, behavior, and risk of eventually developing depression. One study found that the children of mothers who had suffered postpartum depression tended to respond with more anger in mother-infant play than did the babies of nonaffected mothers, even after their mothers had recovered from PPD (Suri & Burt, 1997).

DIAGNOSIS

All the categories of depression are diagnosed on the basis of the patient's history and presenting symptoms. It is important to realize that the symptoms of depression can occur in response to medical illnesses or in response to the use of prescribed medications or nonprescribed substances, such as alcohol or other drugs. The *DSM-IV* (American Psychiatric Association, 1994) differentiates depressive disorders related to medical illness, drug use, or substance use from major depression. When an individual is evaluated for the symptoms of a depressive disorder, the possibility that an illness, a medication, or a substance has triggered the symptoms must be considered. Careful diagnosis by a medical or mental health provider is necessary, because treatment will vary according to these findings and the severity and duration of the depressive symptoms. Screening tools in the form of questionnaires are available and are sometimes used in public health screening programs and by healthcare providers. However, these tools are not meant to replace a good diagnostic evaluation by a well-trained practitioner, such as a psychiatrist, a psychologist, or an advanced practice nurse.

Depression sometimes goes *undiagnosed* for a number of reasons. One is that people tend to seek help from their primary care physicians for the *physical* symptoms that accompany depression, while neglecting to mention the symptoms related to *mood*. Another reason is that individuals sometimes have difficulty *acknowledging* feelings of sadness or depression. They believe that they should be able to pick themselves up and move on with their lives and that failing to do so is a sign of weakness. One of the biggest obstacles to the successful diagnosis and treatment of depression is the *stigma* associated with mental illness (Montano, 1994). Whereas the stigma once associated with diseases such as cancer has all but disappeared, studies of public perception continue to show that the stigma

associated with mental illness persists. For example, a report on attitudes toward mental illness revealed that only 10 percent of those surveyed believed that mental illness has a biological basis; the remaining 90 percent saw mental illness as a result of bad parenting, emotional weakness, or sinful behavior or as the victim's fault (Stahl, 1996). Unfortunately, the stigma of mental illness prevents many from seeking treatment for this very treatable disorder. An additional problem is that some healthcare providers fail to recognize depression in *women* due to their own stereotypical beliefs about women and their own biases related to psychiatric disorders. Given the impact that depression can have on women, their families, and society in general, early recognition of the illness and appropriate treatment are imperative.

TREATMENT

The treatments available for depression can be divided into four main categories: (1) antidepressants and other drugs, (2) electroconvulsive therapy, (3) psychotherapy, and (4) alternative therapies. The nature, severity, timing, and presentation of the depression will influence the selection of one treatment modality over another. Decisions about treatment should be made collaboratively between patients and their healthcare providers.

Antidepressant and Other Drugs The substances most commonly used in the treatment of depression are the antidepressant drugs. These drugs fall into several classifications, according to their effect on the neurotransmitters and receptors in the brain. The broad categories of antidepressants include the *tricyclics (TCAs)*, the *monoamine oxidase inhibitors (MAOIs)*, and the *selective serotonin reuptake inhibitors (SSRIs)*. Newer agents that affect multiple neurotransmitters thought to be involved in depression have been developed, and research into antidepressant therapy is ongoing to find drugs that have maximum benefits and minimal risks.

It is important to realize that most of the studies of the pharmacological effects of medications and dosages have been conducted on *men* (Kornstein & Wojcik, 2000). It was not until 1993 that the Food and Drug Administration required that drugs be tested in women and that their effects on the factors unique to women, such as pregnancy and lactation, be determined (Kornstein & Wojcik, 2000). In general, it has been found that drug metabolism differs somewhat in women and men; women may require lower dosages, and women may experience more side effects than men (Bhati & Bhati, 1999). For example, when male and female volunteers are given the same dose of a given drug, the women are often found to have *higher* blood levels of the drug, which are retained for a *longer* period of time than are the men (Kornstein & Wojcik, 2000).

The physiological changes that occur during *pregnancy* (and those can vary from trimester to trimester) can also alter drug distribution and metabolism in the body, as can *fluctuations in hormone levels,* whether naturally occurring or related to hormone therapies (Kornstein & Wojcik, 2000). When a woman is pregnant or breast-feeding, the treatment of depression is complicated by the need to protect the baby from exposure to any potentially harmful agents. For this reason, pregnant women are not accepted as subjects in drug research. Therefore, animal testing remains the principle means of evaluating the potential effects of medications on an unborn fetus.

Some drugs used to treat depression seem to be more effective in *premenopausal* women, whereas others are more effective in *postmenopausal* women. Premenopausal women tend to respond better, and tolerate better, the SSRIs and MAOIs, whereas postmenopausal women seem to respond better to the TCAs (Kornstein & Wojcik, 2000). The SSRIs have been associated with menstrual disturbances, such as alterations in cycle length and time of ovulation in premenopausal women (Kornstein & Wojcik, 2000). The results of research into the ways in which other medications affect the menstrual cycle have been inconclusive. Some drugs can have an adverse effect on sexual functioning, such as a loss of sex drive or an inability to achieve orgasm. Although both men and women experience these side effects, women tend *not* to report them unless specifically asked (Bhati & Bhati, 1999). Although many of the antidepressants cause sexual side effects, the degree to which they do so varies from individual to individual. In any event, the risks and benefits need to be discussed before an antidepressant is prescribed, and the individual taking the medication must communicate any unpleasant side effects to the prescribing practitioner.

Other types of drugs can be used in addition to the antidepressants to treat certain kinds of depression. *Stimulants,* such as Ritalin, can be used to supplement the treatment of major depression, particularly in elderly or medically ill persons. *Antipsychotic* medications can be used to control the psychotic symptoms that may arise in the course of major depression. Although combining medications in order to achieve a maximal response is not uncommon, such an approach should be taken only by an experienced practitioner in order to avoid a potentially dangerous drug interaction.

Electroconvulsive Therapy Electroconvulsive therapy (ECT) has been used and studied with regard to safety and effectiveness for over 60 years (Fox, 1996). The effectiveness of ECT for major depression (nearly 90 percent) surpasses that of all other treatments (Isenberg & Zorumski, 2000). In ECT, a very small electrical stimulus is administered to the brain of an anesthetized patient in order to produce a *seizure.* The exact mechanism by which ECT works is not understood, but one possibility is that it causes neurotransmitters to be released (Maxmen & Ward, 1995). With current methods of administration, ECT is a safe and effective treatment with minimal side effects. Individuals may experience loss of memory for events immediately preceding ECT and may have some impairment related to the formation of new memories for a few weeks after treatment (Dilts, 2001).

ECT is generally considered the treatment of choice for women who are in their first trimester of pregnancy—a period during which antidepressants are generally contraindicated (Fox, 1996). ECT can also be administered safely during the second and third trimesters, since it does not affect uterine muscles (Fox, 1996). ECT is particularly recommended when depression causes severe symptoms, such as suicidality and psychosis, and when it is linked with eating disorders (Isenberg & Zorumski, 2000). Overall, the data indicate that women who receive ECT have a better response rate and less severe side effects than men who receive ECT (Kornstein & Wojcik, 2000).

Psychotherapy Psychotherapy, also called "talk therapy," is generally used as an adjunctive therapy in the treatment of depression (Maxmen & Ward, 1995). It can provide depressed individuals with an opportunity to learn more about the mechanics of their disorder and allows them to identify early symptoms and triggers. Psychotherapy can help eliminate the feelings of isolation that commonly go along with depression, and it can help individuals learn to cope more effectively and improve their interpersonal relationships. Psychotherapy can also address gender role stereotypes and unrealistic goals and expectations. In short, psychotherapy can help individuals learn to solve problems, build social skills, and gain a greater sense of confidence and control.

In general, psychotherapy alone will not cure a severe depression, although it can alleviate the symptoms in persons with mild to moderate depression. Persons with severe or psychotic depressions are usually unable to benefit from psychotherapy until medications have controlled some of the more severe symptoms (Maxmen & Ward, 1995). When used as an adjunct to pharmacological therapies, however, psychotherapy can improve the outcome for severely depressed individuals.

There are various models of psychotherapy—each based on a particular theory of the etiology of depression (Maxmen & Ward, 1995). *Psychodynamic therapy* targets conflicts in early personality development, focusing on ways in which past experiences are affecting a person's reactions to current situations. *Interpersonal psychotherapy* is a short-term therapy that focuses on current interpersonal problems, such as the need to adapt to changing roles or role expectations and the need to improve social skills in order to eliminate social isolation (Klerman et al., 1996). *Cognitive therapy* focuses on teaching individuals new ways to think about and characterize themselves and their world. It also focuses on identifying the feelings associated with thoughts and actions and helping individuals become conscious of, and perhaps change, their behavioral response to their thoughts and feelings (Maxmen & Ward, 1995). Although psychotherapy can be done with couples, families, or groups, some forms are geared more to individuals.

Alternative Therapies A number of herbs and other food supplements, as well as a few other treatment modalities, have been found to be useful in the treatment of depression, although many are used in conjunction with antidepressant drugs and other traditional therapies. Consumers should keep in mind that some food supplements are contraindicated during pregnancy, and some should not be taken along with standard antidepressant medications. Women should consult a healthcare provider before taking any supplement if they may be pregnant or are already taking an antidepressant. Most of the food supplements and therapies mentioned in this section are addressed more fully in Chapter 11, as are issues related to the quality of herbs and food supplements.

Exercise has been found to have an antidepressant effect similar to that of psychotherapy. This finding may be of particular interest to individuals who resist the idea of seeking therapy. Exercise has been related to improved mood, enhanced self-esteem, a sense of accomplishment, and decreased tension (Clark & Brandman, 1999). Participation in athletics has been shown to improve the confidence, body image, self-esteem, and sense of self-mastery of adolescent girls (Baum, 1998). Exercise has also been shown to increase the levels of neurotransmitters and endorphins in the brain and to increase body temperature, which has a calming effect (Baum, 1998).

St. John's wort (*Hypericum perforatum*), a well-known herbal food supplement, has long been used as an antidepressant in Germany and is gaining popularity in the United States as an alternative to traditional antidepressants (Gaster & Holroyd, 2000). In 1999, the National Institutes of Health Office on Alternative Medicine and the National Institute of Mental Health announced a three-year study of *Hypericum* to be completed by 2002 (Gaster & Holroyd, 2000). This study compares the effectiveness of *Hypericum* to an SSRI antidepressant and to placebo. Many of the substances in the extract of *Hypericum* have been shown to bind neuroreceptors in the brain, thereby interfering with the neurotransmitters believed to be involved in depression (Gaster & Holroyd, 2000). Analyses of 23 randomized studies involving 1,757 outpatients suggest that *Hypericum* is more effective than a placebo and as effective as standard antidepressants in cases of mild to moderate depression and that it has a low rate of side effects (Kiresuk & Trachtenberg, 2000). Recently, though, the FDA has advised healthcare professionals to be aware of potential *interactions* between *Hypericum* and drugs commonly used to treat a variety of diseases (Risk of Drug Interactions with St. John's wort, 2000). St. John's wort should *not* be taken in addition to SSRIs because of the potential for developing toxicity due to an excess of serotonin (Mischoulon, 1999).

Another popular supplement for the treatment of depression is **S-adenosylmethionine,** also known as **SAMe** and previously known as **SAM.** "Sammy" is a modified amino acid that is essential for several biochemical reactions in the body and for the production and use of dopamine, serotonin, and epinephrine (Cerrato & Powell, 1999). Research has shown that levels of S-adenosylmethionine decrease with aging, and persons with a variety of ailments, including depression, have low levels of the enzymes needed to produce SAMe (Cerrato & Powell, 1999). SAMe is reputed to have antidepressant qualities, and a few clinical trials carried out in Europe seem to bear this out (Bottiglieri et al., 1990). Although SAMe seems to be relatively free of side effects, it has been known to precipitate mania in persons with bipolar disorders, and the degree to which it is clinically effective is unclear (Bottiglieri et al., 1990). Early evidence does suggest that the onset of symptoms relief is earlier than with traditional antidepressants, although this has not been clearly demonstrated with clinical trials (Kagan, Sultzer, Rosenlicht, & Gerner, 1999).

A variety of other alternative therapies (see Chapter 11), such as acupuncture, light therapy, transcranial magnetic stimulation, massage therapy, hypnotherapy, relaxation therapy, dance/movement therapy, aromatherapy, homeopathy, and energy therapies, have also been used in the treatment of depression, with varying degrees of effectiveness.

Acupuncture is an ancient Chinese therapy intended to restore the normal flow of energy, or chi, in the body. Western scientists believe that acupuncture may affect neuropeptide levels in the nervous system and/or neuroendocrine function (Kiresuk & Trachtenberg, 2000). In clinical trials, electroacupuncture and computer-controlled electroacupuncture have been shown to produce an improvement in depressive symptoms comparable with that produced by traditional antidepressants (Ernst, Rand & Stevinson, 1998). Case reports and preliminary clinical studies also support the effectiveness of acupuncture technique as adjunctive therapy for depression.

Light therapy involves the therapeutic use of various forms of light. Bright light, provided by panels of full-spectrum light at an intensity of 10,000 Lux or more, has been found to be useful in the treatment of one form of depression, **seasonal affective disorder (SAD)** (Pataki, 2000). SAD is a depressed mood disorder common in northern latitudes, particularly during winter. It is related to insufficient exposure to light. Several other forms of light therapy are available, including colored light and ultraviolet light, but these therapies have not been shown to be effective in clinical studies (Clark & Brandman, 1999).

Transcranial magnetic stimulation (TMS) is a relatively new technique for using brain stimulation to treat depression. This technique was introduced in 1985 as a means of noninvasive and safe stimulation of the cerebral cortex (Klein et al., 1999). TMS involves the application of pulsed magnetic stimulation to the brain through an electromagnet placed on the scalp. Although this stimulation is known to cause neuronal firing, the exact mechanism by which TMS alleviates depression has yet to be identified (Nahas et al., 1999). Although TMS has been found to be effective in the studies done to date, it is still considered an experimental treatment and is not widely used. Isolated case studies suggest that TMS is safe during pregnancy.

Although **massage therapy** has been demonstrated to aid circulation and relaxation, there is little empirical evidence that it is generally effective as a treatment for depression

(Clark & Brandman, 1999). However, in a few recent studies, massage therapy has been found to relieve some symptoms of depression and anxiety and to reduce stress hormone levels (Kiresuk & Trachtenberg, 2000).

Hypnotherapy is conducted while patients are in a state of focused awareness or concentration in conjunction with a deeply relaxed state (Clark & Brandman, 1999). It can be done by therapists or taught to individuals as a self-help modality. Although hypnotherapy has not been shown to *cure* depression, it is sometimes used as an adjunct to cognitive therapy as a means of helping patients restructure negative thought patterns (Ernst et al., 1998). The benefit to using hypnosis as an adjunct to other therapeutic strategies is that the individual can learn to relax and to focus attention on the therapeutic task at hand (Kiresuk & Trachtenberg, 2000).

Relaxation therapy involves the use of techniques such as progressive muscle relaxation, meditation, and yoga which are aimed at reducing muscle tension and inducing the relaxation response. Although research on the efficacy of relaxation therapy is limited, there is some evidence that, like hypnosis, it is a useful adjunctive treatment for depression (Ernst et al., 1998).

Dance/movement therapy in various forms can be provided individually or to groups. Group settings add the element of social interaction (Ernst et al., 1998). The goal of this therapy is to have the individual interact with the environment as a means of gaining inner awareness, releasing tension, and rechanneling anger and frustration (Clark & Brandman, 1999). There is, however, no evidence to date that dance therapy has a significant effect on depression (Ernst et al., 1998).

Aromatherapy is a technique in which essential oils from plants are used to alter the body through the inhalation of sprays, massages, or topical applications (Clark & Brandman, 1999). There is very little evidence to document that aromatherapy is effective for the treatment of depression, although there are anecdotal reports supporting its usefulness (Ernst et al., 1998). In a small study, the application of citrus fragrance reportedly reduced the necessary doses of antidepressants, a finding consistent with other anecdotal reports (Kiresuk & Trachtenberg, 2000).

Homeopathy is based on the belief that illnesses are specific to individuals and that remedies that cause reactions in the body similar to the symptoms of a given disease can cure that disease. The literature on the effectiveness of homeopathy for depression is limited and consists mainly of unsubstantiated case reports (Ernst et al., 1998).

Energy therapies, such as *therapeutic touch* and *healing touch,* are controversial therapies based on the belief that human beings are made up of energy fields, which can be manipulated by practitioners to induce healing. As is the case with many of the alternative therapies, the research findings on the efficacy of therapeutic touch and healing touch have been inconclusive (Clark & Brandman, 1999).

Eating Disorders

Anorexia nervosa (AN), usually characterized by excessively restricted eating, and **bulimia nervosa (BN),** known colloquially as binge-purge syndrome, the two main eating disorders in Western culture, are both characterized by severe disturbances in eating behavior secondary to an extreme preoccupation with *reducing* body weight (American Psychiatric Association, 1994).

Anorexia and bulimia and their variants affect approximately 5 million Americans every year—approximately 90 percent of whom are female (Becker, Grinspoon, Liibanski, & Herzog, 1999). Eating disorders usually arise during adolescence, and their effect on a young woman's psychological and physical health can be devastating (Cooper, 1995). The medical complications of eating disorders can involve every organ of the body and may even be life-threatening (American Psychiatric Association, 1994). All aspects of the woman's reproductive system can be affected, with potentially serious effects on menstruation, ovarian function, fertility, sexuality, and pregnancy (Morgan, 1999). Only about 50 percent of individuals with an eating disorder make a full recovery; 30 percent achieve a partial recovery, and 20 percent show no improvement (Becker et al., 1999). The mortality rate for individuals with anorexia nervosa is between 5 percent and 18 percent, and suicide attempts are as common in women with AN as in women with depression (Bulik, Sullivan, & Joyce, 1999). The mortality rate in the population that suffers from bulimia nervosa is somewhat lower but still significant (Anstine & Grinenko, 2000). Despite their severity, these disorders frequently go unrecognized, and, when they are diagnosed, the individual involved may resist treatment (Becker et al., 1999).

SYMPTOMS

Although anorexia and bulimia have some symptoms in common, they have others that are distinct. The comorbidities in the two eating disorders are also somewhat different.

Anorexia   In anorexia, the individual has an intense *fear of gaining weight,* refuses to maintain what would be considered a normal body weight by accepted standards, and has a *distorted perception* of her own size and shape (American Psychiatric Association, 1994). Some anorectic individuals (the restricting type) attempt to lose weight only by limiting the amount or type of food they eat; others (the binge-eating/purging type) attempt to do so by vomiting after eating, and/or misusing laxatives or diuretics, and/or by exercising excessively (American Psychiatric Association, 1994). Anorectic individuals may weigh less than 85 percent of their normal body weight (American Psychiatric Association, 1994). An important factor in differentiating between someone who is simply striving for thinness and the anorectic is the classic symptom of *denying* the serious consequences of extreme weight loss (Garfinkel, 1995). Another symptom is attempting to *conceal* the eating disorder by refusing to eat in the presence of other people (American Psychiatric Association, 1994). *Amenorrhea,* another symptom of AN, is not completely explained by the loss of body weight and fat, since the cessation of menses may occur before there is any significant weight loss (Garfinkel, 1995).

Eating disorders have a high *comorbidity* with other psychiatric disorders, and there may be a reciprocal relationship between the two. Although the existence of a psychiatric disorder may predispose some individuals to develop an eating disorder, the starvation and malnutrition associated with eating disorders seem to intensify certain symptoms associated with psychiatric disorders—namely, depression, anxiety, and obsessive thinking (Police, Kaye, & Greeno, 1997). Depressive symptoms have been shown to occur in 25 percent to 50 percent of persons with AN, and full-blown mood disorders are present 36 percent to 68 percent of the time (Maser, Weise, & Gwirtsman, 1995). Anorexics who binge and purge are more likely to have impulse control problems and mood instability, to abuse substances, to be more sexually active, and to have more suicide attempts than anorectics who merely restrict food (American Psychiatric Association, 1994). Also, many individuals with AN have personality disturbances indicative of a personality disorder, most commonly borderline personality disorder (American Psychiatric Association, 1994): A personality disorder is an inflexible, deeply ingrained pattern of thinking, perceiving, or relating that is serious enough to cause impaired functioning or distress, and a person with borderline personality disorder is unstable in a number of areas, including mood, behavior, and interpersonal relations. Such individuals tend to have an uncertain sense of their own identities and view various phenomena and people in black-and-white terms—as either all "good" or all "bad" (National Mental Health Association, 2001).

Bulilmia In bulimia, the primary symptom is repeated episodes during which the individual consumes an excessively large amount of food and then begins to feel out of control (American Psychiatric Association, 2000). Two types of bulimia, *purging type* and *nonpurging type,* are differentiated on the basis of what mechanism the individual uses to prevent weight gain. Bulimics who purge use the same mechanisms to eliminate food as anorectic individuals—laxatives, diuretics, or enemas (American Psychiatric Association, 1994). Those who do not purge attempt to compensate for the food binge by fasting or exercising excessively (American Psychiatric Association, 1994). Bulimia is a chronic disorder that can involve both periods of binge eating and normal eating (although rarely) and periods of binge eating and fasting (Maxmen & Ward, 1995). Caloric intake during a binge is generally around 3,000 calories, although the range has been reported to be between 1,200 and 11,500 calories per binge (Maxmen & Ward, 1995). Often, dysphoric moods precede or precipitate the binge, and the binge may initially relieve the mood

symptoms; however, binges typically provoke a fear of gaining weight and discomfort from the amount of food ingested (Garfinkel, 1995).

Bulimia often begins after a stressful event or following a stringent diet (Maxmen & Ward, 1995). Bulimics tend to experience shame about their eating behaviors and frequently attempt to hide their dysfunctional eating behaviors (American Psychiatric Association, 2000). Moreover, unlike anorexics, who lose substantial amounts of weight, bulimics tend to be *near normal* in weight. These factors make it more difficult to detect bulimia than anorexia (American Psychiatric Association, 2000).

Although mood disorders are also common in bulimia nervosa, they tend to be short-lived and related to bingeing and purging episodes (Maser et al., 1995). The symptoms of anxiety may also be present in individuals with BN, but they tend to improve with effective treatments (American Psychiatric Association, 2000). Approximately one-third of bulimic individuals abuse alcohol, and stimulants are often abused as a weight-loss technique (American Psychiatric Association, 2000). The personality traits associated with BN include thrill seeking, excitability, a lack of persistence, and a tendency toward depressive moods in response to rejection or lack of appreciation. All these traits predispose bulimic individuals to seek relief from distressing events through dietary control (Strober, 1995).

ETIOLOGY

The etiology of the eating disorders appears to lie in a combination of various biological, psychological, developmental, and sociocultural factors (Becker et al., 1999). These factors include genetic predisposition, hormone levels, brain activity, dieting, personality, family dynamics, and cultural norms regarding women's bodies.

Genetic Predisposition As yet, the exact mechanism by which genetics contributes to the development of an eating disorder is not known; however, the incidence of AN and BN is *higher* among biological relatives who have those disorders than in the general population (Strober, 1995). Also, the concordant rate of anorexia is higher in identical twins than it is in fraternal twins (American Psychiatric Association, 2000). Anorexia nervosa involves a dysphoric mood, and mood disorders are more common among the first-degree biological relatives of persons who have it than in the general population (American Psychiatric Association, 2000). Similarly, first-degree biological relatives of persons with bulimia nervosa have a higher incidence of mood disorders, substance abuse, and obesity than the general population (American Psychiatric Association, 2000). Finally, persons with anorexia have been found to be more likely to have a variant form of a *gene* related to appetite stimulation than persons without anorexia (Vink et al., 2001). However, people whose genetic makeup puts them at risk may develop an actual disorder only under certain circumstances related to psychological development and environment.

Hormone Levels   Aberrations in the hormonal mechanisms that control appetite and body weight may also play a part in the development of eating disorders. Hormones from the pancreas (insulin), adrenal glands (cortisol), and gonads (estrogen) all influence the ingestion and metabolism of food, and their levels can become unbalanced (Leibowitz, 1995). Even the *normal* developmental shifts in women's hormone profiles may trigger the onset of eating disorders in women who cannot tolerate the normal feminine curves that develop as women mature. Prior to puberty, females demonstrate a preference for carbohydrate-rich foods over fat-rich foods. After puberty, however, this reverses as the hormone estrogen promotes weight gain in preparation for reproduction, which requires larger fat stores (Leibowitz, 1995). The contemporary social mandate that all women acquire the sleek profile of a supermodel is incompatible with the genetic and biological forces intended to prepare women's bodies for reproduction.

Brain Activity   Multiple structures in the brain also influence the amount of food consumed. For example, the *hypothalamus* has a central role in controlling the appetite for carbohydrates, fats, and proteins (Leibowitz, 1995). Also, a large number of neurotransmitters, pathways, and receptors are involved in the processing of information related to appetite control (Blundell, 1995). Alterations in any of these structures, chemicals or pathways can disturb brain neurochemical systems in such a manner that abnormal eating patterns develop (Leibowitz, 1995).

Although the pathophysiology of AN and BN are poorly understood, disturbances related to the neurotransmitter *serotonin* have been implicated in both disorders (Dilts, 2001). Platelet monoamine oxidase (MAO) activity, an index of brain serotonin activity, has been found to be lower in persons with BN. Low MAO activity may reflect impairment of impulse control mechanisms (Carrasco, Diaz-Marsa, Hollander, Cesar, & Saiz-Ruiz, 2000). Moreover, recent studies have shown that persons with AN or BN have an alteration in serotonin receptor function (Spigset, Andersen, Hagg, & Mjondal, 1999), which may contribute to the pathological eating patterns and subsequent weight loss (Kaye, Gendell, & Kye, 1998).

Dieting   Dieting is known to frequently precede the onset of an eating disorder, and individuals who diet are more likely to develop an eating disorder than are those who do not (Wilson, 1995). Dieting is a form of behavioral control that interferes with the normal physiological processes that govern appetite (Blundell, 1995). Under ordinary circumstances, the length of time that eating continues and the amount of food consumed are governed by a complex feedback system, which balances energy consumption with energy requirements (Smith & Gibbs, 1995). Drastic dieting, as well as the bingeing and purging associated with some eating disorders, lead to

an uncontrolled delivery of nutrients, with unpredictable physiological responses (Blundell, 1995).

Personality   Certain personality traits may also foster the development of eating disorders. Traits such as inflexible thinking, perfectionism, restrained initiative and emotional expression, a strong need to control the environment, and feelings of ineffectiveness are common in persons who have AN (American Psychiatric Association, 1994). Internalized anger and ineffective self-control have been found to be important factors in the psychopathology of adolescent anorexic females (Horesh, Zalsman, & Apter, 2000). The low self-esteem, perfectionism, and excessive compliance that are common in anorectic individuals may contribute to their need for a sense of control—which they achieve through abnormal patterns of dieting and weight loss (Cooper, 1995).

Family Dynamics   Undesirable family dynamics have often been implicated as contributors to the development of eating disorders. The family is the first sociocultural environment to which an individual is exposed. It is in the family environment that we acquire beliefs about and attitudes toward body image, relationships, eating patterns, and food (Sobal, 1995).

Certain family characteristics and interaction styles are said to be common in the families of women with eating disorders (Vandereycken, 1995). The characteristics that have been identified as contributing to the development of *eating disorders in general* include unusual eating habits, strong concerns about appearance and weight, and the perception of parental indifference or lack of concern on the part of the child (Cooper, 1995). *Bulimia* has been associated with brittle family attachments. These weak attachments give rise to the stressful events that engender the bulimic person's need to learn methods of self-soothing (Strober, 1995). The families of individuals with *anorexia* are often characterized as emotionally restrained and rigidly controlling—traits often seen in anorectic women prior to the onset of their disorder (Strober, 1995). The families of individuals who eventually develop anorexia are also said to tend to repeatedly invalidate the future anorexic's perceptions, causing the individual to distrust her own perceptions of the world and to have a distorted body image (Norman, 1992). Anorectic women have recently been found to see themselves as having had a low level of parental care and to have experienced more than the usual amount of control by their mothers (Leung, Thomas, & Waller, 2000). They have also reported feeling more antagonism and jealousy toward their sisters (Murphy, Troop, & Treasure, 2000). A decade of research involving the families of women who purge suggests that these families are typically less expressive, less cohesive, and more conflictual than families in which purging does not occur (Laliberte, Boland, & Leichner, 1999).

Some studies suggest that the mother-daughter relationship is important in the etiology of eating disorders. In one study (Moreno, Selby, Aved, & Besse, 2000), eating-disordered women were found to have poorer communica-

tion with their mothers than nondisordered women. The anorectic women had better communication than the bulimic women. In a study comparing Asian American and Euro-American women, the quality of parent-child relationships, particularly the mother-daughter relationship, was found to be an important contributing factor in the development of eating disorders, independent of cultural influence (Haudek, Rorty, & Henker, 1999). However, lest mothers get all the blame, it must be noted that, in a study of women with bulimia, the women perceived more rejection from their *fathers*. This underscores the need to also evaluate the father-daughter relationship (Dominy, Johnson, & Koch, 2000). Having been sexually abused in childhood also increases the likelihood that a girl will develop an eating disorder (Striegel-Moore, 1995).

It is important to remember, however, that, by the time an eating-disordered individual seeks treatment, the family has already become highly stressed by trying to help her with no success. For this reason, in most circumstances, it is difficult to point definitively to the family as a causative factor.

Cultural Norms Regarding Women's Bodies Social scientists have proposed that eating disorders are *culturally bound* disorders that cannot be understood outside of the context of the culture (Wilfley & Rodin, 1995). Culture dictates the appropriate patterns of eating and activity, and it assigns values and social meanings to body weight, especially for women (Leibowitz, 1995). Throughout history, societies have set standards of beauty for women that can be seen as bizarre. For example, in the twelfth and thirteenth centuries, upper-class Chinese girls were intentionally crippled by the practice of foot binding. Fashionable American women in the nineteenth century had to wear corsets, which were laced tightly enough to impair body function. In the twentieth century, women in "advanced" societies routinely resorted to surgery to achieve the culturally prescribed breast size (Wilfley & Rodin, 1995).

Eating disorders are much more common in industrialized nations, in which thinness is associated with both *beauty* and *social prestige* (Wilfley & Rodin, 1995). People in Westernized cultures tend to judge women as more feminine, more attractive, and more likely to be from the upper socioeconomic group if they are thin and if they eat relatively small meals (Striegel-Moore, 1995). It has been documented that, when young women from nonindustrial societies in which eating disorders are all but unknown move to an industrialized one, their risk of developing an eating disorder soon approaches that of women who are native to the industrialized area (American Psychiatric Association, 1994). This is believed to occur because immigrant women soon adopt Western attitudes toward beauty and body weight and size.

From the time they are little girls, playing with dolls such as "Barbie," through adolescence and adulthood, women are exposed to the relentless message that the ideal woman is *thin* and *small* (Lindeman, 1999). The ongoing portrayal of thinness as a standard of beauty by the media has been shown to increase preoccupation with weight and increase eating disturbances in women (Berel & Irving, 1998). The results of one study (Pinhas, Toner, Ali, Garfinkel, & Stuckless, 1999) support the idea that the messages conveyed by the media increase women's dissatisfaction with their bodies. The women in the study were found to experience negative mood changes (to anger and depression) when they viewed images of female fashion models. Women who have the personality traits associated with eating disorders may be especially affected by these messages.

Women's identity and feelings of self-worth are strongly influenced by their ability to form *interpersonal relationships*. This trait makes girls more vulnerable to the opinions of others, leading to the potential for greater identity instability, more social anxiety, and lower self-esteem in girls and women who cannot measure up to others' expectations regarding size and weight (Striegel-Moore, 1995). Social pressure to be thin has increased over recent decades, even as the population as a whole has gotten heavier, and women are judged more on the basis of appearance than on personality or accomplishments (Garner, 1995). This has resulted in more dieting, even among very young girls, and the development of eating disorders in vulnerable individuals (Sobal, 1995). According to Browness, Rodin, and Wilmore (1992), the search for the perfect body is driven by two beliefs: (1) the belief that the perfect body can be achieved by eating the right foods and exercising enough and (2) the belief that having a perfect body will bring greater wealth and happiness and more success in career and interpersonal relationships.

Membership in certain *subcultures* may also predispose women to seek unrealistic levels of thinness (Wilfley & Rodin, 1995). For example, there is strong pressure on women in occupations such as acting, dancing, and modeling and on women who participate in sports, such as gymnastics, to alter their body shape and size.

Some individuals may be at higher risk for developing an eating disorder because they belong to certain ethnic minority groups within the larger culture. For example, in the United States, African American women tend to have higher body weights than Euro-American women. Whereas the misconception has arisen that they are immune to eating disorders (Sobal, 1995), and although African American women do tend to develop eating disorders less frequently than Euro-American women, the exposure to a dominant culture that denigrates their natural features and physiques does cause some African American girls and women to develop anorexia or bulimia (Williamson, 1998). Women who have low self-esteem, together with higher body mass and body dissatisfaction, are known to be at risk for bulimia (Lester & Petrie, 1998).

COMPLICATIONS OF EATING DISORDERS

Both anorexia and bulimia can result in medical complications that damage the body. In anorexia, the damage can be severe or even life-threatening.

Anorexia Anorexia gives rise to more medical complications than any other eating disorder. *Hormonal changes* due to AN may return the individual to prepubertal levels; in females, this may prevent normal breast development and diminish fertility, although reproduction may still be possible (Goldbloom & Kennedy, 1995). Women who become pregnant when their BMI (body mass index) is below 19 have a higher than normal rate of spontaneous abortions, low birth weight babies, and birth defects, especially when ovulation has been induced (Abraham & Llewellyn-Jones, 1995). Hormonal changes may also lead to skeletal problems, such as a reduction in bone mass and bone quality. Even women who have been amenorrheic for only one year sometimes suffer fractures of the long bones, sternum (breastbone), or vertebrae (Goldbloom & Kennedy, 1995). To prevent these skeletal complications from developing, anorectic women are increasingly being placed on hormone replacement therapy (Abraham & Llewellyn-Jones, 1995).

Cardiovascular complications include a slowed heart rate; low blood pressure; cold, mottled extremities; and decreased muscle mass and structural changes in the heart (Goldbloom & Kennedy, 1995). *Gastrointestinal* problems include constipation, abdominal pain and bloating, and irreversible damage to the nerves that stimulate bowel function (Goldbloom & Kennedy, 1995). Vomiting and the abuse of laxatives or diuretics can cause *chronic dehydration, kidney stones,* and *electrolyte imbalances* (Goldbloom & Kennedy, 1995). Chronic dehydration can cause *impaired kidney function* (American Psychiatric Association, 1994). Anorectic individuals may also have a *decreased red blood cell count,* which causes them to be fatigued; a *decreased white blood cell count,* which predisposes them to infection; and a *decreased platelet level,* which puts them at risk for bleeding. However, blood counts return to normal with refeeding (Goldbloom & Kennedy, 1995). Less threatening physical findings in persons with AN include the presence of fine, downy body hair; enlarged salivary glands; a yellowing of the skin; and erosion of the dental enamel (American Psychiatric Association, 1994). AN carries a substantial risk of *death* from medical causes or suicide. The factors associated with a fatal outcome include a longer duration of the illness, the presence of both bingeing and purging, substance abuse, and a co-existing mood disorder (Herzog et al., 2000).

Bulimia The medical complications commonly associated with bulimia are less severe and generally not fatal. Most such complications are related to the fluid and electrolyte imbalances caused by purging (American Psychiatric Association, 1994). Most bulimics continue to menstruate, but their periods may be *irregular* (Mitchell, 1995). *Erosion of dental enamel, tooth decay,* and *gum disease* may be seen in bulimics who have been vomiting for at least four years (Mitchell, 1995). Many individuals who induce vomiting by stimulating the gag reflex have calluses or scars on the top of the hand (American Psychiatric Association, 2000). Those

who induce vomiting with the use of syrup of Ipecac may have *heart muscle damage,* which can compromise the cardiovascular system enough to cause low blood pressure and electrocardiogram abnormalities (Mitchell, 1995). *Gastrointestinal complications* include constipation due to a dependence on laxatives, rectal prolapse, and the rare but potentially fatal complications of esophageal tearing and gastric (stomach) rupture (American Psychiatric Association, 2000). Bulimics who *purge* are more likely to have physical complications than are those who do not purge (American Psychiatric Association, 2000).

TREATMENT

As it is apparent that multiple factors are involved in the development of an eating disorder, an effective treatment plan must address all contributing factors. The goals for the treatment of any eating disorders are three-fold: *to stabilize the individual medically and nutritionally, to resolve the psychological factors that contribute to the disorder,* and to *reestablish healthy patterns of eating and exercise* (Becker et al., 1999). In the treatment of anorexia nervosa, the priorities are to stabilize the malnourished individual and to normalize physiological and endocrine function (Casper, 2000). Whether the treatment is provided in an outpatient or inpatient setting depends on the severity of the symptoms. Inpatient hospitalization is mandatory for patients who are suicidal or at risk for life-threatening medical complications (Maxmen & Ward, 1995). *Family therapy* may be helpful in the early stages of AN, to enhance family support and understanding of the disorder; however, any psychotherapeutic approach will be ineffective if malnutrition has impaired cognitive function (Becker et al., 1999). Carefully monitored programs of *nutritional rehabilitation* are indicated, because starvation can perpetuate the disorder due to changes in physiological and psychosocial functioning (Cooper, 1995).

Once the person is medically stable, other therapies can be implemented. There is some evidence that *antidepressants,* particularly serotonergic agents (drugs such as Prozac), may be useful in treating AN and BN (Dilts, 2001). Psychiatric medications can also be used to treat comorbid psychiatric disorders, such as depression or anxiety, and to treat personality traits, such as obsessionality; however, any of these pharmacological agents will be limited in effect until adequate nutrition has been restored (Becker et al., 1999).

Psychotherapy is aimed at correcting dysfunctional beliefs and abnormal eating behaviors and enhancing self-control, personal identity, and body image (Maxmen & Ward, 1995). Cognitive-behavioral therapy (CBT) has proved most successful in treating bulimia nervosa (Becker et al., 1999). CBT must be continued for a longer period of time with anorectic individuals, because more time is required to modify dysfunctional core beliefs. With bulimic individuals, the treatment can be shorter, focusing only on disorder-specific behaviors and perceptions (Vitousek, 1995). Psychodynamic therapy may be useful in the treatment of eating disorders after behavioral strategies have been used early to control the symptoms (Becker et al., 1999). Interpersonal therapy (IPT) is aimed at addressing the interpersonal sources of stress that may have contributed to the development of the eating disorder (Becker et al., 1999). Feminist therapies generally focus less on gaining insight and more on gaining empowerment, with the goal of self-differentiation and self determination (Wooley, 1995). Last, psychoeducation is a useful therapy and can address issues ranging from the risk factors and complications of the illness to ways to develop a healthy lifestyle related to nutrition, management, and stress management. Psychoeducation can be combined with either individual or group therapy and tailored to assist the individual in meeting her specific treatment goals (Olmsted & Kaplan, 1995).

Although anorexia nervosa and bulimia nervosa are currently the primary eating disorders in the United States, **binge eating disorder (BED)** deserves some mention. Like bulimia nervosa, binge eating disorder involves the periodic consumption of excessive amounts of food. In contrast to women with BN, however, individuals with BED do *not* purge in order to compensate for their overeating (American Psychiatric Association, 2000). People who have BED are more likely to report experiencing *more* pleasure and relaxation around eating, and *less* anxiety and physical discomfort, than people who have bulimia (Mitchell et al., 1999). The course and outcome of BN and BED differ also in that the majority of those with BED recover fully (Fairburn, Cooper, Doll, Norman, & O'Connor, 2000).

Eating disorders continue to present a challenge to the affected individuals, their families, and the treatment teams. Although there has been considerable progress in the understanding and treatment of the disorders, response to treatment has been limited (Kaye, Stober, Stein, & Gendall, 1999). Anorexia is characterized by higher rates of partial recovery and lower rates of full recovery, whereas bulimia tends to have higher rates of partial and full recovery (Herzog et al., 1999). No matter what the type or cause of the eating disorder, *long-term treatment* is required in order to achieve success and prevent relapse. The complexity of the interactions among the various factors associated with eating disorders remains an issue for more research. Until there are more answers, women will continue to be victims of these all too often devastating illnesses.

Anxiety Disorders

The term *anxiety* stems from the Latin word *anxietas,* which means "to vex or trouble." Anxiety is an integral aspect of human nature, and it plays a major role in adaptation and homeostasis. Anxiety is triggered by stress or change and is often confused with fear. However, anxiety differs from fear in that it is a *diffuse, anticipatory* reaction to a perceived potential danger that is not currently manifested, whereas fear is a reaction to an *actual* or *imminent* threat. Experiencing a

sustained, excessive level of anxiety is maladaptive and can greatly limit an individual's ability to enjoy life. A person who does so is said to have an *anxiety disorder.*

Anxiety disorders are among the most common mental disorders in the United States, and they occur more frequently in women than men. The lifetime prevalence (chance that a person will develop something in her lifetime) of any anxiety disorder for women is 30.5 percent, compared with a lifetime prevalence of 24.9 percent for the general population. Many of the predisposing factors and risk factors that pertain to depression pertain to anxiety as well. Like other mental disorders, anxiety disorder tends to be undertreated (Pennington, 1997). The anxiety disorders include, but are not limited to, generalized anxiety disorder, panic disorder, agoraphobia, social phobia, and post-traumatic stress disorder (PTSD) (Pennington, 1997).

GENERALIZED ANXIETY DISORDER

Persons with generalized anxiety disorder (GAD) have *unrealistic* and *excessive* anxiety about a fairly wide range of situations and developments in life, and they have difficulty coping with stress. GAD is twice as common in women as men and slightly more common in young to middle-aged women, nonwhites, unmarried persons, and persons in the lower socioeconomic classes (American Psychiatric Association, 2000). Women often suffer from both GAD and depression at the same time (Kornstein et al., 1995). In order to warrant a diagnosis of GAD, an individual must have experienced anxiety 50 percent of the time for six months (American Psychiatric Association, 2000) and must exhibit at least *three* of the following symptoms: restlessness, fatigue, difficulty with concentration, irritability, muscle tension, or sleep disturbances. Persons with GAD may also experience trembling, twitching, a feeling of shakiness, and muscle aches or soreness (Pennington, 1997).

PANIC DISORDER

Panic disorder is manifested by the occurrence of **panic attacks.** A panic attack is a discrete period of intense fear or discomfort, during which at least *four* of the following symptoms develop abruptly and peak within 10 minutes: palpitations, sweating, trembling, shortness of breath, choking, chest pain, nausea, dizziness, fear of losing control or dying, numbness or tingling, or chills or hot flashes (American Psychiatric Association, 2000). In order to warrant a diagnosis of panic disorder, an individual must experience *recurring* panic attacks, at least one of which is followed by a month or more of persistent concern about having additional attacks. The individual must also have been *worried* about the implications of the attack or its consequences and must exhibit a significant *change in behavior* (such as avoiding crowds) related to the attacks. Panic attacks can co-exist with a variety of other anxiety disorders (American Psychiatric Association, 2000).

Epidemiologic studies suggest that about 3 to 4 percent of the adult U.S. population will, at some time, meet the criteria for panic disorder. Panic disorder is more common among women who are divorced or separated. Panic disorder usually begins in *early adulthood,* although many patients report having had symptoms of anxiety, such as separation anxiety, shyness, or behavioral inhibition in unfamiliar circumstances, in childhood. Patients often report also that a significant life event or psychosocial stressor triggered their initial, or *heraldic,* panic attack. Physiological stimuli, such as illness or substance abuse, can also trigger panic attacks. Once activated, panic disorder frequently persists, even if the initial stressor is no longer present (Pennington, 1997).

Many women report being especially vulnerable to panic attacks when they are premenstrual, and women who have premenstrual syndrome (see Chapter 17) sometimes experience panic attacks as well. Women's greater vulnerability to panic when they are premenstrual suggests that ovarian hormones play a role in modulating anxiety and panic and that similar mechanisms may be responsible for postpartum anxiety and panic (Pennington, 1997).

AGORAPHOBIA

The word *agoraphobia* is derived from the ancient Greek words for fear (*phobia*) of the marketplace (*agora*). It refers to persistent anxiety about being in public places or situations from which escape would be difficult or embarrassing or in which help may not be available if symptoms of panic develop. Persons with agoraphobia experience marked distress in such situations and, so, avoid them. Some agoraphobic persons are not able to leave their homes unless accompanied by trusted companions (American Psychiatric Association, 1994).

Panic disorder can occur with or without agoraphobia, and agoraphobia can be present with or without panic attacks. Agoraphobia occurs mainly in women—specifically, young, married women. The lifetime prevalence of agoraphobia for women is about 8 percent. In the majority of individuals affected, the illness begins before age 25, but it can manifest prior to age 15 (Burgess, 1997).

SOCIAL PHOBIA

Individuals with social phobia have a marked and persistent fear of social or performance situations in which they may be exposed to the scrutiny of unfamiliar people. They fear that their appearance, actions, and the like will cause them to feel *humiliated* or *embarrassed.* People who suffer from social phobia recognize that their fear is excessive but are unable to control it. Their need to avoid social situations and their level of distress make their lives difficult (American Psychiatric Association, 1994). Genetic studies suggest that family members of social phobics are at greater risk of developing the disorder (Fyer, Mannuzza, Chapman, Liebowitz, & Klevin, 1993). Other possible predisposing factors include having been parented by a fearful person and having experienced public embarrassment at

a vulnerable age (Keller et al., 1993; Pollock, 2001). Social phobia occurs in 3 to 13 percent of the population, and women are somewhat more likely to suffer from it (American Psychiatric Association, 2000). The onset of social phobia usually occurs during *adolescence* (Rosenbaum et al., 1993).

POST-TRAUMATIC STRESS DISORDER

Individuals who suffer from post-traumatic stress disorder (PTSD) *re-experience past trauma* in varied ways. They may have recurrent recall of the trauma, nightmares, a sudden feeling that the experience is happening all over again, or intense emotional distress in response to situations that are similar to the original trauma (Copel, 2001). PTSD can develop as a consequence of a wide variety of traumatic events, such as rape, incest, criminal assault, domestic violence, military combat, a concentration camp or cult experience, terrorist or hostage situations, the sudden destruction of one's home or community, and natural disasters. The occurrence of such stressors typically produces feelings of profound fear, terror, and helplessness (Yonkers & Gurguis, 1995). In one epidemiological survey of adult women who had been victims of crime involving assault, the prevalence of PTSD was 38 percent (Burgess, 1997). The risk of developing PTSD after experiencing trauma is high when the person involved is female, has a family history of anxiety or antisocial behavior, was separated from parents at an early age, or has a preexisting disorder of anxiety or depression (Street, 2001). Women are more likely to develop *chronic* PTSD, and the symptoms of PTSD can worsen in certain phases of the menstrual cycle (Kornstein et al., 1995).

SYMPTOMS AND DIAGNOSIS OF ANXIETY DISORDERS

Anxiety generates an array of autonomic, behavioral, motor, and cognitive responses. The involuntary *physical* responses include an increased respiratory rate and heart rate, sweating, and dizziness. The *behavioral* responses include engagement in rituals, avoidance, help seeking, and increased dependency. The *motor* reactions include muscle tension, tremors, stuttering, and restlessness. The *cognitive* symptoms include confusion, a sense of doom or powerlessness, vigilance, and rumination (excessive thinking about something) (Antai-Otong, 1995). Anxiety disorders are diagnosed on the basis of a history of exhibiting the behaviors that meet the criteria for the various disorders.

TREATMENT OF ANXIETY DISORDERS

A combination of *pharmacotherapy* and *psychotherapy* is usually used to treat the various anxiety disorders. The drugs used to treat anxiety include those in the benzodiazepine class, such as Valium and Zanax; antidepressants; and the drug Buspirone (Lehne, 1998). Benzodiazepines have a sedating effect and can be habit-forming in some individuals if taken in substantial dosages for long periods of time. Therefore, they are not generally prescribed for persons who are known to abuse alcohol or other drugs. Buspirone is nonsedating and nonhabit-forming and is an alternative for individuals who cannot tolerate benzodiazepines or have a history of drug abuse.

Multiple forms of psychotherapy—supportive, cognitive, behavioral psychotherapy, or a combination—are often used. Supportive therapy can be used to focus the anxious person's attention on her strengths. Cognitive therapy can help anxious clients focus on realistic thoughts and curtail anxiety-provoking, unrealistic thoughts. A behavioral technique known as *desensitization*, in which phobic individuals are exposed to progressively more realistic replicas of feared objects or situations, is also used (Howell, Browman-Mintzer, Monnier, & Yonkers, 2001).

Some nontraditional therapies seem to be helpful in the management of anxiety disorders. Many therapists teach anxious people how to use relaxation techniques, such as deep breathing and self-hypnosis, to calm themselves. According to a recent overview of Chinese medicine (Ehling, 2001), acupuncture can be useful in the treatment of anxiety. Davidson, Morrison, Shore, Davidson, and Bedayn (1997) found homeopathic treatment to be useful for some individuals suffering from anxiety, and a few clinical studies have shown that dance therapy can be an effective adjunctive treatment, although most have been methodologically flawed (Kiresuk & Trachtenberg, 2000).

Psychological/Emotional Wellness Self-Assessment

Answer the following questions as a means of estimating your level of psychological/emotional wellness.

1. *Do I generally enjoy my life? Do I feel fairly happy more days than not?*
2. *Do I have significant relationships that are emotionally satisfying?*
3. *Do I have hope for good things to come and generally look forward to the future?*
4. *Do I feel a need to conceal my eating patterns from others?*
5. *Does my appearance reflect high self-esteem and good self-care?*
6. *Am I able to listen to feedback from others without feeling threatened?*

New Directions

The 1990s were known as the decade of the brain, because, during that period of time, a number of promising new techniques for investigating neuropsychiatric disorders in hu-

mans were developed. For example, the use of brain imaging techniques, such as CT scanning, MRI, PET scanning, and SPECT, allows the direct viewing of correlating brain structure. This allows functional deficits to be correlated with specific areas of damage or malfunction in the brain and allows physicians to make more accurate diagnoses of psychiatric and neurological problems.

Research into the possible genetic influences on psychological/emotional problems may reveal linkages that will make some of the new genetic therapies, such as gene splicing, useful in the treatment of mental disorders.

The ongoing development of new psychotropic medications gives persons suffering from tenacious mental illnesses reason to hope that relief, or even a cure, may be on the horizon, as does the explosion of research in the field of alternative medicine.

QUESTIONS FOR REFLECTION AND DISCUSSION

1. *Do sociocultural factors influence modern women's mental health less, as much, or more than they influenced the mental health of women who lived in earlier historical periods?*
2. *Are there any societal beliefs about women's bodies that contribute positively to women's psychological/emotional health?*
3. *How might your life be different if you suffered from depression? an eating disorder? an anxiety disorder?*

RESOURCES

Books

Danqueh, M. N. A. (1999). *Willow weep for me: A black woman's journey through depression.* Ballentine Books.

Jamison, K. R. (1997). *An unquiet mind.* Random House.

Jack, D. C. (1993). *Silencing the self: Women and depression.* HarperCollins.

Raskin, V. D. (1997). *When words are not enough: The woman's prescription for depression and anxiety.* Broadway Books.

Rehr-Davis D., & Richardson, B. (2001). *101 ways to help your daughter love her body.* HarperCollins.

Organizations

The American Psychiatric Association
1400 K St. NW, Suite 1050
Washington, DC 20005
Phone: 202-682-6000
www.psych.org

The National Mental Health Association
1021 Prince St.
Alexandria, VA 22314-2971
Phone: 1-800-969-6642
www.nmha.org

Websites

The Depression and Related Affective Disorders Association (DRADA). Nonprofit. Associated with the Department of Psychiatry at the Johns Hopkins School of Medicine. *www.hopkinsmedicine.org/drada.*

The National Anxiety Foundation. Non profit. Provides information and provider lists. *http://www.lexington-on-line.com/naf.html*

REFERENCES

Abraham, S., & Llewellyn-Jones, D. (1995). Sexual and reproductive function in eating disorders and obesity. In K. D. Brownell & C. G. Fairburn (Eds.), *Eating disorders and obesity: A comprehensive handbook* (pp. 281–288). New York: Guilford Press.

Agras, W. S., & Wilson, G. T. (2000). Learning theory. In B.J. Sadock & V. A. Sadock (Eds.), *Comprehensive textbook of psychiatry* (pp. 413–424). Philadelphia: Lippincott, Williams, & Williams.

Akiskal, H. S. (2000). Mood disorders: Introduction and overview. In B. J. Sadock & V. A. Sadock (Eds.),*Comprehensive textbook of psychiatry* (pp. 1284–1297). Philadelphia: Lippincott, Williams, & Williams.

American Psychiatric Association. (1994). *Diagnostic and statistical manual of mental disorders* (4th ed.). Washington, DC: Author.

Angst, J., Angst, F., & Stassen, H. H. (1999). Suicide risk in patients with major depressive disorders. *Journal of Clinical Psychiatry, 60* (Suppl. 2), 57–62.

Anstine, D., & Grinenko, D. (2000). Rapid screening for disordered eating in college aged females in the primary care setting. *Journal of Adolescent Health, 26*(5), 338–342.

Antai-Otong, D. (1995). The client experiencing anxiety. In D. Antai-Otong (Ed.), *Psychiatric nursing, biological & behavioral concepts* (pp. 182–208). Philadelphia: W.B. Saunders.

Baum, A. L. (1998). Young females in the athletic arena. *Child and Adolescent Clinics of North America, 7*(4), 745–755.

Beck, A. T. (1964). Thinking and depression: Theory and therapy. *Archives of General Psychiatry, 10,* 561–571.

Becker, A. E., Grinspoon, S. K., Liibanski, A., & Herzog, D. B. (1999). Eating disorders. *New England Journal of Medicine, 340*(14), 1092–1098.

Berel, S., & Irving, L. M. (1998). Media and disturbed eating: An analysis of media influence and implications for prevention. *Journal of Primary Prevention, 18*(4), 415–430.

Bhati, S. S., & Bhati, S. K. (1999). Depression in women: Diagnostic treatment considerations. *American Family Physician, 60*(1), 225–234, 239–240.

Blazer, D. G. (2000). Mood disorders: Epidemiology. In B. J. Sadock & V. A. Sadock (Eds.), *Comprehensive textbook of psychiatry* (pp. 1298–1307). Philadelphia: Lippincott, Williams & Williams.

Blundell, J. E. (1995). The psychobiological approach to appetite and weight control. In K. D. Brownell & C. G. Fairburn (Eds.), *Eating disorders and obesity: A comprehensive handbook* (pp. 8–13). New York: Guilford Press.

Boland, R. J., & Keller, M. B. (1999). Treatment of chronic depression. *Psychiatric Clinics of North America: Manual of Drug Therapy, 6,* 93–111.

Bottiglieri, T., Godfrey, P., Flynn, T., Carney, M. W. P., Toone, B. K., & Reynolds, E. H. (1990). Cerebro spinal fluid S-adenosylmethionate in depression and dementia: Effects of treatment with parenteral and oral S-adenosylmethionine. *Journal of Neurology, Neurosurgery, and Psychiatry, 53,* 1096–1098.

Briscoe, C. W., & Smith, J. B. (1973). Depression and marital turmoil. *Archives of General Psychiatry, 28,* 811–817.

Browness, K. D., Rodin, J., & Wilmore, J. H. (Eds.). (1992). *Eating, body weight, and performance in athletes.* Philadelphia: Lea & Febiger.

Bulik, C. M., Sullivan, P. F., & Joyce, P. R. (1999). Temperament, character, and suicide attempts in anorexia nervosa, bulimia nervosa and major depression. *Acta Psychiatrica Scandinavica, 100*(1), 27–32.

Burgess, A. (1997). Anxiety disorders. In A. Burgess (Ed.), *Psychiatric nursing, promoting mental health* (pp. 202–221). Stamford, CT: Appleton & Lange.

Carrasco, J. L., Diaz-Marsa, M., Hollander, R., Cesar, J., & Saiz-Ruiz, J. (2000). Decreased platelet monoamine oxidase activity in female bulimia nervosa. *European Neuropsychopharmacology, 10*(2), 113–117.

Casper, R. C. (2000). Updates on the treatment of eating disorders. *Psychiatric Clinics of North America: Annual of Drug Therapy, 7,* 219–233.

Cerrato, P. L., & Powell, N. (1999). SAMe: A dietary remedy for the mind and body? *RN, 62*(12), 61–64.

Clark, C. C., & Brandman, W. (1999). Complementary therapies and practices. In C. A. Shea, L. R. Pelletier, E. C. Poster, G. W. Stuart, & M. P. Verhey (Eds.), *Advanced practice nursing in psychiatric and mental health care* (pp. 243–270). St. Louis: Mosby.

Cooper, Z. (1995). The development and maintenance of eating disorders. In K. D. Brownell & C. G. Fairburn (Eds.), *Eating disorders and obesity: A comprehensive handbook* (pp. 224–229). New York: Guilford Press.

Copel, L. (2001). Anxiety disorders. In L. Copel (Ed.), *Psychiatric and mental health care* (2nd ed., pp. 167–200). Springhouse: Springhouse Corporation.

Davidson, R. T., Morrison, R., Shore, J., Davidson, B. A., & Bedayn, G. (1997). Homeopathic treatment of depression and anxiety. *Alternative Therapies, 3*(1), 46–49.

Dennerstein, L. (2001). *How does women's mental health differ from that of men? 1st world congress on women's mental health* [On-line]. Available: http://www.medscape.com

Dilts, S. L. (2001). *Models of the mind: A framework for biopsychosocial psychiatry.* Philadelphia: Brunner-Routledge.

Dixit, A. R., & Crum, R. M. (2000). Prospective study of depression and the risk of heavy alcohol use in women. *American Journal of Psychiatry, 157,* 751–758.

Dominy, N. L., Johnson, W. B., & Koch, C. (2000). Perception of parental acceptance in women with binge eating disorder. *Journal of Psychology, 134*(1), 23–36.

Ehling, D. (2001). Oriental medicine: An introduction. *Alternative Therapies, 7*(4), 71–82.

Ernst, E., Rand, J. I., & Stevinson, C. (1998). Complementary therapies for depression. *Archives of General Psychiatry, 55,* 1026–1032.

Evans, D. L., Staab, J. P., Petitto, J. M., Morrison, M. F., Szuba, M. P., Ward, H. E., Wingate, B., Luber, M. P., &

O'Reardon, J. P. (1999). Depression in the medical setting: Biopsychological interactions and treatment considerations. *American Journal of Psychiatry, 60*(Suppl. 4), 40–56.

Fairburn, C. G., Cooper, Z., Doll, H. A., Norman, P., & O'Connor, M. (2000). The natural course of bulimia nervosa and binge eating disorder in young women. *Archives of General Psychiatry, 57*(7), 659–665.

Fox, H. A. (1996). Electroconvulsive therapy: An overview. *Journal of Practical Psychiatry and Behavioral Health, 2*(4), 223–230.

Fyder, A. J., Mannuzza, S., Chapman, T. F., Liebowitz, M. R., & Klevin, D. F. (1993). A direct interview study of social phobia. *Archives of General Psychiatry, 50*(4), 286–293.

Gabbard, G. O. (2000). Mood disorders: Psychodynamic aspects. In B. J. Sadock & V. A. Sadock (Eds.), *Comprehensive textbook of psychiatry* (pp. 1328–1337). Philadelphia: Lippincott, Williams, & Williams.

Garfinkel, P. E. (1995). Classification and diagnosis of eating disorders. In K. D. Brownell & C. G. Fairburn (Eds.), *Eating disorders and obesity: A comprehensive handbook* (pp. 125–134). New York: Guilford Press.

Garner, D. M. (1995). Measurement of eating disorder psychopathology. In K. D. Brownell & C. G. Fairburn (Eds.), *Eating disorders and obesity: A comprehensive handbook* (pp. 117–121). New York: Guilford Press.

Gaster, B., & Holroyd, J. (2000). St. John's wort for depression: A systematic review. *Archives of Internal Medicine, 160*(2), 152–156.

Gehlart, S., Chang, C. H., & Hartlage, S. (1999). Symptoms pattern of premenstrual dysphoric disorder as defined in the Diagnostic and Statistical Manual of Mental Disorders—IV. *Journal of Women's Health, 8*(1), 75–85.

Goldbloom, D. S., & Kennedy, S. H. (1995). Medical complications of anorexia nervosa. In K. D. Brownell & C. G. Fairburn (Eds.), *Eating disorders and obesity: A comprehensive handbook* (pp. 271–277). New York: Guilford Press.

Greendale, G. A., Lee, N. P., & Arriola, E. R. (1999). The menopause. *Lancet, 353*(9152), 571–580.

Gullette, E. C. D., & Blumenthal, J. A (1996). Exercise therapy for the prevention and treatment of depression. *Journal of Practical Psychiatry and Behavioral Health, 2*(5), 263–271.

Haudek, C., Rorty, M., & Henker, B. (1999). The role of ethnicity and parental bonding in the eating and weight concerns of Asian-American and Caucasian college women. *International Journal of Eating Disorders, 25*(4), 425–433.

Hendrick, V., Altshuler, L. L., & Suri, R. (1998). Hormonal changes in the postpartum and implications for postpartum depression. *Psychosomatics, 39*(2), 93–99.

Herzog, D. B., Dorer, D. J., Keel, P. K., Selwyn, S. E., Ekeblad, E. R., Flores, A. T., Greenwood, D. N., Burwell, R. A., & Keller, M. B. (1999). Recovery and relapse in anorexia and bulimia nervosa: A 7.5 year follow-up study. *Journal of the American Academy of Child and Adolescent Psychiatry, 38*(7), 829–837.

Herzog, D. B., Greenwood, D. N., Dorer, D. J., Flores, A. T., Ekeblad, E. R., Richards, A., Blais, M. A., & Keller, M. B. (2000). Mortality in eating disorders: A descriptive study. *International Journal of Eating Disorders, 28*(1), 20–26.

Horesh, N., Zalsman, G., & Apter, A. (2000). Internalized anger, self-control, and mastery in inpatient anorexic adolescents. *Journal of Psychosomatic Research, 49*(4), 247–253.

Howell, H. B., Browman-Mintzer, O., Monnier, J., & Yonkers, K. A. (2001). Generalized anxiety disorder in women. *Psychiatric Clinics of North America, 24*(1), 165–178.

Isenberg, K. E., & Zorumski, C. F. (2000). Electroconvulsive therapy. In B. J. Sadock & V. A. Sadock (Eds.), *Comprehensive textbook of psychiatry* (pp. 2503–2515). Philadelphia: Lippincott, Williams, & Williams.

Jenkins, M. A., Westlake, R., & Salloway, S. (1996). The diagnosis and treatment of geriatric depression. *Journal of Practical Psychiatry and Behavioral Health, 2*(6), 336–349.

Kaelber, C. T., Moul, D. E., & Farmer, M. E. (1995). Epidemiology of depression. In E. E. Beckham & W. R. Leber (Eds.), *Handbook of depression* (pp. 30–35). New York: Guilford Press.

Kagan, B. L., Sultzer, D. L., Rosenlicht, N., & Gerner, R. H. (1999). Oral S-adenosylmethionine in depression: A randomized double-blind, placebo-controlled trial. *American Journal of Psychiatry, 147*(5), 591–595.

Kaye, W., Stober, M., Stein, D., & Gendall, K. (1999). New directions in treatment research of anorexia and bulimia nervosa. *Biological Psychiatry, 45*(10), 1285–1292.

Kaye, W. H., Gendell, K., & Kye, C. (1998). The role of the central nervous system in the psychoneuroendocrine disturbances of anorexia and bulimia nervosa. *The Psychiatric Clinics of North America 21*(2), 381–395.

Keller, M. B., Lavori, P. W., Goldenberg, I. M., Baker, L. A., Pollack, M. H., Sachs, G. S., Rosenbaum, J. F., Delito, J. A., Leon, A., & Shear, K. (1993). Influence of depression on the treatment of panic disorder with imipramine, aprazolam and placebo. *Journal of Affective Disorders, 28*(1), 27–38.

Kendler, K. S., & Prescott, C. A. (1999). A population-based twin study of lifetime major depression men and women. *Archives of General Psychiatry, 56*(1), 39–44.

Kiresuk, T. J., & Trachtenberg, A. (2000). Alternative and complementary health practices. In B. J. Sadock & V. A. Sadock (Eds.), *Comprehensive textbook of psychiatry* (pp. 2008–2022). Philadelphia: Lippincott, Williams, & Williams.

Klein, D. N., Schwartz, J. E., Rose, S., & Leader, J. B. (2000). Five-year course and outcome of dysthymic disorder: A prospective, naturalistic follow-up study. *American Journal of Psychiatry, 157*, 931–939.

Klein, E., Krenin, I., Chistyakov, A., Koren, D., Merz, L., Marmur, S., Ben-Shachar, D., & Feinsod, M. (1999). Therapeutic efficacy of right prefrontal slow repetitive transcranial magnetic stimulation in major depression. *Archives of General Psychiatry, 56*, 315–319.

Klerman, G. L., Weissman, M. M, Rounsaville, B., & Chevron, E. S. (1996). Interpersonal psychotherapy for depression. In J. E. Groves (Ed.), *Essential papers on short-term dynamic therapy* (pp. 134–148). New York: Guilford Press.

Kornstein, S. G., Schatzberg, A. F., Yonkers, K. A., Thase, M. E., Keitner, G. I., Ryan, C. E., & Schlager, D. (1995). Gender differences in presentation of major depression. *Psychopharmacological Bulletin, 31*(4), 711–718.

Kornstein, S. G., & Wojcik, B. A. (2000). Gender effects in the treatment of depression. *Psychiatric Clinics of North America: Annual of Drug Therapy, 7*, 23–57.

Laliberte, M., Boland, F. J., & Leichner, P. (1999). Family climates: Family factors specific to disturbed eating and bulimia nervosa. *Journal of Clinical Psychology, 55*(9), 1021–1040.

Lehne, R. (1998). *Pharmacology for nursing care* (3rd ed.). Philadelphia: W. B. Saunders.

Leibowitz, S. F. (1995). Central physiological determinants of eating behavior and weight. In K. D. Brownell & C. G. Fairburn (Eds.), *Eating disorders and obesity: A comprehensive handbook* (pp. 3–7). New York: Guilford Press.

Lester, R., & Petrie, T. A. (1998). Physical, psychological, and societal correlates of bulimic symptomatology among African American college women. *Journal of Counseling Psychology, 45*(3), 315–321.

Leung, N., Thomas, G., & Waller, G. (2000). The relationship between parental bonding and core beliefs in anorexic and bulimic women. *British Journal of Clinical Psychology, 39*(2), 205–213.

Lindeman, A. K. (1999). Quest for ideal weight: costs and consequences. *Medicine and Science in Sports and Exercise, 31*(8), 1135–1140.

Lukse, M. P., & Vass, N. A. (1999). Grief, depression, and coping in women undergoing infertility treatment. *Obstetrics and Gynecology, 93*(2), 245–251.

Maser, J. D., Weise, R., & Gwirtsman, H. (1995). Depression and its boundaries with selected axis I disorders. In E. E. Beckham & W. R. Leber (Eds.), *Handbook of depression* (pp. 86–106). New York: Guilford Press.

Maxmen, J. S., & Ward, N. G. (1995). *Essential psychopathology and its treatment* (2nd ed.). New York: W. W. Norton.

Mischoulon, D. (1999). Herbal remedies for mental illness. *Psychiatric Clinics of North America: Annual of Drug Therapy, 6,* 1–15.

Mitchell, J. E. (1995). Medical complications of bulimia nervosa. In K. D. Brownell & C. G. Fairburn (Eds.), *Eating disorders and obesity: A comprehensive handbook* (pp. 271–277). New York: Guilford Press.

Mitchell, J. E., Mussell, M. P., Peterson, C. B., Crow, S., Wonderlich, S. A., Crosby, R. D., Davis, T., & Weller, C. (1999). Hedonics of binge eating in women with bulimia nervosa and binge eating disorder. *International Journal of Eating Disorders, 26*(2), 165–170.

Montano, C. B. (1994). Recognition and treatment of depression in a primary care setting. *Journal of Clinical Psychiatry (Supplement), 55*(12), 18–34.

Moreno, J. K., Selby, M. J., Aved, K., & Besse, C. (2000). Differences in the family dynamics among anorexic, bulimic, obese and normal women. *Journal of Psychotherapy in Private Practice, 1*(1), 75–87.

Morgan, J. F. (1999). Eating disorders and reproduction. *Australian and New Zealand Journal of Obstetrics and Gynecology, 39*(2), 167–173.

Morse, C. A., Dudley, E., Guthrie, J., & Dennerstein, L. (1998). Relationships between premenstrual complaints and perimenopausal experiences. *Journal of Psychosomatic Obstetrics and Gynecology, 19*(4), 182–191.

Murphy, F., Troop, N. A., & Treasure, J. L. (2000). Differential environmental factors in anorexia nervosa: A sibling pair study. *British Journal of Clinical Psychology, 39*(2), 193–203.

Nahas, Z., Bohning, D. E., Molloy, M. A., Outz, J. A., Risch, R. C., & George, M. S. (1999). Safety and feasibility of repetitive transcranial magnetic stimulation in the treatment of anxious depression in pregnancy: A case report. *Journal of Clinical Psychiatry, 60*(1), 50–52.

National Mental Health Association. (2001). *Other mental illnesses: Personality disorders* [On-line]. Available: http://www.NMHA.org/infoctr/factsheets/91.ofm

Nolen-Hoeksema, S. (1987). *Sex differences in unipolar depression.* Stanford, CA: Stanford University Press.

Norman, K. (1992). Eating disorders. In H. H. Goldman (Ed.), *Review of general psychiatry* (pp. 327–337). Norwalk, CT: Appleton & Lange.

Nyamathi, A., Keenan, C., & Bayley, L. (1998). Differences in personal, cognitive, psychological, and social factors associated with drug and alcohol use and nonuse by homeless women. *Research in Nursing and Health, 21*(6), 525–532.

Olmsted, M. P., & Kaplan, A. S. (1995). Psychoeducation in the treatment of eating disorders. In K. D. Brownell & C. G. Fairburn (Eds.), *Eating disorders and obesity: A comprehensive handbook* (pp. 299–305). New York: Guilford Press.

Paris, B. J. (1994). *Karen Horney: A psychoanalyst's search for self-understanding.* New Haven: Yale University Press.

Pataki, C. S. (2000). Mood disorders and suicide in children and adolescents. In B. J. Sadock & V. A. Sadock (Eds.), *Comprehensive textbook of psychiatry* (pp. 2740–2757). Philadelphia: Lippincott, Williams, & Williams.

Peis, R. W., & Shader, R. I. (1994). Approaches to the treatment of depression. In R. I. Shader (Ed.), *Manual of psychiatric therapeutics* (pp. 217–246). Boston: Little, Brown.

Pennington, A. (1997). Women's health: Anxiety disorders. *Primary Care, 24*(2), 103–111.

Pinhas, L., Toner, B. B., Ali, A., Garfinkel, P. E., & Stuckless, N. (1999). The effects of the ideal of female beauty on mood and body satisfaction. *International Journal of Eating Disorders, 25*(2), 223–226.

Police, C., Kaye, W. H., & Greeno, G. C. (1997). Relationship of depression, anxiety, and obsessionality to state of illness in anorexia nervosa. *International Journal of Eating Disorders, 21,* 367–376.

Pollack, M. H. (2001). Comorbidity, neurobiology, and pharmacology of social anxiety disorder. *Journal of Clinical Psychology, 62* (Suppl. 12), 24–29.

Repetti, R. L., & Crosby, F. (1984). Women and depression: Exploring the adult role explanation. *Journal of Social and Clinical Psychology, 2,* 57–70.

Risk of drug interactions with St. John's wort. (2000). *Journal of the American Medical Association, 283*(13), 1679.

Romans, S. E., Martin, J. L., Morris, E., & Herbison, G. P. (1999). Psychological defense styles in women who report childhood sexual abuse: A controlled community study. *American Journal of Psychiatry, 156*(7), 1080–1085.

Romans, S., Martin, J., & Mullen, P. (1996). Women's self-esteem: A community study of women who report and do not report childhood sexual abuse. *British Journal of Psychiatry, 169*(6), 696–704.

Rosenblatt, E. A. (1995). Emerging concepts of women's development: Implications for psychotherapy. *Psychiatric Clinics of North America, 18*(1), 95–106.

Rosenthal, M. S. (2000). *Women & depression.* Los Angeles: Lowell House.

Sarrel, P. M. (1999). Psychosexual effects of menopause: Role of androgens. *American Journal of Obstetrics and Gynecology, 180,* 319–324.

Smith, G. P., & Gibbs, J. (1995). Peripheral physiological determinants of eating and body weight. In K. D. Brownell & C. G. Fairburn (Eds.), *Eating disorders and obesity: A comprehensive handbook* (pp. 8–13). New York: Guilford Press.

Sobal, J. (1995). Social influences on body weight. In K. D. Brownell & C. G. Fairburn (Eds.), *Eating disorders and obesity: A comprehensive handbook* (pp. 73–77). New York: Guilford Press.

Spigset, O., Andersen, T., Hagg, S., & Mjondal, T. (1999). Enhanced platelet serotonin 5-HT2A receptor binding in anorexia nervosa and bulimia nervosa. *European Neuropsychopharmacology, 9*(6), 469–473.

Stahl, S. M. (1996). *Essential psychopharmacology: Neuroscientific basis and clinical applications.* Cambridge, England: Cambridge University Press.

Steiner, M. (1996). Premenstrual dysphoric disorder: An update. *General Hospital Psychiatry, 18,* 244–250.

Street, A. E. (2001). Psychological abuse and post-traumatic stress disorder in battered women: Examining the roles of guilt and shame. *Violence & Victimology, 16*(1), 65–78.

Striegel-Moore, R. H. (1995). A feminist perspective on the etiology of eating disorders. In K. D. Brownell & C. G. Fairburn (Eds.), *Eating disorders and obesity: A comprehensive handbook* (pp. 224–229). New York: Guilford Press.

Strober, M. (1995). Family-genetic perspectives on anorexia nervosa and bulimia nervosa. In K. D. Brownell & C. G. Fairburn (Eds.), *Eating disorders and obesity: A comprehensive handbook* (pp. 219–223). New York: Guilford Press.

Suri R., & Burt, V. K. (1997). The assessment and treatment of postpartum psychiatric disorders. *Journal of Practical Psychiatry and Behavioral Health, 3*(2), 67–77.

Thase, M. E. (2000). Mood disorders: Neurobiology. In B. J. Sadock & V. A. Sadock (Eds.) *Comprehensive textbook of psychiatry* (pp. 1318–1327). Philadelphia: Lippincott, Williams, & Williams.

Thompson, D. S., & Shear, M. K. (1998). Psychiatric disorders and gynecological oncology: A review of the literature. *General Hospital Psychiatry, 20,* 241–247.

Vandereycken, W. (1995). The families of patients with an eating disorder. In K. D. Brownell & C. G. Fairburn (Eds.), *Eating disorders and obesity: A comprehensive handbook* (pp. 219–223). New York: Guilford Press.

Vink, T., Hinney, A., van Elburg, A. A., van Goozen, S. H. M., Sandkuijl, L. A., Sinke, R. J., Herpetz-Dahlmann, B. M., Hebebrand, J., Remschmidt, H., van Engeland, H., & Adan, R. A. H. (2001). Association between an agouti-related protein gene polymorphism and anorexia nervosa. *Molecular Psychiatry, 6*(3), 325–328.

Vitousek, K. B. (1995). Cognitive-behavioral therapy for anorexia nervosa. In K. D. Brownell & C. G. Fairburn (Eds.), *Eating disorders and obesity: A comprehensive handbook* (pp. 324–329). New York: Guilford Press.

Warren, M. P., & Kulak, J. J. (1998). Is estrogen replacement indicated in perimenopausal women? *Clinical Obstetrics and Gynecology, 41*(4), 976–987.

Wilfley, D. E., & Rodin, J. (1995). Cultural influences on eating disorders. In K. D. Brownell & C. G. Fairburn (Eds.), *Eating disorders and obesity: A comprehensive handbook* (pp. 73–77). New York: Guilford Press.

Williamson, L. (1998). Eating disorders and the cultural faces behind the drive for thinness: Are African American women really protected? *Social Work and Healthcare, 28*(1), 61–73.

Wilson, G. T. (1995). The controversy over dieting. In K. D. Brownell & C. G. Fairburn (Eds.), *Eating disorders and obesity: A comprehensive handbook* (pp. 83–86). New York: Guilford Press.

Wisner, K. L., Peindl, K. S., Gigliotti, T., & Hanusa, B. H. (1999). Obsessions and compulsions in women with postpartum depression. *Journal of Clinical Psychiatry, 60*(3), 176–180.

Wooley, S. G. (1995). Feminist influences on the treatment of eating disorders. In K. D. Brownell & C. G. Fairburn (Eds.), *Eating disorders and obesity: A comprehensive handbook* (pp. 294–298). New York: Guilford Press.

Yonkers, K. A., & Davis, L. L. (2000). Premenstrual dysphoric disorder. In B. J. Sadock & V. A. Sadock (Eds.), *Comprehensive textbook of psychiatry* (pp. 1952–1957). Philadelphia: Lippincott, Williams, & Williams.

27

Spiritual Wellness and Illness

Aline Harrison and Marian C. Condon

CHAPTER OUTLINE

Objectives

1. *Describe three concepts of spirituality.*
2. *Identify several possible explanations for the relationship between religiosity and health.*
3. *Discuss the psychophysiological mechanisms identified by the field of psychoneuroimmunology, including the placebo response.*
4. *Identify the personal characteristics, attitudes, and actions that have been empirically associated with good health.*

Introduction

What is spirituality, and what does it have to do with health? There are, unfortunately, no simple or definitive an-
swers to those questions. The very nature of spirituality is the subject of considerable philosophical debate. Some equate spirituality with religious affiliation, some see it as a broader concept that subsumes religion, and others define *spirit* as the essence of a given person. The lack of agreement as to what spirituality is has made scientific inquiry into its relationship to health difficult, because researchers need concrete definitions, or *conceptualizations,* of what they wish to study. Of the three major conceptualizations of spirituality, one has been studied fairly extensively in terms of its relationship to health, one has been scarcely studied at all, and the third is in an early phase of scientific investigation. The three major conceptualizations of spirituality are as follows:

1. *Spirituality as a belief in and relationship with a deity, expressed as participation in the rituals and practices of an organized religion*

2. *Spirituality as a belief in and relationship with a higher power or anything considered to be transcendent, expressed in a nontraditional or eclectic way*
3. *Spirituality as the essence, or spirit of a person, expressed as the person's total functioning and way of being in the world.*

Spirituality as Religious Orientation

Spirituality conceptualized as religious orientation has been studied more than any other concept of spirituality in terms of its relationship to health. The reasons for that are twofold: For one thing, until fairly recently, to be *spiritual* was to be *religious* in the minds of many, including people who do research. For another, it is much easier to **operationalize,** or find ways to measure, religion than spirituality. Social scientists have used such variables as church or synagogue attendance, adherence to religious doctrines, frequency of scripture study, attendance at religious schools, the watching of religious television and reporting of a religious affiliation as markers of religiosity. It is easier to quantify those things than it is to measure more subtle indicators of an ineffable, loosely defined spirituality.

Religion and Health

There has been curiosity as to whether religious people are healthier and/or longer-lived than other people for a long time. The published research on this topic goes back to the 1800s, but intensive study began in the 1970s, when epidemiologists began to use fairly sophisticated research designs to answer the question, Is there a relationship between religious orientation and health? After 20 years of research, that question is considered to have been answered in the affirmative. Taken together, the many studies that have been done on religion and health suggest that religious people are *healthier* and *generally longer-lived* than nonreligious people (Matthews, Larson, & Barry, 1993). Religious people have been found to have lower rates of many conditions and diseases, including uterine, cervical, and intestinal cancer; ulcer disease, coronary artery disease, and high blood pressure. For example, one study found that those who attended church at least once a week were less likely to become ill than those who did not. The churchgoers were 50 percent less likely to have coronary heart disease, 56 percent less likely to have emphysema, 74 percent less likely to have cirrhosis of the liver, and 53 percent less likely to commit suicide than those in the control group of nonchurchgoers (Levin & Schiller, 1987). However, that study, like many of the early studies, did not control for rates of smoking and drinking, or for dietary differences, between the religious group and the control group. Therefore, no inference could be made as to whether the superior health status of the religious subjects was due to their religiosity per se or to better health habits. Indeed, it is known that religious people do tend to have healthier lifestyles overall than people who are not religious. They smoke less, drink less alcohol, and consume a healthier diet. A study done in the Netherlands found that male Seventh-Day Adventists, who do not smoke, drink, or eat meat, lived an average of nine years longer than their non-Adventist neighbors (Berkel & de Waard, 1983). Adventists are the healthiest among all the religious denominations (Matarazzo, 1984).

Studies have also suggested that religion does have an effect apart from its influence on lifestyle. For example, a longitudinal study of almost 3,000 people (House, Robbins, & Metzner, 1982) controlled for differences in smoking history, overall health history, and diet and still found that individuals who attend church regularly *live longer* than those who attend less frequently or not at all. More recently, in a six-year follow-up study of almost 4,000 older adults, Koenig (1999) found that attendance at religious services was associated with a lower mortality rate. Only 22.9 percent of those who had attended services once a week or more died, whereas 37.4 percent of those who had attended religious services less than once a week did. The relative risk of dying was 46 percent less for frequent attendees than for infrequent attendees. The protective effects of religious observance were more pronounced for women and remained significant, even when such variables as health conditions, social support, and health practices were controlled for.

A few studies have suggested that religion seems to *protect against complications of surgery* as well. A 1995 study of 232 elderly patients who underwent open heart surgery found that the death rate six months after surgery was 5 percent for the group comprising religious observers and 9 percent for the nonobservant group (Oxman, 1995). *Mental health* is also supported by religious orientation. Religious men and women tend to score lower on depression scales than their counterparts who are not religious. Furthermore, one of society's major scourges, addiction to alcohol and/or other drugs, is less common among religious people (Matarazzo, 1984).

Although not all the studies exploring the relationship between religiosity and health have been methodologically sound, there is sufficient evidence to support the positive relationship between religion and health. Jeffry Levin, an epidemiologist at Eastern Virginia Medical School, analyzed more than 375 studies on religion and health and carefully evaluated their results, design, and overall quality. Levin (1996) concluded that 75 percent of the existing body of research is solid enough to support a *scientifically valid positive relationship* between religion and health, regardless of sex or ethnicity. Levin added, however, that there has been little in the way of *interpretation* of these findings. In other words, it is not yet known which of the factors associated with religiosity explain the positive association with health or in what way they may interact with each other or with extrinsic factors. A meta-analysis (McCullough, Hoyt, Larson,

Kpenig, & Thorensen 2000) of data from 42 independent samples that examined a measure of religious involvement and all-cause mortality corroborates Levin's work. These researchers calculated 42 independent effect sizes based on samples of nearly 126,000 people that represented the association of religious involvement with all-cause mortality. The overall odds ratio was 1.29 that people high in religious involvement were more likely to be alive at follow-up than people lower in religious involvement. This means, however, that people high in religious invaluement were only *slightly* more likely to be alive at follow-up, as an equal likelihood would have resulted in an odds ratio of 1.

The primary effect of religious affiliation on health that can be inferred from the existing literature is a *protective* effect against disease. Of course, this does not mean that religious people don't develop diseases, just that they tend to do so less frequently than nonreligious people. The studies that exist do not suggest that religion promotes *healing* from disease once disease has been established. They were not designed to reflect that, and new research in this area is needed. Furthermore, the research does *not* suggest that religious observance is the most important factor in superior health. Other factors, such as diet and activity level, appear to have stronger effects on health than religion does. Finally, there is no justification for assuming that the salutary effects of religious affiliation are due to divine intercession or any other supernatural effect. That may well be the case, of course, but science does not address it, at least not so far (Levin, 1996).

There are a number of factors that may explain religion's salubrious effect on health. For one thing, church or synagogue attendance brings people together and provides them with a network of friends, who may offer practical help, emotional support, and encouragement in time of need. *Social support* is a very well-studied construct, and its positive effect on health is incontrovertible (Levin, 1996).

According to a 1990 Gallup Poll, 95 percent of all Americans say they believe in God, and 76 percent say they pray regularly (Benson, 1996). The act of *praying,* a practice in all religions, may confer health benefits. Prayer likely induces a pleasant and very positive phenomenon called the relaxation response (see Chapter 6). The relaxation response is a body state in which heart rate, respiratory rate, blood pressure, and metabolic rate all decrease. The relaxation response is very restful to the mind and body and has benefited people with hypertension and irritable bowel syndrome, among other health problems (Benson, 1975). The relaxation response can be elicited in a number of ways, but the essential ingredient is a sustained focusing of the mind on one thing—the breath, perhaps, or a word, phrase, or mental image. The elicitation of the relaxation response has another dimension to it, as well. Research by Benson and his colleagues (1974) has suggested that 25 percent of those who regularly achieve this feel more *spiritual.* Exactly what that means varies somewhat from person to person, but most report a sense of the presence of an energy or a force that is beyond themselves but close to them.

People who feel this presence receive greater than average medical benefits from the relaxation response. People who pray often may be realizing considerable benefit from the relaxation response, whatever its mechanism.

Religion also supports *hope,* which, as an independent variable, has been positively associated with both mental and physical health (Magaletta & Oliver, 1999). Studies have shown that religious people tend to have hope for the future and believe that the ultimate rightness of things, however painful or frightening, will eventually become clear.

The emphasis on *love* and *forgiveness* common to most religions may, if taken to heart, do much to foster good health. In his book *Love and Survival,* Dean Ornish (1998) reviewed an impressive body of literature which suggests that considerable health benefits can be realized from participation in loving relationships and that the consequences of alienation, cynicism, and hostility are dire. At Yale University, Seeman and Syme (1987) studied 119 men and 40 women who were having the procedure known as cardiac catheterization—dye was being instilled into their coronary arteries to reveal the presence of blockages (see Chapter 11). The subjects were asked a series of questions about how loved and supported they felt. The researchers found that the degree to which the subjects felt loved and supported in their lives was inversely related to the amount of plaque, in their coronary arteries. The *more* love and support they felt in their lives, the *less* the amount of blockage. The predictive power of the love and support variable was independent of diet, smoking, exercise, cholesterol, and family history. A similar study of 131 women was done in Sweden (Ornish, 1998), and, again, the accessibility of deeply emotional relationships was associated with less coronary blockage as determined by coronary angiography.

Conversely, based on an analysis of more than 45 studies, *hostility* has emerged as one of the most important personality variables in coronary heart disease. Hostility increases the risk of coronary heart disease as much or more than the traditional risk factors, such as smoking, elevated cholesterol levels, and high blood pressure. Fostering understanding, tolerance, appreciation, and love may be one of the ways in which religion supports health (Ornish, 1998).

Within the research literature on religion, there is a concept called **extrinsic religious orientation.** Extrinsically religious people possess only a surface religiosity and use religion as a means to a worldly end, such as social respectability, power, influence, or contacts. They are not truly engaged in a relationship with anything that is transcendent. Interestingly, the relatively small body of research done on extrinsics suggests that they do *not* enjoy the health benefits that intrinsically religious people do (Matthews, 1998).

There is some support in the scientific literature for *prayer as a healing intervention.* Superior outcomes in prayed-for coronary patients, as well as other kinds of patients, have also been reported in numerous studies in the medical literature. Many of those studies, however, are flawed by serious methodological weaknesses. In some cases, subjects in the prayed-for groups knew they were being prayed for; in others, members of the healthcare team knew which patients were being prayed for and which were not. In such circumstances, the effects of *placebo response* (see Chapter 9), or differences in the expectations of the healthcare providers, cannot be ruled out as factors in the results.

A study with a stronger design (Byrd, 1988) was conducted on patients in the coronary care unit of San Francisco General Hospital in the late 1980s. All of the approximately 400 subjects either had had heart attacks or were suspected of having had one. The investigator was Randolph Byrd, a faculty member and staff cardiologist at the University of California Medical School at San Francisco. Dr. Byrd's study was a clinical trial—considered by most Western scientists to be the most valid form of medical research (see Chapter 9). It was randomized and double-blinded, meaning that the subjects were chosen randomly from a pool of acceptable candidates, and neither the subjects nor the investigators knew which subjects were in the control group and which were in the experimental group. The subjects were aware, however, that they were in a study involving prayer. As the patients were admitted to the coronary care unit, they were assigned to one of two groups: the medical treatment only group or the medical treatment plus prayer group. The patients in the first group received only the medical care appropriate to their condition. The patients in the second group received the appropriate medical care, too, but were also prayed for; their names and a brief description of their status was given to Protestant and Catholic prayer groups across the United States. Each patient in the prayer group was prayed for by between five and seven people. Those who prayed did so for several patients and were not given any particular instructions as to how or when to pray. Each patient in both groups was assigned a score on a specially constructed scale (the Byrd Scale), that quantified the patients' complications, their needed treatments, and other aspects of outcome. There were substantial outcome differences between the two groups: Twelve patients assigned to the medical treatment only group required endotrachial intubation (the insertion of an artificial airway with mechanical support for breathing), but no patients in the treatment plus prayer group required such support. Three times as many of the patients in the nonprayed-for group developed pulmonary edema (fluid in the lungs because of heart failure) as those in the prayed-for group. Five times as many patients in the nonprayed-for group required antibiotics, as compared with the patients in the prayed-for group, and fewer of the prayed-for patients died—although the difference in death rate was not statistically significant. Overall, however, the Byrd Scale scores between the two groups were not statistically different.

Although the Byrd (1988) study had a stronger design than its predecessors, it was not without flaws; the conditions under which the study was conducted were not perfectly controlled. For one thing, the patients knew the study to which they had consented was about prayer. Therefore, there were likely prayer-receptive individuals in both groups, who may have assumed they were being prayed for. If so, the well-known placebo effect may have contributed to the outcome similarity between the two groups. Another weakness in the Byrd study was that there was no way to be certain that the patients in the medical treatment only group were not being prayed for by friends or relatives. Still another weakness was that no data were collected on the type of coping strategies used by the patients in the two groups. It is known, for example, that denial has a strongly protective effect in the early period following a heart attack, presumably because it decreases fear and curtails the release of emergency hormones, which foster undesirable effects, such as faster heart rate and higher blood pressure. If, by chance, there were more patients in denial in the treatment plus prayer group, that group would have been expected to do better.

A newer study (Harris et al., 1999) was very similar to the Byrd study but better controlled. It also involved a greater number of patients: 960 overall, with 524 in the control group and 466 in the experimental group. The subjects and caregivers in the Harris study, however, did *not* know the nature of the study they were involved in. Of course, as in the Byrd study, neither the patients nor the researchers knew which patients had been prayed for. The Harris team designed its own instrument for quantifying patient outcomes, and it scored patients according to the Byrd Scale. As in the Byrd study, there were no statistically significant differences on the Byrd Scale between the prayed-for and non-prayed-for groups. On the scale developed by the Harris team, however, the experimental group did 10 percent better overall than the patients in the control group. The patients in both groups spent about the same length of time in the coronary care unit and the hospital overall.

The Patriarchal Aspect of Religion: Implications for Women's Spirituality

As discussed briefly in Chapter 1, the major religions in the contemporary world are overwhelmingly patriarchal. In the scripture of Christianity, Islam, Judaism, and Buddhism, women are described as inferior to men (Mahowald, 1994). In Judaism and the Protestant Christian denominations, women were denied full status as clergy until fairly recently, and the Catholic Church still prohibits women from becoming priests. Nevertheless, women have maintained a strong connection to that which is spiritual since the flowering of the Goddess cultures thousands of years ago (see Chapter 1). For example, women played an important, although subsequently downplayed, role in the development of early Christianity (Torjesen, 1993).

Currently, more women than men affiliate with, and observe the rituals of, organized religions. The past 25 years or so have seen a revitalizing of the woman's force in organized religion. Women have been ordained as priests in several denominations in America and around the world, and as rabbis as well (Torjesen, 1993). Organizations such as Catholics for Free Choice and The Women's Ordination Conference continue to work toward the eradication of masculine bias in the world's religions.

Nontraditional Spirituality

Nontraditional spirituality has been the least studied form of spirituality because it is so hard to pin down. The forms that nontraditional spirituality take are limitless, as are the practices and rituals associated with it. Nontraditional spirituality includes the multifaceted New Age spirituality, as well as older traditions in which everything on the earth (and in the sky) is held to be sacred.

The word *spirituality* is derived from the Latin word *spiritus,* one definition of which is breath. Spirit, then, is that which gives life to, or animates, a person. Apropos of that, some theorists define spirituality rather broadly, saying that spirituality has to do with the process of human unfolding and the search for meaning and purpose in life and that spirituality connotes whatever is at the center of one's life. Others, however, define spirituality more narrowly, in terms of two core concepts: transcendence and connectedness. *Transcendence* refers to a relationship with an ultimate intelligence in the universe, variously referred to as God, the Divine, the Great Unknown, Cosmic Consciousness, and the like. *Connectedness* is a sense of interrelationship among oneself, God, other people, and, in some traditions, with all of creation, including animals, trees, rocks, and so forth. Spirituality subsumes, and can exist apart from, belief systems commonly thought of as religions and can be thought of as the ocean in which religion floats. Social scientists are only now beginning to develop independent variables that will allow them to measure nontraditional manifestations of spirituality, so that they can be correlated with various indicators of health status.

Spirituality as the Essence or Spirit of a Person

Some individuals immediately strike us as energetic, enthusiastic, and full of life. They appear healthy and move briskly and with purpose. A phrase sometimes used to describe such individuals is *spirited.* Conversely, a depressed, apathetic, sluggish person is sometimes referred to as *dispirited.* Both these terms seem to allude to a kind of energy, or essence, that we sense in people, and even in animals. From this standpoint, then, *spirit* is defined as the dynamic state of being within which the mind and body interact. Spirit is a function of the dynamic interaction among all realms of human functioning and, as a totality, affects each of its components. This means that, along with genetic and environmental in-

fluences, everything that constitutes spirit—beliefs, attitudes, mood, body chemistry, and so on—affects our total state of being. Although each factor exerts some influence on the total quality of a person's life, no one factor overrides all of the others.

The conceptualization of spirit as the *essence* of a given person, related to and yet separate from mind and body, arose partly as a result of findings from the relatively new field of **psychoneuroimmunology.** Psychoneuroimmunology is the study of mind/body interactions and has been recognized as an independent field of study for about 20 years. It comprises a large collection of studies about how the mind and body affect one another. The central finding of this discipline is that many health problems, ranging from the common cold to a host of chronic diseases, are affected by the mind and that the mechanism by which such effects take place is a system of *communication* that exists between the mind and the body.

Mind/Body Communication

There are now several studies completed (and many more in progress) that suggest that the mind exerts its influence on the body by making and dispersing what have been called messenger molecules. **Messenger molecules** are chemicals that are generated in the brain and travel to various places in the body, where they attach to special areas (called **receptors**) on the surfaces of cells. These molecules can trigger changes in cells, which ultimately result in chemical and behavioral changes in the body. For example, when we notice a car bearing down on us when we are halfway across a street, the brain perceives a serious threat to our survival and pours out a wide variety of emergency messenger molecules, which travel to many target sites in the body. Ultimately, energy-giving sugar enters our blood and muscle cells, so that we are able to sprint across the street. Other reactions to such a perceived threat include an increase in blood pressure and heart rate. The messenger molecules are used up by the physical reaction to the perceived danger (such as running across the street). When the emergency ends, heart rate, blood pressure, blood sugar level, and so on returns to normal. In some threatening situations, however, messenger molecules may *not* be used up by physical activity; they remain active in the body. For example, if we think we may be fired from a much-needed job, the brain pours forth the *same* emergency molecules it would produce in reaction to a threatening car. There is no explosive physical reaction to use them up, however, and they remain in the body, exerting their effects on it, for a period of time. This is thought to be the mechanism by which chronic stress ultimately results in disease. It causes a steady supply of emergency messenger molecules to be released into the blood and their continuing presence over time can result in high blood pressure, among other problems.

It has been known for a long time that messenger molecules in the form of *stress hormones* have receptor sites in the organs that control blood pressure, heart rate, and blood sugar level. Only recently, however, has it been discovered that receptors for messenger molecules *also* exist in the brain itself, the heart, the immune system, the digestive system, and other places throughout the body. It is the interaction between brain chemicals and organ systems that likely explains the profound effect that thoughts and feelings can have on the body. A fascinating and accessible account of the nature of messenger molecules and mind/body communication may be found in *Molecules of Emotion* (1997) by neuroscientist Dr. Candice Pert. Two phenomena that are functions of mind-body communication are faith healing and the placebo effect.

FAITH HEALING

The term *faith healing* refers to healing seemingly brought about by an appeal to a higher power, or by the intervention of a priest, shaman, or another holy person. An experiment to determine the objective effects of faith healing was conducted in the early 1980s by David McClelland, a noted psychologist at Harvard University, and described by Dreher (1995), as well as in an interview reported in *Advances, the Journal of Mind-Body Health* (Borysenko, 1985). McClelland investigated the healing ability of a well-known healer named Karmu, a middle-aged African American man who lived in a poor neighborhood and maintained the lifestyle of a lower-class man of the people. In truth, he was a highly educated individual whose mother had taught him African mythological traditions. Karmu's mother also told him that, when he was a child, a Tibetan monk had laid hands on him and had declared him a healer of the highest order. Karmu was considered highly charismatic and very dedicated in his eclectic approach to healing. Following a business trip during which McClelland had developed the early symptoms of a cold, he visited Karmu to test his powers. On leaving Karmu's presence, McClelland felt no different; however, by the next morning he was fine, which he found highly unusual. Based on this experience, McClelland devised a controlled study in which he gathered a group of Harvard students, who were instructed to see Karmu within 24 hours of the first symptoms of a cold. He arranged with Karmu that Karmu would actually treat only *half* the students sent to him and would refer the others to another member of his entourage, who would not really perform a healing. The students would not know whether they were in the treated or the untreated group. Within 48 hours of each student's visit, McClelland took a saliva sample and tested for IgA antibodies, the first line of defense against colds. Eighty-five percent of the students seen by Karmu experienced dramatic improvement in their cold symptoms, whereas 85 percent of the students in the referred group developed full-blown respiratory infections. Eighty-two percent of those who experienced a loss of symptoms also showed increases in IgA antibodies, whereas none of the members of the referred group showed elevated IgA levels.

When physicians from the Harvard Health Service heard of the results of McClelland's study, they challenged him to repeat the experiment in a slightly different way. McClelland then designed an experiment wherein half of a population of students who had been voluntarily exposed to rhinovirus (viral strains that cause the common cold) were sent to Karmu and half were sent to the Health Service, where they were assured they would get better. The students' faith in Karmu proved superior to their faith in the health center personnel. None of the students who went to Karmu got sick, whereas most who went to the Health Service did. IgA antibodies increased in many of the students who went to see Karmu but in none of the students who went to the Health Service.

McClelland studied Karmu's work for about 10 years and became convinced that Karmu's success was due to his ability to raise what McClelland defined *affiliative trust* in his patients. Karmu often told his clients that he was not healing them but, rather, was putting them in touch with their ability to heal themselves. Karmu's abilities, and those of other healers, may be explained by the amazing power of *belief* to unleash an innate healing response within individuals.

PLACEBO EFFECT

The placebo effect is the phenomenon of healing, or getting better, in response to something not generally accepted as having an actual effect. An example is a person experiencing pain relief when she has been given a "pain pill," which is actually only a sugar pill. The placebo effect illustrates perfectly how a cognitive state, such as a belief or an expectation, can trigger a chemical change in the body. Researchers have found that the administration of a placebo to a person experiencing pain usually results in the release of **endorphins** and **enkephalins,** the body's natural opiates, within the body. Moreover, when an opiate *antagonist* (anti-opiate) drug is administered, the patient's pain returns. Administering fake medications is not the only way of stimulating the innate ability to heal. Healing takes place, to varying degrees, in response to rituals, amulets, and charms—anything in which the individual believes. A somewhat scary manifestation of the healing effect is its opposite—the "voodoo" death in which an individual believes herself to have been cursed by a powerful shaman or priest and actually dies without having been physically harmed in any way. Accounts of such deaths, not only among tribal members but among average American citizens (Dossey, 1997), provide testimony to the mind's ability to affect the body profoundly.

Individuals vary in the degree to which they respond to placebo and other forms of suggestion. About a third of the population responds very well, with varying levels of response in the remaining two-thirds. The ability to respond to suggestion does *not* correlate with intelligence, educational level, or social status. The power of suggestion is well understood by the advertising industry, which spends billions of dollars yearly on carefully crafted suggestions designed to create a desire for various goods and services.

Markers of Spiritual Wellness

The body and all its chemical processes can be seen as constituting the *physical* manifestation of the totality referred to as spirit, whereas our thoughts and emotions reflect the *mental* manifestation. Because the mind and body are parts of the same whole, it follows that there should be a demonstrable relationship between the state of the mind and the state of the body. The field of psychoneuroimmunology has supplied evidence that this is the case. The immune system, of course, has a profound influence on physical health. A large body of research, starting with publications in the early 1960s, provides convincing evidence that the strength of a person's *spirit,* as evidenced by the degree of mental and emotional well-being and vitality, correlates with the strength of her immune system. Dreher (1995) summarized this research in a book called *The Immune Power Personality—Seven Traits You Can Develop to Stay Healthy.* These traits, as well as some others identified in the mind/body literature, can be considered the markers of spiritual wellness. Intrinsic religiosity (discussed previously) has also been associated with relative resistance to illness and can be considered a marker of spiritual wellness. The seven traits identified by Dreher are the ACE factor, assertiveness, hardiness (discussed in Chapter 7), the capacity to confide, affiliation, altruism, and self-complexity.

ACE Factor

The **ACE factor** is the ability to attend (pay attention to), connect with, and express emotions. Much of the research in this area has been conducted by Gary Schwartz, a professor of psychology at Harvard University. Schwartz decided to investigate the relationship between mental-emotional states and physical states after having become aware, early in his career, that he was having physical symptoms that were clearly a reaction to stress. Over time, he built a body of research that has provided much information about the ways in which various individuals perceive and respond to stress. In one series of experiments, Schwartz (1983) used such physical measures as heart rate, muscle tension, blood pressure, and skin conductance to determine how much stress the subjects were experiencing under a variety of circumstances. He also had the subjects complete tests designed to reveal whether their *perceived* stress matched their *actual* stress. After the studies were complete, Swartz was able to separate his subjects into four groups, depending on their patterns of response to stress. The groups were the true low anxious, the true high anxious, the repressive copers, and the defensive high anxious:

1. True low anxious. *The subjects in this group believed themselves to be calm and relaxed, and objective measurements of their physiological responses showed this to be true. This group was made up of the people strong in what later was called the ACE factor.*

2. True high anxious. *The subjects in this group saw themselves as being anxious a lot of the time, and their physiological responses indicated that this was so.*

3. Repressive copers. *This group consisted of people who believed themselves to be calm but had physiological responses indicatng that they were really quite anxious.*

4. Defensive high anxious. *The subjects in the fourth group believed themselves to be somewhat anxious but were actually even more anxious than they thought they were. They were partially, but not completely, in touch with their feelings.*

Schwartz went on to compare the four groups in terms of certain variables, such as their physiological and cognitive responses to stress and their health patterns. In each experimental situation, the repressive copers had the most *undesirable* response pattern, and the true low anxious (high ACE factor) people had the *best* response. For example, because the repressive copers had strong physiological responses but believed themselves to be calm, Schwartz postulated the members of this group might frequently have high blood pressure. On investigation, he found that the repressive copers consituted only 11 percent of a group of healthy people but 45 percent of a group with high blood pressure.

In another series of studies, Schwartz and a colleague (Jamner & Schwartz, 1986; Jamner, Schwartz, & Leigh, 1988) investigated the effect of the ACE factor on *immunity.* The efficacy of the immune system was assessed in and compared among the four groups. The repressive copers and the defensive high anxious subjects had *poorer* immune function than did the true low anxious and the true high anxious subjects. Of the four groups, the subjects in the true low anxious (high ACE factor) group had the *strongest* and *most balanced* immune systems. This research suggests that it is not negative feelings but, rather, the *suppression* of negative feelings that leads to poorer immune functioning. The repressive copers, not the people in the true high anxious group, had the poorest immune functioning.

Jamner and Schwartz also gathered information about the *physiological mechanism* by which the ACE factor enhances immune function and the similar mechanism by which repression decreases it. They found that strong ACE personalities have *normal* blood glucose levels, whereas repressive copers have *elevated* glucose levels. When people are under stress, sugar enters the bloodstream, presumably to provide energy for coping with the threat. Sugar is also known to *dampen* immune response (Geerling & Hoepelman, 1999). Jamner and Schwartz (1986) also found that repressors have high levels of *endorphins,* painkilling compounds produced by the body that can block or blunt the perception of negative feelings. These researchers administered mild shocks to subjects in all four groups until the subjects became uncomfortable enough to ask that the experiment be stopped. The subjects in the repressive coping group accepted shocks that were *twice* as intense as those tolerated by nonrepressive copers. The subjects in this group were found to have higher levels of endorphins than the subjects in the other groups. Similar to the people who suffer stress-related headaches and reach for an aspirin, repressive copers simply *block* their pain with physiologically generated endorphins (Jamner & Schwartz, 1986).

Endorphins, like sugar, have a *negative* effect on immune functioning, however. In one study (Shavit et al., 1985), mice that had been subjected to electric shock generated high levels of endorphins in their systems. The sudden increase in endorphins was correlated with a substantial *drop* in the numbers of natural killer cells, which provide a first line of defense against cancer. Indeed, the mice subsequently demonstrated a reduced resistance to injected cancerous tumors.

It appears that people who are *high* in the ACE factor release innocuous amounts of sugar and endorphins into their blood and are more likely to have *normal* immune systems, with a normal ability to reject tumors. It also appears that *repressive copers* produce unusually *high* levels of sugar and endorphins, which *dampen* their immune functioning and may reduce their ability to resist tumors. Additional experimentation has suggested that too *little* endorphin also dampens the immune function (Shavit et al, 1984, 1985).

People who are strong in the ACE factor do appear to be less vulnerable to infection and to cancer. A number of disparate studies suggest that an attentive, emotionally connected, expressive spirit really is important to the body's wellness (Abramson, McClelland, Brown, & Kelner 1991; Greer & Morris, 1975; Jensen, 1987; Kneier & Temoshok, 1984; Kreiden et al., 1986; Schwartz, 1990; Solomon, 1981; Spiegel et al., 1989; Temoshok, 1985). Thus, the literature strongly suggests that people who notice their emotions, connect them with their larger lives, and express their needs have the strongest immune systems, the least likelihood of contracting disease, and the greatest likelihood of recovering from the disease most quickly. This is not to say, however, that *all* disease is a disease of the spirit and that genetic and environmental factors play no part. The separation of genetics, environment, and spirit is unfounded and inappropriate. *Disease* involves both the spirit and the body, because they are two expressions of the same whole. The physical manifestation of disease comes about because of physical as well as spiritual changes. However, *wellness* is also both a physical and a spiritual state of being. Modern medicine provides us with medicines or other treatments for disease, thus enabling us to ignore the source of our difficulties and the need to heal the spirit. However, if the spirit is not *also* healed, the disease process is not necessarily halted. For example, bypass surgery must often be *repeated,* because the process of atherosclerosis (see Chapter 12) continues unabated. Those who consistently *disregard* their sensations and feelings and *repress* their emotions will suffer ongoing imbalances in the body/mind system, which are likely to be manifested by physical disease or illness.

Assertiveness

Assertiveness is the capacity to stand up for oneself without disregarding the rights and interests of other people. Assertiveness requires a robust spirit—that is, a healthy overall sense of one's own worth and deservedness combined with a respect and concern for others. Assertiveness allows us to be ourselves and to meet our own needs without inhibiting others from doing the same. Assertiveness also enables us to risk the loss of another's love in order to honor our authentic selves.

Assertiveness has been correlated with immune functioning. Individuals who are assertive tend to have well-balanced immune systems (Kaplan, Greenfield, & Ware, 1989; Moos & Solomon, 1965; Solomon & Moos, 1965; Solomon, Temoshok, O'Leary, & Zich, 1987; Temoshok & Dreher, 1992). That association demonstrates the correlation between spiritual health and physical health. In fact, the quality of assertiveness *within the immune system itself* seems to be necessary for its proper functioning. The immune system must be able to defend the interests of the total organism without overreacting and inadvertently damaging it. If we have an *overly defensive* immune system, we find ourselves plagued by either autoimmune responses or allergies. If we have an *underdefensive* immune system, we find ourselves besieged by cancer or infections. The capacity for assertiveness has been studied in people with AIDS, cancer, rheumatoid arthritis, ulcers, hypertension, and diabetes. The results of such studies indicate that people who are insufficiently assertive tend to be at higher risk for diseases that are associated with the underfunctioning of the immune system, such as AIDS and cancer (Greer & Morris, 1975; Greer, Morris, & Pettingale, 1993). It also suggests that people who are aggressive, rather than assertive, are at higher risk for diseases that are associated with the hyperfunctioning of the immune system, such as rheumatoid arthritis.

Hardiness

Why is it that some of us flourish under stress, whereas others become ill? What enables some of us to deal well with having too much to do and too little time, whereas others become overwhelmed? Suzanne Oulette Kobasa, writing under both the names Oulette and Kobasa, has studied the effects of stress by comparing the personality traits of those who thrive under stress with the personality traits of those who do not. Oulette/Kobasa, who has a background in existential philosophy, has formulated the hypothesis that people who fare well under stress possess a constellation of personality characteristics she calls *hardiness* (Kobasa, 1979). Oulette/Kobasa defines hardiness as comprising three qualities: challenge, commitment, and control. People high in *challenge* see life's problems as something to take on and overcome, rather than as threats to personal well-being. *Commitment* means that the people find meaning and purpose in their work, thus being capable of full-hearted involvement. People high in *control* believe and behave as if they have influence over how events turn out. They approach problems with the confidence that they can devise and implement solutions. To test this thesis, Kobasa studied a group of middle- and upper-level executives at Illinois Bell, fortuitously at a time when the company was undergoing a sweeping reorganization. She used the Homes-Rahe Stress Inventory, a list of stressful life events rated according to severity, to determine the stress levels of the executives willing to be subjects in her study. She identified a cohort that was highly stressed and determined their health status. Kobasa then divided the stressed executives into two groups: healthy and unhealthy. When Kobasa administered the hardiness questionnaire to both groups, the executives in the stressed/healthy group received *higher* hardiness scores than the executives in the stressed/unhealthy group. Seeking substantiation of this outcome, Kobasa set up a prospective study in which she initially determined the stress level, health, and hardiness of 259 executives. She followed them for a period of two years. The results were clear; the hardy executives had significantly *fewer* severe illnesses than those who were not hardy. Statistically, they were half as likely to get sick as their less hardy counterparts, even though their stress levels were about the same (Kobasa, Maddi, & Kahn, 1982). Kobasa controlled for variables such as dietary habits, exercise, smoking, alcohol intake, and social support. When all of those potentially mitigating influences were taken into consideration, however, none had the statistical power to account for the observed effect. Moreover, the hardy executives *stayed* healthier than the less hardy executives even if their family history suggested a higher risk for certain diseases than the histories of less hardy individuals (Kobasa, Maddi, Puccetti, & Zola, 1985). After her prospective study had been completed, Kobasa concluded that hardiness, social support, and exercise all exert a protective effect against stress. She estimated that the likelihood of illness was 92 percent for executives with none of these protective factors, 72 percent for those with one of them, 58 percent for those with two, and only 8 percent for the executives with all three. Of the three factors, hardiness was found to be the most powerful *preventer of illness* and the most powerful *predictor of health*.

More recent studies have disclosed more about the relationship between hardiness and health. For example, hardiness has been found to influence the health and strength of the *immune system;* several researchers have found a positive correlation between hardiness and length or quality of life in AIDS patients. Although the relative importance of the challenge, commitment, and control has varied from one study to another, hardiness has been shown to be a protector of people in all walks of life, cutting across economic and cultural lines (Kobasa, 1984; Oulette, 1993).

Many studies have shown that helplessness suppresses the immune system. In many ways, hardiness is the antithesis of helplessness. Thus, it appears that a helpless spirit correlates with a helpless immune system, and a hardy spirit correlates with a hardy body and a balanced, well-functioning immune system.

Capacity to Confide

Many of us carry untold secrets of past events that we are afraid to tell anyone about for fear of being viewed as less than we are. The effort we expend in holding these secrets within us may use up energy that might otherwise be used for healing. In the early 1980s, James Pennebaker, a psychology professor at Southern Methodist University, developed a theory about the relationship between *self-disclosure* and health. Pennebaker hypothesized that confiding deep feelings about traumatic events confers psychological and physiological benefits, and, over a 10-year period, he conducted a series of studies designed to test his theory. Pennebaker's work revealed that the degree to which the expression of painful feelings is *inhibited* correlates positively with the incidence of ulcers, infections, heart problems, and a number of other illnesses. For example, Pennebaker invited a group of college students to write for 20 minutes on 5 consecutive days, about the most upsetting or traumatic event of their lives. They were to include both *thoughts* and *feelings* about the incident. After completing the experiment, the students were asked to report on how they had felt during and after writing. Typically, the students reported having felt angry and disturbed during the first 3 days but said that, by the fourth day, they had begun to feel better and that, by the fifth, they were calm and had a feeling that the situation had been resolved. Over the next 6 months, the subjects in the experimental group (those who had participated in the 20-minute writing exercises), made significantly *fewer* visits to physicians and reported *fewer* symptoms of illness than subjects in the control groups (Pennebaker & Beall, 1986). Additional studies, wherein students spoke instead of writing about traumatic events, yielded the same results (Pennebaker, 1990; Pennebaker, Hughes, & O'Heeron, 1987). The results of experiments in which the subjects disclosed the details of disturbing incidents, but not their feelings about them, or disclosed feelings, but not details, indicated that, in order for healing to occur, *both facts and feelings must be expressed*.

To demonstrate directly that the recounting of traumatic experiences has an effect on the immune system, Pennebaker collaborated with a leading team of psychoneuroimmunology researchers—Janice Kiecolt-Glaser and Ronald Glaser (Pennebaker, Kiecolt-Glaser, & Glaser, 1988). Pennebaker and the Glasers collected blood samples from participants (students) before and after the participants wrote about traumatic events. They separated immune system cells called lymphocytes from the blood and tested their level of reactivity, or strength, by provoking them with substances called mitogens. The immune cells of the students who had written about their trauma became *stronger* as the exercise progressed and were still stronger when blood was drawn again six weeks later. In contrast, the strength of the immune cells of the control group participants was essentially unchanged. As would be expected, the frequency with which the students who wrote about trauma visited the health center with reports of illness also showed a remarkable drop.

In further studies, Pennebaker invited freshman college students to write about their problems of leaving home, entering a new environment, and adjusting to college life. Those who did so experienced *less illness* than a control group of freshmen who wrote about trivial topics, and their illness rates *remained lower* for about four months. Pennebaker's research suggests that disclosing previously inhibited thoughts and feelings may speed up the coping process and that this process somehow allows the immune system to function at a higher level (Pennebaker, Colder, & Sharp, 1990).

Affiliation

Both the need for power and the need for affiliation (human connections) are highly motivating forces in our lives. David McClelland has studied the relationships between those two motivating forces and health.

McClelland (1979) used the Thematic Apperception Test (TAT) to measure the degree to which power motivated a group of male subjects, as well as the degree to which their desire for power was fulfilled or not fulfilled. Taking the TAT involves answering questions and describing one's thoughts about vague pictures of people in various positions. McClelland also measured the quantity and strength of immune cells and substances isolated from the subject's blood and saliva. McClelland found that the subjects with a *high* power need that was *not* fulfilled tended to have high levels of adrenaline (a stress hormone) in their blood, relatively weak blood immune cells and low levels of IgA (an antibody protective against colds) in their saliva. Additional studies revealed that in general, people with a high but unfulfilled power motivation, whether inhibited internally or by the environment, have relatively *weak* immune systems in comparison with individuals whose power needs are either weak or fulfilled. Interestingly, the men who had a high but unfulfilled power motivation scored low on the need for affiliation.

McClelland's discovery that unfulfilled power motivation has *negative* implications for health led him to wonder whether a fulfilled affiliation motivation has *positive* implications. In a series of studies in which he compared students with an unfulfilled power motivation with students with a fulfilled affiliation motivation, McClelland found that the students with a fulfilled affiliation motivation had superior immune function (McClelland, Floor, Davidson, & Saron, 1980; McClelland & Jemmott, 1980).

McClelland made some other interesting discoveries in the area of love and relationships. The results of studies in which subjects either viewed scenes depicting loving, caring relationships or imagined such scenes, suggest that affiliation does not always correlate positively with immune functioning. Whether a positive correlation is present seems to depend on the presence or absence of what McClelland termed affiliative trust.

AFFILIATIVE TRUST

Affiliative trust is an individual's expectation that she will form loving relationships built on mutual respect and trust. Affiliative trust appears to comprise unconditional love—the ability to love regardless of whether love is returned (McClelland, 1986; McClelland & Kirshnit, 1988). Generally, people who had satisfying and caring relationships early in life develop affiliative trust and have positive expectations about current relationships. However, if early relationships were characterized by abuse, abandonment, or dishonesty, affiliative trust may not develop, and expectations about current relationships may be negative. In a 1988 study, McClelland found that the immune function of subjects *high* in affiliative trust *improved* when they were imagining or viewing loving and caring relationships but that the immune functioning of subjects *low* in affiliative trust became *weaker* when they imagined or viewed similar scenes. McClelland's work suggests that the lingering effects of early relationships may color subsequent relationships throughout our lives.

Later, more extensive studies of immune function indicate that immune function tends to be higher in people who have affiliative trust among their enduring personality traits. For example, McKay (1991) studied affiliative trust and immune function in depressed individuals and found that depressed people *high* in affiliative trust had *stronger* immune systems than depressed people low in affiliative trust. An interesting byproduct of this research was the discovery that *mistrust* or *cynicism* about relationships correlates positively with *lowered* immune function. A leading investigator of personality patterns in heart disease, Dr. Redford Williams, has identified a similar cynicism in people who have suffered heart attacks (Williams, 1989).

Fortunately, individuals who did not develop affiliative trust early in life may be able to acquire it later. In research done by McClelland and Kabat-Zinn at the University of Massachusetts Medical Center's Stress Reduction Program (see Chapter 11), showed that patients who completed the center's spiritually-based, six-week program achieved an increase in affiliative trust, which persisted throughout the two-year follow-up period. Many of the patients who participated in the stress-reduction program developed a sense of belonging to someone or something greater than themselves. This sense of belonging, or movement toward belonging, was called a "motive toward oneness" by the researchers. The patients whose motive toward oneness was enhanced through the mindfulness training showed remarkable improvements in their medical conditions. The sense of oneness, considered to be an aspect of spirituality in many traditions, can be considered a type of affiliative trust (McKay, 1992).

CYNICISM

Cynicism is an attitude of general mistrust regarding the intentions and motives of others; it is the near-opposite of affiliative trust. Affiliative trust is a valuable attitude in the maintenance of high-quality immune functioning and lower incidence of illness. Cynicism, on the other hand, as a component of the psychological construct hostility, has long been known to be a factor in the development of coronary heart disease (Friedman & Rosenman, 1974).

Coronary heart disease (CHD) is a major cause of death among women, especially after menopause (see Chapter 12). Lisspers, Nygren, and Soderman (1998) suggest that patients with CHD are more likely than patients with other diseases to test high in suppressed anger, overall experienced anger, and cynicism. A study of almost 2,000 middle-aged men found cynicism to be associated not only with CHD but with several other disease processes as well (Almada et al., 1991). In a study of 96 women who completed the Cook-Medley Hostility Scale and a measure of perceived availability of social support, cynicism was found to be inversely related to the perceived availability of support (Hart, 1996). The results of a similar study (Lepore, 1995) also suggest that highly cynical individuals tend to benefit *less* from social support. Cynical attitudes may insulate individuals from the stress-buffering potential of support from other people.

The connection between the ability to form meaningful bonds with other people and physical health has been demonstrated most dramatically by cardiologist Dean Ornish. Coronary heart disease had been generally considered irreversible until Ornish (1990) showed that to be false. Ornish put volunteers with demonstrated coronary heart disease on a program that included a very low-fat diet, moderate exercise, training in stress management, and the opportunity to learn to make intimate connections with other people. An impressive number of those who stuck with Ornish's program were able to *reduce* the size of the atherosclerotic lesions in their coronary arteries. In his 1998 book *Love and Survival,* Ornish writes eloquently of coronary heart disease as the physical consequence and manifestation of the lack of intimacy in one's life.

Altruism

Altruism is the inclination to help other people, such as by volunteering. Altruism seems to correlate with superior health and longevity.

In the late 1980s, Luks and Payne (1992) surveyed a group of volunteers and found that those who rated their health as better than that of others were 10 times more likely to be once-a-week rather than once-a-year helpers. Luks also found that helping strangers conferred more benefit than helping friends and that personal contact with the "helpee" is generally beneficial to the helper's health. Luks also identified another benefit of volunteering—a euphoric sensation, which might best be called "the helper's high." This was characterized as initial feelings of warmth, energy, and emotional well-being, which were eventually replaced by a sense of peace, self-worth, and optimism—provided that the helper routinely did helping acts over a period of time. The

volunteers also reported incidents of pain relief and an overall improvement in their health.

A long-term prospective study of volunteerism was included in a 30-year study of women's health and longevity conducted by Dr. Phyllis Moen. Moen found that being a member of a volunteer organization was significantly related to increased longevity (Moen, Dempster-McClain, & Williams, 1989). The data were statistically controlled for education, levels of social support, husband's occupational status, social class, number of children, general life satisfaction, self-esteem, and gender role traditionalism. Moen and her colleagues also found that the women who volunteered had better *health,* as well as greater longevity.

Men also appear to benefit from volunteer activities. In a study of 2,754 men as part of the 10-year Tecumseh Community Health Study (House, Landis, & Umberson, 1988), volunteerism was one of the most powerful predictors of reduced mortality.

Why might volunteerism confer so many health benefits? Volunteerism involves affiliation reward and possibly a sense of connection to something larger than oneself. Choice may play a role as well; volunteers choose their activities and can move on to something different if not satisfied. Volunteering may also increase the degree to which one feels in control of one's life, and it likely involves a sense of commitment. Thus, the health benefits realized by volunteers may be related to affiliative trust and hardiness. Attitude also seems to influence the degree to which volunteers realize health benefits as a result of their activities. If helpers' inner feelings of being rewarded are conditional, the benefits of helping are believed to be lost. Helpers who feel rewarded *only* if the person being helped undergoes specific changes, takes certain actions, or takes the helper's advice, do not realize maximal health benefits (House et al., 1988).

The characteristics of what has been called an "altruistic personality" have been identified (Oliner & Oliner, 1988). People with altruistic personalities just naturally help others. This tendency appears to come from a biologically based empathy (Bower, 1990), although, as with all personality characteristics, it is influenced by experience as well. Psychologist Carl Jung suggested that the impulse toward altruism is part of the collective wisdom that we all have. This is another way of saying that it is an original part of our spirit. The hypothesis that there is truly a genetic basis for empathy is supported by the fact that newborn babies cry in response to the cry of other babies, but not in response to computer simulations or tape recordings of their own cries. The development of empathy seems to occur in stages, which appear at particular ages of life. By age two, however, there are already wide differences in the degree of empathy shown by different babies (Luks & Payne, 1992). However, the fact that all babies exhibit some degree of empathy suggests that the capacity for empathy is innate and that it will someday be found to be located in a particular part of the brain.

Self-Complexity

Self-complexity is the presence of multiple roles in our lives, rather than just one, all-consuming role. The adage "don't put all your eggs in one basket" appears to be a wise one. If an individual has only one focus for her energies—say, her role as a mother—problems in that area will seem to pervade her entire life. If, however, she is also an employee, a volunteer, a neighbor, a friend and a lover, her focus is not so concentrated, and any problems with her children may be balanced by smoother sailing in the other areas of her life. Of course, the taking on of multiple roles can be carried to an extreme—in which case, role overload will occur.

The idea that developing many aspects of the self and spirit helps to protect the body from depression and other effects of stress is supported by a series of studies done by Patricia Linville (1985, 1987), professor of psychology at Duke University. Linville made a list of 33 different descriptors (such as noisy, quiet, outgoing, and playful) and asked a group of male and female students to indicate which descriptors applied to them in their various roles, such as friend, son, daughter, student, and employee. Linville looked at both the number of descriptors students used for themselves and the ways in which the descriptors were distributed over the various roles in order to determine the students' degree of self-complexity. Linville then set up an experiment involving situations wherein the students would experience feelings of both failure and success. Linville found that the individuals who had scored higher in self-complexity experienced fewer highs in their mood following successes and fewer lows in mood following failures. In contrast, the people who had scored lower in self-complexity experienced more severe mood swings in response to successes and failures. Although the students who were low in complexity were not happier or sadder overall, they had less emotional balance in their lives. In a separate study, Linville monitored the health status of a group of high-complexity students and a group of low-complexity students (male and female) for a period of time. She found that the more complex students had fewer symptoms of depression, fewer physical symptoms, and fewer incidences of flu and other illnesses than the less complex students. Linville's findings are thus consistent with those of Moen et al. (1989), who also found that people with multiple roles enjoy greater health, and live longer, than people with less complex lives.

Linville's work led her to postulate that people's self-esteem might vary in regard to the various roles they played. She tested this and determined (1985) that people do, indeed, appear to esteem themselves differently in the disparate aspects of their lives.

Renowned psychologist Lawrence LeShan maintains that becoming our authentic selves supports our biological healing systems. The term *authentic self* refers to a persona that reflects and expresses one's true spirit. It seems unlikely that our authentic selves can be expressed in the context of a one-dimensional being. Piero Ferrucci (1982), a leading psychotherapist, has written:

> Each of us is a crowd. There can be the rebel and the intellectual, the seducer and the housewife, the saboteur and the aesthete, the organizer and the bon vivant—each with its own mythology, and all more or less comfortably crowded into one single person. (p. 244)

It is likely that we are innately complex spirits. As we strive to meet various, and sometimes contradictory, needs, we develop aspects that may, at times, seem incompatible with each other. Thus, our spirit encompasses both loving and assertive aspects, as well as open and self-protective ones. These co-exist in us, making us richer for their presence. We express our authenticity by accessing different aspects of ourselves in different situations and by accepting all of them as part of our wholeness.

Spirit, Socioeconomic Status, and Health

Socioeconomic status is a function of education and income. The positive correlation (Pincus & Callahan, 1985) between poor health and low socioeconomic status (SEC) has been recognized for many years (see Chapter 2). It has been argued that people of low socioeconomic status have inferior health status because they lack access to high-quality medical care (Antonovsky, 1968). However, in the United Kingdom, access to high-quality healthcare is equal among socioeconomic levels, yet disparities in health status continue to widen (Marmot & McDowell, 1986). Although lifestyle choices and risk factors undoubtedly influence the morbidity and mortality among lower SEC people, Pincus and Callahan (1995) reviewed the literature on health and SEC and identified considerable evidence that mind/body factors that can be considered spiritual may be important as well. For example, (Matthews, Kelsey, Meilahn, Kuller, & Wing, 1989) found low SEC to be associated with such negative mental and emotional factors as anger, depression, low self-esteem, job dissatisfaction, low levels of social support, and pessimism—all of which undermine one's spirit and zest for life. Although there are a number of possible causes of poor health among individuals in lower socioeconomic classes, the research suggests that attention must be paid to the emotional/spiritual contributors to morbidity and mortality, as well as to the physical and behavioral ones.

Spiritual Wellness Self-Assessment

The following questions are designed to help you estimate your own degree of spiritual wellness. The more questions for which you have an answer other than "I don't know," the higher your level of spiritual wellness is likely to be.

1. *What is your purpose in life?*
2. *What activities do you do regularly that bring you joy?*
3. *Do you believe in a higher power?*
4. *Who can you count on for encouragement and/or support?*
5. *To whom do you give encouragement and/or support?*
6. *Who loves you?*
7. *Whom do you love or care about?*
8. *In what areas are you growing?*
9. *What activities nurture you?*
10. *Is there something that you do just for yourself every day?*
11. *How do you go about forgiving yourself?*
12. *How do you go about forgiving others?*
13. *To whom do you confide your hopes, dreams, and pain?*
14. *What do you hope for in the future?*
15. *What do you do regularly just for fun?*
16. *When do you reach out to people?*
17. *What goal(s) do you have for six months from now?*
18. *What goal(s) do you have for two years from now?*
19. *Do you look forward to getting up in the morning?*
20. *Would you like to live to be 100?*

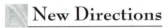

New Directions

Current research efforts are aimed at identifying the mechanisms by which the body, mind, and spirit influence and affect each other. Studies are being conducted that investigate the ways in which the expression of emotion brings about changes in immune function. An example is a study being conducted in California, in conjunction with the University of California and a prestigious medical center. The study is the California Pacific Medical Center's Breast Cancer Personal Support/Lifestyle Intervention Trial. In this clinical trial, the participants are women who were randomly selected from a group of women with breast cancer who volunteered for the study. The women currently participating in the study are assigned to one of two groups: the traditional support group or the integrated support group. The traditional support group meets for 90 minutes each week to share and talk. There is no intended spiritual component to their care. The women in the integrated support group, however, are encouraged to deepen the ways in which they experience themselves. They use such modalities as meditation, prayer, art, movement, and hands-on healing to connect at heart level to an innate life force, which may have the power to heal. Researchers will track the physical, psychological, and emotional well-being of the women in both groups for a number of years, in order to discern whether differences emerge (Kiesling, 1999).

QUESTIONS FOR REFLECTION AND DISCUSSION

1. *What is your personal definition of spirituality?*
2. *What are your views on the effect the organized religions have had on women's welfare?*
3. *To what degree do you think thoughts, emotions, beliefs, and attitudes affect health?*
4. *Would you like to change any aspects of your spirituality? If so, which ones, and why?*
5. *With which major tenets of this chapter do you agree or disagree, and why?*

RESOURCES

Books

Anderson, S., & Hopkins, P. (1992). *The feminine face of god: The unfolding of the sacred in women.* New York: Bantam Doubleday Dell Publishing.

Benson, H. (1997). *Timeless healing: The power and biology of belief.* New York: Simon & Schuster.

Cousins, N. (1983). *The healing heart.* New York: Avon Books.

Domar, A. D., & Dreher, H. (1999). *Healing mind, healthy woman: Using the mind-body connection to manage stress and take control of your life.* New York: Bantam Doubleday Dell.

Dreher, H. (1995). *The immune power personality—Seven traits you can develop to stay healthy.* New York: Dutton (Penguin).

Kidd, S. M. (1996). *The dance of the dissident daughter. A woman's journey from christian tradition to the sacred feminine.* New York: HarperCollins.

Lesser, E. (1999). *The new American spirituality.* New York: Random House.

Ornish, D. (1990). *Dr. Dean Ornish's program for reversing heart disease.* New York: Ivy Books.

Ornish, D. (1998). *Love and survival: 8 pathways to intimacy and health.* New York: HarperPerennial.

Websites

Ontario Consultants for Religious Tolerance, founded by Bruce Robinson. Dedicated to promoting religious tolerance and understanding. Contains numerous essays addressing a wide variety of religions, faith groups, and ethical systems: www.religioustolerance.org

Pluralism Project, founded by Professor Diana Eck of Harvard University. Also dedicated to promoting understanding among people of diverse spiritual backgrounds: www.pluralism.org

Spirituality and Health magazine: www.SpiritualityHealth.com

Under Shekhina's Wings, a cross-cultural and interfaith women's spirituality site. Contains links to organizations seeking the advancement of women in a number of major religions: www.geocities.com/Athens/1501/sheckfil.html

Women's Ordination Conference, a Catholic organization seeking the full ordination of women as priests: www.womensordination.org

REFERENCES

Abramson, L., McClelland, D. C., Brown, D., & Kelner, S. (1991). Alexithymic characteristics and metabolic control in diabetic and healthy adults. *Journal of Nervous and Mental Disease, 179*(8), 490–494.

Almada, S. J., Zonderman, A. B., Shekelle, R. B., Dyer, A. R., Daviglus, M. L., Costa, P. T., & Stamler, J. (1991). Neuroticism and cynicism and risk of death in middle-aged men: The Western Electric Study. *Psychosomatic Medicine, 53,* 165–175.

Antonovsky, A. (1968). Social class and the major cardiovascular diseases. *Journal of Chronic Diseases, 21,* 65–106.

Benson, H. (1975). *The relaxation response.* New York: William Morrow.

Benson, H. (1996). *Timeless healing: The power and biology of belief.* New York: Simon & Schuster.

Benson, H., Beary, J. F., & Carol, M. P. (1974). The relaxation response. *Psychiatry, 37*(1), 37–46.

Berkel, J., & de Waard, F. (1983). Mortality pattern and life expectancy of seventh day adventists in the Netherlands. *International Journal of Epidemiology, 12*(4), 455–459.

Borysenko, J. Z. (1985). Healing motives: An interview with David C. McClelland. *Advances, 2*(2), 29–41.

Bower, B. (1990). Getting out from number one. *Science News, 137,* 266–267.

Byrd, R.C. (1988). Positive therapeutic effects of intercessory prayer in a coronary care unit population. *Southern Medical Journal, 81*(7), 826–829.

Dossey, L. (1997). *Be careful what you pray for; you just might get it: What we can do about the unintentional effects of our thoughts, prayers and wishes.* New York: HarperCollins.

Ferrucci, P. (1982). *What we may be: Techniques for psychological and spiritual growth through psychosynthesis.* Los Angeles: Jeremy P. Tarcher/Perigee Books.

Friedman, M., & Rosenman, R. H. (1974). *Type A behavior and your heart.* New York: Ballentine.

Geerling, S., & Hoepelman, S. E. (1999). Immune dysfunction in patients with diabetes mellitus. *FEMS Immunology in Medicine and Microbiology, 26*(3–4), 259–265.

Greer, S., & Morris, T. (1975). Psychological attributes of women who develop breast cancer: A controlled study. *Journal of Psychosomatic Research, 19,* 147–153.

Greer, S., Morris, T., Pettingale, K. W., & Haybittle, J. (1993). Mental attitudes to cancer: An additional prognostic factor. *Lancet, 1,* 49–50.

Gross, R. M. (1993). *Buddhism after patriarchy: A feminist history, analysis and reconstruction of Buddhism.* Albany: State University of New York Press.

Harris, W. S., Gowda, M., Kolb, J. W., Strychacz, C. P., Vacek, J. L., Jones, P. G., Forker, A., O'Keefe, J. H., & McCallister, B. D. (1999). A randomized, controlled trial of the effects of remote, intercessory prayer on outcomes in patients admitted to the coronary care unit. *Archives of Internal Medicine, 159*(19), 2273–2278.

Hart, K. E. (1996). Perceived availability of different types of social support among cynically hostile women. *Journal of Clinical Psychology, 52,* 383–387.

Herman, B. H., & Panksepp, J. (1978). Effects of morphine and naloxone on separation distress and approach attachment: Evidence for opiate mediation of social affect. *Pharmacology Biochemistry and Behavior, 9,* 213–220.

House, J. S., Landis, K. R., & Umberson, D. (1988). Social relationships and health. *Science, 241,* 540–545.

House, J. S., Robbins, C., & Metzner, H. L. (1982). The association of social relationships and activities with mortality: Prospective evidence from the Tecumseh community health study. *American Journal of Epidemiology, 116,* 123–140.

Jamner, L., Schwartz, G. E., & Leigh, H. (1988).The relationship between repressive and defensive coping styles and monocyte, eosinophil, and serum glucose levels: Support for the opioid peptide hypothesis of repression. *Psychosomatic Medicine, 50,* 567–575.

Jamner, L. D., & Schwartz, G. E. (1986). Self-deception predicts self-report and endurance of pain. *Psychosomatic Medicine, 48,* 211–223.

Jensen, M. R. (1987). Psychobiological factors predicting the course of cancer. *Journal of Personality, 55*(2), 317–342.

Kaplan, S. H., Greenfield, S. S., & Ware, J. E. (1989). Assessing the effects of physician-patient interactions on the outcomes of disease. *Medical Care, 27*(Suppl. 3), S110–S127.

Kiesling, S. (Winter, 1999). The most powerful healing God and women can come up with. *Spirituality and Health,* pp. 22–27.

Kneier, A. W., & Temoshok, L. (1984). Repressive coping reactions in patients with malignant melanoma as compared to cardiovascular disease patients. *Journal of Psychosomatic Medicine, 28*(2), 145–155.

Kobasa, S. C. (1979). Stressful life events, personality and health: An inquiry into hardiness. *Journal of Personality and Social Psychology, 37,* 1–11.

Kobasa, S. C. (1984, September). How much stress can you survive? *American Health,* pp. 14–15.

Kobasa, S. C., Maddi, S., & Kahn, S. (1982). Hardiness and health: A prospective study. *Journal of Personality and Social Psychology, 42,* 168–177.

Kobasa, S. C., Maddi, S. R., Puccetti, M. C., & Zola, M. A. (1985). Effectiveness of hardiness, exercise, and social support as resources against illness. *Journal of Psychosomatic Research, 29,* 525–533.

Koenig, H. G. (1999). Does religious attendence prolong survival? A six year follow-up study of 3,968 adults. *Journal of Gerontological, Biological and Medical Science, 54*(7), 1730–1736.

Kreiden, A. J., et al. (1986). Infective complications of aplastic anemia. *British Journal of Haematology, 63,* 503–506.

Lepore, S. J. (1995). Cynicism, social support, and cardiovascular reactivity. *Health Psychology, 14,* 210–216.

Levin, J. S. (1996). How religion influences morbidity and health: Reflections on natural history, salutogenesis and host resistance. *Social Science and Medicine, 43*(5), 849–864.

Levin, J. S., & Schiller, P. L. (1987). Is there a religious factor in health? *Journal of Religion and Health, 26,* 9–36.

Linville, P. W. (1985). Self-complexity and affective extremity: Don't put all of your eggs in one cognitive basket. *Social Cognition, 3*(1), 94–120.

Linville, P. W. (1987). Self-complexity as a cognitive buffer against stress-related illness and depression. *Journal of Personality and Social Psychology, 52*(4), 663–676.

Lisspers, J., Nygren, A., & Soderman, E. (1998). Psychological patterns in patients with coronary heart disease, chronic pain and respiratory disorder. *Scandinavian Journal of Caring Science, 12,* 25–31.

Luks, A., & Payne, P. (1992). *The healing power of doing good.* New York: Fawcett Columbine.

Magaletta, P. R., & Oliver, J. M. (1999). The hope construct, will, and ways: Their relations with self-efficacy, optimism, and general well-being. *Journal of Clinical Psychology, 55*(5), 539–551.

Mahowald, M. B. (Ed.) (1994). *Philosophy of woman: An anthology of classic to current concepts* (3rd ed.). Indianapolis: Hackett.

Marmot, M. G., & McDowell, M. E. (1986). Mortality decline and widening social inequalities. *Lancet, 2,* 274–276.

Matarazzo, J. D. (1984). Behavioral immunogens and pathogens in health and illness. In B. L. Hammods & C. J. Scheirer (Eds.), *Psychology and health* (pp. 5–43). New York: Viking.

Matthews, D. (1998). *The faith factor.* New York: Viking Penguin.

Matthews, D. A., Larson, D. B., & Barry, C. P. (1993). *The faith factor: An annotated bibliography of clinical research on spiritual subjects* (Vol I). Washington, DC: American Psychological Association.

Matthews, K. A., Kelsey, S. F., Meilahn, E. N., Kuller L. H., & Wing, R. R. (1989). Educational attainment and behavioral and biological risk factors for coronary heart disease in middle-aged women. *American Journal of Epidemiology, 129,* 132–144.

McClelland, D. C. (1979). Inhibited power motivation and high blood pressure in men. *Journal of Abnormal Psychology, 88,* 182–190.

McClelland, D. C. (1986). Some reflections on the two psychologies of love. *Journal of Personality, 54,* 334–353.

McClelland, D. C., Floor, E., Davidson, R. J., & Saron, S. (1980). Stressed power motivation, sympathetic activation, immune function and illness. *Journal of Human Stress, 6*(2), 11–19.

McClelland, D. C., & Jemmott, J. B. (1980). Power motivation, stress and physical illness. *Journal of Human Stress, 6*(4), 6–15.

McClelland, D. C., & Kirshnit, C. (1988). The effect of motivational arousal through films on salivary immunoglobulin A. *Psychology and Health, 2,* 31–52.

McCullough, M. E, Hoyt, W. T., Larson, D. B., Kpenig, H. G., & Thorensen, C. (2000). Religious involvement and mortality: A meta-analytic review. *Health Psychology, 19*(3), 211–222.

McKay, J. R. (1991). Assessing aspects of object relations associated with immune function: Development of the affiliative trust-mistrust coding system. *Psychological Assessment, 3*(4), 641–647.

McKay, J. R. (1992). Affiliative trust-mistrust. In C. P. Smith, J. W. Atkinson, & D. C. McClelland (Eds.), *Motivation and personality: Handbook of thematic content analysis* (pp. 47–54). New York: Cambridge University Press.

Moen, P., Dempster-McClain, D., & Williams, R. M. (1989). Social integration and longevity: An event history analysis of women's roles and resilience. *American Sociological Review, 54,* 635–647.

Moen, P., Dempster-McCain, D., & Williams, R. M. (1992). Successful aging: A life course perspective on women's multiple roles and health. *American Journal of Sociology, 97*(6), 1612–1638.

Moos, R. H., & Solomon, G. F. (1965). Psychologic comparisons between women with rheumatoid arthritis and their non-arthritic sisters: I. Personality test and interview rating data. *Psychosomatic Medicine, 27,* 135–149; II. Content analysis of interviews. *Psychosomatic Medicine, 27,* 150–164.

Oliner, S., & Oliner, P. (1988). *The altruistic personality: Rescuers of Jews in Nazi Europe.* New York: Macmillan/Free Press.

Ornish, D. (1990). *Dr. Dean Ornish's program for reversing heart disease.* New York: Ivy Books.

Ornish, D. (1998). *Love and survival: 8 pathways to intimacy and health.* New York: HarperPerennial.

Oulette, S. C. (1993). Inquiries into hardiness. In L. Goldberger & S. Breznitz (Eds.), *Handbook of stress: Theoretical and clinical aspects* (2nd ed., pp. 242–248). New York: Free Press.

Oxman, T. (1995). Lack of social participation or religious strength and comfort as risk factors for death after cardiac surgery in the elderly. *Psychosomatic Medicine, 57,* 5–15.

Pennebaker, J. W. (1990). *Opening up: The healing power of confiding in others.* New York: William Morrow.

Pennebaker, J. W., & Beall, S. (1986). Confronting a traumatic event: Toward an understanding of inhibition and disease. *Journal of Abnormal Psychology, 95,* 274–281.

Pennebaker, J. W., Colder, M., & Sharp, L. K. (1990). Accelerating the coping process. *Journal of Personality and Social Psychology, 58,* 528–537.

Pennebaker, J. W., Hughes, C., & O'Heeron, R. C. (1987). The psychophysiology of confession: Linking inhibitory and psychosomatic processes. *Journal of Personality and Social Psychology, 52,* 781–793.

Pennebaker, J. W., Kiecolt-Glaser, J. K., & Glaser, R. (1988). Disclosure of traumas and immune function: Health implications for psychotherapy. *Journal of Consulting and Clinical Psychology, 56,* 239–245.

Pert, C. (1997). *Molecules of Emotion.* New York: Scribner.

Pincus, T., & Callahan, L. F. (1985). Formal education as a marker for increased mortality and morbidity in rheumatoid arthritis. *Journal of Chronic Diseases, 38,* 973–984.

Pincus, T., & Callahan, L. F. (1995). What explains the association between socioeconomic status and health: Primarily access to medical care or mind-body variables? *Advances: The Journal of Mind-Body Health, 11*(1), 4–36.

Schwartz, G. E. (1983). Disregulation theory and disease: Applications to the repression/cerebral disconnection/cardiovascular disorder hypothesis. *International Review of Applied Psychology, 32,* 95–118.

Schwartz, G. E. (1990). Psychobiology of repression and health: A systems approach. In J. L. Singer (Ed.), *Repression and dissociation: Implications for personality theory, psychopathology, and health* (pp. 340–347). Chicago: University of Chicago Press.

Shavit, Y., et al. (1984). Opioid peptides mediate the suppressive effect of stress on natural killer cell cytotoxicity. *Science, 223,* 188–190.

Shavit, Y., et al. (1985). Stress, opioid peptides, the immune system, and cancer. *Journal of Immunology, 135*(2), 834–837.

Seeman, T. E., & Syme, S. L. (1987). Social networks and coronary artery disease, a comparison of the structure and function of social relations as predictors of disease. *Psychosomatic Medicine, 49*(4), 341–354.

Solomon, G. F. (1981). Emotional and personality factors in the onset and course of autoimmune disease, particularly rheumatoid arthritis. In R. Ader (Ed.), *Psychoneuroimmunology.* (pp. 361–384). New York: Academic Press.

Solomon, G. F., & Moos, R. H. (1965). The relationship of personality to the presence of rheumatoid factor in asymptomatic relatives of patients with rheumatoid arthritis. *Psychosomatic Medicine, 27,* 350–360.

Solomon, G. F., Temoshok, L., O'Leary, A., & Zich, J. (1987). An intensive psychoimmunologic study of long-surviving persons with AIDS. *Annals of the New York Academy of Sciences, 496,* 647–655.

Spiegel, D., et al. (1989). Effect of psychosocial treatment on survival of patients with metastatic breast cancer. *Lancet, 2,* 888–891.

Temoshok, L. (1985). Biopsychosocial studies on cutaneous malignant melanoma: Psychosocial factors associated with prognostic indicators, progression, psychophysiology, and tumor-host response. *Social Science and Medicine, 20(8),* 833–840.

Temoshok, L., & Dreher, H. (1992). *The type C connection: The behavioral links to cancer and your health.* New York: Random House.

Torjesen, K. J. (1993). *When women were priests: Women's leadership in the early church and the scandal of their subordination in the rise of Christianity.* San Francisco: Harper.

Williams, R. (1989). *The trusting heart.* New York: Times Books.

28

Supporting Body/Mind/Spirit at the End of Life

Rhada Artz Hartman and Marian C. Condon

CHAPTER OUTLINE

 ## Objectives

1. *Identify five elements of a good death.*
2. *List six fears or concerns common to dying people.*
3. *List six obligations healthcare providers have to dying patients.*
4. *List and describe the phases of grief.*
5. *Identify two things friends and relatives can do to be helpful to persons in each phase of the grieving process.*

Introduction

This chapter addresses two inevitable and natural processes that human beings go through: death and grief. It explores the ways in which people commonly respond to these processes, physically, mentally, emotionally, socially, and spir-

itually, and ways in which friends, family, and caregivers can be helpful to those who are dying or grieving.

Death

Death is far less visible in contemporary America than it was in earlier times. In the seventeenth century, for example, sophisticated medical care was nonexistent, communicable diseases abounded, and there were no labor laws protecting workers from dangerous conditions in mines, factories, and other places of employment. Infant and child mortality was high, and the average life expectancy was only around 40 years (Apple, 1990). Death was an all-too-familiar process, as dying individuals were cared for in their homes, and it was family members who prepared the bodies of the dead for burial. Today, however, science and technology allow us to maintain the

---

illusion that we have conquered death. Many once fatal diseases and injuries are merely inconvenient today. Moreover, we are insulated from the realities of death once it has occurred. Eighty percent of people die in hospitals (Stewart, Teno, Patrick, & Lynn, 1999), and, after death, professional morticians preside over death rituals and practices. Consequently, we have become uncomfortable with even the subject of death. The language we use in discussing death both reveals and shapes our attitudes toward it: We say that people have passed on, passed over, passed away, or expired. We say that they are resting in peace or in eternal slumber. We do not say they died and are dead. Our overall unfamiliarity and discomfort with death mean that we are often at a loss when called on to comfort friends or family members who are dying. Worse, we are usually ill prepared for the inevitable end of our own lives. Despite our squeamishness about it, however, death has its positive aspects. For example, the knowledge that we will one day die helps us savor life, and it is the possibility of death that gives meaning to certain forms of courage. Finally, death reveals the importance of intimacy in our lives.

People become aware that they are dying in a number of ways: Sometimes a caregiver, a family member, or a friend simply tells an individual that she is dying. Sometimes, dying people overhear comments made by healthcare personnel or sense changes in the behavior of others: physicians may start to visit less frequently, or distant loved ones may suddenly arrive on the scene. There may be changes in medical care, with different medications being administered or surgery canceled. The person may be moved to another room, sent home, or transferred to an extended care facility. Sometimes there are signals from within the body that are interpreted as fatal on the basis of something the person has read or experienced with another person. Sometimes, future-oriented discussions are suddenly responded to with reluctance or avoided by friends and family. Regardless of how it is revealed, the knowledge of impending death precipitates a *crisis* for the dying person (Weisman, 1988b). In confronting the crisis, the patient faces limit, loss, and change.

Psychological Responses to Terminal Illness

A person newly apprised of her impending death typically experiences a variety of emotional reactions (Heaven & Maguire, 1998). Prominent among such reactions is a sense of *loss:* loss of control, independence, productivity, security, and future existence, as well as loss of various types of psychological, physical, and cognitive abilities. People may also feel they have lost the ability to complete plans and projects, their dreams and hopes for the future, significant others, and aspects of themselves and their identities. Dying people also typically experience *anxiety* and *fear.* They may fear loneliness, loss of self-control, disability, suffering and pain, the process of dying alone, decomposition, or premature burial. Dying individuals may also experience *depression, anger,*

guilt, and *shame.* Dying individuals struggle with many of the same feelings mourners have after a death, and the same process of grieving must occur. There is a need to identify losses, express feelings, and review unfinished business. Like other mourners, dying people require permission to grieve from their loved ones and caregivers. Many achieve resolution and *acceptance,* but some do not.

A person's response to the knowledge of impending death is not linear; it is characterized by waxing and waning emotional and cognitive responses (Chochinov, Tataryn, Clinch, & Dudgeon, 1999). Many people become somewhat ambivalent about dying; fearful avoidance may coexist with the desire for an end to fear and suffering and a wish to begin a new existence in another realm.

Signs of Approaching Death

When a terminally ill person approaches death, she experiences a process that involves all the aspects of her being: physical, mental/emotional, and spiritual. The *body* begins the final process of shutting down, which will end when all its systems stop working. There is a normal, natural progression to the shutting down process, which involves physical and behavioral changes (Long, 1996). The *mind* and *spirit* begin the final process of releasing from the body, and from attachments—to people, roles, the environment, possessions, and so on. This release may be delayed until unfinished business has been completed and permission to let go has been received from loved ones. Caregivers and loved ones can serve the dying person by accepting and encouraging the releasing processes. Death will occur when the body and spirit have finished these processes. Learning about the dying process and what to expect as it unfolds can enable us to be maximally helpful to loved ones and others who have come to the end of their lives.

INWARD FOCUS

Dying persons increasingly withdraw their focus from the external world and refocus inwardly. They lose interest in the details of other people's lives, and become increasingly disinterested in seeing or conversing with all but caregivers and loved ones. Very close friends and family members may have to explain this phenomenon to more distant friends and acquaintances who attempt to visit and are rejected, or who do visit and experience the dying person as remote.

COOLNESS AND COLOR CHANGE

The dying person's hands, arms, feet, and legs may become increasingly cool to the touch. At the same time, the *color* of the skin may change. The underside of the body may become darker, and the skin may become mottled. This is a normal indication that the circulation of blood is decreasing to the body's extremities and is being reserved for the most vital organs. Comfort care should include keeping the dying person *warm* with a blanket. The use of electric blankets should be avoided, however, because excessive heat can damage poorly perfused tissues.

SLEEPING MORE

The dying person may spend an increasing amount of time sleeping and appear to be uncommunicative or unresponsive and at times difficult to arouse. Care should include sitting with the dying person and holding her hand. Caregivers should not shake or speak loudly to the dying person, but rather speak softly and naturally. Others must never assume the person cannot hear; hearing is thought to be the last of the senses to be lost.

DISORIENTATION

Dying people may become confused about the time, place, and identity of the people surrounding them. Caregivers should *identify themselves by name* before they speak and then speak softly, clearly, and truthfully when needing to communicate something important. An example of a concise, clear statement is "Mary, I need to turn you over now, so that your side doesn't get sore."

INCONTINENCE

The person may lose control of urine or bowel matter as the muscles in that area begin to relax. Care should include protection of the skin and frequent cleansing with proper drying. The dying patient's *dignity* should be maintained.

CONGESTION

Gurgling sounds coming from the chest may be heard and may become very loud. This is due to an inability to cough up normal secretions. Care should include allowing gravity to drain the secretions. Gently wiping the mouth with a moist cloth is also helpful. The sound of congestion does not indicate the onset of severe or new pain.

RESTLESSNESS

The dying person may appear restless and make repetitive motions, such as pulling at the bedclothes or clothing. This often happens and is due, in part, to decreasing circulation and oxygen supply to the brain. Caregivers should not interfere with or restrain such motions. Speaking in a calm, quiet manner; reading to the person; playing soothing music; or lightly massaging the forehead may allay the restlessness.

DECREASED INTAKE OF FOOD AND LIQUIDS

The dying person may have a decrease in appetite and thirst, wanting little or nothing to eat or drink. Trying to force nourishment into the person is inappropriate and may result in fear or nausea. Artificial nutrition and hydration are unnecessary and may prolong the dying process.

DECREASED URINATION AND CHANGES IN BREATHING PATTERN

The urine output in the dying person normally decreases and the urine may become darker as the person takes in less liquid.

Breathing may become faster, slower, or irregular. Sometimes, the dying person appears to be panting. A series of shallow breaths followed by an absence of breathing for up to 30 seconds is also not unusual. Elevating the person's head may ease breathing.

Promoting a Good Death

The experience of dying is unique for each individual; however, Weisman (1988a) defines a "good" death as *pain free,* with a minimum of emotional and social impoverishment. The dying person should be able to function as effectively as possible for as long as possible before dying. Conflicts should be recognized and resolved, and remaining wishes should be satisfied. Control should be yielded only to others in whom the dying person has confidence. Care is most effective when the patient's lifestyle is maintained and her philosophy of life is respected. The complexity of treatment and the need for time-consuming procedures can interfere with interactions with family, but the dying person and family need privacy and time to be together. Under no circumstances should a dying person be left to die in isolation. Individuals facing death frequently search for meaning in their lives; spiritual support of a nature acceptable to the person is essential. In their study of correlates of spiritual well-being in terminally ill patients, Pace and Stables (1997) found that the best predictors of spiritual well-being were social support (positive correlation) and loneliness (negative correlation). They also found that, in comparison with patients dying of cancer and other chronic diseases, persons dying from acquired immune deficiency syndrome (AIDS) (see Chapter 20) reported more loneliness, had fewer sources of social support, and were less satisfied with their sources of support. Therefore, attending to the spiritual concerns of a person dying of AIDS may be particularly important. Providing what is known as palliative care is crucial to fostering a good death. Appropriate behaviors on the part of family members and friends is also very important.

Palliative Care

When cure and remission are no longer possible, intervention must shift to palliative care. Palliative care is designed to control physical and emotional pain and provide personal support for the patient and the family. Palliative care requires only a limited use of technology. Extensive personal care and an ordering of the physical and social environment are therapeutic in themselves. Research suggests that many people who are dying of a chronic illness would prefer to die at home, rather than in a hospital, and that some who would prefer to die at home are unable to do so. Older women are less likely to die at home than older men, possibly because men tend to be less efficient than women as caregivers (Grande, Addington-Hall, & Todd, 1998). Dying persons who do not access home-care palliative services, often called hospice services, are more likely to die away from their homes than patients who do. Whatever the setting in which the dying process unfolds, caregivers must remember that a dying person is still alive and should be treated as such.

A series of focus groups held with patients with terminal illnesses, family members, and hospice physicians and nurses has yielded information about how physicians can best meet the needs of their dying patients (Wenrich et al., 2001). The following areas were found to be of central importance: talking with patients in a straightforward and honest way, being willing to discuss death and dying with patients who are ready, being sensitive to patients' readiness, giving bad news in a sensitive manner, and listening to patients and encouraging questions. Unfortunately, however, physicians are often inadequately trained in caring for dying patients (MacCleod, 2001). Medicine has historically been cure-focused, and physicians sometimes feel helpless and withdraw from patients once it becomes obvious that cure is not possible.

The experiences of some groups in American culture may make them less accepting of the palliative care concept. Members of medically underserved groups have long suffered discrimination regarding healthcare (see Chapter 2) and may interpret a recommendation for palliative care as an attempt to deny them optimal medical care. For example, research indicates that black persons suffering a terminal illness are twice as likely as their white counterparts to request life-prolonging treatments that will cause fruitless suffering for them and their families (Mouton, Teno, Mor, & Piette, 1997). Morrison and her colleagues (1998) found that most of the elderly African American and Hispanic participants they interviewed at a senior center in New York City equated less aggressive treatment with abandonment. Gessert, Curry, and Robinson (2001) found that, among a population of nursing home residents with severe cognitive impairment, feeding tubes were used in 10.1 percent of the Euro-American residents and 38.9 percent of the African American residents. Feeding tubes are used to prolong life in persons who can no longer eat.

Adequate pain control is the cornerstone of palliative care, yet pain is inadequately controlled in many dying individuals. Tolle and her colleagues (2000) interviewed 475 family caregivers several months after their loved ones had died. One-third reported that pain had been a problem for the person for whom they had cared. A number of barriers to adequate pain control have been identified. In a study done by Byock and Torma (2000), many of the physicians and nurses surveyed were poorly informed regarding pain assessment techniques and control strategies. On the basis of

their survey of 50 medical textbooks representing multiple specialty areas, Rabow, Hardie, Fair, and McPhee (2000) concluded that medical education regarding end-of-life care is inadequate. Ethnicity can also be a barrier to pain control. For example, in some cultures, pain is seen as a sign that the body is fighting to recover, whereas, in others, it is regarded as a punishment or character builder (Post, Blustein, Gordon, & Dubler, 1996). Members of historically oppressed ethnic groups may reject drug therapy regimens that suppress pain because such regimens may also shorten life (Mitty, 2001). Low socioeconomic status can also be a barrier to adequate pain control. A recent study of pharmacies in low-income neighborhoods revealed that such pharmacies often fail to stock the opioid drugs that are most effective in relieving pain (Morrison, Wallenstein, Natale, Senzel, & Huang, 2000).

The American Medical Association's Institute for Ethics has identified eight elements of good terminal care that dying patients have the right to expect:

1. *The opportunity to discuss end-of-life care, including the opportunity to prepare a living will*
2. *The assurance that physical and mental suffering will be alleviated and that specialists in the control of suffering will be consulted if necessary*
3. *Assurance that preferences for withholding or withdrawing life-sustaining intervention will be honored*
4. *Assurance that the physician will not abandon the patient and that high-quality terminal care will be provided until life has ended*
5. *Assurance that providing for the preservation of dignity will be a priority*
6. *Assurance that a sufficient level of community support will be available to provide for palliative care, including hospice or home care, without an overwhelming burden being placed on family members*
7. *Assurance that patients' personal goals will have reasonable priority, whether they are to communicate with family members or to attend to spiritual needs*
8. *Assurance that care providers will assist the bereaved through the early stages of mourning and adjustment*

Dying persons have other rights as well (see Box 28–1). One such right is to honest answers to questions about diagnosis and prognosis. Although at one time it was commonplace to keep a terminal diagnosis from patients, such deception is no longer considered acceptable, at least among Euro-Americans, as it undermines patients' dignity and autonomy. In some ethnic subcultures, however, persons suffering from fatal illnesses are not told of their condition. Korean Americans and Mexican Americans may believe that to tell a person of her impending death causes unnecessary suffering and the loss of hope. They may also feel that the family, not the patient, bears the burden of making decisions about treatment (Blackhall,

Box 28–1   The Dying Person's Bill of Rights

- I have the right to be treated as a human being as long as I am alive.
- I have the right to maintain an evolving sense of hope.
- I have the right to be cared for by those who can also maintain an evolving sense of hope.
- I have the right to express, in my own way, the unique feelings and emotions related to my approaching death.
- I have the right to participate in decision making concerning my care.
- I have the right to expect continuing care from nurses and physicians, even though "cure" goals must be changed to "comfort" goals.
- I have the right to die in the comforting presence of others, rather than alone.
- I have the right to have my pain controlled.

- I have the right to ask any and all questions and to have them answered honestly.
- I have the right to be told the truth.
- I have the right to help from and for my family in accepting my death.
- I have the right to die in peace and with my dignity respected.
- I have a right to my individuality and to not be judged for making decisions with which others may disagree.
- I have the right to discuss and expand my spiritual experiences in any way I choose, regardless of the views of others.
- I have the right to expect that the sanctity of my body will be respected after death.
- I have the right to be cared for by humane and knowledgeable people who will attempt to understand and meet my needs.

Source: Reprinted/Adapted with permission from Aspen Reference Group. The Dying Patient's Bill of Rights. The palliative care patient and family counseling manual, Copyright 1996, Gaithersburg, MD: Aspen Publishers.

Murphy, Frank, Michel, & Azen, 1995). People from some Asian communities may request that dying persons not be informed of the terminal nature of their illnesses (Tong & Spicer, 1994). A pervasive fear of death, and a reluctance to discuss it, is common in some Native American societies. For example, Navajo people believe that language and thought shape reality and that talking about death may invite it (Carrese & Rhoades, 1995). This belief is also held by many in Greece, China, Italy, Korea, and Mexico.

GUIDELINES FOR FAMILY AND FRIENDS

The two most important things friends and family members can do to support dying persons are to maintain a physical presence, so that the person is *not alone* and to foster honest, open communication (Stewart, Teno, Patrick, & Lynn, 1999). The goal is to create an atmosphere in which the dying person feels free to discuss any topic or to unburden herself in any way, without feeling that the friend or family member is uncomfortable with the process. Those who have not addressed and resolved their own issues related to death and dying are not the ideal persons to assist others in these areas.

Communicating Effectively Before attempting to engage a dying person in conversation, consider whether the person really *wants* to talk at that time. Keep in mind that appearances can be deceiving. Patients with eyes closed and heads buried under covers may perk up when there's a chance to converse, whereas others who appear alert and open may turn away. It is always best to ask whether the person feels like talking. It is also important to provide *privacy* before attempting to initiate a serious conversation. When the dying person indicates that she is open to conversation, sit with her and take care not to appear rushed. Maintain eye contact and remind yourself to remain open and nonjudgmental. Remember that good listeners do not give advice unless asked to. Keep in mind that the person, rather than the illness, should be the focus of the conversation. Try to elicit the person's feelings about what is happening, rather than information related to her physical state. A question such as "How are you feeling about all this, Mary?" is better than "How are you today, Mary?" Dying people must be given every opportunity to express their thoughts, feelings, and ideas about everything connected to their experience of being ill and dying. Spiritual matters, such as what might happen after death and the meaning (or lack of it) of their lives are important to many, but not all, people. It must also be kept in mind that people who did not share their feelings earlier in their lives may not wish to do so when they are dying, either. The dying person must be allowed to set the tone of the discussion. To support the dying means to travel into the world of the dying.

A number of conversational techniques can be used to facilitate conversations with dying people. One such technique is to *provide feedback* to encourage the dying person to express whatever is on her mind. To provide feedback is to repeat to the dying person a bit of what she has just said, in a tone that invites further disclosure. For example, if the dying person says, "I'm so scared," you might reply, "You're feeling scared, Mary?" Feedback shows that the listener is listening closely

Box 28–2   Open-Ended Questions

- What is this illness like for you?
- What is this illness like for your family?
- How did you handle the news that you have a serious illness?
- What do you think will happen?
- What would you like to see happen?

and is willing to hear more on the same topic. A principle to keep in mind is that good listeners help people find their own answers to difficult issues. Another helpful conversational technique is to *use open-ended questions* to initiate conversations with dying persons. Open-ended questions are questions that cannot be answered with a simple yes or no. Some useful open-ended questions are as listed in Box 28–2.

Other techniques that can be used to encourage people to talk are nodding and offering comments such as "I see," "Um hum," "Go on," and "Then what happened?" Never interrupt, but be prepared to listen if the dying person interrupts you. *Rephrasing* ambiguous words or phrases is an effective way to make sure that you understand another person correctly. For example, if a dying person were to say, "I don't want to go on with this any longer," you could say, "You mean you don't want to live any longer?" or "You mean you don't want to have chemotherapy any longer?" Expect to be at a loss for words sometimes. It is perfectly all right to say, "I don't know what to say."

The dying are extremely vulnerable and need to know they can count on others, even if their own behavior is difficult for family and friends to accept (Franklin, 1994–95). For example, the *hostility* sometimes exhibited by dying people is often a manifestation of their fear of loneliness. Ironically, hostility often drives others away. To be helpful to dying persons, you must be able to hear expressions of feelings such as *depression, anxiety* and *hopelessness* without feeling compelled to try to cheer up the person. As death approaches, it is normal for terminally ill people to begin to *withdraw* from the world, and they may disengage from all but the closest loved ones. This often indicates preparation for release and the beginning of letting go. It should not be taken personally; only affirm, support, and give permission to say goodbye.

Nonverbal communication can be an important source of solace to the dying. A gentle touch can be a powerful symbol of caring to someone who has suffered extensive weight loss and other ravages of their illness, which may cause them to feel physically unattractive. Physical touch also helps relieve the fear of being alone. Because people vary widely in their receptiveness to being touched, however, it is important to be sensitive to individual response.

ENCOURAGING LIFE REVIEW

The process known as life review can help dying people find meaning in their lives and identify any unfinished business. Life review can also help people look back on what they have learned over the years, so that those lessons can be passed on to others. Meaning borrowed from the past lends meaning to the present and future. Two essential ingredients for a successful life review are *brevity* and *emphasis on the positive*. Friends and family members can encourage a life review by asking leading questions, such as the following:

- What has life been like this past year?
- When you look back on your life and think about the really fun moments, what comes to mind?
- Do you remember a time when you felt really proud? Describe that to me.
- At what moment in your life were you most aware of the meaning of the word *love*?
- If there were one event you would like to relive, what would it be?

Photographs can also be used to initiate life review. While looking at albums or pictures with dying people, friends and relatives can pose questions such as the following:

- What key family members are not present in any of these photos?
- Are there common themes to all of these photographs?
- Is there a particular significance in the locations?
- Are key periods in your life missing in the photos selected?
- Who took the photographs?

Written messages and recordings are also potential tools for life review. Dying people can be encouraged to leave written or recorded messages for posterity. Messages can include thoughts, feelings, wishes, or desires not previously expressed and can be given to the recipients before or after the author's death. Messages can also be conveyed in the form of poetry, art, or music.

Family members and friends usually want to support dying loved ones in whatever ways they can (Berns & Colvin, 1998). They want to give permission for the loved one to let go, be present at the moment of death, and keep whatever promises they made to the dying person. Family and friends also wish to have honest, thorough communication with professional caregivers. By learning about death, dying, and the responsibilities of caregivers, we can all increase the likelihood that we, as well as people we care about, will have a good death when the time comes.

Advance Directives

An advance directive is a recognized document through which individuals can make known their wishes regarding medical care, in the event they become incapacitated. The most common forms of advance directives are living wills and the durable medical powers of attorney.

LIVING WILLS

Living wills are documents in which preferences regarding medical care in certain situations are recorded. For example, a person can indicate whether she wishes to undergo cardiopulmonary resuscitation in the event that her heart or respiratory function fails. Also, limits can be placed on the type of medical care that can be administered—for example, a person can stipulate that nourishment, but not antibiotics, be provided. Living wills should be discussed with family members and healthcare providers at the time they are prepared, so that everyone fully understands the patient's wishes. Living wills must be kept in a place known and accessible to family members; a living will can do no good if it cannot be located. The provisions of a living will are based on the individual's value system and beliefs. Its function is to speak for a person who can no longer speak for herself. Blank living will forms are available from most healthcare institutions and can be ordered from the organization Choice in Dying (see the Resources section at the end of this chapter).

DURABLE MEDICAL POWERS OF ATTORNEY

A durable medical power of attorney is a legal document that confers the power to make medical decisions on a person other than the patient herself. The individual in whom medical decision-making power has been vested is called the *proxy*. The proxy can be any adult person of the patient's choosing and does not have to be a relative. The proxy must be familiar with the patient's values and wishes concerning medical treatment in the context of a range of life-threatening scenarios.

THE EFFECTIVENESS OF ADVANCE DIRECTIVES

Instruments of patient self-determination in the form of written advance directives, such as living wills and durable medical powers of attorney, are intended to ensure that individuals' desire to accept or refuse life-sustaining treatment is known and respected. In order to be most effective, advance directives must be *known to caregivers, clearly stated,* and *comprehensive* in terms of what scenarios they cover. Unfortunately, these criteria are not always met. Physicians and nurses are sometimes unaware of patients' wishes regarding resuscitation; families may be unable to locate the directive, or it may be lost during transfer from one care setting to another (Tilden, 2000). Even if an advance directive is available, there is no guarantee that family members will fully understand the patient's wishes. Ditto et al. (2001) divided pairs of elderly outpatients and their designated surrogate decision makers (usually spouses or children) into a control group and several experimental groups. The elder-surrogate

pairs in the control group had no advance directives and did not discuss the elder's wishes regarding end-of-life care. In one of four intervention groups, the elders prepared scenario-based advance directives to which the surrogates had access. In the second intervention group, the elders prepared values-based advance directives to which the surrogates had access. In the third intervention group, the elders prepared an advance directive and discussed it with the surrogates, and, in the fourth group, no discussion took place. The elders and the surrogates in all the groups were presented with several written scenarios involving terminal illness. The elders were directed to indicate their wishes regarding treatment in each scenario, and the surrogates were asked to predict their elder's choices. The results of the study indicated that the surrogates in the advance directive groups were *not* significantly more successful at predicting elder's choices than the surrogates in the control group. The surrogates in the discussion group were more accurate in predicting their elders' choices *only* if the elder had not completed an advance directive prior to participation in the study.

Some individuals and families may be unwilling to prepare advance directives, for a variety of reasons. The advance directive form may be written at too high a reading level, or the person may prefer to discuss her wishes with her family. People in the lower socioeconomic groups are accustomed to receiving little or substandard care and may see advance directives as legal devices used by institutions to deny them care (Mitty, 2001). Hispanic persons may be more oriented to the present than the future and may believe that medical personnel are in the best position to make decisions regarding end-of-life care. Deeply religious people may feel that an advance directive would interfere with God's will.

Grief

Grief is a universal response to the loss of a loved one. The grieving process unfolds in stages, and friends and family members of grieving persons can be helpful if they understand the grieving person's needs in each stage, and what behaviors are likely to be experienced as supportive.

The Nature of Grief

Why do people grieve? Grief is a response to *loss,* which is a universally shared experience. Loss binds us together in a common cycle of suffering and healing. Loss occurs whenever we experience a change that requires giving up familiar patterns. Understanding the nature of grief and learning to cope with it ourselves, as well as help others do the same, is very useful—no one escapes loss and grief (Burnett et al., 1994). Some losses are obvious, recognized as severe and generally acknowledged by friends and family. Losses in this category include both the loss of a loved one, job, home, or valued possession and the loss of something that conferred prominence or status in one's community. Less obvious losses, however, can also trigger a grief reaction. We can lose our health, youth, beauty, stamina, energy, dreams, self-esteem, trust, sense of safety in the world, childhood, role as a husband or wife, and so on. Judith Viorst (1986) has written the following:

> For we lose not only through death, but also by leaving and being left, by changing and letting go and moving on. Our losses include not only our separations and departures from those we love, but our conscious and unconscious losses of romantic dreams, impossible expectations, illusions of freedom and power, illusions of safety and the loss of our own younger self, the self that thought it always would be unwrinkled and invulnerable and immortal (p. 68).

Grief is the painful, deeply felt emotional response to the loss of something valued or someone loved (Davis, Nolen-Hoeksema, & Larson, 1998). Grief is a part of all human experience and a natural expression of deep sadness. We feel grief because of attachment, not because of love. Love is merely a sign of attachment. The degree of grief felt is directly proportional to the degree of attachment. Grieving our losses is normal. Loss is a form of injury, and, fortunately, we are designed to heal.

Healing from grief can be a slow, painful process and can take more time to complete than was formerly thought (Steen, 1998). There are four dimensions to the grief process: (1) *physical*—the body and everything related to it; (2) *mental*—cognitive processes, such as thoughts and ideas; (3) *emotional/social*—interpersonal relationships and feelings; and (4) *spiritual*—all matters concerned with meaning and/or a perceived relationship with God or another manifestation of the transcendent. *Mourning* is the term used to describe the external manifestations of the grieving process. Mourning is highly culture-bound. In some societies, grief is experienced more privately, with minimal public crying and limited verbal expression of painful feelings. In other cultures, however, public grieving is encouraged and expected (Kagawa-Singer, 1998). People should not be judged or ridiculed for the outward form their grief takes; moreover, it must be remembered that people who have experienced significant losses are grieving, whether they appear to be or not. *Bereavement* is a term used to describe the grief that follows the death of a loved one.

After a major loss, such as the death of a spouse or child, up to a third of the people most directly affected sustain damage to their physical health, mental health, or both. Severe grief adversely affects many systems of the body, including the immune system (Ornish, 1999). Research suggests that grieving people are at a higher than average risk of developing a catastrophic illness and are nine times more likely to die than people who are not grieving. Bereavement increases the risk of death from coronary heart disease and suicide and contributes to a variety of psychosomatic and psychiatric disorders. Although support from friends and family suffice for most bereaved people, about a third need professional assistance. Many hospitals and other healthcare agencies provide grief counseling and other bereavement services.

The Four Phases of Grief

Four phases, or stages, of grief have been identified: shock and numbness, searching and yearning, disorganization, and reorganization. These phases unfold over time, and the number of days, weeks, months, or years spent in a given phase varies from individual to individual.

SHOCK AND NUMBNESS

News of a severe loss, such as the death of a loved one, usually triggers immediate, severe distress manifested by crying, wailing, and physical collapse. In our society, this initial reaction is often quickly suppressed, although African Americans and members of a number of other ethnic groups may express it more openly and for a longer period of time. Then, a period of shock, numbness, denial, and disbelief sets in. During this shock phase, people may exhibit physical symptoms, such as loss of appetite, shortness of breath, weakness, fatigue, and a feeling of tightness in the chest. They may feel lonely, empty, and often angry. The psychological/emotional/spiritual task in this phase of the grieving process, which can last up to two weeks, is to acknowledge and accept the loss.

People in this phase need support and acceptance, regardless of the manner in which they are manifesting their grief. It is best not to restrain or sedate those experiencing powerful emotions. Encouraging people to tell their story is very helpful, because it makes the experience more real. Questions such as "Where did the death occur?" "How did it happen?" and "Who told you?" are appropriate. Friends and family members must be patient listeners, and should discourage people in this phase of grief from making major decisions. It is important to avoid clichés such as "It was God's will" and "She's in a better place now." No one should suggest, under any circumstances, that a miscarriage or death of a newborn was a good thing. Comments such as "It would probably have been deformed" are not helpful to grieving parents. It is also inappropriate to discard the belongings of the deceased without the permission of the bereaved person.

SEARCHING AND YEARNING

After the shock phase subsides, a period of pining for the lost person, position, body part, and so on begins. The grieving person longs for the return of that which has been lost and may dream about the lost person or thing. It is not unusual for those who have lost a loved one to think they see the deceased person in a crowd. The physical symptoms continue in this phase. There may be headaches, altered sleep patterns, and digestive upsets. Feelings of powerlessness and the fear of an unknown future may persist for as long as four months. *Anger* is also a common symptom in this phase. Anger may

Box 28–3   General Guidelines for Supporting the Bereaved

Do

- Be at peace with your own grief issues.
- Leave all judgments at the door.
- Meet the bereaved with unconditional positive regard and empathy.
- Grant permission to grieve—shared tears are OK.
- Listen, listen, listen—let the bereaved tell their stories.
- Refer to the loved one by name.
- Help the bereaved reminisce, and remember that laughter is OK.
- Help the bereaved remember the good times and the bad.

- Remember the bereaved on anniversaries, birthdays, and death dates.

Don't

- Try to distract the bereaved from her grief.
- Use euphemisms for death.
- Judge the manner in which the bereaved grieves.
- Offer advice.
- Offer meaningless clichés.
- Avoid talking about the loss.
- Dispose of the loved one's things.

---

be directed at God, the deceased, or other people. The anger can be overt or can take the form of general irritability, pessimism, and low self-esteem.

The goal in this phase, which can last as long as four months, is to help the grieving person identify, express, and deal with her feelings. There are no shortcuts through the pain, and avoiding or suppressing it will prolong the course of mourning. Friends and family members should let grieving people know that they are comfortable with crying and other manifestations of grief, and encourage the bereaved person to express her or his feelings. Questions such as "What do you miss most about him?" and "What would you like to say to him now?" encourage the bereaved to express deep feelings. Friends and family members should stay in touch with the bereaved; they should call frequently and schedule visits and outings. The weeks and months after a significant loss are even more difficult if mourning people feel cut off from the support of friends and family. It is essential that grieving people not cut off their feelings, deny their pain, idealize and avoid reminders of the dead, and use alcohol and drugs to numb their pain.

DISORIENTATION

The 3rd phase typically begins five to nine months after a severe loss, such as a death, and is characterized by *increasing acceptance* of the loss. The full reality of the situation becomes apparent to the grieving person, who may experience depression at this time and may have considerable difficulty returning to normal patterns of living. The bereaved may be disorganized, forgetful, and sad and may have difficulty concentrating. They may feel exhausted and ill and lack energy. The psychic task during this stage of the grieving process is to adjust to life without the lost person or thing. This adjustment is particularly hard for *caretakers* who may have organized their entire lives around the deceased. Women are particularly likely to be caretakers in our society. It may also be

hard for widows, especially elderly widows, to learn to make decisions independently.

In this phase, bereaved people need to explore the meaning of the loss and the particular fears and beliefs they are currently struggling with. They need to develop strategies for getting their lives back on track. Friends and family can encourage decision making in such areas as what to do with the deceased's belongings, how often to visit the cemetery, and how to rearrange chairs at the table. Encouraging good nutrition and exercise can hasten adjustment in this phase, as can encouraging the bereaved to join a support group in which they can obtain help and comfort from others who have suffered similar losses.

REORGANIZATION

Approximately 18 to 24 months after a loss, the 4th phase, a reorganization, takes place. Reorganization is characterized by a gradual re-entry into normal life. Although setbacks do occur, the grieving person begins to realize that she is finally beginning to *heal*. Although the memory of what has been lost remains, the pain lessens. The loss has been *integrated* into the bereaved person's life and is no longer immobilizing. There is increased activity and energy, with a return to the normal. There is some renewal of old activities and relationships, as well as formation of new relationships. Emotional energy is withdrawn from the deceased and is reinvested in the living. A sign that this is taking place is the grateful acceptance of condolences. As grief softens, the bereaved become able to discuss the deceased and remember them realistically and with more happiness. They can also encounter grief and pain in another person with compassion and empathy without a re-emergence of their own pain. People commonly worry that detaching themselves from the pain of losing a loved one means dishonoring her memory or, worse, forgetting her, but moving through and out of grief does not involve forgetting. The challenge for the bereaved is to find a treasured place in their lives for the deceased and to move on in old and new relationships. Some people are consciously or unconsciously reluctant to make or strengthen any other attachment for fear of facing another loss. Others try to short circuit the grief process too quickly, attempting to invest their love and energy in a replacement relationship. Until and unless they have *emotionally relocated* their deceased loved one, a healthy relationship with a new person will be complicated and difficult.

Friends and family should encourage the bereaved person to find a new place in her life for the lost loved one—a place that will allow her to move forward with life and to form new relationships. Reminiscing is one way to gradually dissipate the emotional energy tied up with the deceased. Friends and family can help grieving people revisit positive memories of the deceased. Asking questions such as "What gift of the heart will you always keep from this person?" is a helpful strategy. See Box 28–3 for some general guidelines for supporting the bereaved.

QUESTIONS FOR REFLECTION AND DISCUSSION

1. *What information in this chapter was most distressing or surprising to you? Why?*
2. *How prepared are you to offer comfort to a dying person? What would you have to do to become more comfortable?*
3. *What are some ways in which death and grieving are handled in other cultures?*
4. *In what ways might the needs of dying adults and children be the same or different?*

RESOURCES

Organizations

Accord, Inc.
194 Bishop Lane, Suite 202
Louisville, KY 40218
Phone: 1-800-346-3087

Center for Life and Loss Transition
3735 Broken Row Rd.
Fort Collins, CO 80527
Phone: 970-226-6050
Web: http://www.centerforloss.com

Partnership for Caring
1620 Eye Street NW, Suite 202
Washington, DC 20006
Phone: 1-800-989-9455
Web: http://www.partnershipforcaring.org

The Compassionate Friends National Office
P.O. Box 3696
Oak Brook, IL 60522
Phone: 708-990-0010

National SIDS Foundation
8200 Professional Place, Suite 104
Landover, MD 20785
Phone: 1-800-221-SIDS

SHARE Pregnancy and Infant Loss Support, Inc., National Office
St. Joseph Health Center
300 First Capitol Dr.
St. Charles, MO 63301
Phone: 1-800-821-6819
Web: www.NationalSHAREoffice.com

Books

Byock, I. (1998). *Dying well, peace and possibilities at the end of life.* Berkley Publishing Group.
Callanan, M., & Kelly, P. (1997). *Final Gifts: Understanding the special awareness, needs and communications of the dying.* Bantam Books.
Jones, J. W., & Friedman, R. (1998). *The grief recovery handbook: The action program for moving beyond death, divorce and other losses.* HarperCollins.
Mollit, P.-L., Wilkins, I. A., Kohn, I. (1993). *A silent sorrow: Pregnancy loss—Guidance and support for you and your family.* Routledge.

Films

Batesville Management Services
One Batesville Blvd.
Batesville, IN 47006
Phone: 1-800-622-8373

Fanlight Productions
47 Halifax St.
Boston, MA 02130
Phone: 1-800-937-4113
E-mail: fanlight@tiac.net
Web: www.fanlight.com

St. John's Hospital
c/o Care Video Productions
P.O. Box 45132
Cleveland, OH 44145

Terra Nova Films
9848 S. Winchester Ave.
Chicago, IL 60643
Phone: 312-881-8491

Websites

Americans for Better Care of the Dying: www.abcd-caring.com
Center for Loss in Multiple Births (CLIMB)
http://www.geocities.com/Heartland/7479/climb.html
Grief, Loss & Recovery-Loss of a Child:
www.erichad.com/grief/grief2.htm
A Heartbreaking Choice-Information and support for those facing therapeutic termination of pregnancy:
www.erichad.com/ahc.
Pen-Parents, Inc.-Support for those who have lost a child of any age from pregnancy to loss of an adult child:
www.angelfire.com/nv/penparents

REFERENCES

Apple, R. (1990). *Women, health and medicine in America*. New York: Garland.

Berns, R., & Colvin, E. R. (1998). The final story: Events at the bedside of dying patients as told by survivors. *ANNA Journal, 25*(6), 583–587.

Blackhall, L. J., Murphy, S. T., Frank, G., Michel, V., & Azen, S. (1995). Ethnicity and attitudes toward patient autonomy. *Journal of the American Medical Association, 274*(10), 820–825.

Burnett, P., Middleton, W., Raphael, B., Dunne, M., Moylan, A., & Martinek, N. (1994). Concepts of normal bereavement. *Journal of Trauma Stress, 8*(2), 351–353.

Byock, I. R., & Torma, L. M. (2000). Pain as the fifth vital sign research project [On-line]. Missoula Demonstration Project: Available: http://www.missoulademonstration.org/fifth_vital_sign.html

Carrese, J. A., & Rhoades, L. A. (1995). Western bioethics on the Navajo reservation. Benefit or harm? *Journal of the American Medical Association, 274*(10), 826–829.

Chochinov, H. M., Tataryn, D., Clinch, J. J., & Dudgeon, D. (1999). Will to live in the terminally ill. *Lancet, 354*(9181), 816–819.

Davis, C. G., Nolen-Hoeksema, S., & Larson, J. (1998). Making sense of loss and benefiting from the experience: Two construals of meaning. *Journal of Personal and Social Psychology, 75*(2), 561–574.

Ditto, P. H., Danks, J. H., Smucher, W. D., Bookwla, J., Coppola, K. M., Dreser, R., Fagerlin, A., Gready, R. M., Houts, R. M., Lockhart, L. K., & Zyzanski, S. (2001). Advance directives as acts of communication: A randomized controlled trial. *Archives of Internal Medicine, 161*(3), 421–430.

Franklin, M. A. (1994–95). Death and dying fears overcome by progressive strategies. *Journal of Long Term Care Administration, 22*(4), 4–9.

Gessert, C. E., Curry, N. M., & Robinson, A. (2001). Ethnicity and end-of-life care: The use of feeding tubes. *Ethnicity and Disease, 11*(1), 97–106.

Grande, G. E., Addington-Hall, J. M., & Todd, C. J. (1998). Place of death and access to home care services: Are certain patient groups at a disadvantage? *Social Science and Medicine, 47*(5), 565–579.

Heaven, C. M., & Maguire, P. (1998). The relationship between patients' concerns and psychological distress in a hospice setting. *Psychooncology, 7*(6), 502–507.

Kagawa-Singer, M. (1998). The cultural context of death rituals and mourning practices. *Oncology Nursing Forum, 25*(10), 1752–1756.

Long, M. C. (1996). Death and dying and recognizing approaching death. *Clinical Geriatric Medicine, 12*(2), 359–368.

MacCleod, R. D. (2001). On reflection: Doctors learning to care for people who are dying. *Social Science and Medicine, 52*(11), 1719–1727.

Mitty, E. (2001, 1st Quarter). Removing cultural blinders. *Reflections on Nursing Leadership*, pp. 29–31.

Morrison, R. S., Wallenstein, S., Natale, D. K., Senzel, R. S., & Huang, L. L. (2000). We don't carry that—Failure of pharmacies in predominantly nonwhite neighborhoods to stock opioid analgesics. *New England Journal of Medicine, 342*(14), 1023–1026.

Morrison, R. S., Zayas, L. H., Mulvihill, M., Baskin, S. A., & Meie, D. E. (1998). Barriers to completion of healthcare proxy forms: A qualitative analysis of ethnic differences. *Journal of Clinical Ethics, 9*(2), 118–126.

Mouton, C., Teno, J. M., Mor, V., & Piette, J. (1997). Communication of preferences for care among human immunodeficiency virus–infected patients. Barriers to informed decisions? *Archives of Family Medicine, 6*(4), 342–347.

Ornish, D. (1999). *Love and survival: The scientific basis for the healing power of intimacy*. New York: HarperCollins.

Pace, J. C., & Stables, J. L. (1997). Correlates of spiritual wellbeing in terminally ill persons with AIDS and terminally ill persons with cancer. *Journal of the Association of Nurses in AIDS Care, 8*(6), 31–42.

Post, L. F., Blustein, J., Gordon, E., & Dubler, N. N. (1996). Pain: Ethics, culture, and informed consent to relief. *Journal of Law and Medical Ethics, 24*(4), 348–359.

Rabow, M., Hardie, G., Fair, J., & McPhee, J. (2000). End-of-life care content in 50 textbooks from multiple specialties. *Journal of the American Medical Association, 283*(6), 771.

Steen, K. F. (1998). A comprehensive approach to bereavement. *Nurse Practitioner, 23*(3), 54, 59–64, 66–68.

Stewart, A. L., Teno, J., Patrick, D. L., & Lynn, J. (1999). The concept of quality of life of dying persons in the context of health care. *Journal of Pain Symptom Management, 17*(2), 93–108.

Tilden, V. (2000). Advance directives. *American Journal of Nursing, 100*(12), 49–51.

Tolle, S. W., Tilden, V. P., Rosenfeld, A. G., & Hickman, S. E. (2000). Family reports of barriers to optimal care of the dying. *Nursing Research, 49*(6), 310–317.

Tong, K. L., & Spicer, B. J. (1994). The Chinese palliative patient and family in North America: A cultural perspective. *Journal of Palliative Care, 10*(1), 26–28.

Viorst, J. (1986). *Necessary Losses*. New York: Ballentine.

Weisman, A. D. (1980). What do elderly, dying patients want, anyway? *Journal of Geriatric Psychiatry, 13*(1), 63–67.

Weisman, A. D. (1988a). Appropriate death and the hospice program. *Hospital Journal, 4*(1), 65–77.

Weisman, A. D. (1988b). Ultimate questions and existential vulnerability. *Journal of Palliative Care, 4*(1–2), 89–90.

Wenrich, M. D., Curtis, J. R., Shannon, S. E., Carline, J. D., Ambrozy, D. M., & Ramsey, P. G. (2001). Communicating with dying patients within the spectrum of medical care from terminal diagnosis to death. *Archives of Internal Medicine, 161*(6), 868–874.

Index

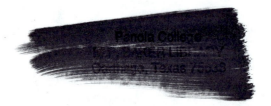